Less managing. More teaching. Greater learning.

 INSTRUCTORS...

Would you like your **students** to show up for class **more prepared**?
(Let's face it, class is much more fun if everyone is engaged and prepared...)

Want an **easy way to assign** homework online and track student **progress**?
(Less time grading means more time teaching...)

Want an **instant view** of student or class performance?
(No more wondering if students understand...)

Need to **collect data and generate reports** required for administration or accreditation?
(Say goodbye to manually tracking student learning outcomes...)

Want to **record and post your lectures** for students to view online?
(The more students can see, hear, and experience class resources, the better they learn...)

With **McGraw-Hill's *Connect*,**

INSTRUCTORS GET:

- Simple **assignment management**, allowing you to spend more time teaching.
- **Auto-graded** assignments, quizzes, and tests.
- **Detailed visual reporting** where student and section results can be viewed and analyzed.
- Sophisticated **online testing** capability.
- A **filtering and reporting** function that allows you to easily assign and report on materials that are correlated to learning objectives and Bloom's taxonomy.
- An easy-to-use **lecture capture** tool.
- The option to **upload course documents** for student access.

core concepts in
Health
canadian edition

Paul M. Insel

Stanford University

Walton T. Roth

Stanford University

Jennifer D. Irwin

University of Western Ontario

Shauna M. Burke

University of Western Ontario

With contributions from

Tara Mantler, *University of Western Ontario*
Don Morrow, *University of Western Ontario*
Heather Clarke Thomas, *University of Western Ontario*
Julie Parsons Tripp, *MD, CCFP*
Patricia Tucker, *University of Western Ontario*

**McGraw-Hill
Ryerson**

Connect. Learn. Succeed.

The McGraw·Hill Companies

McGraw-Hill Ryerson
Connect. Learn. Succeed.

Core Concepts in Health
Canadian Edition

ISBN-13: 978-0-07-096930-8
ISBN-10: 0-07-096930-2

1 2 3 4 5 6 7 8 9 10   DOW   1 9 8 7 6 5 4 3 2

Printed and bound in the United States.

PUBLISHER: Cara Yarzab
SPONSORING EDITOR: Marcia Siekowski
MARKETING MANAGER: Stacey Metz
SENIOR DEVELOPMENTAL EDITOR: Jennifer Cressman
SENIOR EDITORIAL ASSOCIATE: Stephanie Hess
EDITORIAL ASSOCIATE: Erin Catto
PHOTO/PERMISSION RESEARCH: Alison Lloyd-Baker
SUPERVISING EDITOR: Kara Stahl
COPY EDITOR: Dawn Hunter
PRODUCTION COORDINATOR: Tammy Mavroudi
COVER AND INTERIOR DESIGN: Kyle Gell
COVER IMAGE CREDIT: © Kapu/Shutterstock
PAGE LAYOUT: ArtPlus Ltd.
PRINTER: R. R. Donnelley

Library and Archives Canada Cataloguing in Publication

Core concepts in health / Paul M. Insel ... [et al.].
  — Canadian ed.

Includes bibliographical references and index.
ISBN 978-0-07-096930-8

  1. Health. I. Insel, Paul M.

RA776.C66 2012   613   C2011-903389-5

DEDICATION

For Don, Ryan, Lily, and Benjamin, and to each and every student who has and will cross our paths; you inspire us to live fully, choose wisely, and be well. This book is for you.

ABOUT THE AUTHORS

JENNIFER D. IRWIN, PHD

Jennifer D. Irwin is an Associate Professor in the Faculty of Health Sciences at the University of Western Ontario. She received her BA from Wilfrid Laurier University, MA from Dalhousie University, and PhD from the University of Waterloo. She specializes in health promotion from a behavioural perspective. In particular, her work focuses on behaviour change from a positive and empowering approach. Dr. Irwin is passionate about teaching and has received numerous accolades, including the University of Western Ontario's Student's Council/Alumni Teaching Award of Excellence. She is equally passionate about research and has authored or co-authored research papers and book chapters related to physical activity, obesity, body image, nutrition, smoking cessation, and motivational interviewing/health-related coaching.

SHAUNA M. BURKE, PHD

Shauna M. Burke is an Assistant Professor in the Faculty of Health Sciences at the University of Western Ontario. She received her Hons. BSc in Kinesiology from McMaster University, and her MA and PhD from the University of Western Ontario. Her primary research area is the psychology of health and physical activity, with a specific focus on group dynamics and child and youth health. Dr. Burke has published several research articles related to such topics as childhood obesity, physical activity and exercise, group dynamics, and team building. She was also Principle Investigator of a grant that she and a team of researchers received to develop, implement, and assess a group-based lifestyle intervention ("C.H.A.M.P.") for obese children and their families. Since 2006, Dr. Burke has taught the Personal Determinants of Health course to more than 500 first-year Western students each year and has consistently received outstanding teaching evaluations.

BRIEF CONTENTS

CONTENTS

PART TWO

GETTING FIT

PREFACE

Core Concepts in Health has maintained its leadership position in the field of personal health education for more than 30 years. Since Insel and Roth pioneered the concept of self-responsibility for personal health in 1976, millions of students have used the American-based book to become active, informed participants in their own health care. This history of excellence, combined with our own high opinion of the book, motivated us to create *Core Concepts in Health,* Canadian Edition, a decision that filled us with anticipation and excitement from day (and page) one. To offer the best personal health education text for Canadian students, a Canadian-specific book was essential.

Although we share many common experiences with our neighbours to the south, the reality is that differences exist between Canada and the United States (and Canadians and Americans) that make us each unique. We have both subtle and not-so-subtle differences, such as our systems of health care, drug policies, ethnic makeup, and, some even suggest, personality traits. Offering a Canadian edition of *Core Concepts in Health* enables us to continue the high standard of excellence created by Insel and Roth in a book that is tailored *for* Canadian students about Canadian health-related issues, topics, concerns, and resources.

To create *Core Concepts in Health,* Canadian Edition, we conducted a thorough review of the American 11th edition, with input from Canadian instructors and students alike. What works well for Canadians has been maintained; areas that needed to be added, removed, or reordered have been altered accordingly. Using feedback about what would be in the best service of the Canadian audience has enabled us to provide a book that we are both proud of and excited to use in our own classrooms.

OUR GOALS

Our goals and principles for *Core Concepts in Health,* Canadian Edition, are the following:

- To present scientifically based, accurate, up-to-date Canadian information in an accessible format
- To involve Canadian students in taking responsibility for their health and well-being
- To instill a sense of competence and personal power in Canadian students

The first of these goals means making expert knowledge about health and health care available to the individual. *Core Concepts in Health,* Canadian Edition, brings the most current, scientifically based, and accurate information to students about Canadian topics and issues that concern Canadians: exercise, stress, nutrition, weight management, contraception, intimate relationships, HIV infection, drugs, alcohol, and a multitude of others. Current, complete, and straightforward coverage is balanced with user-friendly features designed to make the text appealing. Written in an engaging, easy-to-read style and presented in a colourful, open format, *Core Concepts in Health,* Canadian Edition, invites students to read, learn, and remember. Boxes, tables, artwork, photographs, and many other features highlight areas of special interest throughout the book.

Our second goal is to involve students in taking responsibility for their health. *Core Concepts in Health,* Canadian Edition, uses innovative pedagogy and unique interactive features to get students thinking critically about how the material they're reading relates to their lives. We invite them to examine their emotions about the issues under discussion, consider their personal values and beliefs, develop their critical thinking skills, and analyze their health-related behaviours. Beyond this, for students who want to change behaviours that detract from a healthy lifestyle, we offer guidelines and tools, ranging from samples of health journals and personal contracts, to detailed assessments and behaviour change strategies.

Our third goal is perhaps the most important: to instill a sense of competence and personal power in students who read the book. Everyone has the ability to monitor, understand, and affect his or her health. Although medical and health professionals possess impressive skills and have access to a vast body of knowledge that benefits everyone in our society, people can help to optimize their health and minimize the amount of professional care they require in their lifetime by taking care of themselves—taking charge of their health—from an early age. Our hope is that *Core Concepts in Health,* Canadian Edition, will help Canadians make this exciting discovery—that they have the power to shape their futures.

TEXT ORGANIZATION

The book is divided into seven parts. Part One, Establishing a Basis for Wellness, includes chapters on taking charge of your health (Chapter 1), psychological health (Chapter 2), and stress (Chapter 3). Part Two, Getting Fit, includes a detailed discussion of weight management (Chapter 4), nutrition (Chapter 5), and exercise (Chapter 6).

Part Three, Protecting Yourself from Disease, deals with the most serious health threats facing Canadians today: cardiovascular disease (Chapter 7), cancer (Chapter 8), and infectious diseases (Chapter 9). Part Four, Understanding Sexuality, opens with an exploration of communication and healthy relationships, including friendship, intimate partnerships, marriage, and family (Chapter 10) and then moves on to discuss physical sexuality, contraception, and abortion (Chapter 11), pregnancy and childbirth (Chapter 12), and sexually transmitted infections (Chapter 13).

Part Five, Making Responsible Decisions: Substance Use and Abuse, opens with a discussion of addictive behaviour and the different classes of psychoactive drugs (Chapter 14), followed by chapters on alcohol (Chapter 15) and tobacco (Chapter 16).

Part Six, Accepting Physical Limits, looks at aging (Chapter 17) and dying and death (Chapter 18). Part Seven, Living Well in the World, explores conventional and complementary medicine (Chapter 19), personal safety (Chapter 20), and environmental health (Chapter 21).

Finally, the quick-reference appendix (Nutritional Content of Popular Items from Fast-Food Restaurants) provides information on commonly ordered items at popular Canadian fast-food restaurants. Students can use this handy resource for making healthy food choices when eating out.

Taken together, the text content provides Canadian students with a complete guide to promoting and protecting their health, now and throughout their entire lives.

UNIQUENESS OF THE CANADIAN EDITION

In adapting *Core Concepts in Health* for a Canadian edition, all chapters were carefully reviewed, revised, and updated. Canadian research, content, and examples were integrated throughout each chapter. Additionally, the order of sections and chapters, and the length of the book now reflect Canadian instructors' preferences. *Core Concepts in Health,* Canadian Edition, includes the latest information from scientific and health-related research, and discusses emerging topics and issues of concern to Canadians:

- An introduction to the determinants of health as outlined by the Public Health Agency of Canada and application of these determinants throughout the text
- Unique health challenges among Canadian Aboriginal peoples
- Global warming and climate change, and strategies Canadians can use to reduce their environmental footprint
- The latest recommendations on physical activity and exercise from the Public Health Agency of Canada and the Canadian Society for Exercise

Physiology; new information on the impact of exercise on multiple dimensions of wellness; and guidelines for distinguishing light, moderate, and vigorous exercise

- The continuing overweight and obesity epidemic, with the latest research from Statistics Canada and the Public Health Agency of Canada
- Stress in Canada and the impact of stress on wellness, including current statistics from the Canadian Mental Health Association
- Health challenges specific to students, highlighted by using information from the *Canadian Campus Survey*
- The growing prevalence of diabetes, prediabetes, insulin resistance, and metabolic syndrome among Canadians; their multifaceted causes, warning signs, and health effects; and strategies for prevention
- Food-borne illness and the safety of the Canadian food supply
- Current statistics on sexually transmitted infections, including HIV/AIDS, and on alcohol abuse and tobacco use in Canada
- *Eating Well with Canada's Food Guide* recommendations and simple strategies for incorporating healthy food choices into the lives of all Canadians
- The health implications of drinking diet pop
- The possible role of vitamin D in heart disease and other chronic conditions; the growing use of Aspirin therapy for CVD
- The importance of sleep in health and wellness; sleep disorders; sleep aids and their side effects
- The importance of friendships and social connectedness in overall wellness
- The latest vaccination guidelines from Canada's National Advisory Committee on Immunizations
- Emerging infections and antibiotic resistance, MRSA and *Clostridium difficile*, the H1N1 flu, and strategies for prevention and treatment
- An overview of falls and fall-related injuries among older adults in Canada
- Canadian information pertaining to organ donation and transplantation, and laws on physician-assisted suicide
- The prevalence of and consequences associated with bullying in Canada
- The use of wind power in Canada and a discussion of the potential health impact of noise generated by wind turbines

SPECIAL FEATURES

Core Concepts in Health, Canadian Edition, builds on the features that attracted and held readers' interest in past American editions. One of the most popular features has always been the boxes, which allow for the exploration of a wide range of current topics in greater detail than is possible in the text itself. Each type of box is marked with a distinctive icon and label:

 In the News boxes focus on current Canadian-related health issues that have recently been highlighted in the media. Topics include sleep aids, same-sex marriage, global warming and climate change, trans fats and diet pop, the H1N1 flu pandemic, and the way baby boomers are redefining age and retirement.

 Mind/Body/Spirit boxes focus on spiritual wellness and the close connections among people's feelings, states of mind, and their physical health. Topics include occupational and financial wellness, sexual decision making, the benefits of volunteering, paths to spiritual wellness, the components of a good death, and the effect of stress on pregnancy.

 Take Charge boxes distill from each chapter the practical advice students need in order to apply information to their own lives. By referring to these boxes, students can find ways to foster friendships, stay safe when using online social networking and dating Web sites, perform deep-breathing exercises for stress reduction, help a friend with a drug or tobacco addiction or eating disorder, become more physically active, and cope with grief following the death of a friend or family member.

 Critical Consumer boxes help students develop and apply the critical thinking skills they need to make sound health-related choices. These boxes provide specific guidelines for evaluating health news and advertising, using food and dietary supplement labels to make smart choices, understanding health issues associated with tattooing and body piercing, getting an HIV test, choosing a drug treatment program, and making environmentally friendly shopping choices.

 Dimensions of Diversity boxes reflect on and respond to the diversity of the student population. These boxes give students the opportunity to identify specific health risks that affect them as individuals or as members of a group. One or more determinants of health, as defined by the Public Health Agency of Canada, are highlighted in each of these boxes. Topics include factors contributing to health disparities among rural- versus urban-dwelling Canadians, ethnic and cultural influences on psychological disorders, rates of smoking and alcohol use among ethnic populations, exercise for people with special health concerns, the global pattern of HIV infection, and the link between poverty and environmental health.

 Gender Matters boxes highlight key gender differences related to wellness, as well as areas of particular concern to men or women. An overview of important gender-related wellness concerns is provided in Chapter 1. Topics covered in later chapters include gender differences in anxiety, depression, drug use, cancer, autoimmune disorders, suicide among older Canadians, and unintentional injuries.

 Assess Yourself boxes give students the opportunity to examine their behaviour and identify ways that they can change their habits and improve their health. By referring to these boxes, students can evaluate their fitness levels, discover if they are at increased risk for cancer or cardiovascular disease, measure their emotional intelligence, and determine whether they are aggressive drivers.

In Focus boxes highlight current wellness topics of particular interest. Topics include diabetes, headaches, carpal tunnel syndrome, cellphones and distracted driving, herbal remedies, and organ donation.

Thinking About the Environment boxes highlight specific environmental issues related to chapter topics, such as environmental factors that increase stress, the effect of environmental changes on the global food supply, and the effect of the environment on mood disorders, psychological problems, substance abuse, and the well-being of older adults.

In addition to the boxes, several features and specific learning aids are incorporated in the text:

- Learning objectives labelled **Looking Ahead** appear on the opening page of each chapter, identifying major concepts and helping guide students in their reading and review of the text.

- Each chapter opens with **Test Your Knowledge**— a set of four to six multiple-choice and true-false questions with answers that emphasize important points, highlight common misconceptions, and spark debate on issues of relevance for Canadians.

- **Vital Statistics** tables and figures highlight important facts and figures about Canadian and international health issues in a highly visible format that often reveals surprising contrasts and connections. For students who grasp a subject best when it is displayed graphically, numerically, or in a table, the Vital Statistics feature provides an alternative way of approaching and understanding the material.

- A wealth of attractive and informative **anatomical art**, prepared by medical illustrators, helps students understand important information, such as how blood flows through the heart, how the process of conception occurs, and how cholesterol moves throughout the body. These illustrations will particularly benefit students who learn best from visual images.

- **Quick Stats** highlight striking statistics related to chapter topics.

- **Questions for Critical Thinking and Reflection** prompt students to relate chapter material to their own lives.

- A **Behaviour Change Strategy** concludes many chapters and offers specific behaviour management/modification plans relating to the chapter's topic. Based on the principles of behaviour management that are carefully explained in Chapter 1, these strategies will help students change unhealthy or counterproductive behaviours. Included are strategies for dealing with test anxiety, quitting smoking, developing responsible drinking habits, planning a personal exercise program, phasing in a healthier diet, and many other practical plans for change.

- Important terms appear in boldface type in the text and are defined in a **running glossary**, helping students handle a large and complex new vocabulary.

- **Chapter summaries** offer a concise review of the most important concepts in the chapter.

- **For More Information** sections contain annotated lists of books, newsletters, organizations, and Web sites that Canadian students can use to extend and broaden their knowledge or pursue subjects of interest to them.

- **Selected Bibliographies** can be found at the end of every chapter.

TEACHING AND LEARNING TOOLS

Available with *Core Concepts in Health,* Canadian Edition, is a comprehensive package of supplementary materials designed to enhance teaching and learning.

Mc Graw Hill connect™ McGraw-Hill Connect™ is a Web-based assignment and assessment platform that gives students the means to better connect with their coursework, with their instructors, and with the important concepts that they will need to know for success now and in the future.

With Connect, instructors can deliver assignments, quizzes, and tests online. Questions are presented in an auto-gradable format and tied to the text's learning objectives. Instructors can edit existing questions and author entirely new problems. Track individual student performance—by question, assignment or in relation to the class overall—with detailed grade reports. Integrate grade reports easily with Learning Management Systems (LMS), such as WebCT and Blackboard. And much more!

The Connect Instructor Library provides all the critical resources instructors will need to build their courses, including a Test Bank, Instructor's Manual, and ready-made PowerPoint presentations:

- The **Test Bank** includes more than 3000 multiple-choice, true/false, and short essay questions. Each question is categorized according to learning objective, level of Bloom's taxonomy, correct answer, and text page reference.

  The computerized test bank is also available through EZ Test Online—a flexible and easy-to-use electronic testing program—that allows instructors to create tests from book-specific items. EZ Test accommodates a wide range of question types and allows instructors to add their own questions. Test items are also available in Word format (rich text format).

- The **Instructor's Manual** contains learning objectives, key terms with definitions, a detailed lecture outline, suggested Internet resources, and in-class activities.

- **PowerPoint slides** include key lecture points and images from the text. As an aid for instructors who want to create their own presentations, an **Image Bank** containing all visual elements from the text is also available.

- **Student Handouts** provide additional information and can be used to extend student knowledge on topics such as prediabetes, yoga for relaxation, and dealing with alcohol emergencies.

By choosing Connect, instructors are providing their students with a powerful tool for improving academic performance and truly mastering course material. Connect allows students to practise important skills at their own pace and on their own schedule. Importantly, students' assessment results and instructors' feedback are all saved online—so students can continually review their progress and plot their course to success.

Connect also provides 24/7 online access to an eBook—an online edition of the text—to aid students in successfully completing their work, wherever and whenever they choose.

ⓣegrity Tegrity Campus is a service that makes class time available all the time by automatically capturing every lecture in a searchable format for students to review when they study and complete assignments. With a simple one-click start-and-stop process, you capture all computer screens and corresponding audio. Students replay any part of any class with easy-to-use browser-based viewing on a PC or Mac. Educators know that the more students can see, hear, and experience class resources, the better they learn. With Tegrity Campus, students quickly recall key moments by using Tegrity Campus's unique search feature. This search helps students efficiently find what they need, when they need it across an entire semester of class recordings. Help turn all your students' study time into learning moments immediately supported by your lecture. To learn more about Tegrity, watch a two-minute Flash demo at http://tegritycampus.mhhe.com.

Additional Resources Available with *Core Concepts in Health*

Contact your local representative to find out about packaging the following resources with the text:

- **NutritionCalc Plus Canadian** is a dietary analysis program with an easy-to-use interface that allows users to track their nutrient and food group intakes, energy expenditures, and weight control goals. It generates a variety of personalized reports and graphs for analysis, which can be emailed or downloaded into Excel or Word. The Canadian Edition of NutritionCalc Plus is populated with Canadian food choices and Canadian recommended activity levels and daily intakes for essential nutrients, vitamins, and minerals, and uses metric measurements. The Canadian Nutrient File includes ethnic foods, supplements, fast foods, and convenience foods, and users can add their own foods or recipes to the food list. NutritionCalc Plus is available online at http://www.nutritioncalc.ca.

- The *Daily Fitness and Nutrition Journal* (ISBN 0-07-302988-2) is a handy booklet that guides students in planning and tracking a fitness program. It also helps students assess their current diet and make appropriate changes.

- The **Health and Fitness Pedometer** (ISBN 0-07-320933-3) allows students to count their daily steps and track their level of physical activity.

- The interactive **HealthQuest CD-ROM** (ISBN 0-07-295117-6) helps students explore and change their wellness behaviour. It includes tutorials, assessments, and behaviour change guidelines in such key areas as stress, fitness, nutrition, cardiovascular disease, cancer, tobacco, and alcohol.

SUPERIOR SERVICE

Service takes on a whole new meaning with McGraw-Hill Ryerson and *Core Concepts in Health*. More than just bringing you the textbook, we have consistently raised the bar in terms of innovation and educational research. These investments in learning and the education community have helped us to understand the needs of students and educators across the country, and allowed us to foster the growth of truly innovative, integrated learning.

 Your Integrated iLearning Sales Specialist is a McGraw-Hill Ryerson representative who has the experience, product knowledge, training, and support to help you assess and integrate any of our products, technology, and services into your course for optimal teaching and learning performance. Whether it's helping your students improve their grades, or putting your entire course online, your iLearning Sales Specialist is there to help you do it. Contact your iLearning Sales Specialist today to learn how to maximize all of McGraw-Hill Ryerson's resources!

 McGraw-Hill Ryerson offers a unique iServices package designed for Canadian faculty. Our mission is to equip providers of higher education with superior tools and resources required for excellence in teaching. For additional information, visit www.mcgrawhill.ca/highereducation/iservices.

 The educational environment has changed tremendously in recent years, and McGraw-Hill Ryerson continues to be committed to helping you acquire the skills you need to succeed in this new milieu. Our innovative Teaching & Learning Conference Series brings faculty together from across Canada with 3M Teaching Excellence award winners to share teaching and learning best practices in a collaborative and stimulating environment. Pre-conference workshops on general topics, such as teaching large classes and technology integration, will also be offered. We will also work with you at your own institution to customize workshops that best suit the needs of your faculty.

McGraw-Hill Higher Education and Blackboard have teamed up. Blackboard, the web-based course-management system, has partnered with McGraw-Hill to better allow students and faculty to use online materials and activities to complement face-to-face teaching. Blackboard features exciting social learning and teaching tools that foster more logical, visually impactful and active learning opportunities for students. You'll transform your closed-door classrooms into communities where students remain connected to their educational experience 24 hours a day.

This partnership allows you and your students access to McGraw-Hill's Connect™ and Create™ right from within your Blackboard course—all with one single sign-on. Not only do you get single sign-on with Connect and Create, you also get deep integration of McGraw-Hill content and content engines right in Blackboard. Whether you're choosing a book for your course or building Connect assignments, all the tools you need are right where you want them—inside of Blackboard. Gradebooks are now seamless. When a student completes an integrated Connect assignment, the grade for that assignment automatically (and instantly) feeds your Blackboard grade centre.

McGraw-Hill and Blackboard can now offer you easy access to industry-leading technology and content, whether your campus hosts it, or we do. Be sure to ask your local McGraw-Hill representative for details.

create McGraw-Hill's Create Online places the most abundant resource at your fingertips— literally. With a few mouse clicks, you can create customized learning tools simply and affordably. McGraw-Hill Ryerson has included many of its market-leading textbooks within Create Online for eBook and print customization as well as many licensed readings and cases. For more information, please visit www.mcgrawhillcreate.com.

CourseSmart CourseSmart brings together thousands of textbooks across hundreds of courses in an eTextbook format providing unique benefits to students and faculty. By purchasing an eTextbook, students can save up to 50 percent off the cost of a print textbook, reduce their impact on the environment, and gain access to powerful Web tools for learning, including full text search, notes and highlighting, and email tools for sharing notes among classmates. For faculty, CourseSmart provides instant access to review and compare textbooks and course materials in their discipline area without the time, cost, and environmental impact of mailing print examination copies. For further details, contact your iLearning sales specialist or visit www.coursesmart.com.

A NOTE OF THANKS

The efforts of innumerable people have gone into producing *Core Concepts in Health,* Canadian Edition. The book has benefited immensely from their thoughtful commentaries, expert knowledge and opinions, and many helpful suggestions. We are deeply grateful for their participation in the project.

Canadian Contributors

Heather Clarke Thomas, RD, MSc, PhD(c)
Nutrition Basics

Julie Parsons Tripp, HBSc, MD, CCFP, DPD
Pregnancy and Childbirth

Patricia Tucker, PhD
Cancer

Tara Mantler, MSc, PhD(c)
Toward a Tobacco-Free Self and Society

Don Morrow, BA(Hons), MA, PhD
Conventional and Complementary Medicine

Past Contributors

Paul M. Insel, PhD, Stanford University
Taking Charge of Your Health

Walton T. Roth, MD, Stanford University
Psychological Health; Stress: The Constant Challenge

Judith Sharlin, PhD, RD, Department of Nutrition, Simmons College
Weight Management

R. Elaine Turner, PhD, RD, University of Florida
Nutrition Basics

Thomas D. Fahey, EdD, California State University, Chico
Exercise for Health and Fitness

James V. Freeman, MD, MPH, Stanford University
Cardiovascular Health

Howard Lee, MD, MPH, Hematology and Oncology, San Mateo County General Hospital
Cancer

Martha C. Zúñiga, PhD, University of California, Santa Cruz
Immunity and Infection

Phillip Takakjian, PhD
Healthy Relationships and Communication

Nancy Kemp, MD
Inna Landres, MD, Stanford Hospital and Clinics

Mae Tinklenberg, RN, NP, MS
Healthy Sexuality

Sarah Waller, MD, Stanford University
Pregnancy and Childbirth

Nancy Kemp, MD
Sexually Transmitted Infections

Javier Lopez-Zetina, Associate Professor, Health Science Department, California State University, Long Beach
The Use and Abuse of Psychoactive Drugs

Rachel Stern, MS, RD, Nutrition Consultant
The Responsible Use of Alcohol

Patrick Zickler, Senior Health and Science Writer, Circle Solutions, Inc.
Toward a Tobacco-Free Self and Society

Mary Iten, PhD, University of Nebraska at Kearney
Aging: A Vital Process

Jacob W. Roth, MD, Chief of Adult Psychiatry, Kaiser Permanente San Jose Medical Center Adjunct Clinical Faculty, Stanford University
Dying and Death

Robert Jarski, PhD, Professor, School of Health Sciences, Director, Complementary Medicine and Wellness Program, Oakland University
Conventional and Complementary Medicine

Michael R. Hoadley, PhD, Assistant Vice-President for Academic Affairs, Center for Academic Technology Support, Eastern Illinois University
Personal Safety

John Kowalczyk, PhD, University of Minnesota, Duluth
Environmental Health and Emerging Issues

Reviewers of the Canadian Edition

Monique Bacher, George Brown College
Laurie Bird, North Island College
Brenda Bruner, Queen's University
Antony Card, Memorial University
Jarold Cosby, Brock University
Ann Dodge, Acadia University
Mitchell Fergenbaum, Sheridan Institute of Technology
James Gomes, University of Ottawa
Justin Hall, Queen's University
Corinne Hart, Ryerson University
Sylvia Jennings, Red River College
Sarah Junkin, University of Saskatchewan
Jennifer Kuk, York University
Harry Lendvoy, Langara College
Linda McDevitt, Algonquin College
Norman Naisbitt, Fanshawe College
Barb Pimento, George Brown College
Carolyn Ross, St. Clair College
Brenda Rossow-Kimball, University of Regina
Steve Trujillo, University of Western Ontario
James Wengle, York University

Finally, we would like to thank the members of the *Core Concepts in Health,* Canadian Edition, team at McGraw-Hill Ryerson. We are indebted to Jennifer Cressman for her dedication and steadfast excellence in the role of developmental editor for this edition. Thanks also to Marcia Siekowski, sponsoring editor; Kelly Dickson, managing editor, development; Kara Stahl, supervising editor; Alison Lloyd-Baker, permissions editor; and Dawn Hunter, copy editor. To all we express our deep appreciation.

Jennifer D. Irwin
Shauna M. Burke

SUPERIOR CHAPTER STRUCTURE

The following walkthrough demonstrates the organization of each chapter in Parts One through Five of *Core Concepts in Health*, Canadian Edition. Appropriate background information for each topic is presented in an easily accessible manner, which allows health issues to be more readily understood and a plan for behaviour change to be put into place. Each chapter follows a logical sequence and provides the necessary scientific basis while assuming no previous knowledge. Conquer your personal goals and reach for the top!

INTRODUCTION

The chapter starts with an overview of the topic and an explanation of its importance, such as with a discussion of the prevalence of cardiovascular disease and an introduction to the cardiovascular system.

ANATOMY AND PHYSIOLOGY

The chapter delves into the anatomy and physiology of the topic, using detailed diagrams and visuals to show the inner workings of the body, such as illustrations of the cardiovascular system and circulation in the heart.

RISKS

Next, the chapter describes issues that can adversely affect your health and factors that might increase your susceptibility to these issues. The authors identify which risk factors can be prevented and encourage you to take charge of your behaviour to optimize your health. For example, to help prevent cardiovascular disease, risk factors, such as tobacco use, high blood pressure, and low activity level, can be affected by behaviour change.

DISEASE AND OTHER ISSUES

The chapter outlines what happens when a health issue develops and some options for treatment or management. For example, detection, treatment options, and other important information is given on the major forms of cardiovascular disease, such as atherosclerosis, heart disease, stroke, and congestive heart failure.

PREVENTION

The chapter concludes with preventative measures and efforts for behaviour change, such as eating healthfully and reducing the amount of saturated and trans fats in your diet.

McGraw Hill connect™

Practise and learn online with Connect.

TAKING CHARGE OF YOUR HEALTH

1

LOOKING AHEAD>>>>>

AFTER READING THIS CHAPTER, YOU SHOULD BE ABLE TO

- Describe the dimensions of wellness
- Identify major health problems in Canada today
- Describe the influence of gender, ethnicity, income, disability, family history, and environment on health
- Explain the importance of personal decision making and behaviour change in achieving wellness
- List some available sources of health information and explain how to think critically about them
- Describe the steps in creating a behaviour-management plan to change a health-related behaviour

TEST YOUR KNOWLEDGE

1. **Which of the following lifestyle factors is the leading preventable cause of death for Canadians?**
   a. excess alcohol consumption
   b. cigarette smoking
   c. obesity

2. **The terms *health* and *wellness* mean the same thing.**
   True or false?

3. **Which of the following health-related issues affects the greatest number of university and college students each year?**
   a. stress
   b. colds/flu/sore throat
   c. sleep problems

4. **A person's genetic makeup determines whether he or she will develop certain diseases (such as breast cancer), regardless of that person's health habits.**
   True or false?

ANSWERS

1. **B.** Smoking causes about 37,000 deaths per year; obesity is responsible for more than 8400; and alcohol, more than 4000.

2. **FALSE.** Although the words are used interchangeably, they actually have different meanings. The term *health* refers to the overall condition of the body or mind and to the presence or absence of illness or injury. The term *wellness* refers to optimal health and vitality, encompassing all the dimensions of well-being.

3. **A.** About 34% of university and college students suffer so much stress that it affects their academic performance. High stress levels affect overall health and wellness, making it important to manage stress.

4. **FALSE.** In many cases, behaviour can tip the balance toward good health even when heredity or environment is a negative factor. For example, breast or prostate cancer may run in families, but these diseases are also associated with controllable factors, such as being overweight and inactive.

A first year university student sets the following goals for herself:

- To manage her time to do all of her readings for classes each week
- To exercise every day
- To clean up garbage and plant trees in blighted neighbourhoods in her community

These goals may differ, but they have one thing in common. Each contributes, in its own way, to this student's health and well-being. Not satisfied merely to be free of illness, she wants more. She has decided to live actively and fully—not just to be healthy but to pursue a state of overall wellness.

WELLNESS: THE NEW HEALTH GOAL

Generations of people have viewed health simply as the absence of disease. That view largely prevails today; the word **health** typically refers to the overall condition of a person's body or mind and to the presence or absence of illness or injury. **Wellness** is a relatively new concept that expands our idea of health. Beyond the simple presence or absence of disease, wellness refers to optimal health and vitality—to living life to its fullest. Although we use the words *health* and *wellness* interchangeably in this text, two important differences exist between them:

- Health—or some aspects of it—can be determined or influenced by factors beyond your control, such as your genes, age, the health care system, and the care you received as a young child (i.e., by some of the **determinants of health**, see Table 1.1). For example, consider a 60-year-old man with a strong family history of prostate cancer, who lives in a rural community in the Northwest Territories and has limited access to cancer screening services. These factors place this man at a higher-than-average risk for developing prostate cancer himself.

- Wellness is largely determined by the decisions you make about how you live. That same 60-year-old man can reduce his risk of cancer by eating sensibly, exercising, and having screening tests when they are

TERMS

health The overall condition of body or mind and the presence or absence of illness or injury.

wellness Optimal health and vitality, encompassing all the dimensions of well-being.

determinants of health Twelve factors that influence the health of individuals and groups.

risk factor A condition that increases a person's chances of disease or injury.

health promotion A process of enabling people to increase control over and improve their health.

Table 1.1	Determinants of Health

Canada's Public Health Agency identifies 12 key determinants of health for both populations and individuals, the latter of which is the focus of this text. Some determinants are discussed throughout this chapter, and others are highlighted in the Dimensions of Diversity boxes throughout the entire text.

- Income and social status
- Education and literacy
- Social environments
- Personal health practices and coping skills
- Biology and genetic endowment
- Gender
- Social support networks
- Employment and working conditions
- Physical environments
- Healthy child development
- Health services
- Culture

Source: Public Health Agency of Canada. 2001. *What Determines Health?* (http://www.phac-aspc.gc.ca/ph-sp/determinants/index-eng.php; retrieved September 4, 2009).

available. Even if he develops the disease, he may still rise above its effects to live a rich, meaningful life. This means choosing not only to care for himself physically but also to maintain a positive outlook, keep up his relationships with others, challenge himself intellectually, honour his faith or spirituality, and nurture other aspects of his life.

Enhanced wellness, therefore, involves making conscious decisions to control **risk factors** that contribute to disease or injury. Age and family history are nonmodifiable risk factors that you cannot control. Some behaviours, such as smoking, exercising, and eating a healthy diet, are modifiable factors. The Ottawa Charter for Health Promotion describes **health promotion** as a vehicle for achieving wellness; you must play an active role in the decisions related to each dimension of your wellness rather than deciding simply that your health status happens to you. And it is important to recognize that different people define their level of wellness differently.

The Dimensions of Wellness

Experts have defined six dimensions of wellness:

- Physical
- Emotional
- Intellectual
- Interpersonal
- Spiritual
- Environmental

These dimensions are interrelated; each has an effect on the others, and researchers have found important connections between the wellness of the mind and that of the body (see Chapter 19). The process of achieving wellness is constant and dynamic (Figure 1.1), involving change

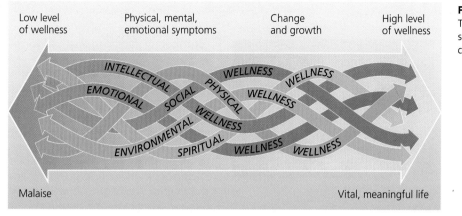

FIGURE 1.1 The wellness continuum.
The concept of wellness includes vitality in six interrelated dimensions, all of which contribute to overall wellness.

Low level of wellness

Physical, mental, emotional symptoms

Change and growth

High level of wellness

INTELLECTUAL WELLNESS WELLNESS
EMOTIONAL SOCIAL PHYSICAL WELLNESS
ENVIRONMENTAL WELLNESS
SPIRITUAL WELLNESS WELLNESS

Malaise

Vital, meaningful life

and growth. Wellness is not static; ignoring any dimension of wellness can have harmful effects on your life. The following sections briefly introduce the dimensions of wellness. Table 1.2 lists some of the specific qualities and behaviours associated with each dimension, and the box "Occupational Wellness" (on p. 6) discusses another important aspect of wellness.

Physical Wellness   Your physical wellness includes not just your body's overall condition and the absence of disease but also your fitness level and your ability to care for yourself. The higher your fitness level, the higher your level of physical wellness will be. Similarly, as you develop the ability to take care of your own physical needs, you ensure a greater level of physical wellness. To achieve optimum physical wellness, you need to make choices that will help you avoid illnesses and injuries. The decisions you make now, and the habits you develop over your lifetime, will largely determine the length and quality of your life.

Emotional Wellness   Your emotional wellness reflects your ability to understand and deal with your feelings. Emotional wellness involves attending to your own

thoughts and feelings, monitoring your reactions, and identifying obstacles to emotional stability. Achieving this type of wellness means finding solutions to emotional problems, with professional help if necessary.

Intellectual Wellness   Those who enjoy intellectual (or mental) wellness constantly challenge their minds. An active mind is essential to wellness because it detects problems, finds solutions, and directs behaviour. People who enjoy intellectual wellness never stop learning; they continue trying to learn new things throughout their lifetime. They seek out and relish new experiences and challenges.

Interpersonal Wellness   Your interpersonal (or social) wellness is defined by your ability to develop and maintain satisfying and supportive relationships. Such relationships are essential to physical and emotional health. Social wellness requires participating in and contributing to your community and to society.

Spiritual Wellness   To enjoy spiritual wellness is to possess a set of guiding beliefs, principles, or values that give meaning and purpose to your life, especially in difficult

Table 1.2	Examples of Qualities and Behaviours Associated with the Dimensions of Wellness				
Physical	**Emotional**	**Intellectual**	**Interpersonal**	**Spiritual**	**Environmental**
• Eating well	• Optimism	• Openness to new ideas	• Communication skills	• Capacity for love	• Having abundant, clean natural resources
• Exercising	• Trust	• Capacity to question	• Capacity for intimacy	• Compassion	• Maintaining sustainable development
• Avoiding harmful habits	• Self-esteem	• Ability to think critically	• Ability to establish and maintain satisfying relationships	• Forgiveness	
• Practising safer sex	• Self-acceptance	• Motivation to master new skills	• Ability to cultivate support system of friends and family	• Altruism	• Recycling whenever possible
• Recognizing symptoms of disease	• Self-confidence	• Sense of humour		• Joy	
• Getting regular checkups	• Ability to understand and accept own feelings	• Creativity		• Fulfillment	• Reducing pollution and waste
• Avoiding injuries	• Ability to share feelings with others	• Curiosity		• Caring for others	
		• Lifelong learning		• Sense of meaning and purpose	
				• Sense of belonging to something greater than yourself	

Occupational Wellness

Many experts contend that occupational (or career) wellness is a seventh dimension of wellness, in addition to the six dimensions described in this chapter. Whether or not occupational wellness appears on every list of wellness dimensions, a growing body of evidence suggests that our daily work has a considerable effect on our overall wellness.

Defining Occupational Wellness

The term *occupational wellness* refers to the level of happiness and fulfillment you gain through your work. Although high salaries and prestigious titles are nice, they alone generally do not bring about occupational wellness. An occupationally well person truly likes his or her work, feels a connection to others in the workplace, and has opportunities to learn and be challenged.

Key aspects of occupational wellness include the following:

- Enjoyable work
- Job satisfaction
- Recognition and acknowledgement from managers and colleagues
- Feelings of achievement
- Opportunities to learn and grow

An ideal job draws on your passions and interests, as well as your vocational skills, and allows you to feel that you are contributing to society in your everyday work.

Financial Wellness

Another important facet of occupational wellness is financial wellness. A person's economic situation is a key factor in his or her overall well-being. People with low socioeconomic status have higher rates of death, injury, and disease; are less likely to have access to preventive health services; and are more likely to engage in unhealthy habits.

Although money and possessions in themselves won't necessarily make you happy, financial security can contribute to your peace of mind. If you are financially secure, you can worry less about daily expenses and focus on personal interests and your future. Conversely, money problems are a source of stress for individuals and families and are a contributing factor in many divorces and suicides.

You don't need to be rich to achieve financial wellness. Instead, you need to be comfortable with your financial situation. Financially well people understand the limits of their income and live within their means by keeping expenses in check. They know how to balance a chequebook and interpret their bank statements. The financially well person may not strive to be wealthy but at least tries to save money for the future.

Achieving Occupational Wellness

How do you achieve such wellness? Career experts suggest setting career goals that reflect your personal values. For example, a career in sales may be a good way to earn a high income but may not be a good career choice for someone whose highest values involve service to others. Such a person might find more personal satisfaction in teaching or nursing.

Aside from career choices, education is a critical factor in occupational and financial wellness. For starters, learn to manage money *before* you start making it. Classes on personal money management are available through many sources and can help you on your way to financial security, whether you dream of being wealthy or not.

times. The spiritually well person focuses on the positive aspects of life and finds spirituality to be an antidote for negative feelings, such as cynicism, anger, and pessimism. Organized religions help many people develop spiritual health. Religion, however, is not the only source or form of spiritual wellness. Many people find meaning and purpose in their lives on their own—through nature, art, meditation, or good works—or with their loved ones.

Environmental Wellness Your environmental wellness is defined by the livability of your surroundings. Personal health depends on the health of the planet—from the safety of the food supply to the degree of violence in society. Your physical environment either supports your wellness or diminishes it. To improve your environmental wellness, you can learn about and protect yourself against hazards in your surroundings and work to make your world a cleaner and safer place.

New Opportunities, New Responsibilities

Wellness is a fairly new concept. A century ago, North Americans considered themselves lucky just to survive to adulthood (Figure 1.2). A child born in 1900, for example, could expect to live only 47 years. Many people died from common **infectious diseases** (such as pneumonia, tuberculosis, or diarrhea) and poor environmental conditions (such as water pollution and poor sanitation).

Since 1900, however, life expectancy has nearly doubled, largely because of the development of vaccines and antibiotics to fight infections and because of public health measures to improve living conditions. Today, a different set of diseases has emerged as our major health threat, and cancer, heart disease, and stroke are now the three leading causes of death for Canadians (Table 1.3, p. 8). Treating such **chronic diseases** is costly and difficult.

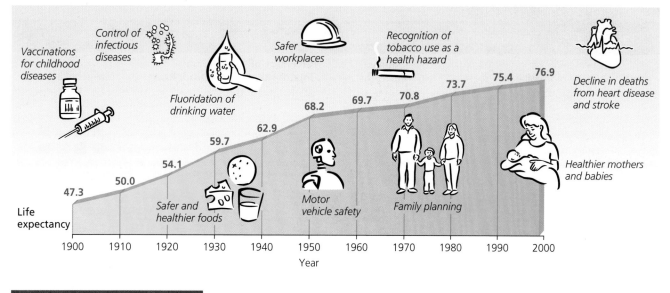

VITAL STATISTICS

FIGURE 1.2 **Public health achievements of the twentieth century.** During the twentieth century, public health achievements greatly improved the quality of life for North Americans. A shift in the leading causes of death also occurred, with deaths from infectious diseases declining from 33% of all deaths to just 2%. Heart disease, cancer, and stroke are now responsible for more than half of all deaths among North Americans.

Sources: National Center for Health Statistics, Centers for Disease Control and Prevention. 1999. Ten great public health achievements—United States, 1900–1999. *Morbidity and Mortality Weekly Report* 48(50): 1141; Statistics Canada. 2005. *Canadian Vital Statistics: Death Database*, CANSIM Table 102-0561 (http://www5.statcan.gc.ca/cansim/a01?lang=eng; retrieved March 4, 2011).

The good news is that people have some control over whether they develop chronic diseases. People make choices every day that increase or decrease their risks for such diseases. These **lifestyle choices** include many different behaviours, such as smoking, diet, exercise, and alcohol use. As Table 1.3 makes clear, lifestyle factors contribute to many deaths in Canada, and people can influence their own health risks.

The need to make good choices is especially true for teens and young adults. For Canadians ages 15 to 24, for example, the top three causes of death are unintentional injuries (accidents), suicide, and cancer (Table 1.4, p. 8).

The Integrated Pan-Canadian Healthy Living Strategy

Wellness is a personal concern, but the Canadian government has humanitarian and financial interests in it, too. In addition to the enormous human suffering caused by our nation's leading chronic diseases, the estimated total cost in Canada of illness, disability, and death attributable to chronic diseases is more than $80 billion annually.

The Integrated Pan-Canadian Healthy Living Strategy was created in 2002 when the federal, provincial, and territorial ministers of health sought a collaborative and coordinated approach to curbing our nation's noncommunicable diseases by addressing their common, preventable risk factors (physical inactivity, unhealthy diet, and tobacco use) and the underlying conditions in society that contribute to them, including income, employment, education, geographic isolation, social exclusion, and other factors.

The Strategy's vision is a healthy nation in which all Canadians experience the conditions that support the attainment of good health. Its goals are to improve overall health outcomes and reduce health disparities in meaningful ways by 2015. More specifically, the Strategy's

> **QUICK STATS**
>
> More than **30%** of drinking drivers involved in fatal car crashes are between the ages of 16 and 24.
>
> —Transport Canada, 2008

> **TERMS**
>
> **infectious disease** A disease that can spread from person to person; caused by microorganisms, such as bacteria and viruses.
>
> **chronic disease** A disease that develops and continues over a long period, such as heart disease or cancer.
>
> **lifestyle choice** A conscious behaviour that can increase or decrease a person's risk of disease or injury; such behaviours include eating a healthy diet, smoking, exercising, and others.

Table 1.3 — Ten Leading Causes of Death in Canada

Rank	Cause of Death	Number of Deaths	Percentage of Total Deaths	Death Rate*	Lifestyle Factors
	All causes	230,132	100.0	712.5	
1	Cancer	67,343	29.3	208.5	D I S A
2	Heart disease	51,574	22.4	159.7	D I S A
3	Stroke	14,054	6.1	43.5	D I S A
4	Chronic lower respiratory diseases	10,515	4.6	32.6	S
5	Unintentional injuries (accidents)	9,506	4.1	29.4	I S A
6	Diabetes mellitus	7,881	3.4	24.4	D I S
7	Influenza and pneumonia	5,845	2.5	18.1	S
8	Alzheimer's disease	5,762	2.5	17.8	
9	Intentional self-harm (suicide)	3,743	1.6	11.6	A
10	Kidney disease	3,643	1.6	11.3	D I S A

Source: Statistics Canada. 2005. *Canadian Vital Statistics: Death Database, CANSIM Table 102-0561* (http://www5.statcan.gc.ca/cansim/a01?lang=eng; retrieved March 4, 2011).

Notes: D Diet plays a part; I Inactive lifestyle plays a part; S Smoking plays a part; A Excessive alcohol use plays a part.

*Age-adjusted death rate per 100,000 people.

Table 1.4 — Five Leading Causes of Death Among Canadians Ages 15 to 24

Rank	Cause of Death	Number of Deaths	Percentage of Total Deaths
	All causes	2,328	
1	Accidents	1,015	43.6
2	Suicide	509	21.9
3	Cancer	156	6.7
4	Homicide	136	5.8
5	Heart disease	67	2.9

Source: Statistics Canada. 2005. *Vital Statistics: Death Database, CANSIM Table 102-0561* (http://www5.statcan.gc.ca/cansim/a01?lang=eng; retrieved March 4, 2011).

aim is to increase healthy eating, physical activity, and healthy weights:

• *Healthy eating objective:* Increase by 20% the proportion of Canadians who make healthy food choices

• *Physical activity objective:* Increase by 20% the proportion of Canadians who participate in regular physical activity based on 30 minutes/day of moderate to vigorous activity (the amount needed for health benefits)

• *Healthy weights objective:* Increase by 20% the proportion of Canadians at a healthy body weight based on a body mass index (BMI) of 18.5 to 24.9

Information is collected for each objective to see if the targets are being met. If all Canadians improve these three areas of their lives, they will be better able to achieve their ideal level of wellness, and the nation as a whole will be much healthier. Table 1.5 outlines how each province and territory is attempting to meet the Strategy's goals. Table 1.6 (p. 10) summarizes the current eating and physical activity habits and smoking rates of each province's and territory's population.

Health Issues for Diverse Populations

Canadians are a diverse people. Statistics Canada lists 29 ethnic origins in the Canadian population, with 8 representing the majority of citizens (Figure 1.3). We live in cities, suburbs, and rural areas and work at every imaginable occupation. We are at heart a nation of diversity, and though we often fall short of our goal, we strive for justice and equality among all.

When it comes to health, most differences among people are insignificant; most health issues concern us all equally. We all need to eat well, exercise, manage stress, and cultivate satisfying personal relationships. We need to know how to protect ourselves from heart disease, cancer, sexually transmitted infections (STIs), and injuries. We need to know how to use the health care system.

But some of our differences, as individuals and as members of groups, have important implications for health. Some of us, for example, have a genetic predisposition for developing certain health problems, such as high cholesterol. Some of us have grown up eating foods that raise our risk of heart disease or obesity. Some of us live in an environment that increases the chance that we will smoke cigarettes or abuse alcohol. These health-related differences

Table 1.5	The Integrated Pan-Canadian Healthy Living Strategy Provincial and Territorial Healthy Living Targets		
Province/Territory	**Physical Activity Goal**	**Healthy Eating Goal**	**Healthy Weight Goal**
British Columbia	↑ by 11.6 percentage points (from 58% to 69.6%)	↑ vegetable/fruit by 8 percentage points (from 40% to 48%)	↓ obesity and overweight by 8.4 percentage points (from 42.3% to 33.9%)
Alberta	↑ by 10 percentage points (from 52% to 62%)	↑ vegetable/fruit by 16 percentage points (from 34% to 50%)	↑ healthy weight by 8 percentage points (from 47% to 55%)
Saskatchewan	↑ by 10 percentage points	not specified	not specified
Manitoba	↑ by 10%	not specified	not specified
Ontario	↑ by 10 percentage points (to 55%)	not specified	not specified
Quebec	become more active	eat more healthily	get weight under control
Newfoundland and Labrador	↓ inactivity by 10 percentage points (from 64% to 54%) ↓ youth inactivity by 10 percentage points (33% to 23%)	not specified	↓ overweight by 5 percentage points (from 60% to 55%)
New Brunswick	↑ by 10%	↑ vegetable/fruit by 10%	↑ healthy weight from 36% to 46%
Nova Scotia	↑ % of active adults by 10 percentage points (from 44% to 54%) ↑ % of children and youth who are active	↑ vegetable/fruit from 29% to 34%	not specified
Prince Edward Island	↑ activity by 10 percentage points	↑ number with good nutritional health	not specified
Yukon	↑ by 10 percentage points	not specified	not specified
Northwest Territories	↑ by 10 percentage points	not specified	not specified
Nunavut	↑ by 10 percentage points	not specified	not specified

Source: Health Canada, 2005. Reproduced with the permission of the Minister of Health, 2011.

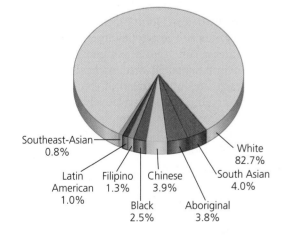

FIGURE 1.3   The ethnic distribution of the Canadian population.

Sources: Statistics Canada. 2010. *Visible Minority Groups, 2006 Counts, for Canada, Provinces and Territories—20% Sample Data* (http://www12.statcan.ca/census-recensement/2006/dp-pd/hlt/97-562/index.cfm?Lang=E; retrieved March 5, 2011); Statistics Canada. 2010. *Aboriginal Identity Population by Age Groups, Median Age and Sex, 2006 Counts for Both Sexes, for Canada, Provinces and Territories—20% Sample Data* (http://www12.statcan.ca/census-recensement/2006/dp-pd/hlt/97-558/index.cfm?Lang=E; retrieved March 5, 2011).

among individuals and groups can be biological—determined genetically—or cultural—acquired as patterns of behaviour through daily interactions with our families, communities, and society. Many health conditions are a function of biology and culture combined. A person can have a genetic predisposition for a disease, for example, but won't actually develop the disease itself unless certain lifestyle factors are present, such as stress or a poor diet.

When we talk about health issues for diverse populations, we face two related dangers. The first is the danger of *stereotyping*, or talking about people as groups rather than as individuals. It's true that every person is an individual with a unique genetic endowment and unique life experiences. But many of these influences are shared with others of similar genetic and cultural background. Statements about these group similarities can be useful; for

Table 1.6	Eating Habits and Physical Activity and Smoking Levels Among Canadians		
	Smoking* (%)	Healthy Eating Habits† (%)	Physically Active‡ (%)
British Columbia	12.3	45.7	53.7
Alberta	17.9	42.7	53.4
Saskatchewan	17.2	39.7	46.1
Manitoba	14.1	38.5	51.8
Ontario	14.4	44.1	48.8
Quebec	17.4	54.0	45.7
New Brunswick	17.9	40.0	42.7
Nova Scotia	18.3	38.3	47.6
Prince Edward Island	15.3	38.9	47.3
Newfoundland and Labrador	18.5	29.9	45.7
Yukon	27.0	45.7	55.4
Northwest Territories	28.9	26.4	49.3
Nunavut	55.6	29.6	

Sources: Statistics Canada. 2007 and 2009. *Health Indicator Profile, Annual Estimates, by Age Group and Sex, Canada, Provinces, Territories, Health Regions and Peer Groups, Occasional, CANSIM Table 105-0501* (http://www5.statcan.gc.ca/cansim/home-accueil?lang=eng; retrieved March 5, 2011); Statistics Canada. 2007 and 2009. *Leisure-Time Physical Activity, by Sex, Household Population Aged 12 and Over, Canada, Provinces and Territories, Occasional, CANSIM Table 105-4033* (http://www5.statcan.gc.ca/cansim/home-accueil?lang=eng; retrieved March 5, 2011).

* Refers to daily smokers
† Refers to consumption of five or more fruit or vegetables a day
‡ Refers to leisure-time activity level

example, they can alert people to areas that may be of special concern for them and their families.

The second danger is that of *overgeneralizing*, or ignoring the extensive biological and cultural diversity that exists among peoples who are grouped together. Groups labelled Latino or Hispanic, for example, include Mexican Canadians, Puerto Ricans, people from South and Central America, and other Spanish-speaking peoples. Similarly, the population labelled Aboriginal peoples includes North American Indians, Metis, and Inuit, each with its own genetic and cultural heritage.

Health-related differences among groups can be identified and described in the context of several different dimensions; well-accepted dimensions are gender, ethnicity, income and education, disability, geographic location, and sexual orientation.

TERMS

sex The biological and physiological characteristics that define men and women.

gender The roles, behaviours, activities, and attributes that a given society considers appropriate for men and women.

Sex and Gender Sex and gender profoundly influence wellness. The World Health Organization (WHO) defines **sex** as the biological and physiological characteristics that define men and women; these characteristics are related to chromosomes and their effects on reproductive organs and the functioning of the body. Menstruation in women and the presence of testicles in men are examples of sex-related characteristics. **Gender** is defined as roles, behaviours, activities, and attributes that a given society considers appropriate for men and women. A person's gender is rooted in biology and physiology, but it is shaped by experience and environment—how society responds to individuals based on their sex. Examples of gender-related characteristics that affect wellness include higher rates of smoking and drinking among men and lower earnings among women (compared with earning for men doing similar work).

Both sex and gender have important effects on wellness, but they can be difficult to separate (see the box "Women's Health/Men's Health"). For example, more women began smoking with changes in culturally defined ideas about women's behaviour (a gender issue). Because women are more vulnerable to the toxins in tobacco smoke (a sex issue), cancer rates also increased. A recent study shows that although men are more biologically likely than women to suffer from certain diseases (a sex issue), men are less likely to visit their physician for regular exams (a gender issue). As a result, more than 70% of Canadian men have not seen their doctor for a checkup in the past year, and many say they wait as long as possible before seeing a doctor—even when they are sick.

Ethnicity Although Canada is recognized for its diversity, little research has been done here about the specific health differences among the various ethnic groups. However, research from elsewhere in North America is relevant, and it shows a variety of health disparities among ethnic groups. These disparities result from a complex mix of genetic variations, environmental factors, and health behaviours.

Some diseases are concentrated in certain gene pools, the result of each ethnic group's relatively distinct history. Sickle-cell disease is most common among people of African ancestry. Tay-Sachs disease affects people of Eastern European Jewish heritage and French-Canadian heritage. Cystic fibrosis is more common among people of Northern European descent. In addition to biological differences, many cultural differences occur along ethnic lines. Ethnic groups may vary in their traditional diets; their family and interpersonal relationships; their attitudes toward tobacco, alcohol, and other drugs; and their health beliefs and practices. All these factors have implications for wellness. (See the box "Health Disparities Among Ethnic Minorities" on p. 12 for more information.)

Within Canada, Aboriginal peoples have been relatively well studied, and these groups represent an important portion of the population in many ways, including cultural richness and historical prominence. Currently, about

Women's Health/Men's Health

In terms of their health, women and men differ in many ways. They have different life expectancies, for one thing, and suffer from various diseases at different rates. Men and women tend to differ in some health-related behaviours, and they respond in dissimilar ways to some medications and medical treatments. The following table highlights some of the gender differences that can affect wellness.

Health Issues	Women	Men
Life expectancy	On average, live about 5 years longer but have higher rates of disabling health problems, such as arthritis, osteoporosis, and Alzheimer's disease	Have a shorter life expectancy but lower rates of disabling health problems
Height and weight	Shorter on average, with a lower proportion of muscle; tend to have a pear shape with excess body fat stored in the hips; obesity is more common in women than men	Taller on average, with a higher proportion of muscle; tend to have an apple shape with excess body fat stored in the abdomen
Skills and fluencies	Score better on tests of verbal fluency, speech production, fine motor skills, and visual and working memory	Score better on tests of visual-spatial ability (such as the ability to imagine the relationships between shapes and objects when rotated in space)
Heart attacks	Experience heart attacks about 10 years later than men, on average, with a poorer 1-year survival rate; more likely to experience atypical heart attack symptoms (such as fatigue and difficulty breathing) or silent heart attacks that occur without chest pain	Experience heart attacks about 10 years earlier than women, on average, with a better 1-year survival rate; more likely to have classic heart attack symptoms (such as chest pain)
Stroke	More likely to have a stroke or die from one but more likely to recover language ability after a stroke that affects the left side of the brain	Less likely to die from a stroke, but more likely to suffer permanent loss of language ability after a stroke that affects the left side of the brain
Immune response	Stronger immune systems; less susceptible to infection by certain bacteria and viruses, but more likely to develop autoimmune diseases, such as lupus	Weaker immune systems; more susceptible to infection by certain bacteria and viruses, but less likely to develop autoimmune diseases
Smoking	Lower rates of smoking than men, but higher risk of lung cancer at a given level of exposure to smoke	Higher rates of smoking and spit tobacco use
Alcohol	Become more intoxicated at a given level of alcohol intake	Become less intoxicated at a given level of alcohol intake, but are more likely to use or abuse alcohol or to develop alcoholism
Stress	More likely to react to stress with a tend-and-befriend response that involves social support; may have a longevity advantage because of a reduced risk of stress-related disorders	More likely to react to stress with aggression or hostility; this pattern may increase the rate of stress-related disorders
Depression	More likely to suffer from depression and to attempt suicide	Lower rates of depression than women and less likely to attempt suicide, but four times as likely to succeed at suicide
Headaches	More commonly suffer migraine and chronic tension headaches	More likely to suffer from cluster headaches
Sexually transmitted infections (STIs)	More likely to be infected with an STI during a heterosexual encounter; more likely to suffer severe, long-term effects from STIs, such as chronic infection and infertility	Less likely to be infected with an STI during a heterosexual encounter

Health Disparities Among Ethnic Minorities

In studying the underlying causes of health disparities, it is often difficult to separate the many potential determinants or contributing factors.

Income and Education

Poverty and low educational attainment are the most important factors underlying health disparities. People with low incomes and less education have higher rates of death from all causes, especially chronic disease and injury, and they are less likely to have preventive health services, such as vaccinations and Pap tests. They are more likely to live in an area with a high rate of violence and many other environmental stressors. They also have higher rates of unhealthy behaviours.

Although ethnic disparities in health are significantly reduced when comparing groups with similar incomes and levels of education, they are not eliminated. For example, people living in poverty report worse health than people with higher incomes; but, within the latter group, minority populations often rate their health as worse than do whites. Infant mortality rates go down as the education level of mothers goes up; but among mothers who have received an education, Canadian Aboriginal peoples have significantly higher rates of infant mortality than whites. These variations point to the complexity of health disparities.

Access to Appropriate Health Care

People with low incomes are more likely to have problems arranging for transportation to access care. They are also more likely to lack information about services and preventive care. Ongoing studies continually find that racial minorities have less access to better health

care (such as complex surgery at high-volume hospitals) and receive lower quality care than whites.

Factors affecting such disparities may include the following:

• *Local differences in the availability of high-tech health care and specialists.* Minorities, regardless of income, may be more likely to live in medically underserved areas.

• *Problems with communication and trust.* People whose primary language is not English or French are more likely to have trouble communicating with health care providers; they may also have problems interpreting health information from public health education campaigns. Language and cultural barriers may be exacerbated by an underrepresentation of minorities in the health professions.

• *Cultural preferences relating to health care.* Groups may vary in their assessment of when it is appropriate to seek medical care and what types of treatments are acceptable.

Culture and Lifestyle

As described in the chapter, ethnic groups may vary in health-related behaviours, such as diet, tobacco and alcohol use, coping strategies, and health practices, and these behaviours can have important implications, both positive and negative, for wellness. Some cultures' nutritional intake, for example, is influenced by their heritage and tradition and this must be honoured and respected when helping groups engage in healthy eating practices. For instance, the Canadian Aboriginal Nutrition Network—a practice group of the Dietitians of Canada—focuses specifically on supporting Aboriginal nutrition. Being sensitive to traditional food preferences, cultural values, and peoples' spiritual connection

with food is an essential part of facilitating healthy choices among Canada's various cultures.

Discrimination

Racism and discrimination are stressful events that can cause psychological distress and increase the risk of physical and psychological problems. Discrimination can contribute to lower socioeconomic status and its associated risks. Bias in medical care can directly affect treatment and health outcomes.

Conversely, recent research shows that better health care results when doctors ask patients detailed questions about their ethnicity. (Most medical questionnaires ask patients to put themselves in a vague racial or ethnic category, such as Asian or Caucasian). Armed with more information on patients' backgrounds, medical professionals may find it easier to detect some genetic diseases or to overcome language or cultural barriers.

Sources: U.S. Department of Health and Human Services, Agency for Healthcare Research and Quality. 2008. *2007 National Healthcare Disparities Report.* Rockville, Md.: U.S. Department of Health and Human Services, Agency for Healthcare Research and Quality, AHRQ Pub. No. 08-0041; National Center for Health Statistics. 2008. *Early Release of Selected Estimates Based on Data from the January–June 2008 National Health Interview Survey* (http://www.cdc.gov/nchs/about/major/nhis/released200812.htm; retrieved December 27, 2008); National Center for Health Statistics. 2007. *Health, United States, 2007, with Chartbook on Trends in the Health of Americans.* Hyattsville, Md.: National Center for Health Statistics; Dietitians of Canada. 2005. *Registered Dietitians in Aboriginal Communities: Feeding Mind, Body and Spirit. Role Paper of the Dietitians of Canada Aboriginal Nutrition Network* (http://www.fsin.com/healthandsocial/childportal/images/Fedding%20Mind%20Body%20and%20Spirit.pdf; retrieved March 5, 2011).

3.8% (almost 1.2 million) of Canadians are Aboriginal people and approximately one-quarter can conduct a conversation in an Aboriginal language (Statistics Canada lists 14 different Aboriginal languages spoken in Canada). No single correct definition exists for the term *Aboriginal*, but Statistics Canada uses questions about ethnic origin (including ancestry), Aboriginal identity, Registered or

Treaty Indian, and Band or First Nation membership to establish its definitions.

Compared with the non-Aboriginal population, Aboriginal people face additional health challenges. This population is about 13 years younger, on average, because of higher birth rates, but those living on reserves have a dramatically higher infant mortality rate than the general population and even in adulthood have a shorter life expectancy. Additional serious health challenges affect First Nations people and Inuit Aboriginal peoples more than non-Aboriginal Canadians:

- About 1.5 times the rate heart disease

- Three to five times the rate of type 2 diabetes mellitus among First Nations people (which is associated with overweight and obesity, a condition affecting about 75% of the First Nations population) and a rising rate among Inuit

- Eight to ten times the rate of infection from tuberculosis (which is caused by a bacteria that is spread through the air)

Lifestyle factors can affect these chronic diseases, including lack of physical activity, excessive alcohol consumption, and poor nutritional intake. For example, Figure 1.4a shows that First Nations people living on reserves struggle to achieve healthy levels of physical activity. And although overall alcohol consumption is less among First Nations than among the general population, First Nations people living on reserves report double the rate of heavy drinking (Figure 1.4b).

Registered Indians on-reserve are also four times as likely to be unemployed and earn about one-half the incomes of non-Aboriginal Canadians. In the next section, we will highlight why the determinants of income and education are so vital to all Canadians' health status.

Recognizing the importance of reducing the health disparities among various group of Canadians, Health Canada's Web site states that the organization "is committed to closing the health status gap between First Nations people and Inuit and non-Aboriginal Canadians by working together to encourage healthy lifestyles, reduce and prevent diseases and provide health care services."

Income and Education   Inequalities in income and education underlie many of the health disparities among Canadians. In fact, poverty and low educational attainment are far more important predictors of poor health than any ethnic factor. Income and education are closely related, and groups with the highest poverty rates and least education have the worst health status. These Canadians have higher rates of infant mortality, traumatic injury and violent death, and many diseases, including heart disease, diabetes, tuberculosis, HIV infection, and some cancers. They are more likely to eat poorly, be overweight, smoke, drink, and use drugs. They are also exposed to more day-to-day stressors (such as the need to hold multiple jobs or deal with unreliable transportation).

A surprising finding from a 2006 study was that poor people living in wealthy neighbourhoods had higher mortality rates than poor people living in lower-income areas, perhaps because of the higher cost of living or psychosocial stressors.

Disability   People with disabilities have activity limitations, need assistance, or perceive themselves as having a disability. About one in seven people in Canada has some level of disability, and the rate is rising, especially among younger segments of the population. People with disabilities are more likely to be inactive and overweight. They report more days of depression than people without disabilities.

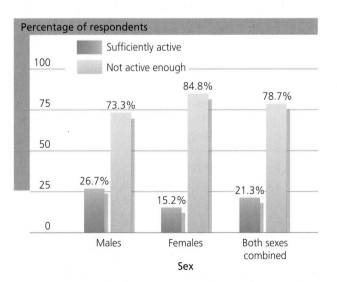

FIGURE 1.4A   Physical activity among First Nations people living on reserves.

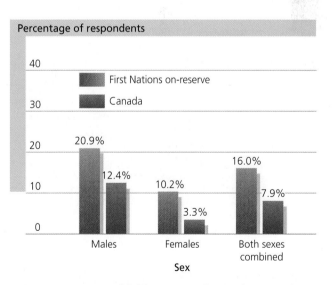

FIGURE 1.4B   Heavy drinking among First Nations people living on reserves.

Sources: Figure 1.4A: Prevalence of self-reported obesity among males and females 18 years and older, by age group, 2007—Obesity in Canada Snapshot. Public Health Agency of Canada. Reproduced with the permission of the Minister of Health, 2006. Figure 1.4B: Survey 2002–03; Results for Adults, Youth and Children Living in First Nations Communities. Assembly of First Nations, November 2005. Health Canada A Statistical Profile on the Health of First Nations in Canada: Determinants of Health, 1999 to 2003. Health Canada February 2009 HC Pub.: 3555 Cat: H34-193/1-2008E-PDF. ISBN: 978-0-662-48920-7 © Her Majesty the Queen in Right of Canada, 2009 Cat.: HP5-82/2009 ISBN: 978-0-662-06799-3.

Geographic Location   About one in five Canadians currently lives in a rural area—a place with fewer than 1000 residents and with less than 400 people per square kilometre. People living in rural areas have higher death rates and are less likely to be physically active, to use seat belts, or to obtain screening tests for preventive health care than are their urban counterparts. They are less likely to finish high school, have less access to timely emergency services, and have much higher rates of some diseases and injury-related death than people living in urban areas (Figure 1.5). But living in a rural community is not all bad; rural Canadians are less likely to be diagnosed with cancer, report feeling less stressed, and have a stronger sense of community belonging than urban dwellers. It is clear that our neighbourhoods matter. In fact, children living in dangerous neighbourhoods—rural or urban—are four times as likely to be overweight as children living in safer areas.

Sexual Orientation   The 1.5% of Canadians aged 18+ who identify themselves as gay, lesbian, or bisexual make up a diverse community with varied health concerns. Their emotional wellness and personal safety are affected by factors relating to personal, family, and social acceptance of their sexual orientation. Gay, lesbian, bisexual, and transgender teens tend to experience increased social pressures, which may help to explain why research has found them to be more likely to engage in risky behaviours, such as unsafe sex and drug use; they are also more likely to be depressed and to attempt suicide. HIV/AIDS is a major concern for gay men, and gay men and lesbians may have higher rates of substance abuse, depression, and suicide.

CHOOSING WELLNESS

Wellness is something everyone can strive toward. Achieving it requires knowledge, self-awareness, motivation, and effort—but the benefits last a lifetime. Optimal health comes mostly from a healthy lifestyle, patterns of behaviour that promote and support your health now and as you get older. In the pages that follow, you'll find current information and suggestions you can use to build a better lifestyle. Of course, your individual health determinants make it easier or more challenging to make wellness-related decisions; it is important that each person make the wellness-enhancing decisions that are within his or her control.

Factors That Influence Wellness

Our behaviour, family health history, environment, and access to health care are all important influences on wellness. These factors, which vary for both individuals and groups, can interact in ways that produce either health or disease.

Health Habits   Scientific research is continually revealing new connections between our habits and health. For example, heart disease is associated with smoking, stress, hostile and suspicious attitudes, a poor diet, and a sedentary way of life. Unfortunately, poor health habits take hold before many Canadians reach adulthood. (See the box "Wellness Matters for Postsecondary Students" for more information on health habits and wellness concerns of university- and college-age North Americans.)

Other habits, however, are beneficial. Regular exercise can help prevent heart disease, high blood pressure, diabetes, osteoporosis, and depression and may reduce the

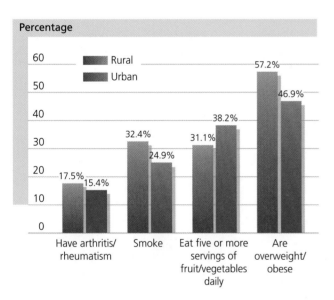

FIGURE 1.5   Selected health-related challenges of rural versus urban Canadians.   Rural dwellers tend to experience poorer health status and engage more often in health-detracting behaviours than urban habitants.

Source: How Healthy Are Rural Canadians? An Assessment of Their Health Status and Health Determinants—2006. Public Health Agency of Canada. Reproduced with the permission of the Minister of Health, 2006.

QUESTIONS FOR CRITICAL THINKING AND REFLECTION
How often do you feel exuberant? Vital? Joyful? What makes you feel that way? Conversely, how often do you feel downhearted, de-energized, or depressed? What makes you feel that way? Have you ever thought about how you might increase experiences of vitality and decrease experiences of discouragement?

Wellness Matters for Postsecondary Students

If you are like most postsecondary students, you probably feel pretty good about your health right now. Most university and college students are in their late teens or early twenties, lead busy lives, have plenty of friends, and look forward to a future filled with opportunity. With all these things going for you, why shouldn't you feel good?

A Closer Look

Although most university- and college-age people look healthy, appearances can be deceiving. Each year, thousands of students lose productive academic time to physical and emotional health problems—some of which can continue for life.

The following table shows the top 10 health issues affecting students' academic performance, according to the 2007 National College Health Assessment.

Health Issue	Students Affected (%)
Stress	32.9
Sleep difficulties	25.4
Cold/flu/sore throat	24.8
Concern for a friend or family member	18.1
Relationship problems	15.5
Depression/anxiety	15.5
Overuse of Internet/games	15.1
Death of a friend or family member	9.8
Sinus or ear infection/bronchitis/strep throat	9.4
Attention deficit disorder	7.0

Each of these issues is related to one or more of the six dimensions of wellness, and most can be influenced by choices students make daily. Although some troubles—such as the death of a friend—cannot be controlled, other physical and emotional concerns can be minimized by choosing healthy behaviours. For example, stress, the top health issue affecting students, can be managed in many ways. By reducing unhealthy choices (such as using alcohol to relax) and by increasing healthy choices (such as using time-management techniques), even busy students can reduce the impact of stress on their lives.

The survey also estimated that, based on students' reporting of their height and weight, more than 36% of university and college students are either overweight or obese. Although heredity plays a role in determining weight, lifestyle is also a factor in weight and weight management. In many studies over the past few decades, a large percentage of students have reported these types of behaviours:

• Overeating

• Snacking on junk food

• Frequently eating high-fat foods

• Using alcohol and binge drinking

Clearly, eating behaviours for students are often a matter of choice. Although students may not see (or feel) the effects of their dietary habits today, the long-term health risks are significant. Overweight and obese people run a higher-than normal risk of developing diabetes, heart disease, and cancer later in life. We now know with certainty that improving your eating habits, even a little, can lead to weight loss and improved overall health.

Other Choices, Other Problems

Students commonly make other unhealthy choices. Here are some examples from the 2007 National College Health Assessment:

• Nearly 50% of students reported that they did not use a condom the last time they had vaginal intercourse.

• About 80% of students had as many as six drinks the last time they partied.

• Almost 19% of students had used tobacco at least once during the past month.

What choices do you make in these situations? Remember: It's never too late to change. The sooner you trade an unhealthy behaviour for a healthy one, the longer you'll be around to enjoy the benefits.

Source: American College Health Association. 2008. *American College Health Association— National College Health Assessment: Reference Group Executive Summary, Fall 2007.* Baltimore, Md.: American College Health Association.

---

risk of colon cancer, stroke, and back injury. A balanced and varied diet helps prevent many chronic diseases. As we learn more about how our actions affect our bodies and minds, we can make informed choices for a healthier life.

Heredity and Family History Your **genome** consists of the complete set of genetic material in your cells; it contains about 25,000 genes, half from each of your parents. **Genes** control the production of proteins that serve both as the structural material for your body and as the regulators of all your body's chemical reactions and metabolic

processes. The human genome varies only slightly from person to person, and many of these differences do not affect health. However, some differences have important implications for health, and knowing your family health

genome The complete set of genetic material in an individual's cells.

gene The basic unit of heredity; a section of genetic material containing chemical instructions for making a particular protein.

TERMS

history can help you determine which conditions may be of special concern for you. Chapter 12 includes more information about creating a family health tree.

Errors in our genes are responsible for about 3500 clearly hereditary conditions, including sickle-cell disease and cystic fibrosis. Altered genes also play a part in heart disease, cancer, stroke, diabetes, and many other common conditions. However, in these more common and complex disorders, genetic alterations serve only to increase an individual's risk, and the disease itself results from the interaction of many genes with other factors. An example of the power of behaviour and environment can be seen in the 100% increase in the incidence of diabetes that has occurred among Canadians since 1997. This huge increase is not due to any sudden change in our genes; it is the result of increasing rates of obesity caused by poor dietary choices and lack of physical activity.

Environment   Your environment includes not only the air you breathe and the water you drink but also substances and conditions in your home, workplace, and community. Are you frequently exposed to environmental tobacco smoke or the radiation in sunlight? Do you live in an area with poor air quality or high rates of crime and violence? Has alcohol or drug abuse been a problem in your family? These and other environmental factors all have an impact on wellness. (See the box "A Planet in Peril: Healing the Environment" for more information on current environmental issues.)

Access to Health Care   Adequate health care helps improve both quality and quantity of life through preventive care and the treatment of disease. For example, vaccinations prevent many dangerous infections, and screening tests help identify key risk factors and diseases in their early, treatable stages. As described earlier in the chapter, inadequate access to the best health care is tied to various factors, such as low income. Cost is one of many issues surrounding the development of advanced health-related technologies.

Behaviour *Can* Make a Difference   In many cases, behaviour can tip the balance toward good health, even

TERMS

behaviour change   A lifestyle-management process that involves cultivating healthy behaviours and working to overcome unhealthy ones.

when heredity or environment is a negative factor. For example, breast cancer can run in families, but it also may be associated with being overweight, having poor nutrition, and being inactive. A woman with a family history of breast cancer is less likely to develop and die from the disease if she controls her weight, eats healthfully, exercises regularly, and has regular mammograms to help detect the disease in its early, most treatable stage.

Similarly, a young man with a family history of obesity can maintain a normal weight by being careful to choose healthier calories and to balance calorie intake against activities that burn calories. If your life is highly stressful, you can lessen the chances of heart disease and stroke by learning ways to manage and cope with stress. If you live in an area with severe air pollution, you can reduce the risk of lung disease by not smoking.

You can also take an active role in improving your environment. Behaviours like these enable you to make a difference in how great an impact heredity and environment will have on your health.

REACHING WELLNESS THROUGH LIFESTYLE MANAGEMENT

As you consider the behaviours that contribute to wellness—being physically active, choosing a healthy diet, and so on—you may be doing a mental comparison with your own behaviours. If you are like most young adults, you probably have some healthy habits and some habits that place your health at risk. For example, you may be physically active and have a healthy diet but indulge in binge drinking on weekends. You may be careful to wear your seat belt in your car but smoke cigarettes or use chewing tobacco. Moving in the direction of wellness means cultivating healthy behaviours and working to overcome unhealthy ones. This approach to lifestyle management is called **behaviour change**.

As you may already know from experience, changing an unhealthy habit can be hard. When you embark on a behaviour change plan, it may seem like too much work at first. But as you make progress, you will gain confidence in your ability to take charge of your life. You will also

A Planet in Peril: Healing the Environment

Our treatment of the environment determines—to a far greater extent than many people want to believe—how Earth will treat us. This lesson has gradually become clear over several generations, but our troubled environment began attracting intensive worldwide attention only in the last few years. Today, the evidence is irrefutable: Our continuing abuse of the environment has led to a natural backlash that includes the extinction of entire species, shifts in global weather patterns, dying oceans, and the disappearance of polar ice fields.

Climate experts are now sounding the alarm. If we don't immediately begin reducing our impact on the environment, the damage may become irreversible. The compounded effects of humanity's environmental neglect could make our planet a much less hospitable and livable place, possibly within two or three decades.

The Root of the Problem

Pollution, of course, is not a new problem. People have contaminated the air by burning coal, wood, and oil for millennia. Age-old industries, such as forestry and mining, have laid waste to vast stretches of land, and such processes as tanning and printing have dumped untold amounts of lethal toxins into the ground and water. People began to take serious notice of pollution even before the Industrial Revolution, when a few scientists reported that the smoke from factories and trains was fouling the air, and that industrial runoff was polluting rivers.

Over time, improvements in technology made manufacturing easier and cheaper, while an increasing population and greater prosperity created an insatiable demand for manufactured goods. Industrial growth gave rise to explosive growth of urban areas—population centres that drove the need for transportation and electricity. As a result, industries and individuals consume ever-larger amounts of fuel and other resources, creating ever more waste and pollution

in the process. Combine this with the pollution generated by our use of fossil-fuelled transportation, and the result is a recipe for global catastrophe.

Global Warming

Human practices affect the environment on every level. Our food chain is contaminated with pesticides, water must be cleaned of sewage and chemicals before we can drink it, and in some cities the air is so polluted with exhaust that it can actually be dangerous to breathe. But the most ravaging—and frightening—consequence of environmental abuse is the phenomenon known as global warming: the gradual rise in Earth's temperature that is causing polar ice caps to shrink, creating unfavourable weather patterns, and contributing to rapid devastation of land and oceans.

What causes global warming? As you will learn in Chapter 21, global warming is largely due to human activity. As we burn fossil fuels (such as coal, oil, and fuels derived from them) to power vehicles and factories, the process releases many kinds of waste gases into the skies. Some of these gases, chiefly carbon dioxide (CO_2), rise up into the air and

stay there, acting as an invisible insulating blanket. These gases create a "greenhouse" effect by trapping some of the heat that radiates from Earth—heat that would normally dissipate through the atmosphere. By defeating the planet's natural temperature controls, CO_2 and other "greenhouse gases" are causing Earth to get warmer.

As already mentioned, this rise in temperature can wreak havoc on Earth, especially if temperatures increase unchecked over a long period. Experts are trying to determine how high Earth's temperature must climb before we reach the tipping point (when damage from climate change becomes irreversible) and how soon that point may be reached.

Reversing the Warming Trend

Until then, however, one fact is obvious. People, industries, societies, and governments must start taking action now to reduce their "imprint" on the environment. Legislation, such as Ontario's Clean Water Act, has helped, but it is important to understand that pollution and global warming are not problems just for governments to solve. The environment affects every person in an individual way. The more we do as individuals, the more benefits will result from our collective efforts.

This is why *Core Concepts in Health*, Canadian edition, has been created with current environmental issues in mind. Not only does Chapter 21 examine the environment in detail, but every chapter also briefly addresses the environment's impact on a specific aspect of your well-being—including the way you exercise, the foods you eat, and your reproductive health. In each chapter, you will see a short feature called "Thinking About the Environment." This feature relates the chapter's main theme to the environment and poses questions for you to consider or suggests actions you can take to improve the environment and promote your personal health and wellness.

Wellness: Evaluate Your Lifestyle

All of us want optimal health. But many of us do not know how to achieve it. Taking this quiz, adapted from one created by the U.S. Public Health Service, is a good place to start. The behaviours covered in the quiz are recommended for most North Americans. (Some of them may not apply to people with certain diseases or disabilities or to pregnant women, who may require special advice from their physician.) After you take the quiz, add up your score for each section.

	ALMOST ALWAYS	SOMETIMES	NEVER

Tobacco Use

If you never use tobacco, enter a score of 10 for this section and go to the next section.

	ALMOST ALWAYS	SOMETIMES	NEVER
1. I avoid using tobacco.	2	1	0
2. I smoke only low-tar/nicotine cigarettes *or* I smoke a pipe or cigars *or* I use smokeless tobacco.	2	1	0

Tobacco Score: _____

Alcohol and Other Drugs

	ALMOST ALWAYS	SOMETIMES	NEVER
1. I avoid alcohol or I drink no more than 1 (women) *or* 2 (men) drinks a day.	4	1	0
2. I avoid using alcohol or other drugs as a way of handling stressful situations or problems in my life.	2	1	0
3. I am careful not to drink alcohol when taking medications, such as for colds or allergies, or when pregnant.	2	1	0
4. I read and follow the label directions when using prescribed and over-the-counter drugs.	2	1	0

Alcohol and Other Drugs Score: _____

Nutrition

	ALMOST ALWAYS	SOMETIMES	NEVER
1. I eat a variety of foods each day, including seven or more servings of fruits and vegetables.	3	1	0
2. I limit the amount of total fat and saturated and trans fat in my diet.	3	1	0
3. I avoid skipping meals.	2	1	0
4. I limit the amount of salt and sugar I eat.	2	1	0

Nutrition Score: _____

Exercise and Fitness

	ALMOST ALWAYS	SOMETIMES	NEVER
1. I engage in moderate exercise for 20–60 minutes, 3–5 times a week.	4	1	0
2. I maintain a healthy weight, avoiding overweight and underweight.	2	1	0
3. I do exercises to develop muscular strength and endurance at least twice a week.	2	1	0
4. I spend some of my leisure time participating in physical activities, such as gardening, bowling, golf, or baseball.	2	1	0

Exercise and Fitness Score: _____

Emotional Health

	ALMOST ALWAYS	SOMETIMES	NEVER
1. I enjoy being a student, and I have a job or do other work that I like.	2	1	0
2. I find it easy to relax and express my feelings freely.	2	1	0

experience the benefits of wellness: more energy, greater vitality, deeper feelings of appreciation and curiosity, and a higher quality of life.

In the rest of this chapter, we outline a general process for changing unhealthy behaviours that is backed by research and that has worked for many people. We also offer many specific strategies and tips for change.

target behaviour An isolated behaviour selected as the subject of a behaviour change program.

Getting Serious About Your Health

Before you can start changing a wellness-related behaviour, you have to know that the behaviour is problematic and that you *can* change it. To make good decisions, you need information about relevant topics and issues, including what resources are available to help you change.

Examine Your Current Health Habits Have you considered how your current lifestyle is affecting your health today and how it will affect your health in the future? Do you know which of your current habits enhance your health and which detract from it? Begin your journey

	ALMOST ALWAYS	SOMETIMES	NEVER
3. I manage stress well.	2	1	0
4. I have close friends, relatives, or others I can talk to about personal matters and call on for help.	2	1	0
5. I participate in group activities (such as church and community organizations) or hobbies that I enjoy.	2	1	0

Emotional Health Score: _____

Safety

1. I wear a seat belt while riding in a car.	2	1	0
2. I avoid driving while under the influence of alcohol or other drugs.	2	1	0
3. I obey traffic rules and the speed limit when driving.	2	1	0
4. I read and follow instructions on the labels of potentially harmful products or substances, such as household cleaners, poisons, and electrical appliances.	2	1	0
5. I avoid smoking in bed.	2	1	0

Safety Score: _____

Disease Prevention

1. I know the warning signs of cancer, diabetes, heart attack, and stroke.	2	1	0
2. I avoid overexposure to the sun and use a sunscreen.	2	1	0
3. I get recommended medical screening tests (such as blood pressure checks and Pap tests), immunizations, and booster shots.	2	1	0
4. I regularly examine my breasts/testicles.	2	1	0
5. I am not sexually active *or* I have sex with only one mutually faithful, uninfected partner *or* I always engage in safer sex (using condoms) *and* I do not share needles to inject drugs.	2	1	0

Disease Prevention Score: _____

What Your Scores Mean

Scores of 9 and 10 Excellent! Your answers show that you are aware of the importance of this area to your health. More important, you are putting your knowledge to work for you by practicing good health habits. As long as you continue to do so, this area should not pose a serious health risk.

Scores of 6 to 8 Your health practices in this area are good, but there is room for improvement.

Scores of 3 to 5 Your health risks are showing.

Scores of 0 to 2 You may be taking serious and unnecessary risks with your health.

toward wellness with self-assessment: Think about your own behaviour, talk with friends and family members about what they've noticed about your lifestyle and your health, and take the quiz in the box "Wellness: Evaluate Your Lifestyle." Challenge any unrealistically optimistic attitudes or ideas you may hold—for example, "To protect my health, I don't need to worry about quitting smoking until I'm 40 years old," or "Being overweight won't put me at risk for diabetes." Health risks are very real, and health habits throughout life are important.

Many people start to consider changing a behaviour when friends or family members express concern, when a landmark event occurs (such as turning 30), or when new

information raises their awareness of risk. If you find yourself reevaluating some of your behaviours as you read this text, take advantage of the opportunity to make a change in a structured way.

Choose a Target Behaviour Changing any behaviour can be demanding. This is why it's a good idea to start small, by choosing one behaviour you want to change—called a **target behaviour**—and working on it until you succeed. Your chances of success will be greater if your first goal is simple, such as resisting the urge to snack between classes. As you change one behaviour, make your next goal a little more significant, and build on your success.

Evaluating Sources of Health Information

Believability of Health Information Sources

A recent survey indicated that university and college students are smart about evaluating health information. They trust the health information they receive from health professionals and educators and are skeptical about popular information sources.

Rank	Source	Rank	Source
1	Health educators	8	Resident assistants or advisers
2	Health centre medical staff	9	Religious centres
3	Parents	10	Internet
4	Faculty or coursework	11	Friends
5	Leaflets, pamphlets, flyers	12	Magazines
6	Campus newspaper articles	13	Television
7	Campus peer educators	14	Other sources

How smart are you about evaluating health information? Here are some tips.

General Strategies

Whenever you encounter health-related information, take the following steps to make sure it is credible:

• *Go to the original source.* Media reports often simplify the results of medical research. Find out for yourself what a study really reported, and determine whether it was based on good science. What type of study was it? Was it published in a recognized medical or health journal? Was it an animal study or did it involve people? Did the study include a large number of people? What did the authors of the study actually report?

• *Watch for misleading language.* Reports that tout "break-throughs" or "dramatic proof" are probably hype. A study may state that a behaviour "contributes to" or is "associated with" an outcome; this does not prove a cause-and-effect relationship.

• *Distinguish between research reports and public health advice.* Do not change your behaviour based on the results of a single report or study. If an agency, such as the Canadian Cancer Society

Research Institute, urges a behaviour change, however, you should follow its advice. Large, publicly funded organizations issue such advice based on many studies, not a single report.

• *Remember that anecdotes are not facts.* A friend may tell you he lost weight on some new diet, but individual success stories do not mean the plan is truly safe or effective. Check with your physician before making any serious lifestyle changes.

• *Be skeptical.* If a report seems too good to be true, it probably is. Be wary of information contained in advertisements. An ad's goal is to sell a product, even if you have no need for it.

• *Make choices that are right for you.* Friends and family members can be a great source of ideas and inspiration, but you need to make health-related choices that work best for you.

Internet Resources

Online sources pose special challenges; when reviewing a health-related Web site, ask these questions:

• *What is the source of the information?* Web sites maintained by government agencies, professional associations, or established academic or medical institutions are likely to present trustworthy information. Many other groups and individuals post accurate information, but it is important to look at the qualifications of the people who are behind the site. (Check the home page or click the "About Us" link.)

• *How often is the site updated?* Look for sites that are updated frequently. Check the "last modified" date of any Web page.

• *Is the site promotional?* Be wary of information from sites that sell specific products, use testimonials as evidence, appear to have a social or political agenda, or ask for money.

• *What do other sources say about a topic?* Be cautious of claims or information that appears at only one site or comes from a chat room, bulletin board, or blog.

• *Does the site conform to any set of guidelines or criteria for quality and accuracy?* Look for sites that identify themselves as conforming to some code or set of principles, such as those set forth by the Health on the Net Foundation or the Canadian Medical Association. These codes include criteria, such as use of information from respected sources and disclosure of the site's sponsors.

Learn About Your Target Behaviour Once you've chosen a target behaviour, you need to learn its risks and benefits for you—both now and in the future. Ask these questions:

• How is your target behaviour affecting your level of wellness today?

• What diseases or conditions does this behaviour place you at risk for?

• What effect would changing your behaviour have on your health?

As a starting point, use this text and the resources listed in the For More Information section at the end of each chapter; see the box "Evaluating Sources of Health Information" for additional guidelines.

Find Help Have you identified a particularly challenging target behaviour or mood, something like alcohol addiction, binge eating, or depression, that interferes with your ability to function or places you at a serious health risk? Help may be needed to change behaviours or conditions that are too deeply rooted or too serious for self-management.

Don't be stopped by the seriousness of the problem; many resources are available to help you solve it. On campus, the student health centre or campus counselling centre can provide assistance. To locate community resources, consult the Yellow Pages, your physician, or the Internet.

Building Motivation to Change

Knowledge is necessary for behaviour change, but it isn't usually enough to make people act. Millions of people have sedentary lifestyles, for example, even though they know it's bad for their health. This is particularly true of young adults, who may not be motivated to change because they feel healthy in spite of their unhealthy behaviours. To succeed at behaviour change, you need strong motivation.

Examine the Pros and Cons of Change   Health behaviours have short-term and long-term benefits and costs. Consider the benefits and costs of an inactive lifestyle:

- In the short term, such a lifestyle allows you more time to watch TV and hang out with friends, but it leaves you less physically fit and less able to participate in recreational activities.

- In the long term, it increases the risk of weight gain, heart disease, cancer, stroke, and premature death.

To successfully change your behaviour, you must believe that the benefits of change outweigh the costs.

Carefully examine the pros and cons of continuing your current behaviour and of changing to a healthier one. Focus on the effects that are most meaningful to you, including those that are tied to your personal identity and values. For example, if you see yourself as an active person who is a good role model for others, then adopting certain behaviours, such as engaging in regular physical activity and getting adequate sleep, will support your personal identity. If you value independence and control over your life, then quitting smoking will be consistent with your values and goals. To complete your analysis, ask friends and family members about the effects of your behaviour on them. For example, a younger sister may tell you that your smoking habit influenced her decision to take up smoking.

The short-term benefits of behaviour change can be an important motivating force. Although some people are motivated by long-term goals, such as avoiding a disease that may hit them in 30 years, most are more likely to be moved to action by shorter-term, more personal goals. Feeling better, looking better, doing better in school, improving at a sport, reducing stress, and increasing self-esteem are common short-term benefits of health behaviour change. Many wellness behaviours are associated with immediate improvements in quality of life. For example, surveys of North Americans have found that nonsmokers feel healthy and full of energy more days each month than do smokers, and they report fewer days of sadness and troubled sleep; the same is true when physically active

people are compared with sedentary people. Over time, these types of differences add up to a substantially higher quality of life for people who engage in healthy behaviours.

Boost Self-Efficacy   When you start thinking about changing a health behaviour, a big factor in your eventual success is whether you have confidence in yourself and in your ability to change. **Self-efficacy** refers to your belief in your ability to successfully take action and perform a specific task. Strategies for boosting self-efficacy include developing an internal locus of control, using visualization and self-talk, and getting encouragement from supportive people.

LOCUS OF CONTROL   Who do you believe is controlling your life? Is it your parents, friends, or school? Is it fate? Or is it you? **Locus of control** refers to the figurative place a person designates as the source of responsibility for the events in his or her life. People who believe they are in control of their own lives are said to have an *internal locus of control*. Those who believe that factors beyond their control determine the course of their lives are said to have an *external locus of control*.

For lifestyle management, an internal locus of control is an advantage because it reinforces motivation and commitment. An external locus of control can sabotage efforts to change behaviour. For example, if you believe that you are destined to die from breast cancer because your mother died from the disease, you may view breast self-exams and regular checkups as a waste of time. In contrast, if you believe that you can take action to reduce your risk of breast cancer in spite of hereditary factors, you will be motivated to follow guidelines for early detection of the disease.

If you find yourself attributing too much influence to outside forces, gather more information about your wellness-related behaviours. List all the ways that making lifestyle changes will improve your health. If you believe you'll succeed, and if you recognize that you are in charge of your life, you're on your way to wellness.

VISUALIZATION AND SELF-TALK   One of the best ways to boost your confidence and self-efficacy is to visualize

self-efficacy   The belief in your ability to take action and perform a specific task.

locus of control   The figurative place a person designates as the source of responsibility for the events in his or her life.

TERMS

yourself successfully engaging in a new, healthier behaviour. Imagine yourself going for an afternoon run three days a week or no longer smoking cigarettes. Also visualize yourself enjoying all the short-term and long-term benefits that your lifestyle change will bring. Create a new self-image: What will you and your life be like when you become a regular exerciser or a nonsmoker?

You can also use self-talk, the internal dialogue you carry on with yourself, to increase your confidence in your ability to change. Counter any self-defeating patterns of thought with more positive or realistic thoughts: "I am a strong, capable person, and I can maintain my commitment to change." See Chapter 2 for more on self-talk.

ROLE MODELS AND OTHER SUPPORTIVE INDIVIDUALS Social support can make a big difference in your level of motivation and your chances of success. Perhaps you know people who have reached the goal you are striving for; they could be role models or mentors for you, providing information and support for your efforts. Gain strength from their experiences, and tell yourself, "If they can do it, so can I." In addition, find a buddy who wants to make the same changes you do and who can take an active role in your behaviour change program. For example, Canadian research has found that an exercise buddy can provide companionship and encouragement when postsecondary students, like you, might be tempted to skip a workout.

IDENTIFY AND OVERCOME BARRIERS TO CHANGE Don't let past failures at behaviour change discourage you; they can be a great source of information you can use to boost your chances of future success. Make a list of the problems and challenges you faced in any previous behaviour change attempts; to this, add the short-term costs of behaviour change that you identified in your analysis of the pros and

THINKING ABOUT THE ENVIRONMENT
As you think about target behaviours you may want to change, consider your behaviour toward the environment. By making simple changes to your daily routine or by using more environmentally friendly products, you can make a positive difference to the planet. For example, do you do any of the following?

- Recycle paper, glass, plastic, and metal products

- Use energy-efficient compact fluorescent light bulbs instead of standard incandescent bulbs

- Keep your car well maintained to get the best possible gas mileage and emit the lowest possible amount of pollution

- Avoid using aerosol products, pesticides, and other chemicals that could pollute the ground, air, or water

For more information on the environment and environmental health, see Chapter 21.

cons of change. Once you've listed these key barriers to change, develop a practical plan for overcoming each one. For example, if you always smoke when you're with certain friends, decide in advance how you will turn down the next cigarette you are offered.

Enhancing Your Readiness to Change

The transtheoretical, or stages of change, model has been shown to be an effective approach to lifestyle self-management. According to this model, you move through distinct stages as you work to change your target behaviour. It is important to determine what stage you are in now so that you can choose appropriate strategies for progressing through the cycle of change. This approach can help you enhance your readiness and intention to change. Read the following sections to determine what stage you are in for your target behaviour. For ideas on changing stages, see the box "Tips for Moving Forward in the Cycle of Behaviour Change."

Precontemplation People at this stage do not think they have a problem and do not intend to change their behaviour. They may be unaware of the risks associated with their behaviour or may deny them. They may have tried unsuccessfully to change in the past and may now think the situation is hopeless. They may also blame other people or external factors for their problems. People in the precontemplation stage believe that they have more reasons or more important reasons not to change than they do to change.

Contemplation People at this stage know they have a problem and intend to take action within six months. They acknowledge the benefits of behaviour change but are also aware of the costs of changing—to be successful, people must believe that the benefits of change outweigh the costs. People in the contemplation stage wonder about possible courses of action but don't know how to proceed. There may also be specific barriers to change that appear too difficult to overcome.

Preparation People at this stage plan to take action within a month or may already have begun to make small changes in their behaviour. They may be engaging in their new, healthier behaviour but not yet regularly or consistently. They may have created a plan for change but may be worried about failing.

Action During the action stage, people outwardly modify their behaviour and their environment. The action stage requires the greatest commitment of time and energy, and people in this stage are at risk for reverting to old, unhealthy patterns of behaviour.

Maintenance People at this stage have maintained their new, healthier lifestyle for at least six months. Lapses

Tips for Moving Forward in the Cycle of Behaviour Change

Precontemplation

• *Raise your awareness.* Research your target behaviour and its effects.

• *Be self-aware.* Look at the mechanisms you use to resist change, such as denial or rationalization. Find ways to counteract these mechanisms.

• *Seek social support.* Friends and family members can help you identify target behaviours and understand their impact on the people around you.

• *Identify helpful resources.* These might include exercise classes or stress-management workshops offered by your school.

Contemplation

• *Keep a journal.* A record of your target behaviour and the circumstances that elicit the behaviour can help you plan a change program.

• *Do a cost-benefit analysis.* Identify the costs and benefits (both current and future) of maintaining your behaviour and of changing it. Costs can be monetary, social, emotional, and so on.

• *Identify barriers to change.* Knowing these obstacles can help you overcome them.

• *Engage your emotions.* Watch movies or read books about people with your target behaviour. Imagine what your life will be like if you don't change.

• *Create a new self-image.* Imagine what you'll be like after changing your target behaviour. Try to think of yourself in new terms right now.

• *Think before you act.* Learn why you engage in the target behaviour. Determine what sets you off, and train yourself not to act reflexively.

Preparation

• *Create a plan.* Include a start date, goals, rewards, and specific steps you will take to change your behaviour.

• *Make change a priority.* Create and sign a contract with yourself.

• *Practise visualization and self-talk.* These techniques can help prepare you mentally for challenging situations.

• *Take short steps.* Successfully practising your new behaviour for a short time—even a single day—can boost your confidence and motivation.

Action

• *Monitor your progress.* Keep up with your journal entries.

• *Change your environment.* Make changes that will discourage the target behaviour—for example, getting rid of snack foods or not stocking the refrigerator with beer.

• *Find alternatives to your target behaviour.* Make a list of things you can do to replace the behaviour.

• *Reward yourself.* Rewards should be identified in your change plan. Give yourself lots of praise, and focus on your success.

• *Involve your friends.* Tell them you want to change, and ask for their help.

• *Don't get discouraged.* Real change can be difficult.

Maintenance

• *Keep going.* Continue using the positive strategies that worked in earlier stages.

• *Be prepared for lapses.* Don't let slip-ups set you back.

• *Be a role model.* Once you have successfully changed your behaviour, you may be able to help someone else do the same thing.

---

may have occurred, but people in maintenance have been successful in quickly reestablishing the desired behaviour. The maintenance stage can last a few months or many years.

Termination For some behaviours, a person may reach the sixth and final stage of termination. People at this stage have exited the cycle of change and are no longer tempted to lapse back into their old behaviour. They have a new self-image and total self-efficacy with regard to their target behaviour.

Dealing with Relapse

People seldom progress through the stages of change in a straightforward, linear way; rather, they tend to move to a certain stage and then slip back to a previous stage before resuming their forward progress. Research suggests that most people make several attempts before they successfully change a behaviour; four out of five people experience some degree of backsliding. For this reason, the stages of change are best conceptualized as a spiral, in which people cycle back through previous stages but are further along in the process each time they renew their commitment (Figure 1.6, p. 24).

If you experience a lapse—a single slip—or a relapse—a return to old habits—don't give up. Relapse can be

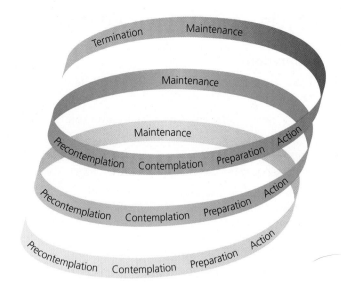

FIGURE 1.6   The stages of change: A spiral model.

Source: Adapted from Prochaska, J. O., C. C. Diclemente, and J. C. Norcross. 1992. In Search of How People Change. *American Psychologist* 47(9): 1102–1114. Copyright © 1992 by the American Psychological Association. Reprinted by permission.

demoralizing, but it is not the same as failure; failure means stopping before you reach your goal and never changing your target behaviour. During the early stages of the change process, it's a good idea to plan for relapse so you can avoid guilt and self-blame and get back on track quickly. Follow these steps:

1. *Forgive yourself.* A single setback isn't the end of the world, but abandoning your efforts to change could have negative effects on your life.

2. *Give yourself credit for the progress you have already made.* You can use that success as motivation to continue.

3. *Move on.* You can learn from a relapse and use that knowledge to deal with potential setbacks in the future.

If relapses keep occurring or if you can't seem to control them, you may need to return to a previous stage of the behaviour change process. If this is necessary, reevaluate your goals and your strategy. A different or less stressful approach may help you avoid setbacks when you try again.

Developing Skills for Change: Creating a Personalized Plan

Once you are committed to making a change, it's time to put together a plan of action. Your key to success is a well-thought-out plan that sets goals, anticipates problems, and includes rewards.

1. Monitor Your Behaviour and Gather Data   Keep a record of your target behaviour and the circumstances surrounding it. Record this information for at least a week or two. Keep your notes in a health journal or notebook or on your computer (see the sample journal entries in Figure 1.7). Record each occurrence of your behaviour, noting the following:

- What the activity was
- When and where it happened
- What you were doing
- How you felt at that time

2. Analyze the Data and Identify Patterns   After you have collected data on the behaviour, analyze the data to identify patterns. When are you most likely to overeat? What events trigger your appetite? Perhaps you are especially hungry at midmorning or when you put off eating dinner until 9 p.m. Perhaps you overindulge in food and drink when you go to a particular restaurant or when you're with certain friends. Note the connections between your feelings and external cues, such as time of day, location, situation, and the actions of others around you.

3. Be SMART About Setting Goals   If your goals are too challenging, you will have trouble making steady progress and will be more likely to give up altogether. If, for example, you are in poor physical condition, it will not make sense to set a goal of being ready to run a marathon within two months. If you set goals you can live with, it will be easier to stick with your behaviour change plan and be successful.

Experts suggest that your goals meet the SMART criteria; that is, your behaviour change goals should be the following:

- *Specific.* Avoid vague goals like "eat more fruits and vegetables." Instead, state your objectives in specific terms, such as "eat 500 millilitres of fruit and 750 millilitres of vegetables every day."

- *Measurable.* Recognize that your progress will be easier to track if your goals are quantifiable, so give your goal a number. You might measure your goal in terms of time (such as "walk briskly for 20 minutes a day"), distance ("run three kilometres, three days per week"), or some other amount ("drink five glasses of water every day").

- *Attainable.* Set goals that are within your physical limits. For example, if you are a poor swimmer, it might not be possible for you to meet a short-term fitness goal by swimming laps. Walking or biking might be better options.

- *Realistic.* Manage your expectations when you set goals. For example, it may not be possible for a long-time smoker to quit cold turkey. As more realistic approach might be to use nicotine-replacement patches or gum for several weeks while getting help from a support group.

Date	November 5				Day	M	TU	W	TH	F	SA	SU	

Time of day	M/S	Food eaten	Cals.	H	Where did you eat?	What else were you doing?	How did someone else influence you?	What made you want to eat what you did?	Emotions and feelings?	Thoughts and concerns?
7:30	M	250 mL Crispix cereal 150 mL skim milk coffee, black 250 mL orange juice	110 40 — 120	3	home	reading newspaper	alone	I always eat cereal in the morning	a little keyed up & worried	thinking about quiz in class today
10:30	S	1 apple	90	1	hall outside classroom	studying	alone	felt tired & wanted to wake up	tired	worried about next class
12:30	M	250 mL chili 1 roll 1 pat butter 1 orange 2 oatmeal cookies 1 soda	290 120 35 60 120 150	2	campus food court	talking	eating w/ friends; we decided to eat at the food court	wanted to be part of group	excited and happy	interested in hearing everyone's plans for the weekend
M/S = Meal or snack			H = Hunger rating (0–3)							

FIGURE 1.7 Sample health journal entries. If your goal is to start an exercise program, track your activities to determine how to make time for workouts.

- *Time-frame specific.* Give yourself a reasonable amount of time to reach your goals, state the time frame in your behaviour change plan, and set your agenda to meet the goal within the given time.

Using these criteria, a sedentary person who wanted to improve his health and build fitness might set a goal of being able to run five kilometre in 30 minutes, to be achieved within six months. To work toward that goal, he might set a number of smaller, intermediate goals that are easier to achieve. For example, his list of goals might look like this:

Week	Frequency (days/week)	Activity	Duration (minutes)
1	3	Walk <2 km	10–15
2	3	Walk 2 km	15–20
3	4	Walk 2–3 km	20–25
4	4	Walk 3–4 km	25–30
5–7	3–4	Walk/run 2 km	15–20
⋮			
21–24	4–5	Run 4–5 km	25–30

Of course, it may not be possible to meet these goals, but you never know until you try. As you work toward meeting your long-term goal, you may find it necessary to adjust your short-term goals. For example, you may find that you can start running sooner than you thought, or you may be able to run farther than you originally estimated. In such cases, it may be reasonable to make your goals more challenging. Otherwise, you may want to make them easier to stay motivated.

For some goals and situations, it may make more sense to focus on something other than your outcome goal. If you are in an early stage of change, for example, your goal may be to learn more about the risks associated with your target behaviour or to complete a cost-benefit analysis. If your goal involves a long-term lifestyle change, such as reaching a healthy weight, it is better to focus on developing healthy habits than to target a specific weight loss. Your goal in this case might be exercising for 30 minutes every day, reducing portion sizes, or eliminating late-night snacks.

52% of Canadians ages 12 and older, and **48%** ages 20 and older engage in physical activity at the level needed for health gains.

—Gilmore, 2007; Canadian Fitness & Lifestyle Research Institute, 2009

QUICK STATS

4. Devise a Plan of Action   Develop a strategy that will support your efforts to change. Your plan of action should include the following steps:

- *Get what you need.* Identify resources that can help you. For example, you can join a community walking club or sign up for a smoking cessation program. You may also need to buy some new running shoes or nicotine-replacement patches. Get the items you need right away; waiting can delay your progress.

Your environment contains powerful cues for both positive and negative lifestyle choices. Identifying and using the healthier options available to you throughout the day is a key part of a successful behaviour change program.

- *Modify your environment.* If cues in your environment trigger your target behaviour, try to control them. For example, if you normally have alcohol at home, getting rid of it can help prevent you from indulging. If you usually study with a group of friends in an environment that allows smoking, try moving to a nonsmoking area. If you always buy a snack at a certain vending machine, change your route so you don't pass by it.
- *Control related habits.* You may have habits that contribute to your target behaviour; modifying these habits can help change the behaviour. For example, if you usually plop down on the sofa while watching TV, try putting an exercise bike in front of the set so you can burn calories while watching your favourite programs.
- *Reward yourself.* Giving yourself instant, real rewards for good behaviour will reinforce your efforts. Plan your rewards; decide in advance what each one will be and how you will earn it. Tie rewards to achieving specific goals or subgoals. For example, you might treat yourself to a movie after a week of avoiding unhealthy snacks. Make a list of items or events to use as rewards; they should be special to you and preferably unrelated to food or alcohol.
- *Involve the people around you.* Tell family and friends about your plan, and ask them to help. To help them respond appropriately to your needs, create a specific list of dos and don'ts. For example, ask them to support you when you set aside time to exercise or avoid second helpings at dinner.
- *Plan for challenges.* Think about situations and people that might derail your program, and develop ways to cope with them. For example, if you think it will be hard to stick to your usual exercise program during exams, schedule short bouts of physical activity (such as a brisk walk) as stress-reducing study breaks.

5. Make a Personal Contract

A serious personal contract—one that commits you to your word—can result in a higher chance of follow-through than a casual, offhand promise. Your contract can help prevent procrastination by specifying important dates and can also serve as a reminder of your personal commitment to change.

Your contract should include a statement of your goal and your commitment to reaching it. The contract should also include details, such as the following:

- The date you will start
- The steps you will take to measure your progress
- The strategies you plan to use to promote change
- The date you expect to reach your final goal

Have someone—preferably someone who will be actively helping you with your program—sign your contract as a witness.

Figure 1.8 shows a sample behaviour change contract for someone who is committing to eating more fruit every day. You can apply the general behaviour change planning framework presented in this chapter to any target behaviour. Additional examples of behaviour change plans appear in the Behaviour Change Strategy sections at the end of many chapters in this text. In these sections, you will find specific plans for quitting smoking, starting an exercise program, and making other positive lifestyle changes.

Behaviour Change Contract

1. I, __Tammy Lau__, agree to _increase my consumption of fruit from_ _250 mL per week to 500 mL per day._

2. I will begin on ____10/5____ and plan to reach my goal of __500 mL__ of fruit per day _____ by __12/7__

3. To reach my final goal, I have devised the following schedule of mini-goals. For each step in my program, I will give myself the reward listed.

I will begin to have 125 mL of fruit with breakfast	10/5	see movie
I will begin to have 125 mL of fruit with lunch	10/26	new cd
I will begin to substitute fruit juice for pop 1 time per day	11/16	concert

   My overall reward for reaching my goal will be _trip to beach_

4. I have gathered and analyzed data on my target behaviour and have identified the following strategies for changing my behaviour: _Keep the fridge stocked with easy-to-carry fruit. Pack fruit in my backpack every day. Buy lunch at place that serves fruit._

5. I will use the following tools to monitor my progress toward my final goal: _Chart on fridge door_ _Health journal_

   I sign this contract as an indication of my personal commitment to reach my goal: ___Tammy Lau___   __9/28__

   I have recruited a helper who will witness my contract and _also increase his consumption of fruit; eat lunch with me twice a week._ _____ _Eric March_ _____ __9/28__

FIGURE 1.8 A sample behaviour change contract.

Putting Your Plan into Action

The starting date has arrived, and you are ready to put your plan into action. This stage requires commitment, the resolve to stick with the plan no matter what temptations you encounter. Remember all the reasons you have to make the change—and remember that *you* are the boss. Use all your strategies to make your plan work. Make sure your environment is change-friendly, and get as much support and encouragement from others as possible. Keep track of your progress in your health journal, and give yourself regular rewards. And don't forget to give yourself a pat on the back—congratulate yourself, notice how much better you look or feel, and feel good about how far you've come and how you've gained control of your behaviour.

Staying with It

As you continue with your program, don't be surprised when you run up against obstacles; they're inevitable. In fact, it's a good idea to expect problems and give yourself time to step back, see how you're doing, and make some changes before going on. If your program is grinding to a halt, identify what is blocking your progress. It may come from one of the sources described in the following sections.

Social Influences   Take a hard look at the reactions of the people you're counting on, and see if they're really supporting you. If they come up short, connect with others who will be more supportive.

A related trap is trying to get your friends or family members to change *their* behaviours. The decision to make a major behaviour change is something people come to only after intensive self-examination. You may be able to influence someone by tactfully providing facts or support, but that's all. Focus on yourself. When you succeed, you may become a role model for others.

Levels of Motivation and Commitment   You won't make real progress until an inner drive leads you to the stage of change at which you are ready to make a personal commitment to the goal. If commitment is your problem, you may need to wait until the behaviour you're dealing with makes you unhappier or unhealthier; then your desire to change it will be stronger. Or you may find that changing your goal will inspire you to keep going. For more ideas, see "Motivation Boosters" in the ▓connect Library.

Choice of Techniques and Level of Effort   If your plan is not working as well as you thought it would, make changes where you're having the most trouble. If you've lagged on your running schedule, for example, maybe it's because you don't like running. An aerobics class might suit you better. There are many ways to move toward your goal. Or you may not be trying hard enough. You do have to push toward your goal. If it were easy, you wouldn't need a plan.

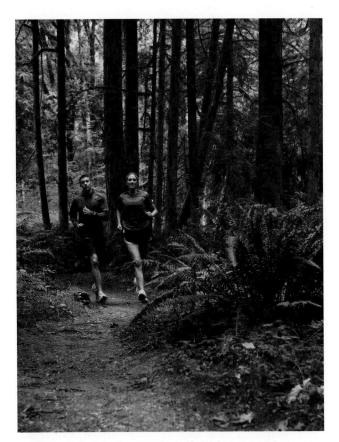

A beautiful day and a spectacular setting contribute to making exercise a satisfying and pleasurable experience. Choosing the right activity and doing it the right way are important elements in a successful health behaviour change program.

Stress Barrier   If you hit a wall in your program, look at the sources of stress in your life. If the stress is temporary, such as catching a cold or having a term paper due, you may want to wait until it passes before strengthening your efforts. If the stress is ongoing, find healthy ways to manage it (see Chapter 3). You may even want to make stress management your highest priority for behaviour change.

Procrastinating, Rationalizing, and Blaming   Be alert to games you might be playing with yourself, so you can stop them. Such games include the following:

• *Procrastinating.* If you tell yourself, "It's Friday already; I might as well wait until Monday to start," you're procrastinating. Break your plan into smaller steps that you can accomplish one day at a time.

• *Rationalizing.* If you tell yourself, "I wanted to go swimming today but wouldn't have had time to wash my hair afterward," you're making excuses. When you "win" by deceiving yourself, it isn't much of a victory.

• *Blaming.* If you tell yourself, "I couldn't exercise because Dave was hogging the elliptical trainer," you're blaming others for your own failure to follow through. Blaming is a way of taking your focus off the real problem and denying responsibility for your own actions.

BEING HEALTHY FOR LIFE

Your first few behaviour change projects may never go beyond the planning stage. Those that do may not all succeed. But as you begin to see progress and changes, you'll start to experience new and surprising positive feelings about yourself. You'll probably find that you're less likely to buckle under stress. You may accomplish things you never thought possible—winning a race, climbing a mountain, quitting smoking. Being healthy takes extra effort, but the paybacks in energy and vitality are priceless.

Once you've started, don't stop. Remember that maintaining good health is an ongoing process. Tackle one area at a time, but make a careful inventory of your health strengths and weaknesses and lay out a long-range plan. Take on the easier problems first, and then use what you have learned to attack more difficult areas. Keep informed about the latest health news and trends; research is constantly providing new information that directly affects daily choices and habits.

Making Changes in Your World

You can't completely control every aspect of your health. At least three other factors—heredity, health care, and environment—play important roles in your well-being. After you quit smoking, for example, you may still be inhaling smoke from other people's cigarettes. Your resolve to eat better foods may suffer a setback when you can't find any healthy choices in vending machines.

But you can make a difference—you can help create an environment around you that supports wellness for everyone. You can help support nonsmoking areas in public places. You can speak up in favour of more nutritious foods and better physical fitness facilities. You can include nonalcoholic drinks at your parties.

You can also work on larger environmental challenges: air and water pollution, traffic congestion, overcrowding and overpopulation, global warming and climate change, toxic and nuclear waste, and many others. These difficult issues need the attention and energy of people who are informed and who care about good health. On every level, from personal to planetary, we can all take an active role in shaping our environment.

What Does the Future Hold?

Sweeping changes in lifestyle have resulted in healthier Canadians in recent years and could have even greater effects in the years to come. In your lifetime, you can choose to take an active role in the movement toward increased awareness, greater individual responsibility and control, healthier lifestyles, and a healthier planet. Your choices and actions will have a tremendous impact on your present and future wellness. The door is open, and the time is now—you simply have to begin.

Practise and learn online with Connect. Connect allows you to practise important skills at your own pace and on your own schedule, with 24/7 online access to an eBook, practice quizzes, interactivities, videos, study tools, additional resources, and more.

SUMMARY

- Wellness is the ability to live life fully, with vitality and meaning. Wellness is dynamic and multidimensional; it incorporates physical, emotional, intellectual, spiritual, interpersonal and social, and environmental dimensions.

- As chronic diseases have become the leading cause of death in Canada, people have recognized that they have greater control over, and greater responsibility for, their health than ever before.

- The Integrated Pan-Canadian Healthy Living Strategy's vision is good health for all Canadians. The broad goals of the Strategy are to improve healthy weights, physical activity, and healthy eating among Canadians.

- Health-related differences among people that have implications for wellness can be described in the context of gender, ethnicity, income and education, disability, geographic location, and sexual orientation.

- Although heredity, environment, and health care all play roles in wellness and disease, behaviour can mitigate their effects.

- To make lifestyle changes, you need information about yourself, your health habits, and resources available to help you change.

- You can increase your motivation for behaviour change by examining the benefits and costs of change, boosting self-efficacy, and identifying and overcoming key barriers to change.

- The stages of change model describes six stages that people move through as they try to change their behaviour: precontemplation, contemplation, preparation, action, maintenance, and termination.

- A specific plan for change can be developed by (1) monitoring behaviour by keeping a journal; (2) analyzing the recorded data; (3) setting specific goals; (4) devising strategies for modifying the environment, rewarding yourself, and involving others; and (5) making a personal contract.

- To start and maintain a behaviour change program, you need commitment, a well-developed plan, social support, and a system of rewards.

- Although we cannot control every aspect of our health, we can make a difference in helping create an environment that supports wellness for everyone.

FOR MORE INFORMATION

BOOKS

American Medical Association. 2006. *American Medical Association Concise Medical Encyclopedia. New York: Random House.* Includes more than 3000 entries on health and wellness topics, symptoms conditions, and treatments.

Claiborn, J., and C. Pedrick. 2001. *The Habit Change Workbook: How to Break Bad Habits and Form Good Ones.* Oakland, Ca.: New Harbinger. Step-by-step instructions for identifying and overcoming a variety of unhealthy behaviours, such as poor eating habits, reluctance to exercise, and addictive behaviour.

Komaroff, A. L. (ed.). 2005. *Harvard Medical School Family Health Guide.* New York: Free Press. Consumer-oriented advice for the prevention and treatment of common health concerns.

Litin, S. C. (ed.) 2004. *Mayo Clinic Family Health Book*, 3rd ed. New York: HarperCollins Publishers. A complete health reference for every stage of life, covering thousands of conditions, symptoms, and treatments.

Murat, B., and G. Stewart. 2009. *Do I Need to See the Doctor? The Home-Treatment Encyclopedia—Written by Medical Doctors— That Lets You Decide*, 2nd ed. New York: John Wiley & Sons. Fully illustrated, easy-to-read guide to hundreds of common symptoms and ailments, designed to help consumers determine whether they can treat themselves or should seek professional medical attention.

O'Neill, M., A., et al. (eds.). 2007. *Health Promotion in Canada: Critical Perspectives*, 2nd ed. Toronto: Canadian Scholars' Press. A profile of the history and evolution of health promotion in Canada.

Prochaska, J. O., J. C. Norcross, and C. C. DiClemente. 1994. *Changing for Good: The Revolutionary Program That Explains the Six Stages of Change and Teaches You How to Free Yourself from Bad Habits.* New York: Morrow. Outlines the authors' model of behaviour change and offers suggestions and advice for each stage of change.

U.S. Government. 2007. 2007 *American Health and Medical Encyclopedia: Authoritative, Practical Guide to Health and Wellness.* FDA, CDC, NIH, Surgeon General Publications (CD-ROM). Washington, D.C.: Progressive Management. Contains thousands of documents from various federal agencies on myriad health issues, as well as links to dozens of health- and wellness-related Web sites.

NEWSLETTERS

Consumer Reports on Health (800-274-7596;
    http://www.consumerreports.org/oh/index.htm)
Harvard Health Publications (877-649-9457;
    http://www.health.harvard.edu)
Harvard Men's Health Watch (877-649-9457)
Harvard Women's Health Watch (877-699-9457)
Mayo Clinic Health Letter (800-291-1128)
University of California, Berkeley, Wellness Letter (800-829-9170;
    http://www.wellnessletter.com)

ORGANIZATIONS, HOTLINES, AND WEB SITES

The Internet addresses listed here were accurate at the time of publication.

Canadian Diabetes Association. Through phone, email, and the Internet, provides a wide variety of diabetes-related information and support.
    http://www.diabetes.ca
Canadian Fitness and Lifestyle Research Institute. Conducts research, monitors trends, and makes recommendations to increase population levels of physical activity and improve the health of all Canadians
    http://www.cflri.ca
Canadian Institute for Health Information. Provides reports and data that inform health policies, support the effective delivery of health services, and raise awareness among Canadians of the factors that contribute to good health.
    http://www.cihi.ca
Centers for Disease Control and Prevention (CDC). Through phone, fax, and the Internet, provides a wide variety of health information.
    http://www.cdc.gov
Health Canada. Includes research articles, summaries, and general information for helping Canadians maintain and improve their health.
    http://www.hc-sc.gc.ca
Healthfinder. A gateway to online publications, Web sites, support and self-help groups, and agencies and organizations that produce reliable health information.
    http://www.healthfinder.gov
MedlinePlus. Provides links to news and reliable information about health from government agencies and professional associations; includes a health encyclopedia and information on prescription and over-the-counter drugs.
    http://www.medlineplus.gov
National Wellness Institute. Serves professionals and organizations that promote optimal health and wellness.
    http://www.nationalwellness.org
National Women's Health Information Center. Provides information and answers to frequently asked questions.
    http://www.4woman.gov

Office of Minority Health Resource Center. Promotes improved health among racial and ethnic minority populations.
    http://www.omhrc.gov
Public Health Agency of Canada. Provides Internet-based information to strengthen Canada's capacity to protect and improve the health of Canadians and to help reduce pressures on the health care system.
    http://www.publichealth.gc.ca
U.S. Federal Trade Commission: Consumer Protection—Health. Includes online brochures about a variety of consumer health topics, including fitness equipment, generic drugs, and fraudulent health claims.
    http://www.ftc.gov/bcp/menus/consumer/health.shtm
U.S. National Health Information Center. Puts consumers in touch with the organizations that are best able to provide answers to health-related questions.
    http://www.health.gov/nhic
U.S. National Institutes of Health. Provides information about all its activities as well as consumer publications, hotline information, and an A to Z listing of health issues with links to the appropriate institute.
    http://www.nih.gov
U.S. Surgeon General. Includes information on activities of the U.S. Surgeon General and the text of many key reports on such topics as tobacco use, physical activity, and mental health.
    http://www.surgeongeneral.gov
World Health Organization. Provides information about health topics and issues affecting people around the world.
    http://www.who.int
The following are just a few of the many sites that provide consumer-oriented information on a variety of health issues:
    CNN Health: http://www.cnn.com/health
    FamilyDoctor.Org: http://www.familydoctor.org
    InteliHealth: http://www.intelihealth.com
    MayoClinic.com: http://www.mayoclinic.com
    Medbroadcast: http://www.medbroadcast.com
    MedlinePlus News: http://www.nlm.nih.gov/medlineplus/newsbydate.html
    MedPage Today Medical News: http://www.medpagetoday.com
    WebMD: http://www.webmd.com
    Yahoo Health News: http://news.yahoo.com/i/751

SELECTED BIBLIOGRAPHY

American Cancer Society. 2008. *Cancer Facts and Figures—2008.* Atlanta: American Cancer Society.
American Heart Association. 2008. *Heart Disease and Stroke Statistics—2009 Update.* Dallas: American Heart Association.
Banks, J., et al. 2006. Disease and disadvantage in the United States and in England. *Journal of the American Medical Association* 295(17): 2037–2045.
Barr, D. A. 2008. *Health Disparities in the United States: Social Class, Race, Ethnicity, and Health.* Baltimore: The Johns Hopkins University Press.
Beckman, M. 2007. Help wanted: In the pursuit of a healthy lifestyle, sheer grit only takes you so far. *Stanford Medicine Magazine* 24(3) (http://stanmed.stanford.edu/2007fall/main.html; retrieved March 6, 2011).
Bren, L. 2005. Does sex make a difference? *FDA Consumer Magazine* 39(4): 10–15.
Canadian Diabetes Association. 2008. *The Prevalence and Costs of Diabetes.* (http://www.diabetes.ca/files/prevalence-and-costs.pdf; retrieved March 6, 2011).

Canadian Fitness and Lifestyle Research Institute. 2009. *Kids CAN PLAY! Bulletin 1: Activity Levels of Canadian Children and Youth* (http://www.cflri.ca/eng/programs/canplay/documents/CANPLAY2009_Bulletin01_PA_levelsEN.pdf; retrieved March 6, 2011).

Casciano, D. A. 2005. Paving the way for safer, more effective drugs, food, and medical products. *FDA Consumer* 39(6): 8–11.

Centers for Disease Control and Prevention. 2008. *Racial and Ethnic Approaches to Community Health (REACH U.S.): Finding Solutions to Health Disparities, 2008* (http://www.cdc.gov/nccdphp/publications/aag/pdf/reach.pdf; retrieved December 27, 2008).

Centers for Disease Control and Prevention. 2008. Racial/ethnic disparities in self-rated health status among adults with and without disabilities—United States, 2004–2006. *Morbidity and Mortality Weekly Report* 57(39): 1069–1073.

Dietitians of Canada. 2005. *Registered Dietitians in Aboriginal Communities: Feeding Mind, Body and Spirit. Role Paper of the Dietitians of Canada Aboriginal Nutrition Network* (http://www.dietitians.ca/resources/resourcesearch.asp; retrieved September 3, 2009).

Finkelstein, E. A., et al. 2008. Do obese persons comprehend their personal health risks? *American Journal of Health Behaviour* 32(5): 508–516.

First Nations Information Governance Centre. 2005. *First Nations Regional Longitudinal Health Survey (RHS) 2002/03: Results for Adults, Youth and Children Living in First Nations Communities* (http://www.fnigc.ca/sites/default/files/ENpdf/RHS_2002/rhs2002-03-technical_report.pdf; retrieved March 12, 2011).

Flegal, K. M., et al. 2005. Excess deaths associated with underweight, overweight, and obesity. *Journal of the American Medical Association* 293(15): 1861–1867.

Flegal, K. M., et al. 2007. Cause-specific excess deaths associated with underweight, overweight, and obesity. *Journal of the American Medical Association* 298(17): 2028–2037.

Garriguet, D. 2008. Obesity and the eating habits of the Aboriginal population. *Health Reports* 19(1): 21–35.

Gilmore, H. 2007. Physically active Canadians. *Health Reports* 18(3): 45–67.

Gorman, B. K., and J. G. Read. 2006. Gender disparities in adult health: An examination of three measures of morbidity. *Journal of Health and Social Behaviour* 47(2): 95–110.

Health Canada. 2009. *A Statistical Profile on the Health of First Nations in Canada: Determinants of Health, 1999 to 2003* (http://www.hc-sc.gc.ca/fniah-spnia/pubs/aborig-autoch/2009-stats-profil/index-eng.php; retrieved March 6, 2011).

Herd, P., et al. 2007. Socioeconomic position and health: The differential effects of education versus income on the onset versus progression of health problems. *Journal of Health and Social Behaviour* 48(3): 223–238.

Horneffer-Ginter, K. 2008. Stages of change and possible selves: Two tools for promoting college health. *Journal of American College Health* 56(4): 351–358.

How to keep those New Year's resolutions. 2006. *Harvard Health Letter*, January, 31.

Irwin, J. D. 2004. Prevalence of university students' sufficient physical activity: a systematic review. *Perceptual and Motor Skills* 98: 927–943.

Irwin, J. D. 2007. The prevalence of physical activity maintenance in a sample of university students: A longitudinal study. *Journal of American College Health* 56(1): 37–41.

Jemal, A., et al. 2008. Cancer statistics, 2008. *CA: A Cancer Journal for Clinicians* 58(2): 71–96.

Martin, G., and J. Pear. 2007. *Behaviour Modification: What It Is and How to Do It*, 8th ed. Upper Saddle River, N.J.: Prentice-Hall.

Mokdad, A. H., et al. 2004. Actual causes of death in the United States, 2000. *Journal of the American Medical Association* 291(10): 1238–1245.

Mokdad, A. H., et al. 2005. Correction: Actual causes of death in the United States, 2000. *Journal of the American Medical Association* 293(3): 293–294.

National Center for Health Statistics. 2006. Health behaviours of adults: United States, 2002–04. *Vital and Health Statistics* 10(230) (http://www.cdc.gov/nchs/data/series/sr_10/sr10_230.pdf; retrieved March 6, 2011).

National Center for Health Statistics. 2007. *Health, United States, 2007, with Chartbook on Trends in the Health of Americans.* Hyattsville, Md.: National Center for Health Statistics.

National Center for Health Statistics. 2008. Deaths: Preliminary data for 2006. *National Vital Statistics Report* 56(16) (http://www.cdc.gov/nchs/data/nvsr/nvsr56/nvsr56_16.pdf; retrieved March 6, 2011).

Nothwehr, F., et al. 2008. Age group differences in diet and physical activity related behaviors among rural men and women. *Journal of Nutrition, Health and Aging* 12(3): 169–174.

Ogden, C. L., et al. 2006. Prevalence of overweight and obesity in the United States, 1999–2004. *Journal of the American Medical Association* 295(13): 1549–1555.

O' Loughlin, J., et al. 2007. Lifestyle risk factors for chronic disease across family origin among adults in multiethnic, low-income, urban neighborhoods. *Ethnicity and Disease* 17(4): 657–663

Secretariat for the Intersectoral Healthy Living Network in partnership with the F/P/T Healthy Living Task Group and the F/P/T Advisory Committee on Population Health and Health Security (ACPHHS). 2005. *The Integrated Pan-Canadian Healthy Living Strategy* (http://www.phac-aspc.gc.ca/hp-ps/hl-mvs/ipchls-spimmvs/pdf/ipchls-spimmvs-eng.pdf; retrieved April 17, 2011).

Statistics Canada. 2005. *Canadian Vital Statistics: Death Database, CANSIM Table 102-0561* (http://www5.statcan.gc.ca/cansim/a01?lang=eng; retrieved March 4, 2011).

Statistics Canada. 2009. *Population Urban and Rural, by Province and Territory* (http://www40.statcan.ca/l01/cst01/demo62a-eng.htm; retrieved March 6, 2011).

Statistics Canada. 2010. Visible Minority Groups, 2006 counts, for Canada, Provinces and Territories—20% Sample Data (table) (http://www12.statcan.ca/census-recensement/2006/dp-pd/hlt/97-562/pages/page.cfm?Lang=E&Geo=PR&Code=01&Table=1&Data=Count&StartRec=1&Sort=2&Display=Page; retrieved March 6, 2011).

Song, J., et al. 2006. Gender differences across race/ethnicity in use of health care among Medicare-aged Americans. *Journal of Women's Health* 15(10): 1205–1213.

Tjepkema, M., and M. Shields. 2004. *Nutrition. Findings from the Canadian Community Health Survey. Issue no.1. Measured Obesity: Adult Obesity in Canada.* Ottawa: Statistics Canada.

Transport Canada. 2008. *A Quick Look at Alcohol-related Crashes in Canada: Fact Sheet* (http://www.tc.gc.ca/eng/roadsafety/tp-tp2436-rs200809-menu-397.htm; retrieved March 6, 2011).

U. C. Berkeley. 2007. Do men get their fair share? University of California, Berkeley, Wellness Letter, April, 1–2.

U. C. Berkeley. 2008. *Evaluating Web Pages: Techniques to Apply and Questions to Ask* (http://www.lib.berkeley.edu/TeachingLib/Guides/Internet/Evaluate. html; retrieved December 27, 2008).

Walker, B., and C. P. Mouton. 2008. Environmental influences on cardiovascular health. *Journal of the National Medical Association* 100(1): 98–102.

U.S. Census Bureau. 2005. *We the People: Women and Men in the United States.* Washington, D.C.: U.S. Census Bureau.

Walsh, T., et al. 2006. Spectrum of mutations in BRCA1, BRCA2, CHEK2, and TP53 in families at high risk of breast cancer. *Journal of the American Medical Association* 295: 1379–1388.

World Health Organization. 2008. *Gender Inequalities and HIV/AIDS* (http://www.who.int/gender/hiv_aids/en; retrieved December 27, 2008).

World Health Organization. 2008. *Why Gender and Health?* (http://www.who.int/gender/genderandhealth/en; retrieved December 27, 2008).

Practise and learn online with Connect.

PSYCHOLOGICAL HEALTH

2

LOOKING AHEAD >>>>>

AFTER READING THIS CHAPTER, YOU SHOULD BE ABLE TO

- Describe what it means to be psychologically healthy

- Explain how to develop and maintain a positive self-concept and healthy self-esteem

- Discuss the importance of an optimistic outlook, good communication skills, and constructive approaches to dealing with loneliness and anger

- Describe common psychological disorders

- List the warning signs of suicide

- Describe the different types of help available for psychological problems

TEST YOUR KNOWLEDGE

1. **Normality is a key component of psychological health.**
   True or false?

2. **Trying to think rationally about what bothers you won't get you very far, because psychological problems usually are due to emotions, not thinking.**
   True or false?

3. **About how many Canadians have a diagnosable psychological disorder at some time during their life?**
   a. 5%
   b. 10%
   c. 20%

4. **People with enough willpower can force themselves to snap out of their depression.**
   True or false?

5. **A person who attempts suicide but survives did not really intend to die.**
   True or false?

ANSWERS

1. **FALSE.** Normality simply means being close to average, and having unusual ideas or attitudes doesn't mean that a person has a mental illness. The fact that people's ideas are varied makes life interesting and helps people respond in creative ways to life's challenges.

2. **FALSE.** Research has shown that getting people to adopt more realistic attitudes and beliefs about themselves and others can alleviate depression.

3. **C.** According to the Canadian Mental Health Association, about 6 million Canadians will have a diagnosable psychological disorder at some point.

4. **FALSE.** Depression, a disorder strongly linked to brain chemistry, can overcome whatever willpower a person has and make it impossible for her or him to make decisions.

5. **FALSE.** A person may intend to die but miscalculate how to successfully commit suicide.

Psychological health (or *mental health*) contributes to every dimension of wellness. It can be very difficult to maintain emotional, social, or even physical wellness if you are not psychologically healthy.

Psychological health, however, is a broad concept—one that is as difficult to define as it is important to understand. That is why the first section of this chapter is devoted to explaining what psychological health is and is not. The rest of the chapter discusses a number of common psychological problems, their symptoms, and their treatments.

If life doesn't bring you the pleasure or happiness you think it should, or if you believe you should be functioning at a higher level, you should know that there are ways of getting help. This chapter will show you how.

DEFINING PSYCHOLOGICAL HEALTH

Psychological or mental health can be defined as our capacity to think, feel, and behave in ways that contribute to our ability to enjoy life and manage challenges. Our psychological wellness can be supported or sabotaged by a variety of factors, such as dietary choices, sleep patterns, and relationship issues. With good psychological health, people have a positive sense of emotional and spiritual well-being that values fairness, culture, dignity, and interpersonal connections. That being said, we must be mindful that if we think of everyone who does not have a severe mental illness as being mentally healthy, we are ignoring common problems that can be addressed. For this reason, psychological health is sometimes defined more negatively as the absence of sickness. Clearly, freedom from disorders is only one factor in psychological wellness.

Maslow's Hierarchy: Striving Toward Self-Actualization

A positive definition—psychological health as the presence of wellness—is a more ambitious outlook that encourages us to fulfil our own potential.

During the 1960s, Abraham Maslow described such an ideal of mental health in his book *Toward a Psychology of Being*. According to Maslow, people have a *hierarchy*

of needs, listed here in order of decreasing importance (Figure 2.1):

- Physiological needs
- Safety
- Being loved
- Maintaining self-esteem
- Self-actualization

When urgent (life-sustaining) needs—such as the need for food and water—are satisfied, less basic needs take priority. Most of us are well fed and feel reasonably safe, and so we are driven by higher-level motives. Maslow's conclusions were based on his study of a group of visibly successful people who seemed to have lived, or be living, at their fullest. He stated that these people had achieved **self-actualization;** they had fulfilled a good measure of their human potential. Maslow suggested that self-actualized people all share certain qualities:

- *Realism.* Self-actualized people are realistic: They know the difference between what is real and what they want. As a result, they can cope with the world as it exists without demanding that it be different; they know what they can and cannot change. Just as important, realistic people accept evidence that contradicts what they want to believe. If the evidence is strong enough, they adapt their belief systems accordingly.
- *Acceptance.* Psychologically healthy people accept themselves as they are. Self-acceptance requires a positive **self-concept,** or *self-image:* a positive but realistic perception

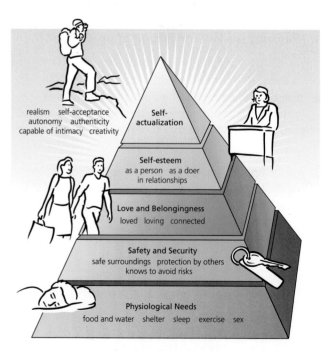

FIGURE 2.1 Maslow's hierarchy of needs.

Source: Maslow, A. 1970. *Motivation and Personality*, 2nd ed. New York: Harper & Row.

of yourself. Similarly, psychological health requires an appropriately high but realistic level of **self-esteem**. People with healthy self-esteem value themselves as people; they feel good about themselves and are likely to live up to their positive self-image and enjoy successes that in turn reinforce these good feelings. Self-acceptance also means being tolerant of your own imperfections, an ability that makes it easier to accept the imperfections of others.

- *Autonomy.* Psychologically healthy people are *autonomous*, meaning they can direct themselves and act independently of their social environment. **Autonomy** is more than physical independence; it is social, emotional, and intellectual independence, as well. Autonomous people are **inner-directed**, finding guidance from within, from their own rules and values. They have an internal locus of control and a high level of self-efficacy (see Chapter 1). By contrast, **other-directed** people often act only in response to what they feel as external pressure from others. Instead of speaking their true feelings, for example, other-directed people are more inclined to say what they believe will make other people happy.

- *Authenticity.* Autonomous people are not afraid to be themselves; sometimes, their capacity for being real may give them a certain childlike quality. They respond in a genuine, spontaneous way to whatever happens, without pretence or self-consciousness. Such people do not worry about being judged by others just for being themselves. This quality of genuineness is sometimes called **authenticity.**

- *Capacity for intimacy.* Healthy people can be physically and emotionally intimate. They are able to share their feelings and thoughts without fear of rejection. A psychologically healthy person is open to the pleasure of physical contact and the satisfaction of being close to others—but without being afraid of the risks involved in intimacy, such as the risk of getting hurt. (Chapters 10 and 11 discuss intimacy in more detail.)

- *Creativity.* Psychologically healthy people continually look at the world with renewed appreciation. Such appreciation can inform a person's creativity, which helps explain why so many mentally healthy people are creative. They may not be great poets or painters, but they live their everyday lives in creative ways. Creative people seem to see more and to be open to new experiences; they don't fear the unknown or avoid uncertainty.

Self-actualization is an ideal to strive for. Rather than dwelling on the past, we need to concentrate on meeting current challenges in ways that lead to long-term mental wellness. We must not consider ourselves failures if we do not achieve our full potential in every way or at every moment.

What Psychological Health Is Not

Psychological health is not the same as psychological **normality**. Being mentally normal simply means being close to average. We can define normal body temperature because a few degrees above or below this temperature means physical sickness. But your ideas and attitudes can vary tremendously without your losing efficiency or feeling emotional distress. In fact, psychological diversity—with the wide range of ideas, lifestyles, and attitudes it brings about—is a valuable asset to society.

Never seeking help for personal problems does not prove you are psychologically healthy, any more than seeking help proves you have a mental illness. Unhappy people may avoid seeking help for many reasons, and people with a severe mental illness may not even realize they need help.

Further, we can't say people have a mental illness or are mentally healthy based solely on the presence or absence of symptoms. Consider the symptom of anxiety, for example. Anxiety can help you face a problem and solve it before it becomes too big. Someone who shows no anxiety may be refusing to recognize problems or to do anything about them. A person who is anxious for good reason is likely to be judged more psychologically healthy in the long run than someone who is inappropriately calm.

Finally, we cannot judge psychological health from the way people look. All too often, a person who seems to be OK and even happy suddenly takes his or her own life.

self-esteem   Satisfaction and confidence in yourself; the valuing of yourself as a person.

autonomy   Independence; the sense of being self-directed.

inner-directed   Guided in behaviour by an inner set of rules and values.

other-directed   Guided in behaviour by the values and expectations of others.

authenticity   Genuineness.

normality   The psychological characteristics attributed to the majority of people in a population at a given time.

TERMS

Usually, such people lack close friends who might have known their desperation. At an early age, we learn to conceal our feelings and even to lie about them. We may believe that our complaints put unfair demands on others. Although silence may sometimes be a virtue, it can also prevent the person from getting help.

MEETING LIFE'S CHALLENGES

Life is full of challenges—large and small. Everyone, regardless of heredity and family influences, must learn to cope successfully with new situations and new people. For emotional and mental wellness, each of us must continue to grow psychologically, developing new and more sophisticated coping mechanisms to suit our current lives. We must develop an adult identity that enhances our spiritual wellness, self-esteem, and autonomy. We must also learn to communicate honestly, handle anger and loneliness appropriately, and avoid being defensive.

Growing Up Psychologically

Our responses to life's challenges influence the development of our personality and identity. Psychologist Erik Erikson proposed that development proceeds through a series of eight stages that extend throughout life. Each stage is characterized by a major crisis or turning point—a time of increased vulnerability as well as increased potential for psychological growth (Table 2.1).

The successful mastery of one stage is a basis for mastering the next; early failures can have repercussions in later life. Fortunately, life provides ongoing opportunities for mastering these tasks. For example, although the development of trust begins in infancy, it is refined as we grow older. We learn to trust people outside our immediate family and to limit our trust by identifying people who are untrustworthy.

Developing an Adult Identity   A primary task beginning in adolescence is the development of an adult identity: a unified sense of self, characterized by attitudes, beliefs, and ways of acting that are genuinely your own. People with adult identities know who they are, what they are capable of, what roles they play, and their place among their peers. They have a sense of their own uniqueness but also appreciate what they have in common with others. They view themselves realistically and can assess their strengths and weaknesses without relying on the opinions of others. Achieving an identity also means being able to form intimate relationships with others while maintaining a strong sense of self.

Our identities evolve as we interact with the world and make choices about what we'd like to do and whom we'd like to model ourselves after. Developing an adult identity is particularly challenging in a heterogeneous, secular, and relatively affluent society like ours, in which many roles are possible, many choices are tolerated, and ample time is allowed for experimenting and making up one's mind.

Table 2.1	Erikson's Stages of Development		
Age	**Conflict**	**Important People**	**Task**
Birth–1 year	Trust vs. mistrust	Mother or other primary caregiver	In being fed and comforted, developing the trust that others will respond to your needs
1–3 years	Autonomy vs. shame and self-doubt	Parents	In toilet training, locomotion, and exploration, learning self-control without losing the capacity for assertiveness
3–6 years	Initiative vs. guilt	Family	In playful talking and locomotion, developing a conscience (based on parental prohibitions) that is not too inhibiting
6–12 years	Industry vs. inferiority	Neighbourhood and school	In school and playing with peers, learning the value of accomplishment and perseverance without feeling inadequate
Adolescence	Identity vs. identity confusion	Peers	Developing a stable sense of who you are—your needs, abilities, interpersonal style, and values
Young adulthood	Intimacy vs. isolation	Close friends, sex partners	Learning to live and share intimately with others, often in sexual relationships
Middle adulthood	Generativity vs. self-absorption	Work associates, children, community	Doing things for others, including parenting and civic activities
Older adulthood	Integrity vs. despair	Humankind	Affirming the value of life and its ideals

Source: Erikson, E. 1963. *Childhood and Society.* New York: Norton.

Early identities are often modelled after parents—or the opposite of parents, in rebellion against what they represent. Over time, peers, rock stars, sports heroes, and religious figures are added to the list of possible models. In high school and university, people often join cliques that assert a certain identity, such as the *jocks*, the *brains*, or the *slackers*. Although much of an identity is internal—a way of viewing ourselves and the world—certain aspects of it can be external, such as styles of talking and dressing; ornaments, such as earrings; and hairstyles.

Early identities are rarely permanent. A student who works for good grades and approval one year can turn into a dropout devoted to hard rock and wild parties a year later. At some point, however, most of us adopt a more stable, individual identity that ties together the experiences of childhood and the expectations and aspirations of adulthood. Erikson's theory does not suggest that one day we suddenly assume our final identity and never change after that. Life is more interesting for people who continue evolving into more distinct individuals, rather than being rigidly controlled by their pasts. Identity reflects a lifelong process, and it changes as a person develops new relationships and roles.

Developing an adult identity is an important part of psychological wellness. Without a personal identity, we begin to feel confused about who we are; Erikson called this situation an **identity crisis**. Until we have found ourselves, we cannot have much self-esteem, because a self is not firmly in place.

How far have you gotten in developing your adult identity? Create a list of characteristics you think a friend who knows you well would use to describe you. Rank them from the most to the least important. Your list might include such elements as gender, socioeconomic status, ethnic and religious identification, choice of university or major, parents' occupations, interests and talents, attitudes toward drugs and alcohol, style of dress, the kinds of people with whom you typically associate, your expected role in society, and aspects of your personality. Which elements of your identity do you feel are permanent, and which do you think may change over time? Are there any characteristics missing from your list that you'd like to add?

Another aid to developing an adult identity is to identify possible role models. Whom do you admire and want to be like? Which characteristics of that person do you want to emulate? How did that person acquire those characteristics, and how could you follow her or his example? Some role models might be willing to be mentors to you, spending time with you and sharing their wisdom.

Developing Intimacy

Erikson's developmental stages don't end with establishing an adult identity. Learning to live intimately with others and finding a productive role for yourself in society are other tasks of adulthood—to be able to love and work.

People with established identities can form intimate relationships and sexual unions characterized by sharing, open communication, long-term commitment, and love. Those who lack a firm sense of self may have difficulty establishing relationships because they feel overwhelmed by closeness and the needs of another person. As a result, they experience only short-term, superficial relationships with others and may remain isolated.

Developing Values and Purpose in Your Life

Erikson assigned his last two stages, generativity versus self-absorption and integrity versus despair, to middle adulthood and older adulthood. But these stages are concerned with values and purpose in life, issues that need to be addressed by young people and reexamined throughout life.

Values are criteria for judging what is good and bad; they underlie our moral decisions and behaviour. The first morality of the young child is to consider *good* to mean what brings immediate and tangible rewards, and *bad*, whatever results in punishment. An older child will explain right and wrong in terms of authority figures and rules. But the final stage of moral development, one that not everyone attains, is being able to conceive of right and wrong in more abstract terms, such as justice and virtue.

As adults we need to assess how far we have evolved morally and what values we actually have adopted. Without an awareness of our personal values, our lives may be hurriedly driven forward by immediate desires and the passing demands of others. Living according to values means doing the following:

- Considering your options carefully before making a choice
- Choosing between options without succumbing to outside pressures that oppose your values
- Making a choice and acting on it rather than doing nothing

Your actions and how you justify them proclaim to others what you stand for.

A practical exercise for clarifying your values and goals is to write a draft of your obituary for a local newspaper. How would you like to be remembered? What would you like to have achieved? What will you have done to meet those goals? This obituary should not be a glorification but an honest, realistic appraisal. End it by summarizing in a few sentences what was most important about your life. In reading what you have written, ask yourself, "How will I have to change to be the person I want to be?"

For more on discovering your values, see the box "Assessing Your Values" (p. 38).

---

identity crisis   Internal confusion about who you are.

values   Criteria for judging what is good and bad, which underlie a person's moral decisions and behaviour.

TERMS

Assessing Your Values

Find out more about your core values by answering these questions.

• What personality traits or characteristics do you most value—for example, being friendly, patient, successful, outgoing, cooperative, loyal to family and friends? These can be characteristics you see in yourself or in others.

• What activities or accomplishments do you most value—for example, making lots of money, getting good grades, spending time with friends, making your own decisions? These can be accomplishments of your own or of others, or goals you have for the future.

• What social ideals, customs, and institutions do you value—for example, education, equality, freedom of speech, tolerance for diverse opinions?

• How well does your current lifestyle reflect your values? Can you think of some recent incidents in which you acted in accordance with your values or in ways that conflict with your values?

Striving for Spiritual Wellness

Spiritual wellness is associated with greater coping skills and higher levels of overall wellness. It is a very personal wellness component, and it can be developed in many ways (see the box "Paths to Spiritual Wellness"). Researchers have linked spiritual wellness to longer life expectancy, reduced risk of disease, faster recovery, and improved emotional health. Although spirituality is difficult to study, and researchers aren't sure how or why spirituality seems to improve health, several explanations have been offered.

• *Social support.* Attending religious services or participating in volunteer organizations helps people feel that they are part of a community with similar values and promotes social connectedness and caring.
• *Healthy habits.* Some of the paths to spiritual wellness may encourage healthy behaviours, such as eating a vegetarian diet or consuming less meat and alcohol, and may discourage harmful habits, such as smoking.
• *Positive attitude.* Spirituality can give people a sense of meaning and purpose in life, and these qualities create a more positive attitude in people, which in turn helps them cope with life's challenges.
• *Moments of relaxation.* Spiritual practices, such as prayer, meditation, and immersion in artistic activities, can reduce stress by eliciting the relaxation response.

Spirituality provides an ethical path to personal fulfillment that includes connectedness with the self, others, and a higher power or larger reality. Spiritual wellness can make you more aware of your personal values and can help clarify them. Without an awareness of personal values, you might be driven by immediate desires and the passing demands of others. Living according to values means considering your options carefully before making a choice, choosing between options without succumbing to outside pressures that oppose your values, and making a choice and acting on it rather than doing nothing.

Achieving Healthy Self-Esteem

Having a healthy level of self-esteem means regarding your self, which includes all aspects of your identity, as good, competent, and worthy of love. It is a critical component of wellness.

Developing a Positive Self-Concept   Ideally, a positive self-concept begins in childhood, based on experiences both within the family and outside it. Children need to develop a sense of being loved and being able to give love and to accomplish their goals. If they feel rejected or neglected by their parents, they may fail to develop feelings of self-worth. They may grow to have a negative concept of themselves.

Another component of self-concept is *integration*. An integrated self-concept is one that you have made for yourself—not someone else's image of you or a mask that doesn't quite fit. Important building blocks of self-concept are the personality characteristics and mannerisms of parents, which children may adopt without realizing it. Later, they may be surprised to find themselves acting like one of their parents. Eventually, such building blocks should be reshaped and integrated into a new, individual personality.

A further aspect of self-concept is *stability*. Stability depends on the integration of the self and its freedom from contradictions. People who have received mixed messages about themselves from parents and friends may have contradictory self-images, which defy integration and make them vulnerable to shifting levels of self-esteem. At times they regard themselves as entirely good, capable, and lovable—an ideal self—and at other times they see themselves as entirely bad, incompetent, and unworthy of love. Neither of these extreme self-concepts allow people to see themselves or others realistically, and their relationships with other people are filled with misunderstandings and ultimately with conflict.

The concepts we have about ourselves and others are an important part of our personalities. And all the components of our self-concept profoundly influence our interpersonal relationships.

Paths to Spiritual Wellness

Spiritual wellness means different things to different people. For many, it involves developing a set of guiding beliefs, principles, or values that give purpose and meaning to life. It helps people achieve a sense of wholeness within themselves and in their relationships with others. Spiritual wellness influences people on an individual level, as well as on a community level, where it can bond people through compassion, love, forgiveness, and self-sacrifice.

Many paths to spiritual wellness exist. One of the most common in our society is organized religion. The major religions provide paths for transforming the self in ways that can lead to greater happiness and serenity and reduce feelings of anxiety and hopelessness. For example, in Christianity, salvation means turning away from the selfish ego and to God's sovereignty and grace, where a joy is found that frees the believer from anxious self-concern and despair. *Islam* is the word for a kind of self-surrender leading to peace with God. Buddhism teaches how to detach the self from selfish desire, leading to compassion for the suffering of others and freedom from fear-engendering illusions. Judaism emphasizes the social and ethical redemption members of the Jewish community can experience if they follow the laws of God.

Religions teach specific techniques for achieving these transformations of the self: prayer, both in groups and in private; meditation; the performance of rituals and ceremonies

symbolizing religious truths; and good works and service to others. Religious organizations also usually offer social and material support to members who might otherwise be isolated.

Spiritual wellness does not require participation in organized religion. Many people find meaning and purpose in other ways. By spending time in nature or working on environmental issues, people can experience continuity with the natural world. Spiritual wellness can come through helping others in the community or by promoting human rights, peace, and harmony among people, and opportunities for human development on a global level. Other people develop spiritual wellness through art or through their personal relationships.

How would you define spiritual wellness and its role in your life? What beliefs and practices do you associate with your sense of spiritual wellness? To achieve overall well-being, it is important to take time out to consider what you can do to help your spiritual side flourish.

Meeting Challenges to Self-Esteem   As an adult, you sometimes run into situations that challenge your self-concept. People you care about may tell you they don't love you or feel loved by you, for example, or your attempts to accomplish a goal may end in failure.

You can react to such challenges in several ways. The best approach is to acknowledge that something has gone wrong and try again, adjusting your goals to your abilities without radically revising your self-concept. Less productive responses are denying that anything went wrong and blaming someone else. These attitudes may preserve your self-concept temporarily, but in the end they keep you from meeting the challenge.

The worst reaction is to develop a lasting negative self-concept in which you feel bad, unloved, and ineffective—in other words, to become demoralized. Instead of coping, the demoralized person gives up, reinforcing the negative self-concept and setting in motion a cycle of bad self-concept and failure. In people who are genetically predisposed to depression, demoralization can progress to additional symptoms, which are discussed later in the chapter.

NOTICE YOUR PATTERNS OF THINKING   One method for fighting demoralization is to recognize and test the negative thoughts and assumptions you may have about yourself and others. Try to note exactly when an unpleasant emotion—feeling worthless, wanting to give up, feeling

depressed—occurs or gets worse, to identify the events or daydreams that trigger that emotion, and to observe whatever thoughts come into your head just before or during the emotional experience. It is helpful to keep a daily journal about such events.

AVOID FOCUSING ON THE NEGATIVE   Imagine that you are waiting for a friend to meet you for dinner, but he's 30 minutes late. What kinds of thoughts go through your head when something like this happens? You might wonder what has happened to cause the delay: Perhaps he is stuck in traffic, you think, or needs to help a roommate who has the flu. This kind of reaction is healthy for several reasons:

• *You aren't jumping to a conclusion or blaming your friend for a failure of any kind.* After all, he probably hasn't forgotten about you or decided to ditch you.

• *You are being reasonable by giving your friend the benefit of the doubt.* Things happen. Your friend probably has a good reason for not being there. He deserves a chance to explain and may even need your help dealing with the situation that made him late.

• *You avoid personalizing the situation in such a way that you feel hurt or betrayed.* Jumping to a negative conclusion (such as "He isn't coming because he doesn't really like me") can make you feel bad unnecessarily. The same thing happens if you place blame—either on your friend or on yourself—without knowing all the facts.

A positive self-concept begins in infancy. Knowing that he's loved and valued by his parents gives this baby a solid basis for lifelong psychological health.

By contrast, people who are demoralized tend to use all-or-nothing thinking. They overgeneralize from negative events. They overlook the positive and jump to negative conclusions, minimizing their own successes and magnifying the successes of others. They take responsibility for unfortunate situations that are not their fault, and then jump to more negative conclusions and more unfounded overgeneralizations. Patterns of thinking that make events seem worse than they are in reality are called **cognitive distortions.**

DEVELOP REALISTIC SELF-TALK When you react to a situation, an important piece of that reaction is your **self-talk**—the statements you make to yourself inside your own mind.

To pick up on our earlier example, suppose your friend is late for a dinner date. As you wait for your friend to arrive, your self-talk has a profound effect on your reaction to his lateness.

Someone who is demoralized or wrestling with a poor self-concept might immediately react with negative self-talk: *"He isn't coming. It's my fault; he probably doesn't like me because I'm boring. I bet he's with someone else."* This type of self-talk assigns blame (not just on your friend but also on you), is judgmental, and jumps to an unverified conclusion about the meaning of your friend's lateness. In fact, you don't know why he is late or what he is thinking.

More rational thinking and self-talk will not only help get you through the situation without feeling upset but will also help you avoid damaging your own self-concept. In this case, helpful self-talk is not negative, but neutral: *"He's never late for dinner. Something must be holding him up. I'll call him and make sure everything is all right."* This thinking recognizes that a problem may exist, but it does not judge or assign blame.

In your own fight against demoralization, it may be hard to think of a rational response until hours or days after the event that upset you. Responding rationally can be especially hard when you are having an argument with someone else, which is why people often say things they don't mean in the heat of the moment or develop hurt feelings even when the other person had no intention of hurting them.

Once you get used to noticing the way your mind works, however, you may be able to catch yourself thinking negatively and change the process before it goes too far. This approach to controlling your reactions is not the same as positive thinking—which means substituting a positive thought for a negative one. Instead, you simply try to make your thoughts as logical and accurate as possible, based on the facts of the situation as you know them, and not on snap judgments or conclusions that may turn out to be false.

Demoralized people can be tenacious about their negative beliefs—so tenacious that they make their beliefs come true in a self-fulfilling prophesy. For example, if you conclude that you are so boring that no one will like you anyway, you may decide not to bother socializing. This behaviour could make the negative belief become a reality.

For additional tips on changing distorted, negative ways of thinking, see the box "Realistic Self-Talk."

Being Less Defensive

Sometimes our wants come into conflict with people around us or with our conscience, and we become frustrated and anxious. If we cannot resolve the conflict by changing the external situation, we try to resolve the conflict internally by rearranging our thoughts and feelings. Some standard **defence mechanisms** are listed in Table 2.2. The drawback of many of these coping mechanisms is that they succeed temporarily but make finding permanent solutions much harder.

Realistic Self-Talk

Do your patterns of thinking make events seem worse than they truly are? Do negative beliefs about yourself become self-fulfilling prophecies? Substituting realistic self-talk for negative self-talk can help you build and maintain self-esteem and cope better with the challenges in your life. Here are some examples of common types of distorted, negative self-talk, along with suggestions for more accurate and rational responses.

Cognitive Distortion	Negative Self-Talk	Realistic Self-Talk
Focusing on negatives	School is so discouraging—nothing but one hassle after another.	School is pretty challenging and has its difficulties, but there certainly are rewards. It's really a mixture of good and bad.
Expecting the worst	Why would my boss want to meet with me this afternoon if not to fire me?	I wonder why my boss wants to meet with me. I guess I'll just have to wait and see.
Overgeneralizing	(After getting a poor grade on a paper) Just as I thought—I'm incompetent at everything.	I'll start working on the next paper earlier. That way, if I run into problems, I'll have time to consult with the TA.
Minimizing	I won the speech contest, but none of the other speakers was very good. I wouldn't have done as well against stiffer competition.	It may not have been the best speech I'll ever give, but it was good enough to win the contest. I'm really improving as a speaker.
Blaming others	I wouldn't have eaten so much last night if my friends hadn't insisted on going to that restaurant.	I overdid it last night. Next time I'll make different choices.
Expecting perfection	I should have scored 100% on this test. I can't believe I missed that one problem through a careless mistake.	Too bad I missed one problem through carelessness, but overall I did very well on this test. Next time I'll be more careful.
Believing you're the cause of everything	Sarah seems so depressed today. I wish I hadn't had that argument with her yesterday; it must have really upset her.	I wish I had handled the argument better, and in the future I'll try to. But I don't know if Sarah's behaviour is related to what I said or even if she's depressed. In any case, I'm not responsible for how Sarah feels or acts; only she can take responsibility for that.
Thinking in black and white	I have to score 10 points in the game today. Otherwise, I don't belong on the team.	I'm a good player or else I wouldn't be on the team. I'll play my best—that's all I can do.
Magnifying events	They went to a movie without me. I thought we were friends, but I guess I was wrong.	I'm disappointed they didn't ask me to the movie, but it doesn't mean our friendship is over. It's not that big a deal.

Source: Adapted from Schafer, W. *Stress Management for Wellness*, 4th ed. Copyright © 2000 Wadsworth, a part of Cengage Learning, Inc. Reproduced by permission. www.cengage.com/permissions.

Table 2.2	Defence and Coping Mechanisms	
Mechanism	**Description**	**Example**
Projection	Reacting to unacceptable inner impulses as if they were from outside the self	A student who dislikes his roommate feels that the roommate dislikes him.
Repression	Expelling from awareness an unpleasant feeling, idea, or memory	The child of an alcoholic, neglectful father remembers him as a giving, loving person.
Denial	Refusing to acknowledge to yourself what you really know to be true	A person believes that smoking cigarettes won't harm her because she's young and healthy.
Passive-aggressive behaviour	Expressing hostility toward someone by being covertly uncooperative or passive	A person tells a co-worker, with whom she competes for project assignments, that she'll help him with a report but then never follows through.
Displacement	Shifting your feelings about a person to another person	A student who is angry with one of his professors returns home and yells at one of his housemates.
Rationalization	Giving a false, acceptable reason when the real reason is unacceptable	A shy young man decides not to attend a dorm party, telling himself he'd be bored.
Substitution	Deliberately replacing a frustrating goal with one that is more attainable	A student having a difficult time passing courses in chemistry decides to change his major from biology to economics.
Humour	Finding something funny in unpleasant situations	A student whose bicycle has been stolen thinks how surprised the thief will be when he or she starts downhill and discovers the brakes don't work.

Recognizing your own defence mechanisms can be difficult, because they've probably become habits, occurring unconsciously. But we each have some inkling about how our mind operates. By remembering the details of conflict situations you have been in, you may be able to figure out which defence mechanisms you used in successful or unsuccessful attempts to cope. Try to look at yourself as an objective, outside observer would and analyze your thoughts and behaviour in a psychologically stressful situation from the past. Having insight into what strategies you typically use can lead to new, less defensive and more effective ways of coping in the future.

Being Optimistic

Many psychologists believe that pessimism is not just a symptom of everyday depression but an important root cause, as well. Pessimists not only expect repeated failure and rejection but also accept it as deserved. Pessimists do not see themselves as capable of success, and they irrationally dismiss any evidence of their own accomplishments. This negative point of view is learned, typically at a young age from parents and other authority figures. But as an optimist would tell you, that means it also has the potential to be unlearned.

Psychologist Martin Seligman points out that we are more used to refuting negative statements, such as "The problem is going to last forever and ruin everything, and it's all my fault," when they come from others rather than from our own mind. But refuting such negative self-talk is exactly what a pessimist must learn to do to avoid chronic unhappiness. Pessimists must first recognize and then dispute the false, negative predictions they generate about themselves.

Maintaining Honest Communication

Another important area of psychological functioning is communicating honestly with others. It can be very frustrating for us and for people around us if we cannot express what we want and feel. Others can hardly respond to our needs if they don't know what those needs are. We must recognize what we want to communicate and then express it clearly. For example, how do you feel about going to the party instead of a movie? Do you care if your roommate talks on the phone late into the night?

Some people know what they want others to do but don't state it clearly because they fear denial of the request, which they interpret as personal rejection. Such people might benefit from **assertiveness** training: learning to insist on their rights and to bargain for what they want. Assertiveness includes being able to say no or yes depending on the situation.

Communicating your feelings appropriately and clearly is important. For example, if you tell people you feel sad, they may have various reactions. If they feel close to you, they may express an intimate thought of their own. Or they may feel guilty because they think you're implying they have caused your sadness. They may even be angry because they feel you expect them to cheer you up.

Depending on your intention and your prediction of how a statement will be taken, you may or may not want to make it. For example, if you say, "I feel like staying home tonight," you may also be implying something different. You could really be saying, "Don't bother me" or opening a negotiation about what you would be willing to do that evening, given the right event or incentive. Although this approach may help you avoid a confrontation (or even a discussion) with someone else, it is unfair because you are not really being clear about what you want.

Good communication means expressing yourself clearly. You don't need any special psychological jargon to communicate effectively. (For tips, see the box "Guidelines for Effective Communication" in Chapter 10.)

Dealing with Loneliness

It can be hard to strike the right balance between being alone and being with others. Some people are motivated to socialize by a fear of being alone—not the best reason to spend time with others. If you discover how to be happy by yourself, you'll be better able to cope with periods when you're forced to be alone—for example, when you've just broken off a romantic relationship or when your usual friends are away on vacation.

Unhappiness with being alone may come from interpreting it as a sign of rejection—that others are not interested in spending time with you. Before you reach such a conclusion, be sure that you give others a real chance to get to know you.

Examine your patterns of thinking: You may harbour unrealistic expectations about other people—for example, that everyone you meet must like you and, if they don't, you must be terribly flawed. You might also consider the possibility that you expect too much from new acquaintances and, sensing this, they start to draw back, triggering your feelings of rejection. Not everyone you meet is a suitable and willing person for a close or intimate relationship.

TERMS

assertiveness Expression that is forceful but not hostile.

University or college offers many antidotes to loneliness, in the forms of clubs, organized activities, sports, and just hanging out with friends.

Feeling pressure to have such a relationship may lead you to take up with someone whose interests and needs are remote from yours or whose need to be cared for leaves you with little time of your own. You will have traded loneliness for potentially worse problems.

Loneliness is a passive feeling state. If you decide that you're not spending enough time with people, take action to change the situation. University or college life provides many opportunities to meet people. If you're shy, you may have to push yourself to join a group. Look for something you've enjoyed in the past or in which you have a genuine interest.

If your loneliness is the result of missing absent friends, remember that communication at a distance is cheaper and easier than ever before. For many people, email and cellphones are immediate and satisfying ways to keep up with people in their lives.

Dealing with Anger

Common wisdom holds that expressing anger is beneficial for psychological and physical health. However, recent studies have questioned this idea by showing that overtly hostile people seem to be at higher risk for heart attacks. Angry words or actions don't contribute to psychological wellness if they damage relationships or produce feelings of guilt or loss of control. Perhaps the best way to resolve this contradiction is to distinguish between a gratuitous expression of anger and a reasonable level of self-assertiveness.

At one extreme are people who never express anger or any opinion that might offend others, even when their own rights and needs are being jeopardized. They may be trapped in unhealthy relationships or chronically deprived of satisfaction at work and at home. If you have trouble expressing your anger, consider training in assertiveness and appropriate expressions of anger to help you learn to express yourself constructively.

At the other extreme are people whose anger is explosive or misdirected—a condition called *intermittent explosive disorder (IED)*. IED is often accompanied by depression or another disorder. Explosive anger or rage, like a child's tantrum, renders individuals temporarily unable to think straight or to act in their own best interest. During an IED episode, a person may lash out uncontrollably, hurting someone else or destroying property. Anyone who expresses anger this way should seek professional help.

Managing Your Own Anger   If you feel explosive anger coming on, consider the following two strategies to head it off.

First, try to *reframe* what you're thinking at that moment. You'll be less angry at another person if it is possible that his or her behaviour was not intentionally directed against you. Imagine that another driver suddenly cuts in front of you. You would certainly be angry if you knew the other driver did it on purpose, but you probably would be less angry if you knew he simply did not see you. You might be even less upset if you consider that other mitigating factors may be present—for example, that the other driver was involved in an urgent situation of his own. If you're angry because you've just been criticized, avoid mentally replaying scenes from the past when you received similar unjust criticisms. Think about what is happening now, and try to act differently than you did in the past—less defensively and more analytically.

Second, until you're able to change your thinking, try to *distract* yourself. Use the old trick of counting to 10 before you respond, or start concentrating on your breathing. If needed, take a longer cooling-off period by

QUESTIONS FOR CRITICAL THINKING AND REFLECTION

Think about the last time you were truly angry. What triggered your anger? How did you express it? Do you typically handle your anger in the same manner? How appropriate does your anger-management technique seem?

leaving the situation until your anger has subsided. This does not mean that you should permanently avoid the issues and people who make you angry. When you've had a chance to think more clearly about the matter, return to it.

Dealing with Anger in Other People Anger can be infectious and disruptive to cooperation and communication. If someone you're with becomes very angry, respond asymmetrically by reacting not with anger but with calm. Try to validate the other person by acknowledging that he or she has some reason to be angry. This does not mean apologizing if you don't think you're to blame, or accepting verbal abuse, which is always inappropriate. Try to focus on solving the problem by allowing the person to explain why he or she is so angry and what can be done to alleviate the situation. Finally, if the person cannot be calmed, it may be best to disengage, at least temporarily. After a time-out, a rational problem-solving approach may become more successful.

PSYCHOLOGICAL DISORDERS

We have all felt anxious at times, and in dealing with the anxiety we may have avoided doing something that we wanted to do or should have done. Most of us have had periods of feeling down when we became pessimistic, less energetic, and less able to enjoy life. Many of us have been bothered at times by irrational thoughts or odd feelings. Such feelings and thoughts can be normal responses to the ordinary challenges of life, but when emotions or irrational thoughts start to interfere with daily activities and rob us of our peace of mind, they can be considered symptoms of a psychological disorder.

Psychological disorders are generally the result of many factors. Genetic differences, which underlie differences in how the brain processes information and experience, are known to play an important role, especially in certain disorders. However, exactly which genes are involved and how they alter the structure and chemistry of the brain is still under study. Learning and life events are important, too: Identical twins often don't have the same psychological disorders in spite of having identical genes. Some people have been exposed to more traumatic events than others, leading either to greater vulnerability to future traumas or, conversely, to the development of better coping skills. Further, what your parents, peers, and others have taught you strongly influences your level of self-esteem and how you deal with frightening or depressing life events (see the box "Ethnicity, Culture, and Psychological Disorders").

This section examines some of the more common psychological disorders, including anxiety disorders, mood disorders, and schizophrenia.

Anxiety Disorders

Fear is a basic and useful emotion. Its value for our ancestors' survival cannot be overestimated; for modern humans, it provides motivation for self-protection and for learning to cope with new or potentially dangerous environmental or social situations. Only when fear is out of proportion to real danger can it be considered a problem. **Anxiety** is another word for fear, especially a feeling of fear that is not in response to any definite threat. When anxiety is experienced almost daily or in life situations that recur and cannot be avoided, then anxiety can be called a disorder. Anxiety disorders are the most common of the psychological disorders among Canadians. This section provides brief descriptions of the major types of anxiety disorders.

Simple Phobia The most common and most understandable anxiety disorder is a **simple** (or **specific**) **phobia,** which is a fear of something definite, such as lightning or a particular animal or location. Nearly 8% of Canadians have a specific phobia. Examples of commonly feared animals are snakes, spiders, and dogs; frightening locations are often high places or enclosed spaces. Simple phobias are believed to result from a combination of biological factors and life events. Sometimes, but not always, these fears originate in bad experiences, such as being bitten by a snake. A special kind of simple phobia is fear of blood, injections, or seeing injured people. These fears usually come from a tendency to faint or become nauseated in such situations.

Social Phobia The 6.7% of Canadians with **social phobia** fear humiliation or embarrassment while being observed by others. Fear of speaking in public is perhaps the most common phobia of this kind. Extremely shy people can have social fears that extend to almost all social situations (see the box "Shyness" on p. 46). People with these kinds of fears may not continue in school as far as they could and may restrict themselves to lower-paying jobs where they do not have to come into contact with new people.

TERMS

anxiety   A feeling of fear that is not directed toward any definite threat.

simple (specific) phobia   A persistent and excessive fear of a specific object, activity, or situation.

social phobia   An excessive fear of being observed in public; speaking in public is the most common example.

Ethnicity, Culture, and Psychological Disorders

DIMENSIONS OF DIVERSITY

Cultural and ethnic backgrounds shape the experience and expression of psychological health and disorders around the world. For example, how symptoms are interpreted and communicated, whether treatment is sought, and whether a social stigma is attached to a particular symptom or disorder can be affected by cultural differences.

Expression of Symptoms

People from different cultures or groups may manifest or describe symptoms differently. For example, in some cultures, people with social phobia may be more distressed about the imagined harm their social clumsiness causes to others than about their own embarrassment. In other cultures depression may be expressed in ways that most Canadians would consider unusual, such as by taking on extra tasks. Some disorders, such as schizophrenia, may manifest with different delusions depending on the local culture.

Differing Attitudes

It is relatively easy for Canadians of northern European descent to regard emotional problems as psychological in nature and to therefore accept a psychological treatment. For other groups, symptoms of psychological distress may be viewed as a spiritual problem, best dealt with by religious figures.

People from some groups may have little hesitation about communicating intimate, personal problems to professional care providers. However, for others,

particularly men and members of certain ethnic groups, loss of emotional control may be seen as a weakness.

In addition, the use of mental health services is viewed negatively in many cultures; this stigma may partly account for the fact that black Canadians and Asian Canadians are only about half as likely as whites to use any type of mental health service.

Assimilation

When people immigrate to Canada, raise their children here, and become more involved in their new community, they sometimes lose aspects of their own cultural heritage. When traditional values become less practiced, or are not honoured in the same ways as they once were, this assimilation can sometimes increase the likelihood for anxiety, depression, and substance abuse. Immigrants are the people in Canada least likely to use mental health services.

Biological Risk Factors

Biology can also be a determinant of the differences seen among people of different ethnic groups. For example, psychotropic drugs are broken down in the body by a specific enzyme called CYP2C19. Reduction of the activity of this enzyme is caused by two mutations, one of which appears to be found only in Asian populations. These poor metabolizers are very sensitive to medications that are broken down by this enzyme. The percentage of poor metabolizers among Asians is about 20%; among

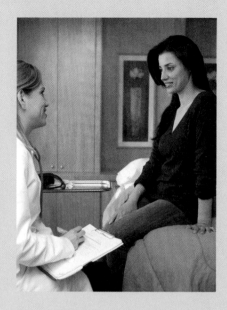

Latinos, about 5%; and among whites, 3%. Asian people thus tend to have more adverse reactions to the doses of drugs standardized principally on white people.

Sources: Alegria, M., et al. 2007. Understanding differences in past year psychiatric disorders for Latinos living in the US. *Social Science & Medicine* 65(2): 214–230; Kleinman, A. 2004. Culture and depression. *New England Journal of Medicine* 351(10): 951–953; Kirmayer, L. J. 2001. Cultural variations in the clinical presentation of depression and anxiety: Implications for diagnosis and treatment. *Journal of Clinical Psychiatry* 62(13 Suppl.): 22–28; Lin, K. M. 2001. Biological differences in depression and anxiety across races and ethnic groups. *Journal of Clinical Psychiatry* 62(13 Suppl.): 13–19; Mood Disorders Society of Canada. 2007; *Quick Facts: Mental Illness and Addiction in Canada* (http://www.mooddisorderscanada.ca/page/quick-facts; retrieved March 7, 2011).

Panic Disorder   People with **panic disorder** experience sudden unexpected surges in anxiety, accompanied by other symptoms, such as rapid and strong heartbeat, shortness of breath, loss of physical equilibrium, and a feeling of losing mental control. Just less than 1% of Canadians experience panic disorders. Such attacks usually begin in a person's early twenties and can lead to a fear of being in crowds or closed places or of driving or flying. These people fear that a panic attack will occur in a situation from which escape is difficult (such as while in an elevator), where the attack could be incapacitating and result in a dangerous or embarrassing loss of control (such as while driving a car or shopping), or where no medical help would be available if needed (such as when a person is alone away

from home). Such fears lead to avoidance of situations that might cause trouble. The fears and avoidance may spread to a large variety of situations until a person is virtually housebound, a condition called **agoraphobia**. People with panic disorder can often function normally in feared situations if someone they trust accompanies them.

> **panic disorder**   A syndrome of severe anxiety attacks accompanied by physical symptoms.
>
> **agoraphobia**   An anxiety disorder characterized by fear of being alone, away from help, and avoidance of many different places and situations; in extreme cases, a fear of leaving home.

TERMS

Shyness

IN FOCUS

Shyness is a form of social anxiety, a fear of what others will think of our behaviour or appearance. Physical signs include a rapid heartbeat, an upset stomach, sweating, cold and clammy hands, blushing, dry mouth, a lump in the throat, and trembling muscles. Shy people are often excessively self-critical, and their self-talk can be very negative. Their feelings of self-consciousness, embarrassment, and unworthiness can be overwhelming.

To avoid situations that make them anxious, shy people may refrain from making eye contact or speaking up in public. They may shun social gatherings and avoid university courses or job promotions that demand interpersonal interaction or public speaking.

Shyness is not the same thing as being introverted. Introverts prefer solitude to society. Shy people often long to be more outgoing, but their own negative thoughts prevent them from enjoying the social interaction they desire.

The consequences of severe shyness can include social isolation, loneliness, and lost personal and professional opportunities. Very shy people also have high rates of other anxiety and mood disorders and of substance abuse.

Shyness may be partly inherited. But for shyness, as for many health concerns, biology is not destiny. Many shy children outgrow their shyness, just as others acquire it later in life. Clearly, other factors are involved. The type of attachment between a child and his or her caregiver is important, as are parenting styles. People's experiences during critical devel-

opmental transitions, such as starting school and entering adolescence, have also been linked to shyness. For adults, the precipitating factor may be an event, such as divorce or the loss of a job.

Shyness is very common, with 40%–50% of North Americans describing themselves as shy. However, only about 3% of Canadian adults experience a severe form of shyness that interferes seriously with daily life. Recent surveys indicate that shyness rates may be rising in North America. With the advent of technologies, such as automatic teller machines, video games, voice mail, faxes, and email, the opportunities for face-to-face interaction are diminishing. Electronic media can be a wonderful way for shy people to communicate, but they can also allow us to hide from social interaction. In fact, one study found that greater use of the Internet was associated with a decline in participants' communication with family members, a reduction in the size of their social circles, and an increase in levels of depression and loneliness.

Shyness is often undiagnosed, but help is available. Shyness classes, assertiveness training groups, and public speaking clinics are available (see the Behaviour Change Strategy at the end of the chapter). For the seriously shy, effective treatments include cognitive behavioural therapy and antidepressant drugs.

If you're shy, try to remember that shyness is widespread. Some degree of shyness has an upside. Shy people tend to be gentle, supportive, kind, and sensitive; they are often exceptional listeners. People who think carefully before they

speak or act are less likely to hurt others' feelings. Shyness may also facilitate co-operation. For any group or society to function well, many roles are required, and quieter, more reflective individuals have a place.

Sources: American Psychological Association. 2007. *Painful Shyness in Children and Adults* (http://www.apahelpcenter.org/featuredtopics/feature.php?id=5; retrieved December 29, 2008); Ebeling-Witte, S., et al. 2007. Shyness, Internet use, and personality. *Cyberpsychology and Behaviour* 10(5): 713–716; Rosenthal, J., et al. 2007. Beyond shy: When to suspect social anxiety disorder. *Journal of Family Practice* 56(5): 369–374; Shields, M. 2004. Social anxiety disorder—Beyond shyness. *Health Reports* 15(Suppl.): 47–91.

Generalized Anxiety Disorder A basic reaction to future threats is to worry about them. **Generalized anxiety disorder (GAD)** is experienced by just more than 1% of Canadians, and this diagnosis is given to people whose worries have taken on a life of their own, pushing out other thoughts and refusing banishment by any effort of will. The topics of the worrying are ordinary concerns: Will I be able to pass the exam next Friday? Where will I get money to get my car fixed?

The worrying of the person with GAD is not completely unjustified—after all, thinking about problems can result in solving them. But this kind of thinking seems to just go around in circles, and the more they try

to stop it, the more they feel at its mercy. The end result is a persistent feeling of nervousness, often accompanied by depression.

Obsessive-Compulsive Disorder The diagnosis of **obsessive-compulsive disorder (OCD)** is given to about 2% of Canadians. They may have obsessions or compulsions or both.

- **Obsessions** are recurrent, unwanted thoughts or impulses. Unlike the worries of GAD, they are not ordinary concerns but improbable fears, such as of suddenly committing an antisocial act or of having been contaminated by germs.

- **Compulsions** are repetitive, difficult-to-resist actions that are usually associated with obsessions. A common compulsion is handwashing, which is typically associated with an obsessive fear of contamination by dirt. Other compulsions are counting and repeatedly checking whether something has been done—for example, whether a door has been locked or a stove turned off.

People with OCD feel anxious, out of control, and embarrassed. Their rituals can occupy much of their time and make them inefficient at work and difficult to live with.

Behavioural Addictions In a **behavioural addiction**, such as to gambling, shopping, or sexual activity, the role of compulsion is small but significant. People experience intense urges to engage in the behaviour, which can create anxiety. The urge intensifies until they carry out the behaviour repeatedly, after which they usually feel relief and elation. As with substance addictions, the behaviour may have negative consequences, but the individual keeps returning to it in spite of them. The behaviour is both maladaptive and persistent. The Centre for Addiction and Mental Health offers treatment options for a wide variety of behavioural and substance-based addictions. (We discuss addiction in greater depth in Part V.)

Post-Traumatic Stress Disorder People who have **post-traumatic stress disorder (PTSD)** are reacting to severely traumatic events (events that produce a sense of terror and helplessness), such as physical violence to themselves or loved ones. Trauma occurs in personal assaults (rape, military combat), natural disasters (floods, hurricanes), and tragedies (fires and airplane or car crashes).

Symptoms include reexperiencing the trauma in dreams and in intrusive memories, trying to avoid anything associated with the trauma, and numbing of feelings. Hyperarousal, sleep disturbances, and other symptoms of anxiety and depression also commonly occur. Such symptoms can last months or even years. PTSD symptoms often decrease substantially within three months, but in up to one-third of PTSD cases, the individual does not fully recover. Recovery may be slower in those who have previously experienced trauma or who have ongoing psychological problems.

The terrorist attacks on September 11, 2001, brought PTSD into the spotlight. Among those affected were survivors, rescue workers, passersby, residents of Manhattan in general, and to some extent, television viewers around the world who saw countless repeated images of the devastation. An estimated 150,000 New Yorkers developed PTSD following the attacks; some were still experiencing symptoms five years later. Hurricane Katrina had a similarly devastating effect; in one survey, 19% of police officers and 22% of firefighters in the Gulf Coast states reported symptoms of PTSD. Canadian soldiers wounded in combat are also at risk for PTSD; among soldiers wounded in Iraq or Afghanistan, rates of PTSD increased during the first year after the injury, suggesting that the emotional impact deepens with time. When symptoms persist, and when daily functioning is disrupted, professional help is needed.

Treating Anxiety Disorders Therapies for anxiety disorders range from medication to psychological interventions concentrating on a person's thoughts and behaviour. Both drug treatments and cognitive behavioural therapies are effective in panic disorder, OCD, and GAD. Simple phobias are best treated without drugs.

Mood Disorders

Daily, temporary mood changes typically don't affect our overall emotional state or level of wellness. A person with a **mood disorder**, however, experiences emotional disturbances that are intense and persistent enough to affect normal functioning. The two most common mood disorders are depression and bipolar disorder.

Depression The Mood Disorders Society of Canada estimates that **depression** affects about 8% of Canadians at some point during their lifetime, with women being twice as likely as their male counterparts to experience depression. Depression affects all ethnic groups although not equally. For example, only 3.1% of Inuit have experienced a major depressive episode, while 16% of First Nations people have experienced major depression.

TERMS

generalized anxiety disorder (GAD) An anxiety disorder characterized by excessive, uncontrollable worry about all kinds of things and anxiety in many situations.

obsessive-compulsive disorder (OCD) An anxiety disorder characterized by uncontrollable, recurring thoughts and the performing of irrational rituals.

obsession A recurrent, irrational, unwanted thought or impulse.

compulsion An irrational, repetitive, forced action, usually associated with an obsession.

behavioural addiction An activity or a behaviour that is maladaptive and persistent despite the negative consequences.

post-traumatic stress disorder (PTSD) An anxiety disorder characterized by reliving traumatic events through dreams, flashbacks, and hallucinations.

mood disorder An emotional disturbance that is intense and persistent enough to affect normal function; two common types of mood disorders are depression and bipolar disorder.

depression A mood disorder characterized by loss of interest, sadness, hopelessness, loss of appetite, disturbed sleep, and other physical symptoms.

Depression takes different forms but usually involves demoralization and can include the following:

- A feeling of sadness and hopelessness
- Loss of pleasure in doing usual activities
- Poor appetite and weight loss
- Insomnia or disturbed sleep
- Restlessness or, alternatively, fatigue
- Thoughts of worthlessness and guilt
- Trouble concentrating or making decisions
- Thoughts of death or suicide

A person experiencing depression may not have all these symptoms. Sometimes instead of poor appetite and insomnia, the opposite occurs: eating too much and sleeping too long. (Depression may contribute to weight gain in young women.) People can have most of the symptoms of depression without feeling depressed, although they usually experience a loss of interest or pleasure in things. (see the box "Could You Have a Mood Disorder?").

In major depression, symptoms are often severe; a diagnosis of *dysthymic disorder* may be applied to people

who experience persistent symptoms of mild or moderate depression for two years or longer. In some cases, depression is a clear-cut reaction to specific events, such as the loss of a loved one or failing in school or work, whereas in other cases no trigger event is obvious.

RECOGNIZING THE WARNING SIGNS OF SUICIDE One of the principal dangers of severe depression is suicide. Although a suicide attempt can occur unpredictably and unaccompanied by depression, the chances are greater if symptoms are numerous and severe. Additional warning signs of suicide include the following:

- The expression of the wish to be dead or the revealing of contemplated methods
- Increasing social withdrawal and isolation
- A sudden, inexplicable lightening of mood (which can mean the person has decided to commit suicide)

Certain risk factors increase the likelihood of suicide:

- A history of previous attempts
- A suicide by a family member or friend
- Readily available means, such as guns or pills
- A history of substance abuse or eating disorders
- Serious medical problems

In Canada, men have much higher suicide rates than women; men between the ages of 45 and 49 have the highest suicide rate (see Figure 2.2). Canadian Aboriginal peoples, and especially Canadian Aboriginal youth, have much higher rates than most other groups, with estimates ranging from two to six times the national average. It is important that culturally sensitive suicide prevention

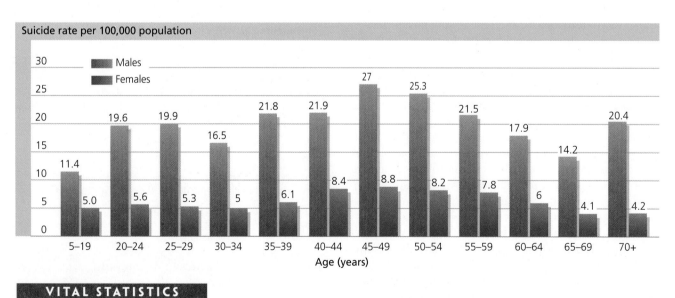

VITAL STATISTICS

FIGURE 2.2 Rates of suicide, by sex and age.

Source: Adapted from Statistics Canada, 2005, CANSIM, table 102-0551 and Catalogue no. 84F0209X. Last modified: 2009-07-06. http://www40.statcan.gc.ca/l01/cst01/hlth66a-eng.htm.

Could You Have a Mood Disorder?

You should be evaluated by a professional if you have any symptoms that are significant enough to interfere with your life, if you've had five or more of the following symptoms for more than two weeks, or if any single symptom causes such a big change that you can't keep up your usual routine.

When You're Depressed

_____ You feel sad or cry a lot, and it doesn't go away.

_____ You feel guilty for no reason; you feel you're no good; you've lost your confidence.

_____ Life seems meaningless, or you think nothing good is ever going to happen again.

_____ You have a negative attitude a lot of the time, or it seems as if you have no feelings.

_____ You don't feel like doing a lot of the things you used to like—music, sports, being with friends, going out, and so on—and you want to be left alone most of the time.

_____ It's hard to make up your mind.

_____ You forget lots of things, and it's hard to concentrate.

_____ You get irritated often. Little things make you lose your temper; you overreact.

_____ Your sleep pattern changes: You start sleeping a lot more or you have trouble falling asleep at night; or you wake up really early most mornings and can't get back to sleep.

_____ Your eating pattern changes: You've lost your appetite or you eat a lot more.

_____ You feel restless and tired most of the time.

_____ You think about death or feel as if you're dying or have thoughts about committing suicide.

When You're Manic

_____ You feel high as a kite, like you're on top of the world.

_____ You get unrealistic ideas about the great things you can do—things that you really can't do.

_____ Thoughts go racing through your head, you jump from one subject to another, and you talk a lot.

_____ You're a nonstop party, constantly running around.

_____ You do too many wild or risky things—with driving, with spending money, with sex, and so on.

_____ You're so up that you don't need much sleep.

_____ You're rebellious or irritable and can't get along at home or school or with your friends.

If you are concerned about depression in yourself or a friend, or if you are thinking about hurting or killing yourself, talk to someone about it and get help immediately.

---

programs be offered. Women attempt suicides three times as often as men, yet men succeed at more than three times the rate of women (see the box "Depression, Anxiety, and Gender" on p. 50). Suicide rates among adolescents and young adults and among adults over 70 have been falling for the last two decades.

Sometimes mistaken for suicide attempts are acts of *self-injury*, including cutting, burning, hitting, and other forms of self-inflicted harm. In a 2007 study, 25% of university-age females surveyed said they had injured themselves intentionally. A maladaptive coping strategy, self-injury is believed to provide relief from unbearable psychological distress or pain, perhaps through the release of endorphins. A variety of psychotherapeutic interventions can help people who injure themselves. Whatever the reason behind it, however, self-harm should be taken very seriously because it may signal an increased risk for

suicide. According to a 2007 British study, young people who purposely hurt themselves were much more likely to commit suicide than were the general population.

HELPING YOURSELF OR A FRIEND If you are severely depressed or know someone who is, expert help from a mental health professional is essential. Don't be afraid to discuss the possibility of suicide with someone you fear is suicidal. You won't give them an idea they haven't already thought of (see the box "Myths About Suicide," p. 51). Asking direct questions is the best way to determine whether someone seriously intends to commit suicide. Encourage your friend to talk and to take positive steps to improve his or her situation (e.g., talk with a mental health professional). If you are feeling unsure about how to help a depressed friend, it may be helpful for you to speak with a mental health professional for support and guidance.

Depression, Anxiety, and Gender

It is evident that gender is a determinant of many aspects of health, including aspects of psychological well-being. The common belief that females are more emotional than males has both a positive and a negative side. On the one hand, women are thought to express positive emotions more clearly than men, especially those related to sympathy and caring. On the other hand, women are more prone to negative emotions, such as depression and worry.

One of the defining characteristics of a psychiatric disorder is that it interferes with daily activities and the ability to live a happy life. Thus, the higher incidence of anxiety and mood disorders in women is convincing evidence that they are more likely to experience psychological distress than are men.

Anxiety Disorders

Panic disorder is more than twice as common in women as in men, whereas obsessive-compulsive disorder occurs in men and women at about the same rate. In population surveys, social anxiety disorder is more common in women than in men, but men are more likely to seek treatment for it—perhaps because men are more likely to find it a barrier to success in white-collar jobs. In some surveys, PTSD is more common in women, but the incidence of PTSD depends on the incidence of traumatic events, which varies in different environments. Men are more often exposed to military combat, and women are more often exposed to rape. Trauma from motor vehicle crashes is a fairly common cause of PTSD in both sexes.

Depression and Suicide

When women are depressed, they are more likely than men to experience guilt, anxiety, increased appetite and weight gain, and increased sleep. When women take antidepressants, they may

need a lower dose than men; at the same dosage, blood levels of medication tend to be higher in women. An issue for women who may become pregnant is whether antidepressants can harm a fetus or newborn. The best evidence indicates that the most frequently prescribed types of antidepressants do not cause birth defects, although several studies have reported withdrawal symptoms in some newborns whose mothers used certain antidepressants.

Although suicidal behaviour is strongly associated with depression, and depression is more prevalent in women, many more men than women commit suicide. Overall, about three times as many women as men attempt suicide, but women's attempts are less likely to be lethal.

Underlying Factors

Why women have more anxiety and depression than men is a matter of debate. Some experts think much of the difference is due to reporting bias: Women are more willing to admit to experiencing negative emotions, being stressed, or having difficulty coping. Women may also be more likely to seek treatment.

Other experts point to biologically based sex differences, particularly in the level and action of hormones. Greater anxiety and depression in women compared with men is most pronounced between puberty and menopause, when female hormones are most active. However, this period of life is also the time in which women's social roles and expectations may be the most different from those of men. Women may put more emphasis on relationships in determining self-esteem, and so the deterioration of a relationship is a cause of depression that can hit women harder than men. In addition, culturally determined gender roles are more likely to place women in situations in which they have less control over key life decisions, and lack of autonomy is associated with depression.

The higher suicide rate among young men may relate to gender norms and expectations that men assert independence and physical prowess—sometimes expressed in risky, dangerous, and potentially self-destructive behaviour. Such behaviour, often involving drugs and alcohol and resulting in motor vehicle crashes, occurs more often in young people who later commit suicide. Even when suicidal intention is never expressed, suicidal impulses are often suspected of contributing to sudden deaths in this age group.

Sources: Sanz, E. J., et al. 2005. Selective serotonin reuptake inhibitors in pregnant women and neonatal withdrawal syndrome. *Lancet* 365(9458): 482–487; Kessler, R. C. 2003. Epidemiology of women and depression. *Journal of Affective Disorders* 74: 5–13; World Health Organization. 2002. *Gender and Mental Health.* Geneva: World Health Organization; Pigott, T. A. 1999. Gender differences in the epidemiology and treatment of anxiety disorders. *Journal of Clinical Psychiatry* 60(18 Suppl.): 4–15.

Most communities have emergency help available, often in the form of a hotline telephone counselling service run by a suicide prevention agency (check the Yellow Pages). If you feel the danger of suicide is immediate, do not leave the person alone. Call for help or take him or her to an emergency room.

TREATING DEPRESSION Although more than 80% of Canadians with depression respond very well to treatment, only about 10% of Canadians with depression seek treatment. Treatment for depression depends on its severity and on whether the depressed person is suicidal. The best initial treatment for moderate to severe depression is usually a

Myths About Suicide

IN FOCUS

Myth People who really intend to kill themselves do not let anyone know about it.

Fact This belief can be an excuse for doing nothing when someone says he or she might commit suicide. In fact, most people who eventually commit suicide have talked about doing it.

Myth People who made a suicide attempt but survived did not really intend to die.

Fact This may be true for certain people, but people who seriously want to end their life may fail because they misjudge what it takes. Even a pharmacist may misjudge the lethal dose of a drug.

Myth People who succeed in suicide really wanted to die.

Fact We cannot be sure of that either. Some people are only trying to make a dramatic gesture or plea for help but miscalculate.

Myth People who really want to kill themselves will do it regardless of any attempts to prevent them.

Fact Few people are single-minded about suicide even at the moment of attempting it. People who are quite determined to take their life today may change their mind completely tomorrow.

Myth Suicide is proof of mental health problems.

Fact Many suicides are committed by people who do not meet ordinary criteria for a mental illness, although people with depression, schizophrenia, and other psychological disorders have a much higher than average suicide rate.

Myth People inherit suicidal tendencies.

Fact Certain kinds of depression that lead to suicide do have a genetic component. But many examples of suicide running in a family can be explained by other factors, such as psychologically identifying with a family member, often a parent, who committed suicide.

Myth All suicides are irrational.

Fact By some standards all suicides may seem irrational. But many people find it at least understandable that someone might want to commit suicide, for example, when approaching the end of a terminal illness or when facing a long prison term.

---

combination of drug therapy and psychotherapy. Newer prescription antidepressants work well, although they may take several weeks to take effect, and patients may need to try multiple medications before finding one that works well. Therefore, when suicidal impulses are strong, hospitalization may be necessary.

Antidepressants work by affecting key neurotransmitters in the brain, including serotonin (Figure 2.3, p. 52). The herbal supplement St. John's wort may also affect serotonin levels, but it is not subject to the same testing and regulation as prescription medications, and recent evidence suggests it is not as effective as previously hoped. Anyone who may be experiencing depression should seek a medical evaluation rather than self-treating with supplements.

Electroconvulsive therapy (ECT) is effective for severe depression when other approaches, including medications and other electronic therapies, such as magnetic stimulation, have failed. In ECT, an epileptic-like seizure is induced by an electrical impulse transmitted through electrodes placed on the head. Patients are given an anaesthetic and a muscle relaxant to reduce anxiety and prevent injuries associated with seizures. A typical course of ECT includes three treatments per week for two to four weeks.

One type of depression is treated by having people sit with their eyes open in front of a bright light source every morning. These people have **seasonal affective disorder (SAD)**; their depression worsens during winter months as the number of hours of daylight diminishes, and then improves with the spring and summer. The Mood Disorders Society of Canada estimates that 15% of Canadians experience the winter blues, and 2%–3% experience

THINKING ABOUT THE ENVIRONMENT

Some depressive disorders, such as SAD, are triggered by environmental factors, such as the long nights and grey skies of winter or job schedules that require people to work at night and sleep during the day. Anxiety disorders, such as social phobia, can be greatly compounded by living or working in a crowded area where the person with the disorder must deal with many other people.

If an environmental factor adds to your depression or anxiety, look for resources in your community that can help. For example, counselling can help with social anxiety, and inexpensive light treatments can relieve seasonal depression for some people. For more information on the environment and environmental health, see Chapter 21.

symptoms severe enough to be diagnosed as SAD. SAD is more common among people who live at higher latitudes, which receive fewer hours of light in winter. Light therapy may work by extending the perceived length of the day and thus convincing the brain that it is summertime even during the winter months.

TERMS

electroconvulsive therapy (ECT) The use of electric shock to induce brief, generalized seizures; used in the treatment of selected psychological disorders.

seasonal affective disorder (SAD) A mood disorder characterized by seasonal depression, usually occurring in winter, when there is less daylight.

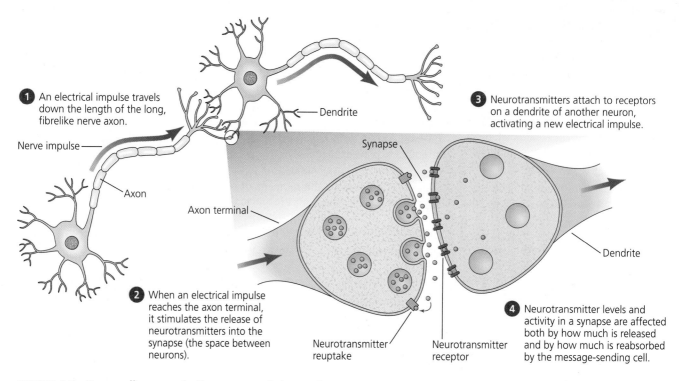

① An electrical impulse travels down the length of the long, fibrelike nerve axon.

Nerve impulse

Axon

② When an electrical impulse reaches the axon terminal, it stimulates the release of neurotransmitters into the synapse (the space between neurons).

Dendrite

Synapse

Axon terminal

Neurotransmitter reuptake

Neurotransmitter receptor

③ Neurotransmitters attach to receptors on a dendrite of another neuron, activating a new electrical impulse.

Dendrite

④ Neurotransmitter levels and activity in a synapse are affected both by how much is released and by how much is reabsorbed by the message-sending cell.

FIGURE 2.3   Nerve cell communication.   Nerve cells (neurons) communicate through a combination of electrical impulses and chemical messages. Neurotransmitters, such as serotonin and norepinephrine, alter the overall responsiveness of the brain and are responsible for mood, level of attentiveness, and other psychological states. Many psychological disorders are related to problems with neurotransmitters and their receptors, and drug treatments frequently target them. For example, the antidepressant drug Prozac increases levels of serotonin by slowing the resorption (reuptake) of serotonin.

Mania and Bipolar Disorder   People who experience **mania**, a less common feature of mood disorders, are restless, have a lot of energy, need little sleep, and often talk nonstop. They may devote themselves to fantastic projects and spend more money than they can afford. Many manic people swing between manic and depressive states, a syndrome called **bipolar disorder** because of the two opposite poles of mood. Bipolar disorder affects men and women equally. Tranquilizers are used to treat individual manic episodes, while special drugs, such as the salt lithium carbonate, taken daily can prevent future mood swings. Anticonvulsants

(drugs used to prevent epileptic seizures) are also prescribed to stabilize moods; examples are Tegretol (carbamazepine) and Lamictal (lamotrigine).

Schizophrenia

Schizophrenia can be severe and debilitating or quite mild and hardly noticeable. Although people are capable of diagnosing their own depression, they usually don't diagnose their own schizophrenia, because they often can't see that anything is wrong. This disorder is not rare; in fact, 1 in every 100 Canadians has a schizophrenic episode in his or her lifetime, most commonly starting in adolescence.

Scientists are uncertain about the exact causes of schizophrenia. Researchers have identified possible chemical and structural differences in the brains of people with the disorder, as well as several genes that appear to increase

TERMS

mania   A mood disorder characterized by excessive elation, irritability, talkativeness, inflated self-esteem, and expansiveness.

bipolar disorder   A mood disorder characterized by alternating periods of depression and mania.

schizophrenia   A psychological disorder that involves a disturbance in thinking and in perceiving reality.

the risk. Schizophrenia is likely caused by a combination of genes and environmental factors that occur during pregnancy and development. For example, children born to a parent with schizophrenia have higher rates of schizophrenia, as do children with prenatal exposure to certain infections or medications.

Some general characteristics of schizophrenia include the following:

- *Disorganized thoughts.* Thoughts may be expressed in a vague or confusing way.
- *Inappropriate emotions.* Emotions may be either absent or strong but inappropriate.
- *Delusions.* People with delusions—firmly held false beliefs—may think that their minds are controlled by outside forces, that people can read their minds, that they are great personages, such as Jesus Christ or the prime minister of Canada, or that they are being persecuted by a group, such as the RCMP.
- *Auditory hallucinations.* People with schizophrenia may hear voices when no one is present.
- *Deteriorating social and work functioning.* Social withdrawal and increasingly poor performance at school or work may be so gradual that they are hardly noticed at first.

None of these characteristics is invariably present. Some people with schizophrenia are quite logical, except on the subject of their delusions. Others show disorganized thoughts but no delusions or hallucinations.

A person with schizophrenia needs help from a mental health professional. Suicide is a risk in schizophrenia, and expert treatment can reduce that risk and minimize the social consequences of the illness by shortening the period when symptoms are active. The key element in treatment is regular medication. At times, medication is like insulin for diabetes—it makes the difference between being able to function or not. Sometimes hospitalization is temporarily required.

MODELS OF HUMAN NATURE AND THERAPEUTIC CHANGE

At least four different perspectives—biological, behavioural, cognitive, and psychodynamic—can be applied to human problems, such as the psychological disorders discussed in this chapter. Each perspective has a distinct view of human nature, and from those views of human nature come distinct therapeutic approaches.

The Biological Model

The *biological model* emphasizes that the mind's activity depends entirely on an organic structure, the brain, whose composition is genetically determined. The activity of neurons, mediated by complex chemical reactions, gives rise to our most complex thoughts, our most ardent desires, and our most pathological behaviour.

Pharmacological therapy (medication) is a common form of treatment for many psychological disorders. Medications can be very effective, but they do have risks and side effects, and they do not work for everyone.

Pharmacological Therapy The most important kind of therapy inspired by the biological model is pharmacological therapy. A list of some of the popular medications currently used for treating psychological disorders follows. All require a prescription from a psychiatrist or other medical doctor. All have been evaluated as being safe and more effective than a **placebo.** Those included in this chapter have received approval from Health Canada but may not necessarily be available in other countries. See the box "Psychiatric Drug Use and the Medication Approval Process in Canada" on p. 54 for more information on Health Canada's approval process. As with all pharmacological therapies, these drugs may cause side effects. For example, the side effects of widely used antidepressants range from diminished appetite to loss of sexual pleasure. In addition, a person may have to try several drugs before finding one that is effective and has acceptable side effects.

1. *Antidepressants:* One group is called the selective serotonin reuptake inhibitors (SSRIs) because of one of their actions. This group includes Prozac (fluoxetine), Paxil (paroxetine), Zoloft (sertraline), Luvox (fluvoxamine), Celexa (citalopram), and Lexapro (escitalopram). Another group is called the tricyclics after their chemical structure; it includes Aventyl (nortriptyline) and Elavil (amitriptyline). Nardil (phenelzine) is a monoamine oxidase inhibitor

placebo A chemically inactive substance that a patient believes is an effective medical therapy for his or her condition. To help evaluate a therapy, medical researchers compare the effects of a particular therapy with the effects of a placebo. The *placebo effect* occurs when a patient responds to a placebo as if it were an active drug.

TERMS

Psychiatric Drug Use and the Medication Approval Process in Canada

Per capita, Canadians use more psychiatric medication than anyone else in the world, with about 51 million prescriptions for them dispensed each year. We are also the second highest users of sedatives and the fourth highest users of prescription narcotics worldwide. But the frequent use of these drugs has caused the Mood Disorders Society of Canada to voice some concerns about how drugs are approved in our country.

In *Quick Facts: Mental Illness and Addiction in Canada* (3rd ed.), the Society notes that 90% of drug trials are created and funded by the same pharmaceutical companies that intend to market the drugs. This fact draws into question the accuracy of the findings being reported, as these companies want favourable results. The duration of the studies is also of concern because most end before any adverse reactions can appear; many longer-term negative side effects may go unreported.

The Society also points out that some physicians prescribe the drugs for purposes other than that approved by Health Canada. That practice may be putting Canadians' health at risk, but the problems arising from these off-label uses have never been studied.

Several organizations, such as the Canadian Agency of Drugs and Technologies in Health (CADTH), can help Canadians make good choices when it comes to taking medications. According to its Web site, the CADTH is "an independent, not-for-profit agency funded by Canadian federal, provincial, and territorial governments to provide credible, impartial advice and evidence-based information about the effectiveness of drugs and other health technologies to Canadian health care decision makers." When you receive a prescription for a medication, be sure to ask your health care provider or pharmacist about the evidence supporting the drug's effectiveness and the conditions for which it has received Health Canada approval.

Sources: Mood Disorders Society of Canada. 2009. *Quick Facts: Mental Illness and Addiction in Canada*, 3rd ed. (http://www.mooddisorderscanada.ca/documents/Quick%20Facts%203rd%20Edition%20Eng%20Nov%2012%2009.pdf; retrieved March 8, 2011); Canadian Agency of Drugs and Technologies in Health. 2011. *Media Centre* (http://www.cadth.ca/index.php/en/media-centre/2011/01/25/238; retrieved March 8, 2011).

(MAOI). Antidepressants that do not fit into these groups include Effexor (venlafaxine), Wellbutrin (buproprion), Remeron (mirtazapine), and Cymbalta (duloxetine). Surprisingly, these antidepressants are as effective in treating panic disorder and certain kinds of chronic anxiety as they are in treating depression. They may also alleviate the symptoms of OCD.

2. *Mood stabilizers:* Lithium carbonate, Depakene (valproic acid), Lamictal (lamotrigine), and Topamax (topiramate) are prescribed as mood stabilizers. They are taken to prevent mood swings that occur in bipolar disorder and certain kinds of schizophrenia.

3. *Antipsychotics:* Older antipsychotics include haloperidol and fluphenazine; newer antipsychotics (sometimes called atypical) are Clozaril (clozapine), Zyprexa (olanzapine), Risperdal (risperidone), Seroquel (quetiapine), Zeldox (ziprasidone), Abilify (aripiprazole), and Invega (paliperidone). These drugs reduce hallucinations and disordered thinking in people with schizophrenia, bipolar disorder, and delirium, and they have a calming effect on agitated patients.

4. *Anxiolytics (antianxiety agents) and hypnotics (sleeping pills):* One of the largest and most prescribed classes of anxiolytics is the benzodiazepines, a group of drugs that includes Valium (diazepam), Librax (chlordiazepoxide), Xanax (alprazolam), and Ativan (lorazepam); Dalmane (flurazepam), Restoril (temazepam), and triazolam are benzodiazepines marketed as sleeping aids. Newer hypnotics include Imovane (zopiclone).

5. *Stimulants:* Ritalin *(methylphenidate)* and Dexedrine *(dextroamphetamine)* are most commonly used for **attention deficit hyperactivity disorder (ADHD)** in children and less often in adults. Drugs of this type are also marketed under the names Adderall (amphetamine aspartate monohydrate), Strattera (atomoxetine), and Concerta (methylphenidate hydrochloride). They are also used for daytime sleepiness in adults, as is Alertec (modafinil).

6. *Anti-dementia drugs:* Dementia is an impairment in memory and thinking that occurs almost exclusively in older adults. The most common type is Alzheimer's disease (see Chapter 17). Many people with this problem are now prescribed Aricept (donepezil) or Ebixa (memantine). Other anti-dementia drugs are Exelon (rivastigmine) and Reminyl (galantamine).

Issues in the Use of Pharmacological Therapy The discovery that many psychological disorders have a biological basis in disordered brain chemistry has led to a revolution in the treatment of many disorders, particularly depression. The new view of depression as based in brain chemistry has also lessened the stigma attached to the

attention deficit hyperactivity disorder (ADHD)
A disorder characterized by persistent, pervasive problems with inattention or hyperactivity, or both, to a degree that is considered inappropriate for a person's developmental stage and that causes significant difficulties in school, work, or relationships.

condition, leading more people to seek treatment, and antidepressants are now among the most widely prescribed drugs in Canada. The development of effective drugs has provided relief for many people, but the widespread use of antidepressants has also raised many questions (see the box "Antidepressant Use in Young People" on p. 56).

Research indicates that for mild cases of depression, psychotherapy and antidepressants are about equally effective. For major depression, combined therapy is significantly more effective than either type of treatment alone. Therapy can help provide insight into factors that precipitated the depression, such as high levels of stress or a history of abuse. A therapist can also provide guidance in changing patterns of thinking and behaviour that contribute to the problem.

The Behavioural Model

The *behavioural model* focuses on what people do—their overt behaviour—rather than on brain structures and chemistry or on thoughts and consciousness. This model regards psychological problems as maladaptive behaviours or bad habits. When and how a person learned the maladaptive behaviour is less important than what makes it continue.

Behaviourists analyze behaviour in terms of **stimulus, response**, and **reinforcement.** The essence of behaviour therapy is to discover what reinforcements keep an undesirable behaviour going and then to try to alter those reinforcements. For example, if people who fear speaking in class (the stimulus) remove themselves from that situation (the response), they experience immediate relief, which acts as reinforcement for future avoidance and escape.

Behavioural therapy can help people overcome many kinds of fears, improving their quality of life.

To change their behaviour, fearful people are taught to practise **exposure**—to deliberately and repeatedly enter the feared situation and remain in it until their fear begins to abate. A student who is afraid to speak in class might begin his behavioural therapy program by keeping a diary listing each time he makes a contribution to a classroom discussion, how long he speaks, and his anxiety levels before, during, and after speaking. He would then develop concrete but realistic goals for increasing his

Canadians spend about **$1.2 billion** each year on antidepressant medications.

—Mood Disorders Society of Canada, 2009

speaking frequency and contract with himself to reward his successes by spending more time in activities he finds enjoyable. This approach is much like the general behaviour change strategy described in Chapter 1.

Although exposure to the real situation works best, exposure in the imagination or through the virtual reality of computer simulation can also be effective. For example, in the case of someone afraid of flying, an imagined scenario would likely be vivid enough to elicit the fear necessary to practise exposure techniques.

The Cognitive Model

The *cognitive model* emphasizes the effect of ideas on behaviour and feeling. According to this model, behaviour results from complicated attitudes, expectations, and motives rather than from simple, immediate reinforcements. When behavioural therapies, such as exposure, work, it is because they change the way a person thinks about the feared situation and his or her ability to cope with it.

Cognitive therapy tries to expose and identify false ideas that produce negative feelings, such as anxiety and depression. For example, a student afraid of speaking in class may harbour such thoughts as "If I begin to speak, I'll say something stupid; if I say something stupid, the teacher and my classmates will lose respect for me; then I'll get a low grade, my classmates will avoid me, and life will be hell." In cognitive therapy, these ideas will be examined critically. If the student prepares, will he or she really sound stupid? Does every sentence said have to be exactly

stimulus   Anything that causes a response.

response   A reaction to a stimulus.

reinforcement   Increasing the future probability of a response by following it with a reward.

exposure   A therapeutic technique for treating fear in which the subject learns to come into direct contact with a feared situation.

Antidepressant Use in Young People

People have become increasingly concerned about the use of antidepressants by youth. On September 14, 2004, a U.S. Food and Drug Administration (FDA) advisory committee recommended a warning label be added to antidepressant drugs based on evidence that their use increases the risk of suicidal thinking and behaviour in children and adolescents. On February 3 of the same year, Health Canada issued a public warning and asked drug manufacturers to provide a review of all (worldwide) safety data pertaining to their drug when used by youth.

Effectiveness

Drug treatment for depression is part of a success story in which people take seriously symptoms of depression and hints of suicidal thinking in children and teens. Over the past decade, the suicide rate among adolescents has fallen. Drug treatment has been considered a key factor in the decline in suicide rates.

A 2005 review of reported childhood depression cases showed that between 1995 and 2002 the number of pediatric psychotherapy sessions declined significantly while prescriptions for antidepressants rose. Most of those prescriptions were for drugs that had not been approved for use in children. In North America, one drug—fluoxetine (Prozac)—has been prescribed regularly for use in children and teens. Studies have found that fluoxetine causes a greater improvement than a placebo, but the combination of drug therapy and cognitive behavioural therapy is more beneficial than either treatment alone. The placebo effect, in which people improve while taking pills containing inactive compounds, is significant in studies of depression and can exceed 30%—meaning almost one-third of people receiving a placebo experience an improvement in their symptoms.

Many antidepressants other than fluoxetine, especially other SSRIs, are also prescribed to young people, but these other drugs haven't been shown to be effective for that age group. Unpublished research data indicate that some SSRIs are not effective in children and teens or are only slightly more effective than a placebo.

Safety

The problem associated with SSRIs is the possibility that they increase the risk of suicide in some young people, particularly in the period immediately following the start of medication use. When study results were pooled, researchers found that in the short term, about 2%–3% of users have an increased risk of suicidal thoughts and actions beyond the risk inherent in depression itself.

Researchers aren't exactly sure what causes this effect. One theory is that SSRIs reverse the lethargy associated with depression more quickly than they relieve the depression itself, giving users the energy to contemplate suicide in the interim. Antidepressants may work differently on the brains of young people than on the brains of adults so as yet unidentified effects may occur.

In February 2004, Health Canada advised that pediatric patients not discontinue their antidepressant medications without consulting their physician. Doctors would make sure the benefits outweighed the potential risks. Depression is a serious illness that can increase the risk of suicide, and mental health professionals and patients must balance the risks of doing nothing against the potential risks and benefits of different types of treatments.

The result of the Health Canada advisory was a 14% reduction in the number of antidepressant prescriptions for this age group. Along with this reduction in prescriptions was a 25% increase in the group's suicide rate. An advisory about antidepressants in children and adolescents was issued in the Netherlands at about the same time, with the same

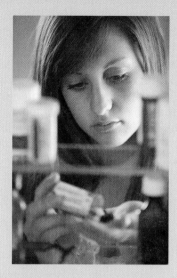

result: SSRI prescriptions dropped but the suicide rate increased. These statistics do not prove a cause-and-effect relationship but certainly are a reason for concern. For some young people, psychological treatment for depression may not have been a practical alternative to medication, because it was not available or not accepted.

Sources: Gibbons, R. D. 2007. Early evidence on the effects of regulators' suicidality warnings on SSRI prescriptions and suicide in children and adolescents. *American Journal of Psychiatry* 164(9): 1356–1363; Newman, T. B. 2004. Treating depression in children: A black-box warning for antidepressants in children? *New England Journal of Medicine* 351(16): 1595–1598; Brent, D. A. 2004. Treating depression in children: Antidepressants and pediatric depression—the risk of doing nothing. *New England Journal of Medicine* 351(16): 1598–1601; Treatment for Adolescents with Depression Study (TADS) Team. 2004. Fluoxetine, cognitive behavioral therapy, and their combination for adolescents with depression. *Journal of the American Medical Association* 292(7): 807–820; Stafford, R. S., et al. 2005. Depression treatment during outpatient visits by U.S. children and adolescents. *Journal of Adolescent Health* 37(6): 434–442; Katz, L. Y., et al. 2008. Effect of regulatory warnings on antidepressant prescription rates, use of health services and outcomes among children, adolescents and young adults. *Canadian Medical Association Journal* 178(8): 1005–1011.

correct and beautifully delivered, or is that an unrealistic expectation? Will classmates' opinions be completely transformed by one presentation? Do classmates even care that much? And why does the student care so much about what they think? People in cognitive therapy are taught to notice their unrealistic thoughts and to substitute more realistic ones, and they are advised to repeatedly test their assumptions.

The Psychodynamic Model

The *psychodynamic model* also emphasizes thoughts. Proponents of this model, however, do not believe thoughts can be changed directly because they are fed by other unconscious ideas and impulses. Symptoms are not isolated pieces of behaviour but the result of a complex set of desires and emotions hidden by active defence mechanisms (see Table 2.2). In psychodynamic therapy, patients speak as freely as possible in front of the therapist and try to understand the basis of their feelings toward the therapist and others. Through this process, patients gain insights that allow them to overcome their maladaptive behaviour. Current therapies of this type tend to focus more on the present (the here and now) than on the past, and the therapist tries to facilitate self-exploration rather than providing explanations.

Evaluating the Models

Ignoring theoretical conflicts among psychological models, therapists have recently developed pragmatic *cognitive behavioural therapies* that combine effective elements of both models in a single package. For example, the package for treating social anxiety emphasizes exposure as well as changing problematic patterns of thinking. Combined therapies have also been developed for panic disorder, obsessive-compulsive disorder, generalized anxiety disorder, and depression. These packages, involving ten or more individual or group sessions with a therapist and homework between sessions, have been shown to produce significant improvement.

Drug therapy and cognitive behavioural therapies are also sometimes combined, especially in the case of depression. For anxiety disorders, both kinds of therapy are equally effective, but the effects of drug therapy last only as long as the drug is being taken, while cognitive behavioural therapies produce longer-term improvement. For schizophrenia, drug therapy is necessary, but a continuing relationship with therapists who give support and advice is also indispensable.

Psychodynamic therapies have been criticized as ineffective and endless. Of course, effectiveness is hard to demonstrate for therapies that do not focus on specific symptoms. But common sense tells us that being able to open yourself up and discuss your problems with a supportive but objective person who focuses on you and lets you speak freely can enhance your sense of self and reduce feelings of confusion and despair.

GETTING HELP

Knowing when self-help or professional help is required for mental health problems is usually not as difficult as knowing how to start or which professional to choose.

Self-Help

If you have a personal problem to solve, a smart way to begin is by finding out what you can do on your own. Some problems are specifically addressed in this book. Behavioural and some cognitive approaches are especially useful for helping yourself. They all involve becoming more aware of self-defeating actions and ideas and combating them in some way: by being more assertive; by communicating honestly; by raising your self-esteem by counteracting negative thoughts, people, and actions that undermine it; and by confronting, rather than avoiding, the things you fear. You can get more information from books in the psychology or self-help sections of libraries

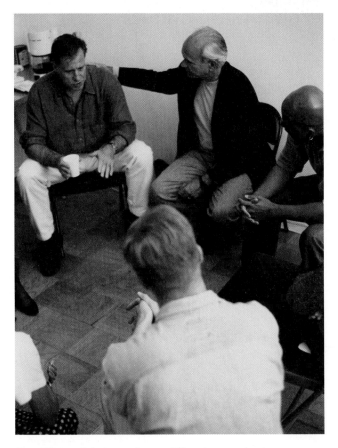

Group therapy is just one of many different approaches to psychological counselling.

and bookstores, but be selective. Watch out for self-help books making fantastic claims that deviate from mainstream approaches.

Some people find it helpful to express their feelings in a journal. Grappling with a painful experience in this way provides an emotional release and can help you develop more constructive ways of dealing with similar situations in the future. Research indicates that using a journal this way can improve physical and emotional wellness.

For some people, religious belief and practice may promote psychological health. Religious organizations provide a social network and a supportive community, and religious practices, such as prayer and meditation, offer a path for personal change and transformation.

Peer Counselling and Support Groups

Sharing your concerns with others is another helpful way of dealing with psychological health challenges. Just being able to share what's troubling you with an accepting, empathetic person can bring relief. Comparing notes with people who have problems similar to yours can give you new ideas about coping.

QUICK STATS

4100 psychiatrists practise in Canada, but the demand for their services far outweighs the supply.

—Canadian Psychiatric Association, 2009

Many universities offer peer counselling through a health centre or through the psychology or education department. Peer counselling is usually done by volunteer students who have received special training that emphasizes confidentiality. Peer counsellors may steer you toward an appropriate campus or community resource or simply offer a sympathetic ear.

Many self-help groups work on the principle of bringing together people with similar problems to share their experiences and support one another. Support groups are typically organized around a specific problem, such as eating disorders or substance abuse. Self-help groups may be listed in the phone book or the campus newspaper.

? QUESTIONS FOR CRITICAL THINKING AND REFLECTION
Have you ever thought professional psychological counselling or therapy might be appropriate for you or a loved one? What circumstances made you think this? Did you or your loved one seek professional help? What was the outcome?

Professional Help

Sometimes self-help or talking to nonprofessionals is not enough. More objective, more expert, or more discreet help is needed. Many people have trouble accepting the need for professional help, and often those who most need help are the most unwilling to get it. You may someday find yourself having to overcome your own reluctance, or that of a friend, about seeking help.

Determining the Need for Professional Help In some cases, professional help is optional. Some people are interested in improving their psychological health in a general way by going into individual or group therapy to learn more about themselves and how to interact with others. Clearly, seeking professional help for these reasons is a matter of individual choice. In some situations, such as friction among family members or between partners, professional help can mean the difference between a painful split and a satisfying relationship.

The following are some strong indications that you or someone you know needs professional help:

- Depression, anxiety, or other emotional problems begin to interfere seriously with school or work performance or in getting along with others.
- Suicide is attempted or is seriously considered (refer to the warning signs earlier in the chapter).
- Such symptoms as hallucinations, delusions, incoherent speech, or loss of memory occur.
- Alcohol or drugs are used to the extent that they impair normal functioning during much of the week, finding or taking drugs occupies much of the week, or reducing the dosage leads to psychological or physiological withdrawal symptoms.

Choosing a Mental Health Professional

Mental health workers belong to several different professions and have different roles. Psychiatrists are medical doctors. They are experts in deciding whether a medical disease lies behind psychological symptoms, and they are usually involved in treatment if medication or hospitalization is required. Clinical psychologists typically hold a PhD degree; they are often experts in behavioural and cognitive therapies. Other mental health workers include social workers, licensed counsellors, and clergy with special training in pastoral counselling. In hospitals and clinics, various mental health professionals may join together in treatment teams.

For more on finding appropriate help, see "Choosing and Evaluating Mental Health Professionals" in the ▇connect Library.

BEHAVIOUR CHANGE STRATEGY

Dealing with Social Anxiety

Shyness is often the result of both high anxiety levels and lack of key social skills. To help overcome shyness, you need to learn to manage your fear of social situations and to develop social skills, such as making appropriate eye contact, initiating topics in conversations, and maintaining the flow of conversations by asking questions and making appropriate responses.

As described in the chapter, repeated exposure to the source of the fear—in this case, social situations—is the best method for reducing anxiety. When you practise new behaviours, they gradually become easier and you experience less anxiety.

A counterproductive strategy is avoiding situations that make you anxious. Although this approach works in the short term— you eliminate your anxiety because you escape the situation—it keeps you from meeting new people and having new experiences. Another counterproductive strategy is self-medicating with alcohol or drugs. Being under their influence actually prevents you from learning new social skills and new ways to handle your anxiety.

To reduce your anxiety in social situations, try some of the following strategies:

- Remember that physical stress reactions are short-term responses to fear. Don't dwell on them—remind yourself that they will pass, and they will.

- Refocus your attention away from the stress reaction you're experiencing and toward the social task at hand. Your nervousness is much less visible than you think.

- Allow a warm-up period for new situations. Realize that you will feel more nervous at first, and take steps to relax and become more comfortable. Refer to the suggestions for deep breathing and other relaxation techniques in Chapter 3.

- If possible, take breaks during anxiety-producing situations. For example, if you're at a party, take a moment to visit the restroom or step outside. Alternate between speaking with good friends and striking up conversations with new acquaintances.

- Watch your interpretations; having a stress reaction doesn't mean that you don't

belong in the group, that you're unattractive or unworthy, or that the situation is too much for you. Try thinking of yourself as excited or highly alert instead of anxious.

- Avoid cognitive distortions and practise realistic self-talk. Replace your self-critical thoughts with more supportive ones: "No one else is perfect, and I don't have to be either." "It would have been good if I had a funny story to tell, but the conversation was interesting anyway."

- Give yourself a reality check: Ask if you're really in a life-threatening situation (or just at a party), if the outcome you're imagining is really likely (or the worst thing that could possibly happen), or if you're the only one who feels nervous (or if many other people might feel the same way).

- Don't think of conversations as evaluations; remind yourself that you don't have to prove yourself with every social interaction. And remember that most people are thinking more about themselves than they are about you.

Starting and maintaining conversations can be difficult for shy people, who may feel overwhelmed by their physical stress reaction. If small talk is a problem for you, try the following strategies:

- Introduce yourself early in the conversation. If you tend to forget names, repeat your new acquaintance's name to help fix it in your mind ("Nice to meet you, Amelia").

- Ask questions, and look for shared topics of interest. Simple, open-ended questions, such as "How's your presentation coming along?" or "How do you know our host?" encourage others to carry the conversation for a while and help bring forth a variety of subjects.

- Take turns talking, and elaborate on your answers. Simple yes and no answers don't move the conversation along. Try to relate something in your life—a course you're taking or a hobby you have—to something in the other person's life. Match self-disclosure with self-disclosure.

- Have something to say. Expand your mind and become knowledgeable about

current events and local or campus news. If you have specialized knowledge about a topic, practise discussing it in ways that both beginners and experts can understand and appreciate.

- If you are stuck for something to say, try giving a compliment ("Great presentation!" or "I love your earrings.") or performing a social grace (pass the chips or get someone a drink).

- Be an active listener. Reward the other person with your full attention and with regular responses. Make frequent eye contact and maintain a relaxed but alert posture. (See Chapter 10 for more on being an active listener.)

At first, your new behaviours will likely make you anxious. Don't give up—things *will* get easier. Create many opportunities to practise your new behaviours; your goal is to make them routine activities. For example, striking up a conversation with someone in a registration or movie line can help you practise your skills at small talk in a nonthreatening setting. Once you are comfortable doing that, you might try initiating brief conversations with classmates about academic topics—the upcoming exams, for example, or an assignment. Following that, you might try something more challenging, such as discussing a more personal topic or meeting new people in a social setting.

Regular practice and stress-management skills are critical. Using these techniques, you can increase your social skills and confidence level at the same time as you decrease your anxiety. Eventually, you'll be able to sustain social interactions with comfort and enjoyment. If you find that social anxiety is a major problem for you and self-help techniques don't work, consider looking into a shyness clinic or treatment program on your campus.

Sources: University of Texas at Dallas, Student Counseling Center. 2008. *Self-Help: Overcoming Social Anxiety* (http://www.utdallas. edu/counseling/selfhelp/social-anxiety.html; retrieved December 29, 2008); Carducci, B. J. 2000. *Shyness: A Bold New Approach*. New York: Harper Paperbacks.

Practise and learn online with Connect. Connect allows you to practise important skills at your own pace and on your own schedule, with 24/7 online access to an eBook, practice quizzes, interactivities, videos, study tools, additional resources, and more.

SUMMARY

- Psychological health encompasses more than a single particular state of normality. Psychological diversity is valuable among groups of people.

- Defining psychological health as the presence of wellness means that to be healthy you must strive to fulfil your potential.

- Maslow's definition of psychological health centred on self-actualization, the highest level in his hierarchy of needs. Self-actualized people have high self-esteem and are realistic, inner-directed, authentic, capable of emotional intimacy, and creative.

- Crucial parts of psychological wellness include developing an adult identity, establishing intimate relationships, and developing values and purpose in life.

- A sense of self-esteem develops during childhood as a result of giving and receiving love and learning to accomplish goals. Self-concept is challenged every day; healthy people adjust their goals to their abilities.

- Using defence mechanisms to cope with problems can make finding solutions harder. Analyzing thoughts and behaviour can help people develop less defensive and more effective ways of coping.

- A pessimistic outlook can be damaging; it can be overcome by developing more realistic self-talk.

- Honest communication requires recognizing what needs to be said and saying it clearly. Assertiveness enables people to insist on their rights and to participate in the give-and-take of good communication.

- People may be lonely if they haven't developed ways to be happy on their own or if they interpret being alone as a sign of rejection. Lonely people can take action to expand their social contacts.

- Dealing successfully with anger involves distinguishing between a reasonable level of assertiveness and gratuitous expressions of anger, heading off rage by reframing thoughts and distracting yourself, and responding to the anger of others with an asymmetrical, problem-solving orientation.

- People with psychological disorders have symptoms severe enough to interfere with daily living.

- Anxiety is a fear that is not directed toward any definite threat. Anxiety disorders include simple phobias, social phobias, panic disorder, generalized anxiety disorder, obsessive-compulsive disorder, and post-traumatic stress disorder.

- Depression is a common mood disorder; loss of interest or pleasure in things seems to be a universal symptom. Severe depression carries a high risk of suicide, and suicidally depressed people need professional help.

- Symptoms of mania include exalted moods with unrealistically high self-esteem, little need for sleep, and rapid speech. Mood swings between mania and depression characterize bipolar disorder.

- Schizophrenia is characterized by disorganized thoughts, inappropriate emotions, delusions, auditory hallucinations, and deteriorating social and work performance.

- The biological model emphasizes that the mind's activity depends on the brain, whose composition is genetically determined. Therapy based on the biological model is primarily pharmacological.

- The behavioural model focuses on overt behaviour and treats psychological problems as bad habits. Behaviour change is the focus of therapy.

- The cognitive model considers how ideas affect behaviour and feelings; behaviour results from complicated attitudes, expectations, and motives, not just from simple reinforcements. Cognitive therapy focuses on changing a person's thinking.

- The psychodynamic model asserts that false ideas are fed by unconscious ideas and cannot be addressed directly. Treatment is based on psychotherapy.

- Help is available in a variety of forms, including self-help, peer counselling, support groups, and therapy with a mental health professional. For serious problems, professional help may be the most appropriate.

BOOKS

Antony, M. M. 2008. *The Shyness & Social Anxiety Workbook: Proven, Step-by-Step Techniques for Overcoming Your Fear*, 2nd ed. Oakland, Calif.: New Harbinger. Practical suggestions for fears of interacting with people you don't know.

Grieco, R. 2009. *The Other Depression: Bipolar Disorder.* New York: Routledge. A complete introduction to bipolar disorder, its symptoms, and its current treatments.

Hayden, J. 2009. *Introduction to Health Behavior Theory.* Sudbury, Mass.: Jones and Bartlett. An introduction to the ways theories are developed and the factors that influence health behaviour theory.

Jenkins, J., D. Keltner, and K. Oatley. 2006. *Understanding Emotions,* 2nd ed. Oxford: Blackwell. A comprehensive guide to emotions, including current research on the neuroscience of emotions, evolutionary and cultural approaches to emotion, and the expression and communication of emotions.

Nathan, P. E., and J. M. Gorman. 2007. *A Guide to Treatments That Work,* 3rd ed. New York: Oxford University Press. A balanced and comprehensive report on various treatments for psychological disorders.

Nutbeam, D., and E. Harris. 1999. *Theory in a Nutshell: A Guide to Health Promotion Theory,* 2nd ed. Sydney, Australia: McGraw-Hill. An overview of some of the central theoretical approaches informing health-related behaviour changes.

Seligman, M. E. 2006. *Learned Optimism: How to Change Your Mind and Your Life.* New York: Vintage. Introduces methods for overcoming feelings of helplessness and building a positive self-image that can contribute to emotional well-being.

Thase, M. E., and S. S. Lang. 2006. *Beating the Blues: New Approaches to Overcoming Dysthymia and Chronic Mild Depression.* New York: Oxford University Press. Describes strategies for changing negative thinking patterns that lead to discouragement and pessimism; also discusses newer medications and alternative therapies.

ORGANIZATIONS, HOTLINES, AND WEB SITES

Canadian Agency for Drugs and Technologies in Health. A national body that provides Canada's health care decision makers with credible, impartial advice and evidence-based information about the effectiveness and efficiency of drugs and other health technologies.
http://www.cadth.ca

Canadian Centre for Addiction and Mental Health. Provides information to help Canadians affected by mental health and addiction issues.
http://www.camh.net

Canada Suicide Support Groups. Provides information about suicide support groups throughout Canada.
http://www.suicide.org

Canadian Mental Health Association. Provides information and resources on many aspects of mental health for Canadians.
http://www.cmha.ca

Centre for Suicide Prevention. Provides knowledge and training in the prevention of suicide.
http://www.suicideinfo.ca

Internet Mental Health. An encyclopedia of mental health information, including medical diagnostic criteria.
http://www.mentalhealth.com

MindZone. Offers information on mental health issues specifically for teens.
http://www.copecaredeal.org

Organization for Bipolar Affective Disorder. Provides information to help people affected directly or indirectly by bipolar disorder, depression, or anxiety live better lives.
http://www.obad.ca

U.S. National Institute of Mental Health. Provides helpful information about anxiety, depression, eating disorders, and other challenges to psychological health.
http://www.nimh.nih.gov

SELECTED BIBLIOGRAPHY

Adams, R. E., and J. A. Boscarino. 2006. Predictors of PTSD and delayed PTSD after disaster: The impact of exposure and psychosocial resources. *Journal of Nervous and Mental Disease* 194(7): 485–493.

Agency for Healthcare Research and Quality. 2007. *Newer Class of Antidepressants Similar in Effectiveness, but Side Effects Differ* (http://www.ahrq.gov/news/press/pr2007/antideppr.htm; retrieved December 29, 2008).

Allard, Y. E., R. Wilkins, and J-M. Berthelot. (2004). Premature mortality in health regions with high Aboriginal populations. *Health Reports* 15(1): 51–60 (http://www.statcan.gc.ca/studies-etudes/82-003/archive/2004/6765-eng.pdf; retrieved March 11, 2011).

American Psychiatric Association. 2000. *Diagnostic and Statistical Manual of Mental Disorders,* 4th ed., Text Revision *(DSM-IV-TR).* Washington, D.C.: American Psychiatric Association Press.

Antidepressants for children and adolescents: An update. 2006. *Harvard Mental Health Letter* 22(12): 4–5.

Avagianou, P. A., and M. Zafiropoulou. 2008. Parental bonding and depression: Personality as a mediating factor. *International Journal of Adolescent Medicine & Health* 20(3): 261–269.

Brenes, G. A. 2006. Age differences in the presentation of anxiety. *Aging and Mental Health* 10(3): 298–302.

Coryell, W. H. 2006. Clinical assessment of suicide risk in depressive disorder. *CNS Spectrums* 11(6): 455–461.

Eranti, S., et al. 2007. A randomized, controlled trial with 6-month follow-up of repetitive transcranial magnetic stimulation and electroconvulsive therapy for severe depression. *American Journal of Psychiatry* 164(1): 73–81.

Favaro, A., et al. 2007. Self-injurious behavior in a community sample of young women: Relationship with childhood abuse and other types of self-damaging behaviors. *Journal of Clinical Psychiatry* 68(1): 122–131.

Fazel, S., and M. Grann. 2006. The population impact of severe mental illness on violent crime. *American Journal of Psychiatry* 163(8): 1397–1403.

Forty, L., et al. 2009. Polarity at illness onset in bipolar I disorder and clinical course of illness. *Bipolar Disorders* 11(1): 82–88.

Gunnell, D., P. K. Magnusson, and F. Rasmussen. 2005. Low intelligence test scores in 18-year-old men and risk of suicide: Cohort study. *British Medical Journal* 330(7484): 167.

Hamilton, B. E., et al. 2007. Annual summary of vital statistics: 2005. *Pediatrics* 119(2): 345–360.

Hettema, J. M., et al. 2006. A population-based twin study of the relationship between neuroticism and internalizing disorders. *American Journal of Psychiatry* 163(5): 857–864.

Jones, S. H., and G. Burrell-Hodgson. 2008. Cognitive-behavioral treatment of first diagnosis bipolar disorder. *Clinical Psychology & Psychotherapy* 15(6): 367–377.

Kasper, S., et al. 2006. Superior efficacy of St. John's wort extract WS(R) 5570 compared to placebo in patients with major depression: A randomized, double-blind, placebo-controlled, multi-center trial. *BMC Medicine* 4(1): 14.

Katz, L. Y. et al. 2008. Effects of regulatory warnings on antidepressant prescription rates, use of health services and outcomes among children, adolescents and young adults. *Canadian Medical Association Journal* 178(8): 1005–1011.

Kendler, K. S., J. Myers, and C. A. Prescott. 2005. Sex differences in the relationship between social support and risk for major depression: A longitudinal study of opposite-sex twin pairs. *American Journal of Psychiatry* 162(2): 250–256.

Licinio, J., and M. L. Wong. 2005. Opinion: Depression, antidepressants and suicidality: A critical appraisal. *Nature Reviews: Drug Discovery* 4(2): 165–171.

Lin, Y. R., et al. 2008. Evaluation of assertiveness training for psychiatric patients. *Journal of Clinical Nursing* 17(21): 2875–2883.

McGirr, A., et al. 2007. An examination of *DSM-IV* depressive symptoms and risk for suicide completion in major depressive disorder: A psychological autopsy study. *Journal of Affective Disorders* 97(1–3): 203–209.

Mood Disorders Society of Canada. 2007. *Quick Facts: Mental Illness and Addiction in Canada,* 2nd ed. (http://www.mooddisorderscanada.ca/documents/Media%20Room/QuickFacts_Edition%202_EN.pdf; retrieved March 11, 2011).

Mood Disorders Society of Canada. 2009. *Quick Facts: Mental Illness and Addiction in Canada,* 3rd ed. (http://www.mooddisorderscanada.ca/documents/Quick%20Facts%203rd%20Edition%20Eng%20Nov%2012%2009.pdf; retrieved March 11, 2011).

Nemeroff, C. B. 2007. The burden of severe depression: A review of diagnostic challenges and treatment alternatives. *Journal of Psychiatric Research* 41(3–4): 189–206. [Epub 2006 Jul 25].

Ozer, D. J., and V. Benet-Martinez. 2006. Personality and prediction of consequential outcomes. *Annual Review of Psychology* 57: 401–421.

Rados, C. 2005. Safeguards for children taking antidepressants strengthened. *FDA Consumer* 39 (http://findarticles.com/p/articles/mi_m1370/is_1_39/ai_n8694498/; retrieved March 11, 2011).

Rothwell, J. D. 2009. *In the Company of Others: An Introduction to Communication,* 3rd ed. New York: McGraw-Hill.

Saewyc, E. M., and R. Tonkin. 2008. Surveying adolescents: Focusing on positive development. *Pediatrics & Child Health* 13(1): 43–47.

Schatzberg, A. F., J. O. Cole, and C. DeBattista. 2007. *Manual of Clinical Psychopharmacology,* 6th ed. Washington, D.C.: American Psychiatric Publishing.

Simon, G. E., and J. Savarino. 2007. Suicide attempts among patients starting depression treatment with medications or psychotherapy. *American Journal of Psychiatry* 164(7): 1029–1034.

Simon, G. 2009. Collaborative care for mood disorders. *Current Opinion in Psychiatry* 22(1): 37–41.

Singh, N. N., et al. 2007. Individuals with mental illness can control their aggressive behavior through mindfulness training. *Behavior Modification* 31(3): 313–328.

Statistics Canada. 2010. *Suicides and Suicide Rate, by Sex and by Age Group* (http://www40.statcan.gc.ca/l01/cst01/hlth66a-eng.htm; retrieved March 11, 2011).

Verhaak, P. F., et al. 2009. Receiving treatment for common mental disorders. *General Hospital Psychiatry* 31(1): 46–55.

Williams, D., et al. 2007. Prevalence and distribution of major depressive disorder in African Americans, Caribbean blacks, and non-Hispanic whites. *Archives of General Psychiatry* 64: 305–315.

Zarit, S. H., and J. M. Zarit. 2006. *Mental Disorders in Older Adults: Fundamentals of Assessment and Treatment,* 2nd ed. New York: Guilford Press.

McGraw Hill **connect**™   Practise and learn online with Connect.

STRESS: THE CONSTANT CHALLENGE

3

LOOKING AHEAD>>>>>

AFTER READING THIS CHAPTER, YOU SHOULD BE ABLE TO

- Explain what stress is and how people react to it—physically, emotionally, and behaviourally
- Describe the relationship between stress and disease
- List common sources of stress
- Describe techniques for preventing and managing stress
- Create a plan for successfully managing the stress in your life

TEST YOUR KNOWLEDGE

1. **Which of the following events can cause stress?**
   a. taking out a loan
   b. failing a test
   c. graduating from university or college

2. **Exercise stimulates which of the following?**
   a. analgesia (pain relief)
   b. birth of new brain cells
   c. relaxation

3. **High levels of stress can impair memory and cause physical changes in the brain.**
   True or false?

4. **Which of the following can result from chronic stress?**
   a. violence
   b. heart attack
   c. stroke

5. **Because eating induces relaxation, it is an excellent means of coping with stress.**
   True or false?

ANSWERS

1. **ALL THREE.** Stress-producing factors can be pleasant or unpleasant and can include physical challenges and goal achievement, as well as events that are perceived as negative.

2. **ALL THREE.** Regular exercise is linked to improvements in many dimensions of wellness.

3. **TRUE.** Low levels of stress may improve memory, but high stress levels impair learning and memory and, over the long term, may shrink an area of the brain called the hippocampus.

4. **ALL THREE.** Chronic—or ongoing—stress can last for years. People who suffer from long-term stress may ultimately become violent toward themselves or others. They also run a greater than normal risk for certain ailments, especially cardiovascular disease.

5. **FALSE.** Eating as a means of coping with stress may lead to weight gain and to binge eating, a risky behaviour associated with eating disorders.

Like the term *wellness*, *stress* is a word many people use without really understanding its precise meaning. Stress is popularly viewed as an uncomfortable response to a negative event, which probably describes *nervous tension* more than the cluster of physical and psychological responses that actually constitute stress. In fact, stress is not limited to negative situations; it is also a response to pleasurable physical challenges and the achievement of personal goals. Whether stress is experienced as pleasant or unpleasant depends largely on the situation and the individual. Because learning effective responses to stress can enhance psychological health and help prevent a number of serious diseases, stress management can be an important part of daily life.

As a postsecondary student, you may be in one of the most stressful times of your life (see the box "How High Is Your Stress Level?"). This chapter explains the physiological and psychological reactions that make up the stress response and describes how these reactions can be risks to good health. The chapter also presents methods of managing stress.

WHAT IS STRESS?

In common usage, the term *stress* refers to two different things: situations that trigger physical and emotional

reactions, *and* the reactions themselves. This text uses the more precise term **stressor** for a situation or event that triggers physical and emotional reactions and the term **stress response** for those reactions. A first date and a final exam are examples of stressors; sweaty palms and a pounding heart are symptoms of the stress response. We'll use the term **stress** to describe the general physical and emotional state that accompanies the stress response. So, a person taking a final exam experiences stress.

Physical Responses to Stressors

Imagine a near miss: As you step off the curb, a car swerves toward you. With just a fraction of a second to spare, you leap safely out of harm's way. In that split second of danger and in the moments following it, you experience a predictable series of physical reactions. Your body goes from a relaxed state to one prepared for physical action to cope with a threat to your life.

Two systems in your body control for your physical response to stressors: the nervous system and the endocrine system. Through rapid chemical reactions affecting almost every part of your body, you are primed to act quickly and appropriately in times of danger.

Actions of the Nervous System The nervous system consists of the brain, spinal cord, and nerves. Part of the nervous system is under voluntary control, as seen when you tell your arm to reach for a banana. The part that is not under conscious supervision—for example, the part that controls the digestion of the banana—is the **autonomic nervous system**. In addition to digestion, it controls your heart rate, breathing, blood pressure, and hundreds of other involuntary functions.

The autonomic nervous system consists of two divisions:

- The **parasympathetic division** is in control when you are relaxed; it aids in digesting food, storing energy, and promoting growth.
- The **sympathetic division** is activated during times of arousal, including exercise, and when there is an emergency, such as severe pain, anger, or fear.

Sympathetic nerves use the neurotransmitter **norepinephrine** to exert their actions on nearly every organ, sweat gland, blood vessel, and muscle to enable your body to handle an emergency. In general, the sympathetic division commands your body to stop storing energy and to use it in response to a crisis.

Actions of the Endocrine System During stress, the sympathetic nervous system triggers the **endocrine system**. This system of glands, tissues, and cells helps control body functions by releasing **hormones** and other chemical messengers into the bloodstream to influence metabolism and other body processes. These chemicals act on a variety of targets throughout the body. Along with the nervous

How High Is Your Stress Level?

Many symptoms of excess stress are easy to self-diagnose. To help determine how much stress you experience on a daily basis, answer the following questions:

1. How many of the symptoms of excess stress listed in Table 3.1 (p. 70) do you experience frequently?
2. Are you easily startled or irritated?
3. Are you increasingly forgetful?
4. Do you have trouble falling or staying asleep?
5. Do you continually worry about events in your future?
6. Do you feel as if you are constantly under pressure to produce?
7. Do you often use tobacco, alcohol, or other drugs to help you relax?
8. Do you often feel as if you have less energy than you need to finish the day?
9. Do you have recurrent stomach aches or headaches?
10. Is it difficult for you to find satisfaction in simple life pleasures?
11. Are you often disappointed in yourself and others?
12. Are you overly concerned with being liked or accepted by others?
13. Have you lost interest in intimacy or sex?
14. Are you concerned that you do not have enough money?

Experiencing some of the stress-related symptoms or answering yes to a few questions is normal. However, if you experience a large number of stress symptoms or you answered yes to a majority of the questions, you are likely experiencing a high level of stress. Take time out to develop effective stress-management techniques. This chapter describes many coping strategies that can aid you in dealing with your stressors. Additionally, your school's counselling centre can provide valuable support.

---

system, the endocrine system prepares the body to respond to a stressor.

The Two Systems Together How do both systems work together in an emergency? Let's go back to your near collision with a car. Both reflexes and higher cognitive areas in your brain quickly make the decision that you are facing a threat—and your body prepares to meet the danger. Chemical messages and actions of sympathetic nerves cause the release of key hormones, including **cortisol** and **epinephrine**. These hormones trigger the physiological changes shown in Figure 3.1 (p. 68), including these:

- Heart and respiration rates accelerate to speed oxygen through the body.
- Hearing and vision become more acute.
- The liver releases extra sugar into the bloodstream to boost energy.
- Perspiration increases to cool the skin.
- The brain releases **endorphins**—chemicals that can inhibit or block sensations of pain—in case you are injured.

Taken together, these almost-instantaneous physical changes are called the **fight-or-flight reaction**. They give you the heightened reflexes and strength you need to dodge the car or deal with other stressors. Although these physical changes vary in intensity, the same basic set of physical reactions occurs in response to any type of stressor: positive or negative, physical or psychological.

The Return to Homeostasis Once a stressful situation ends, the parasympathetic division of your autonomic nervous system takes command and halts the stress response. It restores **homeostasis**, a state in which blood pressure, heart rate, hormone levels, and other vital functions are maintained within a narrow range of normal. Your parasympathetic nervous system calms your body, slowing a rapid heartbeat, drying sweaty palms, and returning breathing to normal. Gradually, your body resumes its normal functions, such as digestion and temperature regulation. Damage that may have been sustained during the fight-or-flight reaction is repaired. The day after you narrowly dodge the car, you wake up feeling fine. In this way, your body can grow, repair itself, and acquire reserves of energy. When the next crisis comes, you'll be ready to respond—instantly—again.

The Fight-or-Fight Reaction in Modern Life The fight-or-flight reaction is a part of our biological heritage, and it's a survival mechanism that has served humans well. In modern life, however, it is often absurdly inappropriate. Many of the stressors we face in everyday life do not require a physical response—for example, an exam, a mess left by a roommate, or a stop light. The fight-or-flight reaction prepares the body for physical action regardless of whether such action is a necessary or appropriate response to a particular stressor.

Pupils dilate to admit extra light for more sensitive vision.

Mucous membranes of nose and throat shrink, while muscles force a wider opening of passages to allow easier airflow.

Secretion of saliva and mucus decreases; digestive activities have a low priority in an emergency.

Bronchi dilate to allow more air into lungs.

Perspiration increases, especially in armpits, groin, hands, and feet, to flush out waste and cool overheating system by evaporation.

Liver releases sugar into bloodstream to provide energy for muscles and brain.

Muscles of intestines stop contracting because digestion has halted.

Bladder relaxes. Emptying of bladder contents releases excess weight, making it easier to flee.

Blood vessels in skin and viscera contract; those in skeletal muscles dilate. This increases blood pressure and delivery of blood to where it is most needed.

Endorphins are released to block any distracting pain.

Hearing becomes more acute.

Heart accelerates rate of beating, increases strength of contraction to allow more blood flow where it is needed.

Digestion, an unnecessary activity during an emergency, halts.

Spleen releases more red blood cells to meet an increased demand for oxygen and to replace any blood lost from injuries.

Adrenal glands stimulate secretion of epinephrine, increasing blood sugar, blood pressure, and heart rate; also spur increase in amount of fat in blood. These changes provide an energy boost.

Pancreas decreases secretions because digestion has halted.

Fat is removed from storage and broken down to supply extra energy.

Voluntary (skeletal) muscles contract throughout the body, readying them for action.

FIGURE 3.1 The fight-or-flight reaction. In response to a stressor, the autonomic nervous system and the endocrine system prepare the body to deal with an emergency.

Emotional and Behavioural Responses to Stressors

We all experience a similar set of physical responses to stressors, which make up the fight-or-flight reaction. These responses, however, vary from person to person and from one situation to another. People's perceptions of potential stressors—and of their reactions to such stressors—also vary greatly. For example, you may feel confident about taking exams but be nervous about talking to people you don't know, while your roommate may love challenging social situations but may be very nervous about taking tests. Many factors, some external and some internal, help explain these differences.

Your cognitive (mental) appraisal of a potential stressor strongly influences how you view it. Two factors that can

reduce the magnitude of the stress response are successful prediction and the perception of control. For instance, receiving course syllabi at the beginning of the term allows you to predict the timing of major deadlines and exams. Having this predictive knowledge also allows you to exert some control over your study plans and can thus help reduce the stress caused by exams.

Cognitive appraisal is highly individual and strongly related to emotions. The facts of a situation—Who? What? Where? When?—typically are evaluated fairly consistently from person to person. Evaluation with respect to personal outcome, however, varies: What does this mean for me? Can I do anything about it? Will it improve or worsen? If an individual perceives a situation as exceeding her or his ability to cope, the result can be negative emotions and an inappropriate stress response. If, however, a person perceives a situation as a challenge that is within her or his ability to manage, more positive and appropriate responses are likely. A certain amount of stress, if coped with appropriately, can help promote optimal performance (Figure 3.2).

Effective and Ineffective Responses   Common emotional responses to stressors include anxiety, depression, and fear. Although emotional responses are determined in part by inborn personality or temperament, we often can moderate or learn to control them. Coping techniques are discussed later in the chapter.

Behavioural responses to stressors—controlled by the **somatic nervous system**, which manages our conscious actions—are entirely under our control. Effective behavioural responses, such as talking, laughing, exercising, meditating, learning time-management skills, and becoming more assertive, can promote wellness and enable us to function at our best. Ineffective behavioural responses to stressors include overeating, expressing hostility, and using tobacco, alcohol, or other drugs.

Let's consider the individual variations demonstrated by two students, David and Amelia, responding to the same stressor—the first exam of the term. David enters the exam with a feeling of dread, and as he reads the exam questions, he responds to his initial anxiety with more anxiety. The more upset he gets, the less he can remember and the more anxious he becomes. Soon he's staring into space, imagining what will happen if he fails the course. Amelia, conversely, takes a deep breath to relax before she reads the questions, wills herself to focus on the answers she knows, and then goes back over the exam to deal with those questions she's unsure of. She leaves the room feeling calm, relaxed, and confident that she has done well.

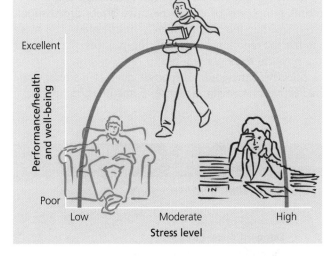

FIGURE 3.2   Stress level, performance, and well-being.
A moderate level of stress challenges individuals in a way that promotes optimal performance and well-being. Too little stress, and people are not challenged enough to improve; too much stress, and the challenges become stressors that can impair physical and emotional health.

As this simple example shows, avoiding destructive responses to stress and adopting effective and appropriate ones can have a direct effect on well-being.

Personality and Stress   Some people seem to be nervous, irritable, and easily upset by minor annoyances; others are calm and composed even in difficult situations. Scientists remain unsure just why this is or how the brain's complex emotional mechanisms work. But **personality**, the sum of cognitive, behavioural, and emotional tendencies, clearly affects how people perceive and react to stressors. To investigate the links among personality, stress, and overall wellness, researchers have looked at different constellations of characteristics, or *personality types*.

- *Type A.* People with type A personality are described as ultracompetitive, controlling, impatient, aggressive, and even hostile. Type A people have a higher perceived stress level and more problems coping with stress. They react explosively to stressors and are upset by events that others would consider only annoyances. Studies indicate that certain characteristics of the type A pattern—anger, cynicism, and hostility—increase the risk of heart disease.
- *Type B.* The type B personality is relaxed and contemplative. Type B people are less frustrated by daily events and more tolerant of the behaviour of others.
- *Type C.* The type C personality is characterized by anger suppression, difficulty expressing emotions, feelings of hopelessness and despair, and an exaggerated response to minor stressors. This heightened response may impair immune functions.
- *Type D.* The type D, or distressed personality is a new personality construct. People with this pattern have a joint tendency to feel (but not express) negative emotions and avoid social contact with others. They tend to be gloomy, socially inept, and anxious worriers, a combination that puts them at risk for heart problems.

Studies of type A, C, and D personalities suggest that expressing your emotions is beneficial, not expressing them is problematic, but habitually expressing exaggerated stress responses or hostility is unhealthy.

somatic nervous system   The branch of the peripheral nervous system that governs motor functions and sensory information, largely under conscious control.

personality   The sum of behavioural, cognitive, and emotional tendencies.

Researchers have also looked for personality traits that enable people to deal more successfully with stress. One such trait is *hardiness*, a particular form of optimism. People with a hardy personality view potential stressors as challenges and opportunities for growth and learning—not as burdens. They see fewer situations as stressful and react less intensely to stress than nonhardy people might. Hardy people are committed to their activities, have a sense of inner purpose and an inner locus of control, and feel at least partly in control of their lives.

The term *resilience* refers to personality traits associated with social and academic success in at-risk populations, such as people from low-income families and those with mental or physical disabilities. Resilience is associated with emotional intelligence and violence prevention. Resilient people tend to set goals and face adversity through individual effort. There are three basic types of resilience, and each one determines how a person responds to stress:

- *Nonreactive resilience*, in which a person does not react to a stressor
- *Homeostatic resilience*, in which a person may react strongly but returns to baseline functioning quickly
- *Positive growth resilience*, in which a person learns and grows from the stress experience

Can you do anything to change your personality traits and become more stress resistant? It isn't likely. You can, however, change some of your typical behaviours and patterns of thinking, and develop positive techniques for coping with stressors. Strategies for successful stress management are described later in this chapter.

Cultural Background Young adults from around the world come to Canada for a higher education; most students finish university or college with a greater appreciation for other cultures and worldviews. The clashing of cultures, however, can be a big source of stress for many students—especially when it leads to disrespectful treatment, harassment, or violence. It is important to remember that everyone's reaction to stress is influenced by his or her family and cultural background. Learning to accept and appreciate the cultural backgrounds of other people is both a mind-opening experience and a way to avoid stress over cultural differences.

Gender Our **gender role**—the activities, abilities, and behaviours our culture expects of us based on our sex—can affect our experience of stress. Some behaviour responses to stressors, such as crying or openly expressing anger, may be deemed more appropriate for one gender than for the other.

Strict adherence to gender roles, however, can limit a person's response to stress and can itself become a source of stress. Gender roles can also affect our perception of a stressor. If a man derives most of his self-worth from his work, for example, retirement may be more stressful for him than for a woman whose self-image is based on several different roles.

See the box "How Women and Men Experience Stress" for more on gender and stress.

Experience Past experiences can profoundly influence the evaluation of a potential stressor. Consider someone who has had a bad experience giving a speech in the past. He or she is much more likely to perceive an upcoming speech as stressful than is someone who has had positive public speaking experiences.

The Stress Experience as a Whole

As Table 3.1 shows, the physical, emotional, and behavioural symptoms of excess negative stress are distinct. Even so, they are also intimately interrelated. The more intense the emotional response, for example, the stronger the physical response will be.

Effective behavioural responses can lessen stress, while ineffective ones make it worse. Sometimes, people have

TERMS

gender role A culturally expected pattern of behaviour and attitudes determined by a person's sex.

Table 3.1	Symptoms of Excess Stress	
Physical Symptoms	**Emotional Symptoms**	**Behavioural Symptoms**
Dry mouth	Anxiety	Crying
Excessive perspiration	Depression	Disrupted eating habits
Frequent illnesses	Edginess	Disrupted sleeping habits
Gastrointestinal problems	Fatigue	Harsh treatment of others
Grinding of teeth	Hypervigilance	Problems communicating
Headaches	Impulsiveness	Sexual problems
High blood pressure	Inability to concentrate	Social isolation
Pounding heart	Irritability	Increased use of tobacco, alcohol, or other drugs
Stiff neck or aching lower back	Trouble remembering things	

How Women and Men Experience Stress

Men and women experience stress, but they experience it differently.

Women and Stress

Research has found that women are more likely than men to find themselves balancing multiple roles, such as those of student, spouse, and parent. Women who work outside the home still do most of the housework—although today's husbands are helping more than previous generations did—and housework isn't limited to cleaning or doing laundry. For example, more than 60% of women make all decisions about their family's health care, including decisions about aging parents. The combined pressures of home, workplace, and school can create very high stress levels. Recent reports suggest these findings apply to people in both Canada and the United States.

Men and Stress

Men who fit a traditional male gender role may feel compelled to be in charge at all times. This may create tension in interpersonal situations and limit men's ability to build a support network. Such men may keenly feel the responsibility to support a family, which can compound existing pressures at home and work.

Perceptions of Stress

The Canadian Heart and Stroke Foundation's *Annual Report Card on Canadians' Health* found that, when it comes to stress, many Canadians feel overwhelmed. Specifically, Canadians received fairly mediocre grades in several areas:

Proportion of Canadians Who	Percentage	Grade
Are not frequently stressed	57%	D
Have enough quality time	47%	F
Feel supported in the workplace	77%	B
Cope well with stress	26%	F

In Canada, employed women are more likely than their male counterparts to report high work stress, although both sexes feel the stress of having too little time in the day to accomplish everything. When it comes to coping, women are more likely than men to cope with stress through unhealthy behaviours, such as overeating or taking prescription medications.

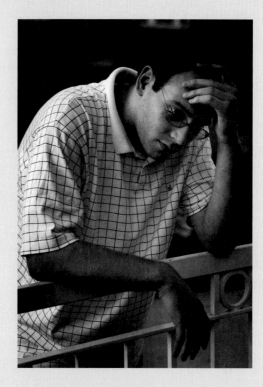

Physiological Differences

Levels of testosterone (the primary male hormone, responsible for many masculine traits) increase from puberty onward, and so men tend to have higher blood pressure than women of the same age. This factor contributes to greater wear on the male circulatory system, sometimes increasing a man's risk for cardiovascular disease. A part of the brain that regulates emotions, the amygdala, is sensitive to testosterone. This may be one reason that men are more likely than women to find certain situations (such as social interactions) to be stressful.

Conversely, women have higher levels of oxytocin (a hormone involved in social interaction and mood regulation) and are more likely to respond to stressors by seeking social support. This coping response may give women a longevity advantage over men by decreasing the risk of some stress-related disorders. It does not, however, free women from stress-related ailments, and women are more likely than men to suffer stress-related hypertensions, depression, and obesity.

such intense responses to stressors or such ineffective coping techniques that they need professional help to overcome the stress in their lives.

This chapter also discusses a variety of ineffective coping behaviours and describes the destructiveness of relying on such habits to deal with stress.

More often, however, people can learn to handle stressors on their own. Strategies for successful stress management are described throughout this chapter. For

QUESTIONS FOR CRITICAL THINKING AND REFLECTION

Think of the last time you faced a significant stressor. How did you respond? List the physical, emotional, and behavioural reactions you experienced. Did these responses help you deal with the stress, or did they interfere with your efforts to handle it?

THINKING ABOUT THE ENVIRONMENT

Environmental problems—whether natural or caused by people—can compound other sources of stress, such as working, commuting, or taking care of a family. Consider the environment where you live, attend school, or work. Do you live with any of the following?

■ Smog or other pollutants, which make the air hard to breathe

■ Crowding, which makes it difficult to move around

■ Poverty, which limits your choices in many aspects of life

■ Crime, which can make you feel unsafe or hypervigilant

If one or more environmental factors make life more stressful for you, look for resources in your community that can help. For example, public transportation may ease your commute while helping to reduce pollution in your city or town. For more information on the environment and environmental health, see Chapter 21.

A person's emotional and behavioural responses to stressors depend on many different factors, including personality, gender, and cultural background. Research suggests that women are more likely than men to respond to stressors by seeking social support, a pattern referred to as tend and befriend.

starters, review the following list of basic stress-management strategies and consider whether any of them has ever worked for you:

• Building greater social support through meaningful relationships

• Participating in and contributing to your family and community in productive ways

• Setting higher expectations for yourself but with clear boundaries and fair, consistent expectations

• Building life skills, such as decision making, effective communication, and conflict management

• Avoiding the urge to control the outcome of every situation

• Knowing your own limits and limitations

• Trusting others

STRESS AND HEALTH

According to the Canadian Mental Health Association, more than 75% of Canadians report feeling very stressed at least once a month, and 43% feel this way a few times each week.

With the economic downturn of 2009, those rates rose even higher, and the associated medical costs are estimated to be in the billions. The role of stress in health is complex, but evidence suggests that stress can increase vulnerability to many ailments. Several theories have been proposed to explain the relationship between stress and disease.

The General Adaptation Syndrome

The term **general adaptation syndrome (GAS)**, coined by Canadian researcher Hans Seyle, describes what many believe is a universal and predictable response pattern to all stressors. As mentioned earlier, some stressors are pleasant (such as attending a party), but others are unpleasant (such as getting a bad grade). In the GAS theory, the stress triggered by a pleasant stressor is called **eustress**; stress brought on by an unpleasant stressor is called **distress**. The sequence of physical responses associated with GAS is the same for eustress and distress and occurs in three stages (Figure 3.3):

• *Alarm.* The alarm stage includes the complex sequence of events brought on by the fight-or-flight reaction. At this stage, the body is more susceptible to disease

FIGURE 3.3 The general adaptation syndrome. During the alarm phase, a lower resistance to injury is evident. With continued stress, resistance to injury is enhanced. With prolonged exposure to repeated stressors, exhaustion sets in, with a return of low resistance levels seen during acute stress.

or injury because it is geared up to deal with a crisis. Someone in this stage may experience headaches, indigestion, anxiety, and disrupted eating or sleep patterns.

• *Resistance.* With continued stress, the body develops a new level of homeostasis in which it is more resistant to disease and injury than usual. In this stage, a person can cope with normal life and added stress.

• *Exhaustion.* The first two stages of GAS require a great deal of energy. If a stressor persists, or if several stressors occur in succession, general exhaustion sets in. This is not the sort of exhaustion you feel after a long, busy day; rather, it's a life-threatening physiological state.

Allostatic Load

Although the GAS model is still viewed as a key conceptual contribution to the understanding of stress, some aspects of it are outdated. For example, increased susceptibility to disease after repeated or prolonged stress is now thought to be due to the effects of the stress response itself rather than to a depletion of resources (exhaustion state). In particular, long-term overexposure to stress hormones, such as cortisol, has been linked with health problems. Further, although physical stress reactions promote homeostasis (resistance stage), they also have negative effects on the body.

The long-term wear and tear of the stress response is called the **allostatic load**. An individual's allostatic load is dependent on many factors, including genetics, life experiences, and emotional and behavioural responses to stressors. A high allostatic load may be due to frequent stressors, poor adaptation to common stressors, an inability to shut down the stress response, or imbalances in the stress response of different body systems. A high allostatic load is linked with heart disease, hypertension, obesity, and reduced brain and immune system functioning. In other words, when your allostatic load exceeds your ability to cope, you are more likely to get sick.

Psychoneuroimmunology

One of the most fruitful areas of current research into the relationship between stress and disease is **psychoneuro-**

immunology (**PNI**). PNI is the study of the interactions among the nervous system, the endocrine system, and the immune system. The underlying premise of PNI is that stress, through the actions of the nervous and endocrine systems, impairs the immune system and thereby affects health. It is important to note, however, that even large stress-induced immune changes can have small clinical (medical) consequences because they are short-term or because the immune system has redundant components and compensates for changes. In short, the immune system is remarkably flexible and capable of substantial change without compromising health. However, chronic stress in individuals predisposed to or experiencing disease may have more substantial consequences.

A complex network of nerve and chemical connections exists between the nervous and endocrine systems and the immune system. In general, increased levels of cortisol are linked to a decreased number of immune system cells called lymphocytes (see Chapter 9 for more on the immune system). Epinephrine appears to promote the release of lymphocytes but at the same time reduces their efficiency. Scientists have identified hormonelike substances called *neuropeptides* that appear to translate stressful emotions into biochemical events, some of which affect the immune system, providing a physical link between emotions and immune function.

Different types of stress may affect immunity in different ways. For instance, during acute stress (typically lasting between 5 and 100 minutes), white blood cells move into the skin, where they enhance the immune response. During a stressful event sequence, such as a personal trauma and the events that follow, however, there are typically no overall significant immune changes. Chronic (ongoing) stressors, such as unemployment, have negative effects on almost all functional measures of immunity. Chronic stress may cause prolonged secretion of cortisol and may accelerate the course of diseases that involve inflammation, including multiple sclerosis, heart disease, and type 2 diabetes.

Mood, personality, behaviour, and immune functioning are intertwined. For example, people who are generally pessimistic may neglect the basics of health care, become passive when ill, and fail to engage in health-promoting behaviours. People who are depressed may reduce physical activity and social interaction, which may in turn affect the immune system and the cognitive appraisal of a stressor. Optimism, successful coping, and positive problem solving, conversely, may positively influence immunity.

allostatic load The long-term negative impact of the stress response on the body.

psychoneuroimmunology (PNI) The study of the interactions among the nervous, endocrine, and immune systems.

TERMS

Ongoing stress has been shown to make people more vulnerable to everyday ailments, such as colds and allergies.

Links Between Stress and Specific Conditions

Although much remains to be learned, it is clear that people who have unresolved chronic stress in their lives or who handle stressors poorly are at risk for a wide range of health problems. In the short term, the problem might be just a cold, a stiff neck, or a stomach ache. Over the long term, the problems can be more severe: cardiovascular disease (CVD), high blood pressure, impaired immune function, or accelerated aging.

Cardiovascular Disease   During the stress response, heart rate increases and blood vessels constrict, causing blood pressure to rise. Chronic high blood pressure is a major cause of atherosclerosis, a disease in which blood vessels become damaged and caked with fatty deposits. These deposits can block arteries, causing heart attacks and strokes. The stress response can precipitate a heart attack in someone with atherosclerosis. The stress response can also cause stress cardiomyopathy ("broken heart syndrome"), a condition that mimics a heart attack but doesn't damage the heart.

Certain types of emotional responses may increase a person's risk of CVD. As described earlier, people who tend to react to situations with anger and hostility are more likely to have heart attacks than are people with a less explosive, more trusting personality.

Stress has also been linked to some of the more recently identified risk factors for CVD, including elevated cholesterol. For example, inflammation is a key component of the damage to blood vessels that leads to heart attacks. Stress increases inflammation throughout the body. Stress-induced increases in inflammatory messenger molecules are also linked to elevated levels of homocysteine and C-reactive protein (CRP), two compounds that appear to be markers for CVD risk. Stress-related depression and anger are associated with elevated homocysteine levels, and job-related exhaustion is linked to high CRP levels in some people. Elevated CRP levels have also been implicated in insulin resistance and the development of diabetes, which is in turn a risk factor for CVD. Clearly, stress reduction can improve cardiovascular health. See Chapter 7 for more on CVD.

Psychological Problems   The hormones and other chemicals released during the stress response cause emotional as well as physical changes (see the box "Stress and Your Brain"). Stress also activates the enzyme PKC, which influences the brain's prefrontal cortex. Excess PKC can negatively affect focus, judgment, and the ability to think clearly. Moreover, many stressors are inherently anxiety producing, depressing, or both. Stress has been found to contribute to psychological problems, such as depression, panic attacks, anxiety, eating disorders, and post-traumatic stress disorder (PTSD). PTSD, which affects war veterans, rape and child abuse survivors, and others who have suffered or witnessed severe trauma, is characterized by nightmares, flashbacks, and a diminished capacity to experience or express emotion. (For more information, see Chapter 2.)

Altered Functioning of the Immune System   PNI research helps explain how stress affects the immune system. Some of the health problems linked to stress-related changes in immune function include vulnerability to colds and other infections, asthma and allergy attacks, susceptibility to cancer, and flare-ups of chronic diseases, such as genital herpes and HIV infection.

Other Health Problems   Many other health problems may be caused or worsened by excessive stress, including the following:

- Digestive problems, such as stomach aches, diarrhea, constipation, irritable bowel syndrome, and ulcers
- Tension headaches and migraines (see the box "Headaches: A Common Symptom of Stress," p. 76)
- Insomnia and fatigue
- Injuries, including on-the-job injuries caused by repetitive strain

Stress and Your Brain

Like a computer that registers information in response to typing on a keyboard, your brain is able to respond to and store information about changes in your environment. Unlike a computer, your brain has the attribute of *plasticity*—it physically changes its structure and function in response to experience. Plasticity allows your brain to be altered by psychological stress.

Moderate stress enhances the ability to acquire and remember information, while high levels of acute stress can impair learning. For example, people can often remember minute details following a fender bender but can't recall the events surrounding a major car crash. Thus, it is good to be a little nervous before an exam—but not too nervous.

The effects of stress on brain form and function are apparent in a structure called the *hippocampus*, which is involved in learning and memory. High levels of chronic stress cause brain cells (neurons) in the hippocampus to shrink in size or die, thus impairing learning and memory. New research in neuroscience has revealed that the hippocampus actually grows new neurons during adulthood. However, stress acts to reduce new cell birth in the hippocampus, reducing the replacement of lost neurons. Together, these effects of stress result in fewer neurons and fewer connections between neurons in the hippocampus, thus decreasing the capacity for information processing.

People who are depressed or who experience post-traumatic stress disorder have higher levels of stress hormones in their bloodstream and smaller hippocampi than others. Even in the absence of a serious disorder, it is thought that the accumulation of stress effects across the lifespan can contribute to brain aging. Thus, the way you cope with stress can affect the way your brain works both immediately and over the long term.

- Menstrual irregularities, impotence, and pregnancy complications
- Loss of interest in previously enjoyable activities

QUESTIONS FOR CRITICAL THINKING AND REFLECTION

Have you ever been so stressed that you felt ill in some way? If so, what were your symptoms? How did you handle them? Did the experience affect the way you reacted to other stressful events?

COMMON SOURCES OF STRESS

Being able to recognize potential sources of stress is an important step in successfully managing the stress in your life.

Major Life Changes

Any major change in your life that requires adjustment and accommodation can be a source of stress. Early adulthood and the postsecondary years are associated with many significant changes, such as moving out of the family home. Even changes typically thought of as positive—graduation, job promotion, marriage—can be stressful.

Clusters of life changes, particularly those that are perceived negatively, may be linked to health problems in some people. Personality and coping skills, however, are important moderating influences. People with a strong support network and a stress-resistant personality are less likely to become ill in response to life changes than people with fewer resources.

Daily Hassles

Although major life changes are undoubtedly stressful, they seldom occur regularly. Researchers have proposed that minor problems—life's daily hassles, such as losing your keys or wallet—can be an even greater source of stress because they occur much more often.

People who perceive hassles negatively are likely to experience a moderate stress response every time they are faced with one. Over time, this can take a significant toll on health. Studies indicate that for some people, daily hassles contribute to a general decrease in overall wellness.

Postsecondary Stressors

University or college is a time of major changes and minor hassles. For many students, university means being away from home and family for the first time. Nearly all students share similar stresses, such as the following:

- *Academic stress.* Exams, grades, and an endless workload await every postsecondary student but can be

Headaches: A Common Symptom of Stress

Many Canadians have chronic, recurrent headaches. Headaches come in various types but are often grouped into three major categories: tension headaches, migraines, and cluster headaches. Other types of headaches have underlying organic causes, such as sinus congestion or infection.

Tension Headaches

Approximately 90% of all headaches are *tension headaches*, characterized by a dull, steady pain, usually on both sides of the head. It may feel as though a band of pressure is tightening around your head, and the pain may extend to your neck and shoulders. Acute tension headaches can last from hours to days, while chronic tension headaches may occur almost every day for months or even years.

Psychological stress, poor posture, and immobility are the leading causes of tension headaches. They have no cure, but the pain can sometimes be relieved with over-the-counter painkillers and with therapies, such as massage, acupuncture, relaxation, hot or cold showers, and rest.

If your headaches are frequent, keep a diary with details about the events surrounding each one. If you can identify the stressors that are consistently associated with your headaches, you can begin to gain more control over the situation. If you have persistent tension headaches, you should consult your physician.

Migraines

About 8% of Canadians ages 12 and older have migraines, which typically progress through a series of stages lasting from several minutes to several days. They can produce a variety of symptoms, including throbbing pain that starts on one side of the head and may spread; heightened sensitivity to light; visual disturbances, such as flashing lights; nausea; and fatigue. About 70% of migraine sufferers are women, with the highest rates among 25- to 54-year-olds,

and migraine headaches may have a genetic component.

Research suggests that people who get migraines may have abnormally excitable nerve cells in their brains. When triggered, these nerve cells send a wave of electrical activity throughout the brain, which in turn causes migraine symptoms. Potential triggers include menstruation, stress, fatigue, atmospheric changes, specific sounds or odours, and certain foods. The frequency of attacks varies from a few in a lifetime to several per week.

Keeping a headache journal can help a person with migraines identify headache triggers—the first step to avoiding them. In addition, many new treatments can help reduce the frequency, severity, and duration of migraines.

Cluster Headaches

Cluster headaches are extremely severe headaches that cause intense pain in and around one eye. They usually occur in clusters of one to three headaches each day over weeks or months, alternating with periods of remission in which no headaches occur. About 90% of people with cluster headaches are male.

There is no known cause or cure for cluster headaches, but a number of treatments are available. During cluster periods, it is important to refrain from smoking cigarettes and drinking alcohol, because these activities can trigger attacks.

---

especially troublesome for young students just out of high school. Test anxiety is a source of stress for many students. To learn some proven techniques for overcoming test anxiety, see the Behaviour Change Strategy at the end of this chapter.

• *Interpersonal stress.* Most students are more than just students; they are also friends, children, employees, spouses, parents, and so on. Managing relationships while juggling the rigors of university or college life can be daunting, especially if some friends or family are less than supportive.

• *Time pressures.* Class schedules, assignments, and deadlines are an inescapable part of postsecondary life. But these time pressures can be drastically compounded for students who also have a job and family responsibilities.

• *Financial concerns.* The majority of postsecondary students need financial aid not just to cover the cost of

tuition but to survive from day to day while in school. For many, this isn't possible without a job, and the pressure to stay afloat financially competes with academic and other stressors.

• *Worries about the future.* As school life comes to an end, students face the reality of life after university or college. This means thinking about a career, choosing a place to live, and leaving the friends and routines of school behind.

Job-Related Stressors

Canadians rate their jobs as a key source of stress in their lives, and the World Health Organization has deemed job-related stress a worldwide epidemic. The Canadian Mental Health Association recently identified the rise in unemployment and job instability as key stressors. And for those who are employed, tight schedules and overtime leave less time to exercise, socialize, and engage in other stress-proofing activities. More than one-half of Canadians report that they regularly feel rushed and stressed. Worries about job performance, salary, and job security, and interactions with bosses, co-workers, and customers can contribute to this experience. High levels of job stress are also common for people who are left out of important decisions relating to their jobs. When workers are given the opportunity to shape how their jobs are performed, job satisfaction goes up and stress levels go down.

If job-related (or school-related) stress is severe or chronic, the result can be **burnout**, a state of physical, mental, and emotional exhaustion. Burnout occurs most often in highly motivated and driven individuals who come to feel that their work is not recognized or that they are not accomplishing their goals. People in the helping professions—teachers, social workers, caregivers, police officers, and so on—are also prone to burnout. For some people who suffer from burnout, a vacation or leave of absence may be appropriate. For others, a reduced work schedule, better communication with superiors, or a change in job goals may be necessary. Improving time-management skills can also help.

Millions of workdays are lost annually because of illness. Stress-related sleep disturbances, headaches, and damaged relationships are quick to arise and easy to identify, but the effects of job stress on chronic diseases are harder to see because they take longer to develop. It's telling, however, that health care costs are nearly 50% greater for workers with high levels of stress. (For some recent statistics on job-related stress, see the box "What Stresses Us Out?" above.)

Social Stressors

Social networks can be real or virtual. Both types can help improve your ability to deal with stress, but any social network can also become a stressor in itself.

Real Social Networks Although social support is a key buffer against stress, your interactions with others can themselves be a source of stress. The postsecondary years, in particular, can be a time of great change in interpersonal relationships. The larger community where you live can also act as a stressor.

Social stressors include prejudice and discrimination. You may feel stress as you try to relate to people of other ethnic or socioeconomic groups. If you are a member of a minority ethnic group, you may feel pressure to assimilate into mainstream society, or to spend as much time as possible with others who share your ethnicity or background. If English is not your first language, you may face the added burden of conducting daily activities in a language with which you are not comfortable. All these pressures can become significant sources of stress. (See the box "Diverse Populations, Discrimination, and Stress" on p. 79 for more information.)

Virtual Social Networks New technologies can potentially be time-savers because we don't have to go home or to the office to check our email or phone messages, and we can make a call on a cellphone instead of jotting down notes to pass on at a later time. Telecommuting can ease the time pressures on people who find it necessary to work from home, such as parents with young children or people with disabilities. Increased electronic interactivity, however, can also impinge on our personal space, waste time, and cause stress. On a typical day, for example, you may check for email or voice mail several times, only to find no messages waiting for you. When you do have messages, you may find that some are of little or no value.

burnout A state of physical, mental, and emotional exhaustion.

Diverse Populations, Discrimination, and Stress

Stress is universal, but in diverse multi-ethnic and multicultural nations, such as Canada, some groups face special stressors and have higher-than-average rates of stress-related physical and emotional problems. These groups include members of ethnic minority groups, the poor, those with disabilities, and gays, lesbians, and transgender people. As you read the information in this box, notice how a variety of the determinants of health introduced in Chapter 1 (particularly culture, gender, and social environments) come together to affect the stress levels of some Canadians.

Discrimination occurs when people act according to their prejudices—biased, negative attitudes toward some group. Blatant examples are painting a swastika on a Jewish studies house or defacing a sculpture depicting a same-sex couple holding hands. More subtle examples include a black Canadian student noticing that white shopkeepers in a mostly white university town tend to keep a close eye on him; a male-to-female transgender individual being treated with less respect by her professors and peers; a student using a wheelchair

finding no accessible bathrooms; or an obese woman overhearing remarks about eating and self-control.

Recent immigrants to Canada have to learn to live in a new society. This requires a balance between assimilating and changing to be like the majority, and maintaining a connection to their own culture, language, and religion. The process of acculturation is generally stressful, especially when the person's background is radically different from that of the people he or she is now living among. Parental expectations generate stress if they are too high or too low. When they are too high, the child may work too hard in an attempt to succeed at everything; when they are too low, the child may not work hard enough to succeed at anything.

Both immigrants and members of minority groups that have lived for generations in Canada can face job-related and school-related stressors because of stereotypes and discrimination. They may make less money in comparable jobs with comparable levels of education and may find it more difficult to achieve leadership positions. However, on a positive note,

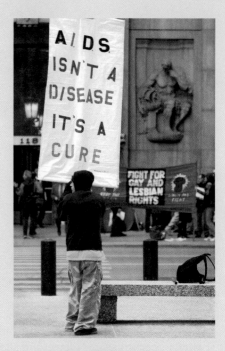

many who experience hardship, disability, or prejudice develop effective, goal-directed coping skills and are successful at overcoming obstacles and managing the stress they face.

If you are "always on" (that is, always available by voice or text messaging), some friends or colleagues may think it's all right to contact you any time, even if you're in class or trying to work. The convenience of staying electronically connected, therefore, comes at a price.

Environmental Stressors

Have you ever tried to eat at a restaurant where the food was great, but the atmosphere was so noisy that it put you on edge? This is an example of a mild environmental stress—a condition or an event in the physical environment that causes stress. Examples of more severe environmental stressors include the following:

- Natural disasters
- Acts of violence
- Industrial accidents

Like the noisy atmosphere of some restaurants, many environmental stressors are mere inconveniences that are easy to avoid. Others, such as pollen or construction noise, may be an unavoidable daily source of stress. For those who live in poor or violent neighbourhoods

or in a war-torn country, environmental stressors can be major stressors (see the box "Coping After Violence on Campus").

Internal Stressors

Some stressors are found not in our environment but within ourselves. We pressure ourselves to reach goals and continually evaluate our progress and performance. Setting goals and striving to reach them can enhance self-esteem if the goals are reasonable. Unrealistic expectations, however, can be a significant source of stress and can damage self-esteem (for example, expecting to earn 100%

QUESTIONS FOR CRITICAL THINKING AND REFLECTION

What are the top two or three stressors in your life right now? Are they new to your life—as part of your postsecondary experience—or are they stressors you've experienced in the past? Do they include both positive and negative experiences (eustress and distress)?

Stories of violence on North American campuses have become all-too familiar:

• In March 2008, an Auburn University student died from gunshot wounds sustained during a robbery. One day later, a University of North Carolina student was killed while being robbed in Chapel Hill, N.C.

• On February 14, 2008, a former Northern Illinois University student walked into one of the school's lecture halls and fatally shot five students before killing himself. Gunfire injured at least 16 other people.

• Just a few days earlier, a student at Louisiana Technical College in Baton Rouge shot two other students to death, then killed herself as classmates watched in horror.

• On April 16, 2007, a student killed 28 students and 5 teachers and injured 29 others during two attacks at Virginia Polytechnic Institute and State University (Virginia Tech). Four Canadian students were among the survivors. The attacker was acting out fantasies of revenge in a drama that held the nation's attention for weeks.

• On September 13, 2006, a young man started shooting people at Dawson College in Montreal, killing 1 woman and injuring 19 others before taking his own life.

• On December 6, 1989, a 25-year-old man killed 13 female students, wounded 13 more, and then killed himself at L'École Polytechnique in Montreal.

People react to news of school violence in different ways, depending on their proximity to the event and its recency. In the case of school massacres, people far from the site may suffer emotional reactions simply from watching endless coverage on television.

Responses to violence or reports of violence include disbelief, shock, fear, anger, resentment, anxiety, mood swings, irritability, sadness, depression, panic, guilt, apathy, feelings of isolation or powerlessness, and many of the symptoms of excess stress. Most of those affected return to normal after a few weeks or months, but a few go on to develop post-traumatic stress disorder (PTSD), a more serious condition.

In the case of the Virginia Tech shootings, the school and community mobilized quickly to respond to the expected surge in behavioural health needs generated by the attack. Hotline calls and emergency room visits increased dramatically, especially during the second and third weeks following the shootings. Information sources and support groups were established for people grieving the loss of friends, family, neighbours, or colleagues. Volunteers contacted each family that was directly affected by the shootings to offer help in making arrangements and other services.

If you are affected by a disastrous event, such as a school shooting or terrorist attack, take these steps:

• Be sure that you have the best information about what happened, whether a continuing risk is present, and what you can do to avoid it. That information

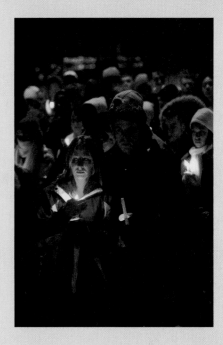

may be posted on Web sites or on local radio or TV stations.

• Don't expose yourself to so much media coverage that you begin to feel overwhelmed by it.

• Take care of yourself. Use the stress-relief techniques discussed in this chapter.

• Share your feelings and concerns with others. Be a supportive listener.

• If you feel able, help others in any way you can, such as by volunteering to work with victims.

• If you feel emotionally distressed days or weeks after the event, consider asking for professional help.

---

on every test or assignment, or being the top performer at work every week). Other internal stressors are physical and emotional states, such as illness and exhaustion (e.g., fighting cancer, having the flu, or even experiencing relationship upsets); these can be both a cause and an effect of unmanaged stress.

MANAGING STRESS

You can control the stress in your life by taking the following steps:

• Shore up your support system.

• Improve your communication skills.

• Develop healthy exercise, eating, and sleeping habits.

• Learn to identify and moderate individual stressors.

The effort required is well worth the time. People who manage stress effectively not only are healthier but also have more time to enjoy life and accomplish goals.

Social Support

The ability to share fears, frustrations, and joys makes life richer. Having the support of friends and family members seems to contribute to the well-being of body and mind.

Research supports this conclusion, as the following examples demonstrate:

- Among university students living in overcrowded apartments, a study revealed that those students with a strong social support system were less distressed by their cramped quarters than were the loners who navigated life's challenges on their own.
- Young adults who have strong relationships with their parents tend to cope with stress better than peers with poor parental relationships.
- Many studies have shown that married people live longer than single people (including those who are divorced, widowed, or never married) and have lower mortality rates from practically all causes of death.

Social support can provide a critical counterbalance to the stress in our lives. Give yourself time to develop and maintain a network of people you can count on for emotional support, feedback, and nurturing. If you believe you don't have enough social support, consider becoming a volunteer to help build your network of friends and to enhance your spiritual wellness.

Communication

How do you communicate your wants and needs to others? Communicating in an assertive way that respects the rights of others—while protecting your own rights—can prevent potentially stressful situations from getting out of control.

Some people have trouble either telling others what they need or saying no to the needs of others. They may suppress their feelings of anger, frustration, and resentment, and they may end up feeling taken advantage of or suffering in unhealthy relationships. At the other extreme are people who express anger openly and directly by being verbally or physically aggressive or indirectly by making critical, hurtful comments to others. Their abusive behaviour pushes other people away, and so they also have problems with relationships.

QUICK STATS

Only **21%** of Canadians deal with stress by talking with others.

—Canadian Mental Health Association, 2001

Better communication skills can help everyone form and maintain healthy relationships. If you typically suppress your feelings, you might want to take an assertiveness training course that can help you identify and change your patterns of communication. If you have trouble controlling your anger, you may benefit from learning anger-management strategies.

Chapter 2 includes a detailed discussion of anger and its impact on health and relationships. Chapter 10 discusses strategies for building healthy relationships, including positive communication techniques.

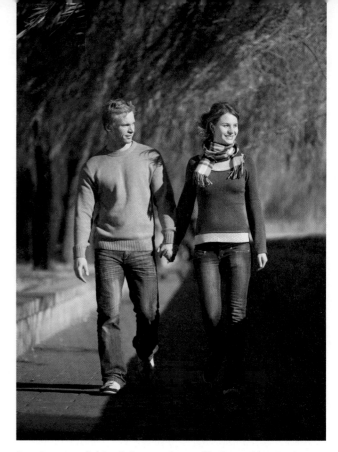

Exercise—even light activity—can be an effective antidote to stress.

Exercise

Exercise helps maintain a healthy body and mind and even stimulates the birth of new brain cells. Regular physical activity can also reduce many of the negative effects of stress. Consider the following examples:

- Taking a long walk can help decrease anxiety and blood pressure.
- A brisk ten-minute walk can leave you feeling more relaxed and energetic for up to two hours.
- People who exercise regularly react with milder physical stress responses before, during, and after exposure to stressors.
- In a study, people who took three brisk 45-minute walks each week for three months reported that they perceived fewer daily hassles. Their sense of wellness also increased.

These findings should not be surprising, because the stress response mobilizes energy resources and readies the body for physical emergencies. If you experience stress and do not physically exert yourself, you are not completing the energy cycle. You may not be able to exercise while your daily stressors occur—during class, for example, or while sitting in a traffic jam—but you can be active at other times of the day. Physical activity allows you to expend the nervous energy you have built up and trains your body to more readily achieve homeostasis following stressful situations.

It isn't hard to incorporate light to moderate exercise into your day. For example, you may be able to walk to class or ride your bike to the store instead of driving. Plan occasional activities with a friend, such as playing tennis or going for a walk. The important thing is to find an activity that you enjoy so that it can become a habit and a regular stress reducer.

One warning: For some people, exercise can become just one more stressor in a highly stressed life. People who exercise compulsively risk overtraining, a condition characterized by fatigue, irritability, depression, and diminished athletic performance. An overly strenuous exercise program can even make you sick by compromising your immune function. (For details on creating a safe and effective exercise program, see Chapter 6.)

Nutrition

A healthy diet gives you an energy bank to draw from whenever you experience stress. Eating wisely also can enhance your feelings of self-control and self-esteem. Learning the principles of sound nutrition is easy, and sensible eating habits rapidly become second nature when practised regularly. (For information on nutrition and healthy eating habits, see Chapter 5.)

For the purposes of managing stress, you may find it especially helpful to limit or avoid caffeine. Although one or two cups of coffee a day probably won't hurt you, caffeine is a mildly addictive stimulant that leaves some people jittery, irritable, and unable to sleep. Consuming caffeine during stressful situations can raise blood pressure and increase levels of cortisol. The following items can contain caffeine, sometimes in high doses:

- Tea
- Cola and some other soft drinks
- Chocolate
- Cold remedies
- Aspirin products
- Weight-loss preparations

If you are concerned about your caffeine intake, read the labels of products you consume daily. You may be surprised at the amount of caffeine you are ingesting, from a variety of sources.

Although your diet has an effect on the way your body handles stress, the reverse is also true. Excess stress can negatively affect the way you eat. Many people, for example, respond to stress by overeating; other people skip meals or stop eating altogether during stressful periods. Both responses are not only ineffective (they don't address the causes of stress) but also potentially unhealthy.

Sleep

Most adults need seven to nine hours of sleep every night to stay healthy and perform their best. Getting enough sleep isn't just good for you physically; adequate sleep also improves mood, fosters feelings of competence and self-worth, enhances mental functioning, and supports emotional functioning.

How Sleep Works Sleep occurs in two phases: **rapid eye movement (REM) sleep** and **non-rapid eye movement (NREM) sleep**. A sleeper goes through several cycles of non-REM and REM sleep each night.

NREM sleep actually includes four stages of successively deeper sleep. As you move through these stages of sleep, a variety of physiological changes occur, including the following:

- Blood pressure drops.
- Respiration and heart rates slow.
- Body temperature declines.
- Growth hormone is released.
- Brain wave patterns become slow and even.

During REM sleep, dreams occur. REM sleep is characterized by the rapid movement of the eyes under closed eyelids. Heart rate, blood pressure, and breathing rate rise, and brain activity increases to levels equal to or greater than those during waking hours. Muscles in the limbs relax completely, resulting in a temporary paralysis. (This total relaxation may prevent you from acting out your dreams while you're asleep.)

Sleep and Stress Stress hormone levels in the bloodstream vary throughout the day and are related to sleep patterns. Peak concentrations occur in the early morning, followed by a slow decline during the day and evening (Figure 3.4 on p. 82). Concentrations return to peak levels during the final stages of sleep and in the early morning hours. Stress hormone levels are low during non-REM sleep and increase during REM sleep. With each successive sleep cycle during the night, REM sleep lasts a little longer. This increase in REM sleep duration with each sleep cycle may underlie the progressive increase in circulating stress hormones during the final stages of sleep.

Even though stress hormones are released during sleep, it is the *lack* of sleep that has the greatest impact on stress. In someone who experiences **sleep deprivation** (not getting enough sleep over time), mental and physical processes steadily deteriorate. A sleep-deprived person has headaches, feels irritable, is unable to concentrate,

rapid eye movement (REM) sleep The portion of the sleep cycle during which dreaming occurs.

non-rapid eye movement (non-REM) sleep The portion of the sleep cycle that involves deep sleep; non-REM sleep includes four states of successively deeper sleep.

sleep deprivation A lack of sleep over time.

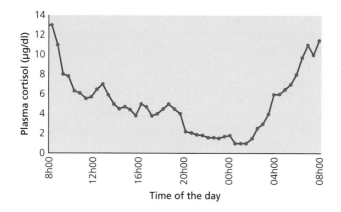

FIGURE 3.4 Changing levels of stress hormones in the bloodstream. Stress hormones, such as cortisol, fluctuate throughout the day and night and reach a high level during the last stages of sleep.

Source: Palma B. D., et al. 2008. Immune outcomes of sleep disorders: The hypothalamic-pituitary adrenal axis as a modulatory factor. *Revista Brasileiro de Psiquiatria*, vol. 29 suppl., Figure 3. 1 São Paulo May 2007.

and is more prone to forgetfulness. Poor-quality sleep has long been associated with stress and depression. A small 2008 study of female university students further associated sleep deprivation with an increased risk of suicide.

Acute sleep deprivation slows the daytime decline in stress hormones, and so evening levels are higher than normal. A decrease in total sleep time also causes an increase in the level of stress hormones. Together, these changes may cause an increase in stress hormone levels throughout the day and may contribute to physical and mental exhaustion. Extreme sleep deprivation can lead to hallucinations and other psychotic symptoms, as well as to a significant increase in heart attack risk.

Sleep Problems According to a study by Statistics Canada, Canadians sleep about eight hours per night, with men sleeping about 11 minutes more than women and women having a harder time falling asleep and staying asleep. Postsecondary students often cite sleep problems, or rather, not enough sleep, as part of the challenge of university or college life. Although many of us can attribute the lack of sleep to long (school and employment) workdays and family responsibilities, many Canadians have chronic sleep disorders—medical conditions that prevent them from sleeping well.

Researchers from the University of Laval in Quebec found that more than one-third of Canadian adults have trouble falling asleep or staying asleep—a condition called **insomnia**. The most common causes of insomnia are lifestyle factors, such as high caffeine or alcohol intake before bedtime (which can actually cause disturbances in sleep quality and duration, even though it can help reduce the time needed to fall asleep); medical problems, such as a breathing disorder; and stress. About 75% of people who suffer from chronic insomnia report some stressful life event at the onset of their sleeping problems. (For more information, see the box "Overcoming Insomnia.")

Another type of chronic sleep problem, called **sleep apnea**, occurs when a person stops breathing while asleep. Apnea can be caused by a number of factors, but it typically results when the soft tissue at the back of the mouth (such as the tongue or soft palate) collapses during sleep, blocking the airway. When breathing is interrupted, so is sleep, as the sleeper awakens repeatedly throughout the night to begin breathing again. In most cases, this occurs without the sleeper's even being aware of it. However, the disruption to sleep can be significant, and over time acute sleep deprivation can result from apnea. Apnea has several treatments, including medications, the use of a special apparatus that helps keep the airway open during sleep, and surgery.

Time Management

Learning to manage your time can be crucial to coping with everyday stressors. Overcommitment, procrastination, and even boredom are significant stressors for many people. Along with gaining control of nutrition and exercise to maintain a healthy energy balance, time management is an important element in a wellness program. Try these strategies for improving your time-management skills:

• *Set priorities.* Divide your tasks into three groups: essential, important, and trivial. Focus on the first two, and ignore the third.

• *Schedule tasks for peak efficiency.* You've undoubtedly noticed you're most productive at certain times of the day (or night). Schedule as many of your tasks for those hours as you can, and stick to your schedule.

• *Set realistic goals and write them down.* Attainable goals spur you on. Impossible goals, by definition, cause frustration and failure. Fully commit yourself to achieving your goals by putting them in writing.

• *Budget enough time.* For each project you undertake, calculate how long it will take to complete. Then tack on another 10%–15%, or even 25%, as a buffer.

TERMS

insomnia A sleep problem involving the inability to fall or stay asleep.

sleep apnea The interruption of normal breathing during sleep.

Overcoming Insomnia

Most people can resolve their insomnia by discovering the cause of their poor sleep and taking steps to remedy it. Insomnia that lasts for more than six months and interferes with daytime functioning requires consultation with a physician. Sleeping pills are not recommended for chronic insomnia because they can be habit forming; they also lose their effectiveness over time.

If you're bothered by insomnia, try the following:

• Determine how much sleep you need to feel refreshed the next day, and don't sleep longer than that.

• Go to bed at the same time every night and, more important, get up at the same time every morning, seven days a week, regardless of how much sleep you got. Don't nap for more than 30 minutes per day.

• Exercise every day, but not too close to bedtime. Your metabolism takes up to six hours to slow down after exercise.

• Avoid tobacco and caffeine late in the day, and avoid alcohol before bedtime (it causes disturbed, fragmented sleep).

• If you take any medications (prescription or not), ask your doctor or pharmacist if they are known to interfere with sleep.

• Use your bed only for sleep. Don't eat, read, study, or watch television in bed.

• Relax before bedtime with a warm bath (again, not too close to bedtime—allow about two hours for your metabolism to slow down afterward), a book, music, or relaxation exercises. Don't lie down in bed until you're sleepy.

• If you don't fall asleep in 15–20 minutes, or if you wake up and can't fall asleep again, get out of bed, leave the room if possible, and do something monotonous until you feel sleepy. Try distracting yourself with imagery instead of counting sheep; imagine yourself on a pleasant vacation or enjoying some beautiful scenery.

• If sleep problems persist, ask your physician for a referral to a sleep specialist in your area. You may be a candidate for a sleep study—an overnight evaluation of your sleep pattern that can uncover many sleep-related disorders.

• *Break up long-term goals into short-term ones.* Instead of waiting for or relying on large blocks of time, use short amounts of time to start a project or keep it moving.

• *Visualize the achievement of your goals.* By mentally rehearsing your performance of a task, you will be able to reach your goal more smoothly.

• *Keep track of the tasks you put off.* Analyze the reasons you procrastinate. If the task is difficult or unpleasant, look for ways to make it easier or more fun. For example, if you find the readings for one of your classes particularly difficult, choose an especially nice setting for your reading, and then reward yourself each time you complete a section or chapter.

• *Consider doing your least-favourite tasks first.* Once you have the most unpleasant ones out of the way, you can work on the tasks you enjoy more.

• *Consolidate tasks when possible.* For example, try walking to the store so that you run your errands and exercise in the same block of time.

• *Identify quick transitional tasks.* Keep a list of five-minute to ten-minute tasks, such as watering your plants, doing the dishes, or checking a homework assignment, that you can do while waiting or between other tasks.

• *Delegate responsibility.* Asking for help when you have too much to do is not a cop-out; it's good time management. Just don't delegate the jobs you know you should do yourself.

• *Say no when necessary.* If the demands made on you don't seem reasonable, say no—tactfully, but without guilt or apology.

• *Give yourself a break.* Allow time for play—free, unstructured time when you can ignore the clock. Don't

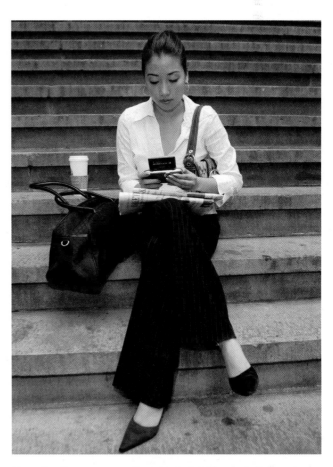

Managing the many commitments of adult life—including work, school, and parenthood—can sometimes feel overwhelming and produce a great deal of stress. Time-management and problem-solving skills, including careful scheduling with a date book or handheld computer, can help people cope with busy days.

consider this a waste of time. Play renews you and enables you to work more efficiently.

- *Avoid your personal time sinks.* You can probably identify your own time sinks—activities such as watching television, surfing the Internet, or talking on the phone that consistently use up more time than you anticipate and put you behind schedule. Some days, it may be best to avoid problematic activities altogether; for example, if you have a big paper due, don't sit down for a five-minute TV break if it is likely to turn into a two-hour break. Try a five-minute walk if you need to clear your head.

- *Stop thinking or talking about what you're going to do, and just do it!* Sometimes the best solution for procrastination is to stop waiting for the right moment and just get started. You will probably find that things are not as bad as you feared, and your momentum will keep you going.

Confiding in Yourself Through Writing

Keeping a diary is analogous to confiding in others, except that you are confiding in yourself. This form of coping with severe stress may be especially helpful for those who are shy or introverted and find it difficult to open up to others. Although writing about traumatic and stressful events may have a short-term negative effect on mood, over the long term, stress is reduced and positive changes in health occur. A key to promoting health and well-being through journaling is to write about your emotional responses to stressful events. Set aside a special time each day or week to write down your feelings about stressful events in your life.

Cognitive Techniques

Some stressors arise in our own minds. Ideas, beliefs, perceptions, and patterns of thinking can add to our stress level. Each of the following techniques can help you change unhealthy thought patterns to ones that will help you cope with stress. As with any skill, mastering these techniques takes practice and patience.

Think and Act Constructively   Think back to the worries you had last week. How many of them were needless? Think about things you *can* control. Try to stand aside from the problem, consider the positive steps you can take to solve it, and then carry them out. Remember, if you can successfully predict that a stressor will occur, you can better control your response to it. In the evening, try to predict stressful events you might encounter the following day. Then decide how to handle them constructively. This may mean dealing positively with an unpleasant person or figuring out how to stay focused during a boring class. By taking a constructive approach, you can prevent stressors from becoming negative events and perhaps even turn them into positive experiences.

Take Control   A situation often feels more stressful if you feel you're not in control of it. Time may seem to be slipping away before a big exam, for example. Unexpected obstacles may appear in your path, throwing you off course. When you feel your environment is controlling you instead of the other way around, take charge! Concentrate on what is possible to control, and set realistic goals. Be confident of your ability to succeed.

Problem Solve   Students with greater problem-solving abilities report easier adjustment to university life, higher motivation levels, lower stress levels, and higher grades. When you find yourself stewing over a problem, sit down and do some problem solving on paper or at your computer. Try this approach:

1. Define the problem in one or two sentences.
2. Identify the causes of the problem.
3. Consider all solutions; don't just stop with the most obvious one.
4. Weigh positive and negative consequences for each solution.
5. Make a decision—choose a solution.
6. List what you will need to do to act on your decision.
7. Begin to carry out your list; if you're unable to do that, temporarily turn to other things.
8. Evaluate the outcome and revise your approach if necessary.

Modify Your Expectations   Expectations are exhausting and restricting. The fewer expectations you have, the more you can live spontaneously and joyfully. The more you expect from others, the more often you will feel let down. And trying to meet the expectations others have of you is often futile.

Stay Positive   If you beat up on yourself—"Late for class again! You can't even cope with university! How do you expect to ever hold down a professional job?"—change your inner dialogue. Talk to yourself as you would to a child you love: "You're a smart, capable person. You've solved other problems; you'll handle this one. Tomorrow you'll simply schedule things so you get to class with a few minutes to spare." (Chapter 2 has more information on self-talk.)

Cultivate Your Sense of Humour   When it comes to stress, laughter may be the best medicine. Even a fleeting smile produces changes in your autonomic nervous system that can lift your spirits. And a few minutes of belly laughing can be as invigorating as brisk exercise. Hearty laughter elevates your heart rate, aids digestion, eases pain, and triggers the release of endorphins and other pleasurable and stimulating chemicals in the brain. After a good laugh, your muscles go slack; your pulse and blood

pressure dip below normal. You are relaxed. Cultivate the ability to laugh at yourself, and you'll have a handy and instantly effective stress reliever.

Focus on What's Important   A major source of stress is trying to store too much data. Forget unimportant details (they will usually be self-evident) and organize important information. One technique you can try is to chunk the important material into categories. If your next exam covers three chapters from your textbook, consider each chapter a chunk of information. Then break down each chunk into its three or four most important features. Create a mental outline that allows you to trace your way from the most general category down to the most specific details. This technique can be applied to managing daily responsibilities as well.

Relaxation Techniques

The **relaxation response** is a physiological state characterized by a feeling of warmth and quiet mental alertness. This is the opposite of the fight-or-flight reaction. When the relaxation response is triggered by a relaxation technique, heart rate, breathing, and metabolism slow down. Blood pressure and oxygen consumption decrease. At the same time, blood flow to the brain and skin increases, and brain waves shift from an alert beta rhythm to a relaxed alpha rhythm. Practised regularly, relaxation techniques can counteract the debilitating effects of stress.

If you decide to try a relaxation technique, practise it daily until it becomes natural to you, and then use it whenever you feel the need. You may feel calmer and more refreshed after each session. You'll know you've mastered a deep relaxation technique when you start to see subtle changes in other areas of your life: You may notice you've been encountering fewer hassles, working more efficiently, or enjoying more free time. None of the techniques takes long to do.

Progressive Relaxation   Unlike most of the others, this simple method requires no imagination, willpower, or self-suggestion. You simply tense, and then relax, the muscles in your body, group by group. The technique, also known as deep muscle relaxation, helps you become aware of the muscle tension that occurs when you're under stress. When you consciously relax those muscles, other systems of the body get the message and ease up on the stress response.

Start, for example, with your right fist. Inhale as you tense it. Exhale as you relax it. Repeat. Next, contract and relax your right upper arm. Repeat. Do the same with your left arm. Then, beginning at your forehead and ending at your feet, contract and relax your other muscle groups. Repeat each contraction at least once, breathing in as you tense, breathing out as you relax. To speed up the process, tense and relax more muscles at one time—both arms simultaneously, for instance. With practice, you'll be able to relax very quickly and effectively by clenching and releasing only your fists.

Visualization   Also known as *imagery*, **visualization** lets you daydream without guilt. Athletes find that the technique enhances sports performance, and visualization is reportedly used by 99% of Canadian Olympic athletes. You can use visualization to help you relax, change your habits, or perform well—whether on an exam, a stage, or a playing field.

Next time you feel stressed, close your eyes. Imagine yourself floating on a cloud, sitting on a mountaintop, or lying in a meadow. Involve all your senses; imagine the sounds, the smells, and the other sensations that would be part of the scene. Your body will respond as if your imagery were real. As an alternative, close your eyes and imagine a deep-purple light filling your body. Now change the colour into a soothing gold. As the colour lightens, so should your distress.

Visualization can also be used to rehearse for an upcoming event and enhance performance. By experiencing an event ahead of time in your mind, you can practise coping with any difficulties that may arise. Think positively, and you can psych yourself up for a successful experience.

Meditation   The need to periodically stop our incessant mental chatter is so great that, since ancient times, hundreds of forms of **meditation** have developed in cultures all over the world. Meditation is a way of telling the mind to be quiet for a while. Because meditation has been at the core of many Eastern religions and philosophies, it has acquired an mys-

tique that has caused some people to shy away from it. Yet meditation requires no special knowledge or background. Whatever the philosophical, religious, or emotional reasons may be given for meditation, it is potentially useful for reducing stress. According to a 2008 study, postsecondary students who learned how to use meditation for stress

relaxation response   A physiological state characterized by a feeling of warmth and quiet mental alertness.

visualization   A technique for promoting relaxation or improving performance that involves creating or re-creating vivid mental pictures of a place or an experience; also called *imagery*.

meditation   A technique for quieting the mind by focusing on a particular word, object (such as a candle flame), or process (such as breathing).

TERMS

management were able to significantly reduce their daily stress levels. Further, those students found it easier to forgive others for perceived wrongdoings and spent less time focusing on negative thoughts.

Meditation helps you tune out the world temporarily, removing you from both internal and external sources of stress. The thinker takes time out to become the observer—calmly attentive, without analyzing, judging, comparing, or rationalizing. Regular practice of this quiet awareness will subtly carry over into your daily life, encouraging physical and emotional balance no matter what confronts you. For a step-by-step description of a basic meditation technique, see "Meditation and the Relaxation Response" in the ▇connect Library.

Another form of meditation, known as *mindfulness meditation*, involves paying attention to physical sensations, perceptions, thoughts, and imagery. Instead of focusing on a word or an object to quiet the mind, you observe any thoughts that occur without evaluating or judging them. Development of this ability requires regular practice but may eventually result in a more objective view of your perceptions. It is believed that a greater understanding of moment-to-moment thought processes (mindful awareness) provides a richer and more vital sense of life and improves coping. Studies also suggest that people who rate high in mindfulness are less anxious and better able to deal with stress; among people with specific health problems, mindfulness can provide substantial benefits.

Deep Breathing   Your breathing pattern is closely tied to your stress level. Deep, slow breathing is associated with relaxation. Rapid, shallow, irregular breathing occurs during the stress response. With practice, you can learn to slow and quiet your breathing pattern, thereby also quieting your mind and relaxing your body. Breathing techniques can be used for on-the-spot tension relief as well as for long-term stress reduction.

The primary goal of many breathing exercises is to change your breathing pattern from chest breathing to diaphragmatic (stomach) breathing. During the day, most adults breathe by expanding their chest and raising their shoulders rather than by expanding their abdomen. Diaphragmatic breathing, which involves free expansion of the diaphragm and lower abdomen, is the pattern of breathing characteristic of children and sleeping adults. (The diaphragm is a sheet of muscle and connective tissue that divides the chest and abdominal cavities.) Diaphragmatic breathing is slower and deeper than chest breathing. For instructions on how to perform diaphragmatic breathing, refer to "Breathing for Relaxation" in the ▇connect Library.

Yoga   Hatha yoga, the yoga style most commonly practised in Canada, emphasizes physical balance and breath control. It integrates components of flexibility, muscular strength and endurance, and muscle relaxation; it also sometimes serves as a preliminary to meditation. A session of yoga typically involves a series of postures, each held for a few seconds to several minutes, which involve stretching and balance and coordinated breathing. Yoga can induce the relaxation response and promote body awareness and flexibility. If you are interested in trying yoga, it's best to take a class from an experienced instructor.

Tai Chi   This martial art (in Chinese, *taijiquan*) is a system of self-defence that incorporates philosophical concepts from Taoism and Confucianism. In addition to self-defence, tai chi aims to bring the body into balance and harmony to promote health and spiritual growth. It teaches practitioners to remain calm and centred, to conserve and concentrate energy, and to manipulate force by becoming part of it— by going with the flow. Tai chi is considered the gentlest of the martial arts. Instead of quick and powerful movements, tai chi consists of a series of slow, fluid, elegant movements, which reinforce the idea of moving *with* rather than *against* the stressors of everyday life. As with yoga, it's best to start tai chi with a class from an experienced instructor.

Listening to Music   Listening to music is another method of inducing relaxation. It can influence pulse, blood pressure, and the electrical activity of muscles. Studies of newborns and people hospitalized with a stroke have shown that listening to soothing, lyrical music can lessen depression, anxiety, and stress levels. Researchers have found that exposure to soothing music leads to reduced levels of the stress hormone cortisol and causes changes in the electrical activity in the brain.

To experience the stress-management benefits of music yourself, set aside a time to listen. Choose music that you enjoy and that makes you feel relaxed.

Taijiquan is one of many techniques for inducing the relaxation response.

Biofeedback   Biofeedback helps people reduce the stress response by enabling them to become more aware of their level of physiological arousal. It involves electrical monitoring of some measure of the physiological stress response, such as perspiration, heart rate, skin temperature, or muscle tension. A person receives feedback about his or her condition through the use of sound (a tone or music), light, or a meter or dial. For example, as heart rate increases, the tone becomes louder; as it decreases, the tone becomes softer. In this way, people can learn to reduce their physiological stress response through conscious control even without biofeedback.

The point of biofeedback training is to learn how relaxation feels, how to induce relaxation, and how to transfer this skill to daily life (without the use of electronic equipment). In addition to monitoring equipment, biofeedback usually also requires the initial help of a therapist, stress counsellor, or technician.

Other relaxation techniques include massage, hypnosis and self-hypnosis, and autogenic training. To learn more about these and other techniques for inducing the relaxation response, refer to For More Information at the end of the chapter.

Counterproductive Coping Strategies

University or college is a time when you'll learn to adapt to new and challenging situations and gain skills that will last a lifetime. It is also a time when many people develop habits, in response to stress, that are counterproductive and unhealthy. Such habits can last well beyond graduation.

Tobacco Use   Many young adults who never smoked in high school smoke their first cigarette in university or college, usually at a party or a bar or in a dorm with friends. Many smokers report that smoking helps them to cope with stress by providing a feeling of relaxation, giving them something to do with their hands in social situations, or breaking up monotony and routine.

Cigarettes and other tobacco products contain nicotine, a chemical that enhances the actions of neurotransmitters. Nicotine can make you feel relaxed and even increase your ability to concentrate, but it is highly addictive, and nicotine dependence itself is considered a psychological disorder. Current research has found that smokers are actually more likely to experience frequent stress than nonsmokers or ex-smokers. Cigarette smoke also contains substances that cause heart disease, stroke, lung cancer, and emphysema. These negative consequences far outweigh any beneficial effects, and tobacco use should be avoided. The easiest thing to do is to not start.

See Chapter 16 for more on the health effects of tobacco use and for tips on how to quit.

Use of Alcohol and Other Drugs   No postsecondary experience is complete without a party or two. Letting loose, dancing, laughing, and interacting with others can

Tobacco and alcohol use may help you relax for a little while, but long-term use is unhealthy and an ineffective way to cope with stress.

be very effective short-term coping strategies. However, partying is usually associated with drinking alcohol. Keg parties and drinking games can be fun, but they contribute to binge drinking and other forms of alcohol abuse. Like nicotine, alcohol is addictive, and many alcoholics find it hard to relax without a drink. Having a

biofeedback   A technique in which monitoring devices help a person become conscious of unconscious body processes, such as body temperature or blood pressure, to exert some control over them.

TERMS

few drinks might make you feel temporarily at ease, and drinking until you're intoxicated may help you forget your current stressors. However, using alcohol to deal with stress places you at risk for all the short-term and long-term problems associated with alcohol abuse. It also does nothing to address the actual causes of stress in your life. Although moderate alcohol consumption may have potential health benefits for some people, many university students have patterns of drinking that detract from wellness. Nearly one-third of Canadian university students recently reported having *at least* one indicator of alcohol dependence. For more on the responsible use of alcohol, refer to Chapter 15.

Using other psychoactive drugs to cope with stress is also counterproductive:

- *Caffeine* raises cortisol levels and blood pressure and can make you feel more stressed; caffeine also disrupts sleep. Other stimulants, such as amphetamine, can activate the stress response, and they affect the same areas of the brain that are involved in regulating the stress response.

- *Marijuana* use is relatively common among post-secondary students, who report that they smoke marijuana in an effort to induce relaxation and for "mind expansion." Use of marijuana causes a brief period of euphoria and decreased short-term memory and attentional abilities. Physiological effects clearly show that marijuana use doesn't cause relaxation; in fact, some neurochemicals in marijuana act to enhance the stress response, and getting high on a regular basis can elicit panic attacks. To compound this, withdrawal from marijuana may also be associated with an increase in circulating stress hormones.

- *Opioids*, such as morphine and heroin, can mimic the effects of your body's natural painkillers and act to reduce anxiety. However, tolerance to opioids develops quickly, and many users become dependent.

For more information on the use of psychoactive drugs, see Chapter 14.

Unhealthy Eating Habits   The nutrients in the food you eat provide energy and the substances needed to maintain your body. Eating is also psychologically rewarding. The feelings of satiation and sedation that follow eating produce a relaxed state. However, regular use of eating as a means of coping with stress may lead to unhealthy eating habits. In fact, the recent Report Card on Canadians' Health revealed that about 75% of Canadians use television, alcohol, cigarettes, and comfort food as a means of coping with stress or anxiety. Comfort eaters are twice as likely as other people to be obese.

Certain foods and supplements are sometimes thought to fight stress. Carbohydrates may reduce the stress response by promoting activity of the parasympathetic nervous system; however, a high-carbohydrate diet can lead to excessive weight gain in sedentary people and is not recommended as a strategy for coping with stressors.

In addition, some evidence suggests that greater ingestion of carbohydrates, simple sugars, and fatty foods may be a predisposing factor for psychological distress. Many dietary supplements are marketed for stress reduction, but supplements are not required to meet the same standards as medications in terms of safety, effectiveness, and manufacturing (see Chapters 5 and 19).

CREATING A PERSONAL PLAN FOR MANAGING STRESS

What are the most important sources of stress in your life? Are you coping successfully with these stressors? No single strategy or program for managing stress will work for everyone, but you can use the principles of behaviour management described in Chapter 1 to tailor a plan specifically to your needs. The most important starting point for a successful stress-management plan is to learn to listen to your body. When you learn to recognize the stress response and the emotions and thoughts that accompany it, you'll be in a position to take charge of that crucial moment and handle it in a healthy way.

Identifying Stressors

Before you can learn to manage the stressors in your life, you have to identify them. Many experts recommend keeping a stress journal for a week or two (see Figure 3.5). Each time you feel or express a stress response, record the time and the circumstances in your journal. Note what you were doing at the time, what you were thinking or feeling, and the outcome of your response.

After keeping your journal for a few weeks, you should be able to identify your key stressors and spot patterns in how you respond to them. Take note of the people, places, events, and patterns of thought and behaviour that cause you the most stress. You may notice, for example, that mornings are usually the most stressful part of your day. Or you may discover that when you're angry at your roommate, you're apt to respond with behaviours that only make matters worse. Keeping a journal allows you to be analytical about what produces the most stress in your life and fills in where your conscious memory fails you.

Designing Your Plan

Once you've identified the key stressors in your life, choose the stress reduction techniques that will work best for you and create an action plan for change. Finding a friend to work with you can make the process more fun and increase your chances of success. Some experts recommend drawing up a formal contract with yourself.

Whether or not you complete a contract, it's important to design rewards into your plan. You might treat yourself to a concert or a movie. It's also important to evaluate

Stress Journal		Date 9-18-12
Time	**Stressor**	**Reaction/Coping Strategy**
7:45 a.m.	Tara wouldn't get out of the shower	Yelled at her, started an argument
8:35 a.m.	Late for class	Slouched in back of room; chewed my nails
11:55 a.m.	Dad called to discuss credit card debt	Cried, skipped lunch and went out to smoke with Greg
5:30 p.m.	Power outage at dorm, couldn't study	Took a walk with Tara, made up for arguing this morning, then went to library to study
7:45 p.m.	Ed called, asked to borrow money	Stayed calm, put down phone, and counted to 10, then explained that he already owes me $50.
8:30 p.m.	Ed called, angry, said he wanted to break up	Argued onphone, then went out withTara for a drink

FIGURE 3.5   A sample stress journal.   Tracking stressful events and reactions can help you understand how you normally cope with stress.

your plan regularly and redesign it as your needs change. Under times of increased stress, for example, you might want to focus on good eating, exercise, and relaxation habits. Over time, your new stress-management skills will become almost automatic. You'll feel better, accomplish more, and reduce your risk of disease.

Getting Help

If the techniques discussed so far don't provide you with enough relief from the stress in your life, you might want to learn more about specific areas you want to work on. Excellent self-help guides can be found in bookstores or the library. Additional resources are listed in the For More Information section at the end of the chapter.

Your student health centre or student affairs office can tell you whether your campus has a peer counselling program. Such programs are usually staffed by volunteer students with special training that emphasizes maintaining confidentiality. Peer counsellors can guide you to other campus or community resources or can simply provide understanding.

Support groups are typically organized around a particular issue or problem. In your area, you might find a support group for first-year students; for older students; for single parents; for students of your ethnicity, religion, or national origin; for people with eating disorders; or for rape survivors. The number of such groups has increased in recent years as more people discover how therapeutic it can be to talk with others who share the same situation.

Short-term psychotherapy can also be tremendously helpful in dealing with stress-related problems. Your student health centre may offer psychotherapy on a sliding-fee scale; the local mental health centre in your area may do the same. If you belong to any type of religious organization, check to see whether pastoral counselling is available. Your physician can refer you to psychotherapists in your community. Not all therapists are right for all people, so be prepared to have initial sessions with several. Choose the one you feel most comfortable with.

Dealing with Test Anxiety

Are you a person who doesn't perform as well as you should on tests? Do you find that anxiety interferes with your ability to study effectively before the test and to think clearly in the test situation? If so, you may be experiencing test anxiety. Two methods that have proven effective in helping people deal with test anxiety are systematic desensitization and success rehearsal.

Systematic Desensitization

Systematic desensitization is based on the premise that you can't feel anxiety and be relaxed at the same time.

Phase I: Constructing an anxiety hierarchy: Begin the first phase by thinking of ten or more situations related to your fear, such as hearing the announcement of the test date in class, studying for the test, sitting in the classroom waiting for the test to begin, reading the test questions, and so on. Write each situation on an index card, using a brief phrase to describe it on one side of the card. On the other side, list several realistic details or prompts that will help you vividly imagine yourself actually experiencing the situation. For example, if the situation is "hearing that 50% of the final grade will be based on the two exams," the prompts might include specific details, such as "sitting in the big lecture auditorium in Baily Hall," "taking notes in my blue notebook," and "listening to Professor Lee's voice."

Next, arrange your cards in order, from least-tense to most-tense situation. Rate each situation to reflect the amount of anxiety you feel when you encounter it in real life, to confirm your anxiety hierarchy. Assign ratings on a scale of 0–100, and make sure the distances between items are fairly small and about equal. When you're sure your anxiety hierarchy is a true reflection of your feelings, number the cards.

Phase II: Learning and practising muscle relaxation: The second phase of the program involves learning to relax your muscles and to recognize when they are relaxed (see the description of progressive relaxation in this chapter). As you become proficient at this technique, you'll be able to go to a deeply relaxed state within just a few minutes. When you can do this, go on to the next phase of the program.

Phase III: Implementing the desensitization program: Use the quiet place where you practised your relaxation exercises. Sit comfortably and place your stack of numbered cards within reach. Take several minutes to relax completely, and then look at the first card, reading both the brief phrase and the descriptive prompts. Close your eyes and imagine yourself in that situation for about 10 seconds. Then put the card down and relax completely for about 30 seconds. Look at the card again, imagine the situation for 10 seconds, and relax again for 30 seconds.

At this point, evaluate your level of anxiety about the situation on the card in terms of the rating scale you devised earlier. If your anxiety level is 10 or lower, relax for 2 minutes and go on to the second card. If it's higher than 10, repeat the routine with the same card until the anxiety decreases.

If you have difficulty with a particular item, go back to the previous item; then try it again. If you still can't visualize it without anxiety, try to construct three new items with smaller steps between them and insert them before the troublesome item. You should be able to move through one to four items per session.

Sessions can be conducted from twice a day to twice a week and should last no longer than 20 minutes. It's helpful to graph your progress in a way that has meaning for you.

After you have successfully completed your program, you should be desensitized to the real-life situations that previously caused anxiety. If you find that you do experience some anxiety in the real situations, take 30 seconds or a minute to relax completely, just as you did when you were practising.

Success Rehearsal

To practise this variation on systematic desensitization, take your hierarchy of anxiety-producing situations and vividly imagine yourself successfully dealing with each one. Create a detailed scenario for each situation, and use your imagination to experience genuine feelings of confidence. Recognize your negative thoughts ("I'll be so nervous I won't be able to think straight") and replace them with positive ones ("Anxiety will keep me alert so I can do a good job").

Proceed one step at a time, thinking as you go of strategies for success that you can later implement. These might include the following:

- Before the test, find out everything you can about it: its format, the material to be covered, the grading criteria. Ask the instructor for practice materials. Study in advance; don't just cram the night before. Avoid all-nighters.

- Devise a study plan. This might include forming a study group with one or more classmates or outlining what you will study, when, where, and for how long. Generate your own questions and answer them.

- In the actual test situation, sit away from possible distractions, listen carefully to instructions, and ask for clarification if you don't understand a direction.

- During the test, answer the easiest questions first. If you don't know an answer and there is no penalty for incorrect answers, guess. If you have difficulty answering several questions, review the ones you have already handled. Figure out approximately how much time you have to cover each remaining question.

- For math problems, try to estimate the answer before doing the precise calculations.

- For true-false questions, look for qualifiers, such as *always* and *never.* Such questions are likely to be false.

- For essay questions, look for key words in the question that indicate what the instructor is looking for in the answer. Develop a brief outline of your answer, sketching out what you will cover. Stick to your outline, and keep track of the time you're spending on your answer. Don't get caught with unanswered questions when time is up.

- Remain calm and focused throughout the test. Don't let negative thoughts rattle you. Avoid worrying about past performance, how others are doing, or the negative consequences of a poor test grade. If you start to become nervous, take some deep breaths and relax your muscles completely for a minute or so.

The best way to counter test anxiety is with successful test-taking experiences. The more times you succeed, the more your test anxiety will recede. If you find that these methods aren't sufficient to get your anxiety under control, you may want to seek professional help.

Practise and learn online with Connect. Connect allows you to practise important skills at your own pace and on your own schedule, with 24/7 online access to an eBook, practice quizzes, interactivities, videos, study tools, additional resources, and more.

SUMMARY

- When confronted with a stressor, the body undergoes a set of physical changes known as the fight-or-flight reaction. The sympathetic nervous system and endocrine system act on many targets in the body to prepare it for action.

- Emotional and behavioural responses to stressors vary among individuals. Ineffective responses increase stress but can be moderated or changed.

- Factors that influence emotional and behavioural responses to stressors include personality, cultural background, gender, and past experiences.

- The general adaptation syndrome (GAS) has three stages: alarm, resistance, and exhaustion.

- A high allostatic load characterized by prolonged or repeated exposure to stress hormones can increase a person's risk of health problems.

- Psychoneuroimmunology (PNI) looks at how the physiological changes of the stress response affect the immune system and thereby increase the risk of illness.

- Health problems linked to stress include CVD, colds and other infections, asthma and allergies, cancer, flare-ups of chronic diseases, psychological problems, digestive problems, headaches, insomnia, and injuries.

- A cluster of major life events that require adjustment and accommodation can lead to increased stress and an increased risk of health problems. Minor daily hassles increase stress if they are perceived negatively.

- Sources of stress associated with postsecondary education may be academic, interpersonal, time-related, or financial pressures.

- Job-related stress is common, particularly for employees who have little control over decisions relating to their jobs. If stress is severe or prolonged, burnout may occur.

- New and changing relationships, prejudice, and discrimination are examples of interpersonal and social stressors.

- Social support systems help buffer people against the effects of stress and make illness less likely. Good communication skills foster healthy relationships.

- Exercise, nutrition, sleep, and time management are wellness behaviours that reduce stress and increase energy.

- Cognitive techniques for managing stress involve developing new and healthy patterns of thinking, such as practising problem solving, monitoring self-talk, and cultivating a sense of humour.

- The relaxation response is the opposite of the fight-or-flight reaction. Techniques that trigger it, including progressive relaxation, imagery, meditation, and deep breathing, counteract the effects of chronic stress. Counterproductive coping strategies include smoking, drinking, and unhealthy eating.

- A successful individualized plan for coping with stress begins with the use of a stress journal or log to identify and study stressors and inappropriate behavioural responses. Completing a contract and recruiting a friend can help your stress-management plan succeed.

- Additional help in dealing with stress is available from self-help books, peer counselling, support groups, and psychotherapy.

FOR MORE INFORMATION

BOOKS

Blonna, R. 2007. *Coping with Stress in a Changing World*, 4th ed. New York: McGraw-Hill. A comprehensive guide to stress management that includes separate chapters on postsecondary stressors and spirituality.

Greenberg, J. 2009. *Comprehensive Stress Management*, 11th ed. New York: McGraw-Hill. Provides a clear explanation of the physical, psychological, sociological, and spiritual aspects of stress and offers numerous stress-management techniques.

Kabat-Zinn, J. 2006. *Coming to Our Senses: Healing Ourselves and the World Through Mindfulness*. New York: Hyperion. Explores the connections among mindfulness, health, and physical and spiritual well-being.

Maté, G. 2004. *When the Body Says No: The Cost of Hidden Stress.* Toronto: Vintage Canada. Explores the connections among emotion, stress, and disease.

McGuigan, F. J. 1999. *Encyclopedia of Stress.* Needham Heights, Mass.: Allyn & Bacon. A reference guide for the broad field of stress and stress-related disorders.

Pennebaker, J. W. 2004. *Writing to Heal: A Guided Journal for Recovering from Trauma and Emotional Upheaval.* Oakland, Calif.: New Harbinger Press. Provides information about using journaling to cope with stress.

Sapolsky, R. M. 2004. *Why Zebras Don't Get Ulcers*, 3rd ed. New York: Henry Holt. A scientific guide to stress, stress-related diseases, and coping.

Seaward, B. L. 2006. *Managing Stress: Principles and Strategies for Health and Well-Being*, 5th ed. Boston: Jones and Bartlett. A comprehensive textbook for postsecondary students.

ORGANIZATIONS, HOTLINES, AND WEB SITES

The Internet addresses listed here were accurate at the time of publication.

American Psychological Association. Provides information on stress management and psychological disorders.
>   http://www.apa.org/helpcenter/ and http://www.apa.org

Association for Applied Psychophysiology and Biofeedback. Provides information about biofeedback and referrals to certified biofeedback practitioners.
>   http://www.aapb.org

Benson-Henry Institute for Mind Body Medicine. Provides information about stress-management and relaxation techniques.
>   http://www.massgeneral.org/bhi/

Canadian Centre for Occupational Health and Safety. Provides information and links on job stress.
>   http://www.ccohs.ca/oshanswers/psychosocial/stress.html

Canadian Mental Health Association. Provides information about mental health issues and offers related services and resources for Canadians.
>   http://www.cmha.ca

Canadian Psychiatric Association. Advocates for the professional needs of its members and promotes excellence in education, research, and clinical practice.
>   http://www.cpa-apc.org

Medical Basis for Stress. Includes information on recognizing stress and on the physiological basis of stress, self-assessments for stress levels, and techniques for managing stress.
>   http://www.teachhealth.com

Public Health Agency of Canada: Mental Health Promotion Unit. Addresses mental health promotion from a population health perspective that takes into account the broad range of determinants of mental health.
>   http://www.phac-aspc.gc.ca/mh-sm/mhp-psm/index-eng.php

Student Counseling Virtual Pamphlet Collection. Links to online pamphlets from student counselling centres; topics include stress, sleep, and time management.
>   http://counseling.uchicago.edu/vpc/virtulets.html

U.S. National Institute of Mental Health (NIMH). Publishes informative brochures about stress and stress management as well as other aspects of mental health.
>   http://www.nimh.nih.gov

U.S. National Sleep Foundation. Provides information about sleep and how to deal with sleep problems, such as insomnia and jet lag.
>   http://www.sleepfoundation.org

SELECTED BIBLIOGRAPHY

Adlaf, E. M., Demers, A., and Gliksman, L. (eds.). 2005. *Canadian Campus Survey 2004.* Toronto: Centre for Addiction and Mental Health.

American College Health Association. 2007. *American College Health Association—National College Health Assessment (ACHA—NCHA) 2007 Web Summary* (http://www.acha-ncha.org/data_highlights.html; retrieved December 27, 2008).

American Psychological Association. 2005. *The Different Kinds of Stress* (http://www.apa.org/helpcenter/stress-kinds.aspx; retrieved March 13, 2011).

American Psychological Association. 2005. *Learning to Deal with Stress* (http://www.apa.org/helpcenter/stress-learning.aspx; retrieved March 13, 2011).

American Psychological Association. 2007. *Stress in America* (http://www.apa.org/pubs/info/reports/2007-stress.doc; retrieved March 13, 2011).

Ano, G. G., and E. B. Vasconcelles. 2005. Religious coping and psychological adjustment to stress: A meta-analysis. *Journal of Clinical Psychology* 61(4): 461–480.

Canadian Institute for Health Information. 2008. *Improving the Health of Canadians: Mental Health, Delinquency and Criminal Activity.* Ottawa: Canadian Institute for Health Information.

Centers for Disease Control. 2005. *Coping with a Traumatic Event: Information for the Public* (http://www.bt.cdc.gov/masscasualties/copingpub.asp; retrieved March 13, 2011).

Cohen, S., W. J. Doyle, and A. Baum. 2006. Socioeconomic status is associated with stress hormones. *Psychosomatic Medicine* 68(3): 414–420.

Constantine, M. G, S. Okazaki, and S. O. Utsey. 2004. Self-concealment, social self-efficacy, acculturative stress, and depression in African, Asian, and Latin American international college students. *American Journal of Orthopsychiatry* 74(3): 230–241.

Daley, M., et al. 2009. The economic burden of insomnia: Direct and indirect costs for individuals with insomnia syndrome, insomnia symptoms, and good sleepers. *Sleep* 32(1): 1–10.

Gilmour, H., and Wilkins, K. 2001. Migraine. *Health Reports* 12(2): 23–40.

Grossman, P., et al. 2004. Mindfulness-based stress reduction and health benefits: A meta analysis. *Journal of Psychosomatic Research* 57(1): 35–43.

Health Canada. 2008. *Mental Health: Coping with Stress* (http://www.hc-sc.gc.ca/hl-vs/alt_formats/pacrb-dgapcr/pdf/iyh-vsv/life-vie/stress-eng.pdf; retrieved September 30, 2010).

Higgins, C., Duxbury, L., and Lyons, S. 2008. *Report 5: Reducing Work-Life Conflict: What Works? What Doesn't?* (http://www.hc-sc.gc.ca/ewh-semt/pubs/occup-travail/balancing-equilibre/index-eng.php; retrieved March 13, 2011).

How stress can make you forgetful, age faster. 2005. *Tufts University Health & Nutrition Letter,* February, 1.

Hurst, M. 2008. *Who Gets Any Sleep These Days? Sleep Patterns of Canadians* (http://www.statcan.gc.ca/pub/11-008-x/2008001/article/10553-eng.htm; Retrieved March 13, 2011).

Institute of Medicine Committee on Sleep Medicine and Research. 2006. *Sleep Disorders and Sleep Deprivation: An Unmet Public Health Problem*, ed. H. R. Colton and B. M. Altevogt. Washington, D.C. National Academies Press.

Lauderdale, D. S., et al. 2006. Objectively measured sleep characteristics among early-middle-aged adults: The CARDIA study. *American Journal of Epidemiology* 164(1): 17–18.

MacGeorge, E. L., et al. 2004. Stress, social support, and health among college students after September 11, 2001. *Journal of College Student Development* 45(6): 655–670.

Mayo Foundation for Medical Education and Research. 2010. *Stress: Constant Stress Puts Your Health at Risk* (http://www.mayoclinic.com/health/stress/SR00001; retrieved December 27, 2008).

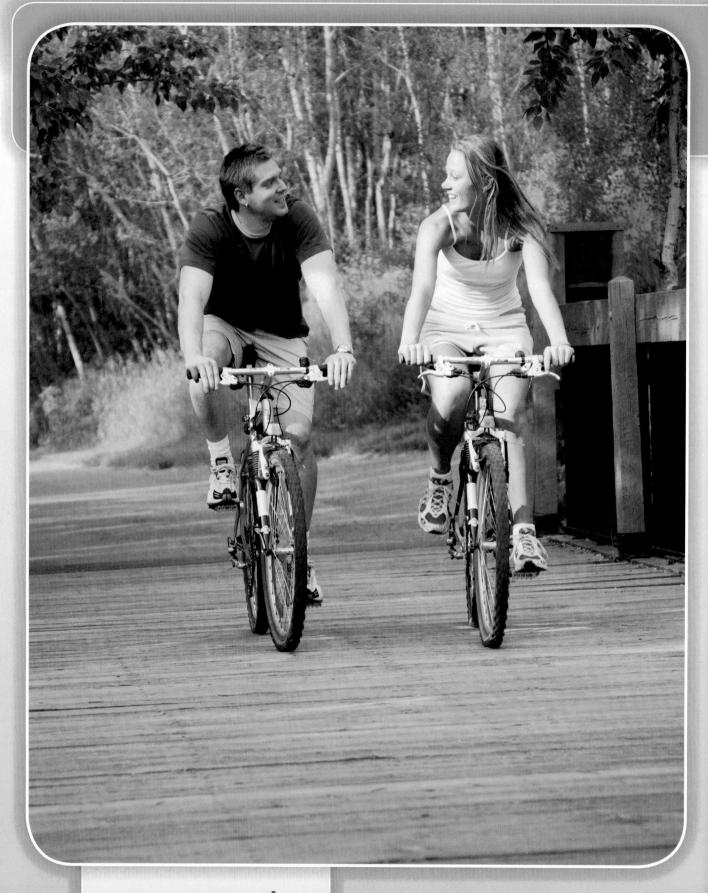

WEIGHT MANAGEMENT

LOOKING AHEAD>>>>>

AFTER READING THIS CHAPTER, YOU SHOULD BE ABLE TO

- Discuss different methods for assessing body weight and body composition
- Explain the health risks associated with overweight and obesity
- Explain factors that may contribute to a weight problem, including genetic, physiological, lifestyle, and psychosocial factors
- Describe lifestyle factors that contribute to weight gain and loss, including the roles of diet, exercise, and emotional factors
- Identify and describe the symptoms of eating disorders and the health risks associated with them
- Design a personal plan for successfully managing body weight

TEST YOUR KNOWLEDGE

1. **About what percentage of Canadian adults have a healthy body weight?**
   a. 58%
   b. 48%
   c. 38%

2. **Genetic factors explain most cases of obesity.**
   True or false?

3. **The consumption of low-calorie sweeteners has helped Canadians control their weight.**
   True or false?

4. **Approximately how many female high school and postsecondary students have either anorexia or bulimia?**
   a. 0%
   b. 1%
   c. 2%

5. **Which of the following is the most significant risk factor for type 2 diabetes (the most common type of diabetes)?**
   a. smoking
   b. low-fibre diet
   c. overweight or obesity
   d. inactivity

ANSWERS

1. **C.** Only 38% of Canadian adults have a healthy body weight; 65% are either overweight or obese (and 1% are underweight).

2. **FALSE.** Genetic factors may increase an individual's tendency to gain weight, but lifestyle is the key contributing factor.

3. **FALSE.** Since the introduction of low-calorie sweeteners, both total calorie intake and total sugar intake have increased, as has the proportion of Canadians who are overweight.

4. **C.** About 2%–4% of female students suffer from bulimia or anorexia, and many more occasionally engage in behaviours associated with these eating disorders.

5. **C.** All four are risk factors for type 2 diabetes, but overweight or obesity is the most significant. It's estimated that 90% of cases of type 2 diabetes could be prevented if people adopted healthy lifestyle behaviours.

Achieving and maintaining a healthy body weight is a serious public health challenge and a source of distress for many Canadians. Under standards developed by Health Canada, about 65% of Canadian adults self-report that they are overweight, including about 15% who identify themselves as obese (Figure 4.1). In Canada, the number of obese adults doubled between 1978 and 2004. Experts say that by 2021, 70% of males and nearly 50% of females in Canada will be either overweight or obese. And while millions struggle to lose weight, others fall into dangerous eating patterns, such as binge eating or self-starvation.

Although not completely understood, management of body weight is not a mysterious process. It's simply a matter of balancing calories consumed with calories expended in daily activities—in other words, eating a moderate diet and exercising regularly. Unfortunately, this is not as exciting as the latest fad diet or "scientific breakthrough" that promises rapid weight loss without effort. Many people fail in their efforts to manage their weight because they focus on short-term weight loss rather than permanent changes in lifestyle. Successful weight management requires the long-term coordination of many aspects of a wellness lifestyle, including proper nutrition, adequate physical activity, and stress management.

This chapter explores the factors that contribute to the development of overweight and to eating disorders. It also takes a closer look at weight management through lifestyle behaviours and suggests specific strategies for reaching and maintaining a healthy weight.

QUICK STATS

Direct physical measurements have found that about 37% of adult Canadians are overweight and 24% are obese.

—*Canadian Health Measures Survey*, 2010

BASIC CONCEPTS OF WEIGHT MANAGEMENT

If you are like most people, you are concerned about your weight. But how do you decide if you are overweight? At what point does being overweight present a health risk? And how thin is too thin?

Body Composition

The human body can be divided into fat-free mass and body fat. Fat-free mass is composed of all the body's non-fat tissues: bone, water, muscle, connective tissue, organ tissues, and teeth. Body fat comes in three types:

- **Subcutaneous fat** is the fat located just beneath the skin. Research has found subcutaneous fat to be protective for a variety of diseases. Subcutaneous fat accumulation represents the normal physiological buffer for excess energy intake. When its storage capacity is exceeded, fat starts to accumulate in other places of the body. About 80% of all body fat is in the subcutaneous area.

- **Visceral fat** is the fat embedded within the mesentery (which is tissue that connects the intestines to the back of the abdominal wall) surrounding the abdominal organs. Excess visceral fat has been linked to cardiovascular and a host of other diseases. Visceral fat accounts for to 10%–20% of total fat in men and 5%–8% in women, and the amount increases with age for both sexes.

- **Ectopic fat** is the fat located on or within organs, such as the liver, heart, and brain. Ectopic fat increases the risk for metabolic syndrome (discussed more fully in Chapter 7), heart disease, and stroke.

One kilogram of body fat is equal to 7000 calories. This means that having only an extra 22 calories each day will cause a 1-kilogram weight gain over the course of a

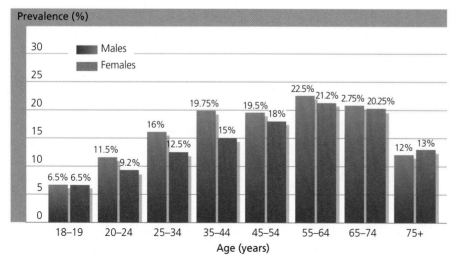

Prevalence (%)

Males
Females

6.5% 6.5% | 11.5% 9.2% | 16% 12.5% | 19.75% 15% | 19.5% 18% | 22.5% 21.2% | 2.75% 20.25% | 12% 13%

18–19   20–24   25–34   35–44   45–54   55–64   65–74   75+

Age (years)

FIGURE 4.1 Prevalence of self-reported obesity among people 18 years and older, by age and sex, 2007. The self-report nature of this information may mean that actual values are higher than reported here; research suggest that people tend to underreport rather than overreport their obesity-related attributes.

Source: Public Health Agency of Canada. 2009. *Obesity in Canada Snapshot*, p. 4 (http://www.phac-aspc.gc.ca/publicat/2009/oc/pdf/oc-eng.pdf; retrieved March 16, 2011).

year. In 10 years, that's 10 kilograms gained. But what is most important for health is not total weight but rather the proportion of the body's total weight that is fat—the **percent body fat**.

For example, two women may both be 1.7 metres tall and weigh 60 kilograms. But one woman, an endurance runner, may have only 15% of her body weight as fat, whereas the other woman, who is sedentary, may have 34% body fat. Although 60 kilograms is not considered overweight for women of this height, the sedentary woman may be overfat. (Methods for measuring and evaluating percent body fat are presented later in this chapter.) Because most people use the word *overweight* to describe the condition of having too much body fat, we use it in this chapter, although *overfat* is actually a more accurate term.

Energy Balance

The key to keeping a healthy ratio of fat-to-fat-free mass is maintaining an energy balance (Figure 4.2). You take in energy (calories) from the food you eat. Your body uses energy (calories) to maintain vital body functions (resting metabolism), to digest food, and to fuel physical activity. When energy in equals energy out, you maintain your current weight. To change your weight and body composition, you must tip the energy balance equation in a particular direction. If you take in more calories daily than your body burns (a *positive* energy balance), the excess calories will be stored as fat and you will gain weight over time. If you eat fewer calories than you burn each day (a *negative* energy balance), you will lose some of the stored fat and probably lose weight.

If we look at the energy balance equation today as expressed for the general Canadian population, the equation is tipped heavily toward the energy-in side. Our environment is rich in large portion sizes; high-fat, high-calorie foods; and palatable, easily available, and inexpensive foods. Unfortunately, the energy-out side of the equation has not compensated for increased energy intake; instead, we've decreased work-related physical activity, decreased activity associated with daily living, and increased time spent in sedentary pastimes, such as TV watching and computer use.

The good news, however, is that you control both parts of the energy balance equation. Specific strategies for altering energy balance are discussed later in the chapter.

Evaluating Body Weight and Body Composition

Overweight is usually defined as total body weight above the recommended range for good health (as determined by large-scale population surveys). **Obesity** is defined as a more serious degree of overweight. Many methods are available for measuring and evaluating body weight and percent body fat; the cut-off points for defining overweight and obesity vary with the method chosen.

Height-Weight Charts   In the past, many people relied on height-weight charts to evaluate body weight. Based on insurance company statistics, these charts list a range of ideal or recommended body weights associated with the lowest mortality for people of a particular sex, age, and height. Although easy to use, height-weight charts can be highly inaccurate for some people, and they provide only an indirect measure of body fat.

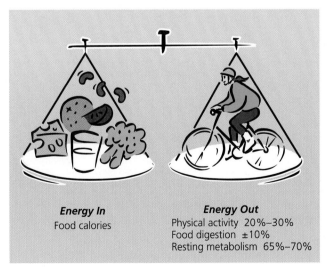

Energy In
Food calories

Energy Out
Physical activity 20%–30%
Food digestion ±10%
Resting metabolism 65%–70%

FIGURE 4.2   The energy balance equation.

Body Mass Index   Body mass index (BMI) is a measure of body weight that is useful for classifying the health risks of body weight if you don't have access to more sophisticated methods. Though more accurate than height-weight tables, BMI is also based on the concept that weight should be proportional to height. Easy to calculate and rate, BMI is a fairly accurate measure of the health risks of body weight for average people. Researchers frequently use BMI in conjunction with waist circumference in studies that examine the health risks associated with body weight.

However, because BMI does not distinguish between fat weight and fat-free weight, it can be very inaccurate for some groups, including short people (under 1.5 metres tall), muscular athletes, and older adults with little muscle mass because of inactivity or an underlying disease. If you are in one of these groups, use one of the methods described in the next section for estimating percent body fat to assess whether your current weight and body composition are healthy. BMI is also not particularly useful for tracking changes in body composition—gains in muscle mass and losses of fat. Women are likely to have more body fat for a given BMI than men.

You can calculate your BMI by dividing your body weight (expressed in kilograms) by the square of your height (expressed in metres). You can look up your BMI by using the chart in Figure 4.3.

Under standards issued by the World Health Organization (WHO), a BMI between 18.5 and 24.9 is considered average, a person with a BMI above 25 is overweight, 25–29.99 is considered pre-obese, 30–34.99 is considered obese class I, 35–39.99 is obese class II, and 40 or higher is obese class III. As obesity classes increase, the risk of associated health problems also increase. A person with a BMI below 18.5 is classified as underweight, although low BMI values may be healthy in some cases if

TERMS

body mass index (BMI)   A measure of relative body weight that takes height into account and is highly correlated with more direct measures of body fat; calculated by dividing total body weight (in kilograms) by the square of height (in metres).

Obese (>30)   Overweight (25–30)   Normal (18.5–25)   Underweight (<18.5)

Height in feet/inches and centimetres

Weight lb	(kg)	4'8" 142 cm	4'9"	4'10" 147	4'11" 150	5'0" 152	5'1" 155	5'2" 157	5'3" 160	5'4" 163	5'5" 165	5'6" 168	5'7" 170	5'8" 173	5'9" 175	5'10" 178	5'11" 180	6'0" 183	6'1" 185	6'2" 188	6'3" 191	6'4" 193	6'5" 196
260	(117.9)	58	56	54	53	51	49	48	46	45	43	42	41	40	38	37	36	35	34	33	32	32	31
255	(115.7)	57	55	53	51	50	48	47	45	44	42	41	40	39	38	37	36	35	34	33	32	31	30
250	(113.4)	56	54	52	50	49	47	46	44	43	42	40	39	38	37	36	35	34	33	32	31	30	30
245	(111.1)	55	53	51	49	48	46	45	43	42	41	40	38	37	36	35	34	33	32	31	31	30	29
240	(108.9)	54	52	50	48	47	45	44	43	41	40	39	38	36	35	34	33	33	32	31	30	29	28
235	(106.6)	53	51	49	47	46	44	43	42	40	39	38	37	36	35	34	33	32	31	30	29	29	28
230	(104.3)	52	50	48	46	45	43	42	41	39	38	37	36	35	34	33	32	31	30	30	29	28	27
225	(102.1)	50	49	47	45	44	43	41	40	39	37	36	35	34	33	32	31	31	30	29	28	27	27
220	(99.8)	49	48	46	44	43	42	40	39	38	37	36	34	33	32	32	31	30	29	28	27	27	26
215	(97.5)	48	47	45	43	42	41	39	38	37	36	35	34	33	32	31	30	29	28	28	27	26	25
210	(95.3)	47	45	44	42	41	40	38	37	36	35	34	33	32	31	30	29	28	28	27	26	26	25
205	(93.0)	46	44	43	41	40	39	37	36	35	34	33	32	31	30	29	29	28	27	26	26	25	24
200	(90.7)	45	43	42	40	39	38	37	35	34	33	32	31	30	30	29	28	27	26	26	25	24	24
195	(88.5)	44	42	41	39	38	37	36	35	33	32	31	31	30	29	28	27	26	26	25	24	24	23
190	(86.2)	43	41	40	38	37	36	35	34	33	32	31	30	29	28	27	26	26	25	24	24	23	23
185	(83.9)	41	40	39	37	36	35	34	33	32	31	30	29	28	27	27	26	25	24	24	23	23	22
180	(81.6)	40	39	38	36	35	34	33	32	31	30	29	28	27	27	26	25	24	24	23	22	22	21
175	(79.4)	39	38	37	35	34	33	32	31	30	29	28	27	27	26	25	24	24	23	22	22	21	21
170	(77.1)	38	37	36	34	33	32	31	30	29	28	27	27	26	25	24	24	23	22	22	21	21	20
165	(74.8)	37	36	34	33	32	31	30	29	28	27	27	26	25	24	24	23	22	22	21	21	20	20
160	(72.6)	36	35	33	32	31	30	29	28	27	27	26	25	24	24	23	22	22	21	21	20	19	19
155	(70.3)	35	34	32	31	30	29	28	27	27	26	25	24	24	23	22	22	21	20	20	19	19	18
150	(68.0)	34	32	31	30	29	28	27	27	26	25	24	23	23	22	22	21	20	20	19	19	18	18
145	(65.8)	33	31	30	29	28	27	27	26	25	24	23	23	22	21	21	20	20	19	19	18	18	17
140	(63.5)	31	30	29	28	27	26	26	25	24	23	23	22	21	21	20	20	19	18	18	17	17	17
135	(61.2)	30	29	28	27	26	26	25	24	23	22	22	21	21	20	19	19	18	18	17	17	16	16
130	(59.0)	29	28	27	26	25	24	23	22	22	21	20	20	19	19	18	18	17	17	16	16	15	15
125	(56.7)	28	27	26	25	24	24	23	22	21	21	20	20	19	18	18	17	17	16	16	16	15	15
120	(54.4)	27	26	25	24	23	23	22	21	21	20	19	19	18	18	17	17	16	16	15	15	15	14
115	(52.2)	26	25	24	23	22	22	21	20	20	19	19	18	17	17	16	16	16	15	15	14	14	14
110	(49.9)	25	24	23	22	21	21	20	20	19	18	18	17	17	16	16	15	15	15	14	14	13	13
105	(47.6)	24	23	22	21	21	20	19	19	18	17	17	16	16	15	15	14	14	13	13	13	13	13
100	(45.4)	22	22	21	20	20	19	18	18	17	17	16	16	15	14	14	14	13	13	12	12	12	12
95	(43.1)	21	21	20	19	19	18	17	17	16	16	15	15	14	14	14	13	13	13	12	12	12	11
90	(40.8)	20	19	19	18	18	17	16	16	15	15	15	14	13	13	13	12	12	12	11	11	11	11
85	(38.6)	19	18	18	17	17	16	16	15	15	14	14	13	13	13	12	12	11	11	11	11	10	10
80	(36.3)	18	17	17	16	16	15	15	14	14	13	13	13	12	12	11	11	11	11	10	10	10	9

Note: BMI values rounded to the nearest whole number. BMI categories based on CDC (Centers for Disease Control and Prevention) criteria.

FIGURE 4.3   Body mass index (BMI).   To determine your BMI, find your height in the left column. Move across the appropriate row until you find the weight closest to your own. The number at the top of the column is the BMI at that height and weight.

Source: © 2009 Vertex42 LLC. BMI chart created by Vertex42.com. Used with permission (http://www.vertex42.com/ExcelTemplates/bmichart.html; retrieved March 16, 2011).

they are not the result of smoking, an eating disorder, or an underlying disease; a BMI of 17.5 or lower is sometimes used as a diagnostic criterion for the eating disorder anorexia nervosa.

Body Composition Analysis   The most accurate and direct way to evaluate body composition is to determine percent body fat. A variety of methods are available, but it is worth noting that the WHO has not established specific guidelines for body composition assessment. See Table 4.1 for body composition ratings based on percent body fat; as with BMI, the percent body fat ratings indicate cut-off points for health risks associated with underweight and obesity.

HYDROSTATIC (UNDERWATER) WEIGHING AND BOD POD   One of the most accurate techniques for analyzing body composition is hydrostatic weighing. In this method, a person is submerged and weighed under water. Percent body fat can be calculated from body density. Muscle has a higher density and fat a lower density than water, and so people with more fat tend to float and weigh less under water, while lean people tend to sink and weigh more under water.

A specialized body composition analysis device called the Bod Pod uses air instead of water. A person sits in a chamber, and computerized pressure sensors determine the amount of air displaced by the person's body. This provides the needed information to calculate body composition density (i.e., lean and fat body mass).

SKINFOLD MEASUREMENTS   The skinfold-thickness technique measures the thickness of fat under the skin. Measurements are taken at several sites and plugged into formulas that calculate body fat percentages.

ELECTRICAL IMPEDANCE ANALYSIS   In this method, electrodes are attached to the body and a harmless electrical current is transmitted from electrode to electrode. The electrical conduction through the body favours the path of the fat-free tissues over fat tissues. A computer can calculate fat percentages from measurements of current.

SCANNING PROCEDURES   High-tech scanning procedures are highly accurate means of assessing body composition,

Calipers are used to perform skinfold measurements, which is a simple and inexpensive way to determine body fat levels. To ensure accuracy, skinfold measurements must be done by someone with appropriate training.

but they require expensive equipment. These procedures include computed tomography (CT), magnetic resonance imaging (MRI), dual-energy X-ray absorptiometry (DEXA), and dual-photon absorptiometry. Other procedures include infrared reactance (Futrex 1100) and total body electrical conductivity (TOBEC).

Excess Body Fat and Wellness

The amount of fat in the body—and its location—can have profound effects on health.

The Health Risks of Excess Body Fat   Obesity doubles mortality rates and can reduce life expectancy by 10–20 years. In fact, if the current trends in overweight and obesity (and their related health problems) continue, scientists believe that the average North American's life expectancy will soon decline by five years. According to the Canadian House of Commons Health Committee, obesity is the reason that, for the first time in history, the current generation of children have shorter life expectancies than their parents.

Obese people have a 50%–100% increased risk of death from all causes, compared with healthy weight people. Obesity is associated with unhealthy cholesterol and triglyceride levels, impaired heart function, and death from cardiovascular disease. Other health risks include hypertension, many kinds of cancer, impaired immune function, gallbladder and kidney diseases, skin problems, impotence, sleep and breathing disorders, back pain, arthritis, and other bone and joint disorders. Obesity is also associated with complications of pregnancy, menstrual irregularities,

Table 4.1	Percentage of Body Fat as the Criterion for Obesity	
Percentage of Body Fat		
Category	Males	Females
Normal	12%–20%	20%–30%
Borderline	21%–25%	31%–33%
Obese	>25%	>33%

Source: Bray, G. A. 2003. *Contemporary Diagnosis and Management of Obesity and the Metabolic Syndrome*, 3rd ed. Newton, Pa.: Handbooks in Health Care.

urine leakage (stress incontinence), increased surgical risk, and psychological disorders and problems (such as depression, low self-esteem, and body dissatisfaction).

A strong association exists between excess body fat and diabetes mellitus, a disease that causes a disruption of normal metabolism. The pancreas normally secretes the hormone insulin, which stimulates cells to take up blood sugar (glucose) to produce energy (Figure 4.4). In diabetes, this process is disrupted, causing a buildup of glucose in the bloodstream. Diabetes is associated with kidney failure; nerve damage; circulation problems and amputations; retinal damage and blindness; and increased rates of heart attack, stroke, and hypertension. Excess body fat is a major risk factor for type 2 diabetes (the most common form of diabetes). Obese people are more than three times as likely to develop type 2 diabetes, and the incidence of type 2 diabetes among Canadians has increased dramatically as the rate of obesity has climbed. Diabetes is currently the sixth leading cause of death in the Canada (see the box "Diabetes" for more information).

The risks from obesity increase with its severity, and they are much more likely to occur in people who are more than twice their desirable body weight. Controversy exists about the precise degree of risk at lower levels of overweight, particularly among overweight individuals who are physically active. The health risks associated with overweight depend in part on an individual's overall health and other risk factors, such as high blood pressure, unhealthy cholesterol levels, body fat distribution, and tobacco use. Weight loss is recommended for people whose BMI places them in the obese category and for those who are overweight *and* have two or more major risk factors for disease. If your BMI is 25 or higher, consult a physician for help in determining a healthy BMI for you.

Many people who are overweight have some of the risk factors associated with obesity. The Nurses' Health Study, in which Harvard researchers have followed more than 120,000 women since 1976, has found that even mildly

Symptoms of diabetes

- Frequent urination
- Extreme thirst and hunger
- Unexplained weight loss
- Extreme fatigue
- Blurred vision
- Frequent infections
- Slow wound healing
- Tingling or numbness in hands and feet
- Dry, itchy skin

Note: In the early stages, diabetes often has no symptoms.

Esophagus
Stomach
Pancreas
Small intestine

Normal
Insulin binds to receptors on the surface of a cell and signals special transporters in the cell to transport glucose inside.

Glucose transporter
Cell
Insulin receptor
Glucose
Insulin

Type 1 diabetes
The pancreas produces little or no insulin. Thus, no signal is sent instructing the cell to transport glucose, and glucose builds up in the bloodstream.

Cell

Type 2 diabetes
The pancreas produces too little insulin or the body's cells are resistant to it. Some insulin binds to receptors on the cell's surface, but the signal to transport glucose is blocked. Glucose builds up in the bloodstream.

Cell

FIGURE 4.4 Diabetes mellitus. During digestion, carbohydrates are broken down in the small intestine into glucose, a simple sugar that enters the bloodstream. The presence of glucose signals the pancreas to release insulin, a hormone that helps cells take up glucose; once inside a cell, glucose can be converted to energy. In diabetes, this process is disrupted, resulting in a buildup of glucose in the bloodstream.

Diabetes

Types of Diabetes

In 2006–2007, 5.5% of Canadian women and 6.2% of Canadian men (almost 2 million people or 1 in 17) had diabetes. The prevalence was lowest in British Columbia, Alberta, and Quebec, and highest in Newfoundland and Labrador, Nova Scotia, and New Brunswick.

More than 240,000 Canadians live with *type 1 diabetes*. In this type of diabetes, the pancreas produces little or no insulin so that daily doses of insulin are required. Type 1 diabetes occurs when the body's immune system, triggered by a viral infection or some other environmental factor, mistakenly destroys the insulin-producing cells in the pancreas. It usually strikes before age 30. The incidence rate of type 1 diabetes is rising by 3%–5% in Canada, and the greatest rise is occurring in five- to nine-year-olds.

The remaining people have *type 2 diabetes*, and its prevalence is rising dramatically. This condition can develop slowly, and about 25% of affected individuals are unaware of their condition. In type 2 diabetes, the pancreas doesn't produce enough insulin, or cells are resistant to insulin, or both. This condition is usually diagnosed in people over age 40, although a tenfold increase in type 2 diabetes in children has occurred in the past two decades. About one-third of people with type 2 diabetes must take insulin; others take medications that increase insulin production or stimulate cells to take up glucose.

A third type of diabetes occurs in some women during pregnancy. *Gestational diabetes* usually disappears after pregnancy, but more than half of women who experience it eventually develop type 2 diabetes. In Canada, the prevalence of gestational diabetes is higher than previously thought, with rates varying from 3.7% in non-Aboriginal women to 8%–18% in Aboriginal women. The number of people with diagnosed diabetes continues to grow, with almost 200,000 new cases of diabetes diagnosed in 2005–2006.

Older Canadians are more likely to have diabetes. In 2005–2006, 22% of people (approximately one in five) who were 75–79 years old had been diagnosed with diabetes. This was almost 10 times the proportion seen in Canadian adults ages 35–39, where the prevalence was 2.3%, or 1 in 43.

Overall, in adults aged 20 and older, death rates for those with diabetes are two to three times those of the general population. Among 20- to 39-year-olds, individuals with diabetes die at a rate more than six times that of the general population, while among 60- to 79-year-olds, the rates are about twice as high.

Research has shown that Aboriginal peoples and certain populations, such as Asians, Hispanics, and Africans, have a significantly higher risk of developing diabetes. Estimates of the prevalence of diabetes in Aboriginal peoples have been found to be as much as three to five times that in non-Aboriginal populations.

Prevention

It is estimated that 90% of cases of type 2 diabetes could be prevented if people adopted healthy lifestyle behaviours, including regular physical activity, a moderate diet, and modest weight loss. For people with pre-diabetes, lifestyle measures are more effective than medication for delaying or preventing the development of diabetes. Studies of people with pre-diabetes show that just a 5%–7% weight loss can lower diabetes onset by nearly 60%. Exercise (endurance and strength training) makes cells more sensitive to insulin and helps stabilize blood glucose levels; it also helps keep body fat at healthy levels.

A moderate diet to control body fat is perhaps the most important dietary recommendation for the prevention of diabetes. However, the composition of the diet may also be important. Studies have linked diets low in fibre and high in sugar, refined carbohydrates, saturated fat, red meat, and high-fat dairy products to increased risk of diabetes; diets rich in whole grains, fruits, vegetables, legumes, fish, and poultry may be protective. Specific foods linked to higher risk of diabetes include soft drinks, white bread, white rice, french fries, processed meats, and sugary desserts.

Treatment

Diabetes has no cure, but it can be successfully managed by keeping blood glucose levels within safe limits through diet, exercise, and, if necessary, medication. Blood glucose levels can be monitored by using a home test; close monitoring and control of glucose levels

can significantly reduce the rate of serious complications. New drug therapies include inhibitors known as DDP-4, which lower blood glucose without causing weight gain.

Nearly 90% of people with type 2 diabetes are overweight when diagnosed, including 55% who are obese. An important step in treatment is weight loss; even a small amount lost can be beneficial. People with diabetes should get their carbohydrates from whole grains, fruits, vegetables, and low-fat dairy products; carbohydrate and monounsaturated fat together should provide 60%–70% of total daily calories. Regular exercise and a healthy diet are often sufficient to control type 2 diabetes.

Warning Signs and Testing

Be alert for the warning signs of diabetes, which include frequent urination and infections, extreme hunger or thirst and fatigue, unexplained weight loss, blurred vision, cuts and bruises that are slow to heal, tingling or numbness in hands or feet, and generalized itching with no rash.

The best way to avoid complications is to recognize these symptoms and get early diagnosis and treatment. Type 2 diabetes is often asymptomatic in the early stages, however, and so routine screening is recommended for people over age 45 and anyone younger who is at high risk. Screening involves a blood test to check glucose levels after either fasting or the administration of a set dose of glucose. A fasting glucose level of 7 mmol/L or higher indicates diabetes; a level of 6.1–6.9 mmol/L indicates pre-diabetes.

Sources: Public Health Agency of Canada. 2008. *National Diabetes Fact Sheet 2008* (http://www.phac-aspc.gc.ca/publicat/2008/ndfs-fnrd-08/ndfs_ff-fnrd_fc-eng.php; retrieved March 17, 2011); Public Health Agency of Canada. 2008. *Diabetes in Canada: Highlights from the National Diabetes Surveillance System, 2004–2005,* Table 2 (http://www.phac-aspc.gc.ca/publicat/2008/dicndss-dacsnsd-04-05/index-eng.php; retrieved March 17, 2011); Juvenile Diabetes Research Foundation of Canada. 2011. *Fact Sheets* http://www.jdrf.ca/index.cfm?fuseaction=home.viewPage&page_id=62495B79-DE19-05A3-5168B63985B9E8B2; retrieved March 17, 2011); Canadian Diabetes Association. 2011. *Gestational Diabetes: Preventing Complications in Pregnancy* (http://www.diabetes.ca/diabetes-and-you/what/gestational/; retrieved March 17, 2011).

to moderately overweight women have an 80% increased risk of developing coronary heart disease compared with leaner women. This study also confirmed that to reduce the risk of dying prematurely of any cause, maintaining a desirable body weight is important. This conclusion was supported by a 10-year study that ended in 2006 after following a half-million people in their fifties. Researchers concluded that subjects who were even slightly overweight were up to 40% more likely to die within the next decade, compared with age-matched people who had a desirable weight. But it is also important to realize that small weight losses—5%–10% of total body weight—can lead to significant health improvements.

Body Fat Distribution and Health The distribution of body fat (that is, the locations of fat on the body) is also an important indicator of health. Men and postmenopausal women tend to store fat in the upper regions of their bodies, particularly in the abdominal area (the apple shape). Premenopausal women usually store fat in hips, buttocks, and thighs (the pear shape). Excess fat in the abdominal area increases risk of high blood pressure, type 2 diabetes, early-onset heart disease, stroke, certain types of cancer, and mortality. This risk is independent of a person's BMI. The reason for this increase in risk is not entirely clear, but it appears that abdominal fat is more easily mobilized and sent into the bloodstream, increasing disease-related blood fat levels.

The risks from body fat distribution are usually assessed by measuring waist circumference (the distance around the abdomen at the level of the hip bone, known as the iliac crest). Waist circumference can be used as a measure of abdominal obesity, an indicator of disease risk, and to monitor changes in body composition over time. More research is needed to determine the precise degree of risk associated with specific values for waist measurement. However, a total waist measurement of more than 102 centimetres for men and 88 centimetres for women is associated with a significantly increased risk of disease.

A person doesn't have to be technically overfat to have fat distribution be a risk factor, nor do all overfat people face this increased risk. The Health Canada guidelines state that large waist circumference can be a marker for increased risk of type 2 diabetes, high blood pressure, and cardiovascular disease (CVD) even in people with a BMI in the normal range. Health Canada recommends measuring waist circumference among people with BMIs between 18.5 and 34.9; for BMIs equal to or great than 35, waist circumference does not seem to provide additional information on health risks. That being said, at any given level of overweight, people with a large waist circumference or additional disease risk factors are considered at greater risk for health problems. For example, a man with a BMI of 27, a waist circumference of more than 102 centimetres, and type 2 diabetes is at greater risk for health problems than another man who has a BMI of 27 but has a smaller waist and no other risk factors. Abdominal obesity and any two other risk factors associated with cardiovascular health put an individual at risk for metabolic syndrome. Abdominal obesity (as measured by waist circumference) is a primary component of metabolic syndrome and a forewarning of type 2 diabetes and heart disease.

Body Image The collective picture of the body as seen through the mind's eye, body image consists of perceptions, images, thoughts, attitudes, and emotions. A negative **body image** is characterized by dissatisfaction with the body in general or some part of the body in particular. Recent surveys indicate that the majority of North Americans, many of whom are not actually overweight, are unhappy with their body weight or with some aspect of their appearance.

Losing weight or getting cosmetic surgery does not necessarily improve body image. However, improvements in body image may occur in the absence of changes in weight or appearance. Many experts now believe that body image issues must be dealt with as part of treating obesity and eating disorders. See the section "Eating Disorders" later in the chapter for more information on body image and eating disorders.

Problems Associated with Very Low Levels of Body Fat Health experts have generally viewed very low levels of body fat—less than 8%–12% for women and 3%–5% for men—as a threat to wellness. Extreme leanness has been linked with reproductive, circulatory, and immune system disorders. Extremely lean people may experience muscle wasting and fatigue; they are also more likely to have dangerous eating disorders.

In physically active women and girls, particularly those involved in sports where weight and appearance are important (ballet, gymnastics, skating, and distance running, for example), a condition called the **female athlete triad** may develop. The triad consists of three interrelated disorders: abnormal eating patterns (see "Eating Disorders" later in this chapter) and excessive exercising, followed by **amenorrhea** (absence of menstruation), followed by decreased bone density (premature osteoporosis). Prolonged amenorrhea can cause bone density to erode to a point that a woman in her twenties will have the bone density of a woman in her sixties. Left untreated, the triad can lead to decreased physical performance, increased incidence of bone fractures, disturbances of heart rhythm and metabolism, and even death.

What Is the Right Weight for You?

BMI, percent body fat, and waist circumference measurement can best serve as general guides or estimates for body weight (Table 4.2).

To answer the question of what you should weigh, let your lifestyle be your guide. Don't focus on a particular weight as your goal. Instead, focus on living a lifestyle that includes eating moderate amounts of healthful foods, getting plenty of exercise, thinking positively, and learning to cope with stress. Then let the kilograms fall where they may. For most people, the result will be close to the recommended weight ranges discussed earlier. For some, their weight will be somewhat higher than societal standards—but right for them. By letting a healthy lifestyle determine your weight, you can avoid developing unhealthy patterns of eating and a negative body image.

FACTORS CONTRIBUTING TO EXCESS BODY FAT

Body weight and body composition are determined by multiple factors that vary with each individual. These factors can be grouped into genetic, physiological, lifestyle, and psychosocial factors.

Genetic Factors

Nutrigenomics is the study of how nutrients and genes interact and how genetic variations can cause people to respond differently to nutrients in food. Estimates of the genetic contribution to obesity vary widely, from 25%–40% of an individual's body fat. Scientists have so far

QUESTIONS FOR CRITICAL THINKING AND REFLECTION

What is important to you about having a healthy body weight? How does your use of food and physical activity reflect your level of respect for yourself? What does it mean to you to be kind to your body?

identified more than 600 genes associated with obesity. Genes influence body size and shape, body fat distribution, and metabolic rate. Genetic factors also affect the ease with which weight is gained as a result of overeating and where on the body extra weight is added. Researchers have suggested a link between a mother's level of obesity and her baby's body-weight-regulating mechanisms while in the womb.

If both parents are obese, their children have an 80% risk of being obese; children with only one obese parent face a 40% risk of becoming obese. In studies that compared adoptees and their biological parents, the weights

body image   The mental representation a person holds about his or her body at any given moment in time, consisting of perceptions, images, thoughts, attitudes, and emotions about the body.

female athlete triad   A condition consisting of three interrelated disorders: abnormal eating patterns and excessive exercising, followed by lack of menstrual periods (amenorrhea) and decreased bone density (premature osteoporosis).

amenorrhea   The absence of menstruation.

Table 4.2	**Body Mass Index (BMI) and Waist Circumference Classification and Disease Risk**				
			Disease Risk Relative to Normal Weight and Waist Circumference[a]		
Classification	**BMI (kg/m^2)**	**Obesity Class**	**Men ≤102 cm Women ≤88 cm**	**Men >102 cm Women >88 cm**
Underweight[b]	<18.5		—	—
Normal[c]	18.5–24.9		—	—
Overweight	25.0–29.9		Increased	High
Obesity	30.0–34.9	I	High	Very high
	35.0–39.9	II	Very high	Very high
Extreme obesity	= 40.0+	III	Extremely high	Extremely high

Sources: Adapted from National Heart, Lung, and Blood Institute. 1998. *Clinical Guidelines on the Identification, Evaluation, and Treatment of Overweight and Obesity in Adults: The Evidence Report.* Bethesda, Md.: National Institutes of Health; *Canadian Guidelines for Body Weight Classification in Adults.* http://www.hc-sc.gc.ca/fn-an/alt_formats/hpfb-dgpsa/pdf/nutrition/cg_quick_ref-ldc_rapide_ref-eng.pdf. Health Canada. Reproduced with the permission of the Minister of Public Works and Government Services Canada, 2011.

[a] Disease risk for type 2 diabetes, hypertension, and cardiovascular disease. The waist circumference cut-offs for increased risk are 102 centimetres for men and 88 centimetres for women.

[b] Research suggests that a low BMI can be healthy in some cases, as long as it is not the result of smoking, an eating disorder, or an underlying disease process. A BMI of 17.5 or lower is sometimes used as a diagnostic criterion for the eating disorder anorexia nervosa.

[c] Increased waist circumference can also be a marker for increased risk, even in people of normal weight.

of the adoptees were found to be more like those of the biological parents than the adoptive parents, again indicating a strong genetic link.

Hereditary influences, however, must be balanced against the contribution of environmental factors. Not all children of obese parents become obese, and non-obese parents may have obese children. Environmental factors, such as diet and exercise, are probably responsible for such differences. Thus, the *tendency* to develop obesity may be inherited, but the expression of this tendency is affected by environmental influences.

The message you should take from this research is that genes are not destiny. It is true that some people have a harder time losing weight and maintaining weight loss than others. However, with increased exercise and attention to diet, even those with a genetic tendency toward obesity can maintain a healthy body weight. And regardless of genetic factors, lifestyle choices remain the cornerstone of successful weight management.

Physiological Factors

Metabolism is a key physiological factor in the regulation of body fat and body weight; hormones and fat cell types also play a role.

Metabolism   Metabolism is the sum of all the vital processes by which food energy and nutrients are made available to and used by the body. The largest component of metabolism, **resting metabolic rate (RMR)**, is the energy required to maintain vital body functions, including respiration, heart rate, body temperature, and blood pressure, while the body is at rest. As was shown in Figure 4.2, RMR accounts for about 65%–70% of daily energy expenditure. The energy required to digest food accounts for an additional ±10% of daily energy expenditure. The remaining 20%–30% is expended during physical activity.

Both heredity and behaviour affect metabolic rate. Men, who have a higher proportion of muscle mass than women, have a higher RMR because muscle tissue is more metabolically active than fat. Also, some individuals inherit a higher or lower RMR than others. A higher RMR means that a person burns more calories while at rest and can therefore take in more calories without gaining weight.

Weight loss or gain also affects metabolic rate. When a person loses weight, both RMR and the energy required to perform physical tasks decrease. The reverse occurs when weight is gained. One of the reasons exercise is so important during a weight-loss program is that exercise, especially resistance training, helps maintain muscle mass and metabolic rate.

Exercise has a positive effect on metabolism. When people exercise, they slightly increase their RMR—the number of calories their bodies burn at rest. They also increase their muscle mass, which is associated with a higher metabolic rate. The exercise itself also burns calories, raising total energy expenditure. The higher the energy expenditure, the more the person can eat without gaining weight. (The role of exercise in weight management is discussed in greater detail later in the chapter.)

Hormones   Hormones clearly play a role in the accumulation of body fat, especially for females. Hormonal changes at puberty, during pregnancy, and at menopause contribute to the amount and location of fat accumulation. For example, during puberty, hormones cause the development of secondary sex characteristics, including larger breasts, wider hips, and a fat layer under the skin.

One hormone thought to be linked to obesity is leptin. Secreted by the body's fat cells, leptin is carried to the brain, where it appears to let the brain know how big or small the body's fat stores are. With this information, the brain can regulate appetite and metabolic rate accordingly. Several other hormones may be involved in the regulation of appetite. Researchers hope to use these hormones to develop treatments for obesity based on appetite control; however, as most of us will admit, hunger is often not the primary reason we overeat. Cases of obesity based solely or primarily on hormone abnormalities do exist, but they are rare. Lifestyle choices still account for the largest proportion of the differences in body weight and body composition among individuals.

Fat Cells   The amount of fat (adipose tissue) the body can store is a function of the number and size of fat (adipose) cells. These fat cells are like little compartments that can inflate to hold body fat; when existing fat cells are filled, the body makes more, thereby increasing its ability to store fat.

Some people are born with an above-average number of fat cells and thus have the potential for storing more energy as body fat. Overeating at critical times, such as in childhood and adolescence, can cause the body to create more fat cells. If a person loses weight, fat cell content is depleted, but it is unclear whether the number of fat cells can be decreased.

Further, it appears that all fat cells are not created equal. As mentioned earlier, visceral adipose tissue is located at waist level, inside the abdominal wall and surrounding the organs. This type of fat contains many biologically active substances, such as inflammatory chemicals and growth factors, which can adhere to the lining of blood vessels, cause insulin resistance, and have a negative influence on cardiovascular health. The more visceral fat and ectopic fat you have, the greater your chances of developing insulin resistance, metabolic syndrome, type 2 diabetes, and heart disease. Researchers consider visceral fat to be an active endocrine organ (like the pancreas), responsible

TERMS   **resting metabolic rate (RMR)**   The energy required to maintain vital body functions, including respiration, heart rate, body temperature, and blood pressure, while the body is at rest.

for many of the pathological conditions of obesity. Visceral fat may also be the reason waist circumference is such a critical indicator of obesity risk.

In contrast, subcutaneous fat carries little or no health risk. Subcutaneous fat lies just under your skin, outside the abdominal wall. This fat tends to be soft and flabby (whereas visceral fat is hard) and is not metabolically active like visceral fat.

Found more often in women than men, subcutaneous fat appears on the lower body—the hips, upper thighs, and buttocks—a trait called *gynoid obesity* (Figure 4.5). As a result of their body shape, people with excess subcutaneous fat are described as "pears." People with excess visceral and ectopic fat tend to carry it on their upper body (*android obesity*) and are called "apples." In terms of health risk, apples are bad and pears are good.

Lifestyle Factors

Although genetic and physiological factors may increase risk for excess body fat, they are not sufficient to explain the increasingly high rate of obesity seen in Canada (see Figure 4.6). The gene pool has not changed in the past 40 years, but the rate of obesity among Canadians has increased dramatically (see Table 4.2, and the box "Overweight and Obesity Among Canadian Ethnic Populations" on p. 106). Clearly, other factors are at work—particularly lifestyle factors, such as increased eating and decreased physical activity.

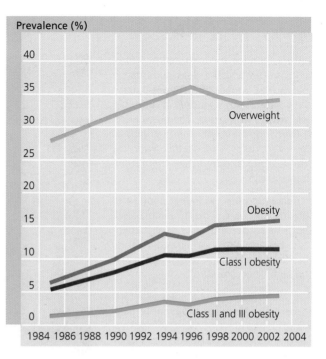

FIGURE 4.6 Prevalence of overweight and obesity (classes I–III) in Canada, 1985–2003.

Source: Katzmarzyk, P. T., and C. Mason. 2006. *CMAJ* 174(2): 156–157, Figure 1 (http://www.cmaj.ca/cgi/reprint/174/2/156; retrieved March 17, 2011). © 2009 Canadian Medical Association or its licensors.

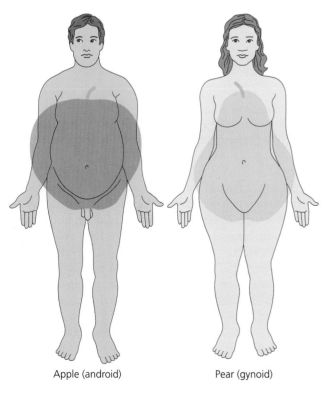

Apple (android)   Pear (gynoid)

FIGURE 4.5 Overweight men tend to have an apple (android) shape; overweight women tend to have a pear (gynoid) shape.

THINKING ABOUT THE ENVIRONMENT

Environmental factors are determinants of obesity and can make weight management even more difficult for many people. In this case, it is the humanmade environment, not the natural one, that creates obstacles to a healthy lifestyle:

- A noisy environment can make it difficult to sleep, and poor sleep quality has been associated with weight gain, difficulty in losing weight, and other conditions, such as depression and high blood pressure.

- In some urban and high-poverty areas, it is not always easy to make ideal food choices because fresh, healthy foods may be more expensive or harder to obtain than cheaper, less healthy fast food or junk food.

- People who live in unsafe environments, such as some inner-city areas, may not get as much physical activity as they need, simply because there are not enough safe places to walk or exercise.

As you create your own weight-management program, remember to account for environmental factors that may interfere with your efforts. You may need creative solutions to keep your program on track.

For more information on health and the environment, see Chapter 21.

Overweight and Obesity Among Canadian Ethnic Populations

DIMENSIONS OF DIVERSITY

Culture, gender, income, and environment are among the determinants of obesity. The impact of culture is particularly interesting. Among all population groups in Canada, the prevalence of overweight and obesity is growing. However, rates and trends vary by ethnic group and by other population characteristics.

• Certain groups, including Aboriginal peoples, and Canadians of Chinese and South Asian descent, may have higher-than-average rates of obesity-related chronic disease (such as heart disease and high blood pressure).

• Cultural factors that influence dietary and exercise behaviours appear to play a role in the development of obesity. Cultural differences also exist in acceptance of larger body size and in body image perception. For example, one study found that black North Americans were more likely to think they were thinner than they really were and whites were more likely to think they were fatter than they really were.

• Rates of overweight and obesity tend to be higher among Canadian females with middle levels of income. However, for Canadian men, higher incomes tend to be associated with higher rates of overweight and obesity.

• In general, low socioeconomic status is associated with higher rates of overweight and obesity. Researchers theorize that people living in poor communities are more greatly affected by a toxic food and exercise environment—meaning they have fewer opportunities to purchase healthy foods and safely engage in regular physical activity. In addition, many foods low in price are high in calorie density (fast food, for example).

• Although overweight and obesity are a problem across Canada, provincial and territorial differences exist with the lowest rates being found in British Columbia, and the highest rates, in both rural areas and in the Atlantic provinces.

• For Asian Canadians or people of Asian descent, waist circumference is a better indicator of relative disease risk than is BMI, and disease risk goes up at a lower level of BMI than it does for individuals of other groups. For Asian populations, WHO guidelines have a lower BMI cut-off for defining overweight (BMI 23).

Sources: Chou, J., and H. S. Juon. 2006. Assessing overweight and obesity risk among Korean Americans in California using World Health Organization body mass index criteria for Asians. *Preventing Chronic Disease* 3(3): A79; Kumanyika, S., and S. Grier. 2006. Targeting interventions for ethnic minority and low-income populations. *The Future of Children* 16(1): 187–207; Whitaker, R. C., and S. M. Orzol. 2006. Obesity among US urban preschool children: Relationships to race, ethnicity, and socioeconomic status. *Archives of Pediatric and Adolescent Medicine* 160(6): 578–584; Goel, M. S., et al. 2004. Obesity among U.S. immigrant subgroups by duration of residence. *Journal of the American Medical Association* 292(23): 2860–2867; Heart and Stroke Foundation of Canada. 2008. *Overweight, Obesity and Heart Disease and Stroke* (http://www.heartandstroke.com/site/c. ikIQLcMWJtE/b.3799193/k.C2EF/Overweight_ obesity_and_heart_disease_and_stroke.htm; retrieved March 17, 2011).

Eating Canadians have access to plenty of calorie-dense foods, and many have eating habits that contribute to weight gain. Most overweight adults admit to eating more than they should of high-fat, high-sugar, high-calorie foods. Canadians eat out more frequently now than in the past, and we rely more heavily on fast food and packaged convenience foods. Restaurant and convenience food portion sizes tend to be large, and the foods themselves are likely to be high in fat, sugar, and calories and low in nutrients. Studies have consistently found that people underestimate portion sizes by as much as 25%.

Canadians' average calorie intake has been climbing since 1995. Many of our extra calories come from carbohydrates, such as refined sugars. The popularity of sugar-free soft drinks does not appear to be helping people lose weight (see the box "Are Diet Soft Drinks Bad for You?"). Levels of physical activity have also been declining. The result has been a substantial increase in the number of overweight and obese Canadians. Eating for weight management is discussed later in this chapter.

Physical Activity Research has shown that activity levels among Canadians are declining, beginning in childhood and continuing throughout life (see Chapter 6). Many schools have cut back on physical education classes and recess. Most adults drive to work, sit all day, and then relax in front of the TV at night. One study found that

QUICK STATS

Between 1981 and 2009 the proportion of boys 15 to 19 years old classified as overweight or obese rose from **14% to 31%.** Among teen girls, it increased from **14% to 25%**.

—*Canadian Health Measures Survey, 2010*

Are Diet Soft Drinks Bad for You?

Soft drink consumption has grown significantly in Canada in the past 30 years, among children, adolescents, and adults. Regular soft drinks, in fact, are now among the leading source of calories in the Canadian diet.

A can of regular pop contains about 150 calories. High consumption of sugary pop has previously been linked with obesity and type 2 diabetes in children and adolescents and with high blood pressure in adults. Further, some studies have shown that the added sweeteners in soft drinks are linked to increased triglycerides in the blood, leading to a greater risk of heart disease.

Why does drinking more pop lead to obesity and insulin resistance? Researchers have attributed this effect to the following factors:

- The consumption of more calories in general

- The high-fructose corn syrup content in pops

- Lower feelings of satiety (satisfaction)

- The general effect of eating a diet that is high in refined carbohydrates, including sugar

Many weight-conscious people have changed to diet pop in the hope that this is a sugar-free, calorie-free alternative to regular pop. But is it? Recent research indicates that drinking more than one soft drink a day, even if it is diet pop, may be associated with an increased incidence of metabolic syndrome. As described else-

where in this text, metabolic syndrome is a cluster of risk factors linked to the development of type 2 diabetes, heart disease, and stroke. The syndrome includes high blood pressure, elevated triglyceride levels, low levels of HDL ("good" cholesterol), high fasting blood glucose levels, and excessive waist circumference.

The news about diet pop came from the Framingham Heart Study, which examined more than 6000 middle-aged people who were initially free of metabolic syndrome. The link between diet soft drink consumption and metabolic syndrome was clear even when the researchers accounted for other factors, such as saturated fat and fibre in the diet, total calories, physical activity, and smoking.

Compared with people who did not drink pop, researchers found that people who consumed more than one soft drink per day—regular or diet—were associated with the following:

- 44% as likely to develop metabolic syndrome

- 31% as likely to be obese

- 25% as likely to have higher-than-average blood pressure

- 18% as likely to have high blood pressure

What is the possible explanation for the association? Some research has suggested that the artificial sweeteners in diet drinks make a person more prone to eating sweet, higher-calorie foods.

Another theory is that the caramel content in both regular and diet pops may play a role in insulin resistance.

Conversely, some contradictory studies show the benefit of diet pop consumption in overweight individuals and suggest that other factors could explain the development of risk factors for heart disease. Regardless, everyone agrees that more research should be done before a final verdict on diet pop consumption is reached.

Meanwhile, nutritionists say that this is a wake-up call for some diet pop drinkers, suggesting that a zero-calorie beverage cannot undo the damage of an otherwise unhealthy diet.

60% of the incidence of overweight can be linked to excessive television viewing. On average, North Americans exercise 15 minutes per day and watch 170 minutes of TV and movies. Modern conveniences, such as remote controls, elevators, and power mowers, have also reduced daily physical activity.

Psychosocial Factors

Many people have learned to use food as a means of coping with stress and negative emotions. Eating can provide a powerful distraction from difficult feelings: loneliness, anger, boredom, anxiety, shame, sadness, inadequacy. It can be used to combat low moods, low energy levels, and low self-esteem (see the box "What Triggers Your Eating?"

on p. 108). When food and eating become the primary means of regulating emotions, binge eating or other disturbed eating patterns can develop.

Obesity is strongly associated with socioeconomic status. In general, the prevalence of obesity goes down as income level goes up. More women than men are obese at lower income levels, but men are somewhat more obese at higher levels. These differences may reflect the greater sensitivity and concern for a slim physical appearance among upper-income women, as well as greater access to information about nutrition, to low-fat and low-calorie foods, and to opportunities for physical activity. It may also reflect the greater acceptance of obesity among certain ethnic groups, as well as different cultural values related to food choices.

ASSESS YOURSELF

What Triggers Your Eating?

Hunger isn't the only reason people eat. Efforts to maintain a healthy body weight can be sabotaged by eating related to other factors, including emotions, environment, and patterns of thinking. This quiz is designed to provide you with a score for five factors that describe many people's eating habits. This information will put you in a better position to manage your eating behaviour and control your weight. Circle the number that indicates to what degree each situation is likely to make you start eating.

Social

	Very Unlikely									Very Likely
1. Arguing or having a conflict with someone	1	2	3	4	5	6	7	8	9	10
2. Being with others when they are eating	1	2	3	4	5	6	7	8	9	10
3. Being urged to eat by someone else	1	2	3	4	5	6	7	8	9	10
4. Feeling inadequate around others	1	2	3	4	5	6	7	8	9	10

Emotional

5. Feeling bad, such as being anxious or depressed	1	2	3	4	5	6	7	8	9	10
6. Feeling good, happy, or relaxed	1	2	3	4	5	6	7	8	9	10
7. Feeling bored or having time on my hands	1	2	3	4	5	6	7	8	9	10
8. Feeling stressed or excited	1	2	3	4	5	6	7	8	9	10

Situational

9. Seeing an advertisement for food or eating	1	2	3	4	5	6	7	8	9	10
10. Passing by a bakery, cookie shop, or other enticement to eat	1	2	3	4	5	6	7	8	9	10
11. Being involved in a party, celebration, or special occasion	1	2	3	4	5	6	7	8	9	10
12. Eating out	1	2	3	4	5	6	7	8	9	10

Thinking

13. Making excuses to myself about why it's OK to eat	1	2	3	4	5	6	7	8	9	10
14. Berating myself for being fat or unable to control my eating	1	2	3	4	5	6	7	8	9	10
15. Worrying about others or about difficulties I'm having	1	2	3	4	5	6	7	8	9	10
16. Thinking about how things should or shouldn't be	1	2	3	4	5	6	7	8	9	10

Physiological

17. Experiencing pain or physical discomfort	1	2	3	4	5	6	7	8	9	10

In some families and cultures, food is used as a symbol of love and caring. It is an integral part of social gatherings and celebrations. In such cases, it may be difficult to change established eating patterns because they are linked to cultural and family values.

? QUESTIONS FOR CRITICAL THINKING AND REFLECTION

How do you view your own body composition? Where do you think you've gotten your ideas about how your body should look and perform? In light of what you've read in this chapter, do the ideals and images promoted in our culture seem reasonable? Do they seem healthy?

ADOPTING A HEALTHY LIFESTYLE FOR SUCCESSFUL WEIGHT MANAGEMENT

The Canadian Medical Association's *Canadian Clinical Practice Guidelines on the Management and Prevention of Obesity in Adults and Children* stress the importance of a lifestyle geared toward healthy bodies. This recommendation is logical, given that when all the research has been assessed, it is clear that most weight problems are lifestyle problems. Even though more and more young people are developing weight problems, most arrive at early adulthood with the advantage of having a normal body weight—neither too fat nor too thin. In fact, many young adults have less than desirable eating and exercise habits

		Very Unlikely									Very Likely	
18.	Experiencing trembling, headache, or light-headedness associated with not eating or consuming too much caffeine	1	2	3	4	5	6	7	8	9	10	
19.	Experiencing fatigue or feeling overtired	1	2	3	4	5	6	7	8	9	10	
20.	Experiencing hunger pangs or urges to eat, even though I've eaten recently	1	2	3	4	5	6	7	8	9	10	

Scoring

Total your scores for each category, and enter them below. Then rank the scores by marking the highest score 1, next highest score 2, and so on. Focus on the highest-ranked categories first, but any score above 24 is high and indicates that you need to work on that category.

Category	Total Score	Rank Order
Social (Items 1–4)	_____	_____
Emotional (Items 5–8)	_____	_____
Situational (Items 9–12)	_____	_____
Thinking (Items 13–16)	_____	_____
Physiological (Items 17–20)	_____	_____

What Your Score Means

Social A high score here means you are very susceptible to the influence of others. Work on better ways to communicate more assertively, handle conflict, and manage anger. Challenge your beliefs about the need to be polite and the obligations you feel you must fulfil.

Emotional A high score here means you need to develop effective ways to cope with emotions. Work on developing skills in stress management, time management, and communication. Practising positive but realistic self-talk can help you handle small daily upsets.

Situational A high score here means you are especially susceptible to external influences. Try to avoid external cues and respond differently to those you cannot avoid. Control your environment by changing the way you buy, store, cook, and serve food. Anticipate potential problems, and have a plan for handling them.

Thinking A high score here means that the way you think—how you talk to yourself, the beliefs you hold, your memories, and your expectations—have a powerful influence on your eating habits. Try to be less self-critical, less perfectionistic, and more flexible in your ideas about the way things ought to be. Recognize when you're making excuses or rationalizations that allow you to eat.

Physiological A high score here means that the way you eat, what you eat, or medications you are taking may be affecting your eating behaviour. You may be eating to reduce physical arousal or deal with physical discomfort. Try eating three meals a day, supplemented with regular snacks if needed. Avoid too much caffeine. If any medication you're taking produces adverse physical reactions, switch to an alternative, if possible. If your medications may be affecting your hormone levels, discuss possible alternatives with your physician.

Source: Adapted from Nash, J. D. 1997. *The New Maximize Your Body Potential.* Boulder, Colorado: Bull. Reprinted with permission from Bull Publishing Company.

and don't develop a weight problem. But as the rapid growth of adolescence slows and family and career obligations increase, maintaining a healthy weight becomes a greater challenge. Slow weight gain is a major cause of overweight and obesity, and so weight management is important for everyone, not just for people who are currently overweight. A good time to develop a lifestyle for successful weight management is during early adulthood, when healthy behaviour patterns have a better chance of taking a firm hold.

Permanent weight loss is not something people can start and stop. They need to adopt healthy behaviours that they can maintain throughout life, including eating habits, level of physical activity, an ability to think positively and manage emotions effectively, and the coping strategies they use to deal with the stresses and challenges.

Diet and Eating Habits

In contrast to dieting, which involves some form of food restriction, the term *diet* refers to your daily food choices. Everyone has a diet, but not everyone is dieting. You need to develop a diet that you enjoy and that enables you to maintain a healthy body composition. Use Health Canada's *Eating Well with Canada's Food Guide* as the basis for a healthy diet (see Chapter 5). For weight management, pay special attention to total calories, portion sizes, energy density, and eating habits.

Total Calories Chapter 5 includes suggestions for approximate daily energy intakes based on gender, age, and activity level. However, energy balance may be a more important consideration for weight management than total calories consumed (refer back to Figure 4.2). To maintain your current weight, the total number of calories you eat must equal the number you burn. To lose weight, you must decrease your calorie intake or increase the number of calories you burn (or both); to gain weight, the reverse is true. (One kilogram of body fat represents 7000 calories.)

The best approach for weight loss is combining an increase in physical activity with moderate calorie restriction. Don't go on a crash diet. To maintain weight loss, you will probably have to maintain some degree of the calorie restriction you used to lose the weight. Therefore, you need to adopt a level of food intake that provides all the essential nutrients and that you can live with over the long term. For most people, maintaining weight loss is more difficult than losing the weight.

Portion Sizes Overconsumption of total calories is closely tied to portion sizes. Many Canadians are unaware that the portions of packaged foods and of foods served at restaurants have increased in size, and most of us significantly underestimate the amount of food we eat. Studies have found that the larger the meal, the greater the underestimation of calories.

People also commonly eat much more of the foods that they perceive as being healthy, but in the process consume far more calories than they need. Limiting portion sizes is critical for maintaining good health. For many people, concentrating on portion sizes is easier than counting calories.

To counteract portion distortion, weigh and measure your food at home for a few days every now and then. In addition, check the serving sizes listed on packaged foods. With practice, you'll learn to judge portion sizes more accurately. When eating out, try to order the smallest-sized items on the menu. It is especially important to limit serving sizes of foods that are high in calories and low in nutrients. Don't supersize your meals and snacks; although huge servings may seem like the best deal, it is more important to order just what you need. Refer to Chapter 5 for more information on choosing appropriate portion sizes.

Energy (Calorie) Density Experts also recommend that you pay attention to *energy density*—the number of calories per gram of food. Studies suggest that it isn't consumption of a certain amount of fat or calories in food that reduces hunger and leads to feelings of fullness and satisfaction; rather, it is consumption of a certain weight of food. Foods that are low in energy density have more volume and bulk—that is, they are relatively heavy but have few calories (see Table 4.3). For example, for the same 100 calories, you could eat 21 baby carrots or 4 pretzel twists; you are more likely to feel full after eating the serving of carrots because it weighs 10 times as much as the serving of pretzels (280 grams versus 28 grams).

Fresh fruits and vegetables, with their high water and fibre content, are low in energy density, as are whole-grain foods. Fresh fruits contain fewer calories and more fibre than fruit juices or drinks. Meat, ice cream, potato chips, croissants, crackers, and cakes and cookies are examples of foods high in energy density. Strategies for lowering the energy density of your diet include the following:

- Eat fruit with breakfast and for dessert.
- Add extra vegetables to sandwiches, casseroles, stir-fry dishes, pizza, pasta dishes, and fajitas.
- Start meals with a bowl of broth-based soup; include a green salad or fruit salad.
- Snack on fresh fruits and vegetables rather than crackers, chips, or other energy-dense snack foods.

Limit serving sizes of energy-dense foods, such as butter, mayonnaise, cheese, chocolate, fatty meats, and croissants, and snack foods that are fried, high in added sugars (including sugar substitutes and reduced-fat products), or contain trans fats. It is also important to watch out for processed foods, which can be high in fat and sodium. Even processed foods labelled "fat free" or "reduced fat" may be high in calories; such products may contain sugar or fat substitutes. And although a number of sugar substitutes (such as Aspartame and Sorbitol) have been approved for use in Canada, controversy about potential long-term side effects continues. Many of the foods containing fat and sugar substitutes are low-nutrient snack foods. Although substituting a lower-fat or lower-sugar version of the same food may be beneficial, fruits, vegetables, and whole grains are healthier snack choices. Otherwise, stick to the calorie and nutrient recommendations offered in *Eating Well with Canada's Food Guide*. These guidelines are described in detail in Chapter 5.

Table 4.3	Examples of Foods Low in Energy Density	
Food	**Amount**	**Calories**
Egg substitute	60 mL (1/4 cup)	30
Plain instant oatmeal	85 g (1/2 cup)	80
Fresh blueberries	130 g (1 cup)	80
Corn on the cob (plain)	1 ear	80
Cantaloupe	1/2 melon	95
Unsweetened apple sauce	250 mL (1 cup)	100
Pear	1 medium	100
Mixed vegetables	130 g (1 cup)	110
Sweet potato	1 medium	120

Eating Habits Equally important to weight management is the habit of eating several small meals—four to five meals per day, including breakfast and snacks—on a regular schedule. Skipping meals leads to excessive hunger, feelings of deprivation, and increased vulnerability to binge eating or snacking. In addition to establishing a regular pattern of eating, set some rules to govern your food choices. Rules for breakfast might be these, for example: Choose a (naturally) sugar-free, high-fibre cereal with fat-free milk on most days; have a hard-boiled egg (no more than three per week); save pancakes and waffles for special occasions, unless they are whole grain. For effective weight management, it is better to consume the majority of calories during the day rather than in the evening.

Decreeing some foods off limits generally sets up a rule to be broken. A more sensible principle is "everything in moderation." If a particular food becomes troublesome, place it off limits until you gain control over it. The ultimate goal is to eat in moderation; no foods need to be entirely off limits, though some should be eaten judiciously.

Physical Activity and Exercise

Regular physical activity is a very important lifestyle factor in weight management. Physical activity and exercise burn calories and keep the metabolism geared to using food for energy instead of storing it as fat. Making *significant* cuts in food intake to lose weight can be a difficult strategy to maintain; increasing your physical activity tends to be a more easily tolerated approach for the long term. Additional good news about physical activity and weight management is that researchers have found that exercise does not automatically prompt increases in feelings of hunger (to replace the energy used from activity). And, in some situations, exercise can suppress appetite. Regular physical activity protects against weight gain, is essential for maintaining weight loss, and improves quality of life (see the box "Exercise, Body Image, and Self-Esteem" on p. 112). The sooner you establish good habits, the better. The key to success is making exercise an integral part of the lifestyle you can enjoy now and in the future. Chapter 6 contains many suggestions for becoming a more active, physically fit person.

Thinking and Emotions

The way you think about yourself and your world influences, and is influenced by, how you feel and how you act. In fact, research on people who have a weight problem indicates that low self-esteem and the negative emotions that accompany it are significant problems. Often, people with low self-esteem mentally compare the actual self to an internally held picture of an ideal self, an image based on perfectionistic goals and beliefs about how they and others should be. The more these two pictures differ, the larger the impact on self-esteem and the more likely the presence of negative emotions.

Along with the internal picture we carry of ourselves, we all carry on an internal dialogue about events happening to us and around us. This *self-talk* can be either self-deprecating or positively motivating, depending on our beliefs and attitudes. Having realistic beliefs and goals, and practising positive self-talk and problem solving support a healthy lifestyle.

Coping Strategies

Appropriate coping strategies help you deal with the stresses of life; they are also an important lifestyle factor in weight management. Many people use eating as a way to cope; others may cope by turning to drugs, alcohol, smoking, or gambling. Those who overeat might use food to alleviate loneliness or to serve as a pickup for fatigue, as an antidote to boredom, or as a distraction from problems. Some people even overeat to punish themselves for real or imagined transgressions.

Those who recognize that they are misusing food in such ways can analyze their eating habits with fresh eyes. They can consciously attempt to find new coping strategies and begin to use food appropriately—to fuel life's activities, to foster growth, and to bring pleasure, but *not* as a way to manage stress. For a summary of the components of weight management through healthy lifestyle choices, see the box "Lifestyle Strategies for Successful Weight Management" on p. 113.

APPROACHES TO OVERCOMING A WEIGHT PROBLEM

What should you do if you are overweight? You have several options.

Doing It Yourself

If you need to lose weight, decide what is important about doing so: Is this a way to be kinder to yourself? Treat yourself with more respect? Reduce potential health risks? All of the above? Once you've decided for yourself why it is important for you to lose weight, focus on adopting the healthy lifestyle described throughout this book. The right weight for you will naturally evolve, and you won't have to diet. Combine modest cuts in energy intake with

Exercise, Body Image, and Self-Esteem

If you gaze into the mirror and wish you could change the way your body looks, consider getting some exercise—not to reshape your contours but to firm up your body image and enhance your self-esteem. In a recent study, 82 adults completed a 12-week aerobic exercise program and had 12 months of follow-up. Compared with the control group, these participants improved their fitness and also benefited psychologically in tests of mood, anxiety, and self-concept. These same physical and psychological benefits were still significant at the one-year follow-up.

One reason for the findings may be that people who exercise regularly often gain a sense of mastery and competence that enhances their self-esteem and body image. In addition, exercise contributes to a more toned look, which many adults prefer.

Research suggests that physically active people are more comfortable with their body and their image than sedentary people are. In one workplace study, 60 employees were asked to complete a 36-session stretching program whose main purpose was to prevent muscle strains at work. At the end of the program, besides the significant increase by all participants in measurements of flexibility, their perceptions of their bodies improved and so did their overall sense of self-worth.

Similar results were obtained in a Norwegian study, in which 219 middle-aged people at risk for heart disease were randomly assigned to one of four groups: (1) diet, (2) diet plus exercise, (3) exercise, and (4) no intervention. The greater the participation of individuals in the exercise component of the program, the higher were their scores in perceived competence and self-esteem and coping.

---

exercise, and avoid very-low-calorie diets. (In general, a low-calorie diet should have 1500–1800 calories per day.) By producing a negative energy balance of 250–1000 calories per day, you will produce the recommended weight loss of 0.25 to 1 kilogram per week.

Don't try to lose weight more rapidly. Most low-calorie diets cause a rapid loss of body water at first. When this phase passes, weight loss slows. As a result, dieters are often misled into believing that their efforts are not working. They then give up, not realizing that smaller, mostly fat, losses later in the diet are actually better than the initial larger, mostly fluid losses. Reasonable weight loss is 8%–10% of body weight over six months.

For many Canadians, maintaining weight loss is a bigger challenge than losing weight. Most weight lost during dieting is regained. When planning a weight-management program, it is extremely important to include strategies that you can maintain over the long term, both for food choices and for physical activity. Weight management is a lifelong project. A registered dietitian or nutritionist can recommend an appropriate plan for you when you want to lose weight on your own. For more tips, refer to the Behaviour Change Strategy at the end of the chapter.

Diet Books and Fad Diets

Many people who try to lose weight by themselves try using one or more of the dozens of diet books on the market or following a fad diet. Although some contain useful advice and motivational tips, most make empty promises. Fad diets are frequently promoted in the media as offering quick and easy weight loss, but weight that is lost quickly is often regained. In many cases, the person gains even more weight back. Typically based on unsound nutrition or the elimination of certain foods or even entire food groups, fad diets may not meet a person's nutrient and calorie requirements. Here are some guidelines for evaluating and choosing a diet book and recognizing a fad diet book:

- Reject books that advocate an unbalanced way of eating, such as a carbohydrate-only diet or a low-carbohydrate, high-protein diet. Also reject books that promote a single food, such as cabbage or grapefruit.

- Reject books that claim to be based on a "scientific breakthrough" or to have the "secret to success."

- Reject books that use gimmicks, such as matching eating to blood type, hyping insulin resistance as the single cause of obesity, combining foods in special ways to achieve weight loss, rotating levels of calories, or purporting that a weight problem is due to food allergies, food sensitivities, yeast infections, or hormone imbalances.

- Reject books that promise quick weight loss, that limit the selection of foods, or that promise more than one kilogram of weight loss each week.

Lifestyle Strategies for Successful Weight Management

Food Choices

• Follow the recommendations in *Eating Well with Canada's Food Guide* for eating a moderate, varied diet. Focus on making good choices from each food group.

• Favour foods with a low energy density and a high nutrient density.

• Check food labels for serving sizes, calories, and nutrient levels.

• Watch for hidden calories. Reduced-fat foods often have as many calories as their full-fat versions. Fat-based condiments, such as butter, margarine, mayonnaise, and salad dressings, provide about 100 calories per tablespoon; added sugars, such as jams, jellies, and syrup, are also packed with calories.

• Drink fewer calories in the form of pop, fruit drinks, sports drinks, alcohol, and specialty coffees and teas.

• For problem foods, try eating small amounts under controlled conditions. Go out for a scoop of ice cream, for example, rather than buying a couple of litres for your freezer.

Planning and Serving

• Keep a log of what you eat. Before you begin your program, your log will provide a realistic picture of your current diet and what changes you can make. Once you start your program, a log will keep you focused on your food choices and portion sizes. Track the food eaten, your hunger level, the circumstances (location, other activities), outside influences (environment, other people), and your thoughts and emotions.

• Eat four to five meals and snacks daily, *including breakfast*, to distribute calories throughout your day. In studies, people who eat breakfast consume fewer calories overall over the course of the day. Make more meals yourself and eat out less often. Keep low-calorie snacks on hand to combat the munchies: baby carrots, popcorn, and fresh fruits and vegetables are good choices.

• When shopping, make a list and stick to it. Don't shop when you're hungry. Avoid aisles that contain problem foods. Generally, the perimeter of the grocery store contains the healthier choices.

• Consume the majority of your daily calories during the day, not in the evening.

• Pay special attention to portion sizes. Use measuring cups and spoons and a food scale to become more familiar with appropriate portion sizes.

• Serve meals on small plates and in small bowls to help you eat smaller portions without feeling deprived.

• Eat only in specifically designated spots. Remove food from other areas of your home.

• When you eat, just eat—don't do anything else, such as reading or watching TV.

• Avoid late-night eating, a behaviour specifically associated with weight gain among university students.

• Eat slowly. It takes time for your brain to get the message that your stomach is full. Take small bites and chew food thoroughly. Pay attention to every bite, and enjoy your food.

Between bites, try putting your fork or spoon down and taking sips of a beverage.

• When you're done eating, remove your plate. Cue yourself that the meal is over; drink a glass of water, suck on a mint, chew gum, or brush your teeth.

Special Occasions

• When you eat out, choose a restaurant where you can make healthy food choices. Ask the server not to put bread and butter on the table before the meal, and request that sauces and salad dressings be served on the side. If portion sizes are large, take half your food home for a meal later in the week. Don't choose supersized meals.

• If you cook a large meal for friends, send leftovers home with your guests.

• If you're eating at a friend's, eat a little and leave the rest. Don't eat to be polite; if someone offers you food you don't want, thank the person and decline firmly.

• Take care during the winter holidays. Research indicates that people gain less than they think during the winter holidays (about a half kilogram) but that the weight isn't lost during the rest of the year, leading to slow, steady weight gain.

Physical Activity and Stress Management

• Increase your level of daily physical activity. If you have been sedentary for a long time or are seriously overweight, increase your level of activity slowly. Start by walking 10 minutes at a time, and work toward 30–60 minutes or more of moderate physical activity per day.

• Begin a formal exercise program that includes cardiorespiratory endurance exercise, strength training, and stretching.

• Develop techniques for handling stress. Try walking, or use a relaxation technique. Practise positive self-talk. Get adequate sleep. (See Chapter 3 for more on stress management.)

• Develop strategies for coping with nonhunger cues to eat, such as boredom, sleepiness, or anxiety. Try calling a friend, taking a shower, or reading a magazine.

• Tell family members and friends that you're changing your eating and exercise habits. Ask them to be supportive.

- Reject books that require you to meet your nutritional needs with supplements instead of food.

- Reject books that advocate diets for men with fewer than 1800 calories a day and for women with fewer than 1500 calories a day.

- Reject books that promote the idea that it is healthy to lose more than one kilogram a week.

- Accept books that advocate a balanced approach to diet along with exercise and sound nutrition advice.

Many diets can cause weight loss if maintained; the real difficulty is finding a safe and healthy pattern of food choices and physical activity that results in long-term maintenance of a healthy body weight and reduced risk of chronic disease (see the box "Is Any Diet Best for Weight Loss?").

Dietary Supplements and Diet Aids

The number of dietary supplements and other weight-loss aids on the market has also increased in recent years. Promoted in advertisements, magazines, direct mail campaigns, infomercials, and Web sites, these products typically promise a quick and easy path to weight loss. Most of these products are marketed as dietary supplements and so are subject to fewer regulations than over-the-counter (OTC) medications. A 2002 report stated that more than half of advertisements for weight-loss products made representations that are likely to be false. In addition, use of OTC products doesn't help in the adoption of lifestyle behaviours that can help people achieve and maintain a healthy weight over the long term.

The bottom line on nonprescription diet aids is caveat emptor—let the buyer beware. There is no quick and easy way to lose weight. The most effective approach is to develop healthy diet and exercise habits and make them a permanent part of your life. The following sections describe some commonly marketed OTC products for weight loss.

Formula Drinks and Food Bars Canned diet drinks, powders used to make shakes, and diet food bars and snacks are designed to achieve weight loss by substituting for some or all of a person's daily food intake. However, most people find it difficult to use these products for long periods, and muscle loss and other serious health problems may result if they are used as the sole source of nutrition for an extended period. Use of such products sometimes results in rapid short-term weight loss, but the weight is typically regained because users don't learn to change their eating and lifestyle behaviours.

Herbal Supplements As described in Chapter 5, herbs are marketed as dietary supplements (natural health products), and so little information is available about effectiveness, proper dosage, drug interactions, and side effects. In addition, labels may not accurately list the ingredients

Many supplements are promoted for weight loss, but few have any research supporting their effectiveness for long-term weight management.

and dosages, and safe manufacturing practices are not guaranteed. For example, the substitution of a toxic herb for another compound during the manufacture of a Chinese herbal weight-loss preparation caused more than 100 cases of kidney damage and cancer among users in Europe.

In 2002, Health Canada issued a health advisory about the sale of ephedra (*ma huang*), stating that it presents a significant and unreasonable risk to human health. Ephedrine, the active ingredient in ephedra, is structurally similar to amphetamine and was widely used in weight-loss supplements. It may suppress appetite, but adverse effects have included elevated blood pressure, panic attacks, seizures, insomnia, and increased risk of heart attack or stroke, particularly when combined with another stimulant, such as caffeine. Products containing ephedra for sale in Canada must be caffeine free and must not have more than 8 milligrams of ephedrine per dose. Other herbal stimulants are described in Table 4.4 on p. 116.

Other Supplements Fibre is another common ingredient in OTC diet aids, promoted for appetite control. However, dietary fibre acts as a bulking agent in the large intestine, not the stomach, and so it doesn't have a pronounced effect on appetite. In addition, many diet aids contain only 3 grams of fibre or fewer, which does not contribute much toward the recommended daily intake of 25–38 grams. Other popular dietary supplements

Is Any Diet Best for Weight Loss?

Experts agree that reducing calorie intake promotes weight loss. However, many popular weight-loss plans include a special hook and promote specific food choices and macronutrient (protein, fat, carbohydrate) combinations as best for weight loss. Research findings have been mixed, but two points are clear. Total calorie intake matters, and the best diet is probably the one you can stick with. It stands to reason that if you go on a diet, you will eventually go off it; you are better off choosing a healthy dietary lifestyle that you can live with over the long term.

Low-Carbohydrate Diets

Some low-carbohydrate diets advocate fewer than 10% of total calories from carbohydrates, compared with the 45%–65% recommended by nutrition experts. Some suggest daily carbohydrate intake below the 130 grams needed to provide essential carbohydrates in the diet. Small studies have found that low-carbohydrate diets can help with short-term weight loss and be safe for relatively short periods of time—although unpleasant effects, such as bad breath, constipation, and headache, are fairly common.

Some low-carbohydrate diets tend to be very high in protein and saturated fat and low in fibre, whole grains, vegetables, and fruits (and thus lack some essential nutrients). Diets high in protein and saturated fat have been linked to an increased risk of heart disease, high blood pressure, and cancer. Other low-carbohydrate diets, though still emphasizing protein, limit saturated fats, allow most vegetables after an initial period, and advocate switching to "healthy carbs." These diets are healthier than the more extreme versions.

Low-Fat Diets

Many experts advocate diets that are relatively low in fat, high in carbohydrates, and moderate in protein. Critics of these diets blame them for rising rates of obesity and note that very-low-fat, very-high-carbohydrate diets can increase triglyceride levels and reduce levels of good (HDL) cholesterol in some people. These negative effects can be counteracted with moderate intensity exercise, however, and low-fat diets combined with physical activity can be safe and effective for many people.

Few experts take the position that low-fat, high-carbohydrate diets, apart from overall diet and activity patterns, are responsible for the increase in obesity among North Americans. However, the debate has highlighted the importance of total calorie intake and the quality of carbohydrate choices. A low-fat diet is not a licence to consume excess calories, even in low-fat foods.

How Do Popular Diets Measure Up?

In one recent study, obese people on a very-low-carbohydrate, high-fat diet lost more weight over six months than did people following a moderate-fat diet. After a year, however, the difference in weight loss between the two groups was no longer significant, and the dropout rate from both groups was high.

A 2005 study followed participants in four popular diets that emphasize different strategies—Weight Watchers (restricted portion sizes and calories), Atkins (low carbohydrate, high fat), the Zone (relatively high protein, moderate fat and carbohydrate), and Ornish (very low fat). Each of these diets modestly reduced body weight and heart disease risk factors. No significant difference in weight loss was found at one year among the

diets, and the more closely people adhered to each diet, the more weight they lost. Dropout rates were high—about 50% for Atkins and Ornish and 35% for Weight Watchers and the Zone.

Energy Balance Counts: The National Weight Control Registry

Future research may determine that certain macronutrient patterns are somewhat more helpful for disease reduction in people with particular risk profiles. In terms of weight loss, however, such differences among diets are likely overshadowed by the importance of total calorie intake and physical activity. Important lessons about energy balance can be drawn from the National Weight Control Registry, an ongoing study of people who have lost significant amounts of weight and kept it off. Although the Registry is based in the United States, it accepts members from anywhere in the world. Participants have lost an average of 32 kilograms and kept the weight off for more than five years. Nearly all participants use a combination of diet and exercise to manage their weight. Most consume diets moderate in calories and relatively low in fat and fried foods; they monitor their body weight and their food intake frequently. Participants engage in an average of 60 minutes of moderate physical activity daily. The National Weight Control Registry study illustrates that to lose weight and keep it off, you must decrease daily calorie intake or increase daily physical activity—and continue to do so over your lifetime.

Sources: Battle of the diet books II. 2006. *Nutrition Action Healthletter*, July/August; Dansinger, M. L., et al. 2005. Comparison of the Atkins, Ornish, Weight Watchers, and Zone diets for weight loss and heart disease risk reduction. *Journal of the American Medical Association* 293(1): 43–53; Hays, N. P., et al. 2004. Effects of an ad libitum low-fat, high-carbohydrate diet on body weight, body composition, and fat distribution in older men and women. *Archives of Internal Medicine* 164(2): 210–217. Hill, J., and R. Wing. 2003. The National Weight Control Registry. *Permanente Journal* 7(3): 34–37; Bravata, D. M., et al. 2003. Efficacy and safety of low-carbohydrate diets. *Journal of the American Medical Association* 289: 1837–1850; Foster, G. D., et al. 2003. A randomized trial of low-carbohydrate diet for obesity. *New England Journal of Medicine* 348: 2082–2090. Screenshot from The National Weight Control Registry reprinted with permission.

Table 4.4 — Ingredients Commonly Found in Weight-Loss Products

Common Name	Use/Claim	Evidence/Efficacy	Safety Issues
Bitter orange extract (Citrus aurantium)	CNS stimulant	Limited evidence	Highly concentrated extracts may increase blood pressure; should not be used by people with cardiac problems
Caffeine	CNS stimulant; increases fat metabolism	Amplifies effects of ephedra	Generally considered safe; caution advised in caffeine-sensitive individuals
Garcinia cambogia	May interfere with fat metabolism or suppress appetite	Inconclusive evidence	Short-term use (<12 weeks) generally considered safe when used as directed
Green tea extract	Diuretic; increases metabolism	Limited evidence	Generally considered safe
Guarana	CNS stimulant; diuretic	Few clinical trials	Same as for caffeine; overdose can cause painful urination, abdominal spasms, and vomiting
Senna, cascara, aloe, buckthorn berries	Stimulant, laxative	Not effective for weight loss	Chronic use decreases muscle tone in large intestine, causes electrolyte imbalances, and leads to dependence on laxatives
Tea, kola, dandelion, bucho, uva-ursi, damiana, juniper	Diuretic	Not effective for weight loss	Chronic use can cause electrolyte imbalance in some people
Yerba mate	Stimulant, laxative, diuretic	Limited evidence	Long-term use as a beverage may increase risk of oral cancer

Source: Adapted from Leslie, K. K. 2003. Herbal weight-loss products: Effective and appropriate? *Today's Dietician* 5(8): 12.

include conjugated linoleic acid, carnitine, chromium, pyruvate, calcium, B vitamins, chitosan, and a number of products labelled "fat absorbers," "fat blockers," and "starch blockers." Research has not found these products to be effective, and many have potentially adverse side effects.

Weight-Loss Programs

Weight-loss programs come in a variety of types, including noncommercial support organizations, commercial programs, Web sites, and clinical programs.

Noncommercial Weight-Loss Programs Noncommercial programs, such as TOPS (Take Off Pounds Sensibly) and Overeaters Anonymous (OA), mainly provide group support. They do not advocate any particular diet but do recommend seeking professional advice for creating an individualized plan. Like Alcoholics Anonymous, OA is a 12-step program with a spiritual orientation that promotes abstinence from compulsive overeating. These types of programs are generally free. Your physician or a registered dietitian can also provide information and support for weight loss.

Commercial Weight-Loss Programs Commercial weight-loss programs typically provide group support, nutrition education, physical activity recommendations, and behaviour modification advice. Some also make available packaged foods to assist in following dietary advice.

A 2005 study evaluated major commercial weight-loss programs, including Weight Watchers, NutriSystem,

Jenny Craig, and LA Weight Loss, for 12 weeks or more with a one-year follow-up assessment. Results showed Weight Watchers to be the only moderately priced commercial program with a mean loss of 5% of initial weight. A responsible and safe weight-loss program should have the following features:

- The recommended diet should be safe and balanced, include all the food groups, and meet the Daily Recommended Intakes (DRIs) for all nutrients. Regular physical activity and exercise should be strongly encouraged.

- The program should promote slow, steady weight loss averaging 0.25–1.0 kilogram per week. (Some greater weight loss may occur initially through fluid loss.)

- If a participant plans to lose more than 10 kilograms, has any health problems, or is taking medication on a regular basis, physician evaluation and monitoring should be recommended. The staff of the program should include qualified counsellors and health professionals.

- The program should include plans for weight maintenance after the weight-loss phase is over.

- The program should provide information on all fees and costs, including those of supplements and prepackaged foods, as well as data on risks and expected outcomes of participating in the program.

In addition, you should consider whether a program fits your lifestyle and whether you are truly ready to make a commitment to it. A strong commitment and a plan for maintenance are especially important because only about 10%–15% of program participants maintain their weight loss—the rest gain back all or more than they had lost. One study of participants found that regular exercise was the best predictor of maintaining weight loss, whereas frequent television viewing was the best predictor of weight gain.

Online Weight-Loss Programs   A recent addition to the weight-loss program scene is the Internet-based program. Most such Web sites provide a cross between self-help and group support through chat rooms, bulletin boards, and e-newsletters. Many sites offer online self-assessment for diet, physical activity habits, and meal plans; some provide access to a staff professional for individualized help. Many are free, but some charge a small weekly or monthly fee.

Preliminary research suggests that this type of program provides an alternative to in-person diet counselling and can lead to weight loss for some people. Studies found that people who logged on to Internet programs more frequently tended to lose more weight; weekly online contact proved most successful for weight loss. The criteria used to evaluate commercial programs can also be applied to Internet-based programs. In addition, the program should offer member-to-member support and access to staff professionals.

Clinical Weight-Loss Programs   Medically supervised clinical programs are usually located in a hospital or other medical setting. Designed to help those who are severely obese, these programs typically involve a closely monitored very-low-calorie diet.

Prescription Drugs

For a medicine to cause weight loss, it must reduce energy consumption, increase energy expenditure, or interfere with energy absorption. The medications most often prescribed for weight loss are appetite suppressants that reduce feelings of hunger or increase feelings of fullness. Appetite suppressants usually work by increasing levels of catecholamine or serotonin, two brain chemicals that affect mood and appetite.

All prescription weight-loss drugs have potential side effects, and some are very dangerous. Most approved by Health Canada are only for short-term use but a few are approved for longer-term use, such as orlistat (Xenical). Orlistat is not an appetite suppressant but rather is considered an anti-obesity drug because it lowers calorie consumption by blocking fat absorption in the intestines; it prevents about 30% of the fat in food from being digested. Because orlistat reduces the absorption of fat-soluble vitamins and antioxidants, taking a vitamin supplement is highly recommended when taking orlistat. Its side effects include diarrhea, cramping, and other gastrointestinal problems if users do not follow a low-fat diet.

All medications work best in conjunction with behaviour modification. Studies have generally found that appetite suppressants produce modest weight loss—about 2–10 kilograms above the loss expected with nondrug obesity treatments. Individuals respond very differently, however, and some experience more weight loss than others. Unfortunately, weight loss tends to level off or reverse after four to six months on a medication, and many people regain the weight they've lost when they stop taking the drug.

Prescription weight-loss drugs are recommended only in certain cases: for people who have been unable to lose weight with nondrug options and who have a BMI higher than 30 (or higher than 27 if two or more additional risk factors, such as diabetes and high blood pressure, are present). For severely obese people who have been unable to lose weight by other methods, prescription drugs may provide a good option.

Surgery

It is estimated that 5.5 million Canadians have a BMI greater than 30 (obese) and 2.7 million have a BMI of 40 or greater (severely, or morbidly, obese). Canadian women are twice as likely as men to be morbidly obese. Severe obesity is a serious medical condition that is often complicated by other health problems, such as diabetes, sleep disorders, heart disease, and arthritis. Surgical intervention may be necessary as a treatment of last

> QUICK STATS
> About **1 in 35** adult Canadians has morbid obesity, meaning the person has a BMI of 40 or higher.
> —*Canadian Community Health Survey,* 2005

resort. According to the U.S. National Institutes of Health, gastric bypass surgery is recommended for patients with a BMI greater than 40, or greater than 35 with obesity-related illnesses. According to a 2010 article in *Canadian Family Physician,* several Canadian provinces are working to improve access to obesity surgery in our country.

Because of the increasing prevalence of severe obesity, surgical treatment of obesity is growing worldwide. Obesity-related health conditions, as well as risk of premature death, generally improve after surgical weight loss. However, lifestyle changes coupled with the surgery are essential for long-term success, and surgery is not without risks. A recent study found that patients with poor cardiorespiratory fitness before surgery experienced more postoperative complications, including stroke, kidney failure, and even death, than patients with higher fitness levels.

Gastric bypass surgery modifies the gastrointestinal tract by changing either the size of the stomach or how the intestine drains, thereby reducing food intake. Two of the most common surgeries are the Roux-en-Y gastric bypass and the vertical banded gastroplasty.

Roux-en-Y Gastric Bypass In the *Roux-en-Y gastric bypass* procedure, the stomach is separated into two pouches, one large and one small. A Y segment of the small intestine is attached to the smaller pouch. The small stomach pouch restricts food intake, and the bypass of the lower stomach and part of the small intestine results in the absorption of fewer calories (and nutrients). Side effects include fat intolerance, nutritional deficiencies, and dumping syndrome, which involves gastrointestinal distress.

Vertical Banded Gastroplasty In *vertical banded gastroplasty (VBG)*, a small gastric pouch is created in the upper part of the stomach by applying a double row of staples that essentially elongates the esophagus. This small pouch empties into the remaining stomach through an outlet that is restricted with a band. The procedure controls the gastric emptying of food and the volume of foods eaten. Common complications associated with this kind of surgery are nausea, vomiting, band slippage, gastroesophageal reflux, and stenosis (constriction of the outlet). When compared with Roux-en-Y gastric bypass, VBG has a lower initial weight loss and a greater weight regain.

In a variation of VGB, called Lap-Band, an adjustable band is placed around the stomach. The band is implanted laparoscopically, via a tube inserted through a small incision in the abdomen. The band ties off a portion of the stomach, creating a small pouch similar to that created in VGB surgery. The band is filled with saline and can be tightened or loosened by adding or removing saline through a small tube that exits through the patient's abdomen. The Lap-Band procedure has about the same success rate as VGB and is generally considered to be safe.

Weight loss from surgery generally ranges between 40% and 70% of total body weight in a year. In a 2006 study that included mild to moderately obese (BMI 30–35) adults, gastric banding surgery was significantly more effective in reducing weight and improving quality of life than nonsurgical methods, even after two years. For surgical procedures, the key to success is to have adequate follow-up and to stay motivated so that lifestyle behaviours and eating patterns are changed permanently. Behavioural counselling should be done in conjunction with surgery—the surgery physically reduces a person's ability to eat large amounts of food, but it doesn't change that person's eating behaviours and food choices or identify psychosocial reasons for overeating or not exercising.

Liposuction Another procedure, *liposuction*, has become popular for removing localized fat deposits. More than 24,000 Canadians underwent liposuction in 2003. This cosmetic procedure does not improve health the way weight loss does and involves considerable pain and discomfort.

Professional Help

Some obesity experts argue that how we eat and whether we exercise can be symptoms of how we feel about ourselves; if we help people deal with other challenges in their lives, weight loss may follow. A recent Canadian study that evaluated the effect of one-on-one life coaching, with a certified coach, on the waist circumference, BMI, self-esteem, physical activity, and functional health status of 20 adults with obesity found that after six to eight sessions, participants experienced significant decreases in their waist circumference and increases in self-esteem and functional health status. Qualitatively, participants reported an increase in daily physical activity and healthier dietary choices, feelings of optimism, and greater self-acceptance. The researchers concluded that the particular form of life coaching used shows promise as an intervention for obesity and that more research should be conducted.

When concern about body weight develops into an eating disorder, the help of a professional is recommended. In choosing a therapist, be sure to ask about credentials and experience (see Chapter 2). The therapist should have experience working with weight management, body image issues, eating disorders, addictions, and abuse issues.

BODY IMAGE

As described earlier in the chapter, body image consists of perceptions, images, thoughts, attitudes, and emotions. Developing a positive body image is an important aspect of psychological wellness and an important component of successful weight management.

Severe Body Image Problems

Poor body image can cause significant psychological distress. A person can become preoccupied with a perceived defect in appearance, thereby damaging self-esteem and interfering with relationships. Adolescents and adults who have a negative body image are more likely to diet restrictively, eat compulsively, or develop some other form of disordered eating.

When dissatisfaction becomes extreme, the condition is called *body dysmorphic disorder (BDD)*. It is estimated that BDD affects about 350,000 Canadians, males and females in equal numbers. BDD usually begins before

QUESTIONS FOR CRITICAL THINKING AND REFLECTION

Why do you think people continue to buy into fad diets and weight-loss gimmicks, even though they are constantly reminded that the key to weight management is lifestyle change? Have you ever tried a fad diet or dietary supplement? If so, what were your reasons for trying it? What were the results?

Does Someone You Know Have an Eating Disorder?

Secrecy and denial are two hallmarks of eating disorders, and so it can be hard to know if someone has anorexia or bulimia. Signs that someone may have anorexia include sudden weight loss, excessive dieting or exercise, guilt or preoccupation with food or eating, frequent weighing, fear of becoming fat despite being thin, and the wearing of baggy or layered clothes to conceal weight loss. Signs that someone may have bulimia include excessive eating without weight gain, secretiveness about food (stealing, hiding, or hoarding food), self-induced vomiting (bathroom visits during or after a meal), swollen glands or a puffy face, erosion of tooth enamel, and use of laxatives, diuretics, or diet pills to control weight.

If you decide to approach a friend with your concerns, here are some tips to follow:

• Find out about treatment resources in your community (see the For More Information section for suggestions). You may want to consult a professional at your school clinic or counselling centre about the best way to approach the situation.

• Arrange to speak with your friend in a private place, and allow enough time to talk.

• Express your concerns, with specific observations of your friend's behaviour. Expect him or her to deny or minimize the problem and possibly to become angry with you. Stay calm and nonjudgmental, and continue to express your concern.

• Avoid giving simplistic advice about eating habits. Listen if your friend wants to talk, and offer your support and understanding. Give your friend the information you found about where he or she can get help, and offer to go along.

• If the situation is an emergency—if your friend has fainted, for example, or attempted suicide—call 911 for help immediately.

• If you are upset about the situation, consider talking to someone yourself. The professionals at the clinic or counselling centre can help you, too. Remember, you are not to blame for another person's eating disorder.

If you suspect you have an eating problem, don't go it alone or delay getting help: Disordered eating habits can develop into a full-blown eating disorder. Check with your student health or counselling centre—nearly all universities and colleges have counsellors and medical personnel who can help you or refer you to a specialist if needed. If you are concerned about the eating habits of a family member or friend, refer to the suggestions in the box "Does Someone You Know Have an Eating Disorder?" above.

Treating Eating Disorders

The treatment of eating disorders must address both problematic eating behaviours and the misuse of food to manage stress and emotions. Treatment for anorexia nervosa first involves averting a medical crisis by restoring adequate body weight, and then the psychological aspects of the disorder can be addressed. The treatment of bulimia nervosa or binge-eating disorder involves first stabilizing the eating patterns, then identifying and changing the patterns of thinking that led to disordered eating, and then improving coping skills. Concurrent problems, such as depression or anxiety, must also be addressed.

In 2006, a study published in the *Journal of the American Medical Association* showed that the antidepressant Prozac, which is widely used to treat anorexia, worked no better than a placebo in preventing recurrence in women recovering from the disorder. However, the anti-seizure drug topiramate has shown promise in the treatment of bulimia by reducing the urges to binge and purge.

Treatment of eating disorders usually involves a combination of psychotherapy and medical management. The therapy may be carried out individually or in a group; sessions involving the entire family may be recommended. A support or self-help group can be a useful adjunct to such treatment. Medical professionals, including physicians, dentists, gynecologists, and registered dietitians, can evaluate and manage the physical damage caused by the disorder. If a patient is severely depressed or emaciated, hospitalization may be necessary.

QUICK STATS

Canadian women hospitalized with an eating disorder are **twice** as likely to have depression than the national average.

—*National Population Health Survey,* 2000

A Weight-Management Program

The behaviour-management plan described in Chapter 1 provides an excellent framework for a weight-management program. The following are some suggestions about specific ways you can adapt that general plan to controlling your weight.

Motivation and Commitment

Make sure you are motivated and committed before you begin. Failure at weight loss is a frustrating experience that can make it more difficult to lose weight in the future. Think about why you want to lose weight. Self-focused reasons, such as to feel good about yourself or to have a greater sense of well-being, are often associated with success. Trying to lose weight for others or out of concern for how others view you is a poor foundation for a weight-loss program. Make a list of your reasons for wanting to lose weight, and post it in a prominent place.

Setting Goals

Choose a reasonable weight you think you would like to reach over the long term, and be willing to renegotiate it as you get further along. Break down your long-term weight and behavioural goals into a series of short-term goals. Develop a new way of behaving by designing small, manageable steps that will get you to where you want to go.

Creating a Negative Energy Balance

When your weight is constant, you are burning approximately the same number of calories as you are taking in. To tip the energy balance toward weight loss, you must either consume fewer calories or burn more calories through physical activity or both. One kilogram of body fat represents 7000 calories. To lose weight at the recommended rate of 0.25–1.0 kilogram per week, you must create a negative energy balance of 1750–7000 calories per week or 250–1000 calories per day. To generate a negative energy balance, it's important to consider increasing your activity level and evaluating your calorie consumption.

Physical Activity

Consider how you can increase your energy output simply by increasing routine physical activity, such as walking or taking the stairs. (Chapter 6 lists some activities that use about 150 calories.) If you are not already involved in a regular exercise routine aimed at increasing endurance and building or maintaining muscle mass, seek help from someone who is competent to help you plan and start an appropriate exercise routine. If you are already doing regular physical exercise, evaluate your program according to the guidelines in Chapter 6.

Don't try to use exercise to spot reduce. Leg lifts, for example, contribute to fat loss only to the extent that they burn calories; they don't burn fat just from your legs. You can make parts of your body appear more fit by exercising them, but the only way you can reduce fat in any specific part of your body is to create an overall negative energy balance.

Diet and Eating Habits

If you can't generate a large enough negative energy balance solely by increasing physical activity, you may want to supplement exercise with modest cuts in your calorie intake. Don't think of this as going on a diet; your goal is to make small changes in your diet that you can maintain for a lifetime. Focus on cutting your intake of saturated and trans fats and added sugars and on eating a variety of nutritious foods in moderation. Don't skip meals, fast, or go on a very-low-calorie diet or a diet that is unbalanced.

Making changes in eating habits is another important strategy for weight management. If your program centres on a conscious restriction of certain food items, you're likely to spend all your time thinking about the forbidden foods. Focus on *how* to eat rather than *what* to eat. Refer to the box "Lifestyle Strategies for Successful Weight Management" (on p. 113) for suggestions.

Self-Monitoring

Keep a record of your weight and behaviour change progress. Try keeping a record of everything you eat. Write down what you plan to eat, in what quantity, *before* you eat. You'll find that just having to record something that is not OK to eat right now is likely to stop you from eating it. If you also note what seems to be triggering your urges to eat (for example, you feel bored, or someone offered you something), you'll become more aware of your triggers and be better able to take corrective action. Also, keep track of your daily activities and your formal exercise program so you can monitor increases in physical activity.

Putting Your Plan into Action

- Examine the environmental cues that trigger poor eating and exercise habits, and devise strategies for dealing with them. For example, you may need to remove problem foods from your house temporarily or put a sign on the refrigerator reminding you to go for a walk instead of having a snack. Anticipate problem situations, and plan ways to handle them more effectively. Create new environmental cues that will support your new healthy behaviours. Put your walking shoes by the front door. Move fruits and vegetables to the front of the refrigerator.

- Get others to help. Talk to friends and family members about what they can do to support your efforts. Find a buddy to join you in your exercise program.

- Give yourself lots of praise and rewards. Think about your accomplishments and achievements and congratulate yourself. Plan special nonfood treats for yourself, such as a walk or a movie. Reward yourself often and for anything that counts toward success.

- If you slip, tell yourself to get back on track immediately, and don't waste time on self-criticism. Think positively instead of getting into a cycle of guilt and self-blame. Don't demand too much of yourself.

- Don't get discouraged. Be aware that although weight loss is bound to slow down after the first loss of body fluid, the weight loss at this slower rate is more permanent than earlier, more dramatic, losses.

- Remember that weight management is a lifelong project. You need to adopt reasonable goals and strategies that you can maintain over the long term.

Practise and learn online with Connect. Connect allows you to practise important skills at your own pace and on your own schedule, with 24/7 online access to an eBook, practice quizzes, interactivities, videos, study tools, additional resources, and more.

SUMMARY

- Body composition is the relative amounts of fat-free mass and fat in the body. *Overweight* and *obesity* refer to body weight or the percentage of body fat that exceeds what is associated with good health.

- The key to weight management is maintaining a balance of calories in (food) and calories out (resting metabolism, food digestion, and physical activity).

- Standards for assessing body weight and body composition include the body mass index (BMI) and percent body fat.

- Too much or too little body fat is linked to health problems; the distribution of body fat can also be a significant risk factor.

- An inaccurate or negative body image is common and can lead to psychological distress.

- Genetic factors help determine a person's weight, but the influence of heredity can be overcome with attention to lifestyle factors.

- Physiological factors involved in the regulation of body weight and body fat include metabolic rate, hormonal influences, and the size and number of fat cells.

- Nutritional guidelines for weight management include consuming a moderate number of calories; limiting portion sizes, energy density, and the intake of fat, simple sugars, refined carbohydrates, and protein to recommended levels; and developing an eating schedule and rules for food choices.

- Activity guidelines for weight management emphasize daily physical activity and regular sessions of cardiorespiratory endurance exercise and strength training.

- Weight management requires developing positive, realistic self-talk and self-esteem and a repertoire of appropriate techniques for handling stress and other emotional and physical challenges.

- Many people are successful at long-term weight loss on their own by combining diet and exercise.

- Diet books, fad diets, OTC diet aids and supplements, and formal weight-loss programs should be assessed for safety and efficacy.

- Professional help is needed in cases of severe or morbid obesity; medical treatments include prescription drugs, surgery, and psychological therapy.

- Dissatisfaction with weight and shape are common to all eating disorders. Anorexia nervosa is characterized by self-starvation, distorted body image, and an intense fear of gaining weight. Bulimia nervosa is characterized by recurrent episodes of uncontrolled binge eating and frequent purging. Binge-eating disorder involves binge eating without regular use of compensatory purging.

FOR MORE INFORMATION

BOOKS

Critser, G. 2004. *Fat Land: How Americans Became the Fattest People in the World.* Boston: Mariner Books. A look at the many factors in American life that have contributed to the rapid increase in obesity rates.

Dillon, E. 2006. *Issues That Concern You: Obesity.* New York: Greenhaven Press. A collection of perspectives on the causes of obesity, its management, and its impact on individuals and society.

Ferguson, J. M., and C. Ferguson. 2003. *Habits Not Diets,* 4th ed. Boulder, Colo.: Bull. A behaviour change approach to changing diet and activity habits that includes many helpful practical tips, assessment worksheets, and tracking forms.

Gaesser, G. A., and K. Kratina. 2006. *It's the Calories, Not the Carbs.* Victoria, B.C.: Trafford. A detailed look at the facts behind successful weight loss that shuns fad diets and encourages sound energy balance.

Hensrud, D. D. 2005. *Mayo Clinic Healthy Weight for Everyone.* Rochester, Minn.: Mayo Clinic. Guidelines for successful weight management.

Ihde, G. M. 2006. *Considering Weight-Loss Surgery: The Facts You Need to Know for a Healthy Recovery.* Victoria, B.C.: Trafford. An easy-to-read guide to the benefits and risks of weight-loss surgery.

Milchovich, S. K., and B. Dunn-Long. 2007. *Diabetes Mellitus: A Practical Handbook,* 9th. ed. Boulder, Colo.: Bull. A user-friendly guide to diabetes.

ORGANIZATIONS, HOTLINES, AND WEB SITES

The Internet addresses listed here were accurate at the time of publication.

Canadian Diabetes Association. Provides information, literature, and guidance for living with and managing diabetes.

   http://www.diabetes.ca

Canadian Fitness and Lifestyle Research Institute. Provides research findings and recommendations to increase population levels of physical activity and improve the health of all Canadians.

   http://www.cflri.ca

Canadian Obesity Network. Provides Canadian obesity-related research, guidelines, and resources for everyone interested in reducing obesity rates.

   http://www.obesitynetwork.ca

Calorie Control Council. Provides a variety of interactive calculators, including an Exercise Calculator that estimates the calories burned from various forms of physical activity.

   http://www.caloriecontrol.org

Directory of Canada Eating Disorder Treatment Programs. Provides a comprehensive list of links to resources on eating disorders throughout Canada.

   http://www.canadadrugrehab.ca/Eating-Disorder-Treatment.html

*MedlinePlus: Eating Disorders.*Contains information from the U.S. National Library of Medicine.

   http://www.nlm.nih.gov/medlineplus/eatingdisorders.html

National Eating Disorders Information Centre. Provides information and resources on eating disorders and food and weight preoccupation.

   http://www.nedic.ca

SmallStep.gov. Provides resources for increasing activity and improving diet through small changes in daily habits.

   http://www.smallstep.gov

Something Fishy: Website on Eating Disorders
   http://www.something-fishy.org

U.S. National Heart, Lung, and Blood Institute: Aim for a Healthy Weight. Provides information and tips on diet and physical activity, as well as a BMI calculator.

   http://www.nhlbi.nih.gov/health/public/heart/obesity/lose_wt

See also the listings in Chapters 5 and 6.

SELECTED BIBLIOGRAPHY

Adams, K. F., et al. 2006. Overweight, obesity, and mortality in a large prospective cohort of persons 50 to 71 years old. *New England Journal of Medicine* 355(8): 763–778.

Baker, B. 2006. Weight loss and diet plans. *American Journal of Nursing* 106(6): 52–59.

Behn, A., and E. Ur. 2006. The obesity epidemic and its cardiovascular consequences. *Current Opinions in Cardiology* 21(4): 353–360.

Blundell, J. E., and King, N. A. 1999. Physical activity and regulation of food intake: current evidence. *Medicine and Science in Sports and Exercise* 31(11 Suppl.): S573-S583.

Bowman, S. A., et al. 2004. Effects of fast-food consumption on energy intake and diet quality among children in a national household survey. *Pediatrics* 113(1 Pt 1): 112–118.

Buchwald, H., et al. 2004. Bariatric surgery: A systematic review and meta-analysis. *Journal of the American Medical Association* 292(14): 1724–1737.

Canadian Medical Association. 2007. 2006 Canadian clinical practice guidelines on the management and prevention of obesity in adults and children, *CMAJ* 176 (8 Suppl.): 1–120 (http://www.cmaj.ca/cgi/content/full/176/8/S1/DC1; retrieved March 20, 2011).

Canada. House of Commons Health Committee. 2007. *Healthy Weights for Healthy Kids* (http://www.ccfn.ca/pdfs/HealthyWeightsForHealthyKids.pdf; retrieved March 17, 2011).

Chandon, P., and B. Wansink. 2007. The biasing health halos of fast-food restaurant health claims: Lower calorie estimates and higher side-dish consumption intentions. *Journal of Consumer Research* 34(3): 301–314.

Dahlman, I., and P. Arner. Obesity and polymorphisms in genes regulating human adipose tissue. *International Journal of Obesity* 31(11): 1629–1641.

Dhingra, R., et al. 2007. Soft drink consumption and risk of developing cardiometabolic risk factors and the metabolic syndrome in middle-aged adults in the community. *Circulation* 116(5): 480–488.

Dietz, W. H. 1994. Critical periods in childhood for the development of obesity. *American Journal of Clinical Nutrition* 59: 955959.

Dong, L., G. Block, and S. Mandel. 2004. Activities contributing to total energy expenditure in the United States: Results from the NHAPS Study. *International Journal of Behavioral Nutrition and Physical Activity* 1(4): 1–11.

Drewnowski, A., and F. Bellisle. 2007. Liquid calories, sugar and body weight. *American Journal of Clinical Nutrition* 85(3): 651–661.

Farshchi, H. R., M. A. Taylor, and I. A. Macdonald. 2005. Deleterious effects of omitting breakfast on insulin sensitivity and fasting lipid profiles in healthy lean women. *American Journal of Clinical Nutrition* 81(2): 388–396.

Flegal, K. M., et al. 2005. Excess deaths associated with underweight, overweight, and obesity. *Journal of the American Medical Association* 293(15): 1861–1867.

Fenicchia, L. M., et al. 2004. Influence of resistance exercise training on glucose control in women with type 2 diabetes. *Metabolism* 53(3): 284–289.

Fung, T. T., et al. 2004. Dietary patterns, meat intake, and the risk of type 2 diabetes in women. *Archives of Internal Medicine* 64(20): 2235–2240.

Graves, B. S., and R. L. Welsh. 2004. Recognizing the signs of body dysmorphic disorder and muscle dysmorphia. *ACSM's Health and Fitness Journal* 8(1): 11–13.

Hamilton, M., et al. 2007. Role of low energy expenditure and sitting in obesity, metabolic syndrome, type 2 diabetes, and cardiovascular disease. *Diabetes* 56(11): 2655–2667.

Health Canada. 2002. *A Report on Mental Illnesses in Canada* (http://www.cmha.ca/data/1/rec_docs/171_full_report_mic.pdf; retrieved March 20, 2011).

Hu, F. B., et al. 2004. Adiposity as compared with physical activity in predicting mortality among women. *New England Journal of Medicine* 351(26): 2694–2703.

Ibrahim, M. M. 2010. Etiology and pathophysiology: Subcutaneous and visceral adipose tissue: Structural and functional differences. *Obesity Reviews* 11: 11–18.

Kaiser Family Foundation. 2004. The role of media in childhood obesity. *Issue Brief*, February (http://www.kff.org/entmedia/upload/The-Role-Of-Media-in-Childhood-Obesity.pdf; retrieved March 20, 2011).

Kumanyika, S. K., et al. 2008. Population-based prevention of obesity: The need for comprehensive promotion of healthful eating, physical activity, and energy balance: A scientific statement from American Heart Association Council on Epidemiology and Prevention, Interdisciplinary Committee for Prevention (formerly the Expert Panel on Population and Prevention Science). *Circulation* 118(4): 428–464.

Karmali, S., et al. 2010. Bariatric surgery: A primer. *Canadian Family Physician* 56(9): 873–879.

Lau, D. C. W., et al. 2007. 2006 Canadian clinical practice guidelines on the management and prevention of obesity in adults and Children. *Canadian Medical Association Journal* 176(8): S1–13.

Le Petit, C. 2005. *How many obese Canadians can we expect by 2010 and 2020?* Presented at the 96th Annual Canadian Public Health Association Conference. Ottawa, Ontario, September 18–21.

Ma, Y., et al. 2005. Association between dietary carbohydrates and body weight. *American Journal of Epidemiology* 161(4): 359–367.

McBride, B. F., et al. 2004. Electrocardiographic and hemodynamic effects of a multicomponent dietary supplement containing ephedra and caffeine. *Journal of the American Medical Association* 291(4): 216–221.

McCullough, P. A., et al. 2006. Cardiorespiratory fitness and short-term complications after bariatric surgery. *CHEST* 130: 517–525.

Muenning, P., et al. 2006. Gender and the burden of disease attributable to obesity. *American Journal of Public Health* 96(9): 1662–1668.

Newnham-Kanas, C., J. D. Irwin, and D. Morrow. 2008. Life coaching as an intervention for individual with obesity. *International Journal of Evidence-Based Coaching and Mentoring* 6(2): 1–12.

Nicklas, B. J., et al. 2004. Association of visceral adipose tissue with incident myocardial infarction in older men and women: "The Health, Aging and Body Composition Study." *American Journal of Epidemiology* 160(8): 741–749.

O'Brien, P., et al. 2006. Treatment of mild to moderate obesity with laparoscopic adjustable gastric banding or an intensive medical program. *Annals of Internal Medicine* 144(9): 625–633.

Ogden, C. L., et al. 2007. Obesity among adults in the United States: No change since 2003–2004. *National Center for Health Statistics Data Brief* 1: 1–8.

Olshansky, S. J., et al. 2005. A potential decline in life expectancy in the United States in the 21st century. *New England Journal of Medicine* 352(11): 1138–1145.

Rubin, C. T., et al. 2007. Adipogenesis is inhibited by brief, daily exposure to high-frequency, extremely low-magnitude mechanical signals. *Proceedings of the National Academy of Sciences* 104(45): 17879–17884.

Shankar, K., et al. 2008. Maternal obesity at conception programs obesity in the offspring. *American Journal of Physiology: Regulatory, Integrative and Comparative Physiology* 294: R528–R523.

Schulze, M. B., et al. 2004. Sugar-sweetened beverages, weight gain, and incidence of type 2 diabetes in young and middle-aged women. *Journal of the American Medical Association* 292(8): 927–934.

Statistics Canada. 2010. *Canadian Health Measures Survey: Cycle 1 Data Tables, 2007–2009* (http://www.statcan.gc.ca/pub/82-623-x/82-623-x2010002-eng.pdf; retrieved March 20, 2011).

Taylor, E. N., et al. 2005. Obesity, weight gain, and risk of kidney stones. *Journal of the American Medical Association* 293(4): 455–462.

Tsai, A. G., and T. A. Wadden. 2005. Systematic review: An evaluation of major commercial weight loss programs in the United States. *Annals of Internal Medicine* 142(1): 56–66.

van Dam, R. M., et al. 2006. The relationship between overweight in adolescence and premature death in women. *Annals of Internal Medicine* 145(2): 91–97.

University of Montreal. 2010. New therapy to overcome body dysmorphic disorder. *ScienceDaily* (http://www.sciencedaily.com/releases/2010/06/100628124605.htm; retrieved March 20, 2011).

Vorona, R. D., et al. 2005. Overweight and obese patients in a primary care population report less sleep than patients with a normal body mass index. *Archives of Internal Medicine* 165: 25–30.

Walsh, T. B., et al. 2006. Fluoxetine after weight restoration in anorexia nervosa. *Journal of the American Medical Association* 295(22): 2605–2612.

Wang, Y., and M. A. Beydoun. 2007. The obesity epidemic in the United States—gender, age, socioeconomic, racial/ethnic and geographical characteristics: A systematic review and meta-regression analysis. *Epidemiologic Reviews* 29: 6–28.

Wansink, B., and P. Chandon. 2006. Meal size, not body size, explains errors in estimating calorie content of meals. *Annals of Internal Medicine* 145: 326–332.

Weinstein, A. R., et al. 2004. Relationship of physical activity vs. body mass index with type 2 diabetes in women. *Journal of the American Medical Association* 292(10): 1188–1194.

Weinstein, P. K. 2006. A review of weight loss programs delivered via the Internet. *Journal of Cardiovascular Nursing* 21(4): 251–258.

Wong, S. L., et al. 2004. Cardiorespiratory fitness is associated with lower abdominal fat independent of body mass index. *Medicine and Science in Sports and Exercise* 36(2): 286–291.

World Health Organization. 1998. *Obesity: Preventing and Managing the Global Epidemic: Report of a WHO Consultation on Obesity.* Geneva, Switzerland: WHO.

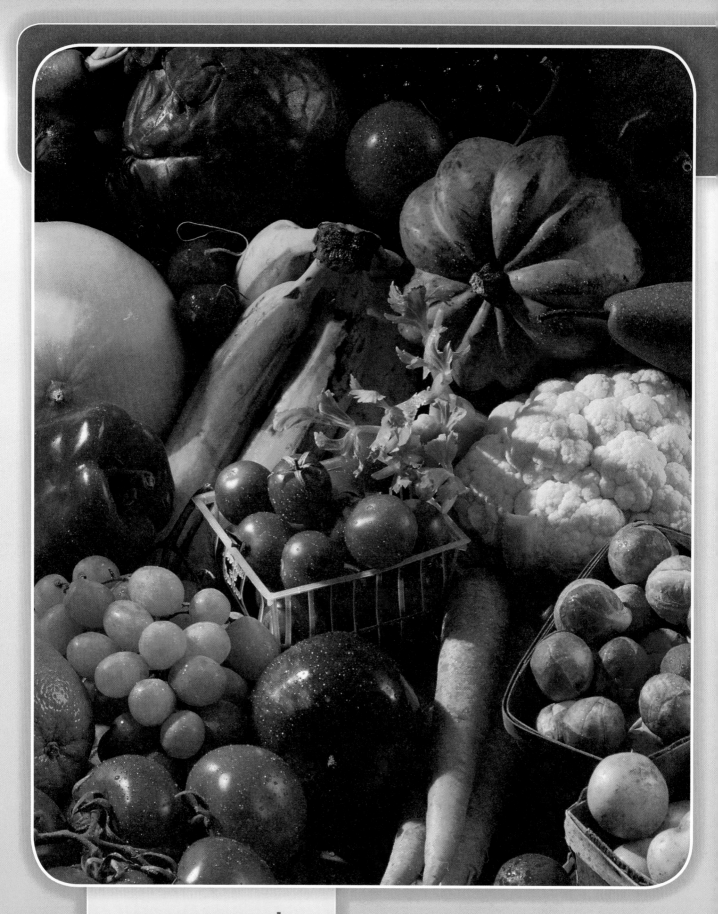

McGraw Hill **connect**™   Practise and learn online with Connect.

NUTRITION BASICS

LOOKING AHEAD>>>>>

AFTER READING THIS CHAPTER, YOU SHOULD BE ABLE TO

- List the essential nutrients, and describe the functions they perform in the body

- Describe the guidelines that have been developed to help people choose a healthy diet, avoid nutritional deficiencies, and reduce their risk of diet-related chronic diseases

- Discuss nutritional guidelines for vegetarians and for special population groups

- Explain how to use food labels and other consumer tools to make informed choices about foods

- Put together a personal nutrition plan based on affordable foods that you enjoy and that will promote wellness, today as well as in the future

TEST YOUR KNOWLEDGE

1. **It is recommended that all adults consume one to two servings of fruits and vegetables every day.**
   True or false?

2. **How many french fries are in one small serving?**
   a. 10
   b. 15
   c. 25

3. **Which of the following is not a whole grain?**
   a. brown rice
   b. wheat flour
   c. popcorn

4. **Registered dietitians advise reduced intake of saturated and trans fats for which of the following reasons?**
   a. They increase the levels of low-density lipoproteins (LDL), or "bad" cholesterol.
   b. They provide more calories than other types of fat.
   c. They increase the risk of heart disease.

ANSWERS

1. **FALSE.** Adult females should consume seven to eight servings of vegetables and fruit daily; adult males should consume eight to ten servings of vegetables and fruit daily.

2. **C.** Many people underestimate the size of the portions they eat, leading to overconsumption of calories and fat. A small serving of french fries (about 75 grams) contains between 20 and 25 fries.

3. **B.** Unless labelled as whole wheat, wheat flour is processed to remove the bran and the germ and is not a whole grain.

4. **A and C.** High intake of saturated and trans fats raises LDL levels and the risk of heart disease. Saturated and trans fats provide the same number of calories as other types of fat: nine calories per gram (compared with four calories per gram for protein and carbohydrate).

In your lifetime, you'll spend about six years eating—about 70,000 meals and 54 metric tons of food. What you eat can have profound effects on your health and well-being. Your nutritional habits help determine your risk of major chronic diseases, including heart disease, cancer, stroke, and diabetes. Choosing foods that provide the nutrients you need while limiting the substances linked to disease should be an important part of your daily life.

Choosing a healthy diet is a two-part process. First, you have to know which nutrients you need and in what amounts. Second, you have to translate those requirements into a diet consisting of foods you like that are both available and affordable. Once you know what constitutes a healthy diet for you, you can adjust your current diet to bring it into line with your goals.

This chapter explains the basic principles of **nutrition**. It introduces the six classes of essential nutrients and explains their roles in the functioning of the body. It also provides guidelines that you can use to design a healthy diet plan. Finally, it offers practical tools and advice to help you apply the guidelines to your own life.

NUTRITIONAL REQUIREMENTS: COMPONENTS OF A HEALTHY DIET

You probably think about your diet in terms of the foods you like to eat. What's important for your health, though, are the nutrients contained in those foods. Your body requires proteins, fats, carbohydrates, vitamins, minerals, and water—about 50 **essential nutrients**. In this context, the word *essential* means that you must get these substances from food because your body is unable to manufacture them, or at least not fast enough to meet your physiological needs. The six classes of nutrients, along with their functions and major sources, are listed in Table 5.1. The body needs some essential nutrients in

relatively large amounts; these **macronutrients** include protein, fat, and carbohydrate. **Micronutrients**, such as vitamins and minerals, are required in much smaller amounts. Your body obtains these nutrients through the process of **digestion**, in which the foods you eat are broken down into compounds your gastrointestinal tract can absorb and your body can use (Figure 5.1). A diet that provides enough essential nutrients is vital because various nutrients provide energy, help build and maintain body tissues, and help regulate body functions (see the box "Eating Habits and Total Wellness" on p. 132).

Calories

The energy in foods is expressed as **kilocalories**. One kilocalorie represents the amount of heat it takes to raise the temperature of one litre of water by one degree Celsius. A person needs about 2000 kilocalories per day to meet his or her energy needs. In common usage, people usually refer to kilocalories as *calories*, which is technically a much smaller energy unit: 1 kilocalorie contains 1000 calories. This text uses the familiar word *calorie* to stand for the larger energy unit; you'll also find the word *calorie* used on food labels.

Of the six classes of essential nutrients, three supply energy:

- Fat = nine calories per gram
- Protein = four calories per gram
- Carbohydrate = four calories per gram

Alcohol, though not an essential nutrient, also supplies energy, providing seven calories per gram. The high caloric content of fat is one reason experts often advise against high fat consumption; most of us do not need the extra calories to meet energy needs. Regardless of their source, calories consumed in excess of energy needs are converted to fat and stored in the body.

Table 5.1	The Six Classes of Essential Nutrients	
Nutrient	**Function**	**Major Sources**
Proteins (4 calories/gram)	Form important parts of muscles, bone, blood, enzymes, some hormones, and cell membranes; repair tissue; regulate water and acid-base balance; help in growth; supply energy	Meat, fish, poultry, eggs, milk products, legumes, nuts
Carbohydrates (4 calories/gram)	Supply energy to cells in brain, nervous system, and blood; supply energy to muscles during exercise	Grains (breads and cereals), fruits, vegetables, milk
Fats (9 calories/gram)	Supply energy; insulate, support, and cushion organs; provide medium for absorption of fat-soluble vitamins	Animal foods, grains, nuts, seeds, fish, vegetables
Vitamins	Promote (initiate or speed up) specific chemical reactions within cells	Abundant in fruits, vegetables, and grains; also found in meat and dairy products
Minerals	Help regulate body functions; aid in growth and maintenance of body tissues; act as catalysts for release of energy	Found in most food groups
Water	Makes up approximately 60% of body weight; provides medium for chemical reactions; transports chemicals; regulates temperature; removes waste products	Fruits, vegetables, liquids

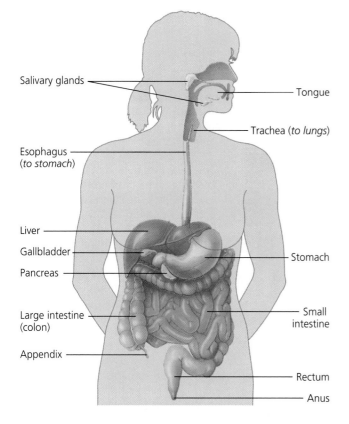

Salivary glands

Tongue

Trachea (*to lungs*)

Esophagus
(*to stomach*)

Liver

Gallbladder

Pancreas

Large intestine
(colon)

Appendix

Stomach

Small
intestine

Rectum

Anus

FIGURE 5.1 The digestive system. Food is partially broken down by being chewed and mixed with saliva in the mouth. After travelling to the stomach via the esophagus, food is broken down further by stomach acids and other secretions. As food moves through the digestive tract, it is mixed by muscular contractions and broken down by chemicals. Most absorption of nutrients occurs in the small intestine, aided by secretions from the pancreas, gallbladder, and intestinal lining. The large intestine reabsorbs excess water; the remaining solid wastes are collected in the rectum and excreted through the anus.

But just meeting energy needs is not enough; our bodies need enough of the essential nutrients to grow and function properly. Practically all foods contain mixtures of nutrients, although foods are commonly classified according to the predominant nutrient; for example, spaghetti is thought of as a carbohydrate. The following sections discuss the function and sources of each class of nutrients.

Proteins: The Basis of Body Structure

Proteins form important parts of the body's main structural components: muscles and bones. Proteins also form important parts of blood, enzymes, some hormones, and cell membranes. As mentioned earlier, proteins also provide energy (four calories per gram) for the body.

Amino Acids The building blocks of proteins are called **amino acids**. Twenty common amino acids are found in food; nine of these are essential: histidine, isoleucine, leucine, lysine, methionine, phenylalanine, threonine,

tryptophan, and valine. The other eleven amino acids can be produced by the body, given the presence of the needed components supplied by foods.

Complete and Incomplete Proteins Individual protein sources are considered *complete* if they supply all the essential amino acids in adequate amounts and are *incomplete* if they do not. Meat, fish, poultry, eggs, milk, cheese, and soy provide complete proteins. Incomplete proteins, which come from other plant sources, such as **legumes** and nuts, are good sources of most essential amino acids but are usually low in one or two.

Certain combinations of vegetable proteins, such as wheat and peanuts in a peanut butter sandwich, allow each vegetable protein to make up for the amino acids missing in the other protein. The combination yields a complete protein. Many traditional Aboriginal food pairings, such as wild turkey, wild rice, potatoes, bannock or cornbread, squash, and beans, emerged as dietary staples because they are complementary proteins.

It was once believed that vegetarians had to complement their proteins at each meal to receive the benefit of a complete protein. It is now known, however, that proteins consumed throughout the day can complement one

TERMS

nutrition The science of food and how the body uses it in health and disease.

essential nutrients Substances the body must get from foods because it cannot manufacture them at all or fast enough to meet its needs; include proteins, fats, carbohydrates, vitamins, minerals, and water.

macronutrient An essential nutrient required by the body in relatively large amounts.

micronutrient An essential nutrient required by the body in minute amounts.

digestion The process of breaking down foods in the gastrointestinal tract into compounds the body can absorb.

kilocalorie A measure of energy content in food; one kilocalorie represents the amount of heat needed to raise the temperature of one litre of water by one degree Celsius; commonly referred to as a *calorie*.

protein An essential nutrient; a compound made of amino acids that contains carbon, hydrogen, oxygen, and nitrogen.

amino acids The building blocks of proteins.

legumes Vegetables, such as peas and beans, that are high in fibre and are also important sources of protein.

Eating Habits and Total Wellness

Healthy eating does more than nourish your body; it enhances your ability to enjoy life to the fullest by improving overall wellness, both physical and mental. One study examined a group of adults who followed a healthy eating plan for four years. At the end of this period, the study subjects were more confident with their food choices and more satisfied with their lives in general than their peers who did not make any dietary changes. The reverse is also true: when people overeat, they often have feelings of guilt, anger, discouragement, and even self-loathing. Out-of-control eating can erode self-confidence and lead to depression.

Can individual foods affect the way we feel? Limited scientific evidence points to some correlation between certain foods and our mood. Many people, especially women, seem to crave chocolate when they feel slightly depressed. Studies show that chocolate, in small quantities, may indeed give you a lift. Sugary foods tend to temporarily raise serotonin levels in the brain, which can improve mood (serotonin is a neurotransmitter associated with a calm, relaxed state). The fat found in chocolate acts to increase endorphins, brain chemicals that reduce pain and increase feelings of well-being. Chocolate also contains a variety of other less studied chemicals that may have a positive impact on mood.

A commonly held belief about the connection between food and the mind is that eating sugary foods makes people (especially children) hyperactive. Parents often comment on the wild behaviour observed at parties and festive events where many sweets are consumed. However, several carefully controlled studies showed no correlation between behaviour and the consumption of sugary foods. Researchers speculate that high-sugar foods tend to be eaten at birthday parties and other exciting occasions when children tend to be highly stimulated regardless of what they eat.

Some recent research shows that eating certain carbohydrate-rich foods, such as a plain baked potato or a bagel with jelly, can have a temporary calming effect. This effect is most pronounced when rapidly digestible carbohydrates are consumed alone, with no fats or proteins in the meal. The practical implications of this research are uncertain.

If you are looking for a mental boost, some scientists think that eating a meal consisting primarily of protein-rich foods may be helpful. The theory is that proteins contain the amino acid tyrosine, which the body uses to make the neurotransmitters dopamine and norepinephrine. Some researchers think that eating protein-rich foods could increase the synthesis of these neurotransmitters, which can speed reaction time and increase alertness. Whether this really works, especially in well-nourished individuals who have not been lacking these nutrients to begin with, remains to be seen. In the meantime, it wouldn't hurt, and might even help, to include some protein in the meal you eat before your next big exam.

What we know about how food affects mood remains limited. But evidence points to the common-sense conclusion that enjoying reasonable portions of a variety of healthy and tasty foods is a great way to optimize your physical and mental health.

Source: Fahey, T. D., P. M. Insel, and W. T. Roth. 2007. *Fit and Well*, 8th ed. New York: McGraw-Hill. Copyright © 2007 The McGraw-Hill Companies, Inc.

---

another and form a pool of amino acids the body can draw from to produce the necessary proteins. Vegetarians should include a variety of vegetable protein sources in their diets to make sure they get all the essential amino acids in adequate amounts. (Healthy vegetarian diets are discussed later in the chapter.) About 30% of the protein in the Canadian comes from animal sources (meat and dairy), making our diet rich in essential amino acids.

Recommended Protein Intake Adequate daily intake of protein for adults is 0.8 gram per kilogram of body weight, corresponding to about 50 grams of protein per day for someone who weighs 63 kilograms and 65 grams of protein for someone who weighs 81 kilograms. Table 5.2 lists some popular food items and the amount of protein each provides.

Table 5.2	Protein Content of Common Food Items
Item	**Protein (grams)**
90 g lean meat, poultry, or fish	20–25
125 mL (½ cup) tofu	20–25
250 mL (1 cup) dried beans	15–20
250 mL (1 cup) milk, yogourt	8–12
45 g cheese	8–12
1 serving of cereals, grains, nuts, vegetables	2–4

Most Canadians meet or exceed the protein intake needed for adequate nutrition. If you consume more protein than your body needs, the extra protein is synthesized into fat for energy storage or burned for energy requirements. A little extra protein is not harmful, but it can contribute fat to the diet because protein-rich foods are often fat-rich as well.

A very high protein intake can also strain the kidneys. A fairly broad range of protein intakes is associated with good health, and Health Canada's Expert Advisory Committee on Dietary Reference Intakes (DRIs) recommends that protein intake should be 10%–35% of total daily caloric intake, depending on the individual's age. The average Canadian diet includes about 17% of total daily calories as protein.

Fats: Essential in Small Amounts

Fats, also known as *lipids*, are the most concentrated source of energy, at nine calories per gram. The fats stored in your body represent usable energy, they help insulate your body, and they support and cushion your organs. Fats in the diet help your body absorb fat-soluble vitamins and add important flavour and texture to foods. Fats are the major fuel for the body during rest and light activity.

Two fats, linoleic acid and alpha-linolenic acid, are essential components of the diet. They are used to make compounds that are key regulators of many body functions, such as the maintenance of blood pressure and the progress of a healthy pregnancy.

Types and Sources of Fats   Most of the fats in foods are fairly similar in composition, generally including a molecule of glycerol (an alcohol) with three fatty acid chains attached to it. The resulting structure is called a *triglyceride* (see Figure 5.2). Animal fat, for example, is made primarily of triglycerides.

Within a triglyceride, differences in the fatty acid structure result in different types of fats. Depending on this structure, a fat may be unsaturated, monounsaturated, polyunsaturated, or saturated. (The essential fatty acids— linoleic and alpha-linolenic acids—are both polyunsaturated.) The different types of fatty acids have different characteristics and different effects on your health.

Food fats are usually composed of both saturated and unsaturated fatty acids; the dominant type of fatty acid determines the fat's characteristics. Food fats containing large amounts of saturated fatty acids are usually solid at room temperature; they are generally found naturally in animal products. The leading sources of saturated fat in the Canadian diet are red meats (hamburger, steak, roasts), homogenized milk, cheese, hot dogs, and lunchmeats. Food fats containing large amounts of monounsaturated and polyunsaturated fatty acids usually come from plant sources and are liquid at room temperature. Olive, canola, safflower, and peanut oils contain mostly monounsaturated fatty acids. Soybean, corn, and cottonseed oils contain mostly polyunsaturated fatty acids.

Hydrogenation   Notable exceptions to these generalizations exist. When unsaturated vegetable oils undergo the process of **hydrogenation**, a mixture of saturated and unsaturated fatty acids is produced, creating a more solid fat from a liquid oil. Hydrogenation also changes some unsaturated fatty acids to **trans fatty acids,** unsaturated fatty acids with an atypical shape that affects their behaviour in the body. Food manufacturers use hydrogenation to increase the stability of an oil so it can be reused for deep frying, to improve the texture of certain foods (to make pastries and pie crusts flakier, for example), and to extend the shelf life of foods made with oil. Hydrogenation is also used to transform a liquid oil into margarine or vegetable shortening.

Many baked and fried foods are prepared with hydrogenated vegetable oils, so they can be relatively high in saturated and trans fatty acids. Leading sources of trans fats in the Canadian diet are processed foods, such as crackers, cookies, doughnuts, cakes, pastries, muffins, croissants, snack foods, and fried foods, such as french fries and breaded foods. In general, the more solid a hydrogenated oil is, the more saturated and trans fats it contains; for example, hard margarines typically contain more saturated and trans

QUICK STATS

Canadians, on average, consume **9.5 grams** of trans fatty acids each day.

—Trans Fat Task Force, 2006

FIGURE 5.2   A triglyceride.

hydrogenation   A process by which hydrogens are added to unsaturated fats, increasing the degree of saturation and turning liquid oils into solid fats. Hydrogenation produces a mixture of saturated fatty acids and standard and trans forms of unsaturated fatty acids.

trans fatty acid   A type of unsaturated fatty acid produced during the process of hydrogenation; trans fats have an atypical shape that affects their chemical activity.

TERMS

fats than do soft margarines. Small amounts of trans fatty acids are found naturally in meat and milk.

Hydrogenated vegetable oils are not the only plant fats that contain saturated fats. Palm and coconut oils, although derived from plants, are also highly saturated. However, fish oils, derived from an animal source, are rich in polyunsaturated fats.

Fats and Health   Different types of fats have very different effects on health. Many studies have examined the effects of dietary fat intake on blood **cholesterol** levels and the risk of heart disease. Saturated and trans fatty acids raise blood levels of **low-density lipoprotein (LDL)**, or "bad" cholesterol, thereby increasing a person's risk of heart disease. Unsaturated fatty acids lower LDL. Monounsaturated fatty acids, such as those found in olive and canola oils, may also increase levels of **high-density lipoproteins (HDL)**, or "good" cholesterol, providing even greater benefits for heart health. In large amounts, trans fatty acids may lower HDL. Saturated fats have been found to impair the ability of HDLs to prevent inflammation of the blood vessels, one of the key factors in vascular disease; they have also been found to reduce the ability of the blood vessels to react normally to stress. Thus, to reduce the risk of heart disease, it is important to choose unsaturated fats instead of saturated and trans fats. (See Chapter 7 for more on cholesterol.)

Health experts are particularly concerned about Canadians' consumption of trans fats because of their triple negative effects on heart health—they raise LDL, lower HDL, and produce inflammation—and because the public is less aware of trans fats than of saturated fats. Since September 2005, food labels have included the trans fat content. Consumers can also check for the presence of trans fats by reading the ingredient list of a food, looking for *partially hydrogenated oil* or *vegetable shortening*.

For heart health, it's important to minimize your consumption of both saturated and trans fats. The best way to reduce saturated fat in your diet is to lower your intake of meat and full-fat dairy products (homogenized milk, cream, butter, cheese, yogourt, ice cream). To lower trans fats, decrease your intake of deep-fried foods and processed foods, such as crackers, cookies, and other baked goods made with hydrogenated vegetable oils; use liquid oils for cooking; and favour soft margarines over hard margarines. Remember, the softer or more liquid a fat is, the less saturated and trans fat it is likely to contain.

Although saturated and trans fats pose health hazards, other fats can be beneficial. When used in place of saturated fats, monounsaturated fatty acids, found in avocados, most nuts, and olive, canola, peanut, and safflower oils, improve blood cholesterol levels and may help protect against some cancers.

Omega-3 fatty acids, a form of polyunsaturated fat found primarily in fish, may be even more healthful. Foods rich in omega-3s are important because they contain the essential nutrient alpha-linolenic acid. Omega-3s and the compounds the body makes from them have a number of heart-healthy effects: They reduce the tendency of blood to clot, inhibit inflammation and abnormal heart rhythms, and reduce blood pressure and risk of heart attack and stroke in some people. Because of these benefits, dietitians recommend that Canadians increase the proportion of omega-3s in their diet by eating at least two servings of fish each week. Serving sizes are based on *Eating Well with Canada's Food Guide*. Salmon, tuna, trout, mackerel, herring, sardines, and anchovies are all good sources of omega-3s; lesser amounts are found in plant foods, including dark-green leafy vegetables; walnuts; flaxseeds; and canola, walnut, and flaxseed oils.

Most of the polyunsaturated fats currently consumed by Canadians are omega-6 fatty acids, primarily from corn oil and soybean oil. Foods rich in omega-6s are important because they contain the essential nutrient linoleic acid. However, some nutritionists recommend that people reduce the proportion of omega-6s they consume in favour of omega-3s. To make this adjustment, use canola oil rather than corn oil in cooking, and check for corn, soybean, or cottonseed oil in such products as mayonnaise, margarine, and salad dressing.

In addition to its effects on heart disease risk, dietary fat can affect health in other ways. Diets high in fatty red meat are associated with an increased risk of certain forms of cancer, especially colon cancer. A high-fat diet can also make weight management more difficult. Because fat is a concentrated source of calories (nine calories per gram versus four calories per gram for protein and carbohydrate), a high-fat diet is often a high-calorie diet that can lead to weight gain. In addition, some evidence shows that calories from fat are more easily converted to body fat than calories from protein or carbohydrate.

Although more research is needed on the precise effects of different types and amounts of fat on overall health, a great deal of evidence points to the fact that most people benefit from keeping their overall fat intake at recommended levels and choosing unsaturated fats instead of saturated and trans fats. The types of fatty acids and their effects on health are summarized in Figure 5.3.

Recommended Fat Intake   To meet the body's demand for essential fats, adult men need about 17 grams

Type of Fatty Acid	Found In[a]	Possible Effects on Health
Keep Intake Low		
SATURATED	Animal fats (especially fatty meats and poultry fat and skin) Butter, cheese, and other high-fat dairy products Palm and coconut oils	Raises total cholesterol and LDL cholesterol levels Increases risk of heart disease May increase risk of colon and prostate cancers
TRANS	French fries and other deep-fried fast foods Stick margarines, shortening Packaged cookies and crackers Processed snacks and sweets	Raises total cholesterol and LDL cholesterol levels Lowers HDL cholesterol levels May increase risk of heart disease and breast cancer
Choose Moderate Amounts		
MONOUNSATURATED	Olive, canola, and safflower oils Avocados, olives Peanut butter (without added fat) Many nuts, including almonds, cashews, pecans, and pistachios	Lowers total cholesterol and LDL cholesterol levels May reduce blood pressure and lower triglyceride levels (a risk factor for CVD) May reduce risk of heart disease, stroke, and some cancers
POLYUNSATURATED (two groups)[b]		
Omega-3 fatty acids	Fatty fish, including salmon, white albacore tuna, mackerel, anchovies, and sardines Lesser amounts in walnut, flaxseed, canola, and soybean oils; tofu; walnuts; flaxseeds; and dark-green leafy vegetables	Reduces blood clotting and inflammation and inhibits abnormal heart rhythms Lowers triglyceride levels (a risk factor for CVD) May lower blood pressure in some people May reduce risk of fatal heart attack, stroke, and some cancers
Omega-6 fatty acids	Corn, soybean, and cottonseed oils (often used in margarine, mayonnaise, and salad dressing)	Lowers total cholesterol and LDL cholesterol levels May lower HDL cholesterol levels May reduce risk of heart disease May slightly increase risk of cancer if omega-6 intake is high and omega-3 intake is low

[a] Food fats contain a combination of types of fatty acids in various proportions; for example, canola oil is composed mainly of monounsaturated fatty acids (62%) but also contains polyunsaturated (32%) and saturated (6%) fatty acids. Food fats are categorized here according to their predominant fatty acid.

[b] The essential fatty acids are polyunsaturated: Linoleic acid is an omega-6 fatty acid and alpha-linolenic acid is an omega-3 fatty acid.

FIGURE 5.3   Types of fatty acids and their possible effects on health.

per day of linoleic acid and 1.6 grams per day of alpha-linolenic acid; adult women need 12 grams of linoleic acid and 1.1 grams of alpha-linolenic acid. It takes only 30–45 mL (2–3 tablespoons) of unsaturated fat per day incorporated into your diet to supply the essential fats. This includes oil used for cooking, salad dressings, margarine, and mayonnaise. Most Canadians consume sufficient amounts of the essential fats; limiting unhealthy fats is a much greater health concern.

Limits for total fat, saturated fat, and trans fat intake have been set by a number of government and research organizations. In 2002, Health Canada adopted recommendations for the balance of energy sources in a healthful diet from the Institute of Medicine. These new recommendations, called Acceptable Macronutrient Distribution Ranges (AMDRs), are based on ensuring adequate intake of essential nutrients while also reducing the risk of chronic diseases, such as heart disease and cancer. As with protein, a range of levels of fat consumption is associated with good health; the AMDR for total fat is 20%–35% of total calories. Although

more difficult for consumers to monitor, AMDRs have also been set for omega-6 fatty acids (5%–10%) and omega-3 fatty acids (0.6%–1.2%) as part of total fat intake. Because any amount of saturated and trans fats increases the risk of heart disease, the Food and Nutrition Board, a committee of the Institute of Medicine, recommends that saturated fat and trans fat intake be kept as low as possible; most fat in a healthy diet should be unsaturated. Canadian adults consume about 31% of their total calories as fat. The best way to minimize the risk of adverse health effects related to trans fat is to reduce your intake of foods that contain trans fatty acids.

QUICK STATS

One hundred grams of Atlantic salmon provides **two grams** of omega-3 fatty acids.

—Marine Harvest Canada, 2010

Setting Intake Goals for Protein, Fat, and Carbohydrate

The Acceptable Macronutrient Distribution Ranges (AMDRs) established by the Institute of Medicine and adopted by Health Canada help ensure adequate intake of the essential amino acids, fatty acids, and carbohydrate. The ranges can help you balance your intake of the energy-providing nutrients in ways that ensure adequate intake while reducing the risk of chronic disease. The AMDRs for protein, total fat, and carbohydrate are as follows:

Protein	10%–35% of total daily calories
Total fat	20%–35% of total daily calories
Carbohydrate	45%–65% of total daily calories

Protein intake goals can be calculated more specifically by multiplying your body weight in kilograms by 0.8. (Refer to the Nutrition Resources section at the end of the chapter for information for specific age groups and life stages.)

To set individual goals, begin by estimating your total daily energy (calorie) needs; if your weight is stable, your current energy intake is the number of calories you need to maintain your weight at your current activity level. Next, select percentage goals for protein, fat, and carbohydrate. You can allocate your total daily calories among the three classes of macronutrients to suit your preferences; just make sure that the three percentages you select total 100% and that you meet the minimum intake AMDR for each macronutrient. Two samples showing different total energy intake and nutrient intake goals are included below.

To translate your own percentage goals into daily intake goals expressed in calories and grams, multiply the appropriate percentages by total calorie intake and then divide the results by the corresponding calories per gram. For example, a fat limit of 35% applied to a 2200-calorie diet would be calculated as follows: 0.35 × 2200 = 770 calories of total fat; 770 ÷ 9 calories per gram = 86 grams of total fat. (Remember that fat has nine calories per gram and that protein and carbohydrate have four calories per gram.)

Two Sample Macronutrient Distributions

Nutrient	AMDR	Sample 1 Individual Goals	Sample 1 Amounts for a 1600-Calorie Diet	Sample 2 Individual Goals	Sample 2 Amounts for a 2800-Calorie Diet
Protein	10%–35%	15%	240 calories = 60 g	30%	840 calories = 210 g
Fat	20%–35%	30%	480 calories = 53 g	25%	700 calories = 78 g
Carbohydrate	45%–65%	55%	880 calories = 220 g	45%	1260 calories = 315 g

Source: Food and Nutrition Board, Institute of Medicine, National Academies. 2002. *Dietary Reference Intakes: Applications in Dietary Planning,* Washington, D.C.: National Academies Press. Reprinted with permission from the National Academies Press, Washington, D.C.

For advice on setting individual intake goals, see the box "Setting Intake Goals for Protein, Fat, and Carbohydrate," above. To determine how close you are to meeting your personal intake goals for fat, keep a running total over the course of the day. For prepared foods, food labels list the number of grams of fat, protein, and carbohydrate; the breakdown for some popular fast-food items can be found in Appendix A. Nutrition information is also available in many grocery stores, in inexpensive published nutrition guides, and online (see For More Information at the end of the chapter). By checking these resources, you can keep track of the total grams of fat, protein, and carbohydrate you eat and assess your current diet.

You can still eat high-fat foods, but it makes sense to limit the size of your portions and to balance your intake with low-fat foods. For example, peanut butter is high in fat: 15 millilitres (one tablespoon) has 90 calories, with 72 of those calories (8 grams) coming from fat. A full serving of peanut butter is 30 millilitres. This amount spread on whole wheat bread and served with a banana, carrot sticks, and a glass of skim milk makes a nutritious lunch, high in protein and carbohydrate, and relatively low in fat (500 calories, 18 grams of total fat, 4 grams of saturated fat). Sixty millilitres (four tablespoons) of peanut butter on high-fat crackers, eaten with potato chips, cookies, and homogenized milk is a far less healthy combination (1000 calories, 62 grams of total fat, 15 grams of saturated fat). So although it's important to evaluate individual food items for their fat content, it is more important to look at them in the context of your overall diet.

Carbohydrates: An Ideal Source of Energy

Carbohydrates are needed in the diet primarily to supply energy for body cells. Some cells, such as those found in the brain and other parts of the nervous system and in blood, use only carbohydrates for fuel. During high-intensity exercise, muscles also use primarily carbohydrates for fuel.

When we don't eat enough carbohydrates to satisfy the needs of the brain and red blood cells, our bodies synthesize carbohydrates from proteins. In situations of extreme deprivation, when the diet lacks a sufficient amount of both carbohydrates and proteins, the body turns to its own organs and tissues, breaking down proteins in muscles, the heart, kidneys, and other vital organs to supply carbohydrate needs. This rarely occurs, however, because consuming the equivalent of just three or four slices of bread supplies the body's daily minimum need for carbohydrates.

Simple and Complex Carbohydrates Carbohydrates are classified into two groups: simple and complex. Simple carbohydrates include sucrose (table sugar), fructose (fruit sugar, honey), maltose (malt sugar), and lactose (milk sugar). Simple carbohydrates provide much of the sweetness in foods and are found naturally in fruits and milk and are added to soft drinks, fruit drinks, candy, and sweet desserts. No evidence suggests that any type of simple carbohydrate is more nutritious than the others.

Complex carbohydrates include starches and most types of dietary fibre. Starches are found in a variety of plants, especially grains (wheat, rye, rice, oats, barley, millet), legumes (dry beans, peas, and lentils), and tubers (potatoes and yams). Most other vegetables contain a mixture of complex and simple carbohydrates. Fibre, discussed in the next section, is found in grains, fruits, and vegetables.

During digestion in the mouth and small intestine, your body breaks down carbohydrates into simple sugar molecules, such as **glucose**, for absorption. Once glucose is in the bloodstream, the pancreas releases the hormone insulin, which allows cells to take up glucose and use it for energy. The liver and muscles also take up glucose to provide carbohydrate storage in the form of **glycogen**. Some people have problems controlling blood glucose levels, a disorder called *diabetes mellitus* (see Chapter 4 for more on diabetes).

Refined Carbohydrates Versus Whole Grains Complex carbohydrates can be further divided between refined, or processed, carbohydrates and unrefined carbohydrates, or **whole grains**. Before they are processed, all grains are whole grains, consisting of an inner layer, the germ; a middle layer, the endosperm; and an outer layer, called bran (see Figure 5.4). During processing, the germ and bran are often removed, leaving just the starchy endosperm. The refinement of whole grains transforms whole wheat flour to white flour, brown rice to white rice, and so on.

Refined carbohydrates usually retain all the calories of their unrefined counterparts, but they tend to be much lower in fibre, vitamins, minerals, and other beneficial compounds. Many refined grain products are enriched or fortified with vitamins and minerals, but often the nutrients lost in processing are not replaced.

Unrefined carbohydrates tend to take longer to chew and digest than refined ones; they also enter the bloodstream more slowly. This slower digestive pace tends to make people feel full sooner and for longer. The slower rise in blood glucose levels following consumption of complex carbohydrates may help in the management of diabetes. Whole grains are also high in dietary fibre and so have all the

FIGURE 5.4 The parts of a whole grain kernel.

benefits of fibre (discussed later). Consumption of whole grains has been linked to a reduced risk of heart disease, diabetes, high blood pressure, stroke, and certain forms of cancer. For all these reasons, whole grains are recommended over those that have been refined. This does not mean that you should never eat refined carbohydrates, such as white bread or white rice, simply that whole-wheat bread, brown rice, and other whole grains are healthier choices. See the box "Choosing More Whole-Grain Foods" on p. 138 for tips on increasing your intake of whole grains.

Glycemic Index and Glycemic Response Insulin and glucose levels rise and fall following a meal or snack containing any type of carbohydrate. Some foods cause a quick and dramatic rise in glucose and insulin levels; others have a slower, more moderate effect. A food that has a rapid effect on blood glucose levels is said to have a high

carbohydrate An essential nutrient; sugars, starches, and dietary fibre are all carbohydrates.

glucose A simple sugar that is the body's basic fuel.

glycogen An animal starch stored in the liver and muscles.

whole grain The entire edible portion of a grain, such as wheat, rice, or oats, consisting of the germ, endosperm, and bran. During milling or processing, parts of the grain are removed, often leaving just the endosperm.

TERMS

Choosing More Whole-Grain Foods

Whole-grain foods are good weapons against heart disease, diabetes, high blood pressure, stroke, and certain cancers. They are also low in fat and so can be a good choice for managing weight. Health Canada recommends that half of your grain products every day should be whole grains.

What Are Whole Grains?

The first step in increasing your intake of whole grains is to correctly identify them. The following are whole grains:

whole wheat	whole-grain corn
whole rye	popcorn
whole oats	brown rice
oatmeal	whole-grain barley

More unusual choices include bulgur (cracked wheat), millet, kasha (roasted buckwheat kernels), quinoa, wheat and rye berries, amaranth, wild rice, graham flour, whole-grain kamut, whole-grain spelt, and whole-grain triticale.

Wheat flour, unbleached flour, enriched flour, and degerminated corn meal are not whole grains. Wheat germ and wheat bran are also not whole grains, but they are the constituents of wheat typically left out when wheat is processed and so are healthier choices than regular wheat flour, which typically contains just the endosperm.

Reading Food Packages to Find Whole Grains

To find packaged foods rich in whole grains, read the list of ingredients and check for special health claims related to whole grains. The *first* item on the list of ingredients should be one of the whole grains listed above. Product names and colours used on food packaging can be misleading. When in doubt, always check the list of ingredients, looking for *whole* as the first word on the list.

Incorporating Whole Grains into Your Daily Diet

Small changes can make a big difference in your fibre intake:

- *Bread:* Look for sandwich breads, bagels, English muffins, buns, and pita breads with a whole grain listed as the first ingredient.

- *Breakfast cereals:* Check the ingredient list for whole grains. Whole-grain choices include oatmeal, muesli, shredded wheat, and some types of raisin bran, bran flakes, wheat flakes, toasted oats, and granola.

- *Rice:* Choose brown rice or rice blends that include brown rice.

- *Pasta:* Look for whole wheat, whole-grain kamut, or whole-grain spelt pasta.

- *Tortillas:* Choose whole wheat or whole-corn tortillas.

- *Crackers and snacks:* Some varieties of crackers are made from whole grains, including some flatbreads or crispbreads, woven wheat crackers, and rye crackers. Other whole-grain snack possibilities include popcorn, popcorn cakes, brown rice cakes, whole-corn tortilla chips, and whole wheat fig cookies. Be sure to check food labels for fat content, as many popular snacks are high in fat.

- *Mixed-grain dishes:* Combine whole grains with other foods to create healthy mixed dishes. Possibilities include tabouli; soups made with hulled barley or wheat berries; and pilafs, casseroles, and salads made with brown rice, whole wheat couscous, kasha, millet, wheat bulgur, or quinoa.

If your grocery store doesn't carry all of these items, try your local health food store.

---

glycemic index. Research findings have been mixed, but some studies have found that a meal containing high glycemic index foods may increase appetite and that over the long term, diets rich in these foods may increase the risk of diabetes and heart disease for some people. High glycemic index foods do not, as some popular diets claim, directly cause weight gain beyond the calories they contain.

Attempting to base food choices on the glycemic index is a difficult task, however. Although unrefined complex carbohydrates and high-fibre foods generally tend to have a low glycemic index, patterns are less clear for other types of foods and do not follow an easy distinction, such as that of simple versus complex carbohydrates. For example, some fruits with fairly high levels of simple carbohydrates have only a moderate effect on blood glucose levels, whereas white rice, potatoes, and white bread, which are rich in complex carbohydrates, have a high glycemic index. Watermelon has a glycemic index more

than twice that of strawberries, and the glycemic index of a banana changes dramatically as it ripens. The acid and fat content of a food also affect its glycemic index; the more acidic and higher in fat a food is, the lower its effect on glucose levels. The body's response to carbohydrates also depends on many other factors, such as how foods are combined and prepared and the fitness status of the individual.

This complexity is one reason major health organizations have not issued specific guidelines for the glycemic index of foods. For people with particular health concerns, a food's glycemic index may be an important consideration; however, it should not be the sole criterion for food choices. For example, ice cream has a much lower glycemic index than brown rice or carrots—but that doesn't make it a healthier choice overall. Remember that most unrefined grains, fruits, vegetables, and legumes are rich in nutrients, have a relatively low energy density, and have a low to moderate glycemic index. Choose a variety of

vegetables daily. Limit foods that are high in added sugars but provide few other nutrients. Some studies have singled out regular soft drinks, with their large dose of rapidly absorbable sugar, as specifically linked to increased risk for diabetes and obesity.

Recommended Carbohydrate Intake Experts recommend that adults consume 45%–65% of their total daily calories as carbohydrate, about 225–325 grams of carbohydrate for someone consuming 2000 calories per day. The focus should be on consuming a variety of foods rich in complex carbohydrates, especially whole grains.

Canada has no specific recommendations for added sugar consumption. That said, foods high in added sugar are generally high in calories and low in nutrients and fibre, thus providing empty calories. Although the Institute of Medicine has set an AMDR for added sugars of 25% or less of total daily calories, many health experts recommend an even lower intake. World Health Organization guidelines suggested a limit of 10% of total daily calories from added sugars; limits set by the United States Department of Agriculture in 2005 are even lower, with a maximum of about 8 teaspoons (32 grams) suggested for someone consuming 2000 calories per day. To reduce your intake of added sugars, limit soft drinks, candy, sweet desserts, and sweetened fruit drinks. The simple carbohydrates in your diet should come mainly from fruits, which are excellent sources of vitamins and minerals, and from low-fat or skim milk and other dairy products, which are high in protein and calcium.

Athletes in training can benefit from high-carbohydrate diets (60%–70% of total daily calories), which enhance the amount of carbohydrates stored in their muscles (as glycogen) and therefore provide more carbohydrate fuel for use during endurance events or long workouts (more than 60 minutes). In addition, carbohydrates consumed during prolonged athletic events can help fuel muscles and extend the availability of the glycogen stored in muscles. Caution is in order, however, because overconsumption of carbohydrates can lead to fatigue and underconsumption of other nutrients. Athletes should focus on complex carbohydrates, such as whole grain breads, cereals, brown rice, whole wheat pastas, and starchy vegetables, such as sweet potatoes, corn, and peas.

Fibre: A Closer Look

Fibre is the term given to nondigestible carbohydrates provided by plants. Instead of being digested, like starch, fibre passes through the intestinal tract and provides bulk for feces in the large intestine, which in turn facilitates elimination. In the large intestine, some types of fibre are broken down by bacteria into acids and gases, which explains why consuming too much fibre can lead to intestinal gas. Because humans cannot digest fibre, it is not a source of carbohydrate in the diet; however, the consumption of fibre is necessary for good health.

Types of Fibre Fibre comes in two types: dietary fibre and functional fibre. **Dietary fibre** refers to the nondigestible carbohydrates (and the noncarbohydrate substance lignin) that are present naturally in plants, such as grains, legumes, and vegetables. **Functional fibre** refers to nondigestible carbohydrates that have been either isolated from natural sources or synthesized in a lab and then added to a food product or dietary supplement. **Total fibre** is the sum of dietary and functional fibre.

Fibres have different properties that lead to different physiological effects in the body. For example, **soluble (viscous) fibre**, such as that found in oat bran or legumes, can delay stomach emptying, slow the movement of glucose into the blood after eating, and reduce absorption of cholesterol. **Insoluble fibre**, such as that found in wheat bran or psyllium seed, increases fecal bulk and helps prevent constipation, hemorrhoids, and other digestive disorders. A diet high in fibre can help reduce the risk of type 2 diabetes and heart disease, and improve gastrointestinal health. Some studies have linked high-fibre diets with reduced risk of colon and rectal cancer; other studies have suggested that other characteristics of diets rich in fruits, vegetables, and whole grains may be responsible for this reduction in risk (see Chapter 8 for more on cancer and diet).

Sources of Fibre All plant foods contain some dietary fibre. Fruits, legumes, oats (especially oat bran), and barley all contain the viscous type of fibre that help lower blood glucose and cholesterol levels. Wheat (especially wheat

glycemic index A measure of how the ingestion of a particular food affects blood glucose levels.

dietary fibre Nondigestible carbohydrates and lignin that are intact in plants.

functional fibre Nondigestible carbohydrates either isolated from natural sources or synthesized; may be added to foods and dietary supplements.

total fibre The total amount of dietary fibre and functional fibre in the diet.

soluble (viscous) fibre Fibre that dissolves in water or is broken down by bacteria in the large intestine.

insoluble fibre Fibre that does not dissolve in water and is not broken down by bacteria in the large intestine.

TERMS

bran), other grains and cereals, and vegetables are good sources of cellulose and other fibres that help prevent constipation. Psyllium, which is often added to cereals or used in fibre supplements and laxatives, improves intestinal health and also helps control glucose and cholesterol levels. The processing of packaged foods can remove fibre, so it is important to rely on fresh fruits and vegetables and foods made from whole grains as your main sources of fibre.

Recommended Fibre Intake   To reduce the risk of chronic disease and maintain intestinal health, the Food and Nutrition Board of the Institute of Medicine recommends a daily fibre intake of 38 grams for adult men and 25 grams for adult women. Canadians, on average, consume about half this amount. Fibre should come from foods, not supplements, which should be used only under medical supervision.

Vitamins: Organic Micronutrients

Vitamins are organic (carbon-containing) substances required in small amounts to regulate various processes within living cells (Table 5.3). Humans need 13 vitamins; four are fat soluble (A, D, E, and K), and nine are water soluble (C, and the eight B-complex vitamins: thiamine, riboflavin, niacin, vitamin B6, folate, vitamin B12, biotin, and pantothenic acid).

Solubility affects how a vitamin is absorbed, transported, and stored in the body. The water-soluble vitamins are absorbed directly into the bloodstream, where they travel freely; excess water-soluble vitamins are detected and removed by the kidneys and excreted in urine. Fat-soluble vitamins require a more complex absorptive process; they are usually carried in the blood by special proteins and are stored in the liver and in fat tissues rather than excreted.

Functions of Vitamins   Many vitamins help chemical reactions take place. They provide no energy to the body directly but help unleash the energy stored in carbohydrates, proteins, and fats. Vitamins are critical in the production of red blood cells and the maintenance of the nervous, skeletal, and immune systems. Some vitamins act as **antioxidants**, which help preserve healthy cells in the body. Key vitamin antioxidants include vitamin E, vitamin C, and the vitamin A precursor beta-carotene. (Antioxidants are described later in the chapter.)

TERMS

vitamins   Carbon-containing substances needed in small amounts to help promote and regulate chemical reactions and processes in the body.

antioxidant   A substance that can lessen the breakdown of food or body constituents by free radicals; actions include binding oxygen, donating electrons to free radicals, and repairing damage to molecules.

Sources of Vitamins   The human body does not manufacture most of the vitamins it requires and must obtain them from foods. Vitamins are abundant in fruits, vegetables, and grains. In addition, many processed foods, such as flour and breakfast cereals, contain added vitamins. A few vitamins are made in certain parts of the body: The skin makes vitamin D when it is exposed to sunlight, and intestinal bacteria make vitamin K. Nonetheless, you still need to obtain vitamin D and vitamin K from foods. Table 5.3 lists good food sources of vitamins.

Vitamin Deficiencies   If your diet lacks a particular vitamin, characteristic symptoms of deficiency can develop. (Table 5.3 lists the signs of certain vitamin deficiencies.) Physicians have known about some common deficiency-related ailments for generations. For example, *scurvy* is a potentially fatal illness caused by a long-term lack of vitamin C. Children who do not get enough vitamin D can develop *rickets*, which leads to potentially disabling bone deformations. Vitamin A deficiency may cause blindness, and seizures can develop in people whose diet lacks vitamin B6. Low intake of folate and vitamins B6 and B12 has been linked to an increased risk of heart disease.

New research is tying vitamin deficiencies with other health risks, as well. For example, two recent studies showed that a lack of vitamin K may contribute to bone brittleness and contribute to bone fractures. A great deal of recent research has focused on vitamin D, with surprising results. Several studies have associated vitamin D deficiency with an increased risk of cardiovascular disease in adults, and show that the vitamin plays an important role in arterial health and blood clotting. A 2008 study also raised the possibility that women with certain types of breast cancer may be more likely to die from their cancer if they do not get enough vitamin D.

Vitamin deficiency diseases are most often seen in developing countries, and they are relatively rare in Canada because vitamins are readily available from our food supply. Still, many Canadians consume less-than-recommended amounts of several vitamins, including vitamins A, C, and E. At the request of Health Canada and several federal agencies in the United States, the Institute of Medicine undertook a study to assess all available data and review the DRIs for vitamin D and calcium. These two essential nutrients have long been known for their important role in bone health, and new research has indicated that they may also play a role in cancer, cardiovascular disease, hypertension, diabetes, metabolic syndrome, falls, immune response, neuropsychological functions, physical performance, preeclampsia, and reproductive outcomes. The Institute of Medicine's report was released at the end of 2010, and although the DRIs were updated for both calcium and vitamin D, additional research is required to determine the benefit of vitamin D and calcium for conditions other than bone health.

Table 5.3	Facts About Vitamins			
Vitamin	**Important Dietary Sources**	**Major Functions**	**Signs of Prolonged Deficiency**	**Toxic Effects of Megadoses**
Fat Soluble				
Vitamin A	Liver, milk, butter, cheese, and fortified margarine; carrots, spinach, and other orange and deep-green vegetables and fruits	Maintenance of vision, skin, linings of the nose, mouth, digestive and urinary tracts, immune function	Night blindness; dry, scaling skin; increased susceptibility to infection; loss of appetite; anemia; kidney stones	Liver damage, miscarriage and birth defects, headache, vomiting and diarrhea, vertigo, double vision, bone abnormalities
Vitamin D	Fortified milk and margarine, fish oils, butter, egg yolks (sunlight on skin also produces vitamin D)	Development and maintenance of bones and teeth, promotion of calcium absorption	Rickets (bone deformities) in children; bone softening, loss, and fractures in adults	Kidney damage, calcium deposits in soft tissues, depression, death
Vitamin E	Vegetable oils, whole grains, nuts and seeds, green leafy vegetables, asparagus, peaches	Protection and maintenance of cellular membranes	Red blood cell breakage and anemia, weakness, neurological problems, muscle cramps	Relatively nontoxic, but may cause excess bleeding or formation of blood clots
Vitamin K	Green leafy vegetables; smaller amounts widespread in other foods	Production of factors essential for blood clotting and bone metabolism	Hemorrhaging	None reported
Water Soluble				
Biotin	Cereals, yeast, egg yolks, soy flour, liver; widespread in foods	Synthesis of fat, glycogen, and amino acids	Rash, nausea, vomiting, weight loss, depression, fatigue, hair loss	None reported
Folate	Green leafy vegetables, yeast, oranges, whole grains, legumes, liver	Amino acid metabolism, synthesis of RNA and DNA, new cell synthesis	Anemia, weakness, fatigue, irritability, shortness of breath, swollen tongue	Masking of vitamin B12 deficiency
Niacin	Eggs, poultry, fish, milk, whole grains, nuts, enriched breads and cereals, meats, legumes	Conversion of carbohydrates, fats, and protein into usable forms of energy	Pellagra (symptoms include diarrhea, dermatitis, inflammation of mucous membranes, dementia)	Flushing of the skin, nausea, vomiting, diarrhea, liver dysfunction, glucose intolerance
Pantothenic acid	Animal foods, whole grains, broccoli, potatoes; widespread in foods	Metabolism of fats, carbohydrates, and proteins	Fatigue, numbness and tingling of hands and feet, gastrointestinal disturbances	None reported
Riboflavin	Dairy products, enriched breads and cereals, lean meats, poultry, fish, green vegetables	Energy metabolism; maintenance of skin, mucous membranes, and nervous system structures	Cracks at corners of mouth, sore throat, skin rash, hypersensitivity to light, purple tongue	None reported
Thiamine	Whole-grain and enriched breads and cereals, organ meats, lean pork, nuts, legumes	Conversion of carbohydrates into usable forms of energy, maintenance of appetite and nervous system function	Beriberi (symptoms include muscle wasting, mental confusion, anorexia, enlarged heart, nerve changes)	None reported
Vitamin B6	Eggs, poultry, fish, whole grains, nuts, soybeans, liver, kidney, pork	Metabolism of amino acids and glycogen	Anemia, convulsions, cracks at corners of mouth, dermatitis, nausea, confusion	Neurological abnormalities and damage
Vitamin B12	Meat, fish, poultry, fortified cereals	Synthesis of blood cells; other metabolic reactions	Anemia, fatigue, nervous system damage, sore tongue	None reported
Vitamin C	Peppers, broccoli, spinach, Brussels sprouts, citrus fruits, strawberries, tomatoes, potatoes, cabbage, other fruits and vegetables	Maintenance and repair of connective tissue, bones, teeth, and cartilage; promotion of healing; aid in iron absorption	Scurvy, anemia, reduced resistance to infection, loosened teeth, joint pain, poor wound healing, hair loss, poor iron absorption	Urinary stones in some people, acid stomach from ingesting supplements in pill form, nausea, diarrhea, headache, fatigue

Sources: Food and Nutrition Board, Institute of Medicine. 2006. *Dietary Reference Intakes: The Essential Guide to Nutrient Requirements.* Washington, D.C.: The National Academies Press. The complete Dietary Reference Intake reports are available from the National Academy Press (http://www.nap.edu); Shils, M. E., et al., eds. 2005. *Modern Nutrition in Health and Disease,* 10th ed. Baltimore: Lippincott Williams & Wilkins.

Vitamin Excesses   Extra vitamins in the diet can also be harmful, especially when taken as supplements. Megadoses of fat-soluble vitamins are particularly dangerous because the excess is stored in the body rather than excreted, increasing the risk of toxicity. Even when vitamins are not taken in excess, relying on supplements for an adequate intake of vitamins can be a problem. Foods have many substances other than vitamins and minerals, and some of these compounds may have important health effects.

As Canadians consume more supplements and eat more foods that have been fortified with vitamin D, they must do so cautiously. Very high levels of vitamin D (more than 10,000 IU per day) are known to cause kidney and tissue damage. High levels have not been shown to provide greater benefits and in fact, have been linked to other health issues. More is not always better, especially in the case of vitamin D.

QUICK STATS

At least **80%** of fractures in people 60 years of age and older are related to osteoporosis.

—Osteoporosis Canada, 2010

Later in the chapter we discuss specific recommendations for vitamin intake and when a vitamin supplement is advisable. For now, keep in mind that it's best to get most of your vitamins from foods rather than from supplements.

Keeping the Nutrient Value in Food   Vitamins and minerals can be lost or destroyed during the storage and cooking of foods. To retain nutrients, consume or process vegetables as soon as possible after purchasing. Store fruits and vegetables in the refrigerator in covered containers or plastic bags to minimize moisture loss; freeze foods that won't be eaten within a few days. Frozen and canned vegetables are usually as high in nutrients as fresh vegetables because nutrients are locked in when produce is frozen or canned. Canned vegetables may have high amounts of sodium added during the processing of the vegetables, so be sure to read the labels. To reduce nutrient losses during food preparation, minimize the amount of water used and the total cooking time. Develop a taste for a crunchier texture in cooked vegetables. Baking, steaming, broiling, grilling, and microwaving are all healthy methods of preparing vegetables.

Minerals: Inorganic Micronutrients

Minerals are inorganic (non-carbon-containing) elements you need in relatively small amounts to help regulate body functions, aid in the growth and maintenance of body tissues, and help release energy (Table 5.4). There are about 17 essential minerals. The major minerals, those that the body needs in amounts exceeding 100 milligrams per day, include calcium, phosphorus, magnesium, sodium, potassium, and chloride. The essential trace minerals, those that you need in minute amounts, include copper, fluoride, iodide, iron, selenium, and zinc.

Characteristic symptoms develop if an essential mineral is consumed in a quantity too small or too large for good health. The minerals commonly lacking in the Canadian diet are calcium, magnesium, potassium, iron, and folate. Iron-deficiency **anemia** is a problem in many age groups, and researchers fear poor calcium intakes in childhood are sowing the seeds for future **osteoporosis**, especially in women. See Chapter 21 for more information on osteoporosis; the box "Eating for Healthy Bones" (p. 144) has tips for building and maintaining bone density.

Water: Vital but Often Ignored

Water is the major component in both foods and the human body: You are composed of about 60% water. Your need for other nutrients, in terms of weight, is much less than your need for water. You can live up to 50 days without food, but only a few days without water.

Water is distributed all over the body, among lean and other tissues and in blood and other body fluids. Water is used in the digestion and absorption of food and is the medium in which most of the chemical reactions take place within the body. Some water-based fluids, such as blood, transport substances around the body, whereas other fluids serve as lubricants or cushions. Water also helps regulate body temperature.

Water is contained in almost all foods, particularly in liquids, fruits, and vegetables. The foods and fluids you consume provide 80%–90% of your daily water intake; the remainder is generated through metabolism. You lose water each day in urine, feces, and sweat and through evaporation from your lungs.

Most people can maintain a healthy water balance by consuming beverages at meals and drinking fluids in response to thirst. Health Canada has set levels of adequate water intake to maintain hydration; all fluids, including those containing caffeine, can count toward your total daily fluid intake. Under these guidelines, men need to consume about 3.7 litres of water; women need 2.7 litres.

TERMS

minerals   Inorganic compounds needed in relatively small amounts for regulation, growth, and maintenance of body tissues and functions.

anemia   A deficiency in the oxygen-carrying material in the red blood cells.

osteoporosis   A condition in which the bones become extremely thin and brittle and break easily.

free radical   An electron-seeking compound that can react with fats, proteins, and DNA, damaging cell membranes and mutating genes in its search for electrons; produced through chemical reactions in the body and by exposure to environmental factors, such as sunlight and tobacco smoke.

Table 5.4   Facts About Selected Minerals

Mineral	Important Dietary Sources	Major Functions	Signs of Prolonged Deficiency	Toxic Effects of Megadoses
Calcium	Milk and milk products, tofu, fortified orange juice and bread, green leafy vegetables, bones in fish	Formation of bones and teeth, control of nerve impulses, muscle contraction, blood clotting	Stunted growth in children, bone mineral loss in adults; urinary stones	Kidney stones, calcium deposits in soft tissues, inhibition of mineral absorption, constipation
Fluoride	Fluoridated water, tea, marine fish eaten with bones	Maintenance of tooth and bone structure	Higher frequency of tooth decay	Increased bone density, mottling of teeth, impaired kidney function
Iodine	Iodized salt, seafood, processed foods	Essential part of thyroid hormones, regulation of body metabolism	Goitre (enlarged thyroid), cretinism (birth defect)	Depression of thyroid activity, hyperthyroidism in susceptible people
Iron	Meat and poultry, fortified grain products, dark-green vegetables, dried fruit	Component of hemoglobin, myoglobin, and enzymes	Iron-deficiency anemia, weakness, impaired immune function, gastrointestinal distress	Nausea, diarrhea, liver and kidney damage, joint pains, sterility, disruption of cardiac function, death
Magnesium	Widespread in foods and water (except soft water); especially found in grains, legumes, nuts, seeds, green vegetables, milk	Transmission of nerve impulses, energy transfer, activation of many enzymes	Neurological disturbances, cardiovascular problems, kidney disorders, nausea, growth failure in children	Nausea, vomiting, diarrhea, central nervous system depression, coma; death in people with impaired kidney function
Phosphorus	Present in nearly all foods, especially milk, cereal, peas, eggs, meat	Bone growth and maintenance, energy transfer in cells	Impaired growth, weakness, kidney disorders, cardio-respiratory and nervous system dysfunction	Drop in blood calcium levels, calcium deposits in soft tissues, bone loss
Potassium	Meats, milk, fruits, vegetables, grains, legumes	Nerve function and body water balance	Muscular weakness, nausea, drowsiness, paralysis, confusion, disruption of cardiac rhythm	Cardiac arrest
Selenium	Seafood, meat, eggs, whole grains	Defence against oxidative stress, regulation of thyroid hormone action	Muscle pain and weakness, heart disorders	Hair and nail loss, nausea and vomiting, weakness, irritability
Sodium	Salt, soy sauce, salted foods, tomato juice	Body water balance, acid-base balance, nerve function	Muscle weakness, loss of appetite, nausea, vomiting; deficiency is rarely seen	Edema, hypertension in sensitive people
Zinc	Whole grains, meat, eggs, liver, seafood (especially oysters)	Synthesis of proteins, RNA, and DNA; wound healing; immune response; ability to taste	Growth failure, loss of appetite, impaired taste acuity, skin rash, impaired immune function, poor wound healing	Vomiting, impaired immune function, decline in blood HDL levels, impaired copper absorption

Sources: Food and Nutrition Board, Institute of Medicine. 2006. *Dietary Reference Intakes: The Essential Guide to Nutrient Requirements.* Washington, D.C.: The National Academies Press. The complete Dietary Reference Intake reports are available from the National Academy Press (http://www.nap.edu); Shils, M. E.,et al., eds. 2005. *Modern Nutrition in Health and Disease,* 10th ed. Baltimore: Lippincott Williams & Wilkins.

(See Table 1 in the Nutrition Resources section at the end of the chapter for information on specific age groups.) If you exercise vigorously or live in a hot climate, you need to consume additional fluids to maintain a balance between water consumed and water lost. Severe dehydration causes weakness and can lead to death.

Other Substances in Food

Many substances in food are not essential nutrients but may influence health.

Antioxidants   When the body uses oxygen or breaks down certain fats or proteins as a normal part of metabolism, it gives rise to substances called **free radicals**. Environmental factors, such as cigarette smoke, exhaust fumes, radiation, excessive sunlight, certain drugs, and stress, can increase free radical production. A free radical is a chemically unstable molecule that reacts with fats, proteins, and DNA, damaging cell membranes and mutating genes. Free radicals have been implicated in aging, cancer, cardiovascular disease, and other degenerative diseases, such as arthritis.

Eating for Healthy Bones

Osteoporosis is a condition in which the bones become dangerously thin and fragile over time. An estimated 2 million Canadians are living with osteoporosis. One in four women and one in eight men over 50 have osteoporosis. Most bone mass is built by age 18. After bone density peaks between ages 25 and 35, bone mass is lost over time. To prevent osteoporosis, the best strategy is to build as much bone as possible during your youth and do everything you can to maintain it as you age. Up to 50% of bone loss is determined by controllable lifestyle factors. Key nutrients for bone health include the following:

• *Calcium.* Consuming an adequate amount of calcium is important throughout life to build and maintain bone mass. Milk, yogourt, and calcium-fortified orange juice, bread, and cereals are all good sources.

• *Vitamin D.* Vitamin D is necessary for bones to absorb calcium; a daily intake of 5 micrograms is recommended for adults ages 19–50. Vitamin D can be obtained from foods and is manufactured by the skin when exposed to sunlight. Candidates for vitamin D supplements include people who don't eat many foods rich in vitamin D; those who don't have incidental exposure to UV radiation from the sun on their face, arms, and hands (without sunscreen) for 5–15 minutes a few times each week; and people who live in northern latitudes throughout Canada where the sun is weaker. Remember that ultraviolet light from the sun can cause skin cancer. Limit your exposure to the sunshine when you are not wearing sunscreen, and do not use tanning beds. Most skin cancers are largely preventable. Regardless of where the melanoma shows up on the body, it is

typically a result of ultraviolet radiation exposure, either from natural sunlight or artificial tanning.

• *Vitamin K.* Vitamin K promotes the synthesis of proteins that help keep bones strong. Broccoli and leafy green vegetables are rich in vitamin K.

• *Other nutrients.* Other nutrients that may play an important role in bone health include vitamin C, magnesium, potassium, manganese, zinc, copper, and boron.

On the other side, several dietary substances may have a *negative* effect on bone health, especially if consumed in excess: alcohol, sodium, caffeine, and retinol (a form of vitamin A). Drinking lots of soft drinks, which often replace milk in the diet and which are high in phosphorus (a mineral that may interfere with calcium absorption), has been shown to increase the risk of bone fracture in teenage girls.

The effect of protein intake on bone mass depends on other nutrients: Protein helps build bone as long as calcium and vitamin D intake are adequate; but if intake of calcium and vitamin D is low, high protein intake can lead to bone loss.

Weight-bearing aerobic exercise helps maintain bone mass throughout life, and strength training improves bone density, muscle mass, strength, and balance. Drinking alcohol only in moderation, refraining from smoking, and managing depression and stress are also important for maintaining strong bones. For people who develop osteoporosis, a variety of medications are available to treat the condition.

Antioxidants found in foods can help protect the body from damage by free radicals in several ways. Some prevent or reduce the formation of free radicals; others remove free radicals from the body; still others repair some types of free radical damage after it occurs. Some antioxidants, such as vitamin C, vitamin E, and selenium, are also essential nutrients. Others—such as the carotenoids found in yellow, orange, and deep-green vegetables—are not. Researchers have identified the top antioxidant-containing foods and beverages as blackberries, walnuts, strawberries, artichokes, cranberries, brewed coffee, raspberries, pecans, blueberries, cloves, grape juice, unsweetened baking chocolate, sour cherries, and red wine. Also high in antioxidants are Brussels sprouts, kale, cauliflower, and pomegranates.

Phytochemicals Antioxidants fall into the broader category of **phytochemicals**, substances found in plant foods that may help prevent chronic disease. Researchers have just begun to identify and study all the different compounds found in foods, and many preliminary findings are promising. For example, certain substances found in soy foods may help lower cholesterol levels. Sulphoraphane, a compound isolated from broccoli and other **cruciferous vegetables**, may render some carcino-

QUESTIONS FOR CRITICAL THINKING AND REFLECTION

Experts say that two of the most important factors in a healthy diet are eating the right kinds of carbohydrates and the right kinds of fats. Based on what you've read so far in this chapter, which are the right carbohydrates and fats? How would you say your own diet stacks up when it comes to carbs and fats?

genic compounds harmless. Allyl sulphides, a group of chemicals found in garlic and onions, appear to boost the activity of cancer-fighting immune cells. Further research on phytochemicals may extend the role of nutrition to the prevention and treatment of many chronic diseases.

If you want to increase your intake of phytochemicals, it is best to eat a variety of fruits, vegetables, and grains rather than relying on supplements. Like many vitamins and minerals, isolated phytochemicals may be harmful if taken in high doses. In addition, it is likely that their health benefits are the result of chemical substances working in combination. The role of phytochemicals in disease prevention is discussed further in Chapters 7 and 8.

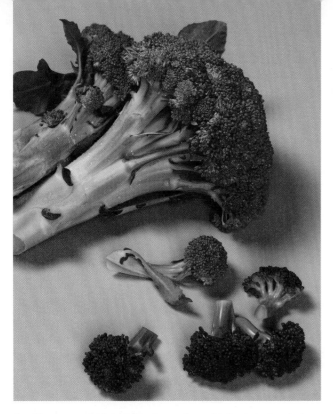

Cruciferous vegetables, such as broccoli, are rich in phytochemicals and essential vitamins and minerals.

NUTRITIONAL GUIDELINES: PLANNING YOUR DIET

Various tools have been created by scientific and government groups to help people design healthy diets. As noted earlier, the **Dietary Reference Intakes (DRIs)** are standards for nutrient intake designed to prevent nutritional deficiencies and reduce the risk of chronic disease. Health Canada has established **Guidelines for Healthy Eating** to promote health and reduce the risk for major chronic diseases through diet and physical activity. *Eating Well with Canada's Food Guide* provides further guidance on daily food intake patterns that meet the DRIs and are consistent with the dietary guidelines.

Dietary Reference Intakes (DRIs)

The Food and Nutrition Board of the Institute of Medicine, in partnership with Health Canada, establishes dietary standards, or recommended intake levels, for Canadians of all ages. The current set of standards, called Dietary Reference Intakes (DRIs), was introduced in 1997. The DRIs are frequently reviewed and updated as new nutrition-related information becomes available. The DRIs present different categories of nutrients in an easy-to-read table format. An earlier set of standards, called the Recommended Nutrient Intakes (RNIs) in Canada, focused on preventing nutritional deficiency diseases, such as anemia. The DRIs have a broader focus because research looked not just at the prevention of nutrient deficiencies but also at the role of nutrients in promoting health and preventing chronic diseases, such as cancer, osteoporosis, and heart disease.

The DRIs include standards for both recommended intakes and maximum safe intakes. The recommended intake of each nutrient is expressed as either a *Recommended Dietary Allowance (RDA)* or *Adequate Intake (AI)*. An AI is set when not enough information is available to set an RDA value; regardless of the type of standard used, however, the DRI represents the best available estimate of intake for optimal health. The *Tolerable Upper Intake Level (UL)* is the maximum daily intake that is unlikely to cause health problems in a healthy person. For example, the AI for calcium for an 18-year-old female is 1300 milligrams per day; the UL is 2500 milligrams per day.

Because of lack of data, ULs have not been set for all nutrients. This does not mean that people can tolerate chronic intakes of these vitamins and minerals above recommended levels (see the box "Should You Take Supplements?" on p. 146. Like all chemical agents, nutrients can produce adverse effects if intakes are excessive. No benefit from consuming nutrients at levels above the RDA or AI has been established. The DRIs can be found in the Nutrition Resources section at the end of the chapter.

The Estimated Average Requirement (EAR) is also part of the DRIs. It is the amount estimated to meet the nutrient needs of half the individuals in a population group. EARs are used to calculate the RDA.

Because the DRIs are too cumbersome to use as a basis for food labels, Health Canada has introduced another set of dietary standards on food labels, the **Daily Values**. The

TERMS

phytochemical A naturally occurring substance found in plant foods that may help prevent and treat chronic diseases, such as cancer and heart disease; *phyto* means "plant."

cruciferous vegetables Vegetables of the cabbage family, including cabbage, broccoli, Brussels sprouts, kale, and cauliflower; the flower petals of these plants form the shape of a cross, hence the name.

Dietary Reference Intakes (DRIs) An umbrella term for four types of nutrient standards. Estimated Average Requirement (EAR) is the amount estimated to meet the nutrient needs of half the individuals in a population group; Adequate Intake (AI) and Recommended Dietary Allowance (RDA) are levels of intake considered adequate to prevent nutrient deficiencies and reduce the risk of chronic disease for most individuals in a population group; Tolerable Upper Intake Level (UL) is the maximum daily intake that is unlikely to cause health problems.

Guidelines for Healthy Eating General principles of good nutrition presented as practical ways that Canadians can follow a healthy diet and reduce their risk for chronic diseases.

Eating Well with Canada's Food Guide A food-group plan that provides practical advice to ensure a balanced intake of the essential nutrients.

Daily Values A simplified version of the RDAs used on food labels; also included are values for nutrients with no RDA.

Should You Take Supplements?

The aim of the Dietary Reference Intakes (DRIs) is to guide you in meeting your nutritional needs primarily with food, rather than with vitamin and mineral supplements. Supplements lack potentially beneficial phytochemicals and fibres that are found only in whole foods. Most Canadians can get the vitamins and minerals they need by eating a nutritionally balanced diet of various foods. The use of supplements to reduce heart disease or cancer risk remains controversial, so experts suggest that you avoid taking any nutrient at a level exceeding the Tolerable Upper Intake Level (UL).

The question of whether to take supplements is a serious one. Some vitamins and minerals are dangerous when taken in excess. Large doses of particular nutrients can also cause health problems by affecting the absorption of certain vitamins or minerals. For this reason, ask your doctor or a dietitian before taking any high-dosage supplement.

In setting the DRIs, Health Canada and the Institute of Medicine recommended supplements of particular nutrients for specific groups:

• Women who are capable of getting pregnant should get 400 micrograms per day of folic acid (the synthetic form

of the vitamin folate) from fortified foods and supplements in addition to folate from a varied diet. This level of folate can reduce the risk of neural tube defects in a developing fetus. Enriched breads, flours, cornmeal, rice, noodles, and other grain products are fortified with folic acid. Folate is found naturally in leafy green vegetables, legumes, oranges, and strawberries.

• Because of the oxidative stress caused by smoking, smokers should get 35 milligrams more vitamin C per day than the RDA set for their age and sex. Supplements aren't usually necessary, however, because this extra vitamin C can easily be found in foods. For example, 250 millilitres (one cup) of orange juice has about 100 milligrams of vitamin C.

• Vitamin D and calcium are important for bone strength and to reduce the risk of osteoporosis and fractures in older adults. Canadians under the age of 71 need 600 IU (IU is the symbol for international units, which vitamin D is measured in) of vitamin D a day, and those 71 and older need 800 IU. Five hundred millilitres (two cups) of milk provide about 200 IU of vitamin D. Because the skin's ability to produce vitamin D decreases with age, men and women 50 and older

need a daily vitamin D supplement of 400 IU, in addition to following *Eating Well with Canada's Food Guide*. People with dark skin and people who are exposed to little sunlight (such as night-shift workers and those living in institutions) may need vitamin D supplements as well.

Supplements may be recommended in other cases. Women with heavy menstrual flows, for example, may need extra iron. Some vegetarians may need supplemental calcium, iron, zinc, and B12, depending on their food choices. Other people may benefit from supplementation based on their physical conditions, the medicines they take, or their dietary habits.

Before deciding whether to take a vitamin or mineral supplement, consider whether you already consume a fortified breakfast cereal every day. Many breakfast cereals contain almost as many nutrients as a multivitamin pill. If you elect to take a supplement, choose one that contains 50%–100% of the Daily Value for vitamins and minerals. Avoid supplements containing large doses of particular nutrients. To determine which supplement may be best for you, consult your doctor or pharmacist.

Daily Values are based on several different sets of guidelines and include standards for fat, cholesterol, carbohydrate, dietary fibre, and selected vitamins and minerals. The Daily Values represent appropriate intake levels for a 2000-calorie diet. The percent Daily Value shown on a food label shows how well that food contributes to your recommended daily intake. Food labels are described in detail later in the chapter.

Guidelines for Healthy Eating

To provide general guidance for choosing a healthy diet, Health Canada has issued Guidelines for Healthy Eating. Most people look for more than just additional information on nutrition to help them decipher the scientific concepts used to establish the Dietary Reference Intakes. The Guidelines for Healthy Eating provide practical, concrete actions that Canadians can take to ensure they follow a healthy diet:

• Enjoy a variety of foods.
• Emphasize cereals, breads, grain products, vegetables, and fruit.

• Choose lower-fat dairy products, leaner meats, and foods prepared with little or no fats.
• Achieve and maintain a healthy weight by enjoying regular physical activity and healthy eating.
• Limit salt, alcohol, and caffeine.

Following these guidelines promotes health and reduces the risk for chronic diseases, including heart disease, cancer, diabetes, stroke, osteoporosis, and obesity. Each of the recommendations Guidelines for Healthy Eating is supported by an extensive review of scientific and medical evidence.

Adequate Nutrients Within Calorie Needs Many people consume more calories than they need while failing to meet recommended intakes for all nutrients. The DRIs provide a foundation not only for current health but also for reducing chronic disease risk.

Following *Eating Well with Canada's Food Guide* can help you to obtain all the nutrients you need by choosing the recommended number of daily servings from basic

IN FOCUS

food groups and following the advice about selecting nutrient-dense foods within the groups.

People's food choices can be affected by individual and cultural preferences, moral beliefs, the cost and availability of food, and food intolerances and allergies. But healthy eating is possible no matter how foods are prepared or combined (see the box "Ethnic Foods" on p. 148). If you avoid most or all foods from any of the major food groups, be sure to get enough nutrients from the other groups. *Eating Well with Canada's Food Guide* can be applied to vegetarian diets.

Weight Management   Overweight and obesity are a major public health problem in Canada. Calorie intake and physical activity work together to influence body weight. Most Canadians need to reduce the number of calories they consume, increase their level of physical activity, and make wiser food choices. Many adults gain weight slowly over time, but even small changes in behaviour can help avoid weight gain. For more information on weight management, see Chapter 4.

Physical Activity   Regular physical activity improves fitness, helps manage weight, promotes psychological well-being, and reduces the risk of heart disease, high blood pressure, cancer, and diabetes. Become active if you are inactive, and maintain or increase physical activity if you are already active. It is important to balance a healthy diet with regular physical activity to maintain optimal

health. The amount of daily physical activity recommended for you depends on your current health status and goals. See Chapter 6 for information on exercise and physical fitness.

Food Groups to Encourage   The Guidelines for Healthy Eating and *Eating Well with Canada's Food Guide* both emphasize eating a wide range of foods. Central to these plans are fruits, vegetables, whole grains, and low-fat and fat-free milk and alternatives. Each of these food groups offers a nearly endless array of choices. The discussion of *Eating Well with Canada's Food Guide* later in this chapter provides detailed information on choices and serving sizes.

Fats   The type and amount of fats consumed can make a difference for health. A diet low in saturated fat, trans fat, and cholesterol helps keep blood cholesterol low and reduces the risk for heart disease. Goals for fat intake for most adults are as follows:

- Total fat: 20%–35% of total daily calories
- Saturated fat: Less than 10% of total daily calories
- Trans fat: Less than 1% of total caloric intake
- Cholesterol: Less than 300 milligrams per day

Most fats in the diet should come from sources of unsaturated fats, such as fish, nuts, and vegetable oils. When selecting and preparing meat, poultry, dry beans, and milk or milk products, make choices that are lean, low fat, or fat free. To reduce trans fat intake, limit intake of foods made with hydrogenated vegetable oils. (See the box "Going Trans Fat Free" on p. 149.)

Cholesterol is found only in animal foods. If you need to reduce your cholesterol intake, limit your intake of foods that are particularly high in cholesterol, including egg yolks, dairy fats, certain shellfish, and liver and other organ meats; watch your serving sizes of animal foods. Food labels list the fat and cholesterol content of foods.

Two servings per week of fish rich in heart-healthy omega-3 fatty acids are also recommended for people at high risk for heart disease. However, for certain groups, intake limits are set for varieties of fish that may contain mercury; see the section "Guidelines for Fish Consumption" later in the chapter for more information. Fish rich in omega-3 fatty acids include salmon, mackerel, and trout.

THINKING ABOUT THE ENVIRONMENT

Environmental issues—including booming populations and changing weather patterns—have coupled with fuel shortages to create a potential global food crisis. In 2008, evidence of such a crisis began to mount, even as worldwide production of many food staples reached all-time highs.

- The growing demand for corn to create ethanol (an alternative to gasoline) has driven up corn prices and greatly reduced the amount of grain used for human and animal consumption.

- Driven by fears of future shortages, the price of rice rose by more than 75% between December 2007 and April 2008. Some rice-producing countries began restricting rice exports to meet their own needs for the staple.

- Riots erupted in Haiti, Egypt, Bangladesh, and other countries in the spring of 2008, as residents protested food shortages and high prices. Many experts warned that if the current trend continues, the world's poorest people soon will not be able to feed themselves.

For more information on the environment and health, see Chapter 21.

Ethnic Foods

No single ethnic diet clearly surpasses all others in providing people with healthful foods. However, every diet has its advantages and disadvantages and, within each cuisine, some foods are better choices. The dietary guidelines described in this chapter can be applied to any ethnic cuisine. For additional guidance, refer to the table below.

	Choose More Often	Choose Less Often
Chinese	• Dishes that are steamed, poached (jum), boiled (chu), roasted (kow), barbecued (shu), or lightly stir-fried • Hoisin sauce, oyster sauce, wine sauce, plum sauce, velvet sauce, or hot mustard • Fresh fish and seafood, skinless chicken, tofu • Mixed vegetables, Chinese greens • Steamed rice, steamed spring rolls, soft noodles	• Fried wontons or egg rolls • Crab rangoon • Crispy (Peking) duck or chicken • Sweet-and-sour dishes made with breaded and deep-fried meat, poultry, or fish • Fried rice • Fried or crispy noodles
French	• Dishes prepared *au vapeur* (steamed), *en brochette* (skewered and broiled), or *grillé* (grilled) • Fresh fish, shrimp, scallops, or mussels or skinless chicken, without sauces • Clear soups	• Dishes prepared *à gratinée* (baked with cream and cheese), or *en croûte* (in pastry crust) • Drawn butter, hollandaise sauce, and remoulade (mayonnaise-based sauce)
Greek	• Dishes that are stewed, broiled, or grilled, including souvlaki • Dolmas (grape leaves) stuffed with rice • Tzatziki (yogourt, cucumbers, and garlic) • Pita bread, especially whole wheat	• Moussaka, saganaki (fried cheese) • Vegetable pies, such as spanakopita and tyropita • Gyros stuffed with ground meat • Baklava
Indian	• Dishes prepared *masala* (curry), *tandoori* (roasted in a clay oven), or *tikke* (pan roasted); kebabs • Raita (yogourt and cucumber salad) and other yogourt-based dishes and sauces • Dal (lentils), pullao or pilau (basmati rice) • Chapati (baked bread)	• Ghee (clarified butter) • Korma (meat in cream sauce) • Samosas, pakoras (fried dishes) • Molee and other coconut milk–based dishes • Poori, bhatura, or paratha (fried breads)
Italian	• Pasta primavera or pasta, polenta, risotto, or gnocchi with marinara, red or white wine, white or red clam, or light mushroom sauce • Dishes that are grilled or prepared *cacciatore* (tomato-based sauce), *marsala* (broth and wine sauce), or *piccata* (lemon sauce) • Cioppino (seafood stew) • Vegetable soup, minestrone or fagioli (beans)	• Antipasto (cheese, smoked meats) • Dishes that are prepared *alfredo*, *frito* (fried), *crema* (creamed), *alla panna* (with cream), or *carbonara* • Veal scaloppini • Chicken, veal, or eggplant parmigiana • Italian sausage, salami, and prosciutto • Buttered garlic bread • Cannoli
Japanese	• Dishes prepared *nabemono* (boiled), *shabu-shabu* (in boiling broth), *mushimono* (steamed), *nimono* (simmered), *yaki* (broiled), or *yakimono* (grilled) • Sushi or domburi (mixed rice dish) • Steamed rice or soba (buckwheat), udon (wheat), or rice noodles	• Tempura (battered and fried) • Agemono (deep fried) • Katsu (fried pork cutlet) • Sukiyaki • Fried tofu
Mexican	• Soft corn or wheat tortillas • Burritos, fajitas, enchiladas, soft tacos, and tamales filled with beans, vegetables, or lean meats • Refried beans, nonfat or low-fat; rice and beans • Ceviche (fish marinated in lime juice) • Salsa, enchilada sauce, and *picante* sauce • Gazpacho, menudo, or black bean soup • Fruit or flan for dessert	• Crispy, fried tortillas • Dishes that are fried, such as chile flautas, and tostadas • Nachos and cheese, chili con queso, and other dishes made with cheese or cheese sauce • Guacamole, sour cream, and extra cheese • Refried beans made with lard • Fried ice cream
Middle Eastern	• Dishes that are stewed, broiled, or grilled, including shish kebabs • Tabouli (bulgur-based salad) • Pita bread, especially whole wheat	• Moussaka • Baba ghanoush (eggplant and olive oil) • Deep-fried falafel (chickpea patties)
Thai	• Dishes that are barbecued, sautéed, broiled, boiled, steamed, braised, or marinated • *Sâté* (skewered and grilled meats) • Fish sauce, basil sauce, chili or hot sauces • Bean thread noodles, Thai salad	• Coconut milk soup • Peanut sauce or dishes topped with nuts • Mee-krob (crispy noodles) • Red, green, and yellow curries, which typically contain coconut milk

Sources: National Heart, Lung, and Blood Institute. 2006. *Guidelines on Overweight and Obesity: Electronic Textbook* (http://www.nhlbi.nih.gov/ guidelines/ obesity/e_txtbk/appndx/6a3b.htm; retrieved February 9, 2009); Duyff, R. L. 2006. *The American Dietetic Association's Complete Food and Nutrition Guide*, 2nd ed. Hoboken, N.J.: Wiley.

In 2005, Health Canada commissioned the Trans Fat Task Force to study ways to reduce or eliminate the trans fats added to our food supply, and in 2006, *TRANSforming the Food Supply*, the Task Force's final report was released. In 2007, the minister of health endorsed the trans fat levels recommended by the Task Force (2% of the total fat content in vegetable oils and soft margarines; and 5% of the total fat in all other foods, including those sold to restaurants) and gave the food industry two years to voluntarily meet those levels. If the levels weren't met, the minister promised regulation of the industry to achieve that goal. Some food companies achieved or bettered these levels, but others have not. Unfortunately, many foods often consumed by children as treats, such as cakes, doughnuts, and brownies, still contain trans fats.

Denmark, Switzerland, California, and many cities in the United States have trans fat regulations. In Canada, British Columbia implemented trans fat regulations in September 2009.

What Are Trans Fats?

Trans fats are unsaturated fatty acids that have at least one double bond in the *trans* configuration. This refers to the way the hydrogen atoms are arranged on either side of the double bond. Normally, these hydrogen atoms are on the same side of the double bond, but in a trans fatty acid, they are on opposite sides. This gives the fatty acid a physical structure more like a saturated fatty acid. Although trans fats are found in small amounts naturally in milk, beef, and lamb, most trans fats are formed through the process of hydrogenation. Many popular food items contain trans fat (see the table at right).

Hydrogenation makes liquid oils into solid or semisolid fats and is the process used to make margarine and shortening. These partially hydrogenated oils have a longer shelf life and ideal physical properties for use in baked goods, such as pastries, pie crusts, pizza dough, biscuits, cookies, and crackers. Partially hydrogenated oils are used for deep-fat frying because they are more stable, don't break down quickly, and therefore are more cost effective than nonhydrogenated oils.

The use of partially hydrogenated oils in restaurant and commercially prepared foods grew throughout the 1960s, 1970s, and 1980s in response to public health recommendations to reduce saturated fat intake from animal fats and tropical oils (such as palm and coconut oil).

Why Worry About Trans Fats?

In the 1990s, studies began to show that trans fats had similar effects in the body as saturated fat. Further research found that trans fats were actually worse for heart health because not only do they raise LDL cholesterol but they also lower HDL cholesterol. A recent study found that a 2% increase in dietary intake from trans fat was associated with a 23% increase in heart disease. Other studies suggest that trans fats may promote obesity and diabetes.

Can Trans Fats Be Eliminated?

Trans fats are not a dietary essential. Health organizations recommend that trans fat intake be as low as possible. Because some trans fats are naturally occurring, unless you are a strict vegetarian, your diet has no room for trans fats from partially hydrogenated oils. More and more products in the grocery store are available without trans fat, and as interest in trans-fat-free restaurants grows, it will be easier for consumers to limit trans fats when eating out.

Denmark has made it illegal for any food to contain more than 2% trans fat, and Canada is considering a nationwide ban on trans fats in restaurants. In the United States in 2004, the Center for Science in the Public Interest petitioned the Food and Drug Administration to ban trans fat as a food ingredient.

Reducing Your Trans Fat Intake

Start by reading food labels; trans fat content is required to be listed. A word of caution, however: A serving of a food can contain up to 0.5 grams of trans fat and still show zero grams on the Nutrition Fact label and the words "trans fat free" on the label. So check the ingredient list. If partially hydrogenated oil is included in the list, then the product contains trans fat.

Next, check the product's calorie and saturated fat content. Foods without trans fat are not healthier if they contain more saturated fat or more calories from added sugars. Ask at restaurants whether trans-fat-free oils are used in cooking. Proposals being considered could require national chain restaurants to include information about the calorie content of their foods, which could also help consumers make smart choices.

Trans Fat Content of Common Food Items

Product	Common Serving Size	Total Fat (g)	Trans Fat (g)
French fries	Medium pkg (147 g)	27	8
Hard margarine	1 tbsp	11	3
Soft margarine	1 tbsp	7	0.5
Shortening	1 tbsp	13	4
Potato chips	Small bag (42.5 g)	11	3
Doughnut	1	18	5
Candy bar	1 (40 g)	10	3
Pound cake	1 slice (80 g)	16	4.5

Sources: Mozaffarian, D., et al. 2006. Trans fatty acids and cardiovascular disease. *New England Journal of Medicine* 354(15): 1601–1613; Eckel, R. H., et al. 2006. Understanding the complexity of trans fatty acid reduction in the American diet. American Heart Association Trans Fat Conference 2006. Report of the *Trans Fat* Conference Planning Group. *Circulation* 115(16): 2231–2246; American Heart Association. 2009. *Trans Fats* (http://www.americanheart.org/presenter.jhtml?identifier=3045792; retrieved February 9, 2009); Center for Science in the Public Interest. 2009. *Trans Fat* (http://www.cspinet.org/transfat; retrieved February 9, 2009); U.S. Food and Drug Administration, Center for Food Safety and Applied Nutrition. 2006 Update. *Questions and Answers about Trans Fat Nutrition Labeling* (http://vm.cfsan.fda.gov/~dms/qatrans2.html; retrieved February 9, 2009); U.S. Food and Drug Administration. 2003. *Revealing Trans Fats* (http://www.fda.gov/FDAC/features/2003/503_fats.html; retrieved February 9, 2009); Trans Fat Task Force. 2006. *TRANSforming the Food Supply* (http://www.hc-sc.gc.ca/fn-an/alt_formats/hpfb-dgpsa/pdf/nutrition/tf-gt_rep-rap-eng.pdf; retrieved April 2, 2011).

Carbohydrates Carbohydrates are an important energy source in a healthy diet. Foods rich in carbohydrates may also be rich in dietary fibre, which promotes healthy digestion and helps reduce the risk of type 2 diabetes and heart disease. Fruits, vegetables, whole grains, and fat-free or low-fat milk can provide the recommended amount of carbohydrate. Choose fibre-rich foods often—for example, whole fruits, whole grains, and legumes.

People who consume foods and beverages high in added sugars tend to consume more calories but smaller amounts of vitamins and minerals than those who limit their intake of added sugars. A food is likely high in sugar if one of the following appears first or second in the list of ingredients or if several are listed: sugar (any type, including beet, brown, invert, raw, and cane), corn syrup or sweetener, fruit juice concentrate, honey, malt syrup, molasses, syrup, cane juice, dextrose, fructose, glucose, lactose, maltose, or sucrose.

To reduce added sugar consumption, cut back on soft drinks, candies, sweet desserts, fruit drinks, and other foods high in added sugars. Watch out for specialty drinks, such as café mochas, chai tea, smoothies, and sports drinks, which can contain hundreds of extra calories from sugar. Drink water rather than sweetened drinks, and don't let pop and other sweets crowd out more nutritious foods, such as low-fat milk. Regular soft drinks are the leading source of both added sugars and calories in the Canadian diet but provide little in the way of nutrients except sugar (Figure 5.5).

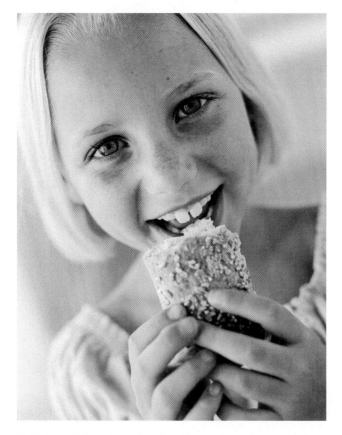

Half of your daily grain servings should come from whole grains. To check whether a food contains whole grains, read the ingredient list on the food label.

Nutrient	Recommended Daily Intake*	Orange Juice	Low-Fat (1%) Milk	Regular Cola	Bottled Iced Tea
Calories	2000 calories	168 calories	150 calories	152 calories	150 calories
Carbohydrate	300 g	40.5 g	18 g	38 g	37.5 g
Added sugars	32 g			38 g	34.5 g
Fat	65 g		3.9 g		
Protein	55 g		12 g		
Calcium	1000 mg	33 mg	450 mg	11 mg	
Potassium	4700 mg	15% 710 mg	12% 570 mg	4 mg	
Vitamin A	700 µg	4% 30 µg	31% 216 µg		
Vitamin C	75 mg	145.5 mg	3.6 mg		
Vitamin D	5 µg		3.7 µg		
Folate	400 µg	160 µg	20 µg		

*Recommended intakes and limits appropriate for a 20-year-old woman consuming 2000 calories per day.

FIGURE 5.5   Nutrient density of 355-millilitre portions of selected beverages.   The coloured bars represent percentage of recommended daily intake or limit for each nutrient.

Sodium and Potassium   Many people can reduce their chance of developing high blood pressure or lower already elevated blood pressure by consuming less salt; reducing blood pressure lowers the risk for stroke, heart disease, and kidney disease. Salt is made up of the minerals sodium and chloride, and although both of these minerals are essential for normal body function, we need only small amounts (1500 milligrams per day for adults). Most Canadians consume much more salt than they need. The goal is to reduce sodium intake to less than 2300 milligrams per day, the equivalent of about one teaspoon of salt. Certain groups, including people with hypertension, blacks, those of South Asian descent, and older adults, benefit from an even lower sodium intake (no more than 1500 milligrams per day).

Salt is found mainly in processed and prepared foods; smaller amounts may also be added during cooking or at the table. To lower your intake of salt, choose fresh or plain frozen meat, poultry, seafood, and vegetables most often; these are lower in salt than processed forms are. Check and compare the sodium content in processed foods, including frozen dinners, cheeses, soups, salad dressings, sauces, and canned mixed dishes. Add less salt during cooking and at the table, and limit your use of high-sodium condiments, such as soy sauce, ketchup, mustard, pickles, and olives. Use lemon juice, herbs, and spices instead of salt to enhance the flavour of foods.

Along with lowering salt intake, increasing potassium intake helps lower blood pressure. Fruits, vegetables, and most milk products are available in forms that contain no salt, and many of these are sources of potassium. Potassium-rich foods include leafy green vegetables, sweet and white potatoes, winter squash, soybeans, tomato sauce, bananas, peaches, apricots, cantaloupes, and orange juice.

Alcoholic Beverages   Alcoholic beverages supply calories but few nutrients. Drinking in moderation—that is, no more than one drink per day for women and no more than two drinks per day for men—is associated with mortality reduction among some groups, primarily males age 45 and older and women age 55 and older. Among younger people, alcohol use provides little if any health benefit, and heavy drinking is associated with motor vehicle injuries and deaths, liver disease, stroke, violence, and other health problems (see Chapter 15 for more on the health risks and potential benefits of alcohol use). If you drink alcohol, follow the low-risk drinking guidelines at all times.

Eating Well with Canada's Food Guide

When the first Canada's food guide was published in 1942, it acknowledged the difficulties of coping with wartime food rationing while still trying to prevent nutritional deficiencies and improve health. Since then, scientists have updated both nutrient recommendations (the DRIs) and the Guidelines for Healthy Eating, and the food guide has had several different names, different looks, and even different messages, but it's core purpose has remained the same:

"guiding food selection to promote the nutritional health of Canadians." In 2002, Health Canada began a revision of the food guide that was evidence based. In 2007, it released *Eating Well with Canada's Food Guide* (Figure 5.6 on p. 152).

Another food plan that has received attention in recent years is the Mediterranean diet, which emphasizes vegetables, fruits, and whole grains; daily servings of beans, legumes, and nuts; moderate consumption of fish, poultry, and dairy products; and the use of olive oil over other types of fat, especially saturated fat. The Mediterranean diet has been associated with lower rates of heart disease and cancer, and recent studies have found a link between the diet and a greatly reduced risk of Alzheimer's disease.

Key Messages of *Eating Well with Canada's Food Guide*   The new food guide has been developed to remind consumers to make healthy food choices and to be active every day. Consuming a balance of servings from each food group will not only meet nutrient needs but also help to reduce chronic disease risk. The key messages include the following:

- *Variety* is represented by the wide range of foods graphically represented in the guide. Many foods, including those typically consumed by different ethic groups living in Canada, are given as examples. Foods from all groups are needed daily for good health.

- *Food guide serving sizes and quantities* are given in both pictures and specific measurements, showing serving sizes of a variety of foods and amounts required by consumers of different ages and sexes.

- *Make each food guide serving count* is represented by directional statements that give consumers ways to ensure they are choosing food with high nutritional quality more often.

- *Advice for different ages and stages* ensures optimal growth, development, and maintenance of health are achieved.

- *Promotion of physical activity* includes recommendations about building physical activity into daily life.

To determine how much and what foods you should be consuming every day, create a personalized version of *Eating Well with Canada's Food Guide* at http://www.myfoodguide.ca. Each food group is described briefly below. Past experiences have shown that many Canadians have trouble identifying serving sizes, so recommended daily intakes from each group are now given; see the box "Judging Portion Sizes" (p. 152) for additional advice.

Judging Portion Sizes

Studies have shown that most people underestimate the size of their food portions, in many cases by as much as 50%. If you need to retrain your eye, try using measuring cups and spoons and an inexpensive kitchen scale when you eat at home. With a little practice, you'll learn the difference between 90 and 225 grams of chicken or meat, and what 125 millilitres of rice really looks like. For quick estimates, use the following equivalents:

• 5 millilitres (1 teaspoon) of margarine = the tip of your thumb

• 30 grams of cheese = two thumbs, four dice stacked together

• 90 grams of chicken or meat = a deck of cards

• 250 millilitres (1 cup) of pasta = a small fist or a baseball

• 125 millilitres (½ cup) of rice or cooked vegetables = a tennis ball

• 30 millilitres (2 tablespoons) of peanut butter = a golf ball

• 1 medium potato = a computer mouse

• 1 small bagel = a hockey puck

• 1 medium fruit (apple or orange) = a baseball or light bulb

• 50 millilitres (¼ cup) of nuts = a golf ball

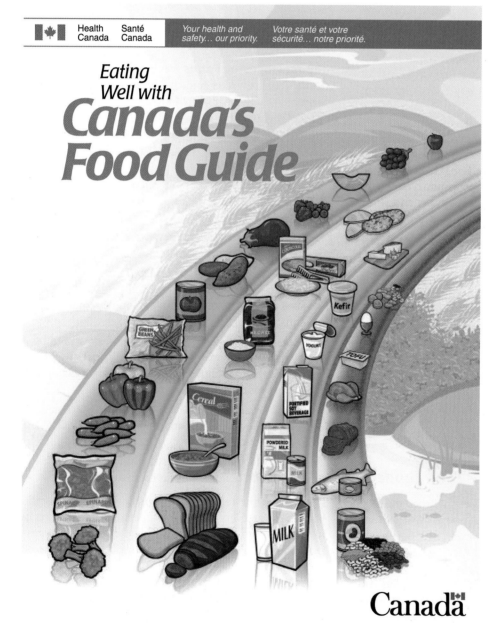

FIGURE 5.6 *Eating Well with Canada's Food Guide.* Health Canada's food guidance system, called *Eating Well with Canada's Food Guide*, can be personalized based on your sex, age, and activity level; visit http://www.myfoodguide.ca to obtain a food plan appropriate for you. *Eating Well with Canada's Food Guide* contains four main food groups. Directional statements, examples of food guide servings, and recommended numbers of servings guide consumers to choose a variety of healthy foods. The guide is available in English, French, Arabic, Chinese (simple), Farsi (Persian), Korean, Punjabi, Russian, Spanish, Tagalog, Urdu, and Tamil.

Source: Eating Well With Canada's Food Guide (2007), Health Canada. Reproduced with the permission of the Minister of Public Works and Government Services Canada, 2011.

Grains Foods from this group are usually low in fat and rich in complex carbohydrates, dietary fibre (if the grains are unrefined), and many vitamins and minerals, including thiamine, riboflavin, iron, niacin, folic acid (if enriched or fortified), and zinc. An adult between the ages of 19 and 50 should include six to eight servings each day, depending on their sex, with half of those servings from whole grains, such as whole-grain bread, whole wheat pasta, high-fibre cereal, and brown rice. The following count as one serving:

- 1 slice of bread
- 1 small (6-centimetre diameter) muffin
- 250 millilitres (1 cup) of ready-to-eat cereal flakes
- 125 millilitres (½ cup) cooked cereal, rice, grains, or pasta
- 1 15-centimetre tortilla

Choose foods that are typically made with little fat or sugar (bread, rice, pasta) over those that are high in fat and sugar (croissants, chips, cookies, doughnuts).

Vegetables and Fruit Vegetables contain carbohydrates, dietary fibre, vitamin A, vitamin C, folate, potassium, and other nutrients. They are also naturally low in fat. Each of the following counts as one serving of vegetables:

- 125 millilitres (½ cup) of raw or cooked vegetables
- 250 millilitres (1 cup) of raw leafy salad greens
- 125 millilitres (½ cup) vegetable juice

Because vegetables vary in the nutrients they provide, it is important to consume a variety of types of vegetables to obtain maximum nutrition. Many Canadians consume only a few types of vegetables, with white potatoes (baked or served as french fries) being the most popular. Canadians should eat at least one dark-green and one orange vegetable each day; should choose vegetables and fruit prepared with little or no added fat, sugar, or salt; and should have vegetables and fruit more often than juice. The following examples will give you ideas to help boost your vegetable intake:

- Dark-green vegetables include spinach, chard, collards, bok choy, broccoli, kale, romaine, turnip greens, and mustard greens.
- Orange and deep-yellow vegetables include carrots, winter squash, sweet potatoes, and pumpkin.
- Starchy vegetables include corn, green peas, and white potatoes.
- Other vegetables, such as tomatoes, bell peppers (red, orange, yellow, or green), green beans, and cruciferous vegetables, such as cauliflower, are also good choices.

Fruits are rich in carbohydrates, dietary fibre, and many vitamins, especially vitamin C. The following each count as one serving of fruit:

- 125 millilitres (½ cup) fresh, canned, or frozen fruit

- 125 millilitres (½ cup) fruit juice (100% juice)
- 1 small whole fruit
- 50 millilitres (½ cup) dried fruit

Good choices from this group are citrus fruits and juices, melons, pears, apples, bananas, and berries. Choose whole fruits often—they are higher in fibre and often lower in calories than fruit juices. Fruit *juices* typically contain more nutrients and less added sugar than fruit *drinks*. For canned fruits, choose those packed in 100% fruit juice or water rather than in syrup.

Milk and Alternatives This group includes all milk, milk products, and milk alternatives, such as yogourt and cheeses (except cream cheese), lactose-free and lactose-reduced products, and soy and rice beverages. Foods from this group are high in protein, carbohydrate, calcium, riboflavin, and vitamin D (if fortified). Each of the following counts as one serving:

- 250 millilitres (1 cup) of milk or fortified soy beverage
- 50 grams of natural cheese
- 175 millilitres (¾ cup) of kefir or yogourt

Meat and Alternatives This group includes meat, poultry, fish, dry beans and peas, eggs, nuts, and seeds. These foods provide protein, niacin, iron, vitamin B6, zinc, and thiamine; the animal foods in the group also provide vitamin B12. Each of the following counts as one serving:

- 75 grams of cooked lean meat, poultry, or fish
- 175 millilitres (¾ cup) of cooked dry beans (legumes) or tofu
- 2 eggs
- 30 millilitres (1 tablespoon) of peanut butter
- 60 millilitres (¼ cup) of nuts or seeds

One egg at breakfast, 175 millilitres of cooked pinto beans at lunch, and a 75-gram (cooked weight) hamburger at dinner would give you 170 grams of lean meat for the day. To limit your intake of fat and saturated fat, choose lean cuts of meat and skinless poultry, and watch your serving sizes carefully. Choose at least one serving of plant proteins, such as black beans, lentils, or tofu, every day.

Discretionary Calories, Solid Fats, and Added Sugars
The suggested intakes from the basic food groups in *Eating Well with Canada's Food Guide* assume that nutrient-dense

You can track your diet and physical activity and create a personal diet plan by using the online tools at MyFoodGuide.ca.

forms are selected from each group; nutrient-dense forms are those that are low in fat, sodium, and sugar. If this pattern is followed, then a small amount of additional calories can be consumed—the *discretionary calorie allowance*.

People who are trying to lose weight may choose not to use discretionary calories. For those wanting to maintain weight, discretionary calories may be used to increase the amount of food from a food group; to consume foods that are not in the lowest-fat form or that contain added sugars; to add oil, fat, or sugars to foods; or to consume alcohol. The values for additional fat suggest no more than 30% of total calories from fat and less than 10% of calories from saturated fat. Examples of discretionary solid fat calories include choosing higher-fat meats, such as sausage or chicken with the skin, drinking whole milk instead of fat-free milk, and topping foods with butter. For example, 250 millilitres (1 cup) of whole milk has 60 calories more than 250 millilitres (1 cup) of skim milk; these 60 calories would be counted as discretionary calories.

TERMS

vegan   A vegetarian who eats no animal products at all.

lacto-vegetarian   A vegetarian who includes milk and cheese products in the diet.

lacto-ovo-vegetarian   A vegetarian who eats no meat, poultry, or fish but does eat eggs and milk products.

partial vegetarian, semivegetarian, or pescovegetarian   A vegetarian who includes eggs, dairy products, and small amounts of poultry and seafood in the diet.

As described earlier in the chapter, added sugars are the sugars added to foods and beverages in processing or preparation, not the naturally occurring sugars in fruits or milk. The suggested amounts of added sugars may be helpful limits for including some sweetened foods or beverages in your daily diet without exceeding your energy needs or underconsuming other nutrients. In the Canadian diet, added sugars are often found in sweetened beverages (regular soft drinks, sweetened teas, fruit drinks), dairy products (ice cream, some yogourts), and grain products (bakery goods). For example, a 591-millilitre bottle of a regular soft drink has 260 calories from added sugars that would be counted as discretionary calories. Remember, to control weight and get enough essential nutrients, it is important to choose nutrient-dense forms of foods for most of your daily servings.

For an evaluation of your diet, complete the activity in the box "Your Diet Versus the *Eating Well with Canada's Food Guide* Recommendations."

The Vegetarian Alternative

Some people choose a diet with one essential difference from the diets we've already described—foods of animal origin (meat, poultry, fish, eggs, milk) are eliminated or restricted. Many do so for health reasons; vegetarian diets tend to be lower in saturated fat and cholesterol, and higher in complex carbohydrates, dietary fibre, folate, vitamins C and E, carotenoids, and phytochemicals. Some people adopt a vegetarian diet out of concern for the environment, for financial considerations, or for reasons related to ethics or religion.

Types of Vegetarian Diets   There are various vegetarian styles; the wider the variety of the diet eaten, the easier it is to meet nutritional needs.

- **Vegans** eat only plant foods.
- **Lacto-vegetarians** eat plant foods and dairy products.
- **Lacto-ovo-vegetarians** eat plant foods, dairy products, and eggs.

Others can be categorized as **partial vegetarians**, **semivegetarians**, or **pescovegetarians**; these individuals eat plant foods, dairy products, eggs, and usually a small selection of poultry, fish, and other seafood. Many other people choose vegetarian meals frequently but are not strictly vegetarian. Including some animal protein (such as dairy products) in a vegetarian diet makes planning easier, but it is not necessary.

Strong evidence links vegetarian diets to the reduction in risk of many chronic diseases. Vegetarian diets often include more potassium, fibre, and antioxidant-rich nutrients, which may play a role in reducing disease risk. Additionally, many people choosing vegetarian diets also choose a healthier lifestyle overall, which includes not smoking, being more physically active, and consuming

Your Diet Versus the *Eating Well with Canada's Food Guide* Recommendations

1. *Keep a food record:* To evaluate your daily diet, begin by keeping a record of everything you eat on a typical day. To help with your analysis, break down each food item into its component parts and note your portion sizes; for example, a turkey sandwich might be listed as 2 slices sourdough bread, 90 grams turkey, 1 tomato, 15 millilitres mayonnaise, and so on.

2. *Compare your servings with the recommendations of* Eating Well with Canada's Food Guide: Complete the chart below to compare your daily diet with *Eating Well with Canada's Food Guide*.

   It may be difficult to track values for added sugars and, especially, oils and fats, but be as accurate as you can. Check food labels for information on fat and sugar. For a more complete and accurate analysis of your diet, keep food records for three days and then average the results. MyFoodGuide.ca has additional guidelines for counting discretionary calories.

3. *Further evaluate your food choices within the groups:* Based on the data you collected and what you learned in the chapter, what were the especially healthy choices you made (for example, whole grains and citrus fruits) and what were your less healthy choices? Identify and list foods in the latter category, as these are areas where you can make changes to improve your diet. In particular, you may want to limit your intake of the following: processed, sweetened grains; high-fat meats and poultry skin; deep-fried fast foods; homogenized milk products; regular soft drinks, sweetened teas, fruit drinks; alcoholic beverages; and other foods that primarily provide sugar and fat and few other nutrients.

4. *Make healthy changes:* Bring your diet in line with *Eating Well with Canada's Food Guide* by adding servings from food groups for which you fall short of the recommendations. To maintain a healthy weight, you may need to balance these additions by reductions in other areas—by eliminating some of the fats, oils, sweets, and alcohol you consume; by cutting extra servings from food groups for which your intake is more than adequate; or by making healthier choices within the food groups. Make a list of foods to add and a list of foods to eliminate; post your lists in a prominent location.

For a more detailed analysis of your current diet, including intakes of specific nutrients, use the online tools for *Eating Well with Canada's Food Guide* available at MyFoodGuide.ca.

Food Group	Recommended Daily, Amounts/Servings for Your Energy Intake	Your Actual Daily Intake (Amounts/Servings)	Serving Sizes and Equivalents
Grain Products (total)			1 serving = 1 slice of bread; 1 small muffin; 250 mL ready-to-eat cereal flakes; or 125 mL cooked cereal, rice, grains, or pasta
Whole grains			
Other grains			
Vegetables and Fruit (total)			1 serving = 125 mL raw or cooked vegetables; 250 mL raw leafy salad greens; 125 mL vegetable juice; 125 mL fresh, canned, or frozen fruit; 125 mL fruit juice; 1 small whole fruit; or 50 mL dried fruit
*Dark green**			
*Deep yellow**			
*Starchy**			
*Other**			
Milk and Alternatives			1 serving = 250 mL milk or 175 mL yogourt; 50 g natural cheese
Meat and Alternatives			1 serving = 75 g lean meat, poultry, or fish; 175 mL cooked dry beans or tofu; 2 eggs; 30 mL peanut butter; or 60 mL nuts or seeds
Oils			
Solid Fats			
Added Sugars			

alcohol in moderation, if at all. This healthy lifestyle also reduces the risk for chronic diseases, such as diabetes, heart disease, cancers, and obesity.

A Food Plan for Vegetarians   *Eating Well with Canada's Food Guide* can be adapted for use by vegetarians with only a few key modifications. For the meat and alternatives group, vegetarians can focus on the nonmeat choices of dry beans (legumes), nuts, seeds, eggs, and soy foods, such as tofu (soybean curd) and tempeh (a cultured soy product). Vegans and other vegetarians who do not consume any dairy products must find other rich sources of calcium (see below). Fruits, vegetables, and whole grains are healthy choices for people following all types of vegetarian diets.

A healthy vegetarian diet emphasizes a wide variety of plant foods. Although plant proteins are generally of lower quality than animal proteins, choosing a variety of plant foods will supply all of the essential amino acids. Choosing minimally processed and unrefined foods will maximize nutrient value and provide ample dietary fibre. Daily consumption of a variety of plant foods in amounts that meet total energy needs can provide all needed nutrients, except vitamin B12 and possibly vitamin D. Strategies for obtaining nutrients of concern include the following:

- *Vitamin B12* is found naturally only in animal foods; if dairy products and eggs are limited or avoided, B12 can be obtained from fortified foods, such as ready-to-eat cereals, soy beverages, meat substitutes, and special yeast products, or from supplements.
- *Vitamin D* can be obtained by consuming vitamin D–fortified products like ready-to-eat cereals and soy or rice milk, or by taking a supplement. Although unprotected exposure to the sun can manufacture vitamin D in your body, it can also increase your risk for skin cancer. It is recommended that people get their vitamin D from fortified foods and supplements rather than by spending time in the sun or in tanning beds.
- *Calcium* is found in legumes, tofu processed with calcium, dark-green leafy vegetables, nuts, and fortified orange juice, soy milk, bread, and other foods.
- *Iron* can be obtained from whole grains, fortified bread and breakfast cereals, dried fruits, green leafy vegetables, nuts and seeds, legumes, and soy foods. The iron in plant foods is more difficult for the body to absorb than is the iron from animal sources; consuming a good source of vitamin C with most meals is helpful because vitamin C improves iron absorption.

- *Zinc* is found in whole grains, nuts, legumes, and soy foods.

If you are a vegetarian or considering becoming one, devote some extra time and thought to your diet. It's especially important to eat as wide a variety of foods as possible to ensure that all your nutritional needs are satisfied. Consulting with a registered dietitian will make your planning even easier. Vegetarian diets for children, teens, and pregnant and lactating women warrant guidance from a health professional.

Dietary Challenges for Special Population Groups

The Guidelines for Healthy Eating and *Eating Well with Canada's Food Guide* provide a basis that everyone can use to create a healthy diet. However, some population groups face special dietary challenges (see the box "How Different Are the Nutritional Needs of Women and Men?").

Children and Teenagers   Young people often simply need to be encouraged to eat. Perhaps the best thing a parent can do for younger children is to provide them with a variety of foods. Add vegetables to casseroles and fruit to cereal; offer fruit and vegetable juices or homemade yogourt or fruit shakes instead of sugary drinks. Allowing children to help prepare meals is another good way to increase overall food consumption and variety. Many children and teenagers enjoy eating at fast-food restaurants; they should be encouraged to select the healthiest choices from fast-food menus (see Appendix A) and to complete the day's diet with low-fat, nutrient-rich foods.

College and University Students   Foods that are convenient for postsecondary students are not always the healthiest choices. It is easy for students who eat in buffet-style dining halls or food courts to overeat, and the foods offered are not necessarily high in essential nutrients and low in fat. The same is true of meals at fast-food restaurants, another convenient source of quick and inexpensive meals for busy students. Although no food is entirely bad, consuming a wide variety of foods is critical for a healthy diet. See the box "Eating Strategies for Postsecondary Students" on p. 158 for tips on making healthy eating convenient and affordable.

Older Adults   Nutrient needs do not change much as people age, but because older adults tend to become less active, they require fewer calories to maintain body weight. At the same time, the absorption of nutrients tends to be lower in older adults because of age-related changes in the digestive tract. Thus, they must consume nutrient-dense foods to meet their nutritional requirements. Because constipation is a common problem, consuming foods high in fibre and getting adequate fluids are important goals.

How Different Are the Nutritional Needs of Women and Men?

GENDER MATTERS

When it comes to nutrition, men and women have a lot in common. Both sexes need the same essential nutrients, and the Guidelines for Healthy Eating apply equally to both. But beyond the basics, men and women need different amounts of essential nutrients and have different nutritional concerns.

Women tend to be smaller and weigh less than men, and thus have lower energy requirements and need to consume fewer calories than men to maintain a healthy weight. For most nutrients, women need the same or slightly lower amounts than men. But because women consume fewer calories, they may have more difficulty getting adequate amounts of all essential nutrients and need to focus on nutrient-dense foods.

Two nutrients of special concern to women are calcium and iron. Low calcium intake may be linked to the development of osteoporosis in later life. Low-fat milk and alternatives and fortified cereal, bread, and orange juice are good choices for calcium-rich foods.

Menstruating women also have higher iron needs than other groups, and low iron intake can lead to iron-deficiency anemia. Lean red meat, green leafy vegetables, and fortified breakfast cereals are good sources of iron. As discussed earlier, all women capable of becoming pregnant should consume adequate folic acid from fortified foods and supplements.

Men are seldom thought of as having nutritional deficiencies because they generally have high-calorie diets. However, many men have a diet that does not follow recommended food intake patterns and includes more red meat and fewer fruits, vegetables, and whole grains than recommended. This dietary pattern is linked to heart disease and some types of cancer. A high intake of calories can lead to weight gain over time if a man's activity level decreases as he ages. To reduce

chronic disease risk, men should focus on increasing their consumption of fruits, vegetables, and whole grains to obtain vitamins, minerals, fibre, and phytochemicals.

The Northern Fruit and Vegetable Program is a provincial initiative that aims to increase fruit and vegetable consumption and increase awareness of the importance of fruits and vegetables among elementary school children in communities in Northern Ontario. It also hopes to educate elementary-school-age children and their families about the importance of eating fruit and vegetables, and the associated benefits of healthy eating and physical activity to overall health. In 2007, only 42% of Canadians ages 12 years and older reported consuming five or more servings of fruits and vegetables each day.

Athletes Key dietary concerns for athletes are meeting their increased energy requirements and drinking enough fluids during practice and throughout the day to remain fully hydrated. Endurance athletes may also benefit from increasing the amount of carbohydrate in the diet to 60%–70% of total daily calories; this increase should come in the form of complex, rather than simple, carbohydrates. Athletes for whom maintaining low body weight and body fat is important—such as skaters, gymnasts, and wrestlers—should consume adequate nutrients and avoid falling into unhealthy patterns of eating. Eating for exercise is discussed in more detail in Chapter 6; refer to Chapter 4 for information on eating disorders.

Low-Income Families Families surviving on low or fixed incomes may have difficulty meeting their nutritional needs. Often, they do not have enough income to support a healthy diet. If they have to use emergency food supports, such as food banks and soup kitchens, their challenge in consistently finding healthy foods is even greater.

First Nations, Inuit, and Metis Aboriginal peoples, especially First Nations living on-reserve, face challenges in maintaining traditional food preparation and eating practices while trying to improve their health. They are also at risk for a variety of chronic diseases (predominantly obesity and diabetes), mental health issues, and addictions. The First Nations, Inuit, and Aboriginal Health Program established by Health Canada supports community-based and community delivered programs, initiatives, and strategies that aim to improve the health of mothers, infants, and families and to support the development of children in an effort to address the gap in life chances between Aboriginal and non-Aboriginal children.

Health Canada has also, for the first time, produced a food guide that specifically addresses the values, traditions, and food choices of Canada's First Nations, Inuit, and Metis. *Eating Well with Canada's Food Guide: First Nations, Inuit and Métis* meshes traditional food choices with those available in stores, especially the sometimes-limited selection available in rural and remote areas. The food guide is available in English, Inuktitut, Ojibwe, Plains Cree, and Woods Cree.

Eating Strategies for Postsecondary Students

General Guidelines

• Eat slowly, and enjoy your food. Set aside a separate time to eat, and don't eat while you study.

• Eat a colourful, varied diet. The more colourful your diet is, the more varied and rich in fruits and vegetables it will be. Many Canadians eat few servings of fruits and vegetables, despite the fact that these foods are typically inexpensive, delicious, rich in nutrients, and low in fat and calories.

• Eat breakfast. You'll have more energy in the morning and be less likely to grab an unhealthy snack later on.

• Choose healthy snacks, such as fruits, vegetables, grains, and cereals.

• Drink water more often than soft drinks or other sweetened beverages. Rent a mini-refrigerator for your dorm room and stock up on healthy beverages, such as milk, water, and 100% fruit juice.

• Pay attention to portion sizes.

• Combine physical activity with healthy eating. You'll feel better and have a much lower risk of many chronic diseases. Even a little exercise is better than none.

Eating in the Dining Hall or Cafeteria

• Choose a meal plan that includes breakfast, and don't skip it.

• Accept that dining hall food is not going to taste the same as home cooking. Find healthy dishes that you like.

• If menus are posted or distributed, decide what you want to eat before you get in line, and stick to your choices. Consider what you plan to do and eat for the rest of the day before making your choices.

• Ask for large servings of vegetables and small servings of meat and other high-fat main dishes. Build your meals around grains and vegetables.

• Try whole grains like brown rice, whole wheat bread, and whole-grain cereals.

• Choose leaner poultry, fish, or bean dishes rather than high-fat meats and fried entrees.

• Ask that gravies and sauces be served on the side; limit your intake.

• Choose broth-based or vegetable soups rather than cream soups.

• At the salad bar, load up on leafy greens, beans, and fresh vegetables. Avoid mayonnaise-coated salads, bacon, croutons, and high-fat dressings. Put dressing on the side, and dip your fork into it rather than pouring it over the salad.

• Drink low-fat milk, water, mineral water, or 100% fruit juice rather than heavily sweetened fruit drinks, whole milk, or soft drinks.

• Choose fruit for dessert rather than pastries, cookies, or cakes.

• Do some research about the foods and preparation methods used in your dining hall or cafeteria. Discuss any suggestions you have with your food-service manager. Students have the ability to advocate for healthy food choices. Make your voice heard if you have concerns.

Eating in Fast-Food Restaurants

• Most fast-food chains can provide a brochure with a nutritional breakdown of the foods on the menu. Ask for it. (See also the information in Appendix A.)

• Order small single burgers with no cheese instead of double burgers with many toppings. If possible, ask for them broiled instead of fried.

• Ask for items to be prepared without mayonnaise, tartar sauce, sour cream, or other high-fat sauces. Ketchup, mustard, and low-fat mayonnaise or sour cream are better choices and are available at many fast-food restaurants.

• Choose whole-grain buns or bread for burgers and sandwiches.

• Choose chicken items made from chicken breast, not processed chicken.

• Order vegetarian pizzas without extra cheese.

• If you order french fries or onion rings, get the smallest size, or share them with a friend. Better yet, get a salad or fruit cup instead.

Eating on the Run

Are you chronically short of time? Pack these items for a quick snack or meal: fresh or dried fruit, fruit juices, raw fresh vegetables, plain bagels, bread sticks, whole wheat fig bars, low-fat cheese sticks or cubes, low-fat crackers or granola bars, fat-free or low-fat yogourt, snack-size cereal boxes, pretzels, rice or corn cakes, plain popcorn, soup (if you have access to a microwave), or water.

QUESTIONS FOR CRITICAL THINKING AND REFLECTION

What factors influence your food choices: convenience, cost, availability, habit? Do you ever consider nutritional content or nutritional recommendations like those found in *Eating Well with Canada's Food Guide*? If not, how big a change would it be for you to think of nutritional content first when choosing food? Is it something you could do easily?

People with Special Health Concerns Many Canadians have special health concerns that affect their dietary needs. For example, women who are pregnant or breastfeeding require extra calories, vitamins, and minerals (see Chapter 12). People with diabetes benefit from a well-balanced diet that is low in simple sugars, high in complex carbohydrates, and relatively rich in monounsaturated fats. People with high blood pressure need to control their weight and limit their sodium consumption. If you have a health problem or concern that may require a special diet, discuss your situation with a physician or registered dietitian.

A PERSONAL PLAN: MAKING INFORMED CHOICES ABOUT FOOD

Now that you understand the basis of good nutrition and a healthy diet, you can put together a diet that works for you. Focus on the likely causes of any health problems in your life, and make specific dietary changes to address them. You may also have some specific areas of concern, such as interpreting food labels and dietary supplement or natural health product labels, avoiding food-borne illnesses and environmental contaminants, and understanding food additives. We turn to these and other topics next.

Reading Food Labels

All processed foods regulated by Health Canada and the Canadian Food Inspection Agency (CFIA) include standardized nutrition information on their labels. Every food label shows serving sizes and the amount of fat, saturated fat, trans fat, cholesterol, sodium, total carbohydrate, dietary fibre, sugars, and protein in each serving. To make intelligent choices about food, learn to read and *understand* food labels (see the box "Using Food Labels" on p. 160).

Fresh meat, poultry, fish, fruits, vegetables, herbs, spices, and alcoholic beverages are not required to have food labels, and many of these products are not packaged. You can find information on the nutrient content of these items from basic nutrition books, registered dietitians, nutrient analysis computer software, the World Wide Web, and the companies that produce or distribute these foods. Supermarkets often have large posters or pamphlets listing the nutrient contents of these foods.

Natural Health Products

In Canada, vitamins and minerals; herbal remedies; homeopathic medicines; traditional medicines, such as traditional Chinese medicines; probiotics; and other products, such as amino acids and essential fatty acids, are called natural health products. They may come in the form of tablets, capsules, liquids, or powders. Although many consumers often consider the use of natural health products to be safe, the products do contain powerful bioactive chemicals that have the potential for harm. About one-quarter of all pharmaceutical drugs are derived from botanical sources: morphine from poppies and digoxin from foxglove, for example. And, as described earlier, even essential vitamins and minerals can have toxic effects if consumed in excess.

The Natural Health Products Directorate, part of Health Canada, is the regulating authority for natural health products for sale in Canada. The role of this directorate is to ensure that Canadians have ready access to natural health products that are safe, effective, and of high quality. Before they are approved by Health Canada and put on the market, all drugs undergo clinical studies to determine safety, effectiveness, side effects and risks, possible interactions with other substances, and appropriate dosages. Although dosage guidelines exist for some of the compounds in natural health products, dosages for many are not well established.

Key differences also exist in how drugs and supplements are manufactured. The potency of herbal natural health products tends to vary widely because of differences in growing and harvesting conditions, preparation methods, and storage. Some manufacturers attempt to standardize their products by isolating the compounds believed to be responsible for a herb's action. However, potency is often still highly variable, and when several compounds are thought to be responsible for a herb's effect, often only one is standardized. In addition, herbs can be contaminated or misidentified at any stage from harvest to packaging. (See Chapter 19 for more on herbal remedies.) Health Canada has recalled several products because of the presence of dangerous contaminants, including heavy metals and pharmaceutical drugs.

To be sold in Canada, a natural health product must have a product licence from Health Canada, and applicants have to provide detailed information about the product, including the medicinal ingredients, source, dose, potency, nonmedicinal ingredients, and recommended uses. If a product is granted a licence, it is also assigned an eight-digit Natural Product Number (NPN) or

Using Food Labels

Food labels are designed to help consumers make food choices based on the nutrients that are most important to good health. In addition to listing nutrient content by weight, the label puts the information in the context of a daily diet of 2000 calories that includes no more than 65 grams of fat (approximately 30% of total calories). For example, if a serving of a particular product has 13 grams of fat, the label will show that the serving represents 20% of the daily fat allowance. If your daily diet contains fewer or more than 2000 calories, you need to adjust these calculations accordingly.

Food labels contain uniform serving sizes. This means that if you look at different brands of salad dressing, for example, you can compare calories and fat content based on the serving amount. (Food label serving sizes may be larger or smaller than *Eating Well with Canada's Food Guide* serving size equivalents, however.) Regulations also require that foods meet strict definitions if their packaging includes the terms *light, low fat,* or *high fibre* (see below). Health claims, such as "good source of dietary fibre" or "low in saturated fat," on packages are signals that those products can wisely be included in your diet. Overall, the food label is an important tool to help you choose a diet that conforms to *Eating Well with Canada's Food Guide* recommendations.

Take 5 to read the facts

Got 5 minutes? Follow these 5 easy steps to read the Nutrition Facts table.

① Serving size
If you eat the serving size shown on the Nutrition Facts table, you will get the amount of Calories and nutrients that are listed. Always compare the serving size on the package to the amount that you eat.

② Calories
Calories tell you how much energy you get from one serving of a packaged food.

③ Percent Daily Value (% Daily Value)
% Daily Value puts nutrients on a scale from 0% to 100%. This scale tells you if there is a *little* or a *lot* of a nutrient in one serving of a packaged food.

④ Get less of these nutrients:
- Fat, saturated fat and trans fat
- Cholesterol
- Sodium

Choose packaged foods with a *low* % Daily Value of fat and sodium, especially if you are at risk for heart disease or diabetes.

⑤ Get more of these nutrients:
- Fibre
- Vitamin A and Vitamin C
- Calcium
- Iron

Choose packaged foods with a *high* % Daily Value of these nutrients. If you have diabetes, watch how much carbohydrate you eat as this will affect your blood glucose levels.

Nutrition Facts

Per 1 cup (55 g)	
Amount	% Daily Value
Calories 220	
Fat 2 g	3 %
Saturated 0 g + Trans 0 g	0 %
Cholesterol 0 mg	
Sodium 270 mg	11 %
Carbohydrate 44 g	15 %
Fibre 8 g	32 %
Sugars 16 g	
Protein 6 g	

Vitamin A	0 %	Vitamin C	0 %
Calcium	4 %	Iron	40 %

Healthy Eating is in Store for You™
Faites provision de saine alimentation™

Selected Nutrient Claims and What They Mean

- *Light:* Reduced in energy or reduced in fat (criteria for "reduced" or "lower in" claims are based on the reference amount of the food)

- *Reduced or fewer:* At least 25% less of a nutrient than a similar product; can be applied to fat ("reduced fat"), saturated fat, cholesterol, sodium, and calories

- *Low in calories:* 40 calories or less per serving

- *High source of fibre:* 4 grams or more of fibre or of each identified fibre

- *Good source of fibre:* 2 grams or more of fibre or of each identified fibre

- *Fat free:* Less than 0.5 grams of fat per serving

- *Reduced fat or low in fat:* 3 grams of fat or less per serving

- *Saturated fatty acid free:* Less than 0.2 grams of saturated fat and 0.2 grams of trans fatty acids per serving

- *Low in saturated fatty acids:* 2 grams or less of saturated fat per serving and no more than 15% of total calories

- *Cholesterol free:* Less than 2 milligrams of cholesterol per serving and "low in saturated fatty acids"

- *Low in cholesterol:* 20 milligrams or less of cholesterol per serving and "low in saturated fatty acids"

- *Low in sodium or salt:* 140 milligrams or less of sodium or salt per serving

- *Sodium free or salt free:* Less than 5 milligrams of sodium or salt per serving

- *Lean:* Cooked seafood, meat, or poultry no more than 17% fat

- *Extra lean:* Cooked seafood, meat, or poultry with no more than 10% fat

Note: Health Canada has not yet defined nutrient claims relating to carbohydrate, so foods labelled low- or reduced-carbohydrate do not conform to any approved standard.

Source: Based on information from Health Canada. 2010. *Nutrition Labelling* (http://www.hc-sc.gc.ca/fn-an/label-etiquet/nutrition/index-eng.php; retrieved May 20, 2011).

Homeopathic Medicine Number (DIN-HM). The number, which must appear on the label, tells you that the product has been reviewed and approved by Health Canada.

In some cases, exceptions are given for products that have had an initial assessment but have not been fully evaluated. The exemption number (EN) will be listed on the product label.

Finally, it is important to remember that natural health products, including dietary supplements, are no substitute for a healthy diet. Supplements do not provide all the known—or yet-to-be-discovered—benefits of whole foods. Supplements should also not be used as a replacement for medical treatment for serious illnesses.

Protecting Yourself Against Food-Borne Illness

Many people worry about additives or pesticide residues in their food, but a greater threat comes from microorganisms that cause food-borne illnesses. Raw or undercooked animal products, such as chicken, hamburger, and oysters, pose the greatest threat, although in recent years contaminated fruits and vegetables have been catching up.

The Public Health Agency of Canada estimates that 11 million to 13 million illnesses are attributed to food-borne illnesses annually. Although most people fully recover, food-borne illnesses can result in chronic health problems in 2%–3% of cases. Some illnesses have long-term consequences for people and for the economy and society as a whole. Health Canada also estimates that the annual cost related to these illnesses is between $12 billion and $14 billion. Symptoms of food-borne illness include diarrhea, vomiting, fever, and weakness. Although the effects of food-borne illnesses are usually not serious, some groups, such as children, pregnant women, older adults, and people with suppressed or weakened immune systems, are more at risk for severe complications, such as rheumatic diseases, seizures, blood poisoning, other ailments, and death.

Causes of Food-Borne Illnesses Most cases of food-borne illness are caused by **pathogens**, disease-causing microorganisms. Food can be contaminated with pathogens through improper handling; pathogens can grow if food is prepared or stored improperly. Causes of food-borne illness in Canada include the following pathogens:

- *Campylobacter jejuni* causes more cases of food-borne illness than any other bacteria. It is most commonly found in contaminated water, raw milk, and raw or undercooked poultry, meat, or shellfish; the majority of chickens sold in Canada test positive for the presence of *C. jejuni*. Symptoms of infection include diarrhea, fever, abdominal and muscle pain, and headache, which resolve in 7–10 days. However, in about 1 in 1000 cases, *Campylobacter* infection triggers Guillain-Barré syndrome, a neurological

disease that can cause numbness, weakness, and (usually temporary) paralysis.

- *Salmonella* bacteria are most often found in raw or undercooked eggs, poultry, and meat; milk and dairy products; seafood; fruits and vegetables, including sprouts; and inadequately refrigerated and reheated leftovers. The recent identification of an antibiotic-resistant strain of *Salmonella* has raised concerns about a potential increase in serious illness from *Salmonella*.

- *Shigella* bacteria are found in the human intestinal tract and usually transmitted via fecal contamination of food and water. Outbreaks are typically traced to foods, especially salads, that have been handled by people with poor personal hygiene. Contaminated water, milk, and dairy products are other possible sources of infection.

- *Escherichia coli* bacteria, found in the intestinal tracts of humans and animals, most commonly contaminate water, raw milk, raw to rare ground beef, unpasteurized juices, and fruits and vegetables. A certain strain, known as *E. coli* O157:H7, is of particular concern because it produces a toxin that causes serious illness and sometimes death. Children are particularly at risk for developing hemolytic uremic syndrome, which causes kidney failure.

- *Listeria monocytogenes* causes listeriosis, which is reported to affect about 100–140 Canadians a year, causing death in about 20% of cases. It is found in soft cheeses, raw milk, improperly processed ice cream, raw leafy vegetables, hot dogs and lunch-meats, and other meat, poultry, and processed foods. For the most part, healthy people who come into contact with *Listeria* are rarely affected by the bacteria. However, *Listeria* is particularly dangerous for pregnant women and their fetuses, babies and children, older adults, and people with weakened immune systems.

- *Staphylococcus aureus* lives mainly in nasal passages and skin sores; it is transferred to food when people handle food or sneeze or cough over food. Foods contaminated with *S. aureus* may include cooked

pathogen A microorganism that causes disease.

TERMS

hams, egg and potato salads, cheese, seafood, whipped cream, and milk. *S. aureus* multiplies rapidly at room temperature to produce a toxin that causes illness.

- *Clostridium botulinum* is widely distributed in nature, but it grows only in environments with little or no oxygen; it produces a toxin that causes illness. Potential sources of *C. botulinum* include improperly canned foods, garlic in oil, sausages and other meat products, and vacuum-packed and tightly wrapped foods. Although rare, botulism is potentially fatal if untreated because the toxin affects the nervous system.

- *Noroviruses*, are a group of viruses that cause gastroenteritis, an illness that usually includes vomiting, diarrhea, and abdominal pain, lasting one to three days. Gastroenteritis is often called the *stomach flu*, although it is not related to the flu (or influenza), which is a respiratory illness caused by the influenza virus. *Novovirus* is the most common viral cause of food-borne illness and may be found in contaminated water, raw or insufficiently cooked shellfish, and salads contaminated by food handlers.

Other causes of food-borne illness include the bacteria *Clostridium perfringens*, *Vibrio vulnificus*, and *Yersinia enterocolitica*; the hepatitis A virus; the parasites *Trichinella spiralis* (found in pork and wild game), *Anisakis* (found in raw fish), *Giardia lamblia*, *Cyclospora cayetanensis*, and tapeworms; and certain moulds.

A potential new threat from food is bovine spongiform encephalopathy (BSE), or mad cow disease, a fatal degenerative neurological disease caused by an abnormal protein (called a prion) that forms deposits in the brain. A variant form that appears in people, known as Creutzfeldt-Jakob disease (CJD), is believed to be caused by eating beef contaminated with central nervous system tissue from BSE-infected cows. To date, there have been about 200 confirmed cases of this variant CJD worldwide, most of them in Great Britain. In 1993, the first case of BSE diagnosed in Canada was in a cow that had been imported from the United Kingdom in 1987, when it was six months old. The animal was destroyed and the Canadian government attempted to trace and destroy all cattle imported from the United Kingdom between 1982 and 1990 (in 1990, cattle imports from the United Kingdom were banned because of BSE). According to Health Canada and the Canadian Food Inspection Agency, the risk to Canadians from BSE is extremely low, but steps are being taken to prevent the BSE protein from entering the food supply.

Preventing and Treating Food-Borne Illnesses Because every teaspoon of the soil that our food grows in contains about 2 billion bacteria (only some of which are pathogenic), we are always exposed to the possibility of a food-borne illness. You can't tell by taste, smell, or sight whether a food is contaminated. Some studies have revealed high levels of contamination. In 2003, for example,

Careful food handling greatly reduces the risk of food-borne illness.

Consumer Reports tested 484 chickens purchased in grocery stores and found that half were contaminated with *Campylobacter* or *Salmonella* or both; many of the strains of bacteria found were resistant to antibiotics.

Although pathogens are usually destroyed during cooking, Health Canada is trying to bring down levels of contamination. In addition to new microbiological testing methods for inspection of meat and poultry processing plants, raw meat and poultry products are now sold with safe handling and cooking instructions, and all packaged, unpasteurized fresh fruit and vegetable juices carry warnings about potential contamination. Food-borne illness outbreaks associated with food-processing plants make headlines, but most cases of illness trace back to poor food handling in the home or in food-service establishments. To decrease your risk of food-borne illness, follow the guidelines in the box "Safe Food Handling."

If you think you may be have a food-borne illness, drink plenty of clear fluids to prevent dehydration and rest to speed recovery. To prevent further contamination, wash your hands often and always before handling food. A fever higher than 38.9 degrees Celsius, blood in the stool, or dehydration deserves a physician's evaluation, especially if the symptoms persist for more than two to three days. In cases of suspected botulism—characterized by such symptoms as double vision, paralysis, dizziness, and vomiting—consult a physician immediately to receive an antitoxin.

Safe Food Handling

- Don't buy food in containers that leak, bulge, or are severely dented. Refrigerated foods should be cold, and frozen foods should be solid.

- Refrigerate perishable items as soon as possible after purchase. Use or freeze fresh meats within three to five days and fresh poultry, fish, and ground meat within one to two days.

- Store raw meat, poultry, fish, and shellfish in containers in the refrigerator so that the juices don't drip onto other foods. Keep these items away from other foods, surfaces, utensils, or serving dishes to prevent cross-contamination.

- Thaw frozen food in the refrigerator or in the microwave oven, not on the kitchen counter. Cook foods immediately after thawing.

- Thoroughly wash your hands with warm soapy water for a minimum of 20 seconds before and after handling food, especially raw meat, fish, shellfish, poultry, or eggs.

- Make sure counters, cutting boards, dishes, utensils, and other equipment are thoroughly cleaned in hot soapy water before and after use. Wash dishcloths and kitchen towels frequently.

- Use separate cutting boards for meat, poultry, and seafood and for foods that will be eaten raw, such as fruits and vegetables. Replace cutting boards once they become worn or develop hard-to-clean grooves.

- Thoroughly rinse and scrub fruits and vegetables with a brush, if possible, or peel off the skin.

- Cook foods thoroughly, especially beef, poultry, fish, pork, and eggs; cooking kills most microorganisms. Use a food thermometer to ensure that foods are cooked to a safe temperature. Hamburgers should be cooked to 71°C. Turn or stir microwaved food to make sure it is heated evenly throughout. When eating out, order hamburger cooked well done and make sure foods are served piping hot.

- Cook stuffing separately from poultry; or wash poultry thoroughly, stuff immediately before cooking, and transfer the stuffing to a clean bowl immediately after cooking. The temperature of cooked stuffing should reach 74°C.

- Keep hot foods hot (60°C or above) and cold foods cold (4°C or below); harmful bacteria can grow rapidly between these two temperatures. Refrigerate foods within two hours of purchase or preparation, and within one hour if the air temperature is above 32°C. Refrigerate foods at or below 4°C and freeze at or below −17°C. Use refrigerated leftovers within three to four days.

- Even for experienced cooks, improper heating and preparation of food means bacteria can survive. Use a food thermometer: You can't tell if food is cooked safely by how it looks. Refer to a temperature chart to see if your food is cooked completely.

- Don't eat raw animal products, including raw eggs in homemade hollandaise sauce or eggnog. Use only pasteurized milk and juice.

- Cook eggs until they're firm, and fully cook foods containing eggs. Store eggs in the coldest part of the refrigerator, not in the door, and use them within three to five weeks.

- Because of possible contamination with *E. coli* O157:H7 and *Salmonella*, avoid raw sprouts. Even sprouts grown under clean conditions in the home can be risky because bacteria may be present in the seeds. Cook sprouts before eating them.

- Read the food label and package information, and follow safety instructions, such as "Keep Refrigerated" and the "Safe Handling Instructions."

- According to the Canadian Food Inspection Agency, "When in doubt, throw it out." Even if a food looks and smells fine, it may not be safe. If you aren't sure that a food has been prepared, served, and stored safely, don't eat it.

Additional precautions are recommended for people at particularly high risk for food-borne illness: pregnant women, young children, older persons, and people with weakened immune systems or certain chronic illnesses. If you are a member of one of these groups, don't eat or drink any of the following products: unpasteurized juices; raw sprouts; unpasteurized (raw) milk and products made from unpasteurized milk; raw or undercooked meat, poultry, eggs, fish, and shellfish; and soft cheeses, such as feta, Brie, Camembert, or blue-veined cheeses. To protect against *Listeria*, it's also important to avoid ready-to-eat foods, such as hot dogs, lunchmeats, and cold cuts, unless they are reheated until they are steaming hot.

Environmental Contaminants and Organic Foods

Contaminants are also present in the food-growing environment, but few of them ever enter the food and water supply in amounts sufficient to cause health problems. Environmental contaminants include various minerals, antibiotics, hormones, pesticides, the industrial chemicals known as **PCBs (polychlorinated biphenyls)**, and naturally occurring substances, such as cyanogenic glycosides (found in lima beans and the pits of some fruits) and certain moulds. Their effects depend on many factors, including concentration, length of exposure, and the age and health status of the person involved. Safety regulations attempt to keep our exposure to contaminants at safe levels, but monitoring is difficult and many substances (such as pesticides) persist in the environment long after being banned from use.

Organic Foods   Some people who are concerned about pesticides and other environmental contaminants choose to buy foods that are **organic**. To be certified as organic by Canadian Food Inspection Agency, foods must meet strict production, processing, handling, and labelling criteria. Organic crops must meet limits on pesticide residues; for meat, milk, eggs, and other animal products to be certified organic, animals must be given organic feed and access to the outdoors and may not be given antibiotics or growth hormones. The use of genetic engineering, ionizing radiation, and sewage sludge is prohibited. General principles of organic production include protection of the environment; maintenance of long-term soil fertility; maintenance of biological diversity; recycling and maintenance of resources to the greatest extent possible; and provision of attentive care to livestock.

Organic foods are not necessarily chemical-free, however. They may be contaminated with pesticides used on neighbouring lands or on foods transported in the same train or truck. However, they do tend to have lower levels of pesticide residues than conventionally grown crops. Some experts recommend that consumers who want to buy organic fruits and vegetables spend their money on those that carry lower pesticide residues than their conventional counterparts (the "dirty dozen"): apples, bell peppers, celery, cherries, imported grapes, nectarines, peaches, pears, potatoes, red raspberries, spinach, and strawberries. Experts also recommend buying organic beef, poultry, eggs, dairy products, and baby food. Fruits and vegetables that carry little pesticide residue whether grown conventionally or organically include asparagus, avocadoes, bananas, broccoli, cauliflower, corn, kiwi, mangoes, onions, papaya, pineapples, and peas. All foods are subject to strict pesticide limits; the debate about the health effects of small amounts of residue is ongoing.

Whether organic foods are better for your health or not, organic farming is better for the environment. It

Government inspectors regularly check Canada's food supply to ensure its safety.

helps maintain biodiversity of crops and replenish Earth's resources; and it is less likely to degrade soil, contaminate water, or expose farm workers to toxic chemicals. As multinational food companies get into the organic food business, however, consumers who want to support environmentally friendly farming methods should look for foods that are not only organic but also locally grown.

Local Foods and Slow Food   New food movements are taking place across Canada, including eating locally the slow food movement. Eating locally promotes the benefits of buying agricultural products grown close to our backyards. Some marketing agencies and companies promoting their local foods identify how far food travels to reach the consumer; others choose to promote the economic and health benefits of purchasing food grown closer to home.

Eating locally grown food supports local agriculture, which in turn supports the local economy while protecting farmland. This benefits both consumers and producers. In addition, local food purchased from nearby farms is often as affordable as nonlocal food but is of higher quality. Price is often the main reason that shoppers purchase imported food, but some consumers in favour of local foods are willing to pay more for foods produced closer to home. Consumers committed to purchasing locally grown food cite the peace of mind that comes with knowing where their food comes from and with making a contribution to the economic stability of the local agricultural industry as their main reasons for purchasing local foods.

The slow food movement is a global, grassroots movement with supporters in 150 countries. According to Slow Food Canada, it is "a national eco-gastronomic organization founded to counteract fast food and fast life and the disappearance of local food traditions."

Guidelines for Fish Consumption   A specific area of concern is possible mercury contamination in fish. Overall, fish and shellfish are healthy sources of protein, omega-3 fats, and other nutrients. Prudent choices can minimize the risk of any possible negative health effects. High mercury concentrations are most likely to be found in predator fish—large fish that eat smaller fish. Mercury can cause brain damage to fetuses and young children.

Health Canada has released an advisory with guidelines for certain groups. To reduce exposure to mercury, women who are or who may become pregnant and breastfeeding mothers should follow these guidelines:

- Some fish contain higher amounts of methylmercury and should be limited to no more than 150 grams per month (that's two servings). These fish include fresh/frozen tuna, shark, swordfish, marlin, orange roughy, and escolar.

- For other varieties of fish and shellfish that are lower in methylmercury, eat up to two servings a week (150 grams total). These varieties include shrimp, canned light tuna, salmon, pollock, and catfish. Albacore tuna (sometimes called white tuna) contains more mercury than light tuna, so you need to watch how much you are eating

- Check advisories about the safety of recreationally caught fish from local lakes, rivers, and coastal areas; if no information is available, limit consumption to two servings (150 grams total) per month.

Children should consume only one serving (75 grams) of fish lower in methylmercury per week.

The levels of mercury in the muscle tissue of salmon are very low. Separate studies have identified other chemicals, such as polychlorinated biphenyls (PCBs), in the fat of both wild-caught and farmed salmon. These chemicals can be found in most fish and in many other foods, but at low levels that do not cause concern for human health. Fish should be labelled with its country of origin and whether it is wild or farmed; most canned salmon is wild.

Additives in Food

Today, some 2800 substances are intentionally added to foods to maintain or improve nutritional quality, to maintain freshness, to help in processing or preparation, or to alter taste or appearance. Additives make up less than 1% of our food. The most widely used are sugar, salt, and corn syrup; these three and citric acid, baking soda, vegetable colours, mustard, and pepper account for 98% by weight of all food additives used in Canada.

Some additives may be of concern for certain people, either because they are consumed in large quantities or because they cause some type of reaction. Additives having potential health concerns include the following:

- *Nitrates and nitrites:* Used to preserve the colour of meats; to enhance their flavour by inhibiting rancidity (in cured meats); and to protect against bacterial growth, specifically, from contamination with botulism.

Consumption of nitrates and nitrites is associated with the synthesis of cancer-causing agents in the stomach, but the cancer risk appears to be low, except for people with low stomach acid output (such as some older adults). That said, a person's overall exposure to nitrosamine-related compounds comes from other substances, such as tobacco smoke, beer and bacon consumption, and exhaust from vehicles.

- *BHA and BHT:* Used to help maintain the freshness of foods. BHT has been shown to reduce the risk of cancer by providing an antioxidant effect similar to that of vitamin E. However, other studies indicate a potential link between BHT and an increased risk of certain cancers when BHT is consumed in very large amounts, but any risk from these agents is considered to be low. Some manufacturers have stopped using BHT and BHA.

- *Sulphites:* Used to keep vegetables from turning brown. They can cause severe allergic reactions in some people. Health Canada severely limits the use of sulphites and requires any foods containing sulphites to be clearly labelled.

- *Monosodium glutamate (MSG):* Typically used as a flavour enhancer. MSG may cause some people to experience episodes of increased blood pressure and sweating. If you are sensitive to MSG, check food labels when shopping, and ask to have it left out of dishes you order at restaurants.

Food additives pose no significant health hazard to most people because the levels used are well below any that could produce toxic effects. To avoid potential problems, eat a variety of foods in moderation. If you are sensitive to an additive, check food labels when you shop, and ask questions when you eat out.

Food Irradiation

Food irradiation is the treatment of foods with gamma rays, X-rays, or high-voltage electrons to kill potentially harmful pathogens, including bacteria, parasites, insects, and fungi that cause food-borne illness. It also reduces spoilage and extends shelf life. For example, irradiated

PCB (polychlorinated biphenyl) An industrial chemical used as an insulator in electrical transformers and linked to certain human cancers.

organic A designation applied to foods grown and produced according to strict guidelines limiting the use of pesticides, nonorganic ingredients, hormones, antibiotics, irradiation, genetic engineering, and other practices.

food irradiation The treatment of foods with gamma rays, X-rays, or high-voltage electrons to kill potentially harmful pathogens and increase shelf life.

strawberries stay unspoiled in the refrigerator up to three weeks, versus only three to five days for untreated berries. The same irradiation process has also been used for decades on many items, such as plastic wrap, milk cartons, teething rings, contact lenses, and medical supplies.

Even though irradiation has been generally endorsed by such agencies as the World Health Organization, the Centers for Disease Control and Prevention, and the American Medical Association, few irradiated foods are on the market because of consumer resistance and skepticism. Currently, onions, potatoes, wheat, flour, whole wheat flour, and whole or ground spices and dehydrated seasonings are approved for irradiation and sale in Canada.

Studies haven't conclusively identified any harmful effects of food irradiation, and the newer methods of irradiation involving electricity and X-rays do not require the use of any radioactive materials.

Studies do indicate that when consumers are given information about the process of irradiation and the benefits of irradiated foods, most want to purchase them. Without such information, many remain skeptical. Irradiated foods are labelled with the flowerlike radura symbol and a brief information label; spices and foods that are merely ingredients do not have to be labelled. It is important to remember that although irradiation kills most pathogens, it does not completely sterilize foods. Proper handling of irradiated foods is still critical for preventing food-borne illness.

Genetically Modified Foods

Genetic engineering involves altering the characteristics of a plant, an animal, or a microorganism by adding, rearranging, or replacing genes in its DNA; the result is a **genetically modified (GM) organism**. New DNA may come from related species or from entirely different types of organisms. About 60% of crops grown in Canada are genetically modified. More than half of North America's soybean crop has been genetically modified to be resistant to a herbicide used to kill weeds. Products made with GM organisms include juice, soft drinks, nuts, tuna, frozen pizza, spaghetti sauce, canola oil, chips, salad dressings, and soup.

The potential benefits of GM foods cited by supporters include improved yields overall and in difficult growing conditions, increased disease resistance, improved nutritional content, lower prices, and less pesticide use. Critics of biotechnology argue that unexpected effects may occur: Gene manipulation could elevate levels of naturally occurring toxins or allergens, permanently change the gene pool and reduce biodiversity, and produce pesticide-resistant insects through the transfer of genes. Experience has shown that GM products are difficult to keep separate from non-GM products; animal escapes, cross-pollination, and contamination during processing are just a few ways GM organisms could potentially appear unexpectedly in the food supply or the environment.

According to the National Academy of Sciences, there is currently no proof that the GM food already on the market is unsafe. However, experts have recommended regulatory changes and further study of key issues, particularly the environmental effects of the escape of GM animals.

Animal Cloning   Cloning allows producers to create animals with highly desirable characteristics, such as disease resistance and more predictable fat-to-lean meat ratios. Cloned animals are similar to identical twins. For example, scientists can produce a cloned cow by taking an egg from a female cow, removing the egg's gene-containing nucleus, and inserting genes from another cow that the scientists want to copy. The egg is then urged to create an embryo, and the embryo is implanted into the uterus of another female cow, which carries it to term and delivers it. (This surrogate cow's DNA does not affect the clone's DNA.)

The recently developed method of animal cloning called somatic cell nuclear transfer (SCNT) has raised potential food safety concerns. At this time, it is unclear if this cloning technique would have an impact on the safety and nutritional quality of foods derived from animals generated by SCNT. SCNT technology is still at the research and development stage, and as a result, very limited data are available to provide answers to these questions. The fact that significant health problems are observed in some animals cloned by using this technology reinforces the fact that questions need to be asked about food products derived from them.

Until more is known about the products of this technology, Health Canada will consider foods produced from livestock developed by using SCNT and the progeny of such livestock to be what is termed "novel food" in the Food and Drug Regulations. At this time, Health Canada does not allow food producers to have cloned animals in the food supply.

Labelling of GM Foods   Labelling has been another major concern, with surveys indicating that most Canadians want to know if their food contains GM ingredients. Health Canada does not require special labelling for foods from genetically modified or cloned sources. Under current rules, Health Canada requires special labelling only when a food's composition or nutrition profile is changed significantly or when a known allergen, such as a peanut gene, is introduced into a food. Health Canada needs to determine what type of information is required on the label to inform Canadians about these changes in the food. The only foods guaranteed not to contain GM ingredients are those certified as organic.

Food Allergies and Food Intolerances

For some people, consuming a particular food causes uncomfortable symptoms, such as itchiness, swollen lips, or abdominal pain. Adverse reactions, such as these, may be due to a food allergy or a food intolerance, and symptoms may range from annoying to life threatening. If you've had an adverse reaction to a food, it's important to determine whether your symptoms are due to an allergy or an intolerance so that you can take appropriate action.

Food Allergies   A true **food allergy** is a reaction of the body's immune system to a food or food ingredient, usually a protein. The immune system perceives the reaction-provoking substance, or allergen, as foreign and acts to destroy it. This immune reaction can occur within minutes of ingesting the food, resulting in symptoms that affect the skin (hives), gastrointestinal tract (cramps or diarrhea), respiratory tract (asthma), or mouth (swelling of the lips or tongue). The most severe response is a systemic reaction called *anaphylaxis*, which involves a potentially life-threatening drop in blood pressure.

Food allergies affect only about 1.3 million Canadians, or 4% of the adult population, and up to 6% of infants; many infants outgrow food allergies. Although numerous food allergens have been identified, just eight foods account for more than 90% of the food allergies in Canada: cow's milk, eggs, peanuts, tree nuts (e.g., walnuts, cashews), soy, wheat, fish, and shellfish. Food labels are now required to state the presence of the eight most common allergens in plain language in the ingredient list. People with food allergies, especially those prone to anaphylaxis, must diligently avoid trigger foods. This involves carefully reading food labels and asking questions about ingredients when eating out. People at risk are usually advised to carry medications to treat anaphylaxis, such as injectable epinephrine. Refer to Chapter 9 for more on allergies.

Food Intolerances   Many people who believe they have food allergies may actually have a much more common source of adverse food reactions: a food intolerance. In the case of a **food intolerance**, the problem usually lies with metabolism rather than with the immune system. Typically, the body cannot adequately digest a food or food component, often because of some type of chemical deficiency; in other cases, the body reacts to a particular compound in a food. Lactose intolerance is a fairly common food intolerance. A more serious condition is intolerance of gluten, a protein component of some grains; in affected individuals, consumption of gluten damages the lining of the small intestine. Sulphite, a common food additive, can produce severe asthmatic reactions in sensitive individuals. Food intolerances have also been attributed to tartrazine (a yellow food colouring), MSG, and the sweetener aspartame.

Food intolerance reactions often produce symptoms similar to food allergies, such as diarrhea or abdominal cramps, but reactions are typically localized and not life threatening. Many people with food intolerances can consume small amounts of the food that affects them; exceptions are gluten and sulphites, which must be avoided by sensitive individuals. Through trial and error, most people with food intolerances can adjust their intake of the trigger food to an appropriate level.

If you suspect that you have a food allergy or intolerance, a good first step is to keep a food diary. Note everything you eat or drink, any symptoms you develop, and how long after eating the symptoms appear. Then make an appointment with your physician to go over your diary and determine if any additional tests are needed.

QUESTIONS FOR CRITICAL THINKING AND REFLECTION
What is the least healthy food you eat every day (either during meals or as a snack)? Identify at least one substitute that would be healthier but just as satisfying.

TERMS

genetically modified (GM) organism   A plant, an animal, or a microorganism in which genes have been added, rearranged, or replaced through genetic engineering.

food allergy   An adverse reaction to a food or food ingredient in which the immune system perceives a particular substance (allergen) as foreign and acts to destroy it.

food intolerance   An adverse reaction to a food or food ingredient that doesn't involve the immune system; intolerances are often caused by a problem with metabolism.

BEHAVIOUR CHANGE STRATEGY

Improving Your Diet by Choosing Healthy Beverages

After reading this chapter and completing the dietary assessment on p. 155, you can probably identify several changes you could make to improve your diet. Here, we focus on choosing healthy beverages to increase intake of nutrients and decrease intake of empty calories from added sugars and fat. However, this model of dietary change can be applied to any modification you'd like to make to your diet. Additional specific plans for improving diet can be found in the Behaviour Change Strategy in Chapter 7 (decreasing saturated and trans fat intake) and Chapter 8 (increasing intake of fruits and vegetables).

Gather Data and Establish a Baseline

Begin by tracking your beverage consumption in your health journal. Write down the types and amounts of beverages you drink, including water. Also note where you were at the time and whether you obtained the beverage there or brought it with you. At the same time, investigate your options. Find out what other beverages you can easily obtain during your daily routine. For example, what drinks are available in the dining hall where you eat lunch or at the food court where you often grab snacks? How many drinking fountains do you walk by over the course of the day? This information will help you put together a successful plan for change.

Analyze Your Data and Set Goals

Evaluate your beverage consumption by dividing your typical daily consumption between healthy and less healthy choices. Use the following guide as a basis, and add other beverages to the lists as needed.

Choose less often:

- Regular soft drinks
- Sweetened iced tea
- Fruit beverages made with little fruit juice (usually labelled fruit drinks, punches, beverages, blends, or ades)
- Homogenized milk

Choose more often:

- Water
- Low-fat or skim milk
- Fruit juice (100% juice)
- Unsweetened herbal tea

How many beverages do you consume daily from each category? What would be a healthy and realistic goal for change? For example, if your beverage consumption is currently evenly divided between the "choose more often" and "choose less often" categories (four from each list), you might set a final goal for your behaviour change program of increasing your healthy choices by two (to six from the "more often" list and two from the "less often" list).

Develop a Plan for Change

Once you've set your goal, you need to develop strategies that will help you choose healthy beverages more often. Consider the following possibilities:

- Keep healthy beverages on hand; if you live in a student dorm, rent a small refrigerator or keep bottled water, juice, low-fat or skim milk, and other healthy choices in the dorm kitchen's refrigerator.
- Plan ahead, and put a bottle of water or 100% juice in your backpack every day.

- Check food labels on beverages for serving sizes, calories, and nutrients; comparison shop to find the healthiest choices, and watch your serving sizes. Use this information to make your "choose more often" list longer and more specific.

- If you eat out frequently, examine all the beverages available at the places you typically eat your meals. You'll probably find that healthy choices are available; if not, bring along your own drink or find somewhere else to eat.

- For a snack, try water and a piece of fruit rather than a heavily sweetened beverage.

- Create healthy beverages that appeal to you; for example, try adding slices of citrus fruit to water or mixing 100% fruit juice with sparkling water.

You may also need to make some changes in your routine to decrease the likelihood that you'll make unhealthy choices. For example, you might discover from your health journal that you always buy a soft drink after class when you pass a particular vending machine. If this is the case, try another route that allows you to avoid the machine. And try to guard against impulse buying by carrying water or a healthy snack with you every day.

To complete your plan, try some of the other behaviour change strategies described in Chapter 1: Develop and sign a contract, set up a system of rewards, involve other people in your program, and develop strategies for challenging situations. Once your plan is complete, take action. Keep track of your progress in your health journal by continuing to monitor and evaluate your beverage consumption.

Practise and learn online with Connect. Connect allows you to practise important skills at your own pace and on your own schedule, with 24/7 online access to an eBook, practice quizzes, interactivities, videos, study tools, additional resources, and more.

SUMMARY

- To function at its best, the human body requires about 50 essential nutrients in specific proportions. People get the nutrients needed to fuel their bodies and maintain tissues and organ systems from foods; the body cannot synthesize most of them.

- Proteins, made up of amino acids, form muscles and bones and help make up blood, enzymes, hormones, and cell membranes. Foods from animal sources provide complete proteins; plants provide incomplete proteins.

- Fats, a concentrated source of energy, also help insulate the body and cushion the organs; 15 mL of vegetable oil per day supplies the essential fats. Dietary fat intake should be 20%–35% of total daily calories. Unsaturated fats should be favoured over saturated and trans fats.

- Carbohydrates supply energy to the brain and other parts of the nervous system as well as to red blood cells.

- Fibre includes nondigestible carbohydrates provided mainly by plants. Adequate intake of fibre (38 grams per day for men and 25 grams per day for women) can help people manage diabetes and high cholesterol levels and improve intestinal health.

- The 13 vitamins needed in the diet are organic substances that promote specific chemical and cell processes within living tissue. Deficiencies or excesses can cause serious illnesses and even death.

- The approximately 17 minerals needed in the diet are inorganic substances that regulate body functions, aid in the growth and maintenance of body tissues, and help in the release of energy from foods.

- Water is used to digest and absorb food, transport substances around the body, lubricate joints and organs, and regulate body temperature.

- Foods contain other substances, such as phytochemicals, which may not be essential nutrients but which reduce chronic disease risk.

- Dietary Reference Intakes (DRIs) are recommended intakes for essential nutrients that meet the needs of healthy people.

- The Guidelines for Healthy Eating address the prevention of diet-related diseases such as heart disease, cancer, and diabetes. The guidelines advise us to consume a variety of foods while staying within calorie needs; manage body weight through calorie control and regular physical activity; eat more fruits, vegetables, whole grains, and reduced-fat dairy products; choose fats and carbohydrates wisely; consume less salt and caffeine; be moderate with alcohol intake; and handle foods safely.

- Choosing foods from each group in *Eating Well with Canada's Food Guide* every day helps ensure the appropriate amounts of necessary nutrients.

- A vegetarian diet can meet our nutritional needs.

- Almost all foods have labels that show how much fat, cholesterol, protein, fibre, and sodium they contain. Serving sizes are standardized, and health claims are carefully regulated.

- Food-borne illnesses are a greater threat to health than additives and environmental contaminants. Other dietary issues of concern to some people include organic foods, food irradiation, genetic modification of foods, and food allergies and intolerances.

FOR MORE INFORMATION

BOOKS

Nestle, M. 2007. *What to Eat*. New York: North Point Press. A nutritionist examines the marketing of food and explains how to interpret food-related information while shopping.

NEWSLETTERS

Nutrition Action Health Letter (613-244-7337; http://www.cspinet.org/nah/canada.htm)
Tufts University Health & Nutrition Letter (800-274-7581; http://www.tuftshealthletter.com)

ORGANIZATIONS, HOTLINES, AND WEB SITES

The Internet addresses listed here were accurate at the time of publication.

Beyond the Basics: Meal Planning for Healthy Eating, Diabetes Management and Prevention. Available online from the Canadian Diabetes Association.

> https://orders.diabetes.ca/cda/

Canadian Council on Food and Nutrition. Provides links to reliable food and nutrition information.

> http://www.ccfn.ca/in_action/links.asp

Canadian Food Inspection Agency. Offers information about many topics, such as food labelling, food additives, dietary supplements, and food-borne illness.

> http://www.inspection.gc.ca

Dietitians of Canada. Provides a wide variety of nutrition-related educational materials, including information related to healthy eating, body image, self-esteem, physical activity. This site also has a tool called EATracker, which allows you to track your day's food and activity choices and compare them with Health Canada guidelines.

> http://www.dietitians.ca

Eat Right Ontario. Offers nutrition information for consumers on a wide-range of topics, in more than 100 languages. Staffed by registered dietitians throughout the weekdays and with extended hours into the evenings.

> http://www.Ontario.ca/EatRight or call toll free 1-877-510-5102

Eating Well with Canada's Food Guide. Provides personalized dietary plans and interactive food and activity tracking tools.

> http://www.myfoodguide.ca

Food Safety Network. Provides information on safe purchase, handling, cooking, and storage of food.

> 1-866-50-FSNET (1-866-503-7638) or e-mail queries to fsnrsn@uoguelph.ca

Health Canada. Provides access to government resources relating to food safety and nutrition.

> http://www.hc-sc.gc.ca

Health Canada: Nutrient Value of Some Common Foods. Provides nutrient breakdowns of individual foods.

> http://www.hc-sc.gc.ca/fn-an/nutrition/fiche-nutri-data/nutrient_value-valeurs_nutritives-eng.php

Health Nexus. Offers health-promotion resources to help organizations and individuals develop and implement prevention and health promotion strategies to enhance well-being and reduce demand on the health care and social service systems.

> http://www.healthnexus.ca

Heart and Stroke Foundation of Canada. Provides basic information about nutrition, tips for shopping and eating out, and heart-healthy recipes.

> http://www.heartandstroke.ca

International Food Information Council. Provides information for consumers, journalists, and educators about food safety and nutrition.

> http://www.foodinsight.org

Institute of Medicine: Food and Nutrition Board. Provides information about the Dietary Reference Intakes and related guidelines.

> http://www.iom.edu/CMS/3788.aspx

Public Health Agency of Canada. Information on promoting health; preventing and controlling chronic diseases and injuries; preventing and controlling infectious diseases; preparing for and responding to public health emergencies, and strengthening Canada's public health capacity.

> http://www.publichealth.gc.ca

Vegetarian Diets. Information for vegetarians and people interested in learning more about vegetarian diets.

> http://www.dietitians.ca/Your-Health/Nutrition-A-Z/Vegetarian-Diets.aspx?categoryID=54

See also the listings for Chapters 4, 6–8, and 17.

SELECTED BIBLIOGRAPHY

Aboriginal Canada Portal. 2010. *Food and Recipes* (http://www.aboriginal-canada.gc.ca/acp/site.nsf/eng/ao35296.html; retrieved January 13, 2010).

Benardot, D. 2005. *Advanced Sports Nutrition: Carbohydrate Requirements* (http://www.healthline.com/hlbook/nut-carbohydrate-requirements; retrieved April 15, 2010).

Bush, M. A., et al. 2007. *Eating Well with Canada's Food Guide*: A tool for the times. *Canadian Journal of Dietetic Practice and Research* 68(2): 92–96.

Canadian Food Inspection Agency. 2007. *Food* (http://www.inspection.gc.ca/english/fssa/fssae.shtml; retrieved April 15, 2010).

Canadian Food Inspection Agency. 2010. *Causes of Foodborne Illness* (http://www.inspection.gc.ca/english/fssa/concen/causee.shtml; retrieved June 15, 2010).

Canadian Food Inspection Agency. 2010. *Food Allergens* (http://www.inspection.gc.ca/english/fssa/labeti/allerg/allerge.shtml; retrieved June 15, 2010).

Canadian Food Inspection Agency. 2010. *Organic Products* (http://www.inspection.gc.ca/english/fssa/orgbio/orgbioe.shtml; retrieved June 15, 2010).

Capital Health, Regional Nutrition and Food Service. 2005. *Canada's Food Guide: Serving size handout* (http://www.capitalhealth.ca/NR/rdonlyres/etgansnparwmjhldsvhl4nmhp6bvkynxnoao2bm3qrcounb6nzu-5jcpqhocw4wk576apdb7v4dmaeywfqk7rdjx6cec/Portion+size+Handout.pdf; retrieved December 12, 2009).

Capital Health. 2007. *Sugar Shocker: An Activity Kit to Help Teach Students About Healthy Drink Choices* (http://www.capitalhealth.ca/nr/rdonlyres/e6nstouxulgpkbvzot7as7dhtyvv6storxwnl57sbz4gl6o2im2rg-wio4tthag2r5vag2aoqodp7fst6zyagrafdccb/sugar+shocker+kit_nov07.pdf; retrieved December 12, 2009).

Cheung, A. M., et al. 2004. Prevention of osteoporosis and osteoporotic fractures in postmenopausal women: Recommendation statement from the Canadian Task Force on Preventive Health Care. *Canadian Medical Association Journal* 170(11): 1665–1667.

Dairy Nutrition. 2010. *Trans Fats in the Canadian Diet* (http://www.dairynutrition.ca/nutrients-in-milk-products/fat/trans-fats-in-the-canadian-diet; retrieved April 10, 2010).

Egg Farmers of Canada. 2008. *Omega-3 Fatty Acids* (http://www.eggs.ca/AllAboutEggs/FAQ_Omega3FattyAcids.aspx; retrieved February 15, 2010).

Garriguet, D. 2004. *Nutrition: Findings from the Canadian Community Health Survey: Overview of Canadians' Eating Habits* (http://www.statcan.gc.ca/pub/82-620-m/82-620-m2006002-eng.pdf; retrieved May 14, 2010).

Government of Alberta. 2004. *Vegetarianism: A Meatless Eating Experience* (http://www1.agric.gov.ab.ca/$department/deptdocs.nsf/all/sis8739; retrieved April 4, 2011).

Hanley, D. M., and K. S. Davison. 2005. Vitamin D insufficiency in North America: A significant risk factor in chronic diseases and potential disease-specific biomarkers of Vitamin D sufficiency. *Journal of Nutrition*, 135: 332–337.

Health Canada. 2003. *Guiding Canadians Towards Healthy Eating: National Nutrition Leadership* (http://www.hc-sc.gc.ca/fn-an/res-rech/res-prog/eat-aliment/guiding_cdn_lead-lead_cdn_inciter-eng.php; retrieved March 5, 2010).

Health Canada. 2003. *Using the Dietary Reference Intakes* (http://www.hc-sc.gc.ca/fn-an/nutrition/reference/dri_using-util_anref-eng.php; retrieved December 9, 2009).

Health Canada. 2006. *Dietary Reference Intakes: Questions and Answers* (http://www.hc-sc.gc.ca/fn-an/nutrition/reference/dri_ques-ques_anref-eng.php; retrieved April 3, 2011).

Health Canada. 2006. *Salmonella Prevention* (http://www.hc-sc.gc.ca/hl-vs/iyh-vsv/food-aliment/salmonella-eng.php; retrieved April 4, 2011).

Health Canada. 2007. *Canada's Food Guide: Questions and Answers for Educators* (http://www.hc-sc.gc.ca/fn-an/food-guide-aliment/educ-comm/faq_educat-eng.php#14; retrieved December 12, 2009).

Health Canada. 2007. *It's Your Health: Trans Fats* (http://www.hc-sc.gc.ca/hl-vs/alt_formats/pacrb-dgapcr/pdf/iyh-vsv/food-aliment/trans-eng.pdf; retrieved March 24, 2010).

Health Canada. 2008. *Eating Well with Canada's Food Guide* (http://www.hc-sc.gc.ca/fn-an/food-guide-aliment/order-commander/eating_well_bien_manger-eng.php; retrieved February 21, 2010).

Health Canada. 2008. *Human Health Risk Assessment of Mercury in Fish and Health Benefits of Fish Consumption* (http://www.hc-sc.gc.ca/fn-an/pubs/mercur/merc_fish_poisson-eng.php; retrieved January 15, 2010).

Health Canada. 2008. *It's Your Health: Sodium* (http://www.hc-sc.gc.ca/hl-vs/alt_formats/pacrb-dgapcr/pdf/iyh-vsv/food-aliment/sodium_eng.pdf; retrieved March 5, 2010).

Health Canada. 2008. *My Food Guide* (http://www.hc-sc.gc.ca/fn-an/food-guide-aliment/myguide-monguide/index-eng.php; retrieved March 5, 2010).

Health Canada. 2010. *Eating Well with Canada's Food Guide: First Nations, Inuit and Métis* (http://www.hc-sc.gc.ca/fn-an/pubs/fnim-pnim/index-eng.php; retrieved April 5, 2010).

Health Canada. 2010. *Food and Nutrition* (http://www.hc-sc.gc.ca/fn-an/index-eng.php; retrieved April 5, 2010).

Health Canada. 2011. *Natural Health Products* (http://www.hc-sc.gc.ca/dhp-mps/prodnatur/index-eng.php; retrieved April 4, 2011).

Health Canada and Statistics Canada. 2004. *Canadian Community Health Survey Cycle 2.2, Nutrition. Nutrient Intakes from Food. Provincial, Regional and National Summary Data Tables: Volume 1*. Ottawa: Health Canada.

Institute of Medicine. 2010. *Dietary Reference Intakes for Calcium and Vitamin D: Report at a Glance* (http://www.iom.edu/Reports/2010/Dietary-Reference-Intakes-for-Calcium-and-Vitamin-D-Report-Brief.aspx; retrieved April 3, 2011).

Katamay, S. W., et al. 2007. *Eating Well with Canada's Food Guide* 2007: Development of the Food Intake Pattern. *Nutrition Reviews* 65(4): 155–166.

L'Abbé, M. R., S. J. Whiting, and D. A. Hanley. 2004. The Canadian health claim for calcium, vitamin D and osteoporosis. *Journal of the American College of Nutrition* 23(4): 303–308.

Lambton Community Health Services Department (n.d.) *New Nutrition Labels* (http://www.lambtonhealth.on.ca/nutrition/readlabels.asp; retrieved February 15, 2010).

Marine Harvest Canada. 2010. *Salmon Nutrition Facts* (http://www.marine-harvestcanada.com/pdf/mics/Nutrition_Facts.pdf; retrieved April 2, 2011).

McDonald, B. E. 2004. The Canadian experience: Why Canada decided against an upper limit for cholesterol. *Journal of the American College of Nutrition* 23(90006): 616S–620S.

National Research Council of Canada. 2006. *Highlights: Missing Ingredients Can Be a Recipe for Disaster* (http://www.nrc-cnrc.gc.ca/eng/news/nrc/2006/12/06/low-folate.html; retrieved February 21, 2010).

Norris, S. 2007. *Trans Fats: The Health Burden* (http://www2.parl.gc.ca/content/LOP/ResearchPublications/prb0521-e.pdf; retrieved February 15, 2010).

Peng, Y. 2004. *Canadian Consumer Trends in Obesity and Food Consumption* (http://www1.agric.gov.ab.ca/$department/deptdocs.nsf/all/sis8438/$file/obesityandnutrition.pdf?OpenElement; retrieved May 14, 2010).

Public Health Agency of Canada. 2009. *Healthy Eating and Healthy Aging* (http://www.phac-aspc.gc.ca/seniors-aines/publications/pro/healthy-sante/haging_newvision/vison-rpt/eating-alimentation-eng.php; retrieved March 5, 2010).

Samra, R. A., and G. H. Anderson. 2007. Insoluble cereal fiber reduces appetite and short-term food intake and glycemic response to food consumed 75 min later by healthy men. *American Journal of Clinical Nutrition* 86(4): 972–979.

Trans Fat Task Force. 2006. *TRANSforming the Food Supply* (http://www.hc-sc.gc.ca/fn-an/alt_formats/hpfb-dgpsa/pdf/nutrition/tf-gt_rep-rap-eng.pdf; retrieved April 2, 2011).

Wolever, T. M., and D. J. Jenkins. 1997. What is a high fiber diet? *Advances in Experimental Medicine and Biology* 427: 35–42.

Nutrition Resources

Table 1	Dietary Reference Intakes (DRIs): Recommended Levels for Individual Intake

Life Stage	Group	Biotin (µg/day)	Choline (mg/day)ᵃ	Folate (µg/day)ᵇ	Niacin (mg/day)	Pantothenic Acid (mg/day)	Riboflavin (mg/day)
Infants	0–6 months	5	125	65	2	1.7	0.3
	7–12 months	6	150	80	4	1.8	0.4
Children	1–3 years	8	200	**150**	**6**	2	**0.5**
	4–8 years	12	250	**200**	**8**	3	**0.6**
Males	9–13 years	20	375	**300**	**12**	4	**0.9**
	14–18 years	25	550	**400**	**16**	5	**1.3**
	19–30 years	30	550	**400**	**16**	5	**1.3**
	31–50 years	30	550	**400**	**16**	5	**1.3**
	51–70 years	30	550	**400**	**16**	5	**1.3**
	>70 years	30	550	**400**	**16**	5	**1.3**
Females	9–13 years	20	375	**300**	**12**	4	**0.9**
	14–18 years	25	400	**400ⁱ**	**14**	5	**1.0**
	19–30 years	30	425	**400ⁱ**	**14**	5	**1.1**
	31–50 years	30	425	**400ⁱ**	**14**	5	**1.1**
	51–70 years	30	425	**400ⁱ**	**14**	5	**1.1**
	>70 years	30	425	**400**	**14**	5	**1.1**
Pregnancy	≤18 years	30	450	**600ⁱ**	**18**	6	**1.4**
	19–30 years	**30**	450	**600ʲ**	**18**	6	**1.4**
	31–50 years	30	450	**600ʲ**	**18**	6	**1.4**
Lactation	≤18 years	35	550	**500**	**17**	7	**1.6**
	19–30 years	35	550	**500**	**17**	7	**1.6**
	31–50 years	35	550	**500**	**17**	7	**1.6**
Tolerable Upper Intake Levels for Adults (19–70)			3500	1000ᵏ	35ᵏ		

Life Stage	Group	Thiamine (mg/day)	Vitamin A (µg/day)ᵈ	Vitamin B-6 (mg/day)	Vitamin B-12 (µg/day)	Vitamin C (mg/day)ᵉ	Vitamin D (µg/day)ᶠ	Vitamin E (mg/day)ᵍ
Infants	0–6 months	0.2	400	0.1	0.4	40	5	4
	7–12 months	0.3	500	0.3	0.5	50	5	5
Children	1–3 years	**0.5**	**300**	**0.5**	**0.9**	**15**	5	**6**
	4–8 years	**0.6**	**400**	**0.6**	**1.2**	**25**	5	**7**
Males	9–13 years	**0.9**	**600**	**1.0**	**1.8**	**45**	5	**11**
	14–18 years	**1.2**	**900**	**1.3**	**2.4**	**75**	5	**15**
	19–30 years	**1.2**	**900**	**1.3**	**2.4**	**90**	5	**15**
	31–50 years	**1.2**	**900**	**1.3**	**2.4**	**90**	5	**15**
	51–70 years	**1.2**	**900**	**1.7**	**2.4ʰ**	**90**	10	**15**
	>70 years	**1.2**	**900**	**1.7**	**2.4ʰ**	**90**	15	**15**
Females	9–13 years	**0.9**	**600**	**1.0**	**1.8**	**45**	5	**11**
	14–18 years	**1.0**	**700**	**1.2**	**2.4**	**65**	5	**15**
	19–30 years	**1.1**	**700**	**1.3**	**2.4**	**75**	5	**15**
	31–50 years	**1.1**	**700**	**1.3**	**2.4**	**75**	5	**15**
	51–70 years	**1.1**	**700**	**1.5**	**2.4ʰ**	**75**	10	**15**
	>70 years	**1.1**	**700**	**1.5**	**2.4ʰ**	**75**	15	**15**
Pregnancy	≤18 years	**1.4**	**750**	**1.9**	**2.6**	**80**	5	**15**
	19–30 years	**1.4**	**770**	**1.9**	**2.6**	**85**	5	**15**
	31–50 years	**1.4**	**770**	**1.9**	**2.6**	**85**	5	**15**
Lactation	≤18 years	**1.4**	**1200**	**2.0**	**2.8**	**115**	5	**19**
	19–30 years	**1.4**	**1300**	**2.0**	**2.8**	**120**	5	**19**
	31–50 years	**1.4**	**1300**	**2.0**	**2.8**	**120**	5	**19**
Tolerable Upper Intake Levels for Adults (19–70)			3000	100		2000	50	1000ᵏ

Note: The table includes values for the type of DRI standard—Adequate Intake (AI) or Recommended Dietary Allowance (RDA)—that has bee n established for that particular nutrient and life stage; RDAs are shown in **bold type**. The final row of the table shows the Tolerable Upper Intake Levels (ULs) for adults; refer to the full DRI report for information on other ages and life stages. A UL is the maximum level of daily nutrient intake that is likely to pose no risk of adverse effects. There is insufficient data to set ULs for all nutrients, but this does not mean that there is no potential for adverse effects; source of intake should be from food only to prevent high levels of intake of nutrients without established ULs. In healthy individuals, there is no established benefit from nutrient intakes above the RDA or AI.

µg is the symbol for micrograms.

ᵃ Although AIs have been set for choline, there are few data to assess whether a dietary supply of choline is needed at all stages of the life cycle, and it may be that the choline requirement can be met by endogenous synthesis at some of these stages.

ᵇ As dietary folate equivalents (DFE): 1 DFE = 1 µg food folate = 0.6 µg folate from fortified food or as a supplement consumed with food = 0.5 µg of a supplement taken on an empty stomach.

ᶜ As niacin equivalents (NE): 1 mg niacin = 60 mg tryptophan.

ᵈ As retinol activity equivalents (RAEs): 1 RAE = 1 µg retinol, 12 µg b-carotene, or 24 µg a-carotene or b-cryptoxanthin. Preformed vitamin A (retinol) is abundant in animal-derived foods; provitamin A carotenoids are abundant in some dark-yellow, orange, red, and deep-green fruits and vegetables. For preformed vitamin A and for provitamin A carotenoids in supplements, 1 RE = 1 RAE; for provitamin A carotenoids in foods, divide the REs by 2 to obtain RAEs. The UL applies only to preformed vitamin A.

Life Stage	Group	Vitamin K (µg/day)	Calcium (mg/day)	Chromium (µg/day)	Copper (µg/day)	Fluoride (mg/day)	Iodine (µg/day)
Infants	0–6 months	2.0	210	0.2	200	0.01	110
	7–12 months	2.5	270	5.5	220	0.5	130
Children	1–3 years	30	500	11	340	0.7	90
	4–8 years	55	800	15	440	1	90
Males	9–13 years	60	1300	25	700	2	120
	14–18 years	75	1300	35	890	3	150
	19–30 years	120	1000	35	900	4	150
	31–50 years	120	1000	35	900	4	150
	51–70 years	120	1200	30	900	4	150
	>70 years	120	1200	30	900	4	150
Females	9–13 years	60	1300	21	700	2	120
	14–18 years	75	1300	24	890	3	150
	19–30 years	90	1000	25	900	3	150
	31–50 years	90	1000	25	900	3	150
	51–70 years	90	1200	20	900	3	150
	>70 years	90	1200	20	900	3	150
Pregnancy	≤18 years	75	1300	29	1000	3	220
	19–30 years	90	1000	30	1000	3	220
	31–50 years	90	1000	30	1000	3	220
Lactation	≤18 years	75	1300	44	1300	3	290
	19–30 years	90	1000	45	1300	3	290
	31–50 years	90	1000	45	1300	3	290
Tolerable Upper Intake Levels for Adults (19–70)			*2500*		*10,000*	*10*	*1100*

Life Stage	Group	Iron (mg/day)[l]	Magnesium (mg/day)	Manganese (mg/day)	Molybdenum (µg/day)	Phosphorus (mg/day)	Selenium (µg/day)	Zinc (mg/day)[m]
Infants	0–6 months	0.27	30	0.003	2	100	15	2
	7–12 months	11	75	0.6	3	275	20	3
Children	1–3 years	7	80	1.2	17	460	20	3
	4–8 years	10	130	1.5	22	500	30	5
Males	9–13 years	8	240	1.9	34	1250	40	8
	14–18 years	11	410	2.2	43	1250	55	11
	19–30 years	8	400	2.3	45	700	55	11
	31–50 years	8	420	2.3	45	700	55	11
	51–70 years	8	420	2.3	45	700	55	11
	>70 years	8	420	2.3	45	700	55	11
Females	9–13 years	8	240	1.6	34	1250	40	8
	14–18 years	15	360	1.6	43	1250	55	9
	19–30 years	18	310	1.8	45	700	55	8
	31–50 years	18	320	1.8	45	700	55	8
	51–70 years	8	320	1.8	45	700	55	8
	>70 years	8	320	1.8	45	700	55	8
Pregnancy	≤18 years	27	400	2.0	50	1250	60	13
	19–30 years	27	350	2.0	50	700	60	11
	31–50 years	27	360	2.0	50	700	60	11
Lactation	≤18 years	10	360	2.6	50	1250	70	14
	19–30 years	9	310	2.6	50	700	70	12
	31–50 years	9	320	2.6	50	700	70	12
Tolerable Upper Intake Levels for Adults (19–70)		*45*	*350*[k]	*11*	*2000*	*4000*	*400*	*40*

[e] Individuals who smoke require an additional 35 mg/day of vitamin C over that needed by nonsmokers; nonsmokers regularly exposed to tobacco smoke should ensure they meet the RDA for vitamin C.

[f] As cholecalciferol: 1 µg cholecalciferol = 40 IU vitamin D. DRI values are based on the absence of adequate exposure to sunlight.

[g] As a-tocopherol. Includes naturally occurring RRR-a-tocopherol and the 2R-stereoisomeric forms from supplements; does not include the 2S-stereoisomeric forms from supplements.

[h] Because 10%–30% of older people may malabsorb food-bound B12, those over age 50 should meet their RDA mainly with supplements or foods fortified with B12.

[i] In view of evidence linking folate intake with neural tube defects in the fetus. It is recommended that all women capable of becoming pregnant consume 400 µg from supplements or fortified foods in addition to consuming folate from a varied diet.

[j] It is assumed that women will continue consuming 400 µg from supplements or fortified food until their pregnancy is confirmed and they enter prenatal care, which ordinarily occurs after the end of the periconceptional period—the critical time for formation of the neural tube.

[k] The UL applies only to intake from supplements, fortified foods, and/or pharmacological agents and not to intake from foods.

[l] Because the absorption of iron from plant foods is low compared with that from animal foods, the RDA for strict vegetarians is approximately 1.8 times as high as the values established for omnivores (14 mg/day for adult male vegetarians; 33 mg/day for premenopausal female vegetarians. Oral contraceptives (OCs) reduce menstrual blood losses, so women taking them need less daily iron; the RDA for premenopausal women taking OCs is 10.9 mg/day. For more on iron requirements for other special situations, refer to *Dietary Reference Intakes for Vitamin A, Vitamin K, Arsenic, Boron, Chromium, Copper, Iodine, Iron, Manganese, Molybdenum, Nickel, Silicon, Vanadium, and Zinc* (visit http://www.nap.edu for the complete report).

[m] Zinc absorption is lower for those consuming vegetarian diets so the zinc requirement for vegetarians is approximately twofold greater than for those consuming a nonvegetarian diet.

Life Stage	Group	Potassium (g/day)	Sodium (g/day)	Chloride (g/day)	Carbohydrate RDA/AI (g/day)	Carbohydrate AMDR (%)	Total Fibre RDA/AI (g/day)	Total Fat AMDR (%)
Infants	0–6 months	0.4	0.12	0.18	60	ND[q]	ND	[r]
	7–12 months	0.7	0.37	0.57	95	ND[q]	ND	[r]
Children	1–3 years	3.0	1.0	1.5	130	45–65	19	30–40
	4–8 years	3.8	1.2	1.9	130	45–65	25	25–35
Males	9–13 years	4.5	1.5	2.3	130	45–65	31	25–35
	14–18 years	4.7	1.5	2.3	130	45–65	38	25–35
	19–30 years	4.7	1.5	2.3	130	45–65	38	20–35
	31–50 years	4.7	1.5	2.3	130	45–65	38	20–35
	51–70 years	4.7	1.3	2.0	130	45–65	30	20–35
	>70 years	4.7	1.2	1.8	130	45–65	30	20–35
Females	9–13 years	4.5	1.5	2.3	130	45–65	26	25–35
	14–18 years	4.7	1.5	2.3	130	45–65	26	25–35
	19–30 years	4.7	1.5	2.3	130	45–65	25	20–35
	31–50 years	4.7	1.5	2.3	130	45–65	25	20–35
	51–70 years	4.7	1.3	2.0	130	45–65	21	20–35
	>70 years	4.7	1.2	1.8	130	45–65	21	20–35
Pregnancy	≤18 years	4.7	1.5	2.3	175	45–65	28	20–35
	19–30 years	4.7	1.5	2.3	175	45–65	28	20–35
	31–50 years	4.7	1.5	2.3	175	45–65	28	20–35
Lactation	≤18 years	5.1	1.5	2.3	210	45–65	29	20–35
	19–30 years	5.1	1.5	2.3	210	45–65	29	20–35
	31–50 years	5.1	1.5	2.3	210	45–65	29	20–35
Tolerable Upper Intake Levels for Adults (19–70)			2.3	3.6				

Life Stage	Group	Linoleic Acid RDA/AI (g/day)	Linoleic Acid AMDR[o] (%)	Alpha-linolenic Acid RDA/AI (g/day)	Alpha-linolenic Acid AMDR[o] (%)	Protein[n] RDA/AI (g/day)	Protein[n] AMDR[o] (%)	Water[p] (L/day)
Infants	0–6 months	4.4	ND[q]	0.5	ND[q]	9.1	ND[q]	0.7
	7–12 months	4.6	ND[q]	0.5	ND[q]	13.5	ND[q]	0.8
Children	1–3 years	7	5–10	0.7	0.6–1.2	13	5–20	1.3
	4–8 years	10	5–10	0.9	0.6–1.2	19	10–30	1.7
Males	9–13 years	12	5–10	1.2	0.6–1.2	34	10–30	2.4
	14–18 years	16	5–10	1.6	0.6–1.2	52	10–30	3.3
	19–30 years	17	5–10	1.6	0.6–1.2	56	10–35	3.7
	31–50 years	17	5–10	1.6	0.6–1.2	56	10–35	3.7
	51–70 years	14	5–10	1.6	0.6–1.2	56	10–35	3.7
	>70 years	14	5–10	1.6	0.6–1.2	56	10–35	3.7
Females	9–13 years	10	5–10	1.0	0.6–1.2	34	10–30	2.1
	14–18 years	11	5–10	1.1	0.6–1.2	46	10–30	2.3
	19–30 years	12	5–10	1.1	0.6–1.2	46	10–35	2.7
	31–50 years	12	5–10	1.1	0.6–1.2	46	10–35	2.7
	51–70 years	11	5–10	1.1	0.6–1.2	46	10–35	2.7
	>70 years	11	5–10	1.1	0.6–1.2	46	10–35	2.7
Pregnancy	≤18 years	13	5–10	1.4	0.6–1.2	71	10–35	3.0
	19–30 years	13	5–10	1.4	0.6–1.2	71	10–35	3.0
	31–50 years	13	5–10	1.4	0.6–1.2	71	10–35	3.0
Lactation	≤18 years	13	5–10	1.3	0.6–1.2	71	10–35	3.8
	19–30 years	13	5–10	1.3	0.6–1.2	71	10–35	3.8
	31–50 years	13	5–10	1.3	0.6–1.2	71	10–35	3.8

[n] Daily protein recommendations are based on body weight for reference body weights. To calculate for a specific body weight, use the following values: 1.5 g/kg for infants, 1.1 g/kg for 1–3 years, 0.95 g/kg for 4–13 years, 0.85 g/kg for 14–18 years, 0.8 g/kg for adults, and 1.1 g/kg for pregnant (using prepregnancy weight) and lactating women.

[o] Acceptable Macronutrient Distribution Range (AMDR), expressed as a percent of total daily calories, is the range of intake for a particular energy source that is associated with reduced risk of chronic disease while providing intakes of essential nutrients. If an individual consumes in excess of the AMDR, there is a potential for increasing the risk of chronic diseases and/or insufficient intakes of essential nutrients.

[p] Total water intake from fluids and food.

[q] Not determinable because of lack of data of adverse effects in this age group and concern with regard to lack of ability to handle excess amounts. Source of intake should be from food only to prevent high levels of intake.

[r] For infants, Adequate Intake of total fat is 31 grams/day (0–6 months) and 30 grams per day (7–12 months) from breast milk and, for infants 7–12 months, complementary food and beverages.

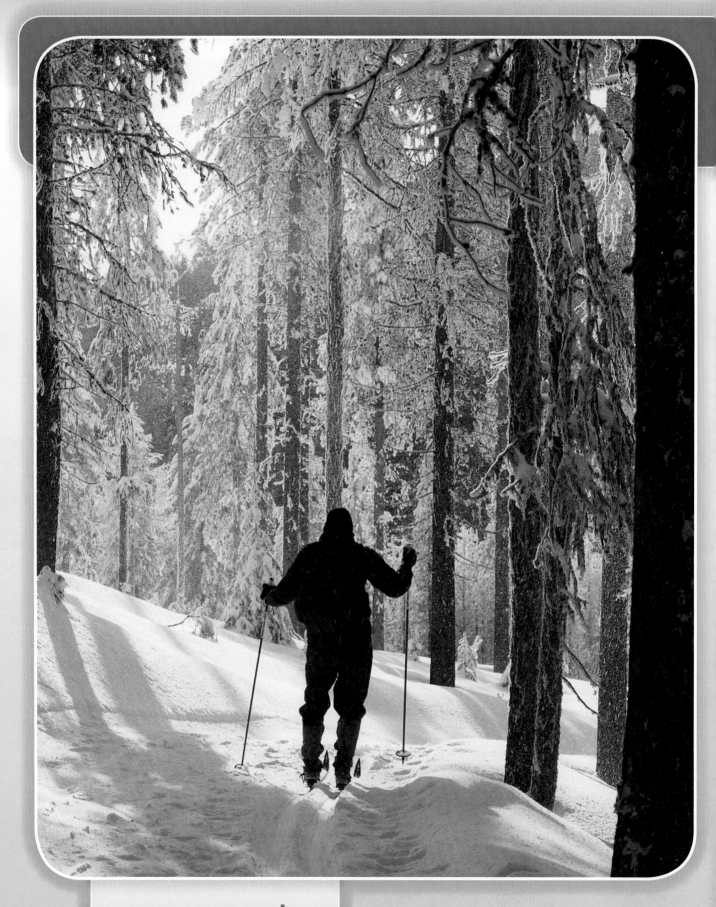

McGraw Hill **connect**™   Practise and learn online with Connect.

EXERCISE FOR HEALTH AND FITNESS

6

LOOKING AHEAD>>>>>

AFTER READING THIS CHAPTER, YOU SHOULD BE ABLE TO

- Define physical fitness, and list the health-related components of fitness
- Explain the wellness benefits of physical activity and exercise
- Describe how to develop each of the health-related components of fitness
- Discuss how to choose appropriate exercise equipment, how to eat and drink for exercise, how to assess fitness, and how to prevent and manage injuries
- Put together a personalized exercise program that you enjoy and that will enable you to achieve your fitness goals

TEST YOUR KNOWLEDGE

1. **To improve your health, you must exercise vigorously for at least 30 minutes straight, five or more days per week.**
   True or false?

2. **Which of the following is considered a form of cardiorespiratory endurance exercise?**
   a. walking
   b. swimming
   c. aerobic dancing

3. **Developing strength in the trunk muscles is the most important way to prevent low-back pain.**
   True or false?

4. **The terms *physical activity* and *exercise* mean the same thing.**
   True or false?

5. **Which principle of fitness states that when you stop exercising, you can lose up to 50% of fitness improvements in two months?**
   a. FITT
   b. reversibility
   c. progressive overload

ANSWERS

1. **FALSE.** Experts recommend about 30 minutes of moderate physical activity five or more days per week, but activity can be done in short bouts—10-minute sessions, for example—spread out over the day.

2. **ALL THREE.** You can develop cardiorespiratory endurance through activities that involve continuous, rhythmic movements of large-muscle groups, such as the legs. Many kinds of activities count as cardiorespiratory endurance exercise.

3. **FALSE.** Although muscular strength is an important factor in low-back health, muscular endurance in the trunk is actually more important to preventing low-back pain.

4. **FALSE.** Physical activity is any body movement carried out by the skeletal muscles that requires energy. Exercise is planned, structured, repetitive movement performed specifically to improve or maintain physical fitness.

5. **B.** The body adapts to any level of physical activity. The harder you exercise, the greater the improvements in fitness you will make. The reverse is also true; as you work less, your fitness drops to lower levels.

Your body is a wonderful moving machine made to work best when it is physically active. It readily adapts to practically any level of activity and exercise: The more you ask of your body—your muscles, bones, heart, lungs—the stronger and fitter it becomes. The opposite is also true. Left unchallenged, bones lose their density, joints stiffen, muscles become weak, and cellular energy systems begin to degenerate. To be truly healthy, human beings must be active.

This chapter gives you the basic information you need to put together a physical fitness program that will work for you. If approached correctly, physical activity and exercise can contribute immeasurably to overall wellness, add fun and joy to life, and provide the foundation for a lifetime of fitness.

WHAT IS PHYSICAL FITNESS?

Physical fitness is the body's ability to respond or adapt to the demands and stress of physical effort—that is, to perform moderate to vigorous levels of physical activity without becoming overly tired.

Some components of fitness are related to specific activities or sports; others relate to general health. **Health-related fitness** includes the following components:

- Cardiorespiratory endurance
- Muscular strength
- Muscular endurance
- Flexibility
- Body composition

Health-related fitness helps you withstand physical challenges and protects you from diseases.

Cardiorespiratory Endurance

Cardiorespiratory endurance is the ability to perform prolonged, large-muscle, dynamic exercise at moderate to high intensity. It depends on such factors as the lungs' ability to deliver oxygen to the bloodstream, the heart's capacity to pump blood, the ability of the nervous system and blood vessels to regulate blood flow, and the body's ability to use oxygen and process fuels for exercise.

When cardiorespiratory fitness is low, the heart has to work hard during normal daily activities and may not be able to work hard enough to sustain high-intensity physical activity in an emergency. Poor cardiorespiratory fitness is linked with heart disease, diabetes, colon cancer, stroke, depression, and anxiety.

QUICK STATS

Less than 50% of Canadian students take physical education classes after grade 9.
—Dwyer et al., 2006

Regular cardiorespiratory **endurance training**, however, conditions the heart. Endurance training makes the heart stronger and improves the function of the entire cardiorespiratory system. As cardiorespiratory fitness improves, related physical functions also improve:

- The heart pumps more blood per heartbeat.
- Resting heart rate slows and resting blood pressure decreases.
- Blood volume increases.
- Blood supply to tissues improves.
- The body can cool itself better.

A healthy heart can better withstand the strains of daily life, the stress of occasional emergencies, and the wear and tear of time.

Endurance training also improves the function of the body's chemical systems, particularly in the muscles and liver, enhancing the body's ability to use energy from food and to do more exercise with less effort.

You can develop cardiorespiratory endurance through activities that involve continuous, rhythmic movements of large-muscle groups, such as the legs. Such activities include walking, jogging, cycling, and aerobic dancing.

Muscular Strength

Muscular strength is the amount of force a muscle can produce with a single maximum effort. It depends on such factors as the size of muscle cells and the ability of nerves to activate muscle cells. Strong muscles are important for everyday activities, such as climbing stairs, as well as for emergencies. They help keep the skeleton in proper alignment, preventing back and leg pain and providing the support necessary for good posture. Muscular strength has obvious importance in recreational activities. Strong people can hit a tennis ball harder, kick a soccer ball farther, and ride a bicycle uphill more easily.

Muscle tissue is an important element of overall body composition. Greater muscle mass makes possible a higher rate of metabolism and faster energy use, which help to maintain a healthy body weight.

Maintaining strength and muscle mass is vital for healthy aging. Older people tend to lose muscle cells (a condition called *sarcopenia*), and many of the remaining muscle cells become nonfunctional because they lose their attachment to the nervous system. Strength training helps maintain muscle mass, function, and balance in older people, which greatly enhances their quality of life and prevents life-threatening injuries. Strength training has also been shown to benefit cardiovascular health and reduce the risk of osteoporosis (bone loss).

Muscular strength can be developed by training with weights or by using the weight of the body for resistance during calisthenic exercises, such as push-ups and curl-ups.

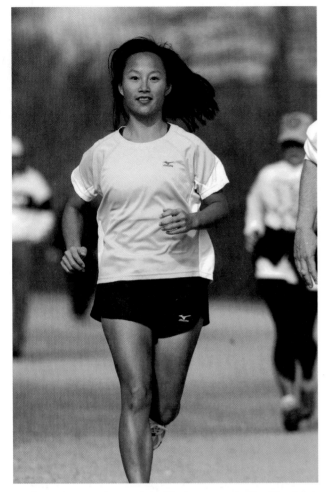
Cardiorespiratory endurance is a critical component of health-related fitness.

Muscular Endurance

Muscular endurance is the ability to resist fatigue and sustain a given level of muscle tension—that is, to hold a muscle contraction for a long time or to contract a muscle over and over again. It depends on such factors as the size of muscle cells, the ability of muscles to store fuel, and the blood supply to muscles.

Muscular endurance is important for good posture and for injury prevention. For example, if abdominal and back muscles cannot hold the spine correctly, the chances of low-back pain and back injury are increased. In fact, good muscular endurance in the trunk muscles is more important than muscular strength for preventing back pain. Muscular endurance helps people cope with the physical demands of everyday life and enhances performance in sports and work.

Like muscular strength, muscular endurance is developed by stressing the muscles with a greater load (weight) than they are used to. The degree to which strength or endurance develops depends on the type and amount of stress that is applied.

Flexibility

Flexibility is the ability to move joints through their full range of motion. It depends on joint structure, the length and elasticity of connective tissue, and nervous system activity. Flexible, pain-free joints are important for good health and well-being. Inactivity causes the joints to become stiffer with age. Stiffness, in turn, can cause people (of any age) to assume unnatural body postures that can stress joints and muscles. Stretching exercises can help ensure a healthy range of motion for all major joints.

Body Composition

Body composition refers to the proportion of fat and **fat-free mass** (muscle, bone, and water) in the body. Healthy body composition involves a high proportion of fat-free mass and an acceptably low level of body fat, for a given age and sex. A person with excessive body fat—especially in the abdomen—is more likely to experience health problems, including heart disease, high blood pressure, stroke, joint problems, diabetes, gallbladder disease, cancer, and back pain.

The best way to lose fat is through a lifestyle that includes a sensible diet and exercise. The best way to add muscle mass is through resistance training, such as weight training. (Body composition is discussed in detail in Chapter 4.)

TERMS

physical fitness   The body's ability to respond or adapt to the demands and stress of physical effort.

health-related fitness   Physical capabilities that contribute to health, including cardiorespiratory endurance, muscular strength, muscular endurance, flexibility, and body composition.

cardiorespiratory endurance   The ability of the body to perform prolonged, large-muscle, dynamic exercise at moderate to high levels of intensity.

endurance training   Exercise intended specifically to improve cardiorespiratory endurance; usually involves prolonged, large-muscle, dynamic exercises.

muscular strength   The amount of force a muscle can produce with a single maximum effort.

muscular endurance   The ability of a muscle or group of muscles to remain contracted or to contract repeatedly for a long time.

flexibility   The ability to move joints through their full range of motion.

body composition   The proportion of fat and fat-free mass (muscle, bone, and water) in the body.

fat-free mass   The nonfat component of the human body, consisting of skeletal muscle, bone, and water.

Skill-Related Components of Fitness

In addition to the five health-related components of physical fitness, the ability to perform a particular sport or activity may depend on **skill-related fitness** components, such as the following:

- *Speed:* the ability to perform a movement in a short time

- *Power:* the ability to exert force rapidly, based on a combination of strength and speed

- *Agility:* the ability to change the body's position quickly and accurately

- *Balance:* the ability to maintain equilibrium while either moving or stationary

- *Coordination:* the ability to perform motor tasks accurately and smoothly by using body movements and the senses

- *Reaction time:* the ability to respond quickly to a stimulus

Skill-related fitness tends to be sport-specific and is best developed through practice. For example, the speed, coordination, and agility needed to play basketball are best developed by playing basketball. Some fitness experts contend that certain sports don't contribute to all the health-related components of physical fitness. Nevertheless, playing a sport can be fun, can help you build fitness, and may contribute to other areas of wellness.

QUICK STATS

Physical inactivity contributes to **more than 21,000** premature deaths in Canada each year and about **$1.6 billion** in direct costs.

—Public Health Agency of Canada, 2007

PHYSICAL ACTIVITY AND EXERCISE FOR HEALTH AND FITNESS

Despite the many benefits of an active lifestyle, levels of physical activity remain low for all populations of Canadians. The physical activities Canadian adults enjoy differ by sex (see Table 6.1). But at all ages, Canadian males are more active than females, with less than half of the population being active enough to trigger health gains. According to the *2010 Canadian Health Measures Survey*, the fitness levels of all Canadians have declined significantly over the last three decades.

Although studies have shown that physical activity helps to boost concentration, memory, and learning in school, a startling 88% of children and youth do not get

QUESTIONS FOR CRITICAL THINKING AND REFLECTION
When you think about exercise, do you think of only one or two of the five components of health-related fitness, such as muscular strength or body composition? If so, where do you think your ideas come from? What role do the media play in shaping your ideas about fitness?

the recommended amount of physical activity every day. As depicted in Figure 6.1, no province's or territory's children are meeting the guidelines. Furthermore, about 80% of Canadian youth between the ages of 12 and 19 are not meeting international physical activity guidelines for optimal growth and development.

Differences also exist among different ethnic groups when it comes to meeting guidelines for moderate physical

VITAL STATISTICS

Table 6.1 — Popularity of Physical Recreation Activities of Adults, Age 20+

Rank 2005	Activity	Percentage of the Population*		
		Total	Men	Women
1	Walking	71%	65%	76%†
2	Gardening, yardwork	49	54†	44
3	Home exercise	33	29	37†
4	Swimming	22	21	22
5	Bicycling	20	24†	16
6	Social dancing	18	15	20†
7	Weight training	17	20	14
8	Jogging, running	16	18†	13
9	Golfing	11	17†	6
10	Exercise classes, aerobics	10	5	16†
11	Fishing	9	14†	5
12	Bowling	8	9	8
13	Skating	6	7†	5
14	Soccer	5	8†	3
15	Basketball	5	8†	2
16	Hockey	5	9†	1
17	In-line skating	4	5	4
18	Baseball, softball	4	7†	2
19	Skiing, snowboarding	4	5†	3
20	Volleyball	4	4	3
21	Tennis	4	5†	3

* Percentage who participated at least once in the last three months.

† *Significantly* greater than other sex.

Source: Popularity of physical recreation activities of adults, age 20+ (Statistics Canada, Canadian *Community Health Survey*, 2000/01). Obtained online at http://www.cflri.ca/eng/levels/popular_pa_adults.php. © Her Majesty the Queen in Right of Canada.

Percentage of children and youth meeting physical activity guidelines

Canada-wide 12%

16
12
8
4
0 NA

Nunavut* | Yukon 14% | Northwest Territories 15% | British Columbia 15% | Alberta 11% | Saskatchewan 13% | Manitoba 13% | Ontario 14% | Quebec 10% | New Brunswick 7% | Nova Scotia 10% | Prince Edward Island 9% | Newfoundland & Labrador 10%

* The percentage of children and youth in Nunavut meeting the guidelines is not able to be determined because of small sample size. Data show that the average number of of steps taken by children and youth in Nunavut is 13,012 as compared with the national average of 11,698 steps.

FIGURE 6.1   Children and youth meeting the physical activity guidelines, by province and territory.

Source: Active Healthy Kids Canada. 2010. Healthy Habits Start Earlier Than You Think. *The Active Healthy Kids Canada Report Card on Physical Activity for Children and Youth.*

activity: White and Aboriginal people are most likely to be moderately active, while black, West Asian and South Asian, and Arab people are least likely to be sufficiently active. Evidence is growing that for many Canadians, becoming more physically active may be the single most important lifestyle change they can make to improve their health and well-being (see the box "Exercise and Total Wellness," on p. 182).

Physical Activity on a Continuum

Physical activity is any body movement carried out by the skeletal muscles and requiring energy. Different types of physical activity can be arranged on a continuum based on the amount of energy they require. Quick, easy movements, such as standing up or walking down a hallway, require little energy or effort; more intense, sustained activities, such as cycling 10 kilometres or running in a race, require considerably more.

Exercise refers to a subset of physical activity—planned, structured, repetitive movement of the body intended specifically to improve or maintain physical fitness. Levels of fitness depend on such physiological factors as the heart's ability to pump blood and the size of muscle fibres. These factors are a function both of genetics—a person's inborn potential for physical fitness—and of behaviour—the amount of exercise a person does to improve fitness. To develop fitness, a person must perform enough physical activity to stress the body and cause long-term physiological changes.

Physical activity is essential to health and confers wide-ranging health benefits, but exercise is necessary to significantly improve physical fitness. This important distinction between physical activity and exercise is a key concept in understanding the guidelines discussed in this chapter.

Increasing Physical Activity to Improve Health and Wellness   In 1998, Health Canada and the Canadian Society for Exercise Physiology (CSEP) worked in partnership to launch *Canada's Physical Activity Guide to Healthy Active Living*. At that time, research indicated that Canadians were unaware that physical inactivity is a serious risk factor for premature death, chronic disease, and disability, with a magnitude of risk comparable with that of smoking. Further, two-thirds of Canadians were inactive, a serious threat to their health and a burden on the public health care system. Canadians were confused by all the data and information available about physical activity and fitness and wanted a valid and practical guide, similar to what is now called *Eating Well with Canada's Food Guide* (discussed in Chapter 5), that would help them judge how much physical activity they needed to achieve better health.

> **Only 12%** of children in Canada get enough physical activity in a day to meet Canadian guidelines.
>
> —Active Healthy Kids Canada, 2010
>
> QUICK STATS

skill-related fitness   Physical abilities that contribute to performance in a sport or activity, including speed, power, agility, balance, coordination, and reaction time.

physical activity   Any body movement carried out by the skeletal muscles and requiring energy.

exercise   Planned, structured, repetitive movement of the body intended to improve or maintain physical fitness.

TERMS

Exercise and Total Wellness

As you will see throughout this chapter, an active lifestyle provides a multitude of benefits. For example, physically active adults live from two to four years longer, on average, than do sedentary adults. The benefits of regular physical activity, however, go beyond longevity. They affect quality of life across multiple dimensions of wellness.

Physical Wellness

In terms of general health, exercise increases your physical capacity so that you are better able to meet the challenges of daily life with energy and vigour. Physical activity can help you do the following:

- Generate more energy
- Increase your stamina
- Control your weight
- Manage stress
- Boost your immune system

Over the long term, even moderate physical activity can help you avoid illnesses, such as heart disease, diabetes, high blood pressure, depression, osteoporosis, and some cancers. Evidence shows that exercise can even prevent premature death from several causes.

Emotional Wellness

Exercise provides psychological and emotional benefits, contributing to your sense of competence and well-being. People

who focus on staying active can also enjoy an improved self-image and a higher level of self-confidence. Such healthy self-esteem can positively affect other aspects of your life. For example, a good self-image can be helpful when dealing with others or when competing.

Intellectual Wellness

Recent studies indicate that regular exercise is good for the brain—literally. One study shows that brain volume actually increases in adults who exercise regularly. Other studies show that exercise helps to reduce mental declines seen with aging. Such valuable impacts in brain mass (growth or replenishment of brain matter) can improve cognitive functions and the overall health of the nervous system. Additionally, the process of mastering physical challenges—such as learning a proper golf swing—can boost intellectual fitness in the same manner as solving puzzles or engaging in other learning experiences.

Interpersonal Wellness

Joining in physical activity with a friend or a group can be a boon to your interpersonal or social wellness, too. By sharing physical challenges with others, you can make new friends, deepen your existing relationships, and build a stronger overall network of support.

In 2011, CSEP released new guidelines with the support of the Public Health Agency of Canada. The new guidelines for Canadian adults (18–64 years old) recommend strength-training activities at least two days per week, and recommend moderate-intensity to vigorous-intensity aerobic physical activity most days per week. Each session of aerobic activity must be at least 10 minutes, and adults should accumulate a total of at least 150 minutes per week. More physical activity provides greater health benefits. Canadians are also encouraged to minimize their sedentary behaviours (such as sitting for long periods) as much as possible. Ideally, Canadians should be active most, if not all, days of the week.

Moderate-intensity activities include brisk walking and bike riding, while vigorous-intensity activities include jogging and cross-country skiing. Moderate activity for 30 minutes uses about 150 calories. Examples of activities

> ### 63% of Canadians are not active enough for health benefits.
>
> —Public Health Agency of Canada, 2009

QUICK STATS

that use about 150 calories are shown in Figure 6.2. You can burn the same number of calories by doing a lower-intensity activity for a longer time or higher-intensity activity for a shorter time. For more examples of light, moderate, and vigorous activities, see the box "Classifying Activity Levels" (p. 184). Research shows that being active for at least 150 minutes every week promotes health and wellness by lowering the risk of high blood pressure, stroke, heart disease, type 2 diabetes, colon cancer, and osteoporosis and by reducing feelings of mild-to-moderate depression and anxiety.

It's easy to fit in the required amount of physical activity because the activities can be done all at once or in 10-minute intervals throughout the week; for example, 10-minute bike rides to and from class and a brisk 10-minute walk to the store each day add up to 150 minutes in a week. In this lifestyle approach to physical activity, people can choose activities that they find enjoyable and that fit into their daily routine; everyday tasks at school, work, and home can be structured to contribute to the daily activity total (see "Making Time for Physical Activity" in the ■connect Library). Public health and individual well-being would receive an enormous benefit if all sedentary Canadians were to increase their lifestyle physical activity to 30 minutes per day.

In addition to the activity guide for adults 18 to 64, CSEP has produced guides for adults 65 and older, for children 5–11 years old, and for youth between the ages of 12 and 17 (Figure 6.3). You can order or download free copies of the guides from the CSEP Web site listed in For More Information at the end of the chapter

Increasing Physical Activity to Manage Weight

Because two-thirds of Canadians are overweight, physical activity guidelines focusing on weight management have also been created by various agencies and health organizations. These guidelines call for more daily physical activity than the guidelines designed for general health promotion. These guidelines do not conflict with those from CSEP, but they do have a different emphasis. They recognize that for people who need to prevent weight gain, lose weight, or maintain weight loss, 150 minutes of physical activity each week may not be enough. Instead, they recommend 45–90 or more minutes of physical activity each day. The different recommendations may seem confusing, but all major international health organizations have the same message: People can improve their health by becoming more active.

Exercising to Improve Physical Fitness
As mentioned earlier, moderate physical activity confers significant health and wellness benefits, especially for those who are currently sedentary and become moderately active.

The leading international physical activity authorities all conclude that people can obtain even greater health and wellness benefits by increasing the duration and intensity of physical activity. With increased activity, they will see more improvements in quality of life and greater reductions in disease and mortality risk.

Activity	Duration (min)	
Washing a car	45–60	**Less Vigorous, More Time**
Washing windows or floors	45–60	
Volleyball	45	
Touch football	30–45	
Gardening	30–45	
Wheeling self in wheelchair	30–40	
Walking 1.75 miles (2.75 km)	35 (20 min/mile)	
Shooting a basketball	30	
Bicycling 5 miles	30 (6 min/mile)	
Dancing fast	30	
Pushing a stroller 1.5 miles (2.5 km)	30	
Raking leaves	30	
Walking 2 miles (3.25 km)	30 (15 min/mile)	
Water aerobics	30	
Swimming laps	20	
Wheelchair basketball	20	
Playing a game of basketball	15–20	
Bicycling 4 miles (6.5 km)	15 (3¾ min/mile)	
Jumping rope	15	
Running 1.5 miles (2.5 km)	15 (10 min/mile)	
Shoveling snow	15	**More Vigorous, Less Time**
Stairwalking	15	

FIGURE 6.2 Examples of moderate amounts of physical activity. Each example uses about 150 calories.

Source: Department of Health and Human Services. 1996. *Physical Activity and Health: A Report of the Surgeon General.* Atlanta: DHHS.

For children 5–11 years

For health benefits, children aged 5–11 years should accumulate at least 60 minutes of moderate- to vigorous-intensity physical activity daily.
This should include:

Vigorous-intensity activities at least 3 days per week.

Activities that strengthen muscle and bone at least 3 days per week.

More daily physical activity provides greater health benefits.

For youth 12–17 years

For health benefits, youth aged 12–17 years should accumulate at least 60 minutes of moderate- to vigorous-intensity physical activity daily.
This should include:

Vigorous-intensity activities at least 3 days per week.

Activities that strengthen muscle and bone at least 3 days per week.

More daily physical activity provides greater health benefits.

For adults 18–64 years

To achieve health benefits, adults aged 18–64 years should accumulate at least 150 minutes of moderate- to vigorous-intensity aerobic physical activity per week, in bouts of 10 minutes or more.

It is also beneficial to add muscle and bone strengthening activities using major muscle groups, at least 2 days per week.

More physical activity provides greater health benefits.

For older adults 65 years and older

To achieve health benefits, and improve functional abilities, adults aged 65 and older should accumulate at least 150 minutes of moderate- to vigorous-intensity aerobic physical activity per week, in bouts of 10 minutes or more.

It is also beneficial to add muscle and bone strengthening activities using major muscle groups, at least 2 days per week.

Those with poor mobility should perform physical activities to enhance balance and prevent falls.

More physical activity provides greater health benefits.

FIGURE 6.3 Canadian Physical Activity Guidelines.

Source: Copyright © 2011 Canadian Society for Exercise Physiology. All rights reserved. Reprinted with permission from the Canadian Society for Exercise Physiology. (http://www.csep.ca/guidelines, retrieved May 19, 2011).

Classifying Activity Levels

Assessing your physical activity level is easier if you know how to classify different kinds of activities. Fitness experts categorize activities into the following three levels:

• *Light activity* includes the routine tasks associated with typical day-to-day life, such as vacuuming or walking to class. You probably perform dozens of light activities every day without even thinking about it. You can gain significant health benefits by turning light activities into moderate activities—by walking briskly instead of slowly, for example.

• *Moderate activity* causes your breathing and heart rate to accelerate but still allows for comfortable conversation. An example is walking at four to five kilometres per hour. It is sometimes described as activity that can be performed comfortably for about 45 minutes. Raking leaves is an example of moderate physical activity, as are most occupational tasks that involve extended periods of moderate effort.

• *Vigorous activity* elevates your heart rate considerably and has other physical effects that improve your fitness level. During vigorous activity you are breathing too heavily to hold a conversation very easily. An example is walking faster than six kilometres per hour.

Here are some examples:

Light	Moderate	Vigorous
Walking slowly	Walking briskly	Walking briskly uphill
Routine tasks:	Cycling moderately on level terrain	Cycling on steep uphill terrain
• Cooking	Social dancing	Heavy housework:
• Shopping	Moderate housework:	• Moving furniture
Light housework:	• Scrubbing floors	• Carrying heavy objects upstairs
• Ironing	• Washing windows	Vigorous yardwork or home activities:
• Dusting	Moderate yardwork or home activities:	• Shovelling snow
• Washing dishes	• Planting	• Trimming trees
Light yardwork or home activities:	• Raking	• Doing construction work
• Pruning	• Painting	• Digging
• Weeding	• Washing car	Fitness activities requiring vigorous effort:
• Plumbing	Fitness activities requiring moderate effort:	• Running
Light fitness activities:	• Low-impact aerobics	• High-impact aerobics
• Light stretching or warm-up	• Frisbee	• Circuit weight training
• Swimming, slow treading	• Swimming	• Swimming laps
	• Tennis, doubles	• Most competitive sports

More vigorous activity, as occurs in a structured, systematic exercise program, is also needed to improve physical fitness; moderate physical activity alone is not enough. Physical fitness requires more intense movement that poses a substantially greater challenge to the body. The American College of Sports Medicine (ACSM), a world leader in exercise science, issued separate guidelines in 2006 for creating a formal exercise program that will develop physical fitness. These guidelines are described in detail later in the chapter.

How Much Physical Activity Is Enough?

Some experts feel that people get most of the health benefits of an exercise program simply by becoming more active during the day; the amount of activity needed depends on an individual's health status and goals. Other experts feel that the activity goal set by the lifestyle approach is too low; they argue that people should exercise long enough and intensely enough to improve their body's capacity for exercise—that is, to improve physical fitness. More research is needed to clarify the health effects of different amounts of lifestyle physical activity, of moderate-intensity versus high-intensity exercise, and of continuous versus intermittent exercise. However, there is probably some truth in both of these positions.

Where does this leave you? Most experts agree that some physical activity is better than none, but that more—as long as it does not result in injury—is better than some. To set a personal goal for physical activity and exercise, consider your current activity level, your health status, and your overall goals. At the very least, strive to become more active and meet the goal set by CSEP of 150 minutes of moderate to vigorous activity each week. Choose to be active whenever you can. If weight management is a concern for you, you may need to start slowly, depending on how long you have been inactive, and raise your activity level gradually to 45–90 minutes per day or more. For even better health and well-being, participate in a structured exercise program that develops physical fitness. This is important for all Canadians—the profile of the typical Canadian has changed (and not necessarily for

	BOY	
1981	**Body Composition**	**2007–2009**
150.9 cm (4'11")	Height	155.8 cm (5'1")*
41.6 kg (92 lb)	Weight	48.0 kg (106 lb)*
18.1 kg/m²	Body mass index	19.2 kg/m²*
64.9 cm (25.6")	Waist circumference	66.2 cm (26.1")
78.0 cm (30.7")	Hip circumference	84.0 cm (33.1")
0.83	Waist-to-hip ratio	0.82*
	Fitness Tests	
49 kg	Grip strength	44 kg*
26.5	Sit-and-reach	21.4 cm*

	GIRL	
1981	**Body Composition**	**2007–2009**
153 cm (5'0")	Height	155.9 cm (5'1")*
42.7 kg (94 lb)	Weight	47.6 kg (105 lb)*
18.4 kg/m²	Body mass index	19.5 kg/m²*
62.4 cm (24.6")	Waist circumference	68.0 cm (26.8")*
81.2 cm (32.0")	Hip circumference	86.0 cm (33.9")*
0.76	Waist-to-hip ratio	0.79*
	Fitness Tests	
43 kg	Grip strength	40 kg*
32.0	Sit-and-reach	28.2 cm*

FIGURE 6.4
Portrait of a typical 12-year-old boy and girl, 1981 and 2007–2009.

Source: M. S. Tremblay, M. Shields, M. Laviolette, et al. 2010. Fitness of Canadian children and youth: Results from the 2007–2009 Canadian Health Measures Survey, *Health Reports* 21(1). Statistics Canada, Catalogue 82-003.

* Significantly different from the estimate for 1981 ($p < .05$)
Note: Estimates are based on median values for boys and girls ages 11 to 13 years. To make estimates more comparable, *Canadian Health Measures Survey* estimates for flexibility and muscular strength exclude respondents screened out of the aerobic fitness test.

QUESTIONS FOR CRITICAL THINKING AND REFLECTION

Does your current lifestyle include enough physical activity—150 minutes of moderate to vigorous activity each week—to support health and wellness? Does your lifestyle go beyond this level to include enough vigorous physical activity and exercise to build physical fitness? What changes could you make in your lifestyle to start developing physical fitness?

the better) over the last 30 years. Figure 6.4, above, illustrates the differences between a typical Canadian 12-year-old boy and girl from 1981 to 2007–2009. The bottom line is that any increase in physical activity will contribute to your health and well-being, now and in the future.

THE BENEFITS OF EXERCISE

As mentioned earlier, the human body is very adaptable. The greater the demands made on it, the more it adjusts to meet the demands—it becomes fit. Over time, immediate, short-term adjustments translate into long-term changes and improvements (Figure 6.5 on p. 186). The goal of regular physical activity is to bring about these kinds of long-term changes and improvements in the body's functioning.

Improved Cardiorespiratory Functioning

Every time you take a breath, oxygen in the air enters your lungs and is picked up by red blood cells and transported to your heart. From there, the heart pumps oxygenated blood throughout the body to organs and tissues that use it. During exercise, the cardiorespiratory system (heart, lungs, and circulatory system) must work harder to meet the body's increased demand for oxygen. Regular endurance exercise improves the functioning of the heart and the ability of the cardiorespiratory system to carry oxygen to body tissues. Exercise directly affects the health of your arteries, keeping them from stiffening or clogging with plaque and reducing the risk of cardiovascular disease. Exercise also improves sexual function and general vitality.

More Efficient Metabolism

Endurance exercise improves metabolism, the process that converts food to energy and builds tissue. This process involves oxygen, nutrients, hormones, and enzymes. A physically fit person can more efficiently generate energy, use carbohydrates and fats for energy, and regulate hormones. Exercise may also protect cells from damage by free radicals, which are destructive chemicals produced during normal metabolism (see Chapter 5), and from inflammation caused by high blood pressure or cholesterol, nicotine, and overeating. Training activates antioxidant enzymes that prevent free radical damage and maintain the health of the body's cells.

Immediate effects

Increased levels of neurotransmitters; constant or slightly increased blood flow to the brain.

Increased heart rate and stroke volume (amount of blood pumped per beat).

Increased pulmonary ventilation (amount of air breathed into the body per minute). More air is taken into the lungs with each breath and breathing rate increases.

Reduced blood flow to the stomach, intestines, liver, and kidneys, resulting in less activity in the digestive tract and less urine output.

Increased energy production in muscles.

Increased blood flow to the skin and increased sweating to help maintain a safe body temperature.

Increased systolic blood pressure; increased blood flow and oxygen transport to working skeletal muscles and the heart; increased oxygen consumption.

Long-term effects

Improved self-image, cognitive functioning, and ability to manage stress; enhanced learning, memory, energy level, and sleep; decreased depression, anxiety, and risk for stroke.

Increased heart size and resting stroke volume; lower resting heart rate. Risk of heart disease and heart attack significantly reduced.

Improved ability to extract oxygen from air during exercise. Reduced risk of colds and upper respiratory tract infections.

Increased sweat rate, earlier onset of sweating, and greater dissipation of sweat, helping to cool the body.

Decreased body fat.

Reduced risk of colon cancer and certain other forms of cancer.

Muscle cell changes that allow for greater energy production and power output during exercise. Insulin sensitivity remains constant or improves, helping to prevent type 2 diabetes. Increase or maintenance of muscle mass.

Increased density and breaking strength of bones, ligaments, and tendons; reduced risk for low-back pain, injuries, and osteoporosis; improved range of motion in joints.

Increased blood volume and capillary density; higher levels of high-density lipoproteins (HDL) and lower levels of triglycerides; lower resting blood pressure; reduced platelet stickiness (a factor in coronary heart disease); improved blood flow control; and reduced blood vessel inflammation.

FIGURE 6.5   Immediate and long-term effects of regular exercise.

Improved Body Composition

Healthy body composition means that the body has a high proportion of fat-free mass and a relatively small proportion of fat. Too much body fat, particularly abdominal fat, is linked to a variety of health problems, including heart disease, cancer, and diabetes. Healthy body composition can be difficult to achieve and maintain because a diet that contains all essential nutrients can be relatively high in calories, especially for someone who is sedentary. Excess calories are stored in the body as fat.

Exercise can improve body composition in several ways. Endurance exercise significantly increases daily calorie expenditure; it can also slightly raise *metabolic rate*, the rate at which the body burns calories, for several hours after an exercise session. Strength training increases muscle mass, thereby tipping the body composition ratio toward fat-free mass and away from fat. It can also help with losing fat because metabolic rate is directly proportional to fat-free mass: The more muscle mass, the higher the metabolic rate.

Physical activity reduces the risk of premature death regardless of its effect on body composition. That is, greater levels of activity are associated with lower death rates among people who are overweight or obese as well as people who are at a healthy weight (Figure 6.6). Physical activity does not eliminate the health risks associated with overweight, but it reduces its negative effects.

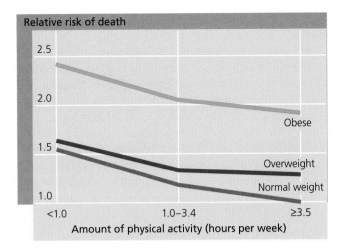

FIGURE 6.6 Relationship among amount of physical activity, body weight, and risk of premature death.

Source: Hu, F. B., et al. 2004. Adiposity compared with physical activity in predicting mortality among women. *New England Journal of Medicine* 351(26): 2694–2703.

Disease Prevention and Management

Regular physical activity lowers your risk of many chronic, disabling diseases.

Cardiovascular Disease A sedentary lifestyle is one of the six major risk factors for cardiovascular disease (CVD), including heart attack and stroke. The other major risk factors are smoking, abnormal blood fats, high blood pressure, diabetes, and obesity. Most of these risk factors are linked by a group of symptoms that scientists call *metabolic syndrome*. These symptoms include insulin resistance, high blood pressure, abnormal blood fats, abdominal fat deposits, type 2 diabetes, blood clotting abnormalities, and blood vessel inflammation (see Chapter 7 for more on metabolic syndrome). Sedentary people have death rates from CVD significantly higher than those of fit individuals. Physical inactivity increases the risk of CVD by 50%–240%.

The benefit of physical activity occurs at moderate levels of activity and rises with increasing levels of activity. Exercise positively affects the risk factors for CVD, including cholesterol levels and high blood pressure. Exercise also directly interferes with the disease process itself, directly lowering risk of heart disease and stroke.

BLOOD FAT LEVELS Endurance exercise and strength training have a positive effect on the balance of lipids (fats) that circulate in the blood. High concentrations of lipids, such as cholesterol and triglycerides, are linked to heart disease because they contribute to the formation of fatty deposits on the linings of arteries. When blood clots block a narrowed artery, a heart attack or stroke can occur.

Cholesterol is carried in the blood by lipoproteins, which are classified according to size and density. Choles-terol carried by low-density lipoproteins (LDLs) sticks to the walls of coronary arteries. High-density lipoproteins (HDLs) pick up excess cholesterol in the bloodstream and carry it back to the liver for excretion from the body. High LDL levels and low HDL levels increase the risk of cardio-vascular disease. High levels of HDL and low levels of LDL are associated with lower risk.

Heart disease is covered in Chapter 7. For our purposes in this chapter, it is important to know only that endur-ance exercise and strength training influence blood lipids in a positive way, by increasing HDL and decreasing LDL and triglycerides—reducing the risk of CVD.

HIGH BLOOD PRESSURE Regular endurance exercise tends to reduce high blood pressure (hypertension), a contributing factor in many diseases, such as coronary heart disease, stroke, heart failure, kidney failure, and blindness. Intense, long-duration exercise works best, but even moderate exercise can produce significant improvements. Strength training also reduces blood pressure.

CORONARY HEART DISEASE Coronary heart disease (CHD), also called coronary artery disease (CAD), involves blockage of one of the coronary arteries. These blood vessels sup-ply the heart with oxygenated blood, and an obstruction in one of them can cause a heart attack. Exercise directly interferes with the disease process that causes coronary artery blockage. It also enhances the function of cells lining the arteries that help regulate blood flow.

STROKE A stroke occurs when a blood vessel leading to the brain is blocked or ruptures, often through the same disease process that leads to heart attacks. Regular exercise reduces the risk of stroke.

Cancer Studies have shown a relationship between increased physical activity and a reduced risk of cancer, but these findings are not conclusive. Evidence suggests that exercise reduces the risk of colon cancer and some studies are showing promising data that it reduces the risk of cancer of the breast and reproductive organs in women and prostate cancer in men. Exercise may decrease the risk of colon can-cer by speeding the movement of food through the gastro-intestinal tract (quickly eliminating potential carcinogens), lowering blood insulin levels, enhancing immune function, and reducing blood fats. The protective mechanism in the case of reproductive system cancers is less clear, but physical activity during the high school and the postsecondary years may be particularly important for preventing breast cancer later in life. Some studies have also found that regular phys-ical activity reduces the risk of pancreatic cancer.

Osteoporosis A special benefit of exercise, especially for women, is protection against osteoporosis, a disease that results in loss of bone density and poor bone strength. Weight-bearing exercise, which includes almost everything except swimming, helps build bone during childhood, the teens, and the twenties. Older people with denser bones can better endure the bone loss that occurs with aging. Strength training and impact exercises, such as jumping rope, can increase bone density throughout life. With stronger bones and muscles and better balance, fit people are less likely to experience debilitating falls and bone fractures. Along with exercise, a well-balanced diet containing adequate calcium and vitamin D and normal hormone function are also essential for strong bones. One caution: Too much exercise can depress levels of estrogen, which helps maintain bone density, thereby leading to bone loss, even in young women.

Type 2 Diabetes People with diabetes are prone to heart disease, blindness, and severe problems of the nervous and circulatory systems. Exercise prevents the development of type 2 diabetes, the most common form of the disease. Exercise burns excess sugar and makes cells more sensitive to insulin. Exercise also helps keep body fat at healthy levels. (Obesity is a key risk factor for type 2 diabetes.) For people who have diabetes, physical activity is an important part of treatment. See Chapter 4 for more on diabetes.

Improved Psychological and Emotional Wellness

People who are physically active experience many social, psychological, and emotional benefits, including the following:

• *Reduced stress.* In response to stressors, physically fit people experience milder physical responses and less emotional distress than sedentary individuals. Physical activity also provides protection against the effects of stress that have been linked to poor cardiorespiratory health. Endurance exercise decreases the secretion of hormones and neurotransmitters triggered by emotional stress. It also can diffuse hostility and alleviate feelings of stress and anxiety by providing an emotional outlet and inducing feelings of relaxation. Regular exercise can also relieve sleeping problems.

• *Reduced anxiety and depression.* Sedentary adults are much more likely to feel fatigue and depression than those who are physically active. Exercise is an effective treatment for people with depression and improves mood in people who aren't experiencing depression.

• *Improved self-image.* Performing physical activities provides proof of skill and self-control, thus enhancing your self-concept. Sticking with an exercise program increases people's belief in their ability to be active, thereby boosting self-efficacy. Exercise also helps you look and feel better, boosting self-confidence and body image.

• *Learning and memory.* Exercise enhances the formation and survival of new nerve cells and the connections between nerves, which in turn improve memory and learning. Physical activity helps maintain mental functioning in older adults and may ward off dementia.

• *Enjoyment.* Exercise is fun. It offers a way to interact with other people, as well as opportunities to strive and excel. Physically fit people can perform everyday tasks with ease. They have plenty of energy and can lead lives that are full and varied.

Improved Immune Function

Exercise can have either positive or negative effects on the immune system, the physiological processes that protect us from disease. It appears that moderate endurance exercise boosts immune function, whereas excessive training depresses it. Physically fit people get fewer colds and upper respiratory tract infections than people who are not fit. The immune system—and ways to strengthen it—is discussed further in Chapter 9.

Prevention of Injuries and Low-Back Pain

Increased muscle strength provides protection against injury because it helps people maintain good posture and appropriate body mechanics when carrying out everyday activities, such as walking, lifting, and carrying. Good muscle endurance in the abdomen, hips, lower back, and legs supports the back in proper alignment and helps prevent low-back pain, which affects a significant majority of Canadians at some time in their lives.

Improved Wellness for Life

Although people differ in the maximum levels of fitness they can achieve through exercise, the wellness benefits of exercise are available to everyone (see the box "Exercise for People with Special Health Concerns"). Exercising regularly may be the single most important thing you can do now to improve the quality of your life in the future. All the benefits of exercise continue to accrue but gain new importance as the resilience of youth begins to wane. Simply stated, exercising can help you live a longer and healthier life.

QUESTIONS FOR CRITICAL THINKING AND REFLECTION
Which benefits of exercise are most important to you, and why? For example, is there a history of heart disease or diabetes in your family? Have you thought about how regular exercise could reduce your risks for specific diseases?

Exercise for People with Special Health Concerns

Regular, appropriate exercise is safe and beneficial for many people with chronic conditions or other special health concerns. For many people with special health concerns, in fact, the risks associated with not exercising are far greater than those associated with a moderate program of regular exercise.

If you have a special health concern and have hesitated becoming more active, one helpful strategy is to take a class or join an exercise group specifically designed for your condition. Many health centres and support groups sponsor specially tailored activity programs. Such a class or group activity can provide you with both expert advice and exercise partners who share your concerns and goals. If you prefer to exercise at home, exercise videos are available for people with a variety of conditions.

The fitness recommendations for the general population presented in this chapter can serve as general guidelines for any exercise program. However, for people with special health concerns, certain precautions and monitoring may be required. *Anyone with special health concerns should consult a physician before beginning an exercise program.* Guidelines and cautions for some common conditions are described below.

Most of the following conditions are influenced by many of the determinants of health noted in Chapter 1; as you read this section, see if you can identify which determinants affect each condition.

Asthma

• Carry medication during workouts and avoid exercising alone. Use your inhaler before exercise, if recommended by your physician.

• Exercise regularly, and warm up and cool down slowly to reduce the risk of acute attacks.

• When starting a fitness program, choose self-paced endurance activities, especially those involving interval training (short bouts of exercise followed by rest periods).

• When possible, avoid circumstances that may trigger an asthma attack, including cold, dry air, or pollen or dust. Drink water to keep your airways moist, and in cold weather, cover your mouth with a mask or scarf to warm and humidify the air you breathe. Swimming is a good activity choice for people with asthma.

Diabetes

• Don't exercise alone; wear a bracelet identifying you as having diabetes.

• If you are taking insulin or another medication, you may need to adjust the timing and amount of each dose as you learn to balance your energy intake and output and your medication dosage.

• To prevent abnormally rapid absorption of injected insulin, inject it over a muscle that won't be exercised and wait at least an hour before exercising.

• Check blood sugar levels before, during, and after exercise, and adjust your diet or insulin dosage if needed. Avoid exercise if your blood sugar level is above 13.5 mmol/L, and ingest carbohydrates before exercise if your blood sugar level is below 5.5 mmol/L. Have high-carbohydrate foods available during a workout.

• Check your skin regularly for blisters and abrasions, especially on your feet.

Obesity

• For maximum benefit and minimum risk, begin with low- to moderate-intensity activities and increase the intensity slowly as your fitness improves.

• To lose weight or maintain lost weight, exercise moderately 60 minutes or more every day; you can exercise all at once or divide your total activity time into sessions of 10 or more minutes.

• At first choose non- or low-weight-bearing activities, such as swimming, water exercises, cycling, or walking.

• Stay alert for symptoms of heat-related problems during exercise.

• Try to include as much lifestyle physical activity in your daily routine as possible.

• Include strength training in your program to build or maintain muscle mass.

Heart Disease and Hypertension

• Warm-up and cool-down sessions should be gradual and should last at least 10 minutes.

• Exercise at a moderate rather than a high intensity; monitor your heart rate during exercise, and stop if you experience dizziness or chest pain.

• Increase exercise frequency, intensity, and time very gradually.

• Don't hold your breath when exercising as this can cause a sudden, steep increase in blood pressure.

• Discuss the effects of your medication with your physician; for example, certain drugs for hypertension affect heart rate. If your physician has prescribed nitroglycerine, carry it with you during exercise.

Arthritis

• Begin an exercise program as early as possible in the course of the disease.

• Warm up thoroughly before each workout to loosen stiff muscles and lower the risk of injury.

• Avoid high-impact activities that may damage arthritic joints; consider swimming or water aerobics.

• In strength training, pay special attention to muscles that support and protect affected joints; add weight very gradually.

• Perform flexibility exercises regularly.

Osteoporosis

• If possible, choose low-impact, weight-bearing activities to help safely maintain bone density.

• To prevent fractures, avoid any activity or movement that stresses the back or carries a risk of falling.

• Weight train to improve strength and balance and reduce the risk of falls and fractures, but avoid lifting heavy weights.

DESIGNING YOUR EXERCISE PROGRAM

The best exercise program has two primary characteristics: It promotes your health, and it's fun for you to do. Exercise does not have to be a chore. On the contrary, it can provide some of the most pleasurable moments of your day, once you make it a habit. A little thought and planning will help you achieve these goals.

Figure 6.7 shows a physical activity pyramid, based on the leading North American research, to guide you in meeting goals for physical activity. If you are sedentary, start at the bottom of the pyramid and gradually increase the moderate-intensity physical activity in your daily life. You don't have to exercise vigorously, but you should experience a moderate increase in your heart and breathing rates; appropriate activities include walking, climbing stairs, doing yardwork, and washing your car. As mentioned earlier, your activity time can be broken up into small blocks over the course of a day. Work up to meeting a goal of 30 minutes of moderate-intensity exercise at least five days per week). Choose to be active whenever you can. If weight management is a concern for you, begin by achieving the goal of 30 minutes per day and then gradually raise your activity level to 60 minutes per day or more.

For even greater benefits, move up to the next two levels of the pyramid, which illustrate parts of a formal exercise program. The American College of Sports Medicine has established guidelines for an exercise program that includes cardiorespiratory endurance (aerobic) exercise, strength training, and flexibility training (Table 6.2). Such a program will develop all the health-related components of physical fitness. The sections of this chapter that follow will show you how to develop a personalized exercise program. For a summary of the health and fitness benefits of different levels of physical activity, see Figure 6.8 on p. 191.

First Steps

Are you thinking about starting a formal exercise program? A little planning can help make it a success.

Medical Clearance   Some people are advised to check with their physicians before increasing their current level of activity or beginning an exercise program. You can use the Physical Activity Readiness Questionnaire (PAR-Q), a self-screening tool, originally designed by the British Columbia Ministry of Health and the Multidisciplinary Board on Exercise to see whether you are in this group. You can take the updated questionnaire on the Public Health Agency of Canada's Web site listed in For More Information at the end of the chapter. In general, it is often recommended that previously inactive men over 40 and women over 50 should get a medical examination before

Sedentary activities
Do infrequently
Watching television, surfing the Internet, talking on the telephone

Strength training
At least 2 days per week, ideally 2–4 (all major muscle groups)
Biceps curls, push-ups, abdominal curls, bench presses, calf raises

Flexibility training
At least 2–3 days per week, ideally most, if not all, days per week (all major joints)
Calf stretches, side lunges, step stretches, modified hurdler stretches

Cardiorespiratory endurance exercise
30 minutes of moderate-intensity exercise most, if not all, days per week or 20 minutes of vigorous-intensity exercise 3 days per week
Walking, jogging, bicycling, swimming, aerobic dancing, in-line skating, cross-country skiing, dancing, basketball

Moderate-intensity physical activity
5 days or more per week (about 30 minutes per day; 60–90 minutes per day for weight loss or prevention of weight regain following weight loss)
Walking to the store or bank, washing windows or your car, climbing stairs, working in your yard, walking your dog, cleaning your room

FIGURE 6.7   Physical activity pyramid.

Table 6.2	ACSM Exercise Recommendations for Fitness Development in Healthy Adults

Exercise to Develop and Maintain Cardiorespiratory Endurance and Body Composition

Frequency of training	3–5 days per week.
Intensity of training	55%/65%–90% of maximum heart rate or 40%/50%–85% of heart rate reserve or maximum oxygen reuptake reserve. The lower intensity values (55%–64% of maximum heart rate and 40%–49% of heart rate reserve) are most applicable to individuals who are unfit. For average individuals, intensities of 70%–85% of maximum heart rate or 60%–80% of heart rate reserve are appropriate; see p. 194 for instructions on determining target heart rate.
Time (duration) of training	20–60 total minutes of continuous or intermittent (in sessions lasting 10 or more minutes) aerobic activity. Duration is dependent on the intensity of the activity; thus, low-intensity activity should be conducted over a longer time (30 minutes or more). Low-to-moderate-intensity activity of longer duration is recommended for nonathletic adults.
Type (mode) of activity	Any activity that uses large-muscle groups, can be maintained continuously, and is rhythmic and aerobic in nature— for example, walking-hiking, running-jogging, cycling-biking, cross-country skiing, aerobic dance, stair climbing, swimming, and skating.

Exercise to Develop and Maintain Muscular Strength and Endurance, Flexibility, and Body Composition

Resistance training	One set of 8–10 exercises that condition the major muscle groups should be performed at least 2 days per week. Most people should complete 8–12 repetitions of each exercise to the point of fatigue; practising other repetition ranges (for example, 3–5 or 12–15) also builds strength and endurance; for older and frailer people (approximately 50–60 and older), 10–15 repetitions with a lighter weight may be more appropriate. Multiple-set regimens will provide greater benefits if time allows. Any mode of exercise that is comfortable throughout the full range of motion is appropriate (for example, free weights, bands, or machines).
Flexibility training	Static stretches should be performed for the major muscle groups at least 2–3 days per week, ideally 5–7 days per week. Stretch to the point of tightness, holding each stretch for 15–30 seconds; perform 2–4 repetitions of each stretch.

Source: Adapted from American College of Sports Medicine. 2006. *ACSM's Guidelines for Exercise Testing and Prescription*, 7th ed. Philadelphia: Lippincott Williams & Wilkins.

FIGURE 6.8   Health and fitness benefits of different amounts of physical activity and exercise.

beginning an exercise program. Diabetes, asthma, heart disease, and extreme obesity are conditions that may call for a modified program. If you have an increased risk of heart disease because of smoking, high blood pressure, or obesity, get a complete physical checkup, including an **electrocardiogram (ECG or EKG)**, before beginning your program.

Basic Principles of Physical Training To put together an effective exercise program, you should first understand the basic principles of physical training.

SPECIFICITY To develop a fitness component, you must perform exercises that are specifically designed for that component. This is the principle of *specificity*. Weight training, for example, develops muscular strength but is less effective for developing flexibility. Specificity also applies to the skill-related fitness components and to the different parts of the body. A well-rounded exercise program includes exercises geared to each component of fitness, to different parts of the body, and to specific activities or sports.

PROGRESSIVE OVERLOAD Your body adapts to the demands of exercise by improving its functioning. When the amount of exercise, also called **overload**, is progressively increased, fitness continues to improve. Too little exercise will have no effect on fitness; too much may cause injury. The appropriate amount depends on your current level of fitness, your fitness goals, and the fitness components being developed. A novice, for example, might experience fitness benefits from jogging two kilometres in 15 minutes, but this level of exercise would cause no physical adaptations in a trained distance runner.

The amount of overload needed to maintain or improve a particular level of fitness is determined in four dimensions, represented by the acronym FITT: **f**requency, **i**ntensity, **t**ime, and **t**ype.

• *Frequency, or how often.* Optimum exercise frequency, expressed in number of days per week, varies with the component being developed, how vigorously you exercise, and your goals. A frequency of three to five days per week is recommended for cardiorespiratory endurance exercise, two or three days per week for strength training, and two to three days per week (ideally five to seven days per week) for stretching.

• *Intensity, or how hard.* Fitness benefits occur when you exercise harder than your normal level of activity. To develop cardiorespiratory endurance, you must raise your heart rate above normal; to develop muscular strength, you must lift a heavier weight than you normally do; to develop flexibility, you must stretch your muscles beyond their normal length. A gradual increase in intensity is recommended to avoid injury.

• *Time (duration), or how long.* If fitness benefits are to occur, exercise sessions must last for an extended time. Depending on the component being developed and your intensity level, a duration of 20–60 minutes is usually recommended.

• *Type or mode of activity.* The type of exercise in which you should engage varies with each fitness component and with your personal fitness goals. To develop cardiorespiratory endurance, you need to engage in continuous activities involving large-muscle groups—walking, cycling, or swimming, for example. Resistive exercises develop muscular strength and endurance; stretching exercises build flexibility. The frequency, intensity, and time of exercise will be different for each type of activity.

These dimensions of overload are described individually as they apply to the health-related components of fitness discussed in this chapter.

REVERSIBILITY The body adjusts to lower levels of physical activity in the same way it adjusts to higher levels—the principle of **reversibility**. When you stop exercising, you can lose up to 50% of fitness improvements within two months. Try to exercise consistently, and don't quit if you miss a few workouts. If you must temporarily curtail your training, you can maintain your fitness improvements by keeping the intensity of your workouts constant while reducing their frequency or duration.

INDIVIDUAL DIFFERENCES There are limits to the potential for improvement and large individual differences in our ability to improve fitness, achieve a desirable body composition, and perform and learn sports skills. Scientists have identified specific genes that influence the capacity to alter body fat, strength, and endurance. In addition, men tend to have higher endurance capacity than women because of higher testosterone levels (which affect oxygen transport and cellular metabolism) and lower levels of body fat. However, men and women have the same capacity for improvement when gains are expressed as a percentage of initial fitness.

Selecting Activities If you have been inactive, you should begin slowly by gradually increasing the amount of moderate physical activity in your life (the bottom of the activity pyramid). Once your body adjusts to your new level of activity, you can choose additional activities for your exercise program.

Be sure the activities you choose contribute to your overall wellness and make sense for you. Are you competitive? If so, try racquetball, basketball, or squash. Do you prefer to exercise alone? Then consider cross-country skiing or road running. Have you been sedentary? A walking program may be a good place to start. If you think you may have trouble sticking with an exercise program, find a structured activity that you can do with a friend or a group.

Be realistic about the constraints presented by some sports, such as accessibility, expense, and time. For example, if you have to travel for hours to get to a ski area, skiing may not be a good choice for your regular exercise program. And if you've never played tennis, it will probably take some time to reach a reasonable skill level; you may be better off with a program of walking or jogging to get good workouts while you're improving your tennis game.

Cardiorespiratory Endurance Exercises

Exercises that condition your heart and lungs should have a central role in your fitness program. The best exercises for developing cardiorespiratory endurance stress a large portion of the body's muscle mass for a prolonged time. These include walking, jogging, running, swimming, bicycling, and aerobic dancing. Many popular sports and recreational activities, such as racquetball, tennis, basketball, and soccer, are also good if the skill level and intensity of the game are sufficient to provide a vigorous workout.

Frequency   The optimal workout schedule for endurance training is three to five days per week. Beginners should start with three and work up to five days. Training more than five days a week often leads to injury for recreational athletes. Although you do get health benefits from exercising very vigorously only one or two days per week, you risk injury because your body never gets a chance to adapt fully to regular exercise training.

Intensity   The most misunderstood aspect of conditioning, even among experienced athletes, is training intensity. Intensity is the crucial factor in attaining a significant training effect—that is, in increasing the body's cardiorespiratory capacity. A primary purpose of endurance training is to increase **maximal oxygen consumption ($\dot{V}O_{2max}$)**. $\dot{V}O_{2max}$ represents the maximum ability of the cells to use oxygen and is considered the best measure of cardiorespiratory capacity. Intensity of training is the crucial factor in improving $\dot{V}O_{2max}$.

One of the easiest ways to determine exactly how intensely you should work involves measuring your heart rate. It is not necessary or desirable to exercise at your maximum heart rate—the fastest heart rate possible before exhaustion sets in—to improve your cardiorespiratory capacity. Beneficial effects occur at lower heart rates with a much lower risk of injury. **Target heart rate range** is the range of rates within which you should exercise to obtain cardiorespiratory benefits. To determine the intensity at which you should exercise, refer to the box "Determining Your Target Heart Rate Range" (p. 194) and Figure 6.9 (p. 194).

After you begin your fitness program, you may improve quickly because the body adapts readily to new exercises; the rate of improvement may slow after the first month or so. The more fit you become, the harder you will have to work to improve. By monitoring your heart rate, you will always know if you are working hard enough to improve, not hard enough, or too hard. For most people, a fitness program involves attaining an acceptable level of fitness and then maintaining that level. There is no need to keep working indefinitely to improve; doing so only increases the chance of injury. After you have reached the level you want, you can maintain fitness by exercising at the same intensity three to five days per week.

Time (Duration)   A total time of 20–60 minutes is recommended; exercise can take place in a single session or several sessions lasting 10 or more minutes. The total duration of exercise depends on its intensity. To improve cardiorespiratory endurance during a low-intensity to moderate-intensity activity, such as walking or slow swimming, you should exercise for 45–60 minutes. For high-intensity exercise performed at the top of your target heart rate zone, a duration of 20 minutes is sufficient. Start with less vigorous activities and gradually increase intensity.

You can use these three dimensions of cardiorespiratory endurance training—frequency, intensity, and time—to develop a fitness program that strengthens your heart and lungs and provides all the benefits described earlier in this chapter. Build your program around at least 20 minutes of endurance exercise at your target heart rate three to five days a week. Then add exercises that develop the other components of fitness.

The Warm-Up and Cool-Down   It is always important to warm up before you exercise and to cool down afterward. Warming up enhances your performance and decreases your chances of injury. Your muscles work better when their temperature is elevated slightly above resting level. Warming up helps your body gradually progress from rest to exercise. Blood needs to be redirected to active muscles, and your heart needs time to adapt to the increased demands of exercise. A warm-up helps spread **synovial fluid** throughout the joints, which helps protect joint surfaces from wear and tear. (It's like warming up a car to spread oil through the engine parts before shifting into gear.)

TERMS

electrocardiogram (ECG or EKG)   A recording of the electrical activity of the heart.

overload   The amount of stress placed on the body; a gradual increase in the amount of overload causes adaptations that improve fitness.

reversibility   The training principle that fitness improvements are lost when demands on the body are lowered.

maximal oxygen consumption ($\dot{V}O_{2max}$)   The body's maximum ability to transport and use oxygen.

target heart rate range   The range of heart rates within which exercise yields cardiorespiratory benefits.

synovial fluid   Fluid found within many joints that provides lubrication and nutrition to the cells of the joint surface.

Determining Your Target Heart Rate Range

TAKE CHARGE

Your target heart rate is the range of rates at which you should exercise to experience cardiorespiratory benefits. Your target heart rate range is based on your maximum heart rate, which can be estimated from your age. (If you are a serious athlete or face possible cardiovascular risks from exercise, you may want to have your maximum heart rate determined more accurately through a treadmill test in a physician's office, hospital, or sports medicine laboratory.) Your target heart rate is a range: The lower value corresponds to moderate-intensity exercise, and the higher value is associated with high-intensity exercise. Target heart rate ranges are shown in the table.

You can monitor the intensity of your workouts by measuring your pulse either at your wrist or at one of your carotid arteries, located on either side of your Adam's apple. Your pulse rate drops rapidly after exercise, so begin counting immediately after you have finished exercising. You will obtain the most accurate results by counting beats for 10 seconds and then multiplying by 6 to get your heart rate in beats per minute (bpm). The 10-second counts corresponding to each target heart rate range are also shown in the table.

Age (years)	Target Heart Rate Range (bpm)*	10-Second Count (beats)*
20–24	127–180	21–30
25–29	124–176	20–29
30–34	121–171	20–28
35–39	118–167	19–27
40–44	114–162	19–27
45–49	111–158	18–26
50–54	108–153	18–25
55–59	105–149	17–24
60–64	101–144	16–24
65+	97–140	16–23

* Target heart rates lower than those shown here are appropriate for individuals with a very low initial level of fitness. Ranges are based on the following formula: Target heart rate = 0.65 to 0.90 of maximum heart rate, assuming maximum heart rate = 220 − age.

A warm-up session should include low-intensity movements similar to those in the activity that will follow. For example, hit forehands and backhands before a tennis game or jog slowly for 400 metres before progressing to 1.6 kilometres in eight minutes. Some people like to include stretching exercises in their warm-up. Experts recommend that you stretch *after* the active part of your warm-up, when your body temperature has been elevated. Studies have found that stretching before exercise can temporarily decrease muscle strength and power, so if a high-performance workout is your goal, it is best to stretch after a workout. See p. 197 for more on stretching.

Cooling down after exercise is important to restore the body's circulation to its normal resting condition. When you are at rest, a relatively small percentage of your total blood volume is directed to muscles, but during exercise, as much as 90% of the heart's output is directed to them. During recovery from exercise, it is important to continue exercising at a low level to provide a smooth transition to the resting state. Cooling down helps regulate the return of blood to your heart.

> **QUICK STATS**
> **5–10** minutes of warming up and cooling down is adequate for a 30-minute workout of brisk walking.
>
> —Mayo Clinic, 2007

When feeling for the carotid pulse under the angle of the jaw, use very light pressure.

The radial pulse is felt on the wrist just under the thumb.

FIGURE 6.9 Checking your pulse. The pulse can be taken at the carotid artery in the neck (top) or at the radial artery in the wrist (bottom). Be sure to not press too hard, particularly on the carotid artery.

Gender Differences in Muscular Strength

At this point in your reading of this book, it should be clear that gender often plays a role as a health determinant, and this is also the case when looking at building muscular strength. Men are generally stronger than women because they typically have larger bodies overall and a larger proportion of their total body mass is made up of muscle. But when strength is expressed per unit of muscle tissue, men are only 1%–2% stronger than women in the upper body and about equal to women in the lower body. Individual muscle cells are larger in men, but the functioning of the cells is the same in both sexes.

Two factors that help explain these disparities are testosterone levels and the speed of nervous control of muscle. Testosterone promotes the growth of muscle tissue in both males and females, but testosterone levels are about 6–10 times as high in men as in women, so men develop larger muscles. Also, because the male nervous system can activate muscles faster, men tend to have more power.

Some women are concerned that they will develop large muscles from strength training. Because of hormonal differ-

ences, most women do not develop large muscles unless they train intensely over many years or take steroids. A study of average women who weight trained two to three days per week for eight weeks found that the women gained about 3.75 kilograms of muscle and lost about 7.7 kilograms of fat. Another study followed women who trained with weights for two years. Not only did the women reduce their overall body fat levels but they ended up with less fat around their midsection.

Losing muscle over time is a much greater health concern for women than small gains in muscle weight in response to strength training, especially as any gains in muscle weight are typically more than balanced with loss of fat weight. Both men and women lose muscle mass and power as they age, but because men start out with more muscle when they are young and don't lose power as quickly as women, older women tend to have greater impairment of muscle function than older men. This may partially explain the higher incidence of life-threatening falls in older women.

Although world authorities recommend strength training two to four days

per week, only 14% of Canadian women and 20% of men do so, underscoring the need for additional programs and campaigns that promote this form of exercise.

Sources: Fahey, T. D. 2007. Basic *Weight Training for Men and Women*, 6th ed. New York: McGraw-Hill; Centers for Disease Control and Prevention. 2006. Trends in strength training—United States, 1998–2004. *Morbidity and Mortality Weekly Report* 55(28): 769–772; Canadian Fitness and Lifestyle Research Institute. 2005. *Physical Activity Levels Among Adults* (http://www.cflri.ca/eng/levels/popular_pa_adults.php; retrieved April 4, 2011).

Developing Muscular Strength and Endurance

Any program designed to promote health should include exercises that develop muscular strength and endurance (see the box "Gender Differences in Muscular Strength," above). Your ability to maintain correct posture and move efficiently depends in part on adequate muscle fitness. Strengthening exercises also increase muscle tone, which improves the appearance of your body.

Types of Strength Training Exercises Muscular strength and endurance can be developed in many ways, from weight training to calisthenics. Common exercises, such as curl-ups, push-ups, pull-ups, and wall-sitting (leaning against a wall in a seated position and supporting yourself with your leg muscles), maintain the muscular strength of most people if they practise them several times a week. To condition and tone your whole body, choose exercises that work the major muscles of the shoulders, chest, back, arms, abdomen, and legs.

To increase muscular strength and endurance, you must do **resistance exercise**—exercises in which your muscles must exert force against a significant amount of

resistance. Resistance can be provided by weights, exercise machines, or your own body weight.

Isometric (static) exercises involve applying force without movement, such as when you contract your abdominal muscles. This static type of exercise is valuable for toning and strengthening muscles. Isometrics can be practised anywhere and do not require any equipment. For maximum strength gains, hold an isometric contraction maximally for six seconds; do five to ten repetitions. Don't hold your breath—that can restrict blood flow to your heart and brain. Within a few weeks, you will notice the effect of this exercise. Isometrics are particularly useful when recovering from an injury.

Isotonic (dynamic) exercises involve applying force with movement, as in weight training exercises, such as

---

resistance exercise   Activities that force muscles to contract against increased resistance; also called *strength training*.

isometric (static) exercise   The application of force without movement.

isotonic (dynamic) exercise   The application of force with movement.

TERMS

Exercise Machines Versus Free Weights

Exercise Machines		Free Weights	
Advantages	Disadvantages	Advantages	Disadvantages
• Are safe and convenient • Don't require spotters	• Have limited availability • Are inappropriate for performing dynamic movements	• Allow dynamic movements • Allow user to develop control of weights	• Are not as safe • Require spotters
• Don't require lifter to balance bar • Provide variable resistance	• Allow limited number of exercises • Train muscles rather than movements	• Allow greater variety of exercises • Are widely available, inexpensive, and convenient for home use	• Require more skill • Cause more blisters and calluses
• Require less skill	• Place minimal stress on core stabilizing muscles (those in torso)	• Train core stabilizing muscles	
• Make it easy to move from one exercise to the next • Allow easy isolation of muscles and muscle groups • Support back (on many machines)		• Are better for building power • Are truer to real-life situations; strength transfers to daily activities	

the bench press. These are the most popular type of exercises for increasing muscle strength and seem to be most valuable for developing strength that can be transferred to other forms of physical activity. They include exercises using barbells, dumbbells, weight machines, and body weight, as in push-ups or curl-ups.

Choosing Equipment   Weight machines are preferred by many people because they are safe, convenient, and easy to use (see the box "Exercise Machines Versus Free Weights," above). You just set the resistance, sit down at the machine, and start working. Machines make it easy to isolate and work specific muscles. Free weights require more care, balance, and coordination to use, but they strengthen your body in ways that are more adaptable to real life. When using free weights, you need to use a spotter, someone who stands by to assist in case you lose control over a weight (see "Safe Weight Training" in the ▣ connect Library).

Choosing Exercises   A complete weight training program works all the major muscle groups: neck, upper back, shoulders, arms, chest, abdomen, lower back, thighs, buttocks, and calves. Different exercises work different muscles, so it usually takes about eight to ten exercises to get a complete workout for general fitness—for example, bench presses to develop the chest, shoulders, and upper arms; pull-ups to work the biceps and upper back; squats to develop the legs and buttocks; toe raises to work the calves; and so on. If you are also training for

a particular sport, include exercises to strengthen the muscles important for optimal performance and those most likely to be injured.

Frequency   For general fitness, the American College of Sports Medicine recommends a frequency of at least two nonconsecutive days per week. This allows your muscles one or more days of rest between workouts to avoid soreness and injury. If you enjoy weight training and would like to train more often, try working different muscle groups on alternate days.

Intensity and Time   The amount of weight (resistance) you lift in weight training exercises is equivalent to intensity in cardiorespiratory endurance training; the number of repetitions of each exercise is equivalent to time. To improve fitness, you must do enough repetitions of each exercise to temporarily fatigue your muscles. The number of repetitions needed to cause fatigue depends on the amount of resistance: the heavier the weight, the fewer repetitions to reach fatigue. In general, a heavy weight and a low number of repetitions (1–5) build strength, whereas a light weight and a high number of repetitions (20–25) build endurance. For a general fitness program to build both strength and endurance, try to do 8–12 repetitions of each exercise; a few exercises, such as abdominal crunches and calf raises, may require more. (For people who are 50–60 years of age and older, 10–15 repetitions of each exercise using a lighter weight is recommended.)

The first few sessions of weight training should be devoted to learning the exercises. To start, choose a weight that you can move easily through 8–12 repetitions. Add weight when you can do more than 12 repetitions of an exercise. If adding weight means you can do only seven or eight repetitions before your muscles fatigue, stay with that weight until you can again complete 12 repetitions. If you can do only four to six repetitions after adding weight, or if you can't maintain good form, you've added too much and should take some off. As a general guideline, try increases of approximately one kilogram of additional weight for each five kilograms you are currently lifting.

For developing strength and endurance for general fitness, a single set (group) of each exercise is sufficient, provided you use enough resistance (weight) to fatigue your muscles. Doing more than one set of each exercise may increase strength development, and most serious weight trainers do at least three sets of each exercise. If you do more than one set of an exercise, rest long enough between sets to allow your muscles to recover. More rapid strength gains occur with one, two, and three sets. If you do more than three sets, you will need to work much harder to get lower results (the law of diminishing returns).

You should warm up before every weight training session and cool down afterward. You can expect to improve rapidly during the first 6–10 weeks of training; gains will then come more slowly. Many factors, such as age, motivation, gender, and heredity, will affect your program. Your ultimate goal depends on you. After you have achieved the level of strength and muscularity that you want, you can maintain your gains by training two to three nonconsecutive days per week.

A Caution About Supplements No nutritional supplement or drug will change a weak person into a strong person. Those changes require regular training that stresses the body and causes physiological adaptations. Supplements or drugs that promise quick, large gains in strength usually don't work and are often either dangerous, expensive, or both (see the box "Drugs and Supplements for Improved Athletic Performance" on p. 198). Over-the-counter supplements are not carefully regulated, and their long-term effects have not been systematically studied.

Flexibility Exercises

Flexibility, or stretching, exercises are important for maintaining the normal range of motion in the major joints of the body. Some exercises, such as running, can actually decrease flexibility because they require only a partial range of motion. Like a good weight training program, a good stretching program includes exercises for all the major muscle groups and joints of the body: neck, shoulders, back, hips, thighs, hamstrings, and calves.

Proper Stretching Technique Stretching should be performed statically. Ballistic stretching (known as *bouncing*) is dangerous and counterproductive. In active stretching,

a muscle is stretched under a person's own power by contracting the opposing muscles. In passive stretching, an outside force or resistance provided by you, a partner, gravity, or a weight helps elongate the targeted muscle. You can achieve a greater range of motion and a more intense stretch by using passive stretching, but there is a greater risk of injury. The safest and most convenient technique may be active static stretching with a passive assist. For example, you might do a seated stretch of your calf muscles both by contracting the muscles on the top of your shin and by grabbing your feet and pulling them toward you.

Frequency Do stretching exercises at least two to three days per week, ideally five to seven days per week. If you stretch after cardiorespiratory endurance exercise or strength training, during your cool-down, you may develop more flexibility, because your muscles are warmer then and can be stretched farther.

Intensity and Time For each exercise, stretch to the point of tightness in the muscle, and hold the position for 15–30 seconds. Rest for 30–60 seconds, then repeat, trying to stretch a bit farther. Relax and breathe easily as you stretch. You should feel a pleasant, mild stretch as you let

When performed regularly, stretching exercises help maintain or improve the range of motion in joints. For each exercise, stretch to the point of tightness in the muscle and hold the position for 15–30 seconds.

Drugs and Supplements for Improved Athletic Performance

Doping scandals have snared athletes in sports as diverse as cycling, baseball, and track and field. In 1988, Canadian sprinter Ben Johnson tested positive for the anabolic steroid stanozolol and was stripped of his gold medal in the 100-metre sprint. In 2007, cyclist Floyd Landis was stripped of his 2006 Tour de France title and banned from cycling for two years after testing positive for synthetic testosterone. Meantime, as baseball legends Barry Bonds and Roger Clemens fought to restore reputations damaged by allegations of steroid abuse, a special congressional report accused nearly 90 professional baseball players of using steroids and other performance-enhancing drugs. That same year, Olympic sprinter Marion Jones admitted to using banned substances before the 2000 Olympic Games. In the wake of these and other events, governments, professional sports leagues, and anti-doping agencies all sought ways to rid sports of banned substances.

Professional and Olympic athletes aren't the only ones using performance-enhancing drugs. About 2%–6% of high school and university students report having used anabolic steroids, and over-the-counter dietary supplements are much more popular. Many such substances are ineffective and expensive, and many are also dangerous. A few of the most widely used compounds are described below.

Anabolic Steroids

These synthetic derivatives of testosterone are taken to increase strength, power, speed, endurance, muscle size, and aggressiveness. **Anabolic steroids** have dangerous side effects, including disruption of the body's hormone system, liver disease, acne, breast development and testicular shrinkage in males, masculinization in women and children, and increased risk of heart disease and cancer. Evidence links steroid use and risk of heart attack, stroke, and sudden death.

Steroid users who inject the drugs face the same health risks as other injection drug users, including increased risk of HIV infection. Steroids have been found to be a gateway to the use of other drugs.

Adrenal Androgens

This group of drugs, which includes dehydroepiandrosterone (DHEA) and androstenedione, are typically taken to stimulate muscle growth and aid in weight control. The few studies of these agents done on humans show that they are of very little value in improving athletic performance, and they have side effects similar to those of anabolic steroids, especially when taken in high doses.

Ephedra and Other Stimulants

These drugs may be taken to increase training intensity, to suppress hunger, to reduce fatigue, and to promote weight loss. They raise heart rate and blood pressure and, at high doses, may increase the risk of heart attack, stroke, and heat-related illness. Several stimulants, including ephedra and phenylpropanolamine, have been banned by government authorities.

Erythropoietin (EPO)

A naturally occurring hormone that boosts the concentration of red blood cells, EPO is used by endurance athletes to improve performance. EPO can cause blood clots and death.

Creatine Monohydrate

Creatine is thought to improve performance in short-term, high-intensity, repetitive exercise and decrease the risk of injury. People vary in their responses to creatine. The long-term effects of creatine use, especially among young people, are not well established.

Protein, Amino Acid, and Polypeptide Supplements

Taking protein supplements after weight training may increase muscle strength and hypertrophy. Little research supports the use of such supplements, however, even in athletes on extremely heavy training regimens. The protein requirements of athletes are not much higher than those of sedentary individuals, and most people take in more than enough protein in their diets. By substituting supplements for food sources of protein, people may risk deficiencies in other key nutrients typically found in such foods, including iron and B vitamins.

Chromium Picolinate

Sold over the counter, chromium picolinate is a more easily digested form of the trace mineral chromium. Although often marketed as a means to build muscle and reduce fat, most studies have found no positive effects. Long-term use of high dosages may have serious health consequences.

	Cardiorespiratory endurance training	Strength training	Flexibility training
Frequency	Most days per week	2–4 nonconsecutive days per week	2–3 days per week (minimum); Most days per week (ideal)
Intensity	55%/65%–90% of maximum heart rate	Sufficient resistance to fatigue muscles	Stretch to the point of tension
Time	20–60 minutes in sessions lasting 10 minutes or more	8–12 repetitions of each exercise, 1 or more sets	2–4 repetitions of each exercise, held for 15–30 seconds
Type	Continuous rhythmic activities using large muscle groups	Resistance exercises for all major muscle groups	Stretching exercises for all major joints

FIGURE 6.10   A summary of the FITT principle for the health-related components of fitness.

the muscles relax; stretching should not be painful. Do two to four repetitions of each exercise. A complete flexibility workout usually takes about 20–30 minutes.

Increase your intensity gradually over time. Improved flexibility takes many months to develop. There are large individual differences in joint flexibility. Don't feel you have to compete with others during stretching workouts.

Training in Specific Skills

The final component in your fitness program is learning the skills required for the sports or activities in which you choose to participate. By taking the time and effort to acquire competence, you can achieve a sense of mastery and add a new physical activity to your repertoire.

The first step in learning a new skill is getting help. Many sports, such as tennis, golf, sailing, and skiing, require mastery of basic movements and techniques, so instruction from a qualified teacher can save you hours of frustration and increase your enjoyment of the sport. Skill is also important in conditioning activities, such as jogging, swimming, and cycling. Even if you learned a sport as a child, additional instruction now can help you refine your technique, get over obstacles, and relearn skills that you may have learned incorrectly.

Putting It All Together

Now that you know the basic components of a fitness program, you can put them all together in a program that works for you. Remember to include the following:

- *Cardiorespiratory endurance exercise:* Do at least 20–60 minutes of aerobic exercise within your target heart rate range three to five days a week.
- *Muscular strength and endurance:* Work the major muscle groups (one or more sets of eight to ten exercises) at least two nonconsecutive days a week.

QUESTIONS FOR CRITICAL THINKING AND REFLECTION
Consider the different activities that have been suggested throughout this chapter. For which ones do you have the necessary fitness prerequisite? Given your current fitness and skill level, which ones could you incorporate into your exercise program?

- *Flexibility exercise:* Do stretches at least two or three days a week, ideally five to seven days a week, preferably after exercise, when your muscles are warm.
- *Skill training:* Incorporate some or all of your aerobic or strengthening exercise into an enjoyable sport or physical activity.

Refer to Figure 6.10 above for a summary of the FITT principle for the health-related fitness components.

GETTING STARTED AND STAYING ON TRACK

Once you have a program that fulfils your basic fitness needs and suits your personal tastes, adhering to a few basic principles will help you improve at the fastest rate, have more fun, and minimize the risk of injury. These principles include buying appropriate equipment, eating and drinking properly, and managing your program so it becomes an integral part of your life.

anabolic steroids   Synthetic male hormones used to increase muscle size and strength.

Selecting Instructors, Equipment, and Facilities

Once you've chosen the activities for your program, you may need to obtain appropriate information, instruction, and equipment or find an appropriate facility.

Finding Help and Advice About Exercise   One of the best places to get help is an exercise class, where an expert instructor can help you learn the basics of training and answer your questions. A qualified personal trainer can also get you started on an exercise program or a new form of training. Make sure that your instructor or trainer has proper qualifications, such as a university degree in exercise physiology, kinesiology, or physical education and certification by such organizations as the Canadian Society for Exercise Physiology (CSEP), the American College of Sports Medicine (ACSM), Can-Fit-Pro, the YMCA, or another professional organization. Don't seek out a person for advice simply because he or she looks fit. You can further your knowledge by reading articles by experts in fitness magazines.

Many Web sites provide fitness programs, including ongoing support and feedback via email. Many of these sites charge a fee, so it is important to review the sites, decide which ones seem most appropriate, and if possible go through a free trial period before subscribing. Also remember to consider the reliability of the information at fitness Web sites, especially those that also advertise or sell products. A few popular sites are listed in For More Information at the end of the chapter.

Selecting Equipment   Try to purchase the best equipment you can afford. Good equipment will enhance your enjoyment and decrease your risk of injury. Appropriate safety equipment, such as pads and helmets for in-line skating, is particularly important. If you shop around, you can often find bargains through mail-order companies and discount or used equipment stores.

Before you invest in a new piece of equipment, investigate it. Try it out at a local gym to make sure that you'll use it regularly. Also check whether you have space to use and store it at home. Ask the experts (coaches, physical educators, and sports instructors) for their opinion. Better yet, educate yourself. Every sport, from running to volleyball, has its own magazine.

Footwear is an important piece of equipment for almost any activity; see "Choosing Exercise Footwear" in the connect Library for shopping strategies.

Choosing a Fitness Centre   Are you thinking of joining a health club or fitness centre? Be sure to choose one that has the right programs and equipment available at the times you will use them. You should feel comfortable with the classes and activities available; the age, fitness level, and dress of others in the club; and the types of music used in classes. The facility and equipment should be clean and well maintained, including the showers and lockers; the staff should be well trained, certified, and helpful.

Ask for a free trial workout, a one-day pass, or an inexpensive one-week to two-week trial membership before committing to a long-term contract. Be wary of promotional gimmicks and high-pressure sales tactics.

Eating and Drinking for Exercise

Most people do not need to change their eating habits when they begin a fitness program. Many athletes and other physically active people are lured into buying aggressively advertised vitamins, minerals, and protein supplements; but, in almost every case, a well-balanced diet contains all the energy and nutrients needed to sustain an exercise program (see Chapter 5).

A balanced diet is also the key to improving your body composition when you begin to exercise more. One of the promises of a fitness program is a decrease in body fat and an increase in muscular body mass. As mentioned earlier, the control of body fat is determined by the balance of energy in the body. If more calories are consumed than are expended through metabolism and exercise, then fat increases. If the reverse is true, fat is lost. The best way to control body fat is to follow a diet containing adequate but not excessive calories and to be physically active.

One of the most important principles to follow when exercising is to drink enough water. Your body depends on water to sustain many chemical reactions and to maintain correct body temperature. Sweating during exercise depletes the body's water supply and can lead to dehydration if fluids are not replaced. Serious dehydration can cause reduced blood volume, accelerated heart rate, elevated body temperature, muscle cramps, heat stroke, and other serious problems.

Drinking fluids before and during exercise is important to prevent dehydration and enhance performance. Thirst receptors in the brain make you want to drink fluids, but during heavy or prolonged exercise or exercise in hot weather, thirst alone isn't a good indication of how much fluid you need to drink. As a general rule, drink at least a half litre of fluid two hours before exercise and then drink enough during exercise to match fluid loss in sweat—at least 250 millilitres (one cup) of fluid every 20–30 minutes of exercise, more in hot weather or if you sweat heavily. To determine if you're drinking the right amount of fluid, weigh yourself before and after an exercise session: Any weight loss is due to fluid loss and needs to be replaced. Any weight gain is due to overconsumption of fluid.

Bring a bottle of water when you exercise so you can replace your fluids when they're depleted. For exercise sessions lasting less than 60–90 minutes, cool water is an excellent fluid replacement. For longer workouts, a sports drink that contains water and small amounts of electrolytes (sodium, potassium, and magnesium) and simple carbohydrates (sugar, usually in the form of sucrose or glucose) is recommended.

Managing Your Fitness Program

How can you tell when you're in shape? When do you stop improving and start maintaining? How can you stay motivated? If your program is going to become an integral part of your life, and if the principles behind it are going to serve you well in the future, these are key questions.

Start Slowly, Get in Shape Gradually   As Figure 6.11 shows, an exercise program can be divided into three phases:

- *Beginning phase:* The body adjusts to the new type and level of activity.
- *Progress phase:* Fitness increases.
- *Maintenance phase:* The targeted level of fitness is sustained over the long term.

FIGURE 6.11   Progression of an exercise program.   This figure shows how the amount of overload is increased gradually over time in a sample walking program. Regardless of the activity chosen, it is important that an exercise program begin slowly and progress gradually. Once you achieve the desired level of fitness, you can maintain it by exercising three to five days a week.

Source: Progression data from American College of Sports Medicine. 2006. *ACSM's Guidelines for Exercise Testing and Prescription*, 7th ed. Philadelphia: Lippincott Williams & Wilkins.

When beginning a program, start slowly to give your body time to adapt to the stress of exercise. Choose activities carefully, according to your fitness status; if you have been sedentary or are overweight, try an activity that won't jar the body or strain your joints, such as walking or swimming.

Exercising Consistently   Consistency is the key to getting into shape without injury. Steady fitness improvement comes when you overload your body consistently over a long time. The best way to ensure consistency is to keep a training journal in which you record the details of your workouts: how far you ran, how much weight you lifted, how many laps you swam, and so on. This record will help you evaluate your progress and plan your workout sessions intelligently. Don't increase your exercise volume by more than 5%–10% per week.

THINKING ABOUT THE ENVIRONMENT

Wherever you see people exercising, you will see bottled water in abundance. For several years, however, a debate has been raging about the quality and safety of commercially bottled water. In recent months, new evidence has emerged showing that most bottled waters are no better for you than regular tap water, and some bottled waters may actually be bad for you.

In a 2008 analysis, the Environmental Working Group (EWG) found 38 different contaminants in ten popular brands of bottled water. Contaminants included heavy metals, such as arsenic, pharmaceutical residues and other pollutants commonly found in urban wastewater, and a variety of industrial chemicals.

In recent years, government and private agencies have revealed that many commercially bottled water products are really just tap water drawn from municipal water systems. These products are priced many times higher than water from a residential tap. They also provide no benefit over standard tap water.

Further, plastic water bottles have become a huge solid waste problem, as millions of bottles end up in landfills each day. Once in a landfill, many kinds of plastic bottles will never decompose at all; at best, some types of plastic take years to biodegrade.

Experts say that when you're exercising, the cheapest and safest way to stay hydrated is to drink filtered tap water. If you need to carry water with you, buy a reusable container (preferably made of stainless steel) that can be cleaned and sterilized after each use. If you drink from plastic bottles, be sure they are recyclable and dispose of them by recycling.

For more information on the environment and environmental health, see Chapter 21.

Assessing Your Fitness When are you in shape? It depends. One person may be out of shape running one to two kilometres in five minutes; another may be in shape running one to two kilometres in 12 minutes. As mentioned earlier, your ultimate level of fitness depends on your goals, your program, and your natural ability. The important thing is to set goals that make sense for you.

If you are interested in finding out exactly how fit you are before you begin a program, the best approach is to get an assessment from a sports medicine laboratory. Such laboratories can be found in university physical education departments and medical centres. Here you will receive an accurate profile of your capacity to exercise. Typically, your endurance will be measured on a treadmill or bicycle, your body fat will be estimated, and your strength and flexibility will be tested. This evaluation will reveal whether your physical condition is consistent with good health, and the staff members at the laboratory can suggest an exercise program that will be appropriate for your level of fitness. To assess your own approximate level of cardiorespiratory endurance, visit the ▣connect Library and take "The 1.5-Mile Run–Walk Test").

Preventing and Managing Athletic Injuries Although annoying, most injuries are neither serious nor permanent. However, an injury that is not cared for properly can escalate into a chronic problem. It is important to learn how to deal with injuries so they don't derail your fitness program (Table 6.3).

Some injuries require medical attention. Consult a physician for head and eye injuries, possible ligament injuries, broken bones, and internal disorders, such as chest pain, fainting, and intolerance to heat. Also seek medical attention for apparently minor injuries that do not get better within a reasonable amount of time.

For minor cuts and scrapes, stop the bleeding and clean the wound with soap and water. Treat soft tissue injuries (muscles and joints) with the R-I-C-E principle:

- *Rest:* Stop using the injured area as soon as you experience pain, protect it from further injury, and avoid any activity that causes pain.

- *Ice:* Apply ice to the injured area to reduce swelling and alleviate pain. Apply ice immediately for 10–20 minutes, and repeat every few hours until

Table 6.3	Care of Common Exercise Injuries and Discomforts	
Injury	**Symptoms**	**Treatment**
Blister	Accumulation of fluid in one spot under the skin	Don't pop or drain it unless it interferes too much with your daily activities. If it does pop, clean the area with antiseptic and cover with a bandage. Do not remove the skin covering the blister.
Bruise (contusion)	Pain, swelling, and discoloration	R-I-C-E: rest, ice, compression, elevation.
Fracture or dislocation	Pain, swelling, tenderness, loss of function, and deformity	Seek medical attention, immobilize the affected area, and apply cold.
Joint sprain	Pain, tenderness, swelling, discoloration, and loss of function	R-I-C-E; apply heat when swelling has disappeared. Stretch and strengthen affected area.
Muscle cramp	Painful, spasmodic muscle contractions	Gently stretch for 15–30 seconds at a time or massage the cramped area. Drink fluids and increase dietary salt intake if exercising in hot weather.
Muscle soreness or stiffness	Pain and tenderness in the affected muscle	Stretch the affected muscle gently; exercise at a low intensity; apply heat. Nonsteroidal anti-inflammatory drugs, such as ibuprofen, help some people.
Muscle strain	Pain, tenderness, swelling, and loss of strength in the affected muscle	R-I-C-E; apply heat when swelling has disappeared. Stretch and strengthen the affected area.
Plantar fasciitis	Pain and tenderness in the connective tissue on the bottom of your feet	Apply ice, take nonsteroidal anti-inflammatory drugs, and stretch. Wear night splints when sleeping.
Shin splint	Pain and tenderness on the front of the lower leg; sometimes also pain in the calf muscle	Rest; apply ice to the affected area several times a day and before exercise; wrap with tape for support. Stretch and strengthen muscles in the lower legs. Purchase good-quality footwear and run on soft surfaces.
Side stitch	Pain on the side of the abdomen	Stretch the arm on the affected side as high as possible; if that doesn't help, try bending forward while tightening the abdominal muscles.
Tendinitis	Pain, swelling, and tenderness of the affected area	R-I-C-E; apply heat when swelling has disappeared. Stretch and strengthen the affected area.

Source: Fahey, T. D., P. M. Insel, and W. T. Roth. 2009. *Fit and Well: Core Concepts and Labs in Physical Fitness and Wellness,* 8th ed. New York: McGraw-Hill. Copyright © 2009 The McGraw-Hill Companies, Inc.

the swelling disappears. Let the injured part return to normal temperature between icings, and do not apply ice to one area for more than 20 minutes (10 minutes if you are using a cold gel pack).

- *Compression:* Wrap the injured area with an elastic bandage or a compression bandage between icings. If the area starts throbbing or begins to change colour, the bandage may be wrapped too tightly. Do not sleep with the bandage on.
- *Elevation:* Raise the injured area above heart level to decrease the blood supply and reduce swelling.

After about 36–48 hours, apply heat, if the swelling has completely disappeared, to help relieve pain, relax muscles, and reduce stiffness. Immerse the affected area in warm water or apply warm compresses, a hot water bottle, or a heating pad.

After a minor athletic injury, gradually reintroduce the stress of the activity until you are capable of returning to full intensity. Before returning to full exercise participation, you should have a full range of motion in your joints; normal strength and balance among your muscles; no injury-compensation movements, such as limping; and little or no pain.

To prevent injuries in the future, follow a few basic guidelines:

- Stay in condition; haphazard exercise programs invite injury.
- Warm up thoroughly before exercise.
- Use proper body mechanics when lifting objects or executing sports skills.
- Don't exercise when you're ill or overtrained (experiencing extreme fatigue because of overexercising).
- Use the proper equipment.
- Don't return to your normal exercise program until athletic injuries have healed.

You can minimize the risk of injury by following safety guidelines, using proper technique and equipment, respecting signals from your body that something may be wrong,

and treating any injuries that occur. Warm up, cool down, and drink plenty of fluids before, during, and after exercise. Use special caution in extreme heat or humidity (over 27°C or 60% humidity): Exercise slowly, rest frequently in the shade, wear clothing with ventilation, and drink plenty of fluids; slow down or stop if you begin to feel uncomfortable. During hot weather, it's best to exercise in the early morning or evening, when temperatures are lowest.

Staying with Your Program Once you have attained your desired level of fitness, you can maintain it by exercising regularly at a consistent intensity, three to five days a week. You must work at the intensity that brought you to your desired fitness level. If you don't, your body will become less fit because less is expected of it. In general, if you exercise at the same intensity over a long period, your fitness will level out and can be maintained easily.

Adapt your program to changes in environment or schedule. Don't use wet weather or a new job as an excuse to give up your fitness program. If you walk in the summer, dress appropriately and walk in the winter as well. (Exercise is usually safe even in very cold temperatures as long as you dress warmly in layers and don't stay out too long.) If you can't walk outside because of darkness or an unsafe neighbourhood, walk in a local shopping mall or on campus or join a gym and walk on a treadmill.

What if you run out of steam? Although good health is an important *reason* to exercise, it's a poor *motivator* for consistent adherence to an exercise program. A variety of specific suggestions for staying with your program are given in the box "Maintaining Your Exercise Program" in the ▣ connect Library and in the Behaviour Change Strategy box at the end of the chapter. It's a good idea to have a meaningful goal, anything from fitting into the same-size jeans you used to wear to successfully skiing down a new slope.

Varying your program is another key strategy. Some people alternate two or more activities—swimming and jogging, for example—to improve a particular component of fitness. The practice, called **cross-training**, can help prevent boredom and overuse injuries. Explore many exercise options. Consider competitive sports at the recreational level: swimming, running, racquetball, volleyball, golf, and so on. Find out how you can participate in an activity you've never done before: canoeing, hang gliding, windsurfing, backpacking. Try new activities, especially ones that you will be able to do for the rest of your life.

cross-training Participating in two or more activities to develop a particular component of fitness.

TERMS

Planning a Personal Exercise Program

BEHAVIOUR CHANGE STRATEGY

Although most people recognize the importance of incorporating exercise into their lives, many find it difficult to do. No single strategy will work for everyone, but the general steps outlined here should help you create an exercise program that fits your goals, preferences, and lifestyle. A carefully designed contract and program plan can help you convert your vague wishes into a detailed plan of action. And the strategies for program compliance outlined here and in Chapter 1 can help you enjoy and stick with your program for the rest of your life.

Step 1: Set Goals

Setting specific goals to accomplish by exercising is an important first step in a successful fitness program because it establishes the direction you want to take. Your goals might be specifically related to health, such as lowering your blood pressure and risk of heart disease, or they might relate to other aspects of your life, such as improving your tennis game or the fit of your clothes. If you can decide why you're starting to exercise, it can help you keep going.

Think carefully about your reasons for incorporating exercise into your life, and then fill in the goals portion of the Personal Fitness Contract.

Step 2: Select Activities

As discussed in the chapter, the success of your fitness program depends on the consistency of your involvement. Select activities that encourage your commitment: The right program will be its own incentive to continue; poor activity choices provide obstacles and can turn exercise into a chore. When choosing activities for your fitness program, consider the following:

- Is this activity fun? Will it hold my interest over time?

- Will this activity help me reach the goals I have set?

- Will my current fitness and skill level enable me to participate fully in this activity?

- Can I easily fit this activity into my daily schedule? Are there any special requirements (facilities, partners, equipment, etc.) that I must plan for?

- Can I afford any special costs required for equipment or facilities?

- If you have special exercise needs because of a particular health problem: Does this activity conform to those exercise needs? Will it enhance my ability to cope with my specific health problem?

Step 3: Make a Commitment

Complete your Fitness Contract and Program Plan by signing your contract and having it signed by someone who can help make you accountable for your progress. By completing a written contract, you will make a firm commitment and will be more likely to follow through until you meet your goals.

Step 4: Begin and Maintain Your Program

Start out slowly to allow your body time to adjust. Be realistic and patient—meeting your goals will take time. The following guidelines may help you start and stick with your program:

- Set aside regular periods for exercise. Choose times that fit in best with your schedule, and stick to them. Allow an adequate amount of time for warm-up, cool-down, and a shower.

- Take advantage of any opportunity for exercise that presents itself (for example, walk to class, take the stairs instead of the elevator).

- Do what you can to avoid boredom. Do stretching exercises or jumping jacks to music, or watch the evening news while riding your stationary bicycle.

- Exercise with a group that shares your goals and general level of competence.

- Vary the program. Change your activities periodically. Alter your route or distance if biking or jogging. Change racquetball partners, or find a new volleyball court.

- Establish minigoals or a point system, and work rewards into your program. Until you reach your main goals, a series of small rewards will help you stick with your program. Rewards should be things you enjoy that are easily obtainable.

Step 5: Record and Assess Your Progress

Keeping a record that notes the daily results of your program will help remind you of your ongoing commitment to your program and give you a sense of accomplishment.

Create daily and weekly program logs that you can use to track your progress. Record the activity frequency, intensity, time, and type. Keep your log handy, and fill it in immediately after each exercise session. Post it in a visible place to remind you of your activity schedule and to provide incentive for improvement.

Personal Fitness Contract

I, _____, am contracting with myself to follow an exercise program to work at the following goals. I will begin my program on _____.

FITNESS GOALS

1. _____   4. _____
2. _____   5. _____
3. _____   6. _____

PROGRAM PLAN

	Activities	Components (Check ✔)					Frequency (Check ✔)							Intensity	Time
		CRE	MS	ME	F	BC	M	Tu	W	Th	F	Sa	Su		
1.															
2.															
3.															
4.															
5.															

Note: You should conduct activities for achieving CRE goals at your target heart rate.

I agree to maintain a record of my activity, assess my progress periodically, and, if necessary, revise my goals.

Signed _____   Date _____

Witness _____   Date _____

Source: Adapted from Kusinitz, I., and M. Fine. 1995. *Your Guide to Getting Fit*, 3rd ed. Mountain View, Calif.: Mayfield.

Practise and learn online with Connect. Connect allows you to practise important skills at your own pace and on your own schedule, with 24/7 online access to an eBook, practice quizzes, interactivities, videos, study tools, additional resources, and more.

SUMMARY

• The five components of physical fitness most important to health are cardiorespiratory endurance, muscular strength, muscular endurance, flexibility, and body composition.

• Exercise improves the functioning of the heart and the ability of the cardiorespiratory system to carry oxygen to the body's tissues. It also increases the efficiency of the body's metabolism and improves body composition.

• Exercise lowers the risk of cardiovascular disease by improving blood fat levels, reducing high blood pressure, and interfering with the disease process that causes coronary artery blockage.

• Exercise reduces the risk of cancer, osteoporosis, and diabetes. It improves immune function and psychological health and helps prevent injuries and low-back pain.

• Everyone should accumulate at least 30–60 minutes per day of moderate endurance-type physical activity. Additional health and fitness benefits can be achieved through longer or more vigorous activity.

• Cardiorespiratory endurance exercises stress a large portion of the body's muscle mass. Endurance exercise should be performed three to five days per week for a total of 20–60 minutes per day. Intensity can be evaluated by measuring the heart rate.

• Warming up before exercising and cooling down afterward improve your performance and decrease your chances of injury.

• Exercises that develop muscular strength and endurance involve exerting force against a significant resistance. A strength training program for general fitness typically involves one set of 8–12 repetitions of 8–10 exercises, at least two nonconsecutive days per week.

• A good stretching program includes exercises for all the major muscle groups and joints of the body. Do a series of active, static stretches two to three days per week, ideally five to seven days per week. Hold each stretch for 15–30 seconds; do two to four repetitions. Stretch when muscles are warm.

• Instructors, equipment, and facilities should be chosen carefully to enhance enjoyment and prevent injuries.

• A well-balanced diet contains all the energy and nutrients needed to sustain a fitness program. When exercising, remember to drink enough fluids.

• Rest, ice, compression, and elevation (R-I-C-E) are treatments for muscle and joint injuries.

• A desired level of fitness can be maintained by exercising three to five days a week at a consistent intensity.

• Strategies for maintaining an exercise program over the long term include having meaningful goals, varying the program, and trying new activities.

FOR MORE INFORMATION

BOOKS

Fahey, T. 2007. *Basic Weight Training for Men and Women*, 6th ed. New York: McGraw-Hill. Weight training and plyometric exercises for fitness, weight control, and improved sports performance.

Fenton, M. 2008. *The Complete Guide to Walking, New and Revised: For Health, Weight Loss, and Fitness*. Guildford, Conn.: Lyons Press. Discusses walking as a fitness method and a way to avoid diseases, such as diabetes.

Gotlin, R. 2007. *Sport Injuries Guidebook*. Champaign, Ill.: Human Kinetics. Provides information and care instructions on many types of sports-related injuries.

Nelson, A. G., et al. 2006. *Stretching Anatomy*. Champaign, Ill.: Human Kinetics. A guide to stretching that features highly detailed illustrations of the muscles affected by each exercise.

Nieman, D. C. 2007. *Exercise Testing and Prescription. A Health-Related Approach*, 6th ed. New York: McGraw-Hill. A comprehensive discussion of the effects of exercise and exercise testing and prescription.

ORGANIZATIONS, HOTLINES, AND WEB SITES

The Internet addresses listed here were accurate at the time of publication.

American College of Sports Medicine. Provides brochures, publications, audiotapes, and videotapes on the positive effects of exercise.
   http://www.acsm.org

Canadian Fitness and Lifestyle Research Institute. Provides research findings and recommendations to increase population levels of physical activity and improve the health of all Canadians.

http://www.cflri.ca

Canadian Diabetes Association. Supports people affected by diabetes by providing information, diabetes research, education, service, and advocacy.

http://www.diabetes.ca

Canadian Society for Exercise Physiology. Provides information about the society, conferences, publications, press releases, and the physical activity guides.

http://www.csep.ca

http://www.csep.ca/guidelines

Can-Fit-Pro. Provides certification and continuing education of group fitness instructors, personal fitness trainers, and allied health professionals.

http://www.canfitpro.com

CDC Physical Activity Information. Provides information on the benefits of physical activity and suggestions for incorporating moderate physical activity into daily life.

http://www.cdc.gov/nccdphp/dnpa

Fitness Industry Council of Canada. Represents the Canadian fitness industry in pursuit of a more physically active and healthy country.

http://www.english.ficdn.ca

Heart and Stroke Foundation of Canada. Provides information about heart disease, stroke, and healthy living in Canada.

http://www.heartandstroke.ca

Mayo Clinic Healthy Living Centers: Fitness. Offers information on incorporating physical activity and exercise into your daily life.

http://www.mayoclinic.com/health/fitness/SM99999

MedlinePlus: Exercise and Physical Fitness. Provides links to news and reliable information about fitness and exercise from government agencies and professional associations.

http://www.nlm.nih.gov/medlineplus/
exerciseandphysicalfitness.html

National Institute on Drug Abuse: Anabolic Steroid Abuse. Provides information and links about the dangers of anabolic steroids.

http://www.steroidabuse.org

Public Health Agency of Canada. Provides physical activity information and tips for active living.

http://www.phac-aspc.gc.ca/hp-ps/hl-mvs/pa-ap/index-eng.php

Public Health Agency of Canada. Provides the Take the Physical Activity Readiness Questionnaire (PAR-Q).

http://www.phac-aspc.gc.ca/sth-evs/english/parq-eng.php

SmallStep.gov. Provides resources for increasing activity and improving diet through small changes in daily habits.

http://www.smallstep.gov

U.S. Federal Trade Commission: Consumer Protection—Diet, Health, and Fitness. Provides several brochures with consumer advice about purchasing exercise equipment.

http://www.ftc.gov/bcp/menus/consumer/health.shtm

World Health Organization (WHO): Move for Health. Provides information about the WHO initiative to promote increased physical activity.

http://www.who.int/moveforhealth/en/

See also the listings for Chapters 4, 5, and 7.

SELECTED BIBLIOGRAPHY

Active Healthy Kids Canada. 2010. *The Active Healthy Kids Canada Report Card on Physical Activity for Children and Youth: Physical Activity and Inactivity* (http://www.activehealthykids.ca/ReportCard/PhysicalActivityand Inactivity.aspx; retrieved April 4, 2011).

American Cancer Society. 2006. *Cancer Prevention and Early Detection: Facts and Figures 2006.* Atlanta, Ga.: American Cancer Society.

American College of Sports Medicine. 2006. *ACSM's Guidelines for Exercise Testing and Prescription,* 7th ed. Philadelphia: Lippincott Williams & Wilkins.

American College of Sports Medicine. 2006. *ACSM's Resource Manual for Guidelines for Exercise Testing and Prescription,* 5th ed. Philadelphia: Lippincott Williams & Wilkins.

American Heart Association. 2008. *Heart Disease and Stroke Statistics—2008 Update.* Dallas: American Heart Association.

Armstrong, L. E., et al. 2007. American College of Sports Medicine position stand: Exertional heat illness during training and competition. *Medicine and Science in Sports and Exercise* 39(3): 556–572.

Bertoli, S., et al. 2006. Nutritional status and dietary patterns in disabled people. *Nutrition Metabolism and Cardiovascular Diseases* 16(2): 100–112.

Brooks, G. A., et al. 2005. *Exercise Physiology: Human Bioenergetics and Its Applications,* 4th ed. New York: McGraw-Hill.

Bryan, S. N., et al. 2006. Physical activity and ethnicity: Evidence from the *Canadian Community Health Survey. Canadian Journal of Public Health* 97(4): 271–276.

Bryan, S., and P. Walsh. 2004. Physical activity and obesity in Canadian women. *BMC Women's Health* 4(1 Suppl.): S6.

Burke, L. M., et al. 2006. Energy and carbohydrate for training and recovery. *Journal of Sports Science* 24(7): 675–685.

Carnathon, M. R., M. Gulati, and P. Greenland. 2006. Prevalence and cardiovascular disease correlates of low cardiorespiratory fitness in adolescents and adults. *Journal of the American Medical Association* 294(23): 2981–2988.

Cooper, C. B. 2006. Exercise testing does not have to be complicated. *Chronic Respiratory Disease* 3(2): 107–108.

Dal Maso, L., et al. 2006. Lifetime occupational and recreational physical activity and risk of benign prostatic hyperplasia. *International Journal of Cancer* 118(10): 2632–2635.

Dishman, R. K., et al. 2006. Neurobiology of exercise. *Obesity* (Silver Spring) 14(3): 345–356.

Dugan, S. 2005. Safe exercise for women. *ACSM Fit Society Page* Winter: 1–2 (http://www.acsm.org/AM/Template.cfm?Section=Home_Page& TEMPLATE=/CM/ContentDisplay.cfm&CONTENTID=5396; retrieved April 5, 2011).

Dunn, A. L., et al. 2005. Exercise treatment for depression: Efficacy and dose response. *American Journal of Preventive Medicine* 28(1): 1–8.

Dwyer, J. J. M., et al. 2006. A provincial study of opportunities for school-based physical activity in secondary schools. *Journal of Adolescent Health* 39: 80–86.

Fahey, T. D., P. M. Insel, and W. T. Roth. 2009. *Fit and Well: Core Concepts and Labs in Physical Fitness and Wellness,* 8th ed. New York: McGraw-Hill.

Fenicchia, L. M., et al. 2004. Influence of resistance exercise training on glucose control in women with type 2 diabetes. *Metabolism* 53(3): 284–289.

Franco, O. H., et al. 2005. Effects of physical activity on life expectancy with cardiovascular disease. *Archives of Internal Medicine* 165(20): 2355–2360.

Gunter, M. J., and M. F. Leitzmann. 2006. Obesity and colorectal cancer: Epidemiology, mechanisms and candidate genes. *Journal of Nutritional Biochemistry* 17(3): 145–156.

Hambrecht, R., and S. Gielen. 2005. Essay: Hunter-gatherer to sedentary lifestyle. *Lancet* 366(1 Suppl.): S60–S61.

Hart, L. 2006. Exercise therapy for nonspecific low-back pain: A meta-analysis. *Clinical Journal of Sports Medicine* 16(2): 189–190.

Haskell, W. L., et al. 2007. Physical activity and public health: Updated recommendations for adults from the American College of Sports Medicine and the American Heart Association. *Circulation* 116(9): 1081–1093.

John, E. M., P. L. Horn-Ross, and J. Koo. 2004. Lifetime physical activity and breast cancer risk in a multiethnic population. *Cancer Epidemiology, Biomarkers & Prevention* 12(11 Pt. 1): 1143–1152.

Katzmarzyk, P. T., N. Gledhill, and R. J. Shephard. 2000. The economic burden of physical inactivity in Canada. *Canadian Medical Association Journal* 163(11): 1435–1440.

Kelly, C. W. 2005. Commitment to Health Scale. *Journal of Nursing Measurement* 13(3): 219–229.

Lakka, T. A., and C. Bouchard. 2005. Physical activity, obesity and cardiovascular diseases. *Handbook of Experimental Pharmacology* 2005(170): 137–163.

Larson, E. B., et al. 2006. Exercise is associated with reduced risk for incident dementia among persons 65 years of age and older. *Annals of Internal Medicine* 144(2): 73–81.

LaRoche, D. P., and D. A. Connolly. 2006. Effects of stretching on passive muscle tension and response to eccentric exercise. *American Journal of Sports Medicine* 34(6): 1000–1007.

Nattiv, A., et al. 2007. American College of Sports Medicine position stand: The female athlete triad. *Medicine and Science in Sports and Exercise* 39(10): 1867–1882.

Nelson, M. E., et al. 2007. Physical activity and public health in older adults: Recommendations from the American College of Sports Medicine and the American Heart Association. *Medicine and Science in Sports and Exercise* 39(8): 1435–1445.

Pescatello, L. S., et al. 2004. American College of Sports Medicine position stand: Exercise and hypertension. *Medicine and Science in Sports and Exercise* 36(3): 533–553.

Physical Activity Guidelines Advisory Committee. 2008. *Physical Activity Guidelines Advisory Committee Report, 2008.* Washington, D.C.: U.S. Department of Health and Human Services.

Public Health Agency of Canada. 2007. *Trends & Impact: The Basis for Investment Decisions* (http://www.phac-aspc.gc.ca/alw-vat/trends-tendances/index-eng.php; retrieved April 4, 2011).

Sawka, M. N., et al. 2005. Human water needs. *Nutritional Reviews* 63(6 Pt. 2): S30–S39.

Sawka, M. N., et al. 2007. American College of Sports Medicine position stand: Exercise and fluid replacement. *Medicine and Science in Sports and Exercise* 39(2): 377–390.

Shehab, R., et al. 2006. Pre-exercise stretching and sports-related injuries: Knowledge, attitudes and practices. *Clinical Journal of Sports Medicine* 16(3): 228–231.

Tremblay, M. S., et al. 2010. Fitness of Canadian children and youth: Results from the 2007–2009 Canadian Health Measures Survey. *Health Reports* 21(1) (http://www.statcan.gc.ca/pub/82-003-x/2010001/article/11065-eng.pdf; retrieved April 5, 2011).

Wheeler, G. 2005. Active living and people with disabilities: The broader context of Access. *Wellspring* 16(4) (http://www.centre4activeliving.ca/publications/wellspring/2005/aug-disabilities.pdf; retrieved April 5, 2011).

CARDIOVASCULAR HEALTH

LOOKING AHEAD >>>>>

AFTER READING THIS CHAPTER, YOU SHOULD BE ABLE TO

- List the major components of the cardiovascular system and describe how blood is pumped and circulated throughout the body

- Describe the controllable and uncontrollable risk factors associated with cardiovascular disease

- Discuss the major forms of cardiovascular disease and how they develop

- List the steps you can take to lower your personal risk of developing cardiovascular disease

TEST YOUR KNOWLEDGE

1. Reducing the amount of cholesterol you eat is the most important dietary change you can make to improve your blood cholesterol levels.
   True or false?

2. Women are about as likely to die of cardiovascular disease as they are to die of breast cancer.
   True or false?

3. Which type of exercise improves cardiovascular health?
   a. weight training
   b. aerobic activities
   c. both

4. Healthy teenagers have no signs of cardiovascular disease.
   True or false?

5. Which of the following foods would be a good choice for promoting heart health?
   a. whole grains
   b. salmon
   c. bananas

ANSWERS

1. **FALSE.** Limiting your intake of saturated and trans fats, which promote the production of cholesterol by the liver, is the key dietary change for improving blood cholesterol levels; dietary cholesterol has much less of an effect on blood cholesterol.

2. **FALSE.** Cardiovascular disease kills far more. Among Canadian women, nearly 1 in 3 deaths is due to cardiovascular disease and about 1 in 25 is due to breast cancer.

3. **C.** Both aerobic exercise and strength training significantly improve cardiovascular health.

4. **FALSE.** Autopsy studies of young trauma victims show that narrowing of the arteries that supply the heart with blood begins in adolescence in many people.

5. **ALL THREE.** Whole grains (such as whole wheat, oatmeal, rye, barley, and brown rice), foods with omega-3 fatty acids (salmon), and foods high in potassium and low in sodium (bananas) all improve cardiovascular health.

cardiovascular disease (CVD) affects about 120,000 Canadians and together, heart disease and stroke surpass cancer as the leading cause of death, claiming one life every seven minutes. Heart attacks and strokes are the second and third leading causes of death in Canada, respectively, making them the most common life-threatening manifestations of CVD. Though we typically think of CVD as primarily affecting men and older adults, heart attack is the number-one killer of Canadian women, and an increasing number of fatal heart attacks occur in people under age 65.

CVD is largely due to our way of life. Too many Canadians eat an unhealthy diet, are overweight and sedentary, smoke, manage stress ineffectively, have uncontrolled high blood pressure or high cholesterol levels, and don't know the signs of CVD. Not all the risk factors for CVD are controllable—for example, the older you are, the greater your risk for CVD. But many key risk factors can be treated or modified, and you can reduce your risk for CVD.

This chapter introduces the workings of the cardiovascular system, explains CVD and its risks, and shows you how to keep your heart healthy for life.

THE CARDIOVASCULAR SYSTEM

The **cardiovascular system** consists of the heart and blood vessels (Figure 7.1); together, they move blood throughout the body.

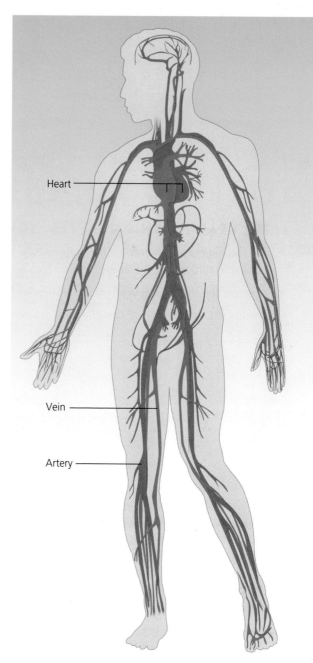

Heart

Vein

Artery

FIGURE 7.1   The cardiovascular system.

The Heart

The heart is a four-chambered, fist-sized muscle located just beneath the sternum (breastbone). It pumps deoxygenated (oxygen-poor) blood to the lungs and delivers oxygenated (oxygen-rich) blood to the rest of the body. Blood actually travels through two separate circulatory systems: The right side of the heart pumps blood to the lungs in what is called **pulmonary circulation**, and the left side pumps blood through the rest of the body in **systemic circulation**.

The following steps describe the path blood follows as it travels through the cardiovascular system (Figure 7.2):

1 Waste-carrying, oxygen-poor blood enters the right atrium from the superior and inferior venae cavae.

Pulmonary artery

Aorta

Left lung

3 In the lungs, blood picks up oxygen and discards carbon dioxide; it then flows through the pulmonary veins into the left atrium.

Superior vena cava

Right lung

Right atrium

Pulmonary vein

Left atrium

4 Oxygen-rich blood flows from the left atrium into the left ventricle; from there it is pumped through the aorta into the rest of the body's blood vessels.

2 Blood flows from the right atrium into the right ventricle; from there, it is pumped through the pulmonary arteries into the lungs.

Left ventricle

Right ventricle

Inferior vena cava

FIGURE 7.2 Circulation in the heart.

1. Waste-laden, oxygen-poor blood travels through large vessels, called **venae cavae**, into the heart's right upper chamber, called the **atrium**.

2. After the right atrium fills, it contracts and pumps blood into the heart's right lower chamber, called the **ventricle**.

3. When the right ventricle is full, it contracts and pumps blood through the pulmonary artery into the lungs.

4. In the lungs, blood picks up oxygen and discards carbon dioxide.

5. The cleaned, oxygenated blood flows from the lungs through the pulmonary veins into the heart's left atrium.

6. After the left atrium fills, it contracts and pumps blood into the left ventricle.

7. When the left ventricle is full, it pumps blood through the **aorta**—the body's largest artery—for distribution to the rest of the body's blood vessels.

The period of the heart's contraction is called **systole**; the period of relaxation is called **diastole**. During systole, the atria contract first, pumping blood into the ventricles.

A fraction of a second later, the ventricles contract, pumping blood to the lungs and the body. During diastole, blood flows into the heart.

Blood pressure, the force exerted by blood on the walls of the blood vessels, is created by the pumping action of the heart; blood pressure is greater during systole than during diastole.

The heartbeat—the split-second sequence of contractions of the heart's four chambers—is controlled by nerve impulses. These signals originate in a bundle of specialized cells in the right atrium called the *sinoatrial node*, or *pacemaker*. Unless it is speeded up or slowed down by the brain in response to stimuli, such as danger or the tissues' need for more oxygen, the heart produces nerve impulses at a steady rate.

The Blood Vessels

Blood vessels are classified by size and function. **Veins** carry blood to the heart. **Arteries** carry blood away from the heart. Veins have thin walls, but arteries have thick elastic walls that enable them to expand and relax with the volume of blood being pumped through them.

After leaving the heart, the aorta branches into smaller and smaller vessels. The smallest arteries branch still further

Aorta

Pulmonary artery

Left atrium

Left coronary artery

Left ventricle

Superior vena cava

Right atrium

Right coronary artery

Right ventricle

Inferior vena cava

FIGURE 7.3   Blood supply to the heart.

QUESTIONS FOR CRITICAL THINKING AND REFLECTION
How often do you think about the health of your heart? Are there certain situations, for example, that make you aware of your heart rate, or make you wonder how strong your heart is?

into **capillaries**, tiny vessels only one cell thick. The capillaries deliver oxygen and nutrient-rich blood to the tissues and pick up oxygen-poor, waste-laden blood. From the capillaries, this blood empties into small veins (*venules*) and then into larger veins that return it to the heart to repeat the cycle.

Blood pumped through the heart does not reach the cells of the heart, so the organ has its own network of arteries, veins, and capillaries (Figure 7.3, above). Two large vessels, the right

A 68-kilogram person has about **five litres** of blood, which circulates about once each minute.

—CDC, 2007

and left **coronary arteries**, branch off the aorta and supply the heart muscle with oxygenated blood. Blockage of a coronary artery is a leading cause of heart attacks.

RISK FACTORS FOR CARDIOVASCULAR DISEASE

Researchers have identified a variety of factors associated with an increased risk of developing CVD. They are grouped into two categories: major risk factors and contributing risk factors. Some risk factors are linked to controllable aspects of lifestyle and can therefore be changed. Others are beyond your control.

Major Risk Factors That Can Be Changed

Six major risk factors for CVD can be changed: tobacco use, high blood pressure, unhealthy blood cholesterol levels, physical inactivity, overweight and obesity, and diabetes.

Tobacco Use   About one in seven (15%) deaths from CVD is attributable to smoking. In 2007, an estimated 5.2 million Canadians were tobacco users, including 343,000 university and college students. Smoking contributes to about 37,000 deaths annually in Canada,

11,000 of which are CVD related. People who smoke a pack of cigarettes a day have twice the risk of heart attack as nonsmokers; smoking two or more packs a day triples the risk. When smokers have heart attacks, they are two to three times as likely as nonsmokers to die from them. Cigarette smoking also doubles the risk of stroke.

Smoking harms the cardiovascular system in several ways:

- It damages the lining of arteries.
- It reduces the level of high-density lipoproteins (HDL), or good cholesterol.
- It raises the levels of triglycerides and low-density lipoproteins (LDL), or bad cholesterol.
- Nicotine increases blood pressure and heart rate.
- The carbon monoxide in cigarette smoke displaces oxygen in the blood, reducing the oxygen available to the body.
- Smoking causes **platelets** to stick together in the blood stream, leading to clotting.
- Smoking speeds the development of fatty deposits in the arteries.

You don't have to smoke to be affected. The risk of death from coronary heart disease increases up to 30% among those exposed to environmental tobacco smoke (ETS) at home or at work. Researchers estimate that about 6300 non-smokers in Canada die from heart disease each year as a result of exposure to ETS. (See Chapter 16 for more information on smoking.)

High Blood Pressure   High blood pressure, or **hypertension**, is a risk factor for many forms of cardiovascular disease, including heart attacks and strokes, and is itself considered a form of CVD.

Blood pressure, the force exerted by the blood on the vessel walls, is created by the pumping action of the heart. High blood pressure occurs when too much force is exerted against the walls of the arteries. Many factors affect blood pressure, such as exercise or excitement. Short periods of high blood pressure are normal, but chronic high blood pressure is a health risk.

Blood pressure is measured with a stethoscope and an instrument called a *sphygmomanometer*. It is expressed as two numbers—for example, 120 over 80—and measured in millimetres of mercury (mm Hg). The first number is the systolic blood pressure; the second is the diastolic blood pressure. Research has found that CVD risk increases when blood pressure rises above 120 over 80. According to Hypertension Canada, although it is important for most people's blood pressure to be less than 140 over 90, people with diabetes or kidney disease should make sure their blood pressure is less than 130 over 80. See Table 7.1 below for a more detailed breakdown of blood pressure categories in adults.

CAUSES   High blood pressure results from an increased output of blood by the heart or from increased resistance to blood flow in the arteries. The latter condition can be caused by constriction of smooth muscle surrounding the arteries or by **atherosclerosis**, a disease process that causes arteries to become clogged and narrowed. (Atherosclerosis is discussed in detail later in this chapter.) High blood pressure also scars and hardens arteries, making them less elastic and further increasing blood pressure. When a person has high blood pressure, the heart must work harder than normal to force blood through the narrowed and stiffened arteries, straining both the heart and the arteries. Eventually, the strained heart weakens and tends to enlarge, which weakens it even more.

Table 7.1	Blood Pressure Classification for Healthy Adults		
Category[a]	Systolic (mm Hg)		Diastolic (mm Hg)
Normal[b]	below 120	and	below 80
Prehypertension	120–139	or	80–89
Hypertension[c]			
Stage 1	140–159	or	90–99
Stage 2	160 and above	or	100 and above

Source: The Seventh Report of the Joint National Committee on Prevention, Detection, Evaluation, and Treatment of High Blood Pressure. 2003. Bethesda, Md.: National Heart, Lung, and Blood Institute. National Institutes of Health (NIH Publication No. 03-5233); Hypertension Canada. 2010. *My BP* (http://hypertension.ca/bpc/wp-content/uploads/2010/03/Brochure_2010.pdf; retrieved May 19, 2011).

[a]When systolic and diastolic pressure fall into different categories, the higher category should be used to classify blood pressure status.

[b]The risk of death from heart attack and stroke begins to rise when blood pressure is above 115/75.

[c]Based on the average of two or more readings taken at different physician visits. In persons over 50, systolic blood pressure greater than 140 is a much more significant CVD risk factor than diastolic blood pressure.

TERMS

capillaries   Very small blood vessels that serve to exchange oxygen and nutrients between the blood and the tissues.

coronary arteries   A system of arteries branching from the aorta that provides blood to the heart muscle.

platelets   Cell fragments in the blood that are necessary for the formation of blood clots.

hypertension   Sustained abnormally high blood pressure.

atherosclerosis   A form of CVD in which the inner layers of artery walls are made thick and irregular by plaque deposits; arteries become narrow, and blood supply is reduced.

HEALTH RISKS High blood pressure is often called a silent killer, because it usually has no symptoms. A person may have high blood pressure for years without realizing it. But during that time, it damages vital organs and increases the risk of heart attack, congestive heart failure, stroke, kidney failure, and blindness. In about 90% of people with high blood pressure, the cause is unknown. This type of high blood pressure is called primary (or *essential*) *hypertension* and is probably due to a mixture of genetic and environmental factors, including obesity, stress, excessive alcohol intake, inactivity, and a high-fat, high-salt diet. In the remaining 10% of people, the condition is caused by an underlying illness and is referred to as *secondary hypertension*.

PREVALENCE Hypertension is common. About 20% of Canadian adults have hypertension, but only 66% of these individuals have it controlled. Another 20% of Canadians have prehypertension. The incidence of high blood pressure increases with age; however, it can occur among children and young adults, and women sometimes develop hypertension during pregnancy (blood pressure usually returns to normal following the pregnancy). High blood pressure is two to three times more common in women taking oral contraceptives, especially in obese and older women; this risk increases with the duration of use. The rate of hypertension is much higher among First Nations Canadian adults, and those of African and South Asian descent, compared with the general population,

TREATMENT Primary hypertension cannot be cured, but it can be controlled. In 2010 a study by researchers with Statistics Canada found that hypertension control has improved considerably over the last two decades. Because hypertension has no early warning signs, it's crucial to have your blood pressure tested at least once every two years (more often if you have other CVD risk factors). In fact, experts now advise that anyone with hypertension or prehypertension monitor their own blood pressure several times each week. Self-monitoring is easy to do, using a low-cost digital home blood pressure monitor. Follow your physician's advice about lifestyle changes and medication.

Lifestyle changes are recommended for everyone with prehypertension and hypertension. In fact, the 2010 Canadian Hypertension Education Program Recommendations stress lifestyle modification as the cornerstone for the prevention and control of hypertension. The specific changes they recommend include reaching a healthy weight, exercising regularly, eating a healthy diet, eating less salt, quitting smoking and avoiding second-hand smoke, and drinking alcohol only moderately. Nutrition experts recommend

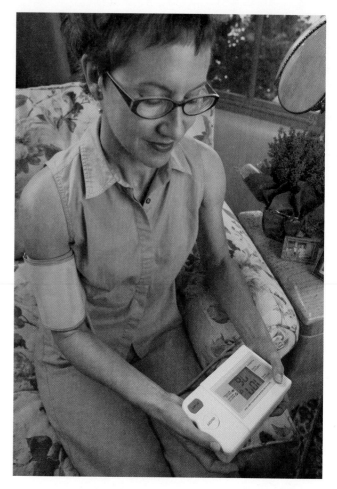

Low-cost, battery-powered home blood pressure monitors make it easy to check and track your blood pressure at home. People who plan to monitor their blood pressure at home should first see their doctor for a baseline reading and specific instructions.

eating more fruits, vegetables, and whole grains and increasing potassium and fibre intake (see Chapter 5). Even small increases in fruit and vegetable intake can create measurable drops in blood pressure.

Sodium restriction is also helpful for most people with hypertension. People with or at risk for hypertension should aim to consume no more than 1500 milligrams of sodium per day. In fact, 1500 milligrams is the amount considered adequate for all adults, and more isn't better. Most Canadians consume more than 3000 milligrams of sodium daily, which is well above Health Canada's recommended maximum of 2300 milligrams (about five millilitres or one teaspoon of salt) per day. Adequate potassium intake is also important. The recommended intake is 4.7 grams per day, which should be obtained through food. Supplements should be taken only when recommended by a physician; excessively high levels of potassium can be lethal.

For people whose blood pressure isn't adequately controlled with lifestyle changes, medication is prescribed. Many different types of antihypertensive drugs are available; the right one lowers blood pressure effectively with few side effects.

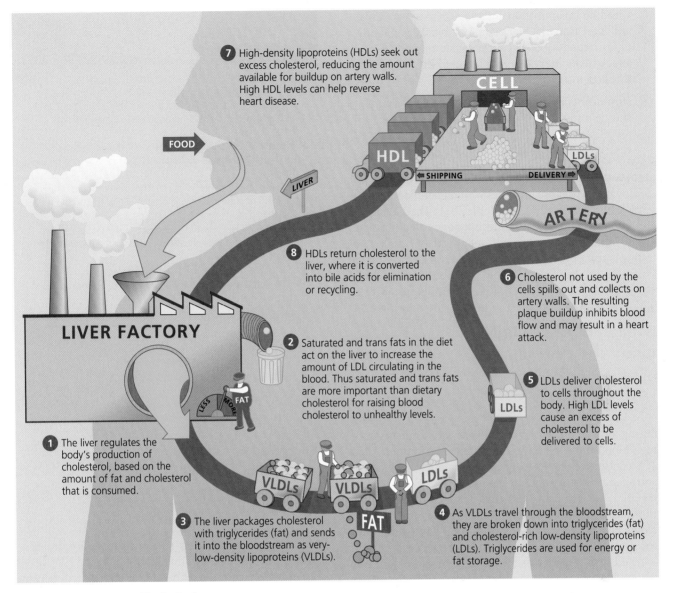

7 High-density lipoproteins (HDLs) seek out excess cholesterol, reducing the amount available for buildup on artery walls. High HDL levels can help reverse heart disease.

FOOD

CELL

HDL

SHIPPING   DELIVERY

LDLs

ARTERY

LIVER

8 HDLs return cholesterol to the liver, where it is converted into bile acids for elimination or recycling.

6 Cholesterol not used by the cells spills out and collects on artery walls. The resulting plaque buildup inhibits blood flow and may result in a heart attack.

LIVER FACTORY

LESS MORE FAT

2 Saturated and trans fats in the diet act on the liver to increase the amount of LDL circulating in the blood. Thus saturated and trans fats are more important than dietary cholesterol for raising blood cholesterol to unhealthy levels.

5 LDLs deliver cholesterol to cells throughout the body. High LDL levels cause an excess of cholesterol to be delivered to cells.

LDLs

1 The liver regulates the body's production of cholesterol, based on the amount of fat and cholesterol that is consumed.

VLDLs   VLDLs   LDLs

FAT

3 The liver packages cholesterol with triglycerides (fat) and sends it into the bloodstream as very-low-density lipoproteins (VLDLs).

4 As VLDLs travel through the bloodstream, they are broken down into triglycerides (fat) and cholesterol-rich low-density lipoproteins (LDLs). Triglycerides are used for energy or fat storage.

FIGURE 7.4   Cholesterol in the body.

Recent research has shed new light on the importance of lowering blood pressure to improve cardiovascular health. Death rates from CVD begin to rise when blood pressure is above 115 over 75, well below the traditional 140 over 90 cut-off for hypertension. People with blood pressure in the prehypertension range are at increased risk of heart attack and stroke and at significant risk of developing full-blown hypertension.

High Cholesterol   Cholesterol is a fatty, wax-like substance that circulates through the bloodstream and is an important component of cell membranes, sex hormones, vitamin D, the fluid that coats the lungs, and the protective sheaths around nerves. Adequate cholesterol is essential for the proper functioning of the body. Excess cholesterol, however, can clog arteries and increase the risk of CVD. Your liver manufactures cholesterol; you also get cholesterol from the foods you eat.

GOOD VERSUS BAD CHOLESTEROL   Cholesterol is carried in the blood in protein-lipid packages called **lipoproteins** (Figure 7.4, above). Two types of lipoproteins influence the risk of heart disease:

- As discussed in Chapter 5, *low-density lipoproteins (LDLs)* shuttle cholesterol from the liver to the organs and tissues that require it. LDL is known as bad cholesterol because if there is more than the body can use, the excess is deposited in the blood vessels. LDL that accumulates and becomes trapped in artery walls may be oxidized by free radicals,

lipoproteins   Protein-and-lipid substances in the blood that carry fats and cholesterol; classified according to size, density, and chemical composition.

TERMS

speeding inflammation and damage to artery walls and increasing the likelihood of a blockage. If coronary arteries are blocked, the result may be a heart attack; if an artery carrying blood to the brain is blocked, a stroke may occur.

- *High-density lipoproteins (HDLs)*, or *good cholesterol*, shuttle unused cholesterol back to the liver for recycling. By removing cholesterol from blood vessels, HDL helps protect against atherosclerosis.

RECOMMENDED BLOOD CHOLESTEROL LEVELS The risk for cardiovascular disease increases with higher blood cholesterol levels, especially LDL (Table 7.2). The College of Family Physicians of Canada recommends all adults over age 20 talk with their physician about whether cholesterol testing is appropriate for them. With no risk factors, routine screening typically beings at age 40 for men, and 50 for women (earlier if they are post-menopausal). The Heart and Stroke Foundation of Canada also suggests cholesterol testing for anybody with heart disease, stroke, diabetes, or high blood pressure; a waist circumference of more than 102 centimetres for men or 88 centimetres for women; and a family history of heart disease or stroke. The recommended test typically measures total cholesterol, LDL cholesterol, HDL cholesterol, and triglycerides (another blood fat). In general, high LDL, total cholesterol, and triglyceride levels combined with low HDL levels, are associated with a higher risk for CVD. You can reduce this risk by lowering LDL, total cholesterol, and triglycerides. Raising HDL is important because a high HDL level seems to offer protection from CVD even in cases where total cholesterol is high. This seems to be especially true for women.

As shown in Table 7.2, LDL levels below 3 mmol/L (millimoles per litre) and HDL levels above 1.0 mmol/L are desirable. The ratio of total cholesterol to HDL (expressed as HDL-C) is also important, and depending on a person's level of risk, the guidelines for this ratio vary. An estimated 10 million Canadian adults have total cholesterol levels higher than are recommended.

The CVD risk associated with elevated cholesterol levels also depends on other factors. For example, an above-optimal level of LDL would be of more concern for an individual who also smokes and has high blood pressure than for someone without these additional CVD risk factors, and it is especially a concern for people with diabetes.

BENEFITS OF CONTROLLING CHOLESTEROL People can cut their heart attack risk by about 2% for every 1% that they reduce their total blood cholesterol levels. People who lower their total cholesterol from about 6.2 to 5.2 mmol/L,

Table 7.2	Cholesterol and Triglyceride Guidelines

Cholesterol Guidelines

- An LDL cholesterol level of less than 3.0 mmol/L is best.
- An HDL above 1.0 mmol/L is best; an HDL cholesterol level of less than 1.0 mmol/L means you're at higher risk for heart disease.
- *If your risk is low*, your LDL cholesterol should be less than 5.0 mmol/L and total cholesterol HDL-C ratio should be less than 6.
- *If your risk is moderate*, your LDL cholesterol should be less than 3.5 mmol/L and total cholesterol HDL-C ratio should be less than 5.
- *If your risk is high*, your LDL cholesterol should be less than 2.0 mmol/L and total cholesterol HDL-C ratio should be less than 4.
- *If you have diabetes*, your LDL should be less than 2.0 mmol/L.
- *If you've already had a heart attack*, your LDL needs to be less than 2.0 mmol/L.

Triglycerides Guidelines

- Less than 1.7 mmol/L is desirable.
- 1.7–2.2 mmol/L is considered borderline high.
- 2.3–5.6 mmol/L is considered high.
- More than 5.6 mmol/L is considered very high.

Sources: The College of Family Physicians of Canada. 2007. *Cholesterol: What You Can Do to Lower Your Level* (http://www.cfpc.ca/ProjectAssets/Templates/Resource.aspx?id=1364&rlangType=4105; retrieved April 6, 2011), used with permission of The College of Family Physicians of Canada; Mayo Clinic. 2010. *Cholesterol Levels: What Numbers Should You Aim For?* (http://www.mayoclinic.com/health/cholesterol-levels/CL00001; retrieved April 6, 2011).

for example, reduce their risk of heart attack by 40%. Studies indicate that lowering LDL and raising HDL levels not only reduces the likelihood that arteries will become clogged but may also reverse deposits on artery walls.

Your primary goal should be to reduce your LDL to healthy levels. Important dietary changes for reducing LDL levels include increasing fibre intake and substituting unsaturated for saturated and trans fats. Decreasing saturated and trans fats is particularly important because they promote the production of cholesterol by the liver. Exercising regularly and eating more fruits, vegetables, fish, and whole grains also help. Many experts believe cholesterol-lowering foods may be most effective when eaten in combination, rather than separately. You can raise your HDL levels by exercising regularly, losing weight if you are overweight, quitting smoking, and altering the amount and type of fat you consume.

See Chapter 5 for detailed information on nutrition and guidelines for heart-healthy eating.

Physical Inactivity As discussed in Chapter 6, many Canadians are very sedentary, so much so that they are at high risk for developing CVD. Exercise is thought to be the closest thing we have to a magic bullet against heart disease. It lowers CVD risk by helping to decrease blood pressure and resting heart rate, increase HDL levels, maintain desirable weight, improve the condition of blood vessels, and prevent or control diabetes. One study found that women who accumulated at least three hours of brisk walking each week cut their risk of heart attack and stroke by more than 50%.

See Chapter 6 for detailed explanations of the benefits of physical activity and for help in creating your own exercise plan.

Obesity   As your weight increases, your risk of CVD increases. The risk of death from CVD is two to three times as likely in obese people (BMI ≥ 30) as it is in lean people (BMI 18.5–24.9), and for every five-unit increment of BMI, a person's risk of death from coronary heart disease increases by 30%. BMI at age 18 predicts mortality from CVD—the higher your BMI at age 18, the more likely you are to eventually die from CVD. Maintaining a healthy weight is also important. Researchers found that middle-aged women who had gained 10 kilograms or more since age 18 had a significantly higher risk of subsequent death from CVD than those who were able to maintain their weight over time.

As explained in Chapter 4, excess body fat is strongly associated with hypertension, high cholesterol levels, insulin resistance, diabetes, physical inactivity, and increasing age. It is also associated with endothelial cell dysfunction and increased inflammatory markers (discussed later in this chapter). **Endothelial cells** line the inside of arteries, including the coronary arteries, and they help regulate blood flow to the heart and keep platelets and other cells from sticking to artery walls. When the endothelial cells are healthy, the coronary arteries dilate (widen) when the heart needs more blood, but when the cells are dysfunctional, the coronary arteries instead constrict, limiting blood flow to the heart. With excess weight, there is also more blood to pump and the heart has to work harder. This causes chronically elevated pressures within the heart chambers that can lead to ventricular **hypertrophy** (enlargement), and eventually the heart muscle can start to fail.

Physical activity and physical fitness have a strong positive influence on cardiovascular health in those who are overweight and obese. People who are obese but have at least moderate cardiorespiratory fitness may have lower rates of cardiovascular disease than their normal-weight but unfit peers. For someone who is overweight, even modest weight reduction—5%–10% of body weight—can reduce CVD risk.

Diabetes   As described in Chapter 4, diabetes is a disorder characterized by elevated blood glucose levels because of an insufficient supply or inadequate action of insulin. Diabetes doubles the risk of CVD for men and triples the risk for women. The most common cause of death in adults with diabetes is CVD, and they usually die at younger ages than people without diabetes. There is an estimated loss of 5–10 years of life in those with diabetes.

People with diabetes have higher rates of other CVD risk factors, including hypertension, obesity, and unhealthy blood lipid levels (typically, high triglyceride levels and low HDL levels). The elevated blood glucose and insulin levels that occur in diabetes can damage the endothelial cells that line the arteries, making them more vulnerable to atherosclerosis; people with diabetes also often have platelet and blood coagulation abnormalities that increase the risk of heart attacks and strokes. People with pre-diabetes also face a significantly increased risk of CVD.

The number of people with diabetes and pre-diabetes continues to climb and is closely linked to obesity. It is estimated that for every kilogram increase in weight, the risk of diabetes increases by approximately 9%. The increase in prevalence of type 2 diabetes over the past decade has been among Canadians of all age groups, and with a particularly alarming increase among children and adolescents. Children who are diagnosed with diabetes typically develop complications in their twenties or thirties.

Complications of diabetes mainly affect the arteries. When the larger arteries are affected, all forms of CVD result, including heart attacks, strokes, and peripheral vascular disease. Having diabetes is considered to be a heart disease risk equivalent, meaning that your CVD morbidity and mortality risk is the same as if you already had coronary artery disease (CAD). People with diabetes who also have CAD fare even worse; they have accelerated atherosclerosis and benefit less from common forms of treatment than people without diabetes.

In addition, evidence suggests that after a heart attack, the risk of diabetes steeply rises. A recent study demonstrated that within 3.5 years after a heart attack, one-third of patients without diabetes will develop diabetes or pre-diabetes. Thus, heart disease and elevated blood glucose are clearly linked, with each being a risk factor for the other.

Routine screening for diabetes is not currently recommended unless a person has symptoms of diabetes or other CVD risk factors. In people with pre-diabetes, a healthy diet and exercise are more effective than medication at preventing diabetes. For people with diabetes, a healthy diet, exercise, and care-

endothelial cells   Cells lining the inside of arteries; they help regulate blood flow and prevent platelets from sticking.

hypertrophy   Abnormal enlargement of an organ secondary to an increase in cell size.

TERMS

Blood glucose monitoring is important in managing diabetes and its associated risks.

ful control of glucose levels are recommended to decrease chances of developing complications. Even people whose diabetes is under control face a high risk of CVD, so control of other risk factors is critical.

Contributing Risk Factors That Can Be Changed

Other factors that can be changed have been identified as contributing to CVD risk, including triglyceride levels and psychological and social factors.

High Triglyceride Levels   Like cholesterol, **triglycerides** are blood fats that are obtained from food and manufactured by the body. High triglyceride levels are a reliable predictor of heart disease, especially if associated with other risk factors, such as low HDL levels, obesity, and diabetes. Factors contributing to elevated triglyceride levels include excess body fat, physical inactivity, cigarette smoking, type 2 diabetes, excess alcohol intake, very high

TERMS

triglyceride   A type of blood fat that can be a predictor of heart disease.

carbohydrate diets, and certain diseases and medications. Much of the picture regarding triglycerides remains unclear, however. Studies have yet to show whether lowering triglyceride levels will actually decrease heart disease. Elevated triglyceride levels are most often seen in people with other lipid abnormalities; and the lifestyle modifications that help lower cholesterol also help decrease triglycerides, making it difficult to identify any potential independent benefit of lowering triglyceride levels.

A full lipid profile should include testing and evaluation of triglyceride levels (see Table 7.2). For people with border-line high triglyceride levels, increased physical activity, reduced intake of added sugars, and weight reduction can help bring levels down into the healthy range; for people with high triglyceride levels, drug therapy may be recommended. Being moderate in the use of alcohol and quitting smoking are also important.

Psychological and Social Factors   Many of the psychological and social factors that influence other areas of wellness are also important risk factors for CVD. The cardiovascular system is affected by both sudden, acute episodes of mental stress and the more chronic, underlying emotions of anger, anxiety, and depression.

STRESS   Excessive stress can strain the heart and blood vessels over time and contribute to CVD. When you experience stress, stress hormones activate the sympathetic nervous system. As described in Chapter 3, the sympathetic nervous system causes the fight-or-flight response; this response increases heart rate and blood pressure so that more blood is distributed to the heart and other muscles in anticipation of physical activity. Blood glucose concentrations and cholesterol also increase to provide a source of energy, and the platelets become activated so that they will be more likely to clot in case of injury. If you are healthy, you can tolerate the cardiovascular responses that take place during stress, but if you already have CVD, stress can lead to adverse outcomes, such as abnormal heart rhythms (arrhythmias), heart attacks, and sudden cardiac death.

Because avoiding all stress is impossible, having healthy mechanisms to cope with it is your best defence. Instead of adopting unhealthy habits, such as smoking or over-eating, use healthier coping strategies, such as exercising, getting enough sleep, and talking to others.

CHRONIC HOSTILITY AND ANGER   Certain traits in the hard-driving type A personality—hostility, cynicism, and anger—are associated with increased risk of heart disease. Men prone to anger have two to three times the heart attack risk of calmer men and are much more likely to develop CVD at young ages. In a 10-year study of young adults ages 18–30 years, those with high hostility levels were more than twice as likely to develop coronary artery calcification (a marker of early atherosclerosis) as those with low hostility levels. See the box "Anger, Hostility, and Heart Disease" on p. 220 for more information.

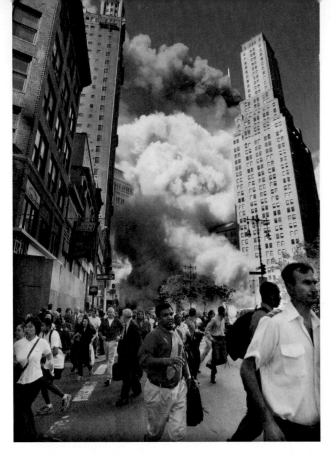
Acute stress is associated with heart rhythm problems and deaths. The rate of arrhythmias in patients with underlying heart disease increased in North America in the month after the September 11, 2001, terrorist attacks in New York City.

SUPPRESSING PSYCHOLOGICAL DISTRESS Consistently suppressing anger and other negative emotions may also be hazardous to a healthy heart. People who hide psychological distress appear to have higher rates of heart disease than people who experience similar distress but share it with others. People with such type D personalities tend to be pessimistic, negative, and unhappy and to suppress these feelings. This type D trait may have physical effects, or it may lead to social isolation and poor communication with physicians.

DEPRESSION Depression appears to increase the risk of CVD in healthy people, and it definitely increases the risk of adverse cardiac events in those who already have heart disease. You do not need to have a major depressive disorder to be affected: For each depressive symptom you have, the risk seems to increase in a linear fashion (see Chapter 2 for symptoms of depression).

Depression is common in people with coronary heart disease (CHD), and patients who are depressed tend to have worse outcomes than those who are not. Up to a third of patients experience major depression within one year of having a heart attack, and those who are depressed after having a heart attack are more likely to have another heart attack or die of a cardiac cause. Even in those with CHD who have not had a recent cardiac event, up to 20%

have depression, and this number may be even higher in women. Major depressive disorder at the time of treatment for coronary artery disease is associated with both short-term and long-term complications, including subsequent heart attack and death.

The relationship between depression and CHD is complex and not fully understood. Depressed people may be more likely to smoke or be sedentary. They may not consistently take prescribed medications, and they may not cope well with having an illness or undergoing a medical procedure. Depression also causes physiological changes; for example, it elevates basal levels of stress hormones, which, as described earlier, induce a variety of stress-related responses.

ANXIETY There is evidence to suggest that chronic anxiety and anxiety disorders (such as phobias and panic disorder) are associated with up to a threefold increased risk of coronary heart disease, heart attack, and sudden cardiac death. There is also some evidence that, similar to people with depression, people with anxiety are more likely to have a subsequent adverse cardiac event after having a heart attack. At the same time, people with anxiety and depression often have medically unexplained chest pain, meaning that no evidence of coronary artery disease can be found. This can create difficulties in diagnosis and disease management, but it is important to always seek medical attention if you experience chest pain.

SOCIAL ISOLATION Social isolation and low social support (living alone, or having few friends or family members) are associated with an increased incidence of CHD and poorer outcomes after the first diagnosis of CHD. Older men and women who report less emotional support from others before they have a heart attack are almost three times as likely to die in the first six months after the attack. A strong social support network is a major antidote to stress. Friends and family members can also promote and support a healthy lifestyle.

LOW SOCIOECONOMIC STATUS Low socioeconomic status and low educational attainment also increase the risk for CVD. These associations are probably due to a variety of factors, including lifestyle and access to health care.

Alcohol and Other Drugs Although moderate drinking (defined as no more than two drinks per day for men and no more than one drink per day for women) may have health benefits for some people, drinking too much alcohol raises blood pressure and can increase the risk of stroke and heart failure. Stimulant drugs, particularly cocaine, can also cause serious cardiac problems, including heart attack, stroke, and sudden cardiac death. Cocaine stimulates the nervous system, promotes platelet aggregation, and can cause spasm in the coronary arteries. Injection drug use can cause infection of the heart and stroke. See Chapters 14–16 for more information on the use of alcohol, tobacco, and other drugs.

Anger, Hostility, and Heart Disease

People with a quick temper, a persistently hostile outlook, and a cynical, mistrusting attitude toward life are more likely to develop heart disease than those with a calmer, more trusting attitude. People who are angry frequently, intensely, and for long periods experience the stress response much more often than more relaxed individuals. Over the long term, the effects of stress may damage arteries and promote CVD.

Are You Too Hostile?

To help answer that question, a short self-test has been devised. It's not a scientific evaluation, but it does offer a rough measure of hostility. Are the following statements true or false for you?

1. I often get annoyed at checkout cashiers or the people in front of me when I'm waiting in line.
2. I usually keep an eye on the people I work or live with to make sure they do what they should.
3. I often wonder how homeless people can have so little respect for themselves.
4. I believe that most people will take advantage of you if you let them.
5. The habits of friends or family members often annoy me.
6. When I'm stuck in traffic, I often start breathing faster and my heart pounds.

7. When I'm annoyed with people, I really want to let them know it.
8. If someone does me wrong, I want to get even.
9. I'd like to have the last word in any argument.
10. At least once a week, I have the urge to yell at or even hit someone.

According to the survey creators, five or more "true" statements suggest that you're excessively hostile and should consider taking steps to learn to deal with it.

Managing Your Anger

Begin by monitoring your angry responses and looking for triggers—people or situations that typically make you angry. Familiarize yourself with the patterns of thinking that lead to angry or hostile feelings, and then try to head them off before they develop into full-blown anger. If you feel your anger starting to build, try reasoning with yourself by asking the following questions:

1. Is this really important enough to get angry about?
2. Am I really justified in getting angry?
3. Is getting angry going to make a real and positive difference in this situation?

If you answer yes to all three questions, then calm but assertive communication may be an appropriate response. If your

anger isn't reasonable, try distracting yourself or removing yourself from the situation. Exercise, humour, social support, and other stress-management techniques can also help (see Chapter 2 for additional anger-management tips). Your heart—and the people around you—will benefit from your calmer, more positive outlook.

Sources: Virginia Williams and Redford Williams. 1999. *Lifeskills: Lifeskills: 8 Simple Ways to Build Stronger Relationships, Communicate More Clearly, and Improve Your Health*. New York: Times Books. Reprinted by permission.

Major Risk Factors That Can't Be Changed

A number of major risk factors, and consequent determinants, for CVD cannot be changed. They include heredity, aging, being male, and ethnicity.

Heredity Multiple genes contribute to the development of CVD and its associated risk factors, such as high cholesterol, hypertension, diabetes, and obesity. Having a favourable set of genes decreases your risk of developing CVD; having an unfavourable set of genes increases your risk. Risk, however, is modifiable by lifestyle factors, such as whether you smoke, exercise, or eat a healthy diet.

Because of the genetic complexity of CVD, genetic screening is usually recommended for only a few specific conditions (for example, certain cholesterol disorders), but you can learn more about your personal risk just by assessing your family history. If you have a first-degree relative (parent,

sibling, child) with CAD, for example, you have a twofold increased risk of someday developing CAD yourself.

Don't forget the role of lifestyle factors, however. Coronary artery disease is usually the result of the interaction of several unfavourable genetic and lifestyle factors, and people with the greatest number of genetic and lifestyle risk factors will face the highest risks. People with favourable genes may not develop CAD despite having an unhealthy lifestyle, and people with many healthy habits may still develop CAD because they have an unfavourable genetic makeup. People who inherit a tendency for CVD are not destined to develop it. They may, however, have to work harder than other people to prevent CVD.

Aging Nearly 85% of people who have a heart attack are 65 or older, and more than 1700 Canadians die each year from heart attacks. For people over 55, the incidence of stroke more than doubles in each successive decade. However,

even people in their thirties and forties, especially men, can have heart attacks. Figure 7.5 shows the percentage of deaths from CVD among Canadians by age and gender.

Being Male   Although CVD is the leading killer of both men and women in Canada, men face a greater risk of heart attack than women, especially earlier in life. Until age 55, men also have a greater risk of hypertension. The incidence of stroke is higher for males than females until age 65, and more Canadian women than men die of stroke each year. Estrogen production, which is highest during the childbearing years, may protect premenopausal women against CVD (see the box "Women and CVD" on p. 222). By age 75, the gender gap nearly disappears.

Ethnicity   Rates of heart disease vary among ethnic groups in Canada, with Canadians of South Asian and African descent, as well as Aboriginal peoples, having much higher rates of hypertension, heart disease, and stroke than other groups.

Inflammation and C-Reactive Protein   Inflammation plays a key role in the development of CVD. When an artery is injured by smoking, cholesterol, hypertension, or other factors, the body's response is to produce inflammation. A substance called *C-reactive protein (CRP)* is released into the bloodstream during the inflammatory response, and high levels of CRP indicate a substantially elevated risk of heart attack and stroke. CRP may also be harmful to the coronary arteries themselves.

Experts recommend testing of CRP levels for people at intermediate risk for CVD because people in this risk category who are found to have high CRP levels may benefit from additional CVD testing or treatment. (This guideline assumes that people at high risk for CVD are already receiving treatment.)

Lifestyle changes and certain drugs can reduce CRP levels. Statin drugs, widely prescribed to lower cholesterol, also decrease inflammation and reduce CRP levels; this may be one reason that statin drugs seem to lower CVD risk even in people with normal blood lipid levels. Patients who receive intensive statin treatment fare better than patients who receive less aggressive treatment that primarily targets LDL levels. The reduction in risk from decreased CRP levels is independent of changes in LDL.

The benefits of statins were confirmed in 2008, when findings were released from a study involving 18,000 patients in 26 countries. Researchers found that volunteers who took statins reduced their risk of CVD by about 50%, even if they had normal cholesterol levels. The patients had undergone a simple blood test that checked for inflammation by measuring levels of CRP; because statins lower CRP regardless of cholesterol levels, researchers concluded that CRP levels and inflammation are important markers of CVD risk.

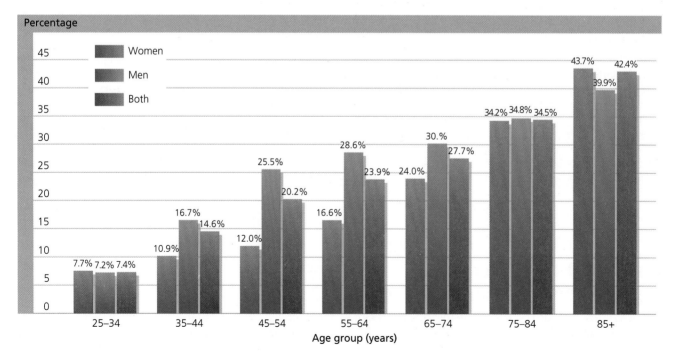

FIGURE 7.5   Percentage of deaths from cardiovascular disease by age group and sex.

Source: Used with the permission of Statistics Canada.

GENDER MATTERS

Women and CVD

CVD has traditionally been thought of as a man's disease, and until recently, this has been the justification for carrying out almost all CVD research on men. It is true that men have a higher incidence of cardiovascular problems than women, especially before age 50. On average, women live 10–15 more years free of coronary heart disease than men do. But heart disease is the leading cause of death among women.

Polls indicate that women vastly underestimate their risk of dying of a heart attack and, in turn, overestimate their risk of dying of breast cancer. In reality, CVD is responsible for seven times as many Canadian women's deaths as breast cancer. Women from minority groups face the highest risk of developing CVD, but their awareness of heart disease as a killer of women is lower than that of white women. Risk factors for CVD are similar for men and women and include age, family history, smoking, hypertension, high cholesterol, and diabetes. There are some gender differences, however. HDL appears to be an even more powerful predictor of CAD risk in women than it is in men. Also, women with diabetes have a greater risk of having CVD events, such as heart attack and stroke, than men with diabetes.

Estrogen: A Heart Protector?

The hormone estrogen, produced naturally by a woman's ovaries until menopause, improves blood lipid concentrations and other CVD risk factors. For the past several decades, many physicians encouraged menopausal women to take hormone replacement therapy (HT) to relieve menopause symptoms and presumably reduce the risk of CVD. However, studies found that HT may actually *increase* a woman's risk for heart disease

and certain other health problems, including breast cancer. Some newer studies have found a reduced risk of CVD in women who start HT in the early stages of menopause (usually the mid-40s), suggesting that outcomes may depend on several factors, including the timing of hormone use. The Heart and Stroke Foundation of Canada currently recommends that HT not be used to protect against CVD.

For younger women, the most common form of hormonal medication is oral contraceptives (OCs). Typical OCs contain estrogen and progestin in relatively low doses and are generally considered safe for most nonsmoking women. But women who smoke and use OCs are up to 32 times as likely to have a heart attack as nonsmoking OC users.

Postmenopausal Women: At Risk

When women have heart attacks, they are more likely than men to die within a year. One reason is that because women develop heart disease at older ages, they are more likely to have other health problems that complicate treatment. Women have smaller hearts and arteries than men, possibly making diagnosis and treatment more difficult. Women may also wait longer before seeking treatment. Unknown biological or psychosocial risk factors may also be contributing to women's mortality.

Medical personnel appear to evaluate and treat women less aggressively than men. Women with positive stress tests and those whose evaluation raises concern about a heart attack are less likely to be referred to further testing than are men. In addition, studies of heart attack patients have found that women usually have to wait longer than

men to receive clot-dissolving drugs in an emergency room.

Women presenting with CHD are just as likely as men to report chest pain, and a recent Canadian study revealed that women experience all of the typical heart attack symptoms that men experience, although other research has suggested additional symptoms, including fatigue, weakness, shortness of breath, nausea, vomiting, and pain in the abdomen, neck, jaw, and back. Women may also have pain at rest, during sleep, or with mental stress. A woman who experiences these symptoms should be persistent in seeking accurate diagnosis and appropriate treatment.

Careful diagnosis of cardiac symptoms is also key in cases of stress-induced cardiomyopathy ("broken heart syndrome"), which occurs much more commonly in women. In this condition, a severe stress response stuns the heart, producing heart-attack-like symptoms and decreased pumping function of the heart, but no damage to the heart muscle. Typically, the condition reverses quickly, and correct diagnosis is important to avoid unnecessary invasive procedures.

Possible Risk Factors Currently Being Studied

In recent years, a number of other possible risk factors for cardiovascular disease have been identified.

Insulin Resistance and Metabolic Syndrome   When you consume carbohydrates, your blood glucose level

increases. This stimulates the pancreas to secrete insulin, which allows body cells to pick up glucose to use for energy (see Chapter 4). The function of insulin is to maintain proper glucose levels in the body, which it does by affecting the uptake of glucose from the blood by muscle and fat tissue and by limiting the liver's production of glucose. As people gain weight and engage in less physical activity, their muscles, fat, and liver become less sensitive to the

effect of insulin—a condition known as insulin resistance (or pre-diabetes). As the body becomes increasingly insulin resistant, the pancreas must secrete more and more insulin (hyperinsulinemia) to keep glucose levels within a normal range. Eventually, however, even high levels of insulin may become insufficient, and blood glucose levels will also start to rise (hyperglycemia), resulting in type 2 diabetes.

Those who have insulin resistance tend to have several other related risk factors; as a group, this cluster of abnormalities is called metabolic syndrome or insulin resistance syndrome (Table 7.3). Metabolic syndrome significantly increases the risk of CVD—more so in women than in men. An estimated 15%–25% of the Canadian population has metabolic syndrome, and even higher rates are estimated for Aboriginal peoples and Canadians of South Asian and African descent.

To reduce your risk for metabolic syndrome, choose a healthy diet and get plenty of exercise. Regular physical activity increases your body's sensitivity to insulin in addition to improving cholesterol levels and decreasing blood pressure. Reducing calorie intake to prevent weight gain or losing weight if needed will also reduce insulin resistance. The amount and type of carbohydrate intake is also important: Diets high in carbohydrates, especially high-glycemic-index foods, can raise levels of glucose and triglycerides and lower HDL, thus contributing to the development or worsening of metabolic syndrome and CVD, particularly in people who are already sedentary and overweight. For people prone to insulin resistance, eating more unsaturated fats, protein, vegetables, and fibre while limiting added sugars and starches may be beneficial.

Homocysteine Elevated levels of homocysteine, an amino acid circulating in the blood, are associated with an increased risk of CVD. Homocysteine appears to damage the lining of blood vessels, resulting in inflammation and the development of fatty deposits in artery walls. These changes can lead to the formation of clots and blockages in arteries, which in turn can cause heart attacks and strokes. High homocysteine levels are also associated with cognitive impairment, such as memory loss.

Men generally have higher homocysteine levels than women, as do individuals with diets low in folic acid, vitamin B12, and vitamin B6. Many genes may cause elevated homocysteine levels, and some genes associated with small-to-moderate elevations are quite common in the general population. A recent study showed that taking folic acid will decrease homocysteine levels, but it does not lower the risk of CVD and may actually be harmful. Therefore, taking folic acid beyond the dose found in a multivitamin is not recommended. Instead, it may be more helpful to follow a diet rich in fruits, vegetables, and whole grains. Also, if your homocysteine level is high, aggressively controlling your other cardiac risk factors is that much more important.

Infectious Agents Several infectious agents have been identified as possible culprits in the development of CVD. *Chlamydia pneumoniae*, a common cause of flulike respiratory infections, has been found in sections of clogged, damaged arteries but not in sections of healthy arteries. It does not appear that antibiotic treatment for *C. pneumoniae* reduces risk, but further research is needed. Other infectious agents may also play a role in CVD.

Lipoprotein(a) A high level of a specific type of LDL called lipoprotein(a), or Lp(a), may be a risk factor for CHD, especially when associated with high LDL or low HDL levels. Lp(a) is thought to contribute to CVD by promoting clots and by delivering cholesterol to a site of vascular injury. Lp(a) levels have a strong genetic component and are difficult to treat. Lp(a) levels tend to increase with age and vary by race. Lifestyle modifications, such as diet, exercise, and weight loss, appear to have little effect in lowering Lp(a). High-dose niacin has been shown to decrease Lp(a), but studies are still needed to see if lower levels actually reduce the risk of CVD. In the meantime, if you have elevated Lp(a), any other cholesterol abnormalities—such as elevated LDL—should be treated even more aggressively.

LDL Particle Size Research has shown that LDL particles differ in size and density and that the concentrations of different particles vary among individuals. LDL cholesterol profiles can be divided into three general types: People with pattern A have mostly large, buoyant LDL particles; people with pattern B have mostly small, dense LDL particles; and people with pattern C have a mixture of particle types. Small, dense LDL particles pose a greater CVD risk than large particles; thus, people with LDL pattern B are at greater risk for CVD. Exercise, a low-fat diet, and certain lipid-lowering drugs may help lower CVD risk in people with LDL pattern B. In a recent study of men who walked or jogged 19–32 kilometres per week, total cholesterol and LDL levels were often unchanged, but the LDL particles became larger and less dense.

Table 7.3	Defining Characteristics of Metabolic Syndrome*
Abdominal obesity (waist circumference)	
Men	>102 cm
Women	>88 cm
Triglycerides	≥1.69 mmol/L
HDL cholesterol	
Men	<1.03 mmol/L
Women	<1.29 mmol/L
Blood pressure	≥130/≥85 mm Hg
Fasting glucose	≥5.6 mmol/L

Sources: S. M. Grundy, B. J. Brewer, J. I. Cleeman, et al. 2004. Definition of metabolic syndrome: Report of the National Heart, Lung, and Blood Institute/American Heart Association conference on scientific issues related to definition. *Circulation* 109: 433–438; National Cholesterol Education Program. 2001. *ATP III Guidelines At-A-Glance Quick Desk Reference.* Bethesda, Md.: National Heart, Lung, and Blood Institute. NIH Publication No. 01-3305.

*A person is diagnosed with metabolic syndrome if she or he has three or more of the risk factors listed here.

Blood Viscosity and Iron High blood viscosity (thickness) may increase the risk of CVD; excess iron stores have also been linked to higher risk, especially for men and postmenopausal women (iron stores are usually lower in younger women because of menstrual blood loss). Regular blood donation, which reduces iron stores and blood viscosity, is associated with lower CVD risk in men. Drinking five or more glasses of water a day may also reduce risk by reducing blood viscosity. On the flip side, high consumption of heme iron—found in meat, fish, and poultry—is associated with an increased risk of heart attack. Men and postmenopausal women should consult a physician before taking iron supplements.

Uric Acid Recent research suggests a link between high blood levels of uric acid and CVD mortality, particularly among those at elevated risk of CVD (i.e., based on diabetes and metabolic syndrome status, ethnicity, obesity). Uric acid may raise CVD risk by increasing inflammation and platelet aggregation or by influencing the development of hypertension; high uric acid levels also cause gout (a type of arthritis), kidney stones, and certain forms of kidney disease. Medications to lower uric acid levels are available, but it is not yet known if they will be useful in preventing CVD.

Time of Day and Time of Year More heart attacks and sudden cardiac deaths occur between 6:00 a.m. and noon than during other times of the day. This trend may be explained by the natural increase in adrenaline and cortisol levels that occurs in the morning and by an increase in the sympathetic nervous system activity as people hurry around at the beginning of their day. Blood pressure is often lowest during sleep and highest in the morning, and endothelial function may be impaired in the early morning.

Heart attacks also follow a seasonal pattern, with up to 50% more occurring in winter months than in summer months. Heart attacks that occur in winter also tend to be more often fatal than those that occur during summer. Possible explanations include low temperature, which can

constrict blood vessels; bursts of exertion, such as snow shovelling; increased rates of smoking; increased stress and depression, including seasonal affective disorder (see Chapter 2); holiday-related episodes of high-fat eating and binge drinking; and physiological factors, including levels of cholesterol and C-reactive protein, which appear to rise in winter. People who have symptoms of heart trouble may also be more reluctant to seek help during the holidays.

MAJOR FORMS OF CARDIOVASCULAR DISEASE

Although deaths from CVD have declined drastically over the past 60 years, it remains the leading cause of death in Canada. According to the Heart and Stroke Foundation of Canada, heart disease killed more than 50,000 Canadians in 2005. Figure 7.6 shows the life-altering limitations experienced by those who have CVD.

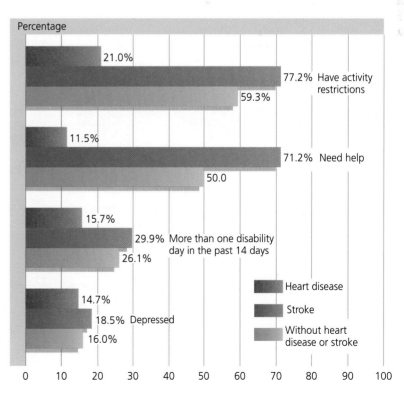

FIGURE 7.6 Limitations experienced by Canadians who have and have not had CVD.

Source: Used with the permission of Statistics Canada.

Plaque buildup begins when endothelial cells lining the arteries are damaged by smoking, high blood pressure, oxidized LDL, and other causes; excess cholesterol particles collect beneath these cells.

In response to the damage, platelets and other types of cells collect at the site; a fibrous cap forms, isolating the plaque within the artery wall. An early-stage plaque is called a fatty streak.

Chemicals released by cells in and around the plaque cause further inflammation and buildup; an advanced plaque contains LDL, white blood cells, connective tissue, smooth muscle cells, platelets, and other compounds.

The narrowed artery is vulnerable to blockage by clots. The risk of blockage and heart attack rises if the fibrous cap cracks (probably because of destructive enzymes released by white blood cells within the plaque).

FIGURE 7.7   Stages of plaque development.

The main forms of CVD are atherosclerosis, heart disease and heart attack, stroke, peripheral arterial disease (PAD), congestive heart failure, congenital heart disease, rheumatic heart disease, and heart valve problems. Many forms are interrelated and have elements in common; we treat them separately here for the sake of clarity. Hypertension, which is both a major risk factor and a form of CVD, was described earlier in the chapter.

Atherosclerosis

Atherosclerosis is a form of arteriosclerosis, or thickening and hardening of the arteries. In atherosclerosis, arteries become narrowed by deposits of fat, cholesterol, and other substances. The process begins when the endothelial cells (cells that line the arteries) become damaged, most likely through a combination of factors, such as smoking, high blood pressure, high insulin or glucose levels, and deposits of oxidized LDL particles. The body's response to this damage results in inflammation and changes in the artery lining that create a sort of magnet for LDL, platelets, and other cells; these cells build up and cause a bulge in the wall of the artery. As these deposits, called **plaques**, accumulate on artery walls, the arteries lose their elasticity and their ability to expand and contract, restricting blood flow. Once narrowed by a plaque, an artery is vulnerable to blockage by blood clots (Figure 7.7, above). The risk of life-threatening clots and heart attacks increases if the fibrous cap covering a plaque ruptures.

If the heart, brain, or other organs are deprived of blood and the oxygen it carries, the effects of atherosclerosis can be deadly. Coronary arteries, which supply the heart with blood, are particularly susceptible to plaque buildup, a condition called **coronary heart disease (CHD)**, or *coronary artery disease (CAD)*. The blockage of a coronary artery causes a heart attack. If a cerebral artery (leading to the brain) is blocked, the result is a stroke. If an artery in a limb becomes narrowed or blocked, it causes *peripheral arterial disease*, a condition that causes pain and sometimes loss of the affected limb.

The main risk factors for atherosclerosis are cigarette smoking, physical inactivity, high levels of blood cholesterol, high blood pressure, and diabetes. Atherosclerosis often begins in childhood; in fact, autopsy studies of young trauma victims have revealed atherosclerosis of the coronary arteries in adolescents.

CAD is responsible for **65%–80%** of deaths among people with diabetes.

—Canadian Diabetes Association, 2009

Heart Disease and Heart Attack

The most common form of heart disease is coronary artery disease caused by atherosclerosis. When one of the coronary arteries becomes blocked, a **heart attack**, or *myocardial infarction (MI)*, results. During a heart attack, the heart muscle (the myocardium) is damaged and part of it may die from lack of blood. Although a heart attack may come without warning, it is usually the end result of a long-term disease process.

Myocardial infarctions are a significant issue in Canada, especially among people ages 65 and older (Table 7.4 on p. 226). The average age for a first heart attack is 65 for men and 70 for women.

plaque   A deposit of fatty (and other) substances on the inner wall of the arteries.

coronary heart disease (CHD)   Heart disease caused by atherosclerosis in the arteries that supply blood to the heart muscle; also called *coronary artery disease*.

heart attack   Damage to, or death of, heart muscle, resulting from a failure of the coronary arteries to deliver enough blood to the heart; also called *myocardial infarction (MI)*.

TERMS

Table 7.4	Percentage of Acute Myocardial Infarctions by Age Group in Canada	
Age	**Percentage**	
20–49	0.3	
50–64	3.4	
65–79	8.2	
80 and older	11.8	

Source: Heart and Stroke Foundation of Canada, 2009. *Statistics: Heart Attack* (http://www.heartandstroke.com/site/c.ikIQLcMWJtE/b.3483991/k.34A8/ Statistics.htm#heartattack; retrieved April 6, 2011).

Heart attack symptoms may include the following:

- Chest pain or pressure (even if it goes away with rest and comes on with exertion)
- Arm, neck, shoulder, back, or jaw pain
- Difficulty breathing or shortness of breath
- Excessive sweating; cool, clammy skin
- Nausea and vomiting
- Loss of consciousness
- Fear, anxiety, or denial

Most people having a heart attack have chest pain, but about one-third do not. Ethnic minorities, older adults, and people with diabetes are the most likely groups to experience heart attack without chest pain. Women may also experience some symptoms differently than men (see the box "Women and CVD" on p. 222).

The Heart and Stroke Foundation of Canada estimates that 70,000 heart attacks occur each year in Canada, which is one every seven minutes. The Canadian Institute for Health Information released a report recently showing that deaths from first heart attacks dropped 2.5% across Canada between 2000 and 2005. An estimated one-third of all attacks are symptomless or "silent" heart attacks.

Angina Arteries narrowed by disease may still be open enough to deliver blood to the heart. At times, however—during stress or exertion, for example—the heart needs more oxygen than can flow through narrowed arteries. When the need for oxygen exceeds the supply, chest pain, called **angina pectoris**, may occur.

Angina pain is usually felt as an extreme tightness in the chest and heavy pressure behind the breastbone or in the shoulder, neck, arm, hand, or back. This pain, although not actually a heart attack, is a warning that the load on the heart must be reduced. The symptoms of angina are often very difficult to distinguish from a heart attack. Any severe chest pain that lasts more than a few minutes should be considered life threatening, and emergency medical help should be obtained immediately. About 2% of Canadians experience angina.

Angina may be controlled in a number of ways (with drugs and surgical or nonsurgical procedures), but its course is unpredictable. Over a period ranging from hours to years, the narrowing may go on to full blockage and a heart attack.

Arrhythmias and Sudden Cardiac Death The pumping of the heart is controlled by electrical impulses from the sinus node that maintain a regular heartbeat of 60–100 beats per minute. If this electrical conduction system is disrupted, the heart may beat too quickly, too slowly, or in an irregular fashion, a condition known as **arrhythmia**. Arrhythmia can cause symptoms ranging from imperceptible to severe and even fatal.

Sudden cardiac death, also called *cardiac arrest*, is most often caused by an arrhythmia called *ventricular fibrillation*, a kind of quivering of the ventricle that makes it ineffective in pumping blood. If ventricular fibrillation continues for more than a few minutes, it is generally fatal. Cardiac defibrillation, in which an electrical shock is delivered to the heart, can be effective in jolting the heart into a more efficient rhythm. Emergency personnel typically carry defibrillators, and automated external defibrillators (AEDs) are becoming increasingly available in public places for use by the general public. AEDs monitor the heart's rhythm and, if appropriate, deliver an electrical shock. Training in the use of AEDs is available from many organizations, such as St. John Ambulance Canada. Sudden cardiac death most often occurs in people with CHD. Serious arrhythmias frequently develop during or after a heart attack and are often the actual cause of death in cases of a fatal MI. In Canada, one cardiac arrest occurs every 12 minutes (about 40,000 a year).

Other potential causes of arrhythmia include congenital heart abnormalities, infections, drug use, chest trauma, and congestive heart failure. Some arrhythmias cause no problems and resolve without treatment; more serious arrhythmias are usually treated with medication or a surgically implanted pacemaker or defibrillator that delivers electrical stimulation to the heart to create a more normal rhythm.

Helping a Person Having a Heart Attack Most people who die from a heart attack do so within two hours from the time they experience the first symptoms. Unfortunately, half of all people having a heart attack wait more than two hours before getting help. If you or someone you are with has any of the warning signs of heart attack listed in the box "What to Do in Case of a Heart Attack, Stroke, or Cardiac Arrest" (p. 228) take immediate action. Get help even if the person denies there is something wrong. Many experts also suggest that the person having the heart attack chew and swallow one adult Aspirin tablet (325 milligrams) as soon as possible after symptoms begin; Aspirin has an immediate anticlotting effect.

If the person loses consciousness, a qualified person should immediately start administering emergency **cardio-pulmonary resuscitation (CPR)**. Damage to the heart muscle increases with time. If the person receives emergency care quickly enough, a clot-dissolving agent can be injected to break up a clot in the coronary artery.

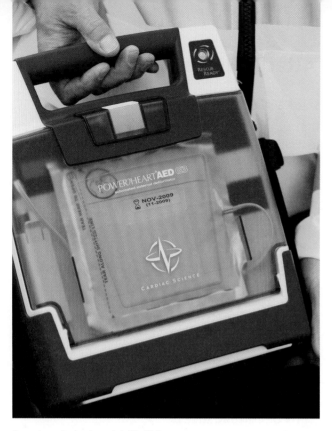

An automated external defibrillator.

Detecting and Treating Heart Disease Physicians have an expanding array of tools to evaluate the condition of the heart and its arteries. Currently, the most common initial screening tool for CAD is the stress, or exercise, test, in which a patient runs or walks on a treadmill or pedals a stationary cycle while being monitored for abnormalities with an electrocardiogram (ECG or EKG). Certain characteristic changes in the heart's electrical activity while under stress can reveal particular heart problems, such as restricted blood flow. Exercise testing can also be performed in conjunction with imaging techniques, such as nuclear medicine or echocardiography that provide pictures of the heart, which can help pinpoint problems.

Other tests for evaluating CHD include the following:

- Electron-beam computed tomography (EBCT) uses a sweeping electron beam to produce computerized cross-sectional images; it can detect calcium in the arteries, a marker for atherosclerosis.

- Echocardiography uses sound waves to examine the heart's pumping function and valves.

- Multi-slice computed tomography (MSCT) is another type of CT that produces very thinly sliced images of the heart, allowing physicians to see very small structures, such as the coronary arteries.

- **Magnetic resonance imaging (MRI)** uses powerful magnets to look inside the body and generate pictures of the heart and blood vessels.

- In nuclear myocardial perfusion imaging, radiotracers, such as thallium-201, are injected into the bloodstream. The radiotracers' location and density in the heart can be imaged and quantified; from this data, physicians can extrapolate the blow flow (perfusion) to various areas of the heart and diagnose coronary artery disease.

- Positron emission tomography (PET) involves the use of positron-emitting isotopes to image and quantify regional blood flow in the heart and diagnose coronary artery disease.

If symptoms or noninvasive tests suggest coronary artery disease, the next step is usually a coronary **angiogram**, performed in a cardiac catheterization lab. In this test, a catheter (a small plastic tube) is threaded into an artery, usually in the groin, and advanced through the aorta to the coronary arteries. The catheter is then placed into the opening of the coronary artery and a special dye is injected. The dye can be seen moving through the arteries under moving X-ray, and any narrowings or blockages can be identified. If a problem is found, it is commonly treated with **balloon angioplasty**, which is performed by specially trained cardiologists (Figure 7.8 on p. 229). Surgeons in Canada performed nearly 37,000 angioplasty procedures in 2001. This technique involves placing a small wire in the artery and feeding a deflated balloon over it. The balloon is advanced to the site of the narrowing and then inflated, flattening the fatty plaque and widening the arterial opening. This is generally followed by placement of a stent, a small metal tube that helps keep the artery open. Repeat clogging of the artery, known as restenosis, can occur, but the introduction of stents coated with medication, which is slowly released over a few months, significantly decreases the chance of restenosis.

Other treatments, ranging from medication to major surgery, are also available. Along with a low-fat diet, regular exercise, and smoking cessation, one frequent

TERMS

angina pectoris   Pain in the chest, and often in the left arm and shoulder, caused by the heart muscle not receiving enough blood.

arrhythmia   A change in the normal pattern of the heartbeat.

sudden cardiac death   A nontraumatic, unexpected death from sudden cardiac arrest, most often from arrhythmia; in most instances, people have underlying heart disease.

cardiopulmonary resuscitation (CPR)   A technique involving mouth-to-mouth breathing and chest compression to keep oxygen flowing to the brain.

magnetic resonance imaging (MRI)   A computerized imaging technique that uses a strong magnetic field and radio frequency signals to examine a thin cross section of the body.

angiogram   A picture of the arterial system taken after injecting a dye that is opaque to X-rays; also called arteriogram.

balloon angioplasty   A technique in which a catheter with a deflated balloon on the tip is inserted into an artery; the balloon is then inflated at the point of obstruction in the artery, pressing the plaque against the artery wall to improve blood supply; also called *percutaneous coronary intervention (PCI)*.

What to Do in Case of a Heart Attack, Stroke, or Cardiac Arrest

Heart Attack Warning Signs

Some heart attacks are sudden and intense—the "movie heart attack," where no one doubts what's happening. But most heart attacks start slowly, with mild pain or discomfort. Often people affected aren't sure what's wrong and wait too long before getting help. Here are signs that can mean a heart attack is happening:

• *Chest discomfort.* Heart attacks often involve discomfort in the chest that lasts more than a few minutes, or that goes away and comes back. It can feel like uncomfortable pressure, squeezing, burning, fullness, or pain.

• *Discomfort in other areas of the upper body.* Symptoms can include pain or discomfort in one or both arms, the back, neck, jaw, or stomach.

• *Shortness of breath.* This may occur with or without chest discomfort.

• *Other signs.* These may include breaking out in a cold sweat, nausea, vomiting, or light-headedness.

If you or someone you're with has chest discomfort, especially with one or more of the other signs, don't wait longer than a few minutes (no more than five) before calling for help. Have the person stop all activity and sit or lie down. It is also recommended that the person take one adult Aspirin (325 milligrams).

Calling 9-1-1 is almost always the fastest way to get lifesaving treatment. Emergency medical services staff can begin treatment when they arrive—up to an hour sooner than if someone gets to the hospital by car. The staff are also trained to revive someone whose heart has stopped. Patients with chest pain who arrive by ambulance usually receive faster treatment at the hospital, too.

If you can't access the emergency medical services, have someone drive you to the hospital right away. If you're the one having symptoms, don't drive yourself, unless you have absolutely no other option.

Stroke Warning Signs

The Heart and Stroke Foundation of Canada says these are the warning signs of stroke:

• Sudden numbness or weakness of the face, arm, or leg (especially on one side of the body)

• Sudden confusion, trouble speaking or understanding

• Sudden trouble seeing in one or both eyes

• Sudden trouble walking, dizziness, or loss of balance or coordination

• Sudden, severe headache with no known cause

If you or someone with you has one or more of these signs (even temporarily), don't delay! Immediately call 9-1-1 or the emergency medical services number so an ambulance (ideally with advanced life support) can be sent for you. Also, check the time so you'll know when the first symptoms appeared. It's very important to take immediate action. If given within three hours of the start of symptoms, a clot-busting drug can reduce long-term disability for the most common type of stroke.

Signs of Cardiac Arrest

Cardiac arrest strikes instantly and without warning. Here are the signs:

• Sudden loss of responsiveness. No response to being called or to gentle shaking. No movement or coughing.

• No normal breathing. The person does not take a normal breath for several seconds.

• No signs of circulation. No pulse or blood pressure.

If cardiac arrest occurs, call 9-1-1 and begin cardiopulmonary resuscitation (CPR) immediately. If an automated external defibrillator (AED) is available and someone trained to use it is nearby, involve her or him.

Source: The Heart and Stroke Foundation of Canada. 2009. *Health Information* (http://www.heartandstroke.com/site/c.ikIQLcMWJtE/b.3479403/k.BF78/Health_Information.htm; retrieved April 6, 2011).

---

recommendation for people at high risk for CVD is to take a low-dose Aspirin tablet (81 milligrams) every day. Aspirin has an anticlotting effect, discouraging platelets in the blood from sticking to arterial plaques and forming clots; it also reduces inflammation. (Low-dose Aspirin therapy appears to help prevent first heart attacks in men, second heart attacks in men and women, and strokes in women over age 65. See the box "Aspirin and CVD" on p. 230 for more information.) Prescription drugs can help control heart rate, dilate arteries, lower blood pressure, and reduce

See the box "Aspirin and CVD" on p. 230 for more information.

> ## QUICK STATS
> ### 50,000 Canadians have strokes each year.
> —Heart and Stroke Foundation of Canada, 2009

the strain on the heart—raising both quality and length of life in heart patients. In patients with coronary artery disease, cholesterol-lowering statins are effective in preventing heart attacks; statins also have beneficial anti-inflammatory effects.

In **coronary bypass surgery** surgeons remove a healthy blood vessel, usually a vein from one of the patient's legs, and graft it from the aorta to one or more coronary arteries to bypass a blockage.

Stroke

For brain cells to function as they should, they must have a continuous supply of oxygen-rich blood. If brain cells are deprived of blood for more than a few minutes, they die. A **stroke**, also called a *cerebrovascular accident (CVA)*, occurs

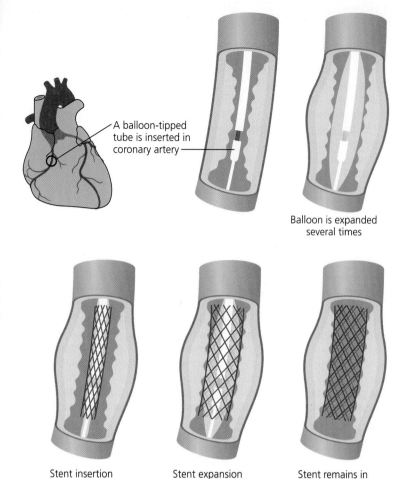

A balloon-tipped tube is inserted in coronary artery

Balloon is expanded several times

Stent insertion

Stent expansion

Stent remains in coronary artery

FIGURE 7.8 Balloon angioplasty and stenting.

Many embolic strokes are linked to a type of abnormal heart rhythm called *atrial fibrillation*; when this arrhythmia occurs, blood may pool in an atrium and form a clot.

Ischemic strokes, which account for 87% of all strokes, are potentially treatable with clot-busting drugs, so immediate medical help is critical to improving the chances of recovery.

HEMORRHAGIC STROKE A **hemorrhagic stroke** occurs when a blood vessel in the brain bursts, spilling blood into the surrounding tissue. Cells normally nourished by the artery are deprived of blood and cannot function. In addition, accumulated blood from the burst vessel may put pressure on surrounding brain tissue, causing damage and even death. There are two types of hemorrhagic strokes:

- In an *intracerebral hemorrhage*, a blood vessel ruptures within the brain. About 10% of strokes are caused by intracerebral hemorrhages.

- In a *subarachnoid hemorrhage*, a blood vessel on the brain's surface ruptures and bleeds into the space between the brain and the skull. About 3% of strokes are of this type.

Hemorrhages can be caused by head injuries or the bursting of a malformed blood vessel or an **aneurysm**, which is a blood-filled pocket that bulges out from a weak spot in an artery wall. Aneurysms in the brain may remain stable and never break. But when they do, the result is a stroke. Aneurysms may be caused or worsened by hypertension.

The Effects of a Stroke The interruption of the blood supply to any area of the brain prevents the nerve cells there from functioning—in some cases causing death.

when the blood supply to the brain is cut off. One study found that about 2 million brain cells died per minute during a stroke and the brain aged about 3.5 years each hour.

In the past, not much could be done for people having a stroke; today, however, prompt treatment of stroke can greatly decrease the risk of permanent disability. Everyone should know the warning signs of a stroke and seek immediate medical help, just as they would at the first sign of a heart attack.

Types of Strokes There are two major types of strokes (Figure 7.9 on p. 231), which are described in the following sections.

ISCHEMIC STROKE An **ischemic stroke** is caused by a blockage in a blood vessel. There are two types of ischemic strokes:

- A *thrombotic stroke* is caused by a **thrombus**, which is a blood clot that forms in a cerebral artery that has been narrowed or damaged by atherosclerosis.

- An *embolic stroke* is cause by an **embolus**, which is a wandering blood clot that is carried in the blood stream and may become wedged in a cerebral artery.

TERMS

coronary bypass surgery Surgery in which a vein is grafted from a point above to a point below an obstruction in a coronary artery, improving the blood supply to the heart.

stroke An impeded blood supply to some part of the brain resulting in the destruction of brain cells; also called *cerebrovascular accident*.

ischemic stroke Impeded blood supply to the brain caused by the obstruction of a blood vessel by a clot.

thrombus A blood clot in a blood vessel that usually remains at the point of its formation.

embolus A blood clot that breaks off from its place of origin in a blood vessel and travels through the bloodstream.

hemorrhagic stroke Impeded blood supply to the brain caused by the rupture of a blood vessel.

aneurysm A sac formed by a distension or dilation of the artery wall.

Aspirin and CVD

There is significant evidence that Aspirin can help decrease the risk of CVD in a wide range of patients.

Aspirin functions by inactivating a clotting component of the blood called platelets. Platelets and their products play a role in virtually all events involving blocked blood vessels, including myocardial infarctions and ischemic strokes. It is believed that when atherosclerotic plaques in the blood vessels become dislodged, platelets begin accumulating at the site and ultimately form a blood clot (thrombus), which can lead to an acute cardiovascular event. Even in small amounts (as little as 75 milligram each day), Aspirin acts as a potent and irreversible inhibitor of platelet clotting function.

The strongest indications for Aspirin are for the acute treatment of thrombotic cardiovascular events and for the prevention of further such events after an initial episode, which is called secondary prevention. There is extremely strong evidence to show that Aspirin should be administered to virtually every patient with an acute MI. The benefits of Aspirin for reducing the risk of subsequent MI, stroke, or vascular death are substantial, and the risks of serious bleeding and other adverse reactions are very low and treatable in an acute care hospital setting. In some patients, prolonged Aspirin use carries side effects, such as gastrointestinal bleeding. Such people, however, are generally able to tolerate different formulations or lower doses of Aspirin.

The use of daily oral Aspirin is recommended in patients with prior MI, unstable angina, chronic stable angina, prior occlusive stroke, and certain other conditions. In addition all patients with chronic stable angina or other clinical or laboratory evidence of coronary artery disease should receive daily oral Aspirin indefinitely.

Aspirin can also be used to prevent an initial thrombotic cardiovascular event, which is called primary prevention. It is vital to remember that when Aspirin is used for primary prevention the benefit is much smaller than for secondary prevention while the risk of major bleeding complication, such as gastrointestinal bleeding or hemorrhagic stroke, is the same. In one meta-analysis looking at multiple trials on this topic, the risk of a major gastrointestinal bleeding event in those treated with Aspirin was 2.30% versus 1.45% percent with placebo at an average of 28 months. Consequently, Aspirin is recommended.

Recent evidence has demonstrated that the use of Aspirin for the primary prevention of CVD events in women is more complicated. Low-dose aspirin is often recommended for women 65 years or older who are at increased risk of CVD. For women under 65 years of age, Aspirin is recommended for the prevention of ischemic stroke in those at risk (for example, patients with TIAs), but not for the prevention of MI. There may be some instances when Aspirin use is not appropriate for some individuals; it is important to consult a physician for individualized recommendations and dosage.

Stroke survivors usually have some lasting disability. Which parts of the body are affected depends on the area of the brain that has been damaged. Nerve cells control sensation and most of our body movements, and a stroke may cause paralysis, walking disability, speech impairment, memory loss, and changes in behaviour. The severity of the stroke and its long-term effects depend on which brain cells have been injured, how widespread the damage is, how effectively the body can restore the blood supply, and how rapidly other areas of the brain can take over. Early treatment can significantly reduce the severity of disability resulting from a stroke.

QUICK STATS

Less than **50%** of Canadians would know to call **9-1-1** if they or someone they knew experienced warning signs of a stroke.

—Heart and Stroke Foundation of Canada, 2009

Detecting and Treating Stroke Death rates from stroke have declined significantly in Canada over the past decades—between 1969 and 1999, death rates from stroke declined by 62%. Effective treatment requires the prompt recognition of symptoms and correct diagnosis of the type of stroke. The signs of a stroke are listed in the box on p. 228; also see "Three Simple Ways to Recognize a Stroke" in the ▪ connect Library.

Many people have strokes, however, without knowing it. These "silent strokes" do not cause any noticeable symptoms while they are occurring. Although they may be mild, having silent strokes leaves people at a higher risk for subsequent and more serious strokes later in life. They also contribute to loss of mental and cognitive skills. In 2008, a study of MRI scans of 2000 older adults revealed that 11% of the subjects had brain damage from one or more strokes but did not realize they had ever had a stroke.

Some people experience a **transient ischemic attack (TIA)**, or ministroke, days, weeks, or months before they have a full-blown stroke. A TIA produces temporary stroke-like symptoms, such as weakness or numbness in an arm or a leg, speech difficulty, or dizziness. These symptoms are brief, often lasting just a few minutes, and do not cause permanent damage. TIAs should be taken as warning signs of a stroke, however, and anyone with a suspected TIA should get immediate medical help.

Strokes should be treated with the same urgency as heart attacks. A person with stroke symptoms should be rushed to the hospital. A **computed tomography (CT)** scan, which uses a computer to construct an image of the brain from X-rays, can assess brain damage and deter-

HEMORRHAGIC STROKE

- 13% of strokes
- Caused by ruptured blood vessels followed by blood leaking into tissue
- Usually more serious than ischemic stroke

ISCHEMIC STROKE

- 87% of strokes
- Caused by blockages in brain blood vessels; potentially treatable with clot-busting drugs
- Brain tissue dies when blood flow is blocked

Subarachnoid hemorrhage

- A bleed into the space between the brain and the skull
- Develops most often from an *aneurysm*, a weakened, ballooned area in the wall of an artery

Embolic stroke

- Caused by *emboli*, blood clots that travel from elsewhere in the body to the brain blood vessels
- 25% of embolic strokes are related to atrial fibrillation

Intracerebral hemorrhage

- A bleed from a blood vessel inside the brain
- Often caused by high blood pressure and the damage it does to arteries

Thrombotic stroke

- Caused by *thrombi*, blood clots that form where an artery has been narrowed by atherosclerosis
- Most often develops when part of a thrombus breaks away and causes a blockage in a downstream artery

FIGURE 7.9   Types of stroke.

Source: Excerpted from *Harvard Health Letter*, April 2000. Reprinted with permission obtained via The Copyright Clearance Center.

mine the type of stroke. Newer techniques using MRI and ultrasound are increasingly available and should improve the speed and accuracy of stroke diagnosis.

If tests reveal that a stroke is caused by a blood clot—and if help is sought within a few hours of the onset of symptoms—the person can be treated with the same kind of clot-dissolving drugs that are used to treat coronary artery blockages. If the clot is dissolved quickly enough, brain damage is minimized and symptoms may disappear. (The longer the brain goes without blood, the greater the risk of permanent damage.) People who have had TIAs or who are at high risk for stroke because of narrowing of the carotid arteries (large arteries on either side of the neck, which carry blood to the head) may undergo a surgical procedure called *carotid endarterectomy*, in which plaque is removed. There is also a nonsurgical procedure, similar to coronary angioplasty and stenting, that can be done in the carotid arteries.

If tests reveal that a stroke was caused by a cerebral hemorrhage, drugs may be prescribed to lower the blood pressure, which will usually be high. Careful diagnosis is crucial, because administering clot-dissolving drugs to a person suffering a hemorrhagic stroke would cause more bleeding and potentially more brain damage.

If detection and treatment of stroke come too late, rehabilitation is the only treatment. Although damaged or destroyed brain tissue does not normally regenerate, nerve cells in the brain can make new pathways, and some

functions can be taken over by other parts of the brain. Some spontaneous recovery starts immediately after a stroke and continues for a few months.

Rehabilitation consists of physical therapy, which helps strengthen muscles and improve balance and coordination; speech and language therapy, which helps those whose speech has been damaged; and occupational therapy, which helps improve hand-eye coordination and every day living skills. Some people recover completely in a matter of days or weeks, but most people who have a stroke and survive must adapt to some disability.

Peripheral Arterial Disease

Peripheral arterial disease (PAD) refers to atherosclerosis in the leg (or arm) arteries, which can eventually limit or completely obstruct blood flow. The same process that

transient ischemic attack (TIA)   A small stroke; usually a temporary interruption of blood supply to the brain, causing numbness or difficulty with speech.

computed tomography (CT)   The use of computerized X-ray images to create a cross-sectional depiction (scan) of tissue density.

peripheral arterial disease (PAD)   Atherosclerosis in arteries in the legs (or, less commonly, arms) that can impede blood flow and lead to pain, infection, and loss of the affected limb.

occurs in the heart arteries can occur in any artery of the body. In fact, patients with PAD frequently also have coronary artery disease and cerebrovascular disease, and they have an increased risk of death from CVD. Approximately 800,000 people in Canada have PAD.

The risk factors associated with coronary atherosclerosis, such as smoking, diabetes, hypertension, and high cholesterol, also contribute to atherosclerosis in the peripheral circulation. The risk of PAD is significantly increased in people with diabetes and people who smoke. The likelihood of needing an amputation is increased in those who continue to smoke, and PAD in people with diabetes tends to be extensive and severe.

Symptoms of PAD include claudication and rest pain. *Claudication* is aching or fatigue in the affected leg with exertion, particularly walking, which resolves with rest. Claudication occurs when leg muscles do not get adequate blood and oxygen supply. Rest pain occurs when the limb artery is unable to supply adequate blood and oxygen even when the body is not physically active. This occurs when the artery is significantly narrowed or completely blocked. If blood flow is not restored quickly, cells and tissues die; in severe cases, amputation may be needed. PAD is the leading cause of amputation in people over age 50.

Congestive Heart Failure

A number of conditions—high blood pressure, heart attack, atherosclerosis, alcoholism, viral infections, rheumatic fever, birth defects—can damage the heart's pumping mechanism. When the heart cannot maintain its regular pumping rate and force, fluids begin to back up. When extra fluid seeps through capillary walls, edema (swelling) results, usually in the legs and ankles, but sometimes in other parts of the body as well. Fluid can collect in the lungs and interfere with breathing, particularly when a person is lying down. This condition is called **pulmonary edema**, and the entire process is known as **congestive heart failure**. About 400,000 Canadians develop heart failure each year.

Congestive heart failure can be controlled. Treatment includes reducing the workload on the heart, modifying salt intake, and using drugs that help the body eliminate excess fluid. Drugs used to treat congestive heart failure improve the pumping action of the heart, lower blood pressure so the heart doesn't have to work as hard, and help the body eliminate excess salt and water. When medical therapy is ineffective, heart transplant is a solution for some patients with severe heart failure, but the need greatly exceeds the number of hearts available.

QUICK STATS

About **160** heart transplants are performed in Canada annually.

—Canadian Institute for Health Information, 2008

The risk of heart failure increases with age, and being overweight is a significant independent risk factor. Experts fear that the incidence of heart failure will increase dramatically over the next few decades as our population ages and becomes increasingly obese.

Other Forms of Heart Disease

Other, less common, forms of heart disease include congenital heart disease, rheumatic heart disease, and heart valve disorders.

Congenital Heart Defects About 8 out of every 1000 children born each year in Canada have a defect or malformation of the heart or major blood vessels. These conditions are collectively referred to as **congenital heart defects**. Most of the common congenital defects can now be accurately diagnosed and treated with medication or surgery. Early recognition of possible heart disease in a newborn is important in saving lives. The most common congenital defects are holes in the wall that divides the chambers of the heart. Such defects cause the heart to produce a distinctive sound, making diagnosis relatively simple. Another common defect is *coarctation of the aorta*, a narrowing, or constriction, of the aorta. Heart failure may result unless the constricted area is repaired by surgery.

Hypertrophic cardiomyopathy (HCM) occurs in 1 out of every 500 people and is the most common cause of sudden death among athletes younger than age 35. It causes the heart muscle to become hypertrophic (enlarged), primarily in the septum, which is the area between the two ventricles. People with hypertrophic cardiomyopathy are at high risk for sudden death, mainly because of serious arrhythmias. Hypertrophic cardiomyopathy may be identified by a **murmur** and then diagnosed by using echocardiography. Possible treatments include medication and a pacemaker or internal defibrillator. If the hypertrophy is mainly in the septum, some of the septum can be surgically removed or a nonsurgical procedure can be done to kill off the extra muscle.

Rheumatic Heart Disease **Rheumatic fever**, a consequence of certain types of untreated streptococcal throat infections, is a leading cause of heart trouble worldwide. Rheumatic fever can permanently damage the heart muscle and heart valves, a condition called *rheumatic heart disease (RHD)*. Many operations on heart valves performed annually are related to RHD, and about 215 Canadians die each year from RHD. The incidence of rheumatic fever has declined significantly in Canada since the introduction of antibiotics.

Symptoms of strep throat include the sudden onset of a sore throat, painful swallowing, fever, swollen glands, headache, nausea, and vomiting. Careful laboratory diagnosis is important because strep throat is treated with antibiotics, which are not useful in the treatment of far more common viral sore throats. If left untreated, up to 3% of strep infections progress into rheumatic fever. Rheumatic fever primarily affects children between the ages of 5 and 15.

Heart Valve Disorders   Congenital defects and certain types of infections can cause abnormalities in the valves between the chambers of the heart. Heart valve problems generally fall into two categories—the valve fails to open fully, or it fails to close completely. In either case, blood flow through the heart is impaired.

Treatment for heart valve disorders depends on their location and severity; serious problems may be treated with surgery to repair or replace a valve. People with certain types of heart valve defects are advised to take antibiotics before some types of dental and surgical procedures to prevent bacteria, which may be dislodged into the bloodstream during the procedure, from infecting the defective valve.

The most common heart valve disorder is **mitral valve prolapse (MVP)**, which occurs in about 2% of the Canadian population. MVP is characterized by a billowing of the mitral valve, which separates the left ventricle and left atrium, during ventricular contraction; in some cases, blood leaks from the ventricle into the atrium. Most people with MVP have no symptoms; they have the same ability to exercise and live as long as people without MVP. The condition is often diagnosed during a routine medical exam when an extra heart sound (a click) or murmur is heard; the diagnosis can be confirmed with echocardiography. Treatment for MVP is usually unnecessary, although surgery may be needed in the rare cases where leakage through the faulty valve is severe.

PROTECTING YOURSELF AGAINST CARDIOVASCULAR DISEASE

You can take steps now to lower your risk of developing CVD (see "Strategies for Reducing Your Risk of Cardiovascular Disease" in the ▤connect Library). CVD can begin very early in life. For example, fatty streaks (very early atherosclerosis) can be seen on the aorta in children younger than age 10. Also, young adults with relatively low cholesterol levels go on to live substantially longer than those with higher levels. Reducing CVD risk factors when you are young can pay off with many extra years of life and health (see the box "Are You at Risk for CVD?" on p. 234).

QUESTIONS FOR CRITICAL THINKING AND REFLECTION
Has anyone you know ever had a heart attack? If so, was the onset gradual or sudden? Were appropriate steps taken to help the person (for example, did anyone call 9-1-1, give CPR, or use an AED)? Do you feel comfortable dealing with a cardiac emergency? If not, what can you do to improve your readiness?

Eat Heart Healthy

For most Canadians, eating a heart-healthy diet involves many of the changes suggested in *Eating Well with Canada's Food Guide*: cutting total fat intake, substituting unsaturated fats for saturated and trans fats, and increasing intake of whole grains and fibre. Such changes can lower blood levels of total cholesterol, LDL cholesterol, and triglycerides. Reducing salt intake and getting enough potassium can help lower blood pressure. A moderate amount of alcohol may also be beneficial for some people.

See Chapter 5 for a detailed discussion of nutrition and dietary guidelines. The following sections briefly discuss specific aspects of nutrition that apply directly to heart health.

Decreased Fat and Cholesterol Intake   Nutritional experts recommend that all people over age two adopt a diet in which total fat consumption is no more than 30% of total daily calories, with no more than one-third of total fat calories (10% of total daily calories) coming from saturated fat. It is best that no more than 7% of daily calories come from saturated fat and less than 1% come from trans fats; this recommendation applies to everyone.

For people with heart disease or high LDL levels, experts recommend a total fat intake of 25%–35% of total daily calories and a saturated fat intake of less than 7% of total calories. The higher total fat allowance is for people with insulin resistance who need to decrease their carbohydrate intake.

It is also recommended that Canadians limit dietary cholesterol intake to no more than 300 milligrams per day; for people with heart disease or high LDL levels, the suggested daily limit is 200 milligrams. Animal products contain cholesterol and saturated fat; vegetable products do not contain cholesterol.

TERMS

pulmonary edema   The accumulation of fluid in the lungs.

congestive heart failure   A condition resulting from the heart's inability to pump out all the blood that returns to it; blood backs up in the veins leading to the heart, causing an accumulation of fluid in various parts of the body.

congenital heart defect   A malformation of the heart or its major blood vessels, present at birth.

hypertrophic cardiomyopathy (HCM)   An inherited condition in which there is an enlargement of the heart muscle, especially between the two ventricles.

murmur   An abnormal heart sound indicating turbulent blood flow through a valve or hole in the heart.

rheumatic fever   A disease, mainly of children, characterized by fever, inflammation, and pain in the joints; often damages the heart valves and muscle, a condition called rheumatic heart disease.

mitral valve prolapse (MVP)   A condition in which the mitral valve billows out during ventricular contraction, possibly allowing leakage of blood from the left ventricle into the left atrium.

Are You at Risk for CVD?

Your chances of suffering an early heart attack or stroke depend on a variety of factors, many of which are under your control. The best time to identify your risk factors and change your behaviour to lower your risk is when you are young. You can significantly affect your future health and quality of life if you adopt healthy behaviours. To help identify your risk factors, circle the response for each risk category that best describes you:

1. Gender and age

    0 Female age 55 or younger; male age 45 or younger

    2 Female age 55 or older or male age 45 or older

2. Heredity

    0 Neither parent suffered a heart attack or stroke before age 60.

    3 One parent suffered a heart attack or stroke before age 60.

    7 Both parents suffered a heart attack or stroke before age 60.

3. Smoking

    0 Never smoked

    3 Quit more than two years ago and lifetime smoking is less than five pack-years*

    6 Quit less than two years ago or lifetime smoking is greater than five pack-years*

    8 Smoke less than half a pack per day

    13 Smoke more than half a pack per day

    15 Smoke more than one pack per day

4. Environmental tobacco smoke

    0 Do not live or work with smokers

    2 Exposed to ETS at work

    3 Live with a smoker

    4 Both live and work with smokers

5. Blood pressure

    If available, average your last three readings:

    0 120/80 or below

    1 121/81–130/85

    3 Don't know

    5 131/86–150/90

    9 151/91–170/100

    13 Above 170/100

6. Total cholesterol (mmol/L)

    Your physician has told you that you have

    0 Low total cholesterol

    3 Minimally high cholesterol

    5 High cholesterol

    6 Very high cholesterol

7. HDL Cholesterol (mmol/L)

    Your physician has told you that you have

    0 Very high HDL levels

    1 High HDL

    3 Moderate HDL

    5 Low HDL

    10 Very low HDL

8. Exercise

    0 Exercise three times a week

    1 Exercise once or twice a week

    2 Occasional exercise less than once a week

    7 Rarely exercise

9. Diabetes

    0 No personal or family history

    2 One parent with diabetes

    6 Two parents with diabetes

    9 Non-insulin-dependent diabetes

    13 Insulin-dependent diabetes

10. Body mass index (using the formula provided in Chapter 4)

    0 <3.0

    1 23.0–24.9

    2 25.0–28.9

    3 29.0–34.9

    5 35.0–39.9

    7 ≥40

11. Stress

    0 Relaxed most of the time

    1 Occasional stress and anger

    2 Frequently stressed and angry

    3 Usually stressed and angry

Scoring

Total your risk factor points. Refer to the list below to get an approximate rating of your risk of suffering an early heart attack or stroke.

Score	Estimated Risk
Less than 20	Low risk
20–29	Moderate risk
30–45	High risk
Over 45	Extremely high risk

*Pack-years can be calculated by multiplying the number of packs you smoked per day by the number of years you smoked. For example, if you smoked a pack and a half a day for 5 years, you would have smoked the equivalent of $1.5 \times 5 = 7.5$ pack-years.

Increased Fibre Intake Fibre traps the bile acids the liver needs to manufacture cholesterol and carries them to the large intestine, where they are excreted. It slows the production of proteins that promote blood clotting. Fibre may also interfere with the absorption of dietary fat and may help you cut total food intake because foods rich in fibre tend to be filling. Studies have shown that a high-fibre diet is associated with a 40%–50% reduction in the risk of heart attack and stroke.

To get the recommended 25–38 grams of dietary fibre per day, eat whole grains, fruits, and vegetables. Good sources of fibre include oatmeal, some breakfast cereals, barley, legumes, and most fruits and vegetables.

Decreased Sodium Intake and Increased Potassium Intake Reducing sodium intake to recommended levels, while also increasing potassium intake, can help reduce blood pressure for many people. The recommended limit for sodium intake is 2300 milligrams per day; for population groups at special risk the recommended limit is 1500 milligrams per day.

Potassium is also important in controlling blood pressure, and many North Americans consume less than recommended amounts of the mineral. Good food sources include leafy green vegetables, such as spinach and beet greens; root vegetables, such as white and sweet potatoes; vine fruits, such as cantaloupe and honeydew melon, winter squash, bananas, many dried fruits, and tomato sauce.

Moderate Alcohol Consumption (For Some) Guidelines for Canadians state that moderate alcohol consumption may lower the risk of CVD among middle-aged and older adults. Moderate means no more than one drink per day for women and two drinks per day for men. Moderate alcohol use may increase HDL cholesterol; it may also reduce stroke risk, possibly by dampening the inflammatory response or by affecting blood clotting.

For most people under age 45, however, the risks of alcohol use probably outweigh any health benefit. Excessive alcohol consumption increases the risk of a variety of serious health problems, including hypertension, stroke, some cancers, liver disease, alcohol dependence, and injuries. See Chapter 15 for a detailed discussion of alcohol use, the effects of alcohol, and the importance of moderation in drinking.

Other Dietary Factors Researchers have identified other dietary factors that may affect CVD risk:

• *Omega-3 fatty acids.* Found in fish, shellfish, and some plant foods (nuts and canola, soybean, and flaxseed oils), omega-3 fatty acids may reduce clotting, abnormal heart rhythms, and inflammation and have other heart-healthy effects, such as lowering triglycerides. Eating fish two or more times a week is often recommended; fish oil capsules may be appropriate for some people who won't eat fish or who have certain CVD risk factors. Note that omega-3 fatty acids may raise LDL levels and some fish sources may be high in mercury. Plant sources of omega-3 fatty acids are also a good choice.

• *Plant stanols and sterols.* Plant stanols and sterols, found in some types of trans-fat-free margarines and other products, reduce the absorption of cholesterol in the body and help lower LDL levels. For people with high LDL levels that do not respond to changes in fat intake, research suggests that an intake of 2 grams per day of plant stanols or sterols may help lower them.

• *Folic acid, vitamin B6, and vitamin B12.* These vitamins lower homocysteine levels, and folic acid has also been found to reduce the risk of hypertension.

• *Calcium.* Diets rich in calcium may help prevent hypertension and possibly stroke by reducing insulin resistance and platelet aggregation. Good sources of calcium are low-fat and fat-free dairy products.

• *Soy protein.* Although soy itself doesn't seem to have much effect on cholesterol, replacing some animal proteins with soy protein (e.g., tofu) may help lower LDL cholesterol.

• *Healthy carbohydrates.* Most of the carbohydrates in the Canadian diet come from added sugars, refined grains, and starchy foods, including soft drinks, sweets, white potatoes (including french fries and chips), white bread, and refined ready-to-eat cereals; these foods are often relatively low in nutrients and have a high glycemic index (see Chapter 5). Healthier carbohydrate choices, including whole grains, fruits, and nonstarchy vegetables, typically provide more nutrients and have a lower glycemic index. Choosing healthy carbohydrates is important for people with insulin resistance, pre-diabetes, or diabetes.

• *Total calories.* Some studies have found that reducing energy intake can improve cholesterol and triglyceride levels as much as reducing fat intake does. Reduced calorie intake also helps control body weight, an extremely important risk factor for CVD.

Most experts recommend against taking nutritional supplements (especially extra folic acid and B vitamins) as a way to prevent heart disease. In fact, a 10-year-long study ending in 2008 revealed that vitamin C and E supplements provided no protection against heart disease in men. In some of the study's subjects, vitamin E supplementation was associated with an increased risk of stroke. An estimated 15% of Canadians take vitamin C and E supplements, and many people do so because of a long-standing yet unproven theory that these antioxidants protect against heart disease. Some evidence suggests that vitamin D deficiency may increase the risk of heart disease, especially in men, but experts do not currently advise taking vitamin D supplements to prevent CVD. If you are concerned about your heart health and may not be getting the nutrition you need, ask your physician or a registered dietitian for advice.

Exercise Regularly

You can significantly reduce your risk of CVD with a moderate amount of physical activity. Follow the guidelines for physical activity and exercise described in Chapter 6. Strength training in addition to aerobic exercise is recommended for building and maintaining cardiovascular health. Strength training helps lower blood pressure, reduce body fat, and improve lipid levels and glucose metabolism.

Avoid Tobacco

The number-one risk factor for CVD that you can control is smoking. If you smoke, quit. If you don't, don't start. If you live or work with people who smoke, encourage them to quit—for their sake and yours. Exposure to ETS raises your risk of CVD, and no level of exposure is safe. If you find yourself breathing in smoke, take steps to prevent or stop the exposure. See Chapter 16 for detailed information on the effects of smoking and strategies for quitting.

Know and Manage Your Blood Pressure

If you have no CVD risk factors, have your blood pressure measured by a trained professional at least once every two years; yearly tests are recommended if you have other risk factors. If your blood pressure is high, follow your physician's advice on how to lower it. For those with hypertension that is not readily controlled with lifestyle changes, many antihypertension medications are available.

QUICK STATS

A stroke survivor has a **20%** chance of having another stroke within 2 years.

—Heart and Stroke Foundation of Canada, 2009

QUESTIONS FOR CRITICAL THINKING AND REFLECTION

Do you know what your blood pressure and cholesterol levels are? If not, is there a reason you don't know? Is there something preventing you from getting this information about yourself? How can you motivate yourself to have these easy but important health checks?

Know and Manage Your Cholesterol Levels

All people ages 20 and older should talk with their physician about having their cholesterol checked. It is a good idea to get a fasting lipoprotein profile that measures total cholesterol, HDL, LDL, and triglyceride levels. Once you know your baseline numbers, you and your physician can develop an LDL goal and lifestyle plan.

Develop Effective Ways to Handle Stress and Anger

To reduce the psychological and social risk factors for CVD, develop effective strategies for handling the stress in your life. Shore up your social support network, and try some of the techniques described in Chapter 3 for managing stress.

Reducing the Saturated and Trans Fats in Your Diet

No more than 7% of the calories in your diet should come from saturated fats, and no more than 1% should come from trans fats. Foods high in saturated fat include meat, poultry skin, full-fat dairy products, coconut and palm oils, and hydrogenated vegetable oils. Hydrogenated fats and products, such as snack foods that are made with them and deep-fried fast food, are high in trans fats.

Monitor Your Current Diet

To see how your diet measures up, keep track in your health journal of everything you eat for three days. Information about the calorie and saturated fat content of foods is available on many food labels, in books, and on the Internet. The list below gives a few average values for foods that are rich sources of trans fats in the Canadian diet. However, food companies are trying to reduce or eliminate trans fats from their products, so it's important to read the labels.

At the end of the monitoring period, write in the calories and grams of saturated and trans fat for as many as possible of the foods you've eaten. Determine the percentage of daily calories as fat that you consumed for each day: Multiply grams of saturated and trans fats by nine (fat has nine calories per gram) and then divide by total calories. For example, if you consumed 30 grams of saturated and trans fats and 2100 calories on a particular day, then your saturated and trans fat consumption as a percentage of total calories would be 30 × 9 = 270 calories of fat ÷ 2100 total calories = 0.13, or 13%. If you have trouble obtaining all the data you need to do the calculations, you can still estimate

whether your diet is high in saturated and trans fats by seeing how many servings of foods high in unhealthy fats you typically consume on a daily basis (see the list).

Making Heart-Healthy Changes

To reduce your intake of unhealthy fats, you may want to set a limit on the number of servings of foods high in saturated and trans fats that you consume each day. Or you may want to set a more precise goal and then continue to monitor your daily consumption. The 7% limit corresponds to 12 grams of saturated and trans fats in a 1600-calorie diet, 17 grams in a 2200-calorie diet, and 22 grams in a 2800-calorie diet.

To plan healthy changes, take a close look at your food record. Do you choose many foods high in saturated and trans fats? Do you limit your portion sizes to those recommended by *Eating Well with Canada's Food Guide*? Try making healthy substitutions. Do you have a salami and cheese sandwich for lunch? Try turkey for a change.

Do you always order french fries when you eat out? Try half a plain baked potato or a different vegetable next time. Do you snack on pastries, cookies, doughnuts, chips, or fatty crackers? Try fresh fruits and vegetables instead. If you frequently eat in fast-food restaurants or other places where the majority of the menu is heavy in saturated and trans fats, trying finding an appealing alternative—and recruit some friends to join you.

When you choose foods that are rich in saturated and trans fats, *watch your portion sizes carefully*. Choose cuts of meat that have the least amount of visible fat, and trim off what you see. And try to balance your choices throughout the day: For example, if your lunch includes a hamburger and fries, choose broiled fish or poultry or a vegetarian pasta dish for dinner. Plenty of delicious choices are low in saturated and trans fats. Plan your diet around a variety of whole grains, vegetables, legumes, and fruits, which are nearly always low in fats and high in nutrients.

	Grams of Trans Fat Per Serving
Pot pie	6
French fries (large)	5
Pound cake	5
Fish sticks	5
Doughnut	4
Biscuit	4
Fried, breaded chicken	3
Danish pastry	3
Vegetable shortening	3
Margarine (stick)	2
Microwave popcorn	2
Sandwich cookies	2
Snack crackers	2
Margarine (tub)	1

Instead of	Try
Butter, stick margarine, vegetable shortening, coconut and palm oils	Vegetable oils, trans-fat-free tub or squeeze margarines
Whole or 2% milk; regular cheese, mayonnaise, and sour cream	Fat-free or 1% milk, low-fat cheese, fat-free or low-fat sour cream, yogourt, or mayonnaise
Chips, cheese puffs, crackers, buttered popcorn	Fruits, vegetables, rice cakes, plain popcorn, pretzels, fat-free chips, baked crackers
Cakes, cookies, pastries, doughnuts, cinnamon rolls, pie, regular ice cream	Fruit or a *small* serving of a low-fat sweet (angel food cake; fat-free ice cream, frozen yogourt, sherbet, or sorbet)
Biscuits, croissants, fried tortillas, regular granola, muffins, coffee cake	Whole-grain breads and rolls, baked tortillas, low-fat granola or cold cereal, English muffin, or bagel
Creamy or cheesy sauces and soups	Tomato- and other vegetable-based sauces, clam sauce, clear soups
Ground beef, hamburger patty, meatloaf, ribs, T-bone or flank steak, prime grades of beef	Ground turkey, veggie burger, extra-lean ground beef, round steak, sirloin, choice or select grades of beef
Pork chops, roast, or ribs; bone-in ham; lamb chops or ribs	Pork sirloin or tenderloin, boneless ham, veal chops and cutlets, leg of lamb
Bacon, sausage, lunch meats, hot dogs	Canadian bacon; turkey ham or pastrami, other low-fat lunch meats
Poultry with skin; fried chicken or fish	Skinless poultry, especially breast or drumstick; baked, broiled, grilled, or roasted poultry or fish; ground turkey
French fries, onion rings	Baked potato or other nonfried vegetable, rice
Pizza, pot pie, macaroni and cheese, and other high-fat convenience foods	Vegetarian or turkey chili, pasta with vegetables, grilled poultry and fish dishes

Sources: New heart dos and don'ts. 2006. *Consumer Reports Health*, March, 49; American Heart Association. 2000. *An Eating Plan for Healthy Americans: The New 2000 Food Guidelines.* Dallas, Tex.: American Heart Association; U.S. Department of Agriculture and U.S. Department of Health and Human Services. 2000. *Nutrition and Your Health: Dietary Guidelines for Americans*, 5th ed. Home and Garden Bulletin No. 232.

BEHAVIOUR CHANGE STRATEGY

McGraw Hill connect™

Practise and learn online with Connect. Connect allows you to practise important skills at your own pace and on your own schedule, with 24/7 online access to an eBook, practice quizzes, interactivities, videos, study tools, additional resources, and more.

SUMMARY

• The cardiovascular system pumps and circulates blood throughout the body. The heart pumps blood to the lungs via the pulmonary artery and to the body via the aorta.

• The exchange of nutrients and waste products takes place between the capillaries and the tissues.

• The six major risk factors for CVD that can be changed are smoking, high blood pressure, unhealthy cholesterol levels, inactivity, overweight and obesity, and diabetes.

• Effects of smoking include lower HDL levels, increased blood pressure and heart rate, accelerated plaque formation, and increased risk of blood clots.

• Hypertension occurs when blood pressure exceeds normal limits most of the time. It weakens the heart, scars and hardens arteries, and can damage the eyes and kidneys.

• High LDL and low HDL cholesterol levels contribute to clogged arteries and increase the risk of CVD.

• Physical inactivity, obesity, and diabetes are interrelated and are associated with high blood pressure and unhealthy cholesterol levels.

• Contributing risk factors that can be changed include high triglyceride levels and psychological and social factors.

• Risk factors for CVD that can't be changed include being over 65, being male, being Aboriginal or of South Asian or African descent, and having a family history of CVD.

• Atherosclerosis is a progressive hardening and narrowing of arteries that can lead to restricted blood flow and even complete blockage.

• Heart attacks are usually the result of a long-term disease process. Warning signs of a heart attack include chest discomfort, shortness of breath, nausea, and sweating.

• A stroke occurs when the blood supply to the brain is cut off by a blood clot or hemorrhage. A transient ischemic attack (TIA) is a warning sign of stroke.

• Congestive heart failure occurs when the heart's pumping action becomes less efficient and fluid collects in the lungs or in other parts of the body.

• Dietary changes that can protect against CVD include decreasing your intake of fat, especially saturated and trans fats, and cholesterol, and increasing your intake of fibre by eating more fruits, vegetables, and whole grains.

• CVD risk can also be reduced by engaging in regular exercise, avoiding tobacco and environmental tobacco smoke, knowing and managing your blood pressure and cholesterol levels, and developing effective ways of handling stress and anger.

FOR MORE INFORMATION

BOOKS

Freeman, M. W., and C. E. Junge. 2005. Harvard *Medical School Guide to Lowering Your Cholesterol*. New York: McGraw-Hill. Information about cholesterol, including lifestyle changes and medication for improving cholesterol levels.

Heller, M. 2005. *The DASH Diet Action Plan, Based on the National Institutes of Health Research: Dietary Approaches to Stop Hypertension*. Northbrook, Ill.: Amidon Press. Provides background information and guidelines for adopting the DASH diet; also includes meal plans to suit differing caloric needs and recipes.

Lipsky, M. S., et al. 2008. *American Medical Association Guide to Preventing and Treating Heart Disease*. New York: Wiley. A team of doctors provides advice for heart health to consumers.

Mostyn, B. 2007. *Pocket Guide to Low Sodium Foods*, 2nd ed. Olympia, Wash.: InData Publishing. Lists thousands of low-sodium products that can be purchased in supermarkets, as well as low-sodium choices available in many restaurants.

Phibbs, B. 2007. *The Human Heart: A Basic Guide to Heart Disease*. Philadelphia: Lippincott Williams & Wilkins. Provides information about heart disease, treatments, and recovery for patients and their families.

Romaine, D. S., and O. S. Randall. 2005. *The Encyclopedia of Heart and Heart Disease*. New York: Facts on File. Includes entries on the functioning of the cardiovascular system, types and causes of heart disease, and prevention and treatment.

ORGANIZATIONS, HOTLINES, AND WEB SITES

The Internet addresses listed here were accurate at the time of publication.

Canadian Hypertension Society. Provides information on the research and management of hypertension in Canada.

http://www.hypertension.ca

Dietary Approaches to Stop Hypertension (DASH). Provides information about the design, diets, and results of the DASH study, including tips on how to follow the DASH diet at home.

http://www.nhlbi.nih.gov/health/public/heart/hbp/dash

Dietitians of Canada. Provides resources for consumers and health professionals, including articles, news events, and nutrition facts.

http://www.dietitians.ca

Health Canada. Provides information and resources for healthy living among Canadians, including *Eating Well with Canada's Food Guide.*

http://www.hc-sc.gc.ca

Heart and Stroke Foundation of Canada. Provides information about heart, stroke, and healthy living in Canada.

http://www.heartandstroke.ca

The Human Heart: An On-Line Exploration. An online museum exhibit containing information on the structure and function of the heart, how to monitor your heart's health, and how to maintain a healthy heart.

http://www.fi.edu/learn/heart/index.html

MyHeartCentral.com. Provides information for heart patients and others interested in learning how to identify and reduce their risk factors for heart disease; includes links to many related sites.

http://www.healthcentral.com/heart-disease

MedlinePlus: Blood, Heart, and Circulation Topics. Provides links to reliable sources of information on many topics relating to cardiovascular health.

http://www.nlm.nih.gov/medlineplus/heartandcirculation.html

Public Health Agency of Canada. Provides information on a variety of diseases in Canada, including population statistics for heart disease and stroke.

http://www.phac-aspc.gc.ca

U.S. National Heart, Lung, and Blood Institute. Provides information on and interactive applications for a variety of topics relating to cardiovascular health and disease, including cholesterol, smoking, obesity, hypertension, and the DASH diet.

http://www.nhlbi.nih.gov

http://rover.nhlbi.nih.gov/health/public/heart/index.htm#chol

U.S. National Stroke Association. Provides information and referrals for people who have had a stroke and their families; the Web site has a stroke risk assessment.

http://www.stroke.org

See also the listings for Chapters 2–6.

SELECTED BIBLIOGRAPHY

Albert, C. M., et al. 2008. Effect of folic acid and B vitamins on risk of cardiovascular events and total mortality among women at high risk for cardiovascular disease: A randomized trial. *Journal of the American Medical Association* 299(17): 2027–2036.

American Heart Association. 2009. *Heart Disease and Stroke Statistics—2009 Update.* Dallas: American Heart Association.

Berger, J. S., et al. 2006. Aspirin for the primary prevention of cardiovascular events in women and men: A sex-specific meta-analysis of randomized controlled trials. *Journal of the American Medical Association* 295(3): 306–313.

Bonaa, K. H., et al. 2006. Homocysteine lowering and cardiovascular events after acute myocardial infarction. *New England Journal of Medicine* 354(15): 1578–1588.

Brien, S. E., and P. T. Katzmarzyk. 2006. Physical activity and the metabolic syndrome in Canada. *Applied Physiology, Nutrition, and Metabolism* 31: 40–47.

Campbell, N. R. C. 2010. *The 2010 Canadian Hypertension Education Program Recommendations* (http://hypertension.ca/chep/wp-content/uploads/2010/08/FullRec2010_BMSbooklet_EN.pdf; retrieved April 6, 2011).

Colihan, D. 2008. *Silent Strokes Take a Toll* (http://www.webmd.com/stroke/news/20080626/silent-strokes-take-a-toll; retrieved November 10, 2008).

Cooper, R. S., et al. 2005. An international comparative study of blood pressure in populations of European vs. African descent. *BMC Medicine* 3(1): 2.

de Torbal, A., et al. 2006. Incidence of recognized and unrecognized myocardial infarction in men and women aged 55 and older: The Rotterdam Study. *European Heart Journal* 27(6): 729–736.

Elliott, P., et al. 2006. Association between protein intake and blood pressure: The INTERMAP study. *Archives of Internal Medicine* 166(1): 79–87.

Forman, J. P., et al. 2005. Folate intake and risk of incident hypertension among U.S. women. *Journal of the American Medical Association* 293(3): 320–329.

Giovannucci, E., et al. 2008. 25-hydroxyvitamin D and risk of myocardial infarction in men; a prospective study. *Archives of Internal Medicine* 168(11): 1174–1180.

Grundy, S. M., et al. 2004. Definition of metabolic syndrome: Report of the National Heart, Lung, and Blood Institute/American Heart Association conference on scientific issues related to definition. *Circulation* 109: 433–438.

Harvard Medical School. 2008. The status of statins. *Harvard Women's Health Watch* 15(6): 1–3.

Jenkins, D. J., et al. 2006. Assessment of the longer-term effects of a dietary portfolio of cholesterol-lowering foods in hypercholesterolemia. *American Journal of Clinical Nutrition* 83(3): 582–591.

Kastrati, A., et al. 2005. Sirolimus-eluting stent or paclitaxel-eluting stent vs. balloon angioplasty for prevention of recurrences in patients with coronary in-stent restenosis. *Journal of the American Medical Association* 293(2): 165–171.

Kelemen, L. E., et al. 2005. Associations of dietary protein with disease and mortality in a prospective study of postmenopausal women. *American Journal of Epidemiology* 161(3): 239–249.

Meadows, M. 2005. Brain attack: A look at stroke prevention and treatment. *FDA Consumer* March/April.

Mozaffarian, D., et al. 2005. Interplay between different polyunsaturated fatty acids and risk of coronary heart disease in men. *Circulation* 111(2): 157–164.

Mukamal, K. J., et al. 2005. Alcohol and risk of ischemic stroke in men: The role of drinking patterns and usual beverage. *Annals of Internal Medicine* 142(1): 11–19.

Nissen, S. E., et al. 2005. Statin therapy, LDL cholesterol, C-reactive protein, and coronary artery disease. *New England Journal of Medicine* 352(1): 29–38.

Ostrom, M. P., et al. 2008. Mortality incidence and the severity of coronary atherosclerosis assessed by computed tomography angiography. *Journal of the American College of Cardiology* 52(16): 1335–1343.

Pickering, T. G., et al. 2008. Call to action on use and reimbursement for home blood pressure monitoring: A joint scientific statement from the American Heart Association, American Society of Hypertension, and Preventive Cardiovascular Nurses Association. *Hypertension* 52(1): 10–29.

Raggi, P., et al. 2008. Coronary artery calcium to predict all-cause mortality in elderly men and women. *Journal of the American College of Cardiology* 52(1): 17–23.

Refsum, H., et al. 2006. The Hordaland Homocysteine Study: A community-based study of homocysteine, its determinants, and associations with disease. *Journal of Nutrition* 136(6 Suppl.): 1731S–1740S.

Ridker, P. M., et al. 2005. C-reactive protein levels and outcomes after statin therapy. *New England Journal of Medicine* 352(1): 20–28.

Ridker, P. M., et al. 2005. A randomized trial of low-dose aspirin in the primary prevention of cardiovascular disease in women. *New England Journal of Medicine,* 7 March [epub].

Ridker, P. M., et al. 2008. Rosuvastatin to prevent vascular events in men and women with elevated C-reactive protein. *New England Journal of Medicine* 359(21): 2195–2207.

Rothwell, P. M., and C. P. Warlow. 2005. Timing of TIAs preceding stroke: Time window for prevention is very short. *Neurology* 64(5): 817–820.

Rozanski, A. S., et al. 2005. The epidemiology, pathophysiology, and management of psychosocial risk factors in cardiac practice: The emerging field of behavioral cardiology. *Journal of the American College of Cardiology* 45(5): 637–651.

Sesso, H. D., et al. 2008. Vitamins E and C in the prevention of cardiovascular disease in men: Physician's Health Study II randomized controlled trial. *Journal of the American Medical Association* 300(18): 2123–2133.

Tufts University. 2006. Pendulum swings on estrogen and women's heart health risk. *Health & Nutrition Newsletter* 24(3): 1–2.

Turhan, H., et al. 2005. High prevalence of metabolic syndrome among young women with premature coronary artery disease. *Coronary Artery Disease* 16(1): 37–40.

University of California, Berkeley. 2008. Heart tests: low- to high-tech. University of California, Berkeley, *Wellness Letter* August, 5.

Webb, D. 2005. Supplements for a healthy heart: What works, what doesn't. *Environmental Nutrition* 28(12): 1, 4.3

Willingham, S. A., and E. S. Kilpatrick. 2005. Evidence of gender bias when applying the new diagnostic criteria for myocardial infarction. *Heart* 91(2): 237–238.

Wilkins, K., et al. 2010. Blood pressure in Canadian adults. *Health Reports* 21(1) (http://www.statcan.gc.ca/pub/82-003-x/2010001/article/11118-eng.pdf; retrieved April 6, 2011).

Wittstein, I. S., et al. 2005. Neurohumoral features of myocardial stunning due to sudden emotional stress. *New England Journal of Medicine* 352(6): 539–548.

Yusuf, S., et al. 2005. Obesity and the risk of myocardial infarction in 27,000 participants from 52 countries: A case-control study. *Lancet* 366(9497): 1640–1649.

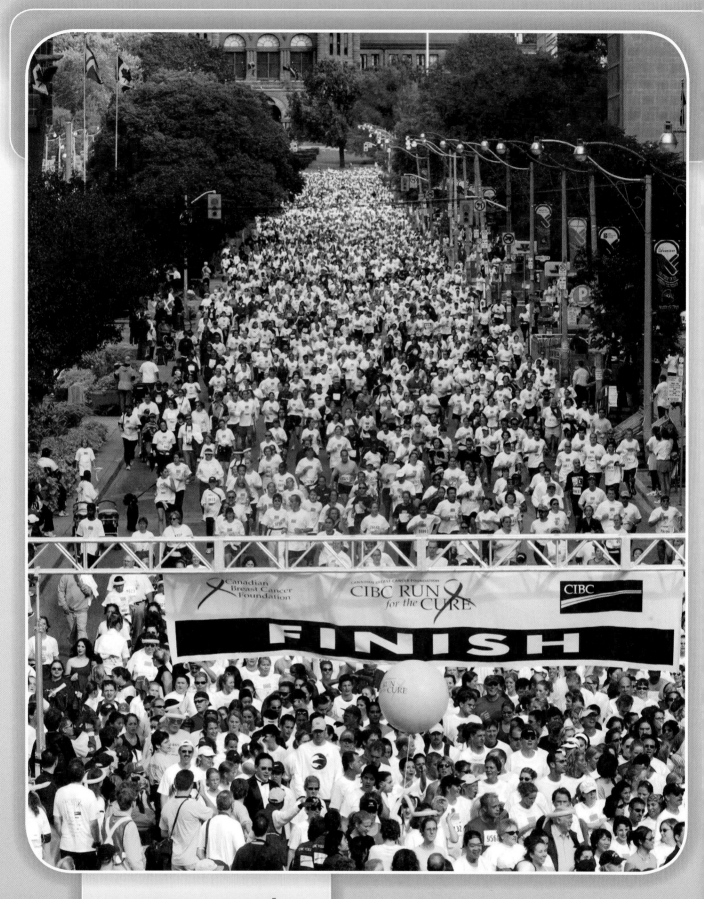

McGraw Hill **connect**™

Practise and learn online with Connect.

CANCER

LOOKING AHEAD>>>>>

AFTER READING THIS CHAPTER, YOU SHOULD BE ABLE TO

- Explain what cancer is and how it spreads
- List and describe common cancers: their risk factors, signs and symptoms, treatments, and approaches to prevention
- Discuss some of the causes of cancer and how they can be avoided or minimized
- Describe how cancer can be detected, diagnosed, and treated
- List specific actions you can take to lower your risk of cancer

TEST YOUR KNOWLEDGE

ANSWERS

1. **Which type of cancer kills the most women each year?**
   a. breast cancer
   b. lung cancer
   c. ovarian cancer

2. **Which type of cancer kills the most men each year?**
   a. prostate cancer
   b. lung cancer
   c. colon cancer

3. **Testicular cancer is the most common cancer in men under age 30.**
   True or false?

4. **The use of condoms during sexual intercourse can prevent cervical cancer in women.**
   True or false?

5. **Eating which of these foods may help prevent cancer?**
   a. chili peppers
   b. broccoli
   c. oranges

1. **B.** There are more cases of breast cancer each year, but lung cancer kills more women. Smoking is the primary risk factor for lung cancer.

2. **B.** There are more cases of prostate cancer, but lung cancer kills about three times as many men as prostate cancer does each year.

3. **TRUE.** Although rare, testicular cancer is the most common cancer in men under age 30. Regular self-exams may aid in its detection.

4. **TRUE.** The primary cause of cervical cancer is infection with human papillomavirus (HPV), a sexually transmitted pathogen. The use of condoms helps prevent HPV infection.

5. **ALL THREE.** These and many other fruit and vegetables are rich in phytochemicals, naturally occurring substances that may have anti-cancer effects.

ancer is the second-leading cause of death, after heart disease. In Canada, cancer is responsible for one in four deaths, claiming approximately 73,500 lives annually—about 1450 each week. In 2009, it was estimated that 171,000 new cases of cancer would be diagnosed; that means 470 Canadians were being diagnosed with some form of cancer each day. Cancer is the leading cause of disease-related death among people under age 65.

Even as medical science struggles to find a cure for cancer, mounting evidence indicates that most cancers can be prevented through simple changes in lifestyle. Tobacco use, for example, is responsible for about 30% of all cancer deaths (Figure 8.1). Poor dietary and exercise habits, and their relationship with obesity, account for another 22% of years of life lost. Such evidence proves that individual behaviour is a significant determinant of cancer risk.

This chapter introduces you to cancer, explains how the disease progresses, and identifies the factors that put people at risk for developing cancer. The following sections also discuss the lifestyle factors that can help you reduce your risk for cancer.

WHAT IS CANCER?

Cancer is the abnormal, uncontrolled multiplication of cells that, if left untreated, can ultimately cause death.

Tumours

Most cancers take the form of tumours, although not all tumours are cancerous. A **tumour** (or *neoplasm*) is simply a mass of tissue that serves no physiological purpose. It can be benign, like a wart, or malignant, like most lung cancers.

Benign (noncancerous) **tumours** are made up of cells similar to the surrounding normal cells and are enclosed in a membrane that prevents them from penetrating neighbouring tissues. They are dangerous only if their physical presence interferes with body functions. A benign brain tumour, for example, can cause death if it blocks the blood supply to the brain.

The term **malignant tumour** is synonymous with cancer. A malignant tumour can invade surrounding structures, including blood vessels, the **lymphatic system**, and nerves. It can also spread to distant sites via the blood and lymphatic circulation, producing invasive tumours in almost any part of the body. A few cancers, such as leukemia (cancer of the blood), do not produce a mass but still

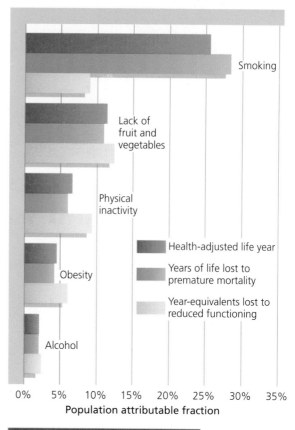

VITAL STATISTICS

FIGURE 8.1   The impact of five risk factors on cancer.

Source: McIntosh, C. N. 2006. *Population Health Impact of Cancer in Canada, 2001* (http://www.statcan.gc.ca/pub/82-005-x/82-005-x2006001-eng.htm; retrieved April 8, 2011). Used with permission of Statistics Canada.

have the fundamental property of rapid, uncontrolled cell multiplication; for this reason, such diseases are malignant and are considered to be a form of cancer.

Every case of cancer begins as a change in a cell that allows it to grow and divide when it should not. Normally (in adults), cells divide and grow at a rate just sufficient to replace dying cells. In contrast, a malignant cell divides without regard for normal control mechanisms and gradually produces a mass of abnormal cells or a tumour. It takes about a billion cells to make a mass the size of a pea, so a single tumour cell must go through many divisions, often taking years, before the tumour grows to a noticeable size (Figure 8.2).

Eventually a tumour produces a sign or symptom that is determined by its location in the body. In the breast, for example, a tumour may be felt as a lump and diagnosed as cancer by an X-ray or a **biopsy**. In less accessible locations, such as the lung, ovary, or intestine, a tumour may be noticed only after considerable growth has taken place and may then be detected only by an indirect symptom—for instance, a persistent cough or unexplained bleeding

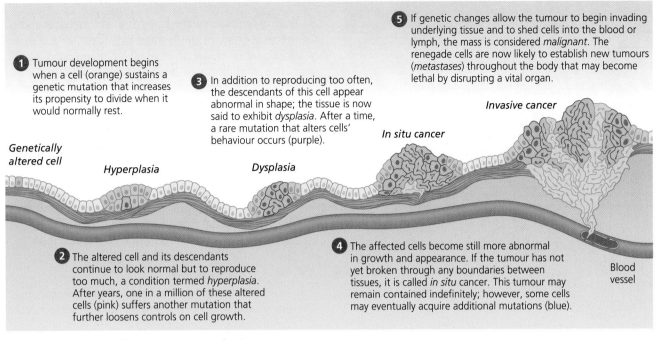

Tumour development begins
when a cell (orange) sustains a
genetic mutation that increases
its propensity to divide when it
would normally rest.

In addition to reproducing too often,
the descendants of this cell appear
abnormal in shape; the tissue is now
said to exhibit *dysplasia*. After a time,
a rare mutation that alters cells'
behaviour occurs (purple).

If genetic changes allow the tumour to begin invading
underlying tissue and to shed cells into the blood or
lymph, the mass is considered *malignant*. The
renegade cells are now likely to establish new tumours
(*metastases*) throughout the body that may become
lethal by disrupting a vital organ.

Invasive cancer

In situ cancer

*Genetically
altered cell*

Hyperplasia

Dysplasia

The altered cell and its descendants
continue to look normal but to reproduce
too much, a condition termed *hyperplasia*.
After years, one in a million of these altered
cells (pink) suffers another mutation that
further loosens controls on cell growth.

The affected cells become still more abnormal
in growth and appearance. If the tumour has not
yet broken through any boundaries between
tissues, it is called *in situ* cancer. This tumour may
remain contained indefinitely; however, some cells
may eventually acquire additional mutations (blue).

Blood
vessel

FIGURE 8.2   Tumour development occurs in stages.

Source: Weinberg, R. A. 1996. How cancer arises. *Scientific American*, September. Copyright © 1996 by Dana Burns-Pizer. Reprinted with permission.

or pain. In the case of leukemia, there is no lump, but the changes in the blood will eventually be noticed as increasing fatigue, infection, or abnormal bleeding.

Metastasis

Metastasis, the spreading of cancer cells from one part of the body to another, occurs because cancer cells do not stick to each other as strongly as normal cells do and therefore may not remain at the site of the *primary tumour* (the cancer's original location). They break away and can pass through the lining of lymph or blood vessels to invade nearby tissue. Once it is established, the tumour can recruit normal cells—such as bone marrow cells—modify them, and use them as envoys to travel to different parts of the body and prepare other sites to receive travelling cancer cells. The envoy cells work by creating proteins that attract the free-floating cancer cells, allowing them to gather at a new site and resume replicating. This travelling and seeding process is called *metastasizing*, and the new tumours are called *secondary tumours*, or *metastases*.

The ability of cancer cells to metastasize makes early cancer detection critical. To control the cancer, every cancerous cell must be removed. Once cancer cells enter either the lymphatic system or the bloodstream, it is extremely difficult to stop their spread to other organs of the body. In fact, counting the number of lymph nodes that contain cancer cells is one of the principal methods of predicting the outcome of the disease; the probability of a cure is much greater when the lymph nodes do not contain cancer cells.

The Stages of Cancer

Once a cancer has been diagnosed, physicians can classify the disease according to the amount of progress it has made in the person's body. The extent or spread of the cancer is described in five **stages**, as shown in Table 8.1 (on p. 246).

To identify a cancer's stage, physicians assess the size or extent of the primary tumour, whether the cancer has invaded nearby lymph nodes, and whether any metastases are present. By judging the extent of each criterion,

cancer   Abnormal, uncontrolled cellular multiplication.

tumour   A mass of tissue that serves no physiological purpose; also called a *neoplasm*.

benign tumour   A mass of tissue that is not cancerous.

malignant tumour   A mass of tissue that is cancerous and capable of spreading.

lymphatic system   A network of vessels that returns proteins, lipids, and other substances from fluid in the tissues to the circulatory system.

biopsy   The removal and examination of a small piece of body tissue; a needle biopsy uses a needle to remove a small sample, but some biopsies require surgery.

metastasis   The spread of cancer cells from one part of the body to another.

staging   A method of classifying the progress or extent of a cancer in a person.

TERMS

Table 8.1	Cancer Stages
Stage	**Description**
0	Early cancer, present only in the layer of cells where it originated
I, II, III	More extensive cancer, with higher numbers indicating greater tumour size and/or the degree to which the cancer has spread to nearby lymph nodes or organs adjacent to the primary tumour.
IV	Advanced cancer that has spread to another organ

Source: U.S. National Institutes of Health, National Cancer Institute. 2004. Staging: Questions and Answers (http://www.cancer.gov/cancertopics/factsheet/detection/staging; retrieved February 15, 2009).

physicians can determine the cancer's current stage and choose the most appropriate treatment based on the disease's progress.

Types of Cancer

The behaviour of tumours arising in different body organs is characteristic of the tissue of origin. (Figure 8.3 shows the major cancer sites and the incidence of each type.)

Because each cancer begins as a single altered cell with a specific function in the body, the cancer retains some of the properties of the normal cell for a time. For instance, cancer of the thyroid gland may produce too much thyroid hormone and cause hyperthyroidism as well as cancer. Usually, however, cancer cells lose their resemblance to normal tissue as they continue to multiply, becoming groups of rogue cells with increasingly unpredictable behaviour.

Malignant tumours are classified according to the types of cells that give rise to them:

- **Carcinomas** arise from **epithelia**, tissues that cover external body surfaces, line internal tubes and cavities, and form the secreting portion of glands. They are the most common type of cancers; major sites include the skin, breast, uterus, prostate, lungs, and gastrointestinal tract.

- **Sarcomas** arise from connective and fibrous tissues, such as muscle, bone, cartilage, and the membranes covering muscles and fat.

- **Lymphomas** are cancers of the lymph nodes, part of the body's infection-fighting system.

- **Leukemias** are cancers of the blood-forming cells, which reside chiefly in the **bone marrow**.

New cases	Deaths	Male	Female	New cases	Deaths
1,500	1,000	Brain	Brain	1,150	750
2,200	750	Oral	Oral	1,150	390
2,900	580	Skin (melanoma)	Skin (melanoma)	2,300	350
12,900	11,200	Lung	Lung	11,200	9,400
180	50	Breast	Breast	23,200	5,300
1,900	1,100	Stomach	Stomach	1,050	720
1,400	590	Liver	Liver	440	160
1,950	1,850	Pancreas	Pancreas	2,100	2,000
12,400	5,000	Colorectal	Colorectal	10,100	4,100
5,300	1,300	Bladder	Bladder	1,800	550
24,600	4,300	Prostate	Ovary	2,600	1,750
930	n/a	Testes	Uterus	4,500	790
1,250	780	Myeloma	Cervix	1,300	370
2,800	1,450	Leukemia	Myeloma	1,000	650
510	n/a	Hodgkin lymphoma	Leukemia	2,000	1,000
4,100	1,750	Non-Hodgkin lymphoma	Hodgkin lymphoma	420	n/a
6,900	5,400	Other	Non-Hodgkin lymphoma	3,400	1,450
90,000	40,000	Total*	Other	7,600	5,300
			Total*	83,900	36,200

*Column totals may not sum to row totals because of rounding; n/a = not available.

VITAL STATISTICS

FIGURE 8.3   Cancer cases and deaths by site and sex.   The "New cases" column indicates the number of cancers that occur annually in each site; the "Deaths" column indicates the number of cancer deaths that are annually attributed to each type.

Source: Canadian Cancer Society's Steering Committee. 2010. *Canadian Cancer Statistics 2010.* Toronto: Canadian Cancer Society.

Cancers vary greatly in how easily they can be detected and how well they respond to treatment. For example, certain types of skin cancer are easily detected, grow slowly, and are very easy to remove; virtually all of these cancers are cured. Cancer of the pancreas, conversely, is very difficult to detect or treat, and very few patients survive the disease. In general, it is very difficult for an **oncologist** or a **hematologist** to predict how a specific cancer will behave, because each one arises from a unique set of changes in a single cell.

The Incidence of Cancer

In 2010, about 83,900 women and 90,000 men were diagnosed with cancer in Canada—this translates into approximately 3300 Canadians being diagnosed with cancer each week. Most were cured or were able to live years longer. In fact, the Canadian Cancer Society estimates that the five-year survival rate for all cancers that were diagnosed between 2002 and 2004 is 62%. This is a 4.5% increase over the five-year relative survival rate for all cancers diagnosed between 1992 and 1994. These statistics exclude more than 1 million cases of the curable types of skin cancer. At current Canadian incident rates, nearly 45% of men and 40% of women will develop cancer at some point in their lives (see the box "Gender and Cancer" on p. 248).

Until 1991, the number of cancer deaths increased fairly steadily in North America, largely because of a wave of lethal lung cancers among men caused by smoking. In 1991, the death rate began to fall slowly; since then it has dropped more than 18% in men and 10% in women. This trend suggests that efforts at prevention, early detection, and improved therapy are all bearing fruit. However, death rates from cancer are not declining as fast as those from heart disease, in large part because of the differing effects that quitting smoking has on disease risk. Heart damage from smoking reverses more quickly and more significantly than the cancer-related damage from smoking. Smoking-related gene mutations cannot be reversed, although other mechanisms can sometimes control cellular changes. Heart disease also has other risk factors, such as high cholesterol and blood pressure, that can be tested for and controlled. If heart disease death rates continue to decline faster than cancer death rates, cancer may overtake heart disease as the leading cause of death among Canadians of all ages.

Still, many more people could be saved from cancer. Researchers estimate that 90% of skin cancer could be prevented by protecting the skin from the rays of the sun, and 87% of lung cancer could be prevented by avoiding exposure to tobacco smoke. Thousands of cases of colon, breast, and uterine cancer could be prevented by improving diet and controlling body weight. Regular screenings and self-examinations have the potential to save an additional 100,000 lives per year. Although cancer may seem like a mysterious disease, many concrete strategies can reduce the risk.

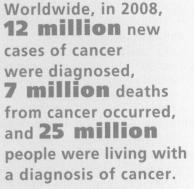

COMMON CANCERS

A discussion of all types of cancer is beyond the scope of this book. In this section we look at some of the most common cancers and their causes, prevention, and treatment.

Lung Cancer

Lung cancer accounts for approximately 14% of all new cancer diagnoses and is the most common cause of cancer death in Canada; it is responsible for about 394 deaths each week. Since the early 1990s lung cancer has surpassed breast cancer as the leading cause of cancer death in women.

TERMS

carcinoma Cancer that originates in epithelial tissue (skin, glands, and lining of internal organs).

epithelia Tissue that covers a surface or lines a tube or cavity of the body, enclosing and protecting other parts of the body.

sarcoma Cancer arising from bone, cartilage, or striated muscle.

lymphoma A tumour originating from lymphatic tissue.

leukemia Cancer of the blood or the blood-forming cells.

bone marrow Soft vascular tissue in the interior cavities of bones that produces blood cells.

oncologist A medical specialist in the study of tumours.

hematologist A medical specialist in the study of blood disorders, including cancers, such as leukemia and lymphoma.

GENDER MATTERS

Gender and Cancer

Men and women share most major risk factors for cancer, but they have a different experience because more than a third of all cancers occur in sex organs (prostate, testes, breast, ovary, uterus, cervix).

For women, this means that in addition to lifestyle factors, such as smoking, diet, and exercise, hormonal factors relating to their menstrual and childbearing history are also important risk considerations. Women may also have a greater biological vulnerability to certain carcinogens, such as those in cigarettes.

Overall, however, men are more likely than women to have cancer and to die of cancer. For some cancers, the differences are especially significant. For example, men are much more likely than women to die from oral cancer, skin cancer, lung cancer, liver cancer, and urinary cancer. Here are some of the factors underlying the higher death rates among men:

• *Higher rates of tobacco use:* Particularly in the past, men had significantly higher rates of smoking than women, leading to much higher rates of the many cancers linked to smoking. Men also have much higher rates of spit tobacco and cigar use. Lung cancer rates among men increased dramatically following

significantly increased smoking rates beginning in the early 1900s (inexpensive machine-produced cigarettes were developed in the late 1800s). The lung cancer rate levelled off and (for men) started to decline after smoking rates began dropping. The smoking-related increase in lung cancer among women occurred about 20–30 years after that seen in men, as smoking among women became more socially acceptable and widespread beginning in the 1930s and 1940s.

• *Higher rates of alcohol use and abuse:* Alcohol abuse is more common in men and is a risk factor for several cancers, including oral and liver cancers.

• *Greater occupational exposure to carcinogens:* Men are more likely to work in jobs where they are exposed to chemicals—including asbestos, arsenic, coal tar, pitch, and dyes—or radiation, and such exposure is a risk factor for cancers of the bladder, lung, and skin. Men are also more likely to have outdoor jobs involving frequent sun exposure.

• *Less use of preventive measures and less contact with health care providers:* Traditional gender roles may make men more likely to minimize symptoms and

less likely to seek help or to discuss cancer-related worries with a health care provider. Men may place a low status on preventive care or screenings, such as using sunscreen and wearing hats to protect the skin from the sun or performing self-exams.

Many of the factors underlying men's greater risk for cancer are controllable. It is important for both men and women to remember that there are many concrete steps they can take to significantly reduce their risk of cancer.

Risk Factors   The chief risk factor for lung cancer is tobacco smoke, which currently accounts for 30% of all cancer deaths and more than 85% of lung cancer deaths. When smoking is combined with exposure to other carcinogens, such as asbestos particles or certain pollutants, the risk of cancer can be multiplied by a factor of 10 or more.

The smoker is not the only one at risk. Environmental tobacco smoke (ETS) is a human carcinogen; even brief exposure can cause serious harm. Long-term exposure to ETS increases the risk of lung cancer. It is estimated that exposure to ETS increases a nonsmoker's risk of developing lung cancer by 20% as compared with people who are not exposed.

Detection and Treatment   Lung cancer is difficult to detect at an early stage and hard to cure even when detected early. Symptoms of lung cancer do not usually appear until the disease has advanced to the invasive stage. Signals such as a persistent cough, chest pain, or recurring bronchitis may be the first indication of a tumour's presence.

Studies suggest that spiral CT (computed tomography) scans, a computer-assisted body imaging technique, can detect lung cancer significantly earlier than chest X-rays.

Smoking is responsible for about 30% of all cancer deaths. The benefits of quitting are substantial: Lung cancer risk decreases significantly after one smoke-free year and drops to half that of continuing smokers after 10 smoke-free years.

In cases where CT scanning is not available, a diagnosis can usually be made by chest X-ray or by studying the cells in sputum. Because almost all lung cancers arise from the cells that line the bronchi, tumours can sometimes be visualized by fibre-optic bronchoscopy, a test in which a flexible lighted tube is inserted into the windpipe and the surfaces of the lung passages are directly inspected.

Treatment for lung cancer depends on the type and stage of the cancer. If caught early, localized cancers can be treated with surgery. But because only about 16% of lung cancers are detected before they spread, radiation and **chemotherapy** are often used in addition to surgery. For cases detected early, 49% of patients are alive five years after diagnosis; but overall, the five-year survival rate is only 15%. Phototherapy, gene therapy, and immuno-therapy (a vaccine) are being studied in the hope of improving these statistics.

In addition, one form of lung cancer, known as small-cell lung cancer and accounting for about 13% of cases, can be treated fairly successfully with chemotherapy, alone or in combination with radiation. A large percentage of cases go into **remission**, which in some cases lasts for years.

Colon and Rectal Cancer

Another common cancer in Canada is colon and rectal cancer (also called *colorectal cancer*). Although we have effective screening methods for colorectal cancer, it is the third most common type of cancer in Canada.

Risk Factors Age is a key risk factor for colon and rectal cancer, with more than half of cases diagnosed in people age 70 and older. Heredity also plays a role. Many cancers arise from preexisting **polyps**, small growths on the wall of the colon that may gradually develop into malignancies. The tendency to form colon polyps appears to be determined by specific genes, so many colon cancers may be due to inherited gene mutations. Chronic bowel inflammation and type 2 diabetes increase the risk of colon cancer.

Lifestyle is also a risk factor for colon and rectal cancer. Excessive alcohol use and smoking may increase the risk of colorectal cancer. Regular physical activity appears to reduce a person's risk, whereas obesity increases it. A diet rich in red and processed meats increases risk, whereas eating fruit, vegetables, and whole grains is associated with lower risk. However, research findings on whether dietary fibre prevents colon cancer have been mixed. Studies have suggested a protective role for folic acid, magnesium, vitamin D, and calcium; in contrast, high intake of refined carbohydrates, simple sugars, and smoked meats and fish may increase risk.

Use of oral contraceptives or hormone replacement therapy may reduce risk in women. Regular use of non-steroidal anti-inflammatory drugs, such as Aspirin and ibuprofen, may decrease the risk of colon cancer and other cancers of the digestive tract.

Detection and Treatment If identified early, precancerous polyps and early-stage cancers can be removed before they become malignant or spread. Because polyps may bleed as they progress, the standard warning signs of colon cancer are bleeding from the rectum and a change in bowel habits.

Regular screening tests are recommended beginning at age 50 (earlier for people with a family history of the disease). A yearly stool blood test can detect small amounts of blood in the stool long before obvious bleeding would be noticed. More involved screening tests are recommended at 5-year or 10-year intervals. In sigmoidoscopy or colonoscopy (Figure 8.4), a flexible fibre-optic device is inserted through the rectum; the colon can be examined and polyps can be biopsied or removed without major surgery. Screening is effective; studies show it could reduce the occurrence of colorectal cancer by 80%. Still, only about one-half of adults have undergone any of these tests.

Surgery is the primary treatment for colon and rectal cancer. Radiation and chemotherapy may be used before surgery to shrink a tumour or after surgery to destroy any remaining cancerous cells. For advanced cancer, treatment with chemotherapy or monoclonal antibodies in

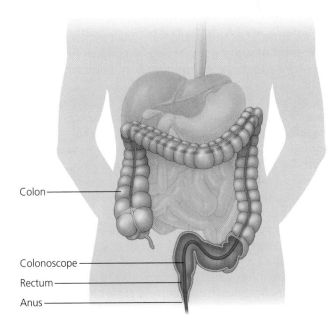

Colon
Colonoscope
Rectum
Anus

FIGURE 8.4 Colonoscopy.

TERMS

chemotherapy The treatment of cancer with chemicals that selectively destroy cancerous cells.

remission A period during the course of cancer in which there are no symptoms or other evidence of disease.

polyp A small, usually harmless, mass of tissue that projects from the inner surface of a mucous membrane, such as the colon or rectum.

combination is an option. This treatment inhibits the growth of new blood vessels (angiogenesis) in tumours. The five-year survival rate for colorectal cancer is 61% for men and 62% for women.

Breast Cancer

Breast cancer is the most common cancer in women and causes almost as many deaths in women as lung cancer. In men, breast cancer occurs only rarely. In Canada, about 1 woman in 9 will develop breast cancer during her lifetime, and 1 woman in 28 will die from the disease. About 22,700 Canadian women will be diagnosed with breast cancer, and about 5400 women will die from it, in the next year.

Less than 1% of breast cancer cases occur in women under age 30, but a woman's risk doubles every five years between ages 30 and 45 and then increases more slowly, by 10%–15% every five years after age 45. More than 75% of breast cancers are diagnosed in women over 50.

Risk Factors   Breast cancer has a strong genetic component. A woman who has two close relatives with breast cancer is four to six times as likely to develop the disease as a woman who has no close relatives with it. However, even though genetic factors are important, only about 15% of cancers occur in women with a family history of breast cancer.

Other risk factors include early onset of menstruation, late onset of menopause, having no children or having a first child after age 30, current use of hormone replacement therapy (HT), obesity, and alcohol use. Estrogen may be a unifying element for many of these risk factors. Estrogen circulates in a woman's body in high concentrations between puberty and menopause. Fat cells also produce estrogen, and estrogen levels are higher in obese women. Alcohol can interfere with estrogen metabolism in the liver and increase estrogen levels in the blood. Estrogen promotes the growth of cells in responsive sites, including the breast and the uterus, so any factor that increases estrogen exposure may raise breast cancer risk. A dramatic drop in rates of breast cancer between 2001 and 2004 was attributed in part to reduced use of HT by women over 50 beginning in July 2002. Millions of women stopped taking the hormones after research linked HT with an increased risk of breast cancer and heart disease.

Although some of the risk factors for breast cancer cannot be changed, important lifestyle risk factors can be controlled. Eating a low-fat, vegetable-rich diet, exercising regularly, limiting alcohol intake, and maintaining a healthy body weight can minimize the chance of developing breast cancer, even for women at risk from family history or other factors. Some research has also found that long-term use of Aspirin and other nonsteroidal anti-inflammatory drugs reduces risk, possibly by affecting estrogen synthesis.

Early Detection   A cure is most likely if breast cancer is detected early, so regular screening is a good idea, even for younger women. The Canadian Cancer Society advises the use of the following guidelines for the early detection of breast cancer:

- *A **mammogram** (low-dose breast X-ray) at least every two years for women over 50* (Figure 8.5). Mammography is especially valuable as an early detection tool because it can identify about 85% of breast cancers at an early stage, before physical symptoms develop. Studies show that magnetic resonance imaging (MRI) may be better than mammography at detecting breast abnormalities in some women, specifically those at high risk, or those with dense breast tissue. A number of factors determine a woman's risk for developing breast cancer, and every woman should discuss her risk factors with a physician to determine what kinds of screening tests are warranted.

Unlike traditional mammography, digital mammograms are recorded on a computer disk rather than film. Digital mammograms can be enhanced and analyzed in more ways than traditional mammograms. Although digital mammography has not yet proved to be more effective at catching breast cancer in all women, there is evidence that it is more effective at spotting tumours in dense breast tissue. A National Cancer Institute study showed that digital mammography might be a better screening tool for women under age 50 who have dense breasts. Although the benefits of early detection and treatment of breast cancer are apparent, mammography is not without risk: It exposes women to X-rays, and X-ray radiation is linked to cancer. A woman's exposure to radiation from screening mammograms depends on the number of tests she has; however, X-ray technicians are well positioned to reduce women's radiation exposure.

FIGURE 8.5   Mammograms can detect breast cancer in women with no symptoms.

Research suggests the incidence of a new cancer forming because of radiation from breast screening mammography is very low. Therefore, the benefits of mammograms (i.e., early diagnosis and management of breast cancer) dramatically outweigh the potential threat associated with the small exposure to radiation resulting from a mammogram.

Ultrasound technology uses sound waves to create images of soft tissue. Although ultrasound is not often used as a standard screening tool for breast cancer, it is sometimes used as a follow-up investigational tool if a mammogram reveals an abnormality in breast tissue.

- *Clinical breast exam:* Women between 40 and 49 should have a clinical breast exam completed by a health professional every two years. Women age 40 and older should have one every year before their scheduled mammogram.

- *Breast awareness:* Breast self-exam (BSE) allows a woman to become familiar with her breasts, so she can alert her health care provider to any changes. For decades, BSE was heavily promoted as a way to detect breast cancer early. However, in 2007, the Canadian Cancer Society stopped recommending routine BSEs as a means of finding cancer. Research indicates that in the absence of mammography, BSE is not likely to reduce breast cancer mortality and can increase the number of benign breast biopsies conducted. In addition to the possible physical risks of biopsies, women face the emotional distress of undergoing a medically invasive procedure only to receive a benign result. Women who choose to continue practising BSE should be informed of its limitations. Beginning at age 20, women are now encouraged to become familiar with their breasts and to recognize what looks and feels normal for them. Women should become "breast aware," know the early symptoms of breast cancer, and notify their doctor of any changes. Unlike with BSE, women do not need to follow a particular technique or schedule.

Breast pain or tenderness is usually associated with benign conditions, such as menstruation, rather than with breast cancer. The first physical signs of breast cancer are more likely to be a lump, swelling, or thickening; skin irritation or dimpling; or nipple pain, scaliness, or retraction. Although most breast lumps are benign, any breast lump should be brought to the attention of a health care provider.

Treatment If a lump is detected, it may be scanned by **ultrasonography** and biopsied to see if it is cancerous. In 90% of cases, the lump is found to be a cyst or other harmless growth, and no further treatment is needed. If the lump contains cancer cells, a variety of surgeries may be called for, ranging from a lumpectomy (removal of the lump and surrounding tissue) to a mastectomy (removal of the breast). For small tumours, lumpectomy is as effective as mastectomy. To determine whether the cancer has spread, lymph nodes from the armpit may be removed and examined. If cancer cells are found, tumour cells remaining in the body can often be slowed or killed by additional therapy, such as radiation, chemotherapy, or both.

Survival of breast cancer varies, depending on the nature of the tumour and whether it has metastasized. If the tumour is discovered before it has spread to the adjacent lymph nodes, the patient has about a 98% chance of surviving more than five years. The survival rate for all stages is 89% at five years and 80% at ten years.

New Strategies for Treatment and Prevention A number of new drugs have been developed for the treatment or prevention of breast cancer. A family of drugs called selective estrogen-receptor modulators, or SERMs, act like estrogen in some tissues of the body but block estrogen's effects in others. One SERM, tamoxifen, has long been used in breast cancer treatment because it blocks the action of estrogen in breast tissue. In 1998, tamoxifen was approved to reduce the risk of breast cancer in healthy women who are at high risk for the disease. However, the drug has serious potential side effects, including increased risk of blood clots and uterine cancer, and its long-term effects are unknown. Another SERM currently being tested as a potential preventive agent is raloxifene, an osteoporosis drug that has fewer side effects than tamoxifen. Although still controversial, the use of SERMs in the prevention of breast cancer is a major breakthrough.

Women may take tamoxifen, anastrozole, or other drugs or undergo chemotherapy to help reduce the risk of recurrence. A genetic test can help predict the risk of breast cancer recurrence and help identify women who will benefit most from chemotherapy; women can then make more informed treatment decisions. For advanced cancer, treatment with trastuzumab, a monoclonal antibody, is an option for some women. Antibodies, discussed in Chapter 9, are proteins produced by the immune system that recognize and bind to foreign substances, such as bacteria; monoclonal antibodies are a special type of antibody that is produced in the laboratory and designed to bind to a specific cancer-related target.

---

mammogram Low-dose X-ray of the breasts used to check for early signs of breast cancer.

ultrasonography An imaging method in which sound waves are bounced off body structures to create an image on a TV monitor; also called *ultrasound*.

TERMS

Prostate Cancer

The prostate gland is situated at the base of the bladder in men and completely surrounds the male's urethra. It produces seminal fluid; if enlarged, it can block the flow of urine. Prostate cancer is the most common cancer in men and the third leading cause of cancer death in men. Approximately 25,500 new cases are diagnosed, and more than 4400 Canadian men die from the disease each year.

Risk Factors   Age is the strongest predictor of the risk, with about 80% of cases of prostate cancer diagnosed in men over age 65. Inherited genetic predisposition may be responsible for 5%–10% of cases, and men with a family history of the disease should be particularly vigilant about screening.

Diets high in calories, dairy products, and animal fats and low in plant foods have also been implicated as possible culprits, as have obesity, inactivity, and a history of sexually transmitted diseases. Type 2 diabetes and insulin resistance are also associated with prostate cancer. Soy foods, tomatoes, and cruciferous vegetables are being investigated for their possible protective effects.

Detection   Early prostate cancer usually has no symptoms. Warning signs of prostate cancer can include changes in urinary frequency, weak or interrupted urine flow, painful urination, and blood in the urine.

Techniques for early detection include a digital rectal examination and the **prostate-specific antigen (PSA) blood test**. The Canadian Cancer Society recommends that men be provided information about the benefits and limitations of the tests and that men over 50 years talk with their doctor about screening for prostate cancer. For men at high risk, including North Americans of African descent and those with a family history of the disease, speak with your doctor about the appropriateness of being tested earlier.

During a digital rectal exam, a physician feels the prostate gland through the rectum to determine if the gland is enlarged or if lumps are present. The PSA blood test may detect an elevated level or a rapid increase in PSA. The PSA test can help catch early prostate cancer, but it also can register benign conditions (more than half of men over 50 have benign prostate disease) and very slow-growing cancers that are unlikely to kill affected individuals. Further, it is not rare for men with normal PSA levels to have prostate cancer.

Because PSA tests can yield false-positive results, they may lead men to receive further testing or treatment that is not needed. Researchers are looking for ways to make the PSA test more sensitive. A new approach involves measuring the percentage of PSA that is free floating in the blood. PSA made by cancer cells is more likely to circulate bound to other proteins, whereas PSA from healthy prostate cells is more likely to be unbound. Thus, a low proportion of unbound or free PSA indicates greater risk, while a high proportion of free PSA is associated with lower risk.

PSA testing has been a subject of controversy among experts for several years because of its tendency to yield misleading results, leading to further testing that can lead to harm. This is especially a concern for men over 75, who are more likely to die of other causes even if they have slow-growing prostate cancer. In older men, most prostate cancers are not deadly, making treatments pointless and potentially harmful.

The Canadian Task Force on Preventive Health Care recommends against PSA screening; however, the Canadian Cancer Society recommends that men over 50 should talk to their doctor about getting tested for prostate cancer.

Ultrasound is used increasingly as a follow-up, to detect lumps too small to be felt and to determine their size, shape, and properties. A needle biopsy of suspicious lumps can be performed relatively painlessly, and whether the biopsied cells are malignant or benign can be determined by examining them under a microscope.

Treatment   Treatments vary based on the stage of the cancer and the age of the patient. A small, slow-growing tumour in an older man may be treated with watchful waiting because he is more likely to die from another cause before his cancer becomes life threatening; however, a recent study shows that older men who undergo treatment live longer than those who don't. More aggressive treatment would be indicated for younger men or those with more advanced cancers. Treatment usually involves radical prostatectomy, in which the prostate is removed surgically. Although radical surgery has an excellent cure rate, it is major surgery and often results in **incontinence** or erectile dysfunction.

A less-invasive alternative involves surgical implantation of radioactive seeds. Radiation from the seeds destroys the tumour and much of the normal prostate tissue but leaves surrounding tissue relatively untouched. Alternative or additional treatments include external radiation, hormones that shrink tumours, cryotherapy, and chemotherapy. Survival rates for all stages of this cancer have improved steadily over the last two decades; the five-year survival rate is now 95%.

Cancers of the Female Reproductive Tract

Because the uterus, cervix, and ovaries are subject to similar hormonal influences, the cancers of these organs can be discussed as a group.

Cervical Cancer   Cancer of the cervix occurs frequently in women in their thirties or even twenties. In Canada, more than 1300 women are diagnosed with cervical cancer each year; the disease kills 370 annually.

Cervical cancer is at least in part a sexually transmitted infection. Almost all cases of cervical cancer stem from infection by the human papillomavirus (HPV), a group of about 100 related viruses that cause both common warts and genital warts. When certain types of HPV are introduced into the cervix, usually by an infected sex partner, the virus infects cervical cells, causing the cells to divide and grow. If unchecked, this growth can develop into cervical cancer. Cervical cancer is associated with multiple sex partners and is extremely rare in women who have not had heterosexual intercourse. Of those men and women who are sexually active, it is estimated that approximately 75% will develop at least one HPV infection during their lifetime. The regular use of condoms can reduce the risk of transmitting HPV. Studies also suggest that women whose sexual partners are circumcised may be at reduced risk because circumcised men are less likely to be infected with HPV and to pass it to their partners.

Because only a very small percentage of HPV-infected women ever get cervical cancer, other factors must be involved. Two of the most important seem to be smoking and infection with genital herpes (discussed in Chapter 13 with other STIs). Both smoking and herpes infection can cause cancerous changes in cells in the laboratory and can speed and intensify the cancerous changes begun by HPV. Research suggests that women with high levels of HPV 16, a specific form of HPV, are at particularly high risk for the infection to develop into cancer. Some studies show that past exposure to the bacterium that causes the STI chlamydia may be a risk factor for cervical cancer that operates independently of HPV.

Screening for the changes in cervical cells that precede cancer is done chiefly by means of the **Pap test**. During a pelvic exam, cells are scraped from the cervix and examined under a microscope to see whether they are normal. If cells are abnormal but not yet cancerous, a condition commonly referred to as *cervical dysplasia*, the Pap test is repeated at intervals. Sometimes cervical cells spontaneously return to normal, but in about one-third of cases, the cellular changes progress toward malignancy. If this happens, the abnormal cells must be removed, either surgically or by destroying them with a cryoscopic (ultra-cold) probe or localized laser treatment. When the abnormal cells are in a precancerous state, the small patch of dangerous cells can be completely removed.

Without timely surgery, the malignant patch of cells goes on to invade the wall of the cervix and spreads to adjacent lymph nodes and to the uterus. At this stage, chemotherapy may be used with radiation to kill the fast-growing cancer cells, but chances for a complete cure are lower. Even when a cure can be achieved, it often means surgical removal of the uterus.

Because the Pap test is highly effective, all sexually active women and women between ages 18 and 65 should be tested. The recommended schedule for testing depends on risk factors, the type of Pap test performed, and whether the Pap test is combined with HPV testing.

A vaccine called Gardasil that protects against four types of HPV viruses, including two that cause about 70% of cervical cancer cases, has been approved for use in Canada. Studies show that the vaccine, given in three doses over six months, also protects against cancers of the vagina and vulva. Vaccination works best when given to girls before they become sexually active, but the recommendation also allows for vaccination of girls and women ages 9–26. In 2010, Health Canada also approved the Gardasil vaccine for boys and men ages 9–26 to prevent genital warts. Cervarix, which prevents certain types of HPV, has also been approved for use in Canada among females ages 10–25.

Preliminary studies are providing good support for Gardasil's ability to prevent HPV among vaccinated females. However, vaccinated females are still encouraged to have a Pap test at regular intervals since the vaccine does not protect against all types of HPV. In March 2007, the Government of Canada announced $300 million for provinces and territories to establish an HPV immunization program. In Ontario, the government has created an immunization program that entitles all grade 8 students to receive the vaccine free (Gardasil is an expensive vaccine at $135/dose).

Uterine, or Endometrial, Cancer   Cancer of the lining of the uterus, or endometrium, most often occurs after the age of 55. Uterine cancer affects about 4500 Canadian women annually and kills about 790 women each year.

The risk factors are similar to those for breast cancer, including prolonged exposure to estrogen, early onset of menstruation, late menopause, never having been pregnant, and obesity. Type 2 diabetes is also associated with increased risk. The use of oral contraceptives, which combine estrogen and progestin, appears to provide protection.

Endometrial cancer is usually detectable by pelvic examination. It is treated surgically, commonly by hysterectomy, or removal of the uterus. Radiation treatment, hormones, and chemotherapy may be used in addition to surgery. Of those diagnosed with uterine cancer, about 85% of patients are alive and disease-free five years later.

prostate-specific antigen (PSA) blood test   A diagnostic test for prostate cancer that measures blood levels of prostate-specific antigen (PSA).

incontinence   The inability to control the flow of urine.

Pap test   A scraping of cells from the cervix for examination under a microscope to detect cancer.

TERMS

Ovarian Cancer   Although ovarian cancer is rare compared with cervical or uterine cancer, it causes more deaths than the other two combined. Ovarian cancer often has no warning signs. Early clues may include increased abdominal size and bloating, urinary urgency, and pelvic pain. It cannot be detected by Pap tests or any other simple screening method and is often diagnosed only late in its development, when surgery and other therapies are unlikely to be successful.

The risk factors are similar to those for breast and endometrial cancer: increasing age (most ovarian cancer occurs after age 60), never having been pregnant, a family history of breast or ovarian cancer, obesity, and specific genetic mutations. A high number of ovulations appears to increase the chance that a cancer-causing genetic mutation will occur, so anything that lowers the number of lifetime ovulation cycles—pregnancy, breastfeeding, or use of oral contraceptives—reduces a woman's risk of ovarian cancer. A diet rich in fruit and vegetables may be associated with reduced risk.

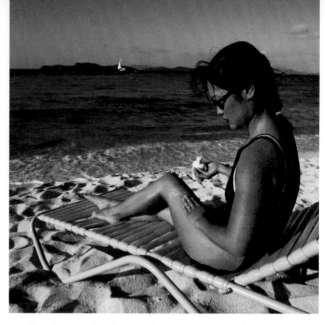

Tanning, either under direct sunlight or in a tanning bed, is a known cause of skin cancer.

Women with symptoms or who are at high risk because of family history or because they harbour a mutant gene should have thorough pelvic exams at regular intervals, as recommended by their physician. Pelvic exams may include the use of ultrasound to view the ovaries.

Ovarian cancer is treated by surgical removal of both ovaries, the fallopian tubes, and the uterus. Radiation and chemotherapy are sometimes used in addition to surgery. The five-year survival rate is only 40%, reflecting the difficulty of early detection.

Skin Cancer

Skin cancer is the most common cancer when cases of the highly curable forms are included in the count. (Usually these forms are not included, precisely because they are easily treated. Treatments are usually simple and successful when the cancers are caught early.) But of the 81,100 cases of skin cancer diagnosed each year, 5000 are of the most serious type, **melanoma**.

Risk Factors   Almost all cases of skin cancer can be traced to excessive exposure to **ultraviolet (UV) radiation** from the sun, including longer-wavelength ultraviolet A (UVA) and shorter-wavelength ultraviolet B (UVB) radiation. UVB radiation causes sunburns and can damage the eyes and the immune system. UVA is less likely to cause an immediate sunburn, but by damaging connective tissue it leads to premature aging of the skin, giving it a wrinkled, leathery appearance. (Tanning lamps and tanning-salon beds emit mostly UVA radiation.) Both UVA and UVB radiation have been linked to the development of skin cancer, and both solar and artificial sources of UV radiation, including sunlamps and tanning beds, are known human carcinogens.

Both severe, acute sun reactions (sunburns) and chronic low-level sun reactions (suntans) can lead to skin cancer. People with fair skin have less natural protection against skin damage from the sun and a higher risk of developing skin cancer; people with naturally dark skin have a considerable degree of protection (see the box "Sun Sensitivity Test"). Melanoma is more common among Caucasians, particularly those with light-coloured skin. For example, in the United States, the annual average incidence rates for melanoma in 2000–2004 were 0.9 per 100,000 for black people, 3.8 per 100,000 for Hispanics, and 19.1 per 100,000 for white people. Although the statistics are likely similar in Canada, the Canadian Cancer Registry does not record ethnicity, and so race-specific rates cannot be estimated for the Canadian population. In general, men are more likely to develop and die from melanoma.

Severe sunburns in childhood have been linked to a greatly increased risk of skin cancer in later life, so children in particular should be protected. The risk of skin cancer increases in people who have had sunburns during childhood, in fact, the earlier in life a child is burned, the greater their risk for developing skin cancer later in life. Because of damage to the ozone layer of the atmosphere (discussed in Chapter 21), we may all be exposed to increasing amounts of UV radiation in the future.

QUICK STATS

People with more than 50 moles are at increased risk for skin cancer.

—Canadian Cancer Society, 2009

QUICK STATS

Melanoma in an immediate family member increases your risk by 50% over people who do not have a family history of the disease.

—Alberta Health Services, 2008

Sun Sensitivity Test

Your risk for developing skin cancer depends on:

- How much sun you get at work and during recreation
- How much your skin reacts to the sun

Try the **Sun Sensitivity Test**, below, to determine your risk of developing skin cancer.

	Yes	No
I have red or blonde hair	☐	☐
I have light-coloured eyes—blue, green, or grey	☐	☐
I freckle easily	☐	☐
I always burn before I tan	☐	☐
I have many moles	☐	☐
I had two or more blistering sunburns before the age of 18	☐	☐
I lived or had long vacations in a tropical climate as a child	☐	☐
There is a family history of skin cancer	☐	☐
I work outdoors in spring and summer	☐	☐
I spend a lot of time in outdoor recreation	☐	☐

Score 10 points for each Yes.

Scores

70 to 100   You are in the high-risk zone for skin cancer and other skin damage. Be careful and protect your skin from the sun.

40 to 60   You are increased risk for skin cancer. Pick up tips on sun protection.

10 to 30   You are still at risk. Carry on being careful.

Source: Canadian Dermatology Association. n.d. *Fact Sheet: Sun Sensitivity Test* (http://www.dermatology.ca/files/SunSensitivityTest_eng.pdf; retrieved April 9, 2011). Used with permission of The Canadian Dermatology Association.

Other risk factors for skin cancer include having many moles, particularly large ones; spending time at high altitudes; and a family history of the disease. Skin cancer may also be caused by exposure to coal tar, pitch, creosote, arsenic, and radioactive materials; but compared with sunlight, these agents account for only a small proportion of cases.

Types of Skin Cancer   There are three main types of skin cancer, named for the types of skin cells from which they develop. **Basal cell** and **squamous cell carcinomas** together account for about 94% of the skin cancers diagnosed each year. They are usually found in chronically sun-exposed areas, such as the face, neck, hands, and arms. They usually appear as pale, waxlike, pearly nodules or red, scaly, sharply outlined patches. These cancers are often painless, although they may bleed, crust, and form an open sore on the skin.

Melanoma is by far the most dangerous skin cancer because it spreads so rapidly. It can occur anywhere on the body, but the most common sites are the back, chest, abdomen, and lower legs. A melanoma usually appears at the site of a preexisting mole. The mole may begin to enlarge, become mottled or varied in colour (colours can include grey or blue, pink or red, and white), or develop an irregular surface or irregular borders. Tissue invaded by melanoma may also itch, burn, or bleed easily.

Prevention   One of the major steps you can take to protect yourself against all forms of skin cancer is to avoid overexposure to sunlight. Blistering, peeling sunburns from unprotected sun exposure are particularly dangerous, but suntans—whether from sunlight or tanning lamps—also increase your risk of developing skin cancer later in

TERMS

melanoma   A malignant tumour of the skin that arises from pigmented cells, usually a mole.

ultraviolet (UV) radiation   Light rays of a specific wavelength emitted by the sun; most UV rays are blocked by the ozone layer in the upper atmosphere.

basal cell carcinoma   Cancer of the deepest layers of the skin.

squamous cell carcinoma   Cancer of the surface layers of the skin.

life. People of every age, especially babies and children, need to be protected from the sun with **sunscreens** and protective clothing. For a closer look at sunlight and skin cancer, see the box "Choosing and Using Sunscreens and Sun-Protective Clothing."

Detection and Treatment   The only sure way to avoid a serious outcome from skin cancer is to make sure it is recognized and diagnosed early. More than half of all melanomas are brought to a physician's attention by patients themselves. Make it a habit to examine your skin regularly. Most of the spots, freckles, moles, and blemishes on your body are normal; you were born with some of them, and others appear and disappear throughout your life. But if you notice an unusual growth, discoloration, a sore that does not heal, or a mole that undergoes a sudden or progressive change, see your physician or a dermatologist immediately.

The characteristics that may signal a skin lesion as a melanoma—asymmetry, border irregularity, colour change, and a diameter greater than 0.5 centimetres—are shown in Figure 8.6. A mole that changes in size, shape, or colour is also of concern. In addition, if someone in your family has had numerous skin cancers or melanoma, consult a dermatologist for a complete skin examination and discussion of your particular risk.

Melanoma is a less common but most dangerous form of skin cancer since it can spread in the body.

MELANOMA SKIN CANCER
KNOW THE SIGNS, SAVE A LIFE

ABCDEs of Melanoma

A ASYMMETRY
The shape on one side is different than the other side.

B BORDER
The border or visible edge is irregular, ragged and imprecise.

C COLOUR
There is a colour variation with brown, black, red, grey or white within the lesion.

D DIAMETER
Growth is typical of melanoma. It is usually more than 6 mm although it can be less.

E EVOLUTION
Look for change in colour, size, shape or symptom such as itching, tenderness or bleeding.

Photos provided by Dr Joël Claveau

5 steps to SKIN CANCER SELF-EXAM

1   Using a mirror in a well lit room, check the front of your body - face, neck, shoulders, arms, chest, abdomen, thighs and lower legs.

2   Turn sideways, raise your arms and look carefully at the right and left sides of your body, including the underarm area.

3   With a hand-held mirror, check your upper back, neck and scalp. Next, examine your lower back, buttocks, backs of thighs and calves.

4   Examine your forearms, palms, back of the hands, fingernails and in between each finger.

5   Finally, check your feet - the tops, soles, toenails, toes and spaces in between.

PROTECT YOURSELF!
The best ways to protect yourself are to:
• Find out your risk factors
• Learn the early signs, the ABCDEs of melanoma
• Protect yourself from the sun from spring to fall and avoid sunbeds
• Check your skin once a month
• Take action if you see any suspicious spots

Dermatologists Your **SKINexperts**
CDA-ACD
Canadian Dermatology Association
Association canadienne de dermatologie

For further information, visit www.dermatology.ca

FIGURE 8.6   The ABCDE test for melanoma.   To see a variety of photos of melanoma and benign moles, visit SkinCancerGuide.ca (http://www.skincancerguide.ca/ sitemap.html).

Source: Canadian Dermatology Association. 2009. *Melanoma Skin Cancer: Know the Signs, Save a Life* (http://www.dermatology.ca/patients_ public/info_patients/skin_cancer/ Melanoma-poster2009_e.pdf; retrieved April 9, 2011).

Table 8.2 Foods with Phytochemicals

Food	Phytochemical	Potential Anti-cancer Effects
Chili peppers (the hotter the pepper, the more capsaicin it contains)	Capsaicin	Neutralizes effect of nitrosamines; may block carcinogens in cigarette smoke from acting on cells
Oranges, lemons, limes, onions, apples, berries, eggplant	Flavonoids	Act as antioxidants; block access of carcinogens to cells; suppress malignant changes in cells; prevent cancer cells from multiplying
Citrus fruit, cherries	Monoterpenes	Help detoxify carcinogens; inhibit spread of cancer cells
Cruciferous vegetables (broccoli, cabbage, bok choy, cauliflower, kale, Brussels sprouts, collards)	Isothiocyanates	Boost production of cancer-fighting enzymes; suppress tumour growth; block effects of estrogen on cell growth
Garlic, onions, leeks, shallots, chives	Allyl sulphides	Increase levels of enzymes that break down potential carcinogens; boost activity of cancer-fighting immune cells
Grapes, red wine, peanuts	Resveratrol	Acts as an antioxidant; suppresses tumour growth
Green, oolong, and black teas (note that drinking very hot tea may *increase* the risk of some cancers), grapes, wine, turmeric	Polyphenols	Increase antioxidant activity; prevent cancer cells from multiplying; help speed excretion of carcinogens from body
Orange, deep yellow, red, pink, and dark green vegetables; some fruit	Carotenoids	Act as antioxidants; reduce levels of cancer-promoting enzymes; inhibit spread of cancer cells
Soy foods, whole grains, flax seeds, nuts	Phytoestrogens	Block effects of estrogen on cell growth; lower blood levels of estrogen
Whole grains, legumes	Phytic acid	Binds iron, which may prevent it from creating cell-damaging free radicals

healthy weight if you are currently overweight or obese. Being overweight or obese is linked with increased risk of several kinds of cancer, including breast and colon cancer (Figure 8.7). See Chapters 4 and 6 for detailed information on weight management, physical activity, and exercise.

One expert estimates that if we were all to exercise for 20 minutes each day and make the dietary changes discussed in this chapter, about 40,000 cancer deaths could be prevented each year. Many people are unaware of the link between obesity and cancer; see the box "Cancer Myths and Misperceptions" on p. 264 for more facts on cancer.

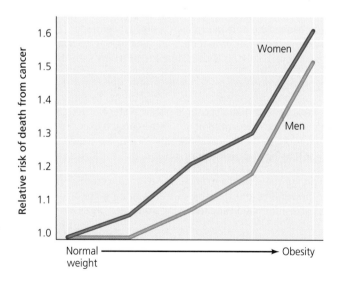

FIGURE 8.7 Body weight and cancer mortality.

Source: Calle, E. E., et al. 2003. Overweight, obesity, and mortality from cancer in a prospectively studied cohort of U.S. adults. *New England Journal of Medicine* 348(17): 1625–1638.

Carcinogens in the Environment

Some carcinogens occur naturally in the environment, such as viruses and the sun's UV rays. Others are manufactured or synthetic substances that show up occasionally in the general environment but more often in the work environments of specific industries.

Microbes It is estimated that about 15% of the world's cancers are caused by microbes, including viruses, bacteria, and parasites, although the percentage is much lower in developed countries, such as Canada. As discussed earlier, certain types of human papillomavirus cause many cases of cervical cancer, and the *Helicobacter pylori* bacterium has been definitely linked to stomach cancer.

Viruses seem to be the main cancer causers. The Epstein-Barr virus, best known for causing mononucleosis, is also suspected of contributing to Hodgkin's disease, cancer of the pharynx, and some stomach cancers. Human herpes-virus 8 has been linked to Kaposi's sarcoma and certain types of lymphoma. Hepatitis viruses B and C together cause as many as 80% of the world's liver cancers.

Ingested Chemicals The food industry uses preservatives and other additives to prevent food from becoming

anticarcinogen An agent that destroys or otherwise blocks the action of carcinogens.

carotenoid Any of a group of yellow-to-red plant pigments that can be converted to vitamin A by the liver; many act as antioxidants or have other anti-cancer effects. The carotenoids include beta-carotene, lutein, lycopene, and zeaxanthin.

TERMS

Cancer Myths and Misperceptions

Almost daily, cancer receives wide-ranging media coverage as it affects the lives of its victims and as breakthroughs create new hope for a cure. During regular checkups, doctors and dentists routinely look for signs of cancer and are quick to discuss the risks of developing cancer.

Remarkably, even as we are being inundated with information about cancer, studies show that many North Americans do not understand basic facts about the disease. Indeed, many still believe myths about cancer that were disproved long ago. Such misperceptions are leading North Americans to ignore good advice on cancer prevention and to continue lifestyle habits that increase the risk of cancer.

Healthier Cigarettes?

Scientists have concluded that so-called low-tar, low-nicotine, and light cigarettes are no safer than regular cigarettes. In fact, some brands of light cigarettes contain just as much nicotine and additives as regular cigarettes. Further, users of light cigarettes tend to smoke more frequently and inhale more deeply than smokers of regular cigarettes—often in the misguided belief that their chosen brand won't hurt them. In a 2006 survey, 72% of women and 63% of men said they believed light cigarettes were not as harmful as regular cigarettes. Meantime, smoking remains the leading preventable cause of cancer.

Similarly, many smokers have switched to smokeless tobacco products (such as chewing tobacco), thinking they pose no health risks. Smokeless tobacco products contribute to head, throat, and oral cancers.

Obesity and Cancer

A recent survey conducted showed that only 8% of North Americans are aware of the link between obesity and cancer. (Only about 15% of respondents knew their own BMI; most overweight and obese people surveyed did not view themselves as being too heavy.)

As is the case with heart disease, maintaining a healthy weight and body composition can help reduce the risk of cancer. Although scientists aren't sure how body fat works to increase cancer risk, evidence shows that overweight and obese people are in greater danger of breast, prostate, colorectal, and other cancers. In fact, obesity is the second most preventable cause of death.

Prevailing Myths

In light of such findings, it may not be surprising to learn that many Canadians accept some myths about cancer, such as the following:

• *Antiperspirants and breast cancer.* The Canadian Cancer Society holds that no direct causal relationship has been found between antiperspirant use and breast cancer incidence.

• *Bras and breast cancer.* Currently, no reliable, scientific evidence shows a link between wearing a bra and developing breast cancer.

• *Microwaves and plastic containers.* Canadians believe that heating food in a microwave by using plastic dishes or plastic wrap will increase the risk of developing cancer. Some scientific evidence suggests that substances used to manufacture plastic products may transfer from the container into the food and that some of these products may be carcinogenic. Health Canada recommends not using plastic bowls or wrap in the microwave unless they are labelled as microwave safe.

• *Oyster sauce and soy sauce.* The production process for these products can lead to the formation of 3-MCPD, a chemical that has been identified as a possible carcinogen in humans. After completing its research, Health Canada has concluded that there is no immediate health risk to Canadians from consumption of soy and oyster sauces. However, Health Canada has identified that lifetime exposure to high levels of 3-MCPD could pose a health risk. Consequently, Health Canada has established 1.0 part per million (ppm) guideline for manufacturers of these sauces to reduce Canadians' long-term exposure to this chemical (this is considered to be a very safe level).

• *Reusing disposable water bottles.* Although many people are using nonplastic water bottles for environmental reasons, some people believe that disposable plastic water bottles can cause cancer if they are frozen or left in the car and exposed to heat. According to the Canadian Cancer Society, no evidence shows that reusing disposable plastic water bottles causes cancer.

Belief in these myths may be cause for concern. The first step in preventing and treating cancer is finding good sources of reliable information and following a qualified physician's advice.

---

spoiled or stale (see Chapter 5). Some of these compounds are antioxidants and may actually decrease any cancer-causing properties the food might have.

Other compounds, such as the nitrates and nitrites found in processed meat, are potentially more dangerous. The nitrites inhibit the growth of bacteria, which could

otherwise cause food poisoning. They also preserve the pink colour of the meat, which has no bearing on taste but looks more appetizing to many people. While nitrates and nitrites are not themselves carcinogenic, they can combine with dietary substances in the stomach and be converted to nitrosamines, which are highly potent carcinogens. Foods cured with nitrites, as well as those cured by salt or smoke, have been linked to esophageal and stomach cancer, and they should be eaten only in modest amounts.

Environmental and Industrial Pollution   Pollutants in urban air have long been suspected of contributing to the incidence of lung cancer. Fossil fuels and their combustion products, such as complex hydrocarbons, have been of special concern.

The best available data indicate that less than 2% of cancer deaths are caused by general environmental pollution, such as substances in our air and water. Exposure to carcinogenic materials in the workplace is a more serious problem. Occupational exposure to specific carcinogens may account for up to 5% of cancer deaths. With increasing industry and government regulation, we can anticipate that the industrial sources of cancer risk will continue to diminish, at least in North America. In contrast, in the former Soviet Union and Eastern European countries, where environmental concerns were sacrificed to industrial productivity for decades, cancer rates from industrial pollution continue to climb.

Radiation   All sources of radiation are potentially carcinogenic, including medical X-rays, radioactive substances (radioisotopes), and UV rays from the sun. Most physicians and dentists are quite aware of the risk of radiation, and successful efforts have been made to reduce the amount of radiation needed for mammograms, dental X-rays, and other necessary medical X-rays. Full-body CT scans are sometimes advertised for routine screening in otherwise well individuals to look for tumours. Such screening is not recommended; it is typically expensive and may have false-positive findings that lead to unnecessary and invasive additional tests. Also, the radiation in these full-body X-rays may itself raise the risk of cancer; the radiation dose of one full-body CT scan is nearly 100 times that of a typical mammogram.

Sunlight is a very important source of radiation, but because its rays penetrate only a millimetre or so into the skin, it could be considered a surface carcinogen. Most

cases of skin cancer are the relatively benign and highly curable basal cell carcinomas, but a substantial minority are the potentially deadly malignant melanomas. As discussed earlier, all types of skin cancer are increased by early and excessive exposure to the sun, and severe sunburn early in childhood appears to carry with it an added risk of melanoma later in life.

DETECTING, DIAGNOSING, AND TREATING CANCER

Early cancer detection often depends on our willingness to be aware of changes in our own body and to make sure we keep up with recommended diagnostic tests. Although treatment success varies with individual cancers, cure rates have increased—sometimes dramatically—in this century.

Detecting Cancer

Unlike those of some other diseases, early signs of cancer are usually not apparent to anyone but the person who has them. Even pain is not a reliable guide to early detection, because the initial stages of cancer may be painless. Self-monitoring is the first line of defence, and you can watch for the seven major warning signs shown in Figure 8.8. Remember them by the acronym CAUTION.

Although none of the warning signs is a sure indication of cancer, the appearance of any one should send you to

QUESTIONS FOR CRITICAL THINKING AND REFLECTION
What do you think your risks for cancer are? Do you have a family history of cancer, or have you been exposed to carcinogens? How about your diet and exercise habits? What can you do to reduce your risks?

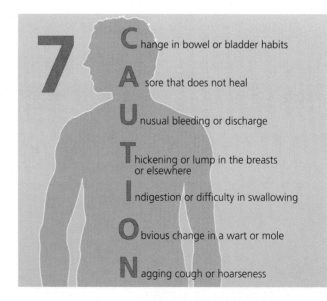

FIGURE 8.8   The seven major warning signs of cancer.

see your physician. By being aware of the risk factors in your own life, your immediate family's cancer history, and your own history, you may bring a problem to the attention of a physician long before it would have been detected at a routine physical.

In addition to self-monitoring, the Canadian Cancer Society recommends routine cancer checkups, as well as specific screening tests for certain cancers (Table 8.3).

Diagnosing Cancer

Detection of a cancer by physical examination is only the beginning. Methods for determining the location, type, and degree of malignancy of a cancer continue to improve. Knowledge of the precise location and size of a tumour is necessary for effective surgery or radiation therapy. This is especially true in cases where the tumour may be hard to reach, as in the brain.

Imaging studies or exploratory surgery may be performed to identify a cancer's stage. A biopsy may be performed to confirm the type of tumour. Several diagnostic imaging techniques have replaced exploratory surgery for some patients. In magnetic resonance imaging (MRI), a huge electromagnet is used to detect hidden tumours by mapping, on a computer screen, the vibrations of different atoms in the body. Computed tomography (CT) scanning uses X-rays to examine the brain and other parts of the body. The process allows the construction of cross-sections, which show a tumour's shape and location more accurately than is possible with conventional X-rays. For patients undergoing radiation therapy, CT scanning

enables the therapist to pinpoint the tumour more precisely, thereby providing more accurate radiation dosage while sparing normal tissue.

Table 8.3	Early Detection Screening Guidelines
Site	**Recommendation**
Breast	• Mammograms every second year are recommended starting at age 50. The age at which screening should be stopped should be individualized by considering the potential risks and benefits of screening in the context of overall health status and longevity. • A clinical breast exam should be part of a health exam about every 2 years for women 40 and older. • Women should know how their breasts normally feel and report any breast change promptly to their health care providers. Breast self-exam is an option for women starting in their twenties.
Cervix	Annual screening is recommended for women who are sexually active or at age 18; after 2 normal smears, pap test should be completed every 3 years to age 69. The HPV vaccine prevents HPV infection but should occur in addition to, not instead of, cervical cancer screening.
Colon and rectum	Beginning at age 50, men and women should begin screening with one of the examination schedules below: • A fecal occult blood test (FOBT) or fecal immunochemical test (FIT) every 2 years. • If a test is positive for blood, a colonoscopy should be performed to determine the cause of bleeding.
Prostate	Men over 50 should talk to their doctor about being tested for prostate cancer. The PSA test and the digital rectal examination are methods to screen for prostate cancer. Men at high risk (black men and men with a strong family history of one or more first-degree relatives diagnosed with prostate cancer at an early age) should talk to their doctor to see if they should be examined at an earlier age. For men at both average risk and high risk, information should be provided about what is known and what is uncertain about the benefits and limitations of early detection and treatment of prostate cancer so that they can make an informed decision about testing.

Sources: Canadian Cancer Society. 2009. Various pages on site (http://www.cancer.ca; retrieved April 12, 2011).

Ultrasonography has also been used increasingly in the past few years to view tumours. It has several advantages: It can be used in the physician's office, it is less expensive than other imaging methods, and it is completely safe. Prostate ultrasound (a rectal probe that uses ultrasonic waves to produce an image of the prostate gland) is being investigated for its ability to detect small, hidden tumours that would be missed by a digital rectal exam.

Treating Cancer

The ideal cancer therapy would kill or remove all cancerous cells while leaving normal tissue untouched. Sometimes this is almost possible, as when a surgeon removes a small superficial tumour of the skin. Usually the tumour is less accessible, and some combination of surgery, radiation therapy, and chemotherapy must be applied instead. Some patients choose to combine conventional therapies with alternative treatments (see the box "Including Complementary Cancer Care" on p. 268).

Surgery   For most cancers, surgery is the most useful treatment. In many cases, the organ containing the tumour is not essential for life and can be partially or completely removed. This is true especially for localized breast, prostate, or testicular cancer, where the surgical removal of one breast, the prostate gland, or one testicle may give a long-lasting cure. Surgery is less effective when the tumour involves cells of the immune system, which are widely distributed throughout the body, or when the cancer has already metastasized. In such cases, surgery must be combined with other techniques.

Chemotherapy   Chemotherapy, or the use of cell-killing drugs to destroy rapidly growing cancer cells, has been in use since the 1940s. Many of these drugs work by interfering with DNA synthesis and replication in rapidly dividing cells. Normal cells, which usually grow slowly, are not destroyed by these drugs. However, some normal tissues, such as intestinal, hair, and blood-forming cells, are always growing, and damage to these tissues produces the unpleasant side effects of chemotherapy, including nausea, vomiting, diarrhea, and hair loss.

Chemotherapy drugs are often used in combinations or with surgery. Recently, in a procedure called **induction chemotherapy**, physicians have begun to use chemotherapy before surgery, both to shrink the tumour and to kill any existing small metastases as soon as possible.

Radiation   In cancer radiation therapy, a beam of X-rays or gamma rays is directed at the tumour, and the tumour cells are killed. Occasionally, when an organ is small enough, radioactive seeds are surgically placed inside the cancerous organ to destroy the tumour and then removed later if necessary. Radiation destroys both normal and cancerous cells, but because it can be precisely directed at the tumour

it is usually less toxic for the patient than either surgery or chemotherapy, and it can often be performed on an outpatient basis. Radiation may be used as an exclusive treatment or in combination with surgery and chemotherapy.

New and Experimental Techniques   Many new and exciting possibilities for cancer therapy promise alternatives to the options of surgery, radiation, and chemotherapy. The research into alternatives is ongoing. One Canadian devoted to finding a cure for cancer was Terry Fox. Terry Fox's cancer journey raised awareness and money and left a lasting legacy (see the box "Cancer Research in Canada: The Efforts of Terry Fox" on p. 269). Although it is impossible to predict which of these new approaches will be most successful, researchers hope that cancer therapy overall will become increasingly safer and more effective:

• *Gene therapy.* Completion of the sequencing of the human genome in 2000 offered many new insights into cancer. Scientists have already discovered important new subtypes of tumours for breast cancer, melanoma, leukemia, and lymphomas based on patterns of gene expression. **Gene therapy** is the manipulation of gene expression in human cells. Gene therapy offers a potential treatment or cure for cancer, as well as for various genetic diseases. For gene therapy to succeed, new genes must be delivered to defective cells without disturbing the overall functioning of the cells. In the treatment of cancer, gene therapy would turn off the genes responsible for causing cells to divide rapidly and become malignant. By using this approach, researchers hope to develop targeted therapies for specific cancers.

• *Bone marrow and stem cell transplants.* In cancers of the blood-forming cells or lymph cells, a patient's own bone marrow may have to be eliminated by radiation or chemotherapy to rid the body of cancer cells. Bone marrow can then be restored by transplanting healthy bone marrow cells from a compatible donor. Transplant incompatibility can be a problem, but progress on this

---

induction chemotherapy   The use of chemotherapy before surgery to shrink a cancerous tumour and prevent metastasis; sometimes eliminates the need for radical surgery.

gene therapy   The manipulation of gene expression in human cells; offers a potential treatment or cure for cancer by turning off the genes responsible for causing cells to divide rapidly and become malignant.

TERMS

Including Complementary Cancer Care

Sometimes conventional treatments for cancer are simply not enough. A patient may be told that there is little conventional therapy can do, other than providing medication to ease pain. When therapy is available, it may be painful and even intolerable to some people. Not surprisingly, many people with cancer look for complementary and alternative therapies. As many as 80% of cancer patients report combining conventional treatments with some type of mind-body technique. A much smaller number of patients look for alternatives to the more conventional therapies. These may be therapies within the bounds of legitimate medical practice that have not yet proven themselves in clinical trials. Or, at the extreme, alternative therapies may be scientifically unsound and dangerous, as well as expensive.

Complementary therapies, such as yoga, massage, acupuncture, meditation, music therapy, tai chi, and prayer, can have positive physical and psychological benefits for patients and improve quality of life as people deal with illness and the often difficult treatments for cancer. Mind-body practices can reduce pain and anxiety, improve sleep, and give people a sense of control and participation in their treatment; such practices may also enhance the immune system. (See Chapter 3 for more on stress and relaxation techniques.) Mind-body practices typically can be used in combination with conventional cancer therapies. There is some proof that these techniques may be helpful as complementary therapies to conventional cancer treatment.

For other types of therapies, the Canadian Cancer Society suggests several ways people with cancer can make safe and informed decisions:

• Understand the differences among conventional, complementary, integrative, and alternative therapies.

• Find out as much as you can about complementary or alternative therapies you are thinking about, including the possible benefits and risks.

• Talking to your health care team about complementary therapy or alternative therapies and how they may interact with the care you are receiving.

• Be especially cautious when evaluating cancer remedies promoted online; one recent study found that as many as one-third of cancer-related alternative medicine sites offered advice that was harmful or potentially dangerous.

One danger of alternative medicine is the very real possibility that proven therapies will be neglected while unproven, faddish alternative approaches are pursued; if alternate therapies delay proven therapies, lives may be lost. Another danger is that complementary therapies may counteract or affect conventional therapies; for example, some herbal supplements have been found to affect how cancer drugs are absorbed and used by the body. Further, some of these alternative therapies are expensive, and many patients are concerned about the cost of unproven therapies. A recent study revealed that 70% of patients using complementary therapies did not inform their physicians. However, it is essential for physicians to have this information so any side effects or harmful interactions can be prevented.

Sources: Canadian Cancer Society. 2009. *Complementary and Alternative Therapies* (http://www.cancer.ca/Canada-wide/About%20cancer/Treatment/ Complementary%20and%20alternative%20therapies.aspx?sc_lang=en; retrieved November 21, 2009); National Cancer Institute. 2006. *Complementary and Alternative Medicine in Cancer Treatment: Questions and Answers* (http://www.cancer.gov/cancertopics/factsheet/therapy/ CAM; retrieved February 15, 2009).

---

front has been made through the use of **stem cells**. These unique, unspecialized cells can divide and produce more specialized cell types, including bone marrow cells (see Chapter 17). These stem cells can be identified, purified, and grown outside the body and then transplanted back into the person with cancer. This technique would allow for safe repopulation of bone marrow after radiation.

• *Biological therapies.* Biological therapies are based on enhancing the immune system's reaction to a tumour. Techniques include cancer vaccines, genetic modification of the body's immune cells, and the use of genetically engineered cytokines, which enhance immune cell function. Melanomas seem particularly susceptible to these biological approaches. Cancer vaccines are also under study for kidney cancer, lymphoma, lung cancer, and other cancers.

• *Proteasome inhibitors.* Proteasomes help control the cell cycle—the process through which cells divide. If proteasomes malfunction, as is often the case in cancer cells, then cells may begin multiplying out of control. Proteasome inhibitors block the action of proteasomes, halting cell division and killing the cells. One proteasome inhibitor is now being used against certain cancers, and other such drugs are in development.

• *Anti-angiogenesis drugs.* To obtain nutrients, cancer cells signal the body to produce new blood vessels, a process called angiogenesis. Drugs that block angiogenesis could keep tumours from growing and spreading.

• *Enzyme activators/blockers.* Normal cells die after dividing a given number of times. Scientists believe that the enzyme caspase triggers the death of normally functioning cells. In cancer cells, caspase activity may be blocked. Conversely, if the enzyme telomerase becomes active in cancer cells, the life-death cycle stops and the cells duplicate indefinitely. In effect, inactive caspase or active telomerase may keep cancer cells alive. Researchers are studying compounds that can either activate caspase or deactivate telomerase; either type of drug might lead cancer cells to self-destruct. No such drugs are now in clinical use.

Cancer Research in Canada: The Efforts of Terry Fox

In 1977, at the age of 18, a young sports enthusiast named Terry Fox was diagnosed with osteogenic sarcoma (bone cancer). As a result of his cancer, Terry had his right leg amputated 15 centimetres above the knee. But rather than dwelling on his own circumstances, he found himself moved by the stories of other people with cancer and the terrible treatments they endured. His compassion motivated Terry to run across Canada and raise money for cancer research. His goal was a lofty one: to raise $1 million.

Terry started his journey on April 12, 1980, in St. John's, Newfoundland, running with one strong leg and one artificial leg. In the beginning, not many people were aware of the run, but it soon began to attract attention and donations. His journey was quickly named the Marathon of Hope.

But after running 5373 kilometres in 143 days, and crossing six provinces, Terry's journey came to an end in Thunder Bay, Ontario. His cancer had metastasized to his lungs. Although he couldn't finish his run across Canada, his spirit had touched Canadians and the donations continued.

On his return to British Columbia, Terry was honoured with numerous awards, including those from the American Cancer Society and the Province of British Columbia. Terry is also the youngest Champion of the Order of Canada. On June 28, 1981, at the age of 22, Terry lost his battle with cancer. His Marathon of Hope had raised $24.17 million.

More than 30 years later, Terry's legacy lives on. To date, more than $500 million has been raised for cancer research in Terry's name.

Sources: The Terry Fox Foundation. 2011. *Terry Fox and the Terry Fox Foundation* (https://www.terryfox.org/Foundation/index.html; retrieved April 8, 2011); The Terry Fox Foundation. 2011. (https://www.terryfox.org/Foundation/Facts.html; retrieved April 8, 2011); Mayo Clinic. 2009. *Bone Cancer* (http://www.mayoclinic.com/health/bone-cancer/DS00520; retrieved April 8, 2011).

QUESTIONS FOR CRITICAL THINKING AND REFLECTION

Do you know how to perform self-examinations? Has your doctor ever suggested that you do so, or given you instructions on proper technique? Given what you know about yourself and your family's medical history, do you think self-exams could be important for you?

Living with Cancer

Nearly 695,049 people in Canada have survived cancer. However, the fear of cancer never disappears; recurrence is always a possibility.

Psychological support is an important factor during treatment for cancer (see the box "Coping with Cancer" on p. 270). For some patients, family, friends, and a caring physician or nurse provide all the support that is necessary. For many people, an organized support group can help provide needed social and psychological support.

PREVENTING CANCER

As mentioned throughout this chapter, your lifestyle choices can radically lower your cancer risks (see Figure 8.9 on p. 270). Here are some guidelines:

• *Avoid tobacco.* The bloodstream carries carcinogens from tobacco smoke throughout the body, making smoking a risk for many forms of cancer other than lung cancer.

The use of spit tobacco increases the risk of cancers of the mouth, larynx, throat, and esophagus. It is also important to avoid exposure to environmental tobacco smoke.

• *Control diet and weight.* About one-third of all cancers are in some way linked to what we eat. Choose a low-fat, plant-based diet containing a wide variety of fruit, vegetables, and whole grains rich in phytochemicals. Drink alcohol only in moderation, if at all. Maintain a healthy weight.

• *Exercise.* Regular exercise is linked to lower rates of some cancers. It also helps control weight and reduce risk factors for other diseases.

• *Protect your skin.* Almost all cases of skin cancer are sun related. Wear protective clothing when you're out in the sun, and use a sunscreen with an SPF rating of 15 or higher. Don't go to tanning salons or use tanning booths.

• *Avoid environmental and occupational carcinogens.* Try to avoid exposure to cancer-causing agents in the environment, especially in the workplace. These agents can range from second-hand smoke to pesticides and other chemicals.

Also, follow the Canadian Cancer Society's recommendations for cancer screenings. Your doctor can help you determine the most appropriate timing and methods for screenings.

stem cells Unspecialized cells that can divide and produce cells that differentiate into the many different types of specialized cells in the body (brain cells, muscle cells, skin cells, blood cells, and so on).

Coping with Cancer

A cancer diagnosis was once viewed as a death sentence, and patients and families were often left to face their fears alone. People were sometimes reluctant to admit to the diagnosis of cancer or share it with others because of feelings of hopelessness or irrational guilt.

Since about the 1970s, a cultural shift has taken place. Improved diagnostic methods and therapies have increased survival times and cures. Media attention on positive developments has created a better understanding of the scientific basis of cancer. Some of the mystery about and dread of cancer have begun to abate, leading to a more positive atmosphere for people with cancer and their families.

If You Have Cancer

Each person's experience with cancer is unique, based on his or her own personality and values. Some people turn to their friends and family members for support, whereas others prefer help from other people with cancer, professional counsellors, or faith-based groups. If you have cancer, it is important to do what is right for you. Here are some strategies for dealing with the difficult emotions that may accompany a cancer diagnosis:

• Remember that cancer doesn't always mean death. Many cancers are curable or controllable for long periods, and people return to a normal, healthy life. Hope and optimism are important elements in cancer survival.

• Focus on controlling what you can. Be informed and involved with your medical care, keep your appointments, and make healthy changes in your lifestyle.

• Work toward having a positive attitude, but don't feel guilty if you can't maintain it all the time. Having cancer is difficult, and low moods will occur no matter how good you are at coping. If they become frequent or severe, seek help.

• Use strategies that have helped you solve problems and manage your emotions in the past. Some people respond to information gathering, talking with others, and prayer or meditation. Physical activity, music, art, and sharing personal stories may help lessen stress.

• Confide feelings and worries to someone close to you. Don't bottle up your feelings to spare your loved ones. If you don't feel comfortable sharing with others, consider expressing your emotions in a journal.

Finding a Support Group

Support groups may be led by cancer survivors, group members, or trained professionals. These groups typically present information, teach coping skills, and give people with cancer a place to share common concerns and obtain emotional support. Support groups may focus on education, behavioural training, or group interaction. Behavioural training can involve meditation and other techniques

to reduce stress or the effects of chemotherapy or radiation therapy.

Research has shown that support groups can enhance quality of life in very practical ways. For instance, patients in breast cancer support groups were found to have improved psychological symptoms, less pain, and improved family relationships compared with patients in a control group.

Support groups vary in quality, and people with cancer may find that a support group fails to discuss topics relevant to their personal situation. Some people

---

Do More

• Eat a varied, plant-based diet that is high in fibre-rich foods, such as legumes and whole grains.

• Eat five to ten servings of fruits and vegetables every day, favouring foods from the following categories:
> Cruciferous vegetables
> Citrus fruits
> Berries
> Dark green leafy vegetables
> Dark yellow, orange, or red fruits and vegetables

• Be physically active.

• Maintain a healthy weight.

• Practise safer sex (to avoid HPV infection).

• Protect your skin from the sun with appropriate clothing and sunscreen.

• Perform regular self-exams (testicular self-exam, skin self-exam).

• Obtain recommended screening tests and discuss with your physician any family history of cancer.

Do Less

• Don't use tobacco in any form:
> Cigarettes
> Spit tobacco
> Cigars and pipes
> Bidis and clove cigarettes

• Avoid exposure to environmental tobacco smoke.

• Limit consumption of fatty meats and other sources of saturated fat.

• Avoid excessive alcohol consumption.

• Limit consumption of salt.

• Don't eat charred foods, and limit consumption of cured and smoked meats and meat and fish grilled in a direct flame.

• Limit exposure to UV radiation from sunlight or tanning lamps or beds.

• Avoid occupational exposure to carcinogens.

FIGURE 8.9   Strategies for reducing your risk of cancer.

may find a support group upsetting because it stirs up too many uncomfortable feelings or because the leader is not skilled. Find a group that is right for you.

Online support groups can be very helpful for people living in rural areas or confined to their homes. Medical information on the Internet is highly variable in quality, however; you should check with your physician before making any decisions based on online information.

Supporting a Person with Cancer

There is no one right way to act with a person facing cancer. Reassure the person of your love, and let him or her know that you are available for both practical and emotional support. A person with cancer may want you to be very involved in treatment or coping, or he or she may want your help in maintaining a more normal routine. Guidelines for visiting a person with cancer include the following:

• Before you visit, call to ask if it's a good time. Surprise visits are often not welcome. Don't overstay.

• Be a good listener. Allow the person to express all his or her feelings, and don't discount fears or minimize the seriousness of the situation. Let the person with cancer decide whether the two of you talk about the illness. It's human to want to laugh and talk about other things sometimes.

• Ask "What can I get you?" or "How can I help?" instead of saying "Let me know if I can help." Make specific offers: to clean the bathroom, go grocery shopping, do laundry, or give caregivers a break.

• Refrain from offering advice. You may have heard about the latest treatment or hottest physician, but unless you are asked for suggestions, keep them to yourself.

• If you want to take food, ask about dietary restrictions ahead of time. Use a disposable container so the person won't have to return it.

• Don't be put off if your first visit gets a lukewarm reception. Many people with cancer are on an emotional roller coaster, and their feelings and needs will change over time.

Support groups also exist for friends and family members of people with cancer. These groups give people a place to express their fears about many issues, such as relationship changes, financial problems, and ways to provide emotional support for the person with cancer.

Palliative Care

Palliative care, while not postponing death, enhances the quality of life for people who have been diagnosed with terminal cancer and their families. An essential component of cancer management, it provides pain and symptom relief, along with psychosocial support.

This holistic approach to end-of-life care begins at diagnosis and continues through to death, where dying is considered a normal part of life. Drawing on music, relaxation, and art therapy, palliative care strives to enhance emotional well-being. As a result, studies show that palliative care can positively influence a patient's disease progression. A comprehensive, multidisciplinary approach, involving both family and community resources, is required for effective palliative care.

Sources: Kissane, D. W., et al. 2004. Effect of cognitive-existential group therapy on survival in early-stage breast cancer. *Journal of Clinical Oncology* 22(21): 4255–4260; National Cancer Institute. 2002. *Your Mind and Your Feelings After Cancer Treatment* (http://www.cancer.gov/cancerinfo/life-after-treatment/page6; retrieved February 15, 2009); Goodwin, P. J., et al. 2001. The effect of group psychosocial support on survival in metastatic breast cancer. *New England Journal of Medicine* 345(24): 1719–1726; Life with cancer: How to provide support. 1996. *Women's Health Advocate*, September; Holland, J. C. 1996. Cancer's psychological challenges. *Scientific American*, September; Nainis, N., et al. 2006. Relieving symptoms in cancer: Innovative use of art therapy. *Journal of Pain and Symptom Management* 31(2): 162–169; World Health Organization. 2010. *Cancer: Palliative Care* (http://www.who.int/cancer/palliative/en/; retrieved April 12, 2011).

QUESTIONS FOR CRITICAL THINKING AND REFLECTION

Review the guidelines just listed for preventing cancer. How many of these things do you do regularly? How often do you think about them? For example, do you often forget to use sunscreen before going outdoors or do you ever hang out in places where people smoke?

Incorporating More Fruit and Vegetables into Your Diet

When we think about the health benefits of fruit and vegetables, we usually focus on the fact that they are rich in carbohydrates, dietary fibre, and vitamins and low in fat. A benefit that we may overlook is that they contain specific cancer-fighting compounds, phytochemicals that help slow, stop, or even reverse the process of cancer. In line with *Eating Well with Canada's Food Guide*, the Canadian Cancer Society recommends eating five to ten servings of fruit and vegetables each day, in an effort to reduce a person's risk of cancer. However, most Canadians are not meeting these guidelines. In 2001, more than 60% of Canadians did not consume the suggested number of fruit and vegetables each day, varying from 55% in Quebec to 72% in NWT. Fruit and vegetable consumption also varies with age and sex. Consistently, men tend to eat fewer servings than their female counterparts in all age groups; those 55 years of age and older consume the largest amount of fruit and vegetables.

Most Canadians need to increase the amount of fruit and vegetables they eat every day. Begin by monitoring your diet for one to two weeks to assess your current intake; then look for ways to incorporate these foods into your diet in easy and tasty ways. Here are some tips to get you started.

Breakfast

- Drink 100% juice every morning.
- Add raisins, berries, or sliced fruit to cereal, pancakes, or waffles. Top bagels with tomato slices.
- Try a fruit smoothie made from fresh or frozen fruit and orange juice or low-fat yogourt.

Lunch

- Choose vegetable soup or salad with your meal.

- Replace potato chips or french fries with cut-up vegetables.
- Add extra chunks of fruit or vegetables to salads.
- Try adding vegetables, such as roasted peppers, cucumber slices, shredded carrots, avocado, or salsa, to sandwiches.
- Drink tomato or vegetable juice instead of soda (watch for excess sodium).

Dinner

- Choose a vegetarian main course, such as stir-fry or vegetable stew. Have at least two servings of vegetables with every dinner.
- Microwave vegetables and sprinkle them with a little bit of Parmesan cheese.
- Substitute vegetables for meat in casseroles and pasta and chilli recipes.
- At the salad bar, pile your plate with healthy vegetables and use low-fat or non-fat dressing.

Snacks and On the Go

- Keep ready-to-eat-fruit and vegetables on hand (apples, plums, pears, and carrots).
- Keep small packages of dried fruit in the car (try dried apricots, peaches, and pears and raisins).
- Make ice cubes from 100% fruit juice and drop them into regular or sparkling water.
- Freeze grapes for a cool summer treat.

In the Grocery Store

- Stock up on canned, frozen, and dried fruit and vegetables when they go on sale.
- Buy fresh fruit and vegetables in season; they'll taste best and be less expensive.
- To save on preparation time, buy pre-cut vegetables and fruit and packaged salads.

- Try a new fresh fruit or vegetable every week.

The All-Stars

Different fruit and vegetables contribute different vitamins, phytochemicals, and other nutrients, so be sure to get a variety. The following types of produce are particularly rich in nutrients and phytochemicals:

- Cruciferous vegetables (broccoli, cauliflower, cabbage, kale, etc.)
- Citrus fruit (oranges, lemons, limes, grapefruit, tangerines, etc.)
- Berries (strawberries, raspberries, blueberries, etc.)
- Dark green leafy vegetables (spinach, chard, collards, beet greens, kale, mustard greens, romaine and other dark lettuces, etc.)
- Deep yellow, orange, and red fruit and vegetables (carrots, pumpkin, sweet potatoes, winter squash, red and yellow bell peppers, apricots, cantaloupe, mangoes, papayas, etc.)

Sources: BC Cancer Agency. 2002. *Phytochemicals: The "Super Nutrients" of the 21st Century* (http://www.bccancer.bc.ca/NR/rdonlyres/10C9D76D-9390-4825-BDAF-FB011502FF0A/9333/Phytochemicals1.pdf; retrieved November 21, 2009); The produce prescription. 2000. *Consumer Reports on Health,* December; Welland, D. 1999. Fruits and vegetables: Easy ways to five-a-day. *Environmental Nutrition,* June; Canadian Cancer Society. 2004. *Continue to Eat 5 to 10 Servings of Fruit and Vegetables a Day* (http://www.cancer.ca/Canada-wide/About%20us/Media%20centre/CW-Media%20releases/CW-2004/Continue%20to%20eat%205%20to%2010%20servings%20of%20fruit%20and%20vegetables%20a%20day.aspx?sc_lang=en; retrieved November 11, 2009).

McGraw Hill connect™

Practise and learn online with Connect. Connect allows you to practise important skills at your own pace and on your own schedule, with 24/7 online access to an eBook, practice quizzes, interactivities, videos, study tools, additional resources, and more.

SUMMARY

- A malignant tumour can invade surrounding structures and spread to distant sites via the blood and lymphatic system, producing additional tumours.

- A malignant cell divides without regard for normal growth. As tumours grow, they produce signs or symptoms that are determined by their location in the body.

- One in two men and one in three women will develop cancer.

- Lung cancer kills more people than any other type of cancer. Tobacco smoke is the primary cause.

- Colon and rectal cancer are linked to age, heredity, obesity, and a diet rich in red meat and low in fruit and vegetables. Most colon cancers arise from preexisting polyps.

- Breast cancer affects about one in nine women in Canada. Although breast cancer has a genetic component, diet and hormones are also risk factors.

- Prostate cancer is chiefly a disease of aging; diet and lifestyle probably are factors in its occurrence. Early detection is possible through rectal examinations, PSA blood tests, and sometimes ultrasound.

- Cancers of the female reproductive tract include cervical, uterine, and ovarian cancer. The Pap test is an effective screening test for cervical cancer.

- Abnormal cellular changes in the epidermis, often a result of exposure to the sun, cause skin cancer, as does chronic exposure to certain chemicals. Skin cancers occur as basal cell carcinoma, squamous cell carcinoma, and melanoma.

- Oral cancer is caused primarily by smoking, excess alcohol consumption, and use of spit tobacco. Oral cancers are easy to detect but often hard to treat.

- Testicular cancer can be detected early through self-examination.

- Mutational damage to a cell's DNA can lead to rapid and uncontrolled growth of cells; mutagens include radiation, viral infection, and chemical substances in food and air.

- Cancer-promoting dietary factors include meat, certain types of fats, and alcohol.

- Diets high in fruit and vegetables are linked to a lower risk of cancer.

- Other possible causes of cancer include inactivity and obesity, certain types of infections and chemicals, and radiation.

- Self-monitoring and regular screening tests are essential to early cancer detection.

- Methods of cancer diagnosis include magnetic resonance imaging, computed tomography, and ultrasound.

- Treatment methods usually consist of some combination of surgery, chemotherapy, and radiation. Gene therapy, bone marrow and stem cell transplants, proteasome inhibitors, biological therapies, and drugs that inhibit angiogenesis or telomerase also hold promise as effective treatments.

- Strategies for preventing cancer include avoiding tobacco; eating a varied, moderate diet and controlling weight; exercising regularly; protecting skin from the sun; avoiding exposure to environmental and occupational carcinogens; and getting recommended cancer screening tests.

FOR MORE INFORMATION

BOOKS

Beliveau, R., and D. Gingras, 2006. *Foods That Fight Cancer: Preventing Cancer through Diet.* New York: DK Publishing. Provides information about appropriate foods to fight cancer.

Cotter, A. 1999. *From This Moment On: A Guide for Those Recently Diagnosed with Cancer.* MacMillan Canada. Provides information on the experience of having cancer.

Hartmann, L. C., C. L. Loprinzi, and B. S. Gostout. 2005. *Mayo Clinic: Guide to Women's Cancers.* New York: Kensington. Provides information about a variety of women's cancers.

McKinnell, R. G., et al. 2006. *The Biological Basis of Cancer,* 2nd ed. Boston: Cambridge University Press. Examines the underlying causes of cancer and discusses actual cases of the disease and its impact on patients and families.

Oh, W. 2006. *Prostate Cancer: An Issue of Hematology/Oncology Clinics.* Toronto: Elsevier Canada. Provides information on prostate cancer.

Rosenbaum, E., et al. 2008. *Everyone's Guide to Cancer Therapy,* rev. 5th ed. Riverside, N.J.: Andrews McMeel. Reviewed by a panel of more than 100 oncologists; provides articles on the known causes, diagnoses, and treatments for many types of cancer.

Servan-Schreiber, D. 2008. *The Anti-Cancer Life: A New Way of Life.* Toronto: HarperCollins Publishers. Provides information on both the personal experience and the research of a physician diagnosed with cancer, discussing both conventional treatments and alternative therapies.

Turkington, C., and W. LiPera. 2005. *The Encyclopedia of Cancer.* New York: Facts on File. Includes entries on a variety of topics relating to cancer causes, prevention, diagnosis, and treatment.

Williams, P. 2006. *Breast Cancer.* Toronto: Penguin Group Canada. Provides information about breast cancer.

ORGANIZATIONS, HOTLINES, AND WEB SITES

The Internet addresses listed here were accurate at the time of publication.

Breast Cancer Society of Canada. Provides information on breast cancer.
  http://www.bcsc.ca
Canadian Breast Cancer Foundation. Provides information about breast cancer.
  http://www.cbcf.org
Cancer Care Ontario. Provides information on the prevention and care of cancer in Ontario.
  http://www.cancercare.on.ca
Canadian Cancer Research Alliance. Provides information about organizations devoted to cancer work.
  http://www.ccra-acrc.ca
Canadian Cancer Society. Provides information on cancer, treatments, prevention, and research.
  http://www.cancer.ca
Canadian Dermatology Association. Provides information on skin cancer.
  http://www.dermatology.ca
Cancer Guide: Steve Dunn's Cancer Information Page. Links to many good online cancer resources and advice about how to make the best use of information.
  http://www.cancerguide.org
Cancer News. Provides links to news and information on many types of cancer.
  http://www.cancernews.com
Clinical Trials. Information about clinical trials for new cancer treatments can be accessed at the following sites:
  http://www.cancer.gov/clinicaltrials
  http://www.centerwatch.com
Colorectcal Cancer Association of Canada. Provides information on treatment, screening, and statistics.
  http://www.colorectal-cancer.ca
Harvard School of Public Health: Disease Risk Index. Includes interactive risk assessments and tips for preventing common cancers.
  http://www.diseaseriskindex.harvard.edu/update
Lung Cancer Canada. Provides detailed information about lung cancer.
  http://www.lungcancercanada.ca
MedlinePlus Cancer Information. Provides news and links to reliable information on a variety of cancers and cancer treatment.
  http://www.nlm.nih.gov/medlineplus/cancers.html

National Comprehensive Cancer Network. Presents treatment guidelines for physicians and patients related to the treatment of various cancers; these guidelines were developed by a group of leading cancer centres.
  http://www.nccn.org
Ovarian Cancer Canada. Presents information on ovarian cancer and treatment options.
  http://www.ovariancanada.org
Prostate Cancer Canada. Contains facts, statistics, and treatment on prostate cancer.
  http://www.prostatecancer.ca
Public Health Agency of Canada. Provides information about the various forms of cancer.
  http://www.phac-aspc.gc.ca/cd-mc/cancer/index-eng.php
U.S. National Cancer Institute. Provides information on treatment options, screening, and clinical trials.
  http://www.cancer.gov
U.S. National Toxicology Program. The national U.S. program that creates regular reports listing those substances that are known or reasonably assumed to cause cancer in humans.
  http://ntp-server.niehs.nih.gov

See also the listings in Chapters 4–6, 15, and 16.

SELECTED BIBLIOGRAPHY

Abbasi, N. R., et al. 2004. Early diagnosis of cutaneous melanoma. *Journal of the American Medical Association* 292(22): 2771–2776.

Alberta Health Services. 2008. *Melanoma* (http://www.albertahealthservices.ca/2273.asp; retrieved April 9, 2011).

Baker, S., and J. Kaprio. 2006. Common susceptibility genes for cancer: Search for the end of the rainbow. *British Medical Journal* 332(7550): 1150–1152.

Bjorge, T., S. Tretli, and A. Engeland. 2004. Relation of height and body mass index to renal cell carcinoma in two million Norwegian men and women. *American Journal of Epidemiology* 60(12): 1168–1176.

Brand, T. C., et al. 2006. Prostate cancer detection strategies. *Current Urology Reports* 7(3): 181–185.

Brenner, D. J., et al. 2004. Estimated radiation risks potentially associated with full-body CT screening. *Radiology* 232(3): 735–738.

Canadian Cancer Society. 2003. *21,000 Cancer Deaths Could Be Prevented If People Had Quit Smoking Sooner* (http://www.cancer.ca/Canada-wide/About%20us/Media%20centre/CW-Media%20releases/CW-2003/21%20000%20cancer%20deaths%20could%20be%20prevented%20if%20people%20had%20quit%20smoking%20sooner.aspx?sc_lang=en; retrieved April 10, 2011).

Canadian Cancer Society. 2006. *Media Backgrounder: Tobacco Facts and What We're Doing* (http://www.cancer.ca/Canada-wide/About%20us/Media%20centre/CW-Media%20releases/CW-2006/Media%20backgrounder%20Tobacco%20facts%20and%20what%20were%20doing.aspx?sc_lang=en; retrieved April 10, 2011).

Canadian Cancer Society's Steering Committee. 2009. *Canadian Cancer Statistics 2009.* Toronto: Canadian Cancer Society (http://www.cancer.ca/canada-wide/about%20cancer/cancer%20statistics/~/media/CCS/Canada%20wide/Files%20List/English%20files%20heading/pdf%20not%20in%20publications%20section/Stats%202009E%20Cdn%20Cancer.ashx; retrieved April 8, 2011).

Canadian Dermatology Association. 2009. *Canadian Dermatology Association 2009 Skin Cancer Fact Sheet* (http://www.dermatology.ca/patients_public/info_patients/skin_cancer/2009-SkinCancer-factsheet_e.pdf; retrieved April 13, 2011).

Canadian Women's Health Network. 2007. *Abnormal Pap Tests* (http://www.cwhn.ca/en/node/40773; retrieved April 9, 2011).

Chao, A., et al. 2005. Meat consumption and risk of colorectal cancer. *Journal of the American Medical Association* 293(2): 172–182.

Chia, K. S., et al. 2005. Profound changes in breast cancer incidence may reflect changes into a Westernized lifestyle: A comparative population-based study in Singapore and Sweden. *International Journal of Cancer* 113(2): 302–306.

de Vries, S. H., et al. 2004. Prostate cancer characteristics and prostate specific antigen changes in screening detected patients initially treated with a watchful waiting policy. *Journal of Urology* 172(6 Pt 1): 2193–2196.

Elmore, J. G., et al. 2005. Screening for breast cancer. *Journal of the American Medical Association* 293(10): 1245–1256.

Flood, A., et al. 2005. Calcium from diet and supplements is associated with reduced risk of colorectal cancer in a prospective cohort of women. *Cancer Epidemiology, Biomarkers and Prevention* 14(1): 126–132.

Garland, S. 2006. Efficacy of a quadrivalent HPV (types 6, 11, 16, 18) L1 VLP vaccine against external genital disease: Future 1 analysis. *European Journal of Obstetrics, Gynecology, and Reproductive Biology* 107(1): 18–27.

Goff, B. A., et al. 2004. Frequency of symptoms of ovarian cancer in women presenting to primary care clinics. *Journal of the American Medical Association* 291(22): 2705–2712.

Harper, D. M., et al. 2004. Efficacy of a bivalent L1 virus-like particle vaccine in prevention of infection with human papillomavirus types 16 and 18 in young women: A randomised controlled trial. *Lancet* 364(9447): 1757–1765.

Health Canada. 2008. *Sleeping with a Killer: A Report from Health Canada's Tobacco Control Programme* (http://www.hc-sc.gc.ca/hc-ps/pubs/tobac-tabac/swk-dat/intro01-eng.php; retrieved November 21, 2009).

Hou, L., et al. 2004. Computing physical activity and risk of colon cancer in Shanghai, China. *American Journal of Epidemiology* 160(9): 860–867.

Jee, S. H., et al. 2005. Fasting serum glucose level and cancer risk in Korean men and women. *Journal of the American Medical Association* 293(2): 194–202.

Jemal, A., et al. 2005. Cancer Statistics, 2005. *CA: A Cancer Journal for Clinicians* 55(1): 10–30.

Kaplan, R. N., et al. 2005. VEGFR1-positive haematopoietic bone marrow progenitors initiate the pre-metastatic niche. *Nature* 438(7069): 820–827.

Kauff, N. D., et al. 2008. Risk-reducing salpingo-oophorectomy for the prevention of *BRCA1*- and *BRCA2*-associated breast and gynecologic cancer: A multicenter, prospective study. *Journal of Clinical Oncology* 26(8): 1331–1337.

Kroenke, C. H., et al. 2005. Weight, weight gain, and survival after breast cancer diagnosis. *Journal of Clinical Oncology* 23(7): 1370–1378.

Laaksonen, D. E., et al. 2004. Serum linoleic and total polyunsaturated fatty acids in relation to prostate and other cancers: A population-based cohort study. *International Journal of Cancer* 111(3): 444–450.

Martinez, M. E. 2005. Primary prevention of colorectal cancer: Lifestyle, nutrition, exercise. *Recent Results in Cancer Research* 166: 177–211.

Mayo Clinic. 2006. Skin cancer epidemic. Take steps to avoid sun damage. *Mayo Clinic Health Letter* 24(4): 1–3.

Mayo Clinic. 2008. Bladder cancer: Early discovery, vigilance are key. *Mayo Clinic Health Letter* 26(10): 1–3.

Mayo Clinic. 2008. Breast imaging: Advances in earlier cancer detection. *Mayo Clinic Health Letter* 26(2): 1–3.

McIntosh, C. N. 2006. *Population Health Impact of Cancer in Canada, 2001* (http://www.statcan.gc.ca/pub/82-005-x/82-005-x2006001-eng.htm; retrieved April 8, 2011).

Meadows, M. 2004. Cancer vaccines: Training the immune system to fight cancer. *FDA Consumer*, September/October.

Melanoma. 2004. *Journal of the American Medical Association* 292(22): 2800.

Mor, G., et al. 2005. Serum protein markers for early detection of ovarian cancer. *Proceedings of the National Academy of Sciences USA*, May 12 [epub].

Nainis, N., et al. 2006. Relieving symptoms in cancer: Innovative use of art therapy. *Journal of Pain and Symptom Management* 31(2): 162–169.

National Toxicology Program. 2005. *Report on Carcinogens,* 11th ed. Research Triangle Park, N.C.: National Toxicology Program.

New treatments for colorectal cancer. 2004. *FDA Consumer,* May/June.

Ontario Ministry of Health and Long-Term Care. 2005. *Costs of Tobacco Use and Tax Revenues* (http://www.health.gov.on.ca/english/public/updates/archives/hu_04/tobacco/tobacco_revenue.html; retrieved April 10, 2011).

Osborn, N. K., and D. A. Ahlquist. 2005. Stool screening for colorectal cancer: Molecular approaches. *Gastroenterology* 128(1): 192–206.

Paik, S., et al. 2004. A multigene assay to predict recurrence of tamoxifen-treated, node-negative breast cancer. *New England Journal of Medicine* 351(27): 2817–2826.

Parmet, S. 2004. Genetics and breast cancer. *Journal of the American Medical Association* 292(4): 522.

Pelucchi, C., et al. 2004. Fibre intake and prostate cancer risk. *International Journal of Cancer* 109(2): 278–280.

Prostate cancer: Should you still have a PSA test? 2005. *University of California, Berkeley Wellness Letter,* January (http://www.wellnessletter.com/html/wl/2005/wlFeatured0105.html; retrieved April 13, 2011).

Public Health Agency of Canada. 2004. *Progress Report on Cancer Control in Canada.* (http://www.phac-aspc.gc.ca/publicat/prccc-relccc/index-eng.php; retrieved November 21, 2009).

Public Health Agency of Canada. 2007. *Trends & Impact: The Basis for Investment Decisions* (http://www.phac-aspc.gc.ca/alw-vat/trends-tendances/index-eng.php#cancer; retrieved April 8, 2011).

Putt, K. S., et al. 2006. Small-molecule activation of procaspase-3 to caspase-3 as a personalized anticancer strategy. *Nature Chemical Biology* 2: 543–550 (http://www.nature.com/nchembio/journal/v2/n10/full/nchembio814.html; retrieved April 13, 2011).

Roden, R. B., et al. 2004. Vaccination to prevent and treat cervical cancer. *Human Pathology* 35(8): 971–982.

Seeff, L. C., et al. 2004. How many endoscopies are performed for colorectal cancer screening? Results from CDC's survey of endoscopic capacity. *Gastroenterology* 127(6): 1670–1677.

Statistics Canada. 2006. *Population Health Impact of Cancer in Canada, 2001* (http://www.statcan.gc.ca/daily-quotidien/060307/dq060307b-eng.htm; retrieved November 21, 2009).

Terry, M. B., et al. 2004. Association of frequency and duration of aspirin use and hormone receptor status with breast cancer risk. *Journal of the American Medical Association* 291(20): 2433–2440.

Trimble, C. L., et al. 2005. Active and passive cigarette smoking and the risk of cervical neoplasia. *Obstetrics and Gynecology* 105(1): 174–181.

U.S. Preventive Services Task Force. 2008. Screening for prostate cancer: U.S. Preventive Services Task Force recommendation statement. *Annals of Internal Medicine* 149(3): 185–191.

Van Gils, C. H., et al. 2005. Consumption of vegetables and fruits and risk of breast cancer. *Journal of the American Medical Association* 293(3): 183–193.

Velicer, C. M., et al. 2004. Antibiotic use in relation to the risk of breast cancer. *Journal of the American Medical Association* 291(7): 827–835.

Weinstein, S. J., et al. 2005. Serum alpha-tocopherol and gamma-tocopherol in relation to prostate cancer risk in a prospective study. *Journal of the National Cancer Institute* 97(5): 396–399.

Wellness facts. 2006. *Wellness Letter* 22(5): 1.

World Health Organization. 2005. *Cancer: Diet and Physical Activity's Impact* (http://www.who.int/dietphysicalactivity/publications/facts/cancer/en/; retrieved February 15, 2009).

World Health Organization. 2010. *Cancer: Palliative Care* (http://www.who.int/cancer/palliative/en/; retrieved December 11, 2010).

World Health Organization. 2011. *Cancer* (http://www.who.int/cancer/en/; retrieved April 12, 2011).

World Health Organization: International Agency for Research on Cancer. 2008. *World Cancer Report 2008* (http://www.iarc.fr/en/publications/pdfs-online/wcr/2008/index.php; retrieved April 8, 2011).

Practise and learn online with Connect.

IMMUNITY AND INFECTION

9

LOOKING AHEAD>>>>>

AFTER READING THIS CHAPTER, YOU SHOULD BE ABLE TO

- Describe the step-by-step process by which infectious diseases are transmitted
- Identify the body's physical and chemical barriers to infection
- Explain how the immune system responds to an invading microorganism
- Identify the major types of pathogens and describe the common diseases they cause
- Discuss steps you can take to prevent infections and strengthen your immune system

TEST YOUR KNOWLEDGE

1. Which of the following can transmit disease-causing pathogens (such as bacteria or viruses) from one person to another?

   a. mosquitoes
   b. doorknobs
   c. soil

2. When taking a prescription antibiotic, you should always finish the entire course of medication, even if you start feeling better before running out of medicine.
   True or false?

3. Which of the following can recognize and eliminate specific microbes (such as bacteria) that invade the body?

   a. antigens
   b. antibodies
   c. antidotes

4. Because medical facilities are sanitary, patients rarely catch bacterial infections in hospitals.
   True or false?

5. You can reduce your chances of getting sick by doing which of the following?

   a. washing your hands frequently
   b. keeping your immunizations up to date
   c. getting enough sleep

ANSWERS

1. **ALL THREE.** Pathogens can be transmitted directly (by contact with a sick person) or indirectly (by contact with an infected animal or insect or a contaminated object like a doorknob).

2. **TRUE.** Failing to take all your medication can lead to a relapse of the illness; taking antibiotics incorrectly also contributes to the development of antibiotic-resistant bacteria.

3. **B.** Antibodies are specialized proteins produced by the immune system, which can recognize and target specific invading organisms.

4. **FALSE.** Thousands of people die each year from infections contracted in health care settings.

5. **ALL THREE.** Frequent handwashing prevents the spread of many disease-causing agents. Immunizations prime the body to tackle an invading organism. Sleep helps support a healthy immune system.

Countless microscopic organisms live around, on, and in us. Although most microbes are beneficial, many of them can cause disease. But the constant vigilance of our immune system keeps them at bay and our bodies intact and healthy. The immune system works to keep the body from being overwhelmed not just by external invaders that cause **infections** but also by internal changes, such as cancer.

Most people don't notice these internal skirmishes unless they become sick. But people today are more knowledgeable about the complexities of immunity because they have heard about or had experience with *human immunodeficiency virus (HIV)* infection, which directly attacks the immune system. The rise in other infections has caught the public's attention, too. Old scourges, such as tuberculosis, are making comebacks—in stronger, drug-resistant forms.

This chapter introduces you to the mechanisms of immunity and infection and shows how to keep yourself well in a world of disease-causing microorganisms.

THE CHAIN OF INFECTION

Infectious diseases are transmitted from one person to another through a series of steps—a chain of infection (Figure 9.1). New infections can be prevented by interfering with any step in this process.

Links in the Chain

The chain of infection has six major links: the pathogen, its reservoir, a portal of exit, a means of transmission, a portal of entry, and a new host.

Pathogen The infectious disease cycle begins with a pathogen, a microorganism that causes disease. HIV (the virus that causes acquired immune deficiency syndrome, commonly known as *AIDS*) and the tuberculosis bacterium are examples of pathogens. Many pathogens cause illness because they produce **toxins** that harm human tissue; others do so by directly invading body cells.

Reservoir The pathogen has a natural environment—called a **reservoir**—in which it typically lives. This reservoir can be a person, an animal, or an environmental component, such as soil or water. A person who is the reservoir for a pathogen may be ill or may be an asymptomatic carrier who, although having no symptoms, can spread infection.

Portal of Exit To transmit infection, the pathogen must leave the reservoir through some portal of exit. In the case of a human reservoir, portals of exit include saliva (for mumps, for example), the mucous membranes (for many sexually transmitted infections), blood (for HIV and hepatitis), feces (for intestinal infections), and nose and throat discharges (for colds and influenza).

Means of Transmission Transmission can occur directly or indirectly. In direct transmission, the pathogen is passed from one person to another without an intermediary. Direct transmission usually requires fairly close association with an infected host but not necessarily physical contact. For example, sneezing and coughing can discharge infectious particles into the air, where they can be inhaled by someone nearby. Most common respiratory infections and many intestinal infections are passed directly—for example, when a person with an infectious agent on his or her hands touches someone else. In addition to coughing

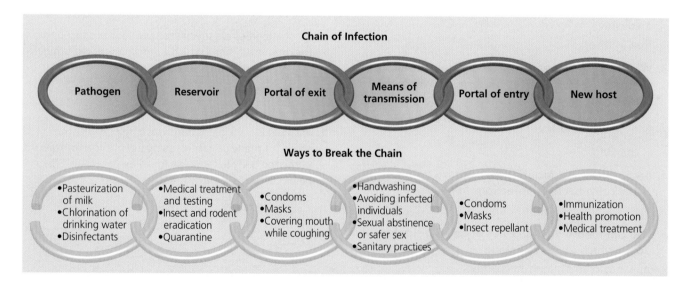

FIGURE 9.1 The chain of infection. Any break in the chain of infection can prevent disease.

and sneezing into the crook of the arm, proper hand-washing is also key. See Figure 9.2 for proper handwashing techniques to help reduce transmission opportunities. Other means of direct transmission include sexual contact and contact with blood.

Transmission can also occur indirectly. Animals and insects, such as rats, ticks, and mosquitoes, can serve as **vectors**, carrying the pathogen from one host to another. Pathogens can also be transmitted via contaminated soil, food, or water or from inanimate objects, such as eating utensils, doorknobs, and handkerchiefs. Some pathogens float in the air for long periods, suspended on tiny particles of dust or droplets that can travel long distances before they are inhaled and cause infection.

Portal of Entry   To infect a new host, a pathogen must have a portal of entry into the body. Pathogens can enter in one of three general ways:

1. Direct contact with or penetration of the skin

TERMS

infection   Invasion of the body by a microorganism.

toxin   A poisonous substance.

reservoir   A natural environment in which a pathogen typically lives.

vector   An insect, a rodent, or another organism that carries and transmits a pathogen from one host to another.

Handwashing with soap and water

1. Remove jewellery and wet hands and wrists with warm water.
2. Use 1 or 2 squirts of liquid or foam soap.
3. Lather soap and scrub hands well, palm to palm.
4. Scrub in between and around fingers.
5. Scrub back of each hand with palm of other hand.
6. Scrub fingertips of each hand in opposite palm.
7. Scrub each thumb clasped in opposite hand.
8. Scrub each wrist clasped in opposite hand.
9. Rinse thoroughly under running water.
10. Pat hands dry with paper towel.
11. Turn off water using same paper towel.

Cleaning with alcohol-based hand rub

1. Apply 1 to 2 pumps of product to palms of dry hands.
2. Rub hands together, palm to palm.
3. Rub in between and around fingers.
4. Rub back of each hand with palm of other hand.
5. Rub fingertips of each hand in opposite palm.
6. Rub each thumb clasped in opposite hand.
7. Rub each wrist clasped in opposite hand.
8. Rub hands until product is dry. Do not use paper towels.

FIGURE 9.2   Proper handwashing technique.

Source: Ontario Ministry of Health and Long-Term Care. 2007. *Handwashing* (http://www.health.gov.on.ca/english/public/pub/pubhealth/pdf/handwash_tech.pdf; retrieved April 14, 2011). Catalogue No. CIB-4446797 March 2007. © Queen's Printer for Ontario, 2007. Reproduced with permission.

2. Inhalation through the mouth or nose
3. Ingestion of contaminated food or water

Pathogens that enter the skin or mucous membranes can cause a local infection of the tissue, or they may penetrate into the bloodstream or lymphatic system, thereby causing a more extensive **systemic infection**. Agents that cause sexually transmitted infections (STIs) usually enter the body through the mucous membranes lining the urethra (in males) or the cervix (in females). Organisms that are transmitted via respiratory secretions may cause upper respiratory infections or pneumonia, or they may enter the bloodstream and cause systemic infection. Food-borne and water-borne organisms enter the mouth and travel to the location that will best support their reproduction. They may attack the cells of the small intestine or the colon, causing diarrhea, or they may enter the bloodstream via the digestive system and travel to other parts of the body.

The New Host   Once in the new host, a variety of factors determine whether the pathogen will be able to establish itself and cause infection. People with a strong immune system or resistance to a particular pathogen are less likely to become ill than people with poor immunity (the concept of immunity will be discussed later in the chapter). The number of pathogens that enter the new host is also important; the body's defences may be able to overcome a few bacteria, for example, but may be overwhelmed by thousands. If conditions are right, the pathogen will multiply and produce disease in the new host. In such a case, the new host may become a reservoir from which a new chain of infection can be started.

Breaking the Chain

Interrupting the chain of infection at any point can prevent disease. Strategies for breaking the chain include a mix of public health measures and individual action. For example, a pathogen's reservoir can be isolated or destroyed, as when a sick individual is placed under quarantine or when insects or animals carrying pathogens are killed. Public sanitation practices, such as sewage treatment and the chlorination of drinking water, can also kill pathogens. Transmission can be disrupted through various strategies, such as handwashing and the use of facemasks. Immunization and the treatment of infected hosts can stop the pathogen from multiplying, producing a serious disease, and being passed on to a new host. Some methods of breaking the chain of infection are listed in Figure 9.1.

THE BODY'S DEFENCE SYSTEM

Our bodies have very effective ways of protecting themselves against invasion by foreign organisms, especially pathogens. The body's first line of defence is a formidable array of physical and chemical barriers. When these barriers are breached, the body's **immune system** comes into play. Together, these defences provide an effective response to nearly all the challenges and invasions our bodies will ever experience.

Physical and Chemical Barriers

The skin, the body's largest organ, prevents many microorganisms from entering the body. Although many bacterial and fungal organisms live on the surface of the skin, very few can penetrate it except through a cut or break.

Wherever there is an opening in the body, or an area without skin, other barriers exist. The mouth is lined with mucous membranes, which contain cells designed to prevent the passage of unwanted organisms and particles. Body openings and the fluids that cover them (for example, tears, saliva, and vaginal secretions) are rich in antibodies (discussed in detail later in the chapter) and in enzymes that break down and destroy many microorganisms.

The respiratory tract is lined not only with mucous membranes but also with cells that have hairlike protrusions called *cilia*. The cilia sweep foreign matter up and out of the respiratory tract. Particles that are not caught by this mechanism may be expelled from the system by a cough. If the ciliated cells are damaged or destroyed, a cough is the body's only way of ridding the airways of foreign particles. This is one reason smokers generally have a chronic cough—to compensate for damaged airways.

The Immune System

The immune system operates through a remarkable information network involving billions of cellular defenders that rush to protect the body when a threat arises. Once the body has been invaded by a foreign organism, an elaborate system of responses is activated. Two of these responses are the inflammatory response and the immune response.

QUESTIONS FOR CRITICAL THINKING AND REFLECTION
Think about the last time you were sick with a cold, the flu, or an intestinal infection. Can you identify the reservoir from which the infection came? What vector, if any, transmitted the illness to you? Did you pass the infection to anyone else? If so, how?

Immunological Defenders The immune response is carried out by different types of white blood cells, which are continuously being produced in the bone marrow.

- **Neutrophils**, one type of white blood cell, travel in the bloodstream to areas of invasion, attacking and ingesting pathogens.
- **Macrophages**, or "big eaters," take up stations in tissues and act as scavengers, devouring pathogens and worn-out cells.
- **Natural killer cells** directly destroy virus-infected cells and cells that have turned cancerous.
- **Dendritic cells**, which reside in tissues, eat pathogens and activate lymphocytes.
- **Lymphocytes**, of which there are several types, are white blood cells that travel in both the bloodstream and the lymphatic system.

At various places in the lymphatic system are lymph nodes (or glands), where macrophages and dendritic cells congregate and filter bacteria and other substances from the lymph (Figure 9.3 on p. 282). When these nodes are actively involved in fighting an invasion of microorganisms, they fill with cells; physicians use the location of swollen lymph nodes as a clue to the location and cause of an infection.

The two main types of lymphocytes are **T cells** and **B cells**. T cells are further differentiated into **helper T cells**, **killer T cells**, and **suppressor T cells** (also called *regulatory T cells*). B cells are lymphocytes that produce **antibodies**. The first time T cells and B cells encounter a specific invader, some of them are reserved as **memory T and B cells**, enabling the body to mount a rapid response should the same invader appear again in the future. These cells and cell products—macrophages, natural killer cells, dendritic cells, T cells, B cells and antibodies, and memory cells—are the primary players in the body's immune response.

The immune system is built on a remarkable feature of these defenders: the ability to distinguish foreign cells from the body's own cells. Because lymphocytes are capable of great destruction, it is essential that they not attack the body itself. When they do, they cause **autoimmune diseases**, such as lupus and rheumatoid arthritis.

All the cells in your body display markers on their surfaces—tiny molecular shapes—that identify them as "self" to lymphocytes that encounter them. Invading microorganisms also display markers on their surface; lymphocytes identify these as foreign, or "nonself." Nonself markers that trigger the immune response are known as **antigens**.

Antibodies have complementary surface markers that work with antigens like a lock and key. When an antigen appears in the body, it eventually encounters an antibody with a complementary pattern. The antibody locks onto the antigen, triggering a series of events designed to destroy the invading pathogen. The truly astonishing thing is that the body does not synthesize the appropriate antibody lock after it comes into contact with the antigen key. Rather, antibodies already exist for millions, if not billions, of possible antigens.

The Inflammatory Response When the body has been injured or infected, one of the body's responses is the inflammatory response. Special cells in the area of invasion or injury release **histamine** and other substances that cause blood vessels to dilate and fluid to flow out of capillaries into the injured tissue. This produces increased heat, swelling, and redness in the affected area. White blood cells, including neutrophils, dendritic cells, and

TERMS

systemic infection An invasion by a microorganism that spreads though the blood or lymphatic system to large portions of the body.

immune system The body's collective physical and chemical defences against foreign organisms and pathogens.

neutrophil A type of white blood cell that engulfs foreign organisms and infected, damaged, or aged cells; particularly prevalent during the inflammatory response.

macrophage A large phagocytic (cell-eating) cell that devours foreign particles.

natural killer cell A type of white blood cell that directly destroys virus-infected cells and cancer cells.

dendritic cell A white blood cell specialized to activate T and B cells.

lymphocyte A white blood cell that works in both the bloodstream and the lymphatic system.

T cell A lymphocyte that arises in bone marrow and matures in the thymus (thus its name).

B cell A lymphocyte that matures in the bone marrow and produces antibodies.

helper T cell A lymphocyte that helps activate other T cells and may help B cells produce antibodies.

killer T cell A lymphocyte that kills body cells that have been invaded by foreign organisms; also can kill cells that have turned cancerous.

suppressor T cell A lymphocyte that inhibits the growth of other lymphocytes; also called *regulatory T cells*.

antibody A specialized protein produced by white blood cells that can recognize and neutralize specific microbes.

memory T and B cells Lymphocytes generated during an initial infection that circulate in the body for years, remembering the specific antigens that caused the infection and quickly destroying them if they appear again.

autoimmune disease A disease in which the immune system attacks the person's own body.

antigen A marker on the surface of a foreign substance that immune system cells recognize as nonself and that triggers the immune response.

histamine A chemical responsible for the dilation and increased permeability of blood vessels in allergic reactions.

FIGURE 9.3 The lymphatic system. The lymphatic system consists of a network of vessels and organs, including the spleen, lymph nodes, thymus, and tonsils. The vessels pick up excess fluid and proteins, lipids, and other particles from body tissues. These pass through the lymph nodes, where macrophages and dendritic cells help clear the lymph (fluid) of debris and bacteria and other pathogens. The cleansed lymph is then returned to the bloodstream. The lymphatic organs are production centres for infection-fighting cells and sites for some immune responses.

The Immune Response The immune system makes two types of responses to invading pathogens: natural (innate) and acquired (adaptive).

Neutrophils, macrophages, dendritic cells, and natural killer cells are part of the natural response. They recognize pathogens as "foreign" but have no memory of past infections; they respond the same way no matter how many times a pathogen invades. These cells essentially eat the invaders, destroying them internally. Natural killer cells also destroy infected body cells, breaking the chain of reproduction of a pathogen and helping to stop an infection.

T and B cells are part of the acquired response. They change after one contact with the pathogen, developing a memory for the antigen. If the body is invaded again, they recognize the pathogen and mount a much more potent response.

Think of the immune response as having four phases (Figure 9.4). In each phase, the system takes steps to destroy the invader and restore the body to health.

- *Phase 1.* Dendritic cells are drawn to the site of the injury and consume the foreign cells; they then provide information about the pathogen by displaying its antigen on their surfaces. Helper T cells read this information and rush to respond.
- *Phase 2.* Helper T cells multiply rapidly and trigger the production of killer T cells and B cells in the spleen and lymph nodes. **Cytokines**, chemical messengers secreted by lymphocytes, help regulate and coordinate the immune response; *interleukins* and *interferons* are two examples of cytokines. They stimulate increased production of T cells, B cells, and antibodies; promote the activities of natural killer cells; produce fever; and have special antipathogenic properties themselves.

macrophages, are drawn to the area and attack the invaders—in many cases, destroying them. At the site of infection there may be *pus*, a collection of dead white blood cells and debris resulting from the encounter.

Dendritic cells are white blood cells that engulf foreign cells and display their antigens, thereby activating T and B cells. The dendritic cell shown in this scanning electron micrograph is magnified 2700 times.

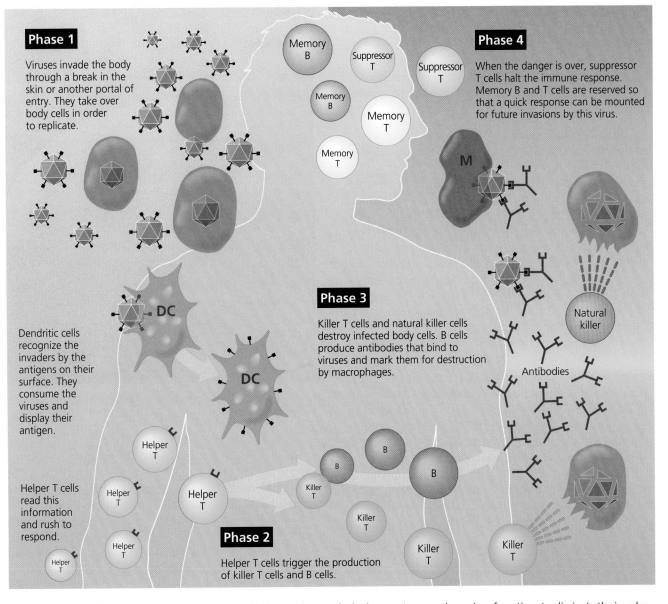

Phase 1

Viruses invade the body through a break in the skin or another portal of entry. They take over body cells in order to replicate.

Dendritic cells recognize the invaders by the antigens on their surface. They consume the viruses and display their antigen.

Helper T cells read this information and rush to respond.

Phase 2

Helper T cells trigger the production of killer T cells and B cells.

Phase 3

Killer T cells and natural killer cells destroy infected body cells. B cells produce antibodies that bind to viruses and mark them for destruction by macrophages.

Phase 4

When the danger is over, suppressor T cells halt the immune response. Memory B and T cells are reserved so that a quick response can be mounted for future invasions by this virus.

FIGURE 9.4 **The immune response.** Once invaded by a pathogen, the body mounts a complex series of reactions to eliminate the invader. Pictured here are the principal elements of the immune response to a virus; not shown are the many types of cytokines that help coordinate the actions of different types of defenders.

• *Phase 3.* Killer T cells strike at foreign cells and body cells that have been invaded and infected, identifying them by the antigens displayed on the cell surfaces. Puncturing the cell membrane, they sacrifice body cells to destroy the foreign organism within. This type of action is known as a *cell-mediated immune response*, because the attack is carried out by cells. Killer T cells also trigger an amplified inflammatory response and recruit more macrophages to help clean up the site.

B cells work in a different way. Stimulated to multiply by helper T cells, they produce large quantities of antibody molecules, which are released in the bloodstream and tissues. Antibodies are Y-shaped protein molecules that bind to antigen-bearing targets and mark them for destruction by

macrophages. This type of response is known as an *antibody-mediated immune response*. Antibodies work against bacteria and against viruses and other substances when they are in the body but outside cells. They do not work against infected body cells or viruses that are replicating inside cells.

• *Phase 4.* The last phase of the immune response is a slowdown of activity. During the course of the immune response, regulatory molecules and cells inhibit lymphocyte proliferation and induce lymphocyte death; this process restores resting levels of B and T cells. The dead cells, killed pathogens, and other debris that result from the immune response are scavenged by certain types of white blood cells; filtered out of circulation by the liver, spleen, and kidneys; and excreted from the body.

Immunity After an infection, survival often confers **immunity**; that is, an infected person will never get the same illness again. This is because some of the lymphocytes created during the second phase of the immune response are reserved as memory T and B cells. As part of the acquired immune response, they continue to circulate in the blood and lymphatic system for years or even for the rest of the person's life. If the same antigen enters the body again, the memory T and B cells recognize and destroy it before it can cause illness. This subsequent response takes only a few days to initiate and prevents illness. The ability of memory lymphocytes to remember previous infections is known as **acquired immunity.**

Symptoms and Contagion The immune system is operating at the cellular level at all times, maintaining its vigilance when you're well and fighting invaders when you're sick. How does it all feel to you, the host for these activities? How do your symptoms relate to the course of the infection and the immune response?

During **incubation**, when viruses are multiplying in the body or when bacteria are actively multiplying before the immune system has gathered momentum, you may not have any symptoms of the illness, but you may be contagious. During the second and third phases of the immune response, you may still be unaware of the infection, or you may "feel a cold coming on." Symptoms first appear during the *prodromal period*, which follows incubation. If the infected host has acquired immunity, the infection may be eradicated during the incubation period or the prodromal period. In this case, although you may have felt you were coming down with a cold, for example, it does not develop into a full-blown illness.

Many symptoms of an illness are actually due to the immune response of the body rather than to the actions or products of the invading organism. For example, fever is caused by the release and activation of certain cytokines in macrophages and other cells during the immune response. These cytokines travel in the bloodstream to the brain and cause the body's thermostat to be reset to a higher level. The resulting elevated temperature helps the body in its fight against pathogens by enhancing immune responses.

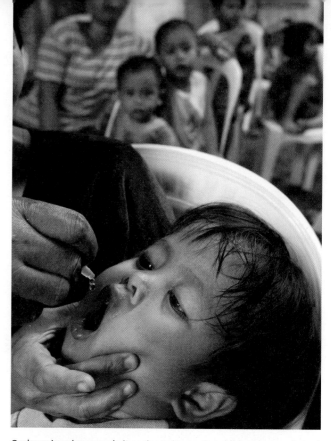

Oral vaccines have made it easier to immunize children in remote and impoverished areas of the world.

During an illness, it is necessary to lower a fever only if it is uncomfortably high (more than 38.6°C) or if it occurs in an infant who is at risk for seizures from fever.

Similarly, you get a runny nose when your lymphocytes destroy infected mucosal cells, leading to increased mucus production. The malaise and fatigue of the flu are caused by pro-inflammatory cytokines.

You are contagious when you have infectious microbes in your body and they can gain access to another person. This may be before a vigorous immune response has occurred, so at times you may be contagious before experiencing any symptoms. This means that you can transmit an illness without knowing you're infected or catch an illness from someone who doesn't appear to be sick. Conversely, your symptoms may continue after the pathogens have been mostly destroyed, when you are no longer infectious.

Immunization

The ability of the immune system to remember previously encountered organisms and retain its strength against them is the basis for **immunization**. When a person is immunized, the immune system is primed with an antigen similar to the pathogenic organism but not as dangerous. The body responds by producing antibodies, which prevent serious infection when and if the person is exposed to the disease organism itself. The preparations used to manipulate the immune system are known as **vaccines** (Table 9.1).

Table 9.1   Immunizations for Canadian Children and Adults

Vaccine	People for Whom Immunization Is Recommended
Diphtheria, tetanus, acellular pertussis, and inactivated polio virus vaccine (DTAP-IPV)	All children up to 6 years. Infants receive it starting at 2 months. Booster shots are recommended every 10 years.
Haemophilus influenzae type b conjugate (Hib)	All children up to 5 years of age. All infants starting at 2 months up till 18 months. Older children and adults who have had a splenectomy or bone marrow transplant, have sickle-cell disease or HIV/AIDS, or are undergoing immunosuppressant drug therapy
HPV vaccine	Females between 9 and 13 years of age, before the onset of sexual intercourse; Females between the ages of 14 and 26 years of age, even if they are already sexually active, have had previous pap abnormalities, or have had a previous HPV infection.
Measles, mumps and rubella (MMR)	All children. First dose is given when the child is 12 months old. For convenience should be given at school entry (4–6 years). All children at age 11–18 years or at high-school entry, unvaccinated first-year postsecondary students living in dormitories, military recruits, and others at increased risk. Booster is recommended every 10 years.
Varicella (Var)	Children aged 12 months to 12 years should receive one dose. Susceptible individuals 13 years of age should receive two doses at least 28 days apart. All adults if no record or unclear, doses 1 and 2, at least 4 weeks apart for susceptible adults (no history of natural disease or seronegativity)
Hepatitis A	Occupational risk, lifestyle, travel, and living in areas lacking adequate sanitation. Outbreak control, post-exposure immunoprophylaxis. Patients with chronic liver disease.
Hepatitis B	All children. For infants that are born to chronic carriers first dose should be given at birth, otherwise first dose is given at 2 months. For those with occupational risk, lifestyle, post-exposure immunoprophylaxis. Patients with chronic liver disease. Health care workers.
Pneumococcal conjugate-7-valent (Pneu-C-7)	All children under 2 years of age. First dose is given at 2 months.
Pneumococcyl polysaccharide	Adults 65 years; adults <65 who have conditions putting them at increased risk of pneumococcal disease.
Meningococcal C conjugate (Men-C)	Recommended for children under 5 years of age, adolescents, and young adults. The recommended schedule depends on the age of the individual.
Influenza (Inf)	Recommended for all children 6–23 months of age and all persons (stressed for those at risk for complication or working with those at risk).
Diphtheria, tetanus (Td)	All adults. Booster is recommended every 10 years. If no record, or unclear then doses 1 and 2, 4–8 weeks apart and dose 3 at 6–12 months later; one of the doses should be given as Tdap for pertussis protection.

Source: Immunizations for Canadian Children and Adults (*Canadian Immunization Guide,* 7th ed. 2006. National Advisory Committee on Immunization.) http://www.phac-aspc.gc.ca/publicat/cig-gci/p03-02-eng.php. © Her Majesty the Queen in Right of Canada.

Types of Vaccines   Vaccines can be made in several ways. In some cases, microbes are cultured in the laboratory in a way that attenuates (weakens) them. These live, attenuated organisms are used in vaccines against several diseases, such as measles, mumps, and rubella (German measles). In other cases, when it is not possible to breed attenuated organisms, vaccines are made from pathogens that have been killed in the laboratory but that still retain their ability to stimulate the production of antibodies. Vaccines composed of killed viruses are used against influenza viruses, among others.

Vaccines confer what is known as *active immunity*—that is, the vaccinated person produces his or her own antibodies to the microorganism. Another type of injection confers *passive immunity*. In this case, a person exposed to a disease is injected with the antibodies themselves, produced

immunity   Mechanisms that defend the body against infection; specific defences against specific pathogens.

acquired immunity   The body's ability to mobilize the cellular memory of an attack by a pathogen to throw off subsequent attacks; acquired through vaccination and the normal immune response.

incubation   The period when bacteria or viruses are actively multiplying inside the body's cells; usually a period without symptoms of illness.

immunization   The process of conferring immunity to a pathogen by administering a vaccine.

vaccine   A preparation of killed or weakened microorganisms, inactivated toxins, or components of microorganisms that is administered to stimulate an immune response; a vaccine protects against future infection by the pathogen.

TERMS

by other human beings or animals who have recovered from the disease. Injections of gamma globulin—a product made from the blood plasma of many individuals containing all the antibodies they have ever made—are sometimes given to people to create a rapid but temporary immunity to a particular disease. Gamma globulin is also sometimes used to treat antibody deficiency syndromes.

VACCINE SAFETY Side effects from immunization, such as soreness at the injection site, are usually mild. It is estimated that an allergic reaction may occur in 1 in 1.5 million doses. Any risk from vaccines must be balanced against the risk posed by the diseases they prevent; for example, the death rate from diphtheria is about 5%–10%.

The Public Health Agency of Canada monitors reports of adverse reactions to vaccines, and new formulations or types of vaccines are being developed to increase safety. For example, oral polio vaccine, which contains live but weakened poliovirus, has been replaced by inactivated poliovirus, which contains killed virus. The oral vaccine is somewhat more effective, but in about 1 in 2.4 million cases, it causes polio; because of the low risk for polio in Canada, the oral vaccine is no longer used.

A possible link has also been proposed between immunization and autism, a severe developmental disorder characterized by behavioural problems and impaired social and communication skills. However, a 2004 Institute of Medicine report concluded that evidence does not support such a link; a large 2006 study confirmed this conclusion. Thimerosal, a mercury-containing preservative, was withdrawn from most pediatric vaccines in Canada, although no clear link has been found between thimerosal-containing vaccines and autism.

Allergy: The Body's Defence System Gone Haywire

Many Canadians are affected by **allergies**. Allergies result from a hypersensitive and overactive immune system. The immune system typically defends the body against only genuinely harmful pathogens, such as viruses and bacteria. However, in someone with an allergy, the immune system also mounts a response to a harmless substance, such as pollen or animal dander. Allergy symptoms—stuffy nose, sneezing, wheezing, skin rashes, and so on—result primarily from the immune response rather than from the substances that provoke the response.

Allergens Substances that provoke allergies are known as **allergens**; they may cause a response if they are inhaled or swallowed or if they come in contact with the skin. Different people have allergic reactions to different substances, but many Canadians react to at least one common allergen, such as one of the following:

• *Pollen:* Referred to as hay fever or allergic rhinitis, pollen allergies are widespread; weeds, grasses, and trees are common producers of allergenic pollen.

• *Animal dander:* People with animal allergies are usually allergic not to fur but to dander (dead skin flakes), urine, or a protein found in saliva; allergies to mice, dogs, and cats are common.

• *Dust mites and cockroaches:* The droppings of cockroaches and microscopic dust mites can trigger allergies; mites live in carpets, upholstered furniture, and bedding.

• *Moulds and mildew:* The small spores produced by these fungi can trigger allergy symptoms; moulds and mildew thrive in damp areas of buildings.

• *Foods:* The most common food allergens in adults include peanuts, tree nuts, fish, and shellfish.

• *Insect stings:* The venom of insects, such as yellow jackets, honeybees, hornets, paper wasps, and fire ants, causes allergic reactions in some people.

People may also be allergic to certain medications; plants, such as poison oak; latex; metals, such as nickel; and compounds found in cosmetics.

The Allergic Response Most allergic reactions are due to the production of a special type of antibody known as immunoglobulin E (IgE). Initial exposure to a particular allergen may cause little response, but it sensitizes the immune system by causing the production of allergen-specific IgE, which binds to mast cells (Figure 9.5, p. 288). Mast cells are part of the immune system and play a role in healing, the immune response, and allergic reactions. When the body is subsequently exposed to the allergen, the allergen binds to IgE, causing the mast cells to release large amounts of histamine and other compounds into surrounding tissues.

Histamine has many effects, including increasing the inflammatory response and stimulating mucus production. The precise symptoms depend on what part of the body is affected. In the nose, histamine may cause congestion and sneezing; in the eyes, itchiness and tearing; in the skin, redness, swelling, and itching; in the intestines, bloating and cramping; and in the lungs, coughing, wheezing, and shortness of breath. In some people, an allergen can trigger an asthma attack (see the box "Environment, Ethnicity, and Asthma"). Symptoms often occur immediately, within minutes of exposure, but inflammatory reactions may take hours or days to develop and then may persist for several days.

The most serious, but rare, kind of allergic reaction is **anaphylaxis**, which results from a release of histamine

Environment, Ethnicity, and Asthma

Asthma is caused by both inflammation of the airways and spasm of the muscles surrounding the airways. The spasm causes constriction, and the inflammation causes the airway linings to swell and secrete extra mucus, which further obstructs the passages. The inflammation can become chronic, making airways even more sensitive to triggers. The symptoms of asthma—wheezing, tightness in the chest, and shortness of breath—may be mild and occur only occasionally, or they may be severe and occur daily.

An asthma attack begins when something sets off inflammation of the bronchial tubes. Usually it's an allergic reaction to an inhaled allergen, most commonly dust mites, mould, animal dander, or pollen. Anything that irritates or overtaxes the bronchial airways can also trigger spasms: exercise, cold air, pollutants, tobacco smoke, infection, or stress. In females with asthma, hormonal changes that occur as menstruation starts may increase vulnerability to attacks.

Patterns and Prevalence

The prevalence of asthma is increasing. In Canada, more than 2.3 million adults and nearly 2 million children have asthma; each year asthma is responsible for almost 150,000 emergency department visits and somewhere between 250 and 500 deaths. Between 1994 and 2001, the number of Canadian children with asthma increased by 2%, representing 70,000 children, and despite better treatment options, the death rate remains worrisome.

The tendency to develop asthma may be hereditary, but some patterns appear to link it to the increased Westernization of environmental factors, such as changes in maternal diet, increased exposures to

household allergens, pets, environmental tobacco smoke, and environmental pollution. Although research is ongoing, it is clear that the environment is an important determinant of asthma.

With regard to ethnicity, Canadian researchers recently found that children of Asian and African descent are at greater risk of being misdiagnosed with asthma and, therefore, being overmedicated for the condition. The reason for this misdiagnosis has to do with an increasingly popular diagnostic test—assessing the amount of nitric oxide in exhaled breath—to detect and manage the disease. Children of Asian and African descent have higher levels of nitric oxide than other children, leading to a diagnosis of asthma in some children who do not actually have it. More research is needed to better identify the typical levels of nitric oxide among various groups, thus avoiding potential misdiagnosis and treatment.

Treatment and Prevention of Attacks

Inhaling a muscle-relaxing medication from a bronchodilator can relieve an

asthma attack immediately by opening the bronchial tubes. Inhaling an anti-inflammatory drug can treat the underlying inflammation. Both types of treatments may be needed to get asthma under control. Other medications for asthma block the actions of molecules involved in the body's inflammatory response. Asthmatics can monitor their condition by testing their peak airflow several times a day; a drop in peak airflow can signal an upcoming attack.

It's also a good idea to avoid allergens when possible. A recent study of urban children found that relatively small changes can reduce asthma symptoms and health care visits. In this study, allergen exposures were reduced by covering the mattresses and pillows with special covers; using HEPA filters in vacuum cleaners and room air purifiers; and employing professional pest control. Other researchers have found that many children with asthma live in households in which simple allergen control methods haven't been taken, including closing windows to keep pollen out, avoiding environmental tobacco smoke, and reducing or eliminating exposure to pets.

Sources: Asthma Society of Canada. 2005. *Asthma Facts and Statistics* (http://www.asthma.ca/corp/newsroom/pdf/asthmastats.pdf; retrieved April 15, 2011); Kovesi, T., Y. Kulka, and R. Dales. 2008. Exhaled nitric oxide concentration is affected by age, height, and race in healthy 9–12-year-old children. *CHEST* 133: 169–175; Garner, R., and D. Kohen. 2008. Changes in the prevalence of asthma among Canadian children. *Health Reports* 19(2) (http://www.statcan.gc.ca/pub/82-003-x/2008002/article/10551-eng.htm; retrieved April 15, 2011); Wang, H.-Y., et al. 2008. Prevalence of asthma among Chinese adolescents living in Canada and in China. *Canadian Medical Association Journal* 179(11): 1133–1142 (http://www.cmaj.ca/cgi/content/full/179/11/1133; retrieved April 15, 2011).

throughout the body. Anaphylactic reactions can be life threatening because symptoms may include swelling of the throat, extremely low blood pressure, fainting, heart arrhythmia, and seizures. Anaphylaxis is a medical emergency, and treatment requires immediate injection of epinephrine. People at risk for anaphylaxis should wear MedicAlert identification and keep self-administrable epinephrine readily available.

allergy   A disorder caused by the body's exaggerated response to foreign chemicals and proteins; also called *hypersensitivity*.

allergen   A substance that triggers an allergic reaction.

anaphylaxis   A severe systemic hypersensitive reaction to an allergen characterized by difficulty breathing, low blood pressure, heart arrhythmia, seizure, and sometimes death.

During sensitization, allergens, such as pollen, trigger the production of IgE antibodies, which bind to mast cells.

During an allergic reaction, the allergens enter the bloodstream and are recognized and bound by the IgE antibodies.

The IgE-allergen combination causes mast cells to release histamine and other compounds into surrounding tissue, producing allergy symptoms.

FIGURE 9.5 The allergic response.

Dealing with Allergies   If you suspect you might have an allergy, visit your physician or an allergy specialist. You have three general strategies for dealing with allergies:

• *Avoidance:* You may be able to avoid or minimize exposure to allergens by making changes in your environment or behaviour. For example, removing carpets from the bedroom and using special bedding can reduce dust mite contact. Pollen exposure can be limited by avoiding outdoor activities during peak pollination times, keeping windows shut, and showering and changing clothes following outdoor activities. If you can't part with a pet, keep pets out of bedrooms and frequently vacuum or damp-mop floors.

• *Medication:* A variety of medications are available for allergy sufferers. Many over-the-counter antihistamines are effective at controlling symptoms, such as blocked nasal, sinus, or middle ear passages. Prescription corticosteroids delivered by aerosol markedly reduce allergy symptoms, increase effectiveness, and help limit systemic absorption and side effects.

• *Immunotherapy:* Referred to as allergy shots, immunotherapy desensitizes a person to a particular allergen through the administration of gradually increasing doses of the allergen over months or years.

PATHOGENS AND DISEASE

When pathogens enter body tissue, they can cause illness and sometimes death to the host. Worldwide, infectious diseases are responsible for more than 11 million deaths each year (Table 9.2).

Pathogens include bacteria, viruses, fungi, protozoa, parasitic worms, and prions (Figure 9.6). Infections can occur almost anywhere in or on the body. Common types of infection include bronchitis, infection of the airways (bronchi); meningitis, infection of the tissue surrounding

Table 9.2	Most Prevalent Infectious Diseases Worldwide
Disease	**Approximate Number of Deaths per Year**
Pneumonia	3,884,000
HIV/AIDS	2,777,000
Diarrheal diseases	1,798,000
Tuberculosis	1,566,000
Malaria	1,272,000
Measles	611,000
Pertussis (whooping cough)	294,000
Tetanus	214,000
Meningitis	173,000
Syphilis	157,000

Many of the 618,000 deaths from liver cancer each year can be traced to viral hepatitis. Overall, infectious diseases kill more than 11 million people each year, representing nearly 19% of all deaths.

Source: World Health Organization. 2004. *The World Health Report 2004*; Geneva: World Health Organization.

the brain and spinal cord; conjunctivitis, infection of the layer of cells surrounding the eyes; pharyngitis, or sore throat; pneumonia, infection of the lung; gastroenteritis, infection of the gastrointestinal tract; cellulitis, infection of the soft tissues; osteomyelitis, infection of the bones; and so on, for every tissue and organ.

Type of Organism	Selected Pathogens	Associated Diseases
Bacteria Microscopic single-celled organisms 	*Bordetella pertussis* *Borrelia burgdorferi* *Chlamydia* *Clostridium tetani* *Helicobacter pylori* *Legionella pneumophila* *Mycobacterium tuberculosis* Mycoplasma *Neisseria* Rickettsia Staphylococcus Streptococcus	Pertussis (whooping cough) Lyme disease Pneumonia (*C. pneumoniae*), chlamydia (*C. trachomatis*) Tetanus Peptic ulcers Legionnaire's disease Tuberculosis Pneumonia, ear infections, sore throat, urethritis Gonorrhea (*N. gonorroeae*), meningitis (*N. meningitidis*) Rocky Mountain spotted fever, typhus Boils and other skin infections, toxic shock syndrome Strep throat, skin infections, pneumonia, rheumatic fever and rheumatic heart disease, necrotizing fasciitis
Viruses Infectious agents consisting of a protein shell enclosing DNA or RNA	Coronavirus, rhinovirus Epstein-Barr virus Hepatitis viruses Herpes simplex 1 and 2 Human immunodeficiency virus Human papillomaviruses Influenza viruses A and B Paramyxovirus Rhabdovirus Togavirus Varicella-zoster	Severe acute respiratory syndrome (SARS), common cold Infectious mononucleosis Hepatitis (inflammation of the liver) Cold sores, genital herpes HIV/AIDS Warts, cervical cancer Flu Measles, mumps Rabies Rubella Chicken pox, shingles
Fungi Single- or multicelled organisms (e.g., yeasts, moulds)	*Candida albicans* *Cryptococcus neoformans* Dermatophyte fungi *Histoplasma capsulatum* *Coccidioides immitis*	Yeast infections, thrush Pneumonia, meningitis Athlete's foot, jock itch, ringworm, nail infections Histoplasmosis Coccidioidomycosis
Protozoa Single-celled organisms	*Entamoeba histolytica* *Giardia lamblia* *Plasmodia* *Trichomonas vaginalis* *Trypanosoma brucei*	Amoebic dysentery Giardiasis Malaria Trichomoniasis African sleeping sickness
Parasitic worms Worms that feed and live on or in a host	*Ancylostoma duodenale* *Ascaris lumbricoides* Beef, pork, or fish tapeworms *Enterobius vermicularis* *Necator americanus* Schistosoma	Ancylostomiasis (hookworm infection) Ascariasis (roundworm infection) Tapeworm infection Pinworm infection Hookworm infection Cercarial dermatitis (swimmer's itch), schistosomiasis
Prions Proteinaceous infectious particles	PrP^{Sc}	Creutzfeldt-Jakob disease (CJD)

FIGURE 9.6 Pathogens and associated infectious diseases.

Bacteria

The most abundant living things on Earth are **bacteria**, single-celled organisms that usually reproduce by splitting in two to create a pair of identical cells. Many species of bacteria feed on dead matter and play an important role in the recycling of nutrients for other organisms; other species feed on living things and may cause disease. Bacteria are often classified according to their shape: They may be bacilli (rod shaped), cocci (spherical), spirochete (spiral), or vibrios (comma shaped).

We harbour both helpful and harmful bacteria on our skin and in our gastrointestinal and reproductive tracts. The human colon contains friendly bacteria that produce certain vitamins and help digest nutrients. (A large portion of feces consists of bacteria.) Friendly bacteria also

bacterium (bacteria, plural) A microscopic single-celled organism; about 100 bacterial species can cause disease in humans.

TERMS

keep harmful bacteria in check by competing for food and resources and secreting substances toxic to pathogenic bacteria. For example, *Lactobacillus acidophilus* resides in the vagina and produces chemicals that kill yeast and bacteria that cause vaginal infections.

Not all bacteria found in the body are beneficial, however. Pathogenic bacteria in food or drink can disrupt the normal harmony in the intestines by invading cells or producing damaging toxins. Sexual activity can introduce pathogenic bacteria into the reproductive tract. Within the bloodstream, tissues, and organs, the human body is usually aseptic—devoid of bacteria. If bacteria find their way into these areas, infection may result.

Pneumonia Inflammation of the lungs, called **pneumonia**, may be caused by infection with bacteria, viruses, or fungi or by contact with chemical toxins or irritants. Pneumonia can be serious if the alveoli (air sacs) become clogged with fluid, thus preventing oxygen from reaching the bloodstream. Pneumonia often follows another illness, such as a cold or the flu, but the symptoms are typically more severe: fever, chills, shortness of breath, increased mucus production, and cough. Pneumonia grouped with influenza ranks seventh among the leading causes of death for Canadians; people most at risk for severe infection include those under age 2 and over age 75 and those with chronic health problems, such as heart disease, asthma, or HIV. Bacterial pneumonia can be treated with antibiotics.

Pneumococcus bacteria are the most common cause of bacterial pneumonia; a vaccine is available and recommended for all adults age 65 and older and others at risk. Other bacteria that may cause pneumonia include *Streptococcus pneumoniae*, *Chlamydia pneumoniae*, and

mycoplasmas. Outbreaks of infection with mycoplasmas are relatively common among young adults, especially in crowded settings, such as dormitories.

Meningitis Infection of the *meninges*, the membranes covering the brain and spinal cord, is called **meningitis**. Viral meningitis is usually mild and goes away on its own; bacterial meningitis, however, can be life threatening and requires immediate treatment with antibiotics. Symptoms of meningitis include fever, a severe headache, stiff neck, sensitivity to light, and confusion. Before the 1990s, *Haemophilus Influenzae* type b (Hib) was the leading cause of bacterial meningitis, but routine vaccination of children has reduced the occurrence of Hib meningitis. Today, *Neisseria meningitidis* and *Streptococcus pneumoniae* are the leading causes of bacterial meningitis.

In Canada, about 1000 cases of meningitis are reported each year, although the actual number is probably higher. The disease is fatal in 10% of cases, and about 10%–20% of people who recover have permanent hearing loss or other serious effects. Worldwide, meningitis kills about 170,000 people each year, particularly in the so-called meningitis belt in sub-Saharan Africa.

A vaccine is available, but it is not effective against all strains of meningitis-causing bacteria.

Strep Throat and Other Streptococcal Infections The **streptococcus** bacterium is spherical and often grows in chains. Streptococcal pharyngitis, or strep throat, is characterized by a red, sore throat with white patches on the tonsils, swollen lymph nodes, fever, and headache. It is typically spread through close contact with an infected person via respiratory droplets (sneezing or coughing). If left untreated, strep throat can develop into the more serious rheumatic fever (see Chapter 7). Other streptococcal infections include scarletina (scarlet fever), characterized by a sore throat, fever, bright red tongue, and a rash over the upper body; impetigo, a superficial skin infection most common among children; and erysipelas, inflammation of skin and underlying tissues.

A particularly virulent type of streptococcus can invade the bloodstream, spread to other parts of the body, and produce dangerous systemic illness. It can also cause a serious but rare infection of the deeper layers of the skin, a condition called necrotizing fasciitis, or "flesh-eating strep." This dangerous infection is characterized by tissue death and is treated with antibiotics and removal of the infected tissue or limb. Other species of streptococci are implicated in pneumonia, endocarditis (infection of the heart lining and valves), and serious infections in pregnant women and newborns.

Toxic Shock Syndrome and Other Staphylococcal Infections The spherical **staphylococcus** bacterium often grows in small clusters. It is commonly found on the skin and in the nasal passages of healthy people. Occasionally, staphylococci enter the body and cause an infection,

TERMS

pneumonia Inflammation of the lungs, typically caused by infection or exposure to chemical toxins or irritants.

mycoplasma A small bacterium with an incomplete cell wall that may cause sore throats, ear infections, and pneumonia.

meningitis Infection of the meninges (membranes covering the brain and spinal cord).

streptococcus Any of a genus (Streptococcus) of spherical bacteria; streptococcal species can cause skin infections, strep throat, rheumatic fever, pneumonia, scarlet fever, and other diseases.

staphylococcus Any of a genus (Staphylococcus) of spherical, clustered bacteria commonly found on the skin or in the nasal passages; staphylococcal species may enter the body and cause several conditions, such as boils, pneumonia, and toxic shock syndrome.

MRSA: The Superbug?

Staphylococcus (often shortened to staph) infections are certainly nothing new; people have been dealing with minor staph infections for generations. In fact, it is estimated that as many as 30% of people carry the staph bacteria in their bodies. Most of us come into contact with the germ many times during our lives, usually with little or no consequences.

In recent years, however, an antibiotic-resistant strain of staph—called methicillin-resistant *Staphylococcus aureus* (MRSA)—has changed the public's perception of staph as a relatively harmless germ. Medical experts have dubbed MRSA a *superbug* because it is highly resistant to several first-line medicines normally used to treat staph infections. These drugs include methicillin, penicillin, oxacillin, and amoxicillin, among others. MRSA is virulent, and it can be deadly.

In Canada, just fewer than 6000 cases of MRSA are reported annually. About 85% of these infections affect patients in health care facilities or those who have recently left a health care setting. People who contract health-care-associated MRSA typically have undergone an invasive surgical procedure or have an immune system weakened by illness or treatment for another disease. Experts say invasive MRSA is now the leading cause of surgical site infections, bloodstream infections, and pneumonia in hospitals and nursing homes.

Although less common, MRSA also affects people who have not been exposed to a health care facility; such infections

are called *community-associated MRSA (CA-MRSA)* infections. CA-MRSA usually is not invasive, meaning it doesn't enter the soft tissues under the skin. Instead, most community-associated infections take the form of surface abscesses and pus-filled lesions. Even though their numbers are low, community-based infections are a growing concern because they may indicate that MRSA is gaining strength "in the wild," making it more difficult to manage.

In the age of antibiotics, it's hard to imagine being infected by a germ that can't be killed. But epidemiologists say the overuse of antibiotics is one of the main reasons that bugs, such as MRSA, have become so strong. When people take antibiotics inappropriately or incorrectly, as North Americans have been doing for decades, bacteria have an opportunity to adapt. As a result, they can become resistant to antibiotics and the drugs lose their effectiveness.

Doctors also say that MRSA is a powerful reminder of a valuable lesson: Wash your hands. Frequent handwashing may be the most effective way to avoid infections—not just from MRSA but also from a host of other germs. Other simple but important methods for preventing infections also apply to MRSA:

• When washing your hands, use lots of soap and scrub briskly for at least 20 seconds.

• If soap and water aren't available, carry an alcohol-based hand sanitizer with you and use it often.

• Keep your hands away from your face.

• If you have an open wound, keep it clean, dry, and covered with a bandage.

• Don't share personal items, such as towels, razors, and tweezers; they can harbour germs and spread infection.

• If you have a skin lesion that resembles a spider bite, have it checked by a physician right away.

Sources: Centers for Disease Control and Prevention. 2007. *Invasive MRSA* (http://www.cdc.gov/ncidod/dhqp/ar_mrsa_Invasive_FS.html; retrieved February 16, 2009); Klevens, R. M., et al. 2007. Invasive methicillin-resistant *Staphylococcus aureus* infections in the United States. *Journal of the American Medical Association* 298(15): 1763–1771. Public Health Agency of Canada. 2008. *Canadian Nosocomial Infection Surveillance Program (CNISP)* (http://www.phac-aspc.gc.ca/nois-sinp/survprog-eng.php; retrieved October 30, 2009).

---

ranging from minor skin infections, such as boils, to very serious conditions, such as blood infections and pneumonia. The strain known as methicillin-resistant *Staphylococcus aureus* (MRSA) has become the most common cause of skin infections treated in emergency rooms (see the box "MRSA: The Superbug?" above, for more information). This antibiotic-resistant strain causes painful skin lesions that resemble infected spider bites.

Staphylococcus aureus is also responsible for many cases of toxic shock syndrome (TSS). The bacteria produce a deadly toxin that causes shock (potentially life-threatening low blood pressure), high fever, a peeling skin rash, and inflammation of several organ systems. TSS was first diagnosed in women using highly absorbent

tampons, which appear to allow the growth of staphylococci; however, about half of all cases occur in men and in women not using tampons. (See Chapter 11 for information on TSS as it relates to contraception.)

Tuberculosis Caused by the bacterium *Mycobacterium tuberculosis*, **tuberculosis (TB)** is a chronic bacterial infection that usually affects the lungs. TB is spread via the

tuberculosis (TB) A chronic bacterial infection that usually affects the lungs.

TERMS

respiratory route. Symptoms include coughing, fatigue, night sweats, weight loss, and fever.

About 1500 Canadians are infected with TB annually. Only about 10% of people with latent TB infections actually develop an active case of the disease; their immune system prevents the disease from becoming active. In Canada, active TB is most common among Aboriginal peoples and foreign-born immigrants from countries where TB is **endemic**. TB accounts for only about 10 deaths each year. Worldwide, about 2 billion people—one-third of the population—are infected with TB, and each year about 8.9 million develop active TB and more than 1.5 million die.

Many strains of tuberculosis respond to antibiotics, but only over a course of treatment lasting 6–12 months. Failure to complete treatment can lead to relapse and the development of strains of antibiotic-resistant bacteria. Of particular concern is the emergence of *M. tuberculosis* with extensive resistance to second-line drugs. These drugs are more toxic than first-line drugs—the drugs primarily used against bacterial infections. From 2000 to 2004, 20% of TB bacteria isolated in labs were multidrug resistant (MDR) and 2% were extensively drug resistant (XDR). XDR TB is geographically widespread, occurring even in North America, and is a serious threat to public health.

Tick-Borne Infections   Some diseases are transmitted via insect vectors. Lyme disease is one such infection, and it accounts for more than 95% of all reported vector-borne illness in North America. It is spread by the bite of a tick of the genus *Ixodes* that is infected with the spiral bacterium *Borrelia burgdorferi*. Ticks acquire the spirochete by ingesting the blood of an infected animal; they can then transmit the microbe to their next host. The deer tick is responsible for transmitting Lyme disease bacteria to humans in the northeastern and north-central areas of North America; on the Pacific Coast, the culprit is the western black-legged tick (Figure 9.7). Lyme disease is not a nationally reported disease in Canada, which makes incidence rates difficult to determine. It is thought to be uncommon here, with, for example, only 172 cases being reported in Ontario between 1999 and 2004.

Symptoms of Lyme disease vary but typically occur in three stages. In the first stage, about 80% of victims develop a bull's-eye-shaped red rash expanding from the area of the bite, usually about two weeks after the bite occurs. The second stage occurs weeks to months later in 10%–20% of untreated patients; symptoms may involve the nervous and cardiovascular systems and can include impaired coordination, partial facial paralysis, and heart rhythm abnormalities. These symptoms usually disappear on their own within a few weeks. The third stage, which occurs in about half of untreated people, can develop months or years after the tick bite and usually consists of chronic or recurring arthritis. Lyme disease can also cause fetal damage or death at any stage of pregnancy. Lyme disease is treatable at all stages, although arthritis symptoms may

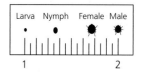

FIGURE 9.7   Deer tick (actual size).

not completely resolve. Lyme disease is preventable by avoiding contact with ticks or by removing a tick before it has had the chance to transmit the infection.

Rocky Mountain spotted fever and typhus are caused by the *rickettsias* bacterium and are also transmitted via tick bites. Rocky Mountain spotted fever is characterized by sudden onset of fever, headache, and muscle pain, followed by development of a spotted rash. Ehrlichiosis, another tick-borne disease, typically causes less severe symptoms.

Ulcers   About 10% of Canadians have ulcers, sores in the lining of the stomach or the first part of the small intestine (duodenum). Some ulcers are caused by long-term use of nonsteroidal anti-inflammatory drugs (NSAIDs). In addition, up to 90% of ulcers are caused by infection with *Helicobacter pylori*. Ulcer symptoms include gnawing or burning pain in the abdomen, nausea, and loss of appetite. If tests show the presence of *H. pylori*, antibiotics often cure the infection and the ulcers.

Other Bacterial Infections   The following are a few of the many other infections caused by bacteria:

• *Tetanus:* Also known as *lockjaw*, tetanus is caused by the bacterium *Clostridium tetani*, which thrives in deep puncture wounds and produces a deadly toxin. The toxin causes muscular stiffness and spasms, and infection is fatal in about 30% of cases. Because of widespread vaccination, tetanus is rare in the Canada. Worldwide, however, more than 200,000 people die from tetanus each year, primarily newborns infected through the unsterile cutting of the umbilical cord.

• *C. diff:* Another type of *Clostridium bacteria*, called *Clostridium difficile (C. diff)*, has joined MRSA as a major emerging threat in North American health care settings. Several varieties of *C. diff* have been known for decades to exist, and they generally cause illnesses ranging from diarrhea to life-threatening colitis. Most *C. diff* bugs do their harm by damaging the mucous lining of the intestine. Since 2000, however, one specific strain of *C. diff*—named NAP1—has emerged as a growing problem in hospitals. The NAP1 variant of *C. diff* is especially dangerous because it produces multiple toxins and generates them many times faster than other types of *C. diff*. Further, NAP1 is resistant to a wide range of antibiotics. Some experts describe the trend in *C. diff* NAP1 infections as an **epidemic** because infections are increasing at a rate of about 10% annually. Most *C. diff* infections occur in hospitals and commonly affect people who are already being treated with antibiotics for other infections. However, community-based infections are also on the rise, indicating that *C. diff* is spread via person-to-person contact. More than 2% of infected people die from the disease, and the death rate has doubled over the past five years. The infection can be treated with a few powerful antibiotics, and treatment is most successful when the infection is caught early. The best ways to avoid *C. diff* infection are to wash your hands frequently and take antibiotics only when absolutely necessary.

• *Pertussis:* Also known as *whooping cough,* pertussis is a highly contagious respiratory illness caused by a toxin produced by the bacterium *Bordetella pertussis.* Pertussis is characterized by bursts of rapid coughing, followed by a long attempt at inhalation that is often accompanied by a high-pitched whoop; symptoms may persist for two to eight weeks. Over the past decade, cases of pertussis in Canada have ranged from 2400 to 10,000. Those at high risk include infants and children who are too young to be fully vaccinated and those who have not completed the primary vaccination series. One to three Canadian infants die each year from whooping cough. Adolescents and adults become susceptible when immunity from vaccination wanes, so a booster shot is recommended every 10 years. Adults account for about 28% of whooping cough cases.

• *Urinary tract infections (UTIs):* Infection of the bladder and urethra is most common among sexually active women but can occur in anyone. The bacterium *Escherichi coli* is the most common infectious agent, responsible for about 80% of all UTIs. Infection most often occurs when bacteria from the digestive tract that live on the skin around the anus get pushed toward the opening of the urethra during sexual intercourse; then, the bacteria travel up the urethra and into the bladder. Women who are particularly susceptible may be given a supply of antibiotics to use after intercourse or at the first sign of infection; urinating before and after intercourse may also help prevent UTIs.

Bacteria responsible for food-borne illness are described in Chapter 5; Chapter 13 discusses sexually transmitted bacterial infections, such as chlamydia.

Antibiotic Treatments The body's immune system can fight off many, if not most, bacterial infections. However, while the body musters its defences, some bacteria can cause a great deal of damage: Inflammation, caused by the gathering of white blood cells, may lead to scarring and permanently damaged tissues. To help the body deal with these infections, science and medicine have made a considerable contribution: antibiotics.

ACTIONS OF ANTIBIOTICS **Antibiotics** are both naturally occurring and synthetic substances that can kill bacteria. Most antibiotics work in a similar fashion: They interrupt the production of new bacteria by damaging some part of their reproductive cycle or by causing faulty parts of new bacteria to be made. Penicillin inhibits the formation of the cell wall when bacteria divide to form new cells. Other antibiotics inhibit the production of certain proteins by the bacteria, and still others interfere directly with the

One of the dangers of antibiotic overuse is the development of bacteria resistant to drugs. Cultures of *E. coli* (a bacterium normally present in the human intestine) in this laboratory dish are sensitive to four different types of antibiotics, as indicated by the wide circles where no bacteria are growing, but they are resistant to two other types, which have no effect on their growth.

reading of genetic material (DNA) during the process of bacterial reproduction. Antibiotics are among the most widely prescribed and effective drugs.

ANTIBIOTIC RESISTANCE When antibiotics are misused or overused, the pathogens they are designed to treat can become resistant to their effects. A bacterium can become resistant from a chance genetic mutation or through the transfer of genetic material from one bacterium to another. When exposed to antibiotics, resistant bacteria can grow and flourish, while the antibiotic-sensitive bacteria die off. Eventually, an entire colony of bacteria can become resistant to one or more antibiotics and can become very difficult to treat. Antibiotic-resistant strains of many common bacteria have developed, including strains of gonorrhea (an STI) and salmonellosis (a food-borne illness). One strain of tuberculosis is resistant to seven different antibiotics. Antibiotic resistance is a major factor contributing to the recent rise in problematic infectious diseases.

The more often bacteria encounter antibiotics, the more likely they are to develop resistance. Resistance is promoted when people fail to take the full course of an

endemic Persistent and relatively widespread in a given population.

epidemic The occurrence in a particular community or region of more than the expected number of cases of a particular disease.

antibiotics Synthetic or naturally occurring substances used as drugs to kill bacteria.

TERMS

antibiotic or when they inappropriately take antibiotics for viral infections. Another possible source of resistance is the substantial use of antibiotics in agriculture. At least four species of antibiotic-resistant bacteria are documented to have been transmitted from food animals to humans. Limits may be placed on the use in animals of drugs used in human medicine as last resorts for serious or life-threatening disease.

You can help prevent the development of antibiotic-resistant strains of bacteria by using antibiotics properly:

- Don't take an antibiotic every time you get sick. They are mainly helpful for bacterial infections; they are ineffective against viruses.

- Use antibiotics as directed, and finish the full course of medication even if you begin to feel better. This helps ensure that all targeted bacteria are killed off.

- Never take an antibiotic without a prescription. If you take an antibiotic for a viral infection, take the wrong one, or take an insufficient dose, your illness will not improve, and you'll give bacteria the opportunity to develop resistance.

Viruses

Visible only with an electron (high-magnification) microscope, **viruses** lack all the enzymes essential to energy production and protein synthesis in normal animal cells, and they cannot grow or reproduce by themselves. Viruses are **parasites**; they take what they need for growth and reproduction from the cells they invade. Once a virus is inside the host cell, it sheds its protein covering, and its genetic material takes control of the cell and manufactures more viruses like itself (Figure 9.8). To fight viruses, the cellular immunity system produces several substances, such as interferon; these same substances are also responsible for most of the symptoms of a viral illness.

Illnesses caused by viruses are the most common forms of **contagious disease**. Different viruses affect different kinds of cells, and the seriousness of the disease they cause depends greatly on which kind of cell is affected. The viruses that cause colds, for example, attack upper respiratory tract cells, which are constantly cast off and replaced; the disease is therefore mild. Poliovirus, in contrast, attacks nerve cells that cannot be replaced, and the consequences, such as paralysis, are severe. HIV infection, a viral illness that destroys immune system cells, can destroy the body's ability to fight infectious diseases (see Chapter 13).

The Common Cold Although generally brief, lasting only one to two weeks, colds are nonetheless irritating and often interfere with our normal activities. A cold may be caused by any of more than 200 different viruses

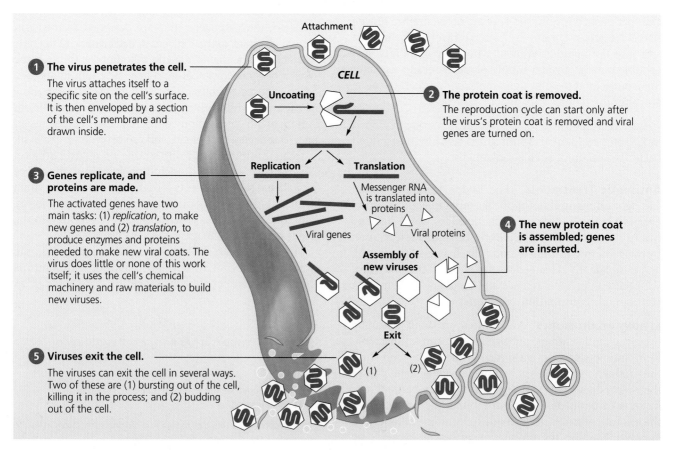

FIGURE 9.8 Life cycle of a virus.

① **The virus penetrates the cell.**
The virus attaches itself to a specific site on the cell's surface. It is then enveloped by a section of the cell's membrane and drawn inside.

② **The protein coat is removed.**
The reproduction cycle can start only after the virus's protein coat is removed and viral genes are turned on.

③ **Genes replicate, and proteins are made.**
The activated genes have two main tasks: (1) *replication*, to make new genes and (2) *translation*, to produce enzymes and proteins needed to make new viral coats. The virus does little or none of this work itself; it uses the cell's chemical machinery and raw materials to build new viruses.

④ **The new protein coat is assembled; genes are inserted.**

⑤ **Viruses exit the cell.**
The viruses can exit the cell in several ways. Two of these are (1) bursting out of the cell, killing it in the process; and (2) budding out of the cell.

Attachment

CELL

Uncoating

Replication   Translation

Messenger RNA is translated into proteins

Viral genes   Viral proteins

Assembly of new viruses

Exit

(1)   (2)

that attack the lining of the nasal passages; rhinoviruses and coronaviruses cause a large percentage of all colds among adults.

Cold viruses are almost always transmitted by hand-to-hand contact. To lessen your risk of contracting a cold, wash your hands frequently; if you touch someone else, avoid touching your face until after you've washed your hands. Colds are not caused by exposure to cold weather or by being chilled or overheated; more colds occur in the fall and winter months, probably because of the opening of school season (children contract more colds than adults) and because people spend more time indoors in the fall and winter months, making person-to-person transmission of viruses more likely.

If you catch a cold, over-the-counter cold remedies may help treat your symptoms but do not directly attack the viral cause (see the box "Preventing and Treating the Common Cold" on p. 296). Sometimes it is difficult to determine whether your symptoms are due to a virus (as for colds, flu, and some sinus infections), a bacterium (as for other sinus infections), or an allergy, but this information is important for appropriate treatment (Table 9.3). For example, antibiotics will not help treat a cold but will help treat a bacterial sinus infection.

Influenza Commonly called *the flu*, **influenza** is an infection of the respiratory tract caused by the influenza virus. (Many people use the term "stomach flu" to describe gastrointestinal illnesses, but these infections are actually caused by organisms other than influenza viruses). Compared with the common cold, influenza is a more serious illness, usually including a fever and extreme fatigue. Most people who get the flu recover within one to two weeks, but some develop potentially life-threatening

complications, such as pneumonia. The highest rates of infection occur in children. Influenza is highly contagious and is spread via respiratory droplets (see the box "The H1N1 Flu Pandemic" on p. 297).

The most effective way of preventing the flu is through annual vaccination. The influenza vaccine consists of killed virus and provides protection against the strains of the virus currently circulating; it is updated each year in response to changes in the virus. Vaccination can be appropriate for anyone age six months or older

virus A very small infectious agent composed of nucleic acid (DNA or RNA) surrounded by a protein coat; lacks an independent metabolism and reproduces only within a host cell.

parasite An organism that lives on or in a living host; the relationship benefits the parasite and harms the host.

contagious disease A disease that can be transmitted from one person to another; most are viral diseases, such as the common cold and flu.

influenza Infection of the respiratory tract by the influenza virus, which is highly infectious and adaptable; the form changes so easily that every year new strains arise, making treatment difficult; commonly known as *the flu*.

Table 9.3	What's Causing My Symptoms?			
Symptoms	**Influenza**	**Common Cold**	**Allergy**	**Sinusitis**
Headache	Usually	Occasionally	Occasionally	Usually
Muscle aches	Usually (severe)	Usually (mild)	Rarely	Rarely
Fatigue, weakness	Usually (severe; sudden onset; may last several weeks)	Usually (mild)	Rarely	Rarely
Fever	Usually (high, typically 38.8°C–40°C; sudden onset; lasts 3–4 days)	Occasionally (mild)	Never	Occasionally
Cough	Usually (often severe)	Occasionally	Occasionally	Usually
Runny, stuffy nose	Occasionally	Usually	Usually	Usually (stuffy)
Nasal discharge	Occasionally	Usually (thick, clear to yellowish green)	Usually (watery, clear)	Usually (thick, yellowish green)
Sneezing	Occasionally	Occasionally	Usually	Rarely
Sore throat	Occasionally	Usually	Occasionally	Rarely
Itchy eyes, nose, throat	Rarely	Rarely	Usually	Never

Source: Is it the flu? 2000. *Consumer Reports*, November. Copyright © 2000 by Consumers Union of U.S., Inc. Yonkers, NY 10703-1057, a nonprofit organization. Reprinted with permission from the November 2000 issue of *Consumer Reports* for educational purposes only. No commercial use or reproduction permitted. http://www.consumerreports.org/oh/index.htm.

Preventing and Treating the Common Cold

Prevention

Colds are usually spread by hand-to-hand contact with another person or with objects, such as doorknobs and telephones, which an infected person may have handled. The best way to avoid transmission is to wash your hands frequently with warm water and soap. Keeping your immune system strong is another good prevention strategy (see the guidelines provided later in the chapter).

Home Treatments

• Get some extra rest. It isn't usually necessary to stay home in bed, but you will need to slow down a little from your usual routine to give your body a chance to fight the infection.

• Drink plenty of liquids to prevent dehydration. Hot liquids, such as herbal tea and clear chicken soup, will soothe a sore throat and loosen secretions; gargling with a glass of slightly salty water may also help. Avoid alcoholic beverages when you have a cold.

• Hot showers or the use of a humidifier can help eliminate nasal stuffiness and soothe inflamed membranes.

Over-the-Counter Treatments

Avoid multisymptom cold remedies. Because these products include drugs to treat symptoms you may not even have, you risk suffering from side effects from medications you don't need. It's better to treat each symptom separately:

• *Analgesics*—Aspirin, acetaminophen (Tylenol), ibuprofen (Advil or Motrin), and naproxen sodium (Aleve)—all help lower fever and relieve muscle aches. Use of Aspirin is associated with an increased risk of a serious condition called Reye's syndrome in children and teenagers; for this reason, Aspirin should be given only to adults.

• *Decongestants* shrink nasal blood vessels, relieving swelling and congestion. However, they may dry out mucous membranes in the throat and make a sore throat worse. Nasal sprays shouldn't be used for more than two or three days to avoid rebound congestion.

• *Cough medicines* may be helpful when your cough is non-productive (not bringing up mucus) or if it disrupts your sleep or work. Expectorants make coughs more productive by increasing the volume of mucus and decreasing its thickness, thereby helping remove irritants from the respiratory airways. Suppressants (antitussives) reduce the frequency of coughing.

• *Antihistamines* decrease nasal secretions caused by the effects of histamine, so they are much more useful in treating allergies than colds. *Caution:* Many antihistamines can make you drowsy.

Antibiotics will not help a cold unless a bacterial infection, such as strep throat, is also present, and overuse of antibiotics leads to the development of drug resistance. The jury is still out on whether other remedies, including zinc gluconate lozenges, echinacea, and vitamin C, will relieve symptoms or shorten the duration of a cold. Researchers are also studying antiviral drugs that target the most common types of cold viruses.

Sometimes a cold leads to a more serious complication, such as bronchitis, pneumonia, or strep throat. If a fever of 38.8°C or higher persists, or if cold symptoms don't get better after two weeks, see your health care provider.

who wants to reduce his or her risk of the flu. A number of medications are used to treat influenza, but in most cases they can shorten the duration of illness by little more than a day and then only if treatment begins within one to two days after onset of symptoms. Several medications are also effective in reducing the risk of illness from influenza; however, they are less effective than the vaccine.

Measles, Mumps, and Rubella   Three childhood viral illnesses that have waned in Canada because of effective vaccines are measles, mumps, and rubella (German measles). Measles and rubella are generally characterized by rash and fever. Measles can occasionally cause more severe illness, including liver or brain infection or pneumonia; worldwide, more than 600,000 people die each year from measles. Measles is a highly contagious disease, and before the introduction of vaccines, 300,000–400,000 Canadians contracted the measles annually. Now, only about 200 cases are reported each year.

Rubella, if it infects a pregnant woman, can be transmitted to a fetus, causing miscarriage, stillbirth, and severe birth defects, including deafness, eye and heart defects, and mental impairment.

Mumps generally causes swelling of the parotid (salivary) glands, located just below and in front of the ears. This virus can also cause meningitis and, in males, inflammation of the testes.

Chicken Pox, Cold Sores, and Other Herpesvirus Infections   The **herpesviruses** are a large group of viruses. Once infected, the host is never free of the virus. The virus lies latent within certain cells and becomes active periodically, producing symptoms. Herpesviruses are particularly dangerous for people with a depressed immune system, as in the case of HIV infection. The family of herpesviruses includes the following:

• *Varicella-zoster virus*, which causes chicken pox and shingles. Chicken pox is a highly contagious childhood disease characterized by an itchy rash made up of small blisters; the infection is usually mild, although complications are more likely to occur in young infants and adults. After the rash resolves, the virus becomes latent, living in

The H1N1 Flu Pandemic

In April 2009, the H1N1 flu virus emerged as a new strain of **pandemic** influenza, which differed from the seasonal flu. People had no natural immunity to protect against virus. Surveillance of its spread showed that it affected more young and healthy people than the regular seasonal flu, which normally affects seniors and young children. People with underlying medical conditions and pregnant women were at a greater risk for severe illness.

H1N1 flu virus has been reported around the world and was a strain of the influenza virus that had previously primarily affected pigs. In the spring of 2009, it emerged in people in North America and spread to humans in regions around the world. This was a new strain of influenza and humans had little to no natural immunity to this virus. The WHO declared H1N1 a pandemic in June 2009.

Like seasonal influenza strains, the H1N1 flu virus is contagious and can be spread when an infected person coughs or sneezes and the germs enter the nose, eyes, or throat of another person. These germs can also rest on hard surfaces, like counters and doorknobs, and can be picked up on hands and transmitted to the respiratory system when someone touches their mouth and/or nose. It is not possible to catch it through blood transfusions.

Symptoms

Almost Always	Common	Sometimes
Cough and fever	Fatigue	Nausea
	Muscle aches	Vomiting
	Sore throat	Diarrhea
	Headache	
	Decreased appetite	
	Runny nose	

More investigation is needed on how long a person can be infectious (be able to spread the virus to others); however, it is believed that this period is for one day before the onset of symptoms and continues for approximately seven days after symptoms have started.

Prevention

To help minimize the spread of influenza, the Public Health Agency advises Canadians to:

• Wash hands often with soap and warm water for at least 20 seconds, or use hand sanitizer.

• Keep your hands away from your face.

• Cough and sneeze into your arm, not your hand. If you use a tissue, dispose of it as soon as possible and wash your hands.

• Get immunized.

• Keep common surface areas—for example, doorknobs, light switches, telephones, and keyboards—clean and disinfected.

• Eat healthy foods and stay physically active to keep your immune system strong.

• Keep doing what you normally do, but if you get sick, stay home.

Treatment

If you get flu-like symptoms and are otherwise healthy, you should stay home to recover. If your symptoms worsen or you experience difficulty breathing or serious shortness of breath, it is important to seek medical attention.

Antivirals

Antivirals are prescription medications used to treat viral illnesses, including the flu. If taken shortly after getting sick (within the first 24 to 48 hours), they can reduce flu symptoms, shorten the length of illness and may reduce serious complications. They are available in two forms: a pill (called oseltamivir or Tamiflu) or an inhaler (called zanamivir or Relenza).

Antivirals are recommended for the treatment of moderate to severe illness, and for people at risk of severe disease. Your doctor will decide if treatment is right for you.

Vaccination

As the circulation of H1N1 influenza in Canada is very low at this time, vaccination against H1N1 is only recommended for travellers visiting areas where H1N1 is circulating. If travellers have previously received the H1N1 vaccine, no further vaccine is needed.

During the H1N1 outbreak in Canada, adjuvanted vaccine was recommended for most Canadians as it provided better protection against H1N1 influenza. However, the adjuvanted vaccine has now expired and is not currently available in Canada.

The H1N1 vaccine currently available in Canada is the Influenza A (H1N1) 2009 Pandemic Monovalent Vaccine (Without Adjuvant).

Source: Key Facts on H1N1 Flu Virus. Public Health Agency of Canada. Reproduced with the permission of the Minister of Health, 2011.

---

sensory nerves. Many years later, the virus may reactivate and cause shingles; symptoms of shingles include pain in the affected nerves and a rash on the skin that follows the pattern of the nerve pathways (often a band over the ribs on one side of the body). A vaccine is available that prevents chicken pox in the majority of cases and results in milder illness if the disease does occur.

herpesvirus   A family of viruses responsible for cold sores, mononucleosis, chicken pox, and the STI known as herpes; frequently causes latent infections.

pandemic   A disease epidemic that is unusually severe or widespread; often used to refer to worldwide epidemics affecting a large proportion of the population.

- *Herpes simplex virus (HSV) types 1 and 2*, which cause cold sores and the STI herpes (Chapter 13). Herpes infections are characterized by small, painful ulcers in the area around the mouth or genitals, at the site where a person first contracts the virus. Following the initial infection, HSV becomes latent and may reactivate again and again over time. Many infected people do not know they are infected, and the virus can be transmitted even when sores are not apparent. Antiviral medications are available to prevent recurrences of genital herpes.
- *Epstein-Barr virus (EBV)*, which causes infectious mononucleosis. Mono, as it is commonly called, is characterized by fever, sore throat, swollen lymph nodes, and fatigue. It is usually spread by intimate contact with the saliva of an infected person—hence the name "kissing disease." Mono most often affects adolescents and young adults. Although EBV does reactivate throughout life, it generally does not cause any further symptoms. In a few people, especially those with HIV infection, EBV is associated with the development of cancers of the lymph system (see "Are All Diseases Infectious?" in the ■connect Library).

Two herpes viruses that can cause severe infections in people with a suppressed immune system are cytomegalovirus (CMV), which infects the lungs, brain, colon, and eyes, and human herpesvirus 8 (HHV-8), which has been linked to Kaposi's sarcoma.

Viral Encephalitis HSV type 1 is a possible cause of viral **encephalitis**, inflammation of brain tissue caused by a viral infection. Other possible causes include HIV and several mosquito-borne viruses, including Japanese encephalitis virus, equine encephalomyelitis virus, and West Nile virus. Mild cases of encephalitis may cause fever, headache, nausea, and lethargy; severe cases are characterized by memory loss, delirium, diminished speech function, and seizures, and they may result in permanent brain damage or death. Although rare, it is difficult to determine the exact prevalence of encephalitis because it is often underreported.

Viral Hepatitis Viral **hepatitis** is a term used to describe several different infections that cause inflammation of the liver. Hepatitis is usually caused by one of the three most common hepatitis viruses.

- *Hepatitis A virus (HAV)* causes the mildest form of the disease and is usually transmitted by food or water contaminated by sewage or an infected person.
- *Hepatitis B virus (HBV)* is usually transmitted sexually; it is discussed in detail in Chapter 13.

Body art procedures, such as tattooing, can lead to infection unless they are done with care.

- *Hepatitis C virus (HCV)* can also be transmitted sexually, but it is much more commonly passed through direct contact with infected blood via injection drug use or, before the development of screening tests, blood transfusions. HBV and, to a lesser extent, HCV can also be passed from a pregnant woman to her child.

There are effective vaccines for hepatitis A and B, but new cases of hepatitis occur in Canada each year. Symptoms of acute hepatitis infection can include fatigue, **jaundice**, abdominal pain, loss of appetite, nausea, and diarrhea. Most people recover from hepatitis A within a month or so. However, 5%–10% of people infected with HBV and 85%–90% of people infected with HCV become chronic carriers of the virus, capable of infecting others for the rest of their lives. Some chronic carriers remain asymptomatic, while others slowly develop chronic liver disease, cirrhosis, or liver cancer. An estimated 500 million people worldwide may be chronic carriers of hepatitis.

The extent of HCV infection has only recently been recognized, and many infected people are unaware of their condition. To ensure proper treatment and prevention, testing for HCV may be recommended for people at risk, including people who have ever injected drugs (even once), who received a blood transfusion or a donated organ

Tattoos and Body Piercing

Because tattooing and body piercing involve the use of needles, they carry health risks. If you are considering either procedure, you can reduce the risks by carefully choosing a body artist and following aftercare directions.

Tattoos are permanent marks applied with an electrically powered instrument that injects dye into the second layer of the skin. Pain and a little bleeding are common; a tattoo typically takes a week or two to heal and should be protected from sun exposure until then.

In piercing, the artist pushes a needle through the skin; a piece of jewellery holds the piercing open. Earlobe piercing is the most common, but people also pierce the upper ear, eyebrow, tongue, lip, nose, navel, nipples, and genitals. Healing time varies depending on the site of the piercing and other factors. Some pain and swelling are common; prolonged bleeding may follow oral piercing because the tongue contains so many blood vessels.

Potential Health Issues

• *Infection:* People are at risk from the transmission of blood-borne infectious agents, such as hepatitis and HIV, if instruments are not sterilized properly. No cases of HIV infection have been traced to tattooing or piercing. In 2006, an outbreak of MRSA occurred among customers of tattoo parlours in several U.S. states. In most cases, investigators found that the tattooists had not followed proper hygiene procedures, such as changing gloves between customers. Because of the potential risks of infection, people currently cannot donate blood for 12 months following application of body art, including tattoos and some body piercings. People with heart valve problems should check with a physician before body piercing to determine if they should take antibiotics before the procedure.

• *Allergic reactions:* Some people may be allergic to pigments used in tattooing or to metals used in body-piercing jewellery. All jewellery should be of noncorrosive materials, such as stainless steel or titanium; avoid jewellery that contains nickel.

• *Nodules and scars:* Some people may develop granulomas (nodules) or keloids (a type of scar) following tattooing or body piercing.

• *Problems relating to placement:* Tattoos may become swollen or burn if the wearer undergoes magnetic resonance imaging (MRI), and tattoos may also interfere with the quality of MRI images. Oral ornaments may obscure dental problems in dental X-rays; they may also damage teeth and fillings and interfere with speech and chewing. Navel piercings may become infected more easily because tight-fitting clothes allow moisture to collect in the area.

Tattoos are meant to be permanent and so are expensive and very difficult (or impossible) to remove completely. Tattoo removal may involve scraping or cutting off the layers of tattooed skin or using a laser to break up the pigment in the tattoo; some scarring can occur. Body piercings may close and heal once the jewellery is removed, but they may leave a permanent scar.

Choosing a Body Artist and Studio

A body art studio should be clean and have an autoclave for sterilizing instruments. Needles should be sterilized and disposable; piercing guns should not be used, as they cannot be adequately sterilized. The body artist should wear disposable latex gloves throughout the procedure. Leftover tattoo ink should be thrown away and not reused. Ask to see references and aftercare instructions beforehand.

---

before July 1992, who have engaged in high-risk sexual behaviour, or who have had body piercing, tattoos, or acupuncture involving unsterile equipment (see the box "Tattoos and Body Piercing," above). Antiviral drugs are available to treat chronic hepatitis, but they are not completely effective and may have significant side effects.

Poliomyelitis   An infectious viral disease that affects the nervous system, **poliomyelitis** (polio) can cause irreversible paralysis and death in some affected individuals. As with other vaccine-preventable diseases, the incidence of polio declined dramatically in Canada following the introduction of the vaccine, and North and South America are now considered free of the disease.

Rabies   Caused by a rhabdovirus, rabies is a potentially fatal infection of the central nervous system that is most often transmitted through an animal bite Canadian rabies-related deaths among humans declined dramatically during the twentieth century because of the widespread vaccina-

tion of domestic animals and the development of a highly effective vaccine regimen that provides immunity following exposure (post-exposure prophylaxis, or PEP).

Although rabies is rare in Canada (only 22 cases have been reported over the last 56 years), most recent cases have been traced to bats. It is recommended that PEP be considered for anyone who has had direct contact with a

encephalitis   Inflammation of the brain; fever, headache, nausea, and lethargy are common initial symptoms, followed in some cases by memory loss, seizures, brain damage, and death.

hepatitis   Inflammation of the liver, which can be caused by infection, drugs, or toxins.

jaundice   Increased bile pigment levels in the blood, characterized by yellowing of the skin and the whites of the eyes.

poliomyelitis   A disease of the nervous system, sometimes crippling; vaccines now prevent most cases of polio.

bat, including someone who has been in the same room with a bat and who might be unaware that contact has occurred (a sleeping child, for example). PEP consists of one dose of immunoglobulin and five doses of rabies vaccine over a 28-day period.

Human Papillomavirus (HPV)   The more than 100 different types of HPV cause a variety of warts (noncancerous skin tumours), including common warts on the hands, plantar warts on the soles of the feet, and genital warts around the genitalia. Depending on their location, warts may be removed by using over-the-counter preparations or professional methods, such as laser surgery or cryosurgery. Because HPV infection is chronic, warts can reappear despite treatment. As described in Chapter 8, HPV causes the majority of cases of cervical cancer. A vaccine was approved for use by Health Canada in 2006 for females ages 9–26 and in 2010 for males in the same age range. A second vaccine option is now available for females only, ages 10–25.

Treating Viral Illnesses   Antiviral drugs typically work by interfering with some part of the viral life cycle; for example, they may prevent a virus from entering body cells or from successfully reproducing within cells. Antivirals are currently available to fight infections caused by HIV, influenza, herpes simplex, varicella-zoster, HBV, and HCV. Most other viral diseases must simply run their course.

Fungi

A **fungus** is an organism that absorbs food from organic matter. Fungi may be multicellular (like moulds) or unicellular (like yeasts). Mushrooms and the moulds that form on bread and cheese are all fungi. Only about 50 fungi out of many thousands of species cause disease in humans, and these diseases are usually restricted to the skin, mucous membranes, and lungs. Some fungal diseases are extremely difficult to treat because some fungi form spores, an especially resistant dormant stage of the organism.

Candida albicans is a common fungus found naturally in the vagina of most women. When excessive growth occurs, the result is itching and discomfort, commonly known as a *yeast infection*. Factors that increase the growth of *C. albicans* include the use of antibiotics, clothing that keeps the vaginal area excessively warm and moist, pregnancy, oral contraceptive use, and certain diseases, including diabetes and HIV infection. The most common symptom is usually a thick white or yellowish discharge. Prescription and OTC treatments are available. Women should not self-treat unless they are certain from a past medical diagnosis that they have a yeast infection. (Misdiagnosis could mean that a different and more severe infection goes untreated.) *C. albicans* overgrowth can occur in other areas of the body, especially in the mouth in infants (a condition known as thrush).

Other common fungal conditions, including athlete's foot, jock itch, and ringworm, affect the skin. These three conditions are usually mild and easy to cure.

Fungi can also cause systemic diseases that are severe, life threatening, and extremely difficult to treat. Histoplasmosis, or valley fever, causes pulmonary and sometimes systemic disease and is most common in the St. Lawrence River Valley where 20%–30% of people test positive. In North America, more than 50 million people have tested positive. Fungal infections can be especially deadly in people with an impaired immune system.

Protozoa

Another group of pathogens is single-celled organisms known as **protozoa**. Millions of people in developing countries have protozoal infections.

Malaria, caused by a protozoan of the genus *Plasmodium*, is characterized by recurrent attacks of severe flulike symptoms (chills, fever, headache, nausea, and vomiting) and may cause anemia. The protozoan is injected into the bloodstream via a mosquito bite. Although relatively rare in Canada, malaria is a major killer worldwide; each year, 350 million to 500 million new cases of malaria and more than 1 million deaths occur, mostly among infants and children. Drugs are available to prevent and treat malaria, but in the poorest, most remote areas, conditions make it difficult to distribute drugs. Drug-resistant strains of malaria have emerged, requiring new medicines.

Giardiasis is caused by *Giardia lamblia*, a single-celled parasite that lives in the intestines of humans and animals. Giardiasis is characterized by nausea, diarrhea, bloating, and abdominal cramps, and it is among the most common waterborne diseases in North America. People may become infected with *Giardia* if they consume contaminated food or water or pick up the parasite from the contaminated surface of an object, such as a bathroom fixture, diaper pail, or toy. People at risk include child care workers, children who attend day care, international travellers, and hikers and campers who drink untreated water. Giardiasis is rarely serious and can be treated with prescription medications.

Other protozoal infections include the following:

- *Trichomoniasis (trich)*, a common vaginal infection. Although usually mild and treatable, trich may increase the risk of HIV transmission (see Chapter 13).

- *Trypanosomiasis (African sleeping sickness)*, which is transmitted through the bite of an infected tsetse fly and causes extreme fatigue, fever, rash, severe headache, central nervous system damage, and death.

- *Amoebic dysentery*, a severe form of amebiasis, infection of the intestines with the parasite *Entamoeba histolytica*. It is characterized by bloody diarrhea, stomach pain, and fever.

Parasitic Worms

The **parasitic worms** are the largest organisms that can enter the body to cause infection. The tapeworm, for example, can grow several metres long. Worms, including intestinal parasites, such as the tapeworm and hookworm, cause a variety of relatively mild infections. Pinworm, the most common worm infection in Canada, primarily affects young children. Pinworms are white and about the size of a staple and live in the rectum of humans; they can cause itching and difficulty sleeping. Smaller worms known as flukes infect organs, such as the liver and lungs, and in large numbers can be deadly. Worm infections generally originate from contaminated food or drink and can be controlled by careful attention to hygiene.

Prions

In recent years, several fatal degenerative disorders of the central nervous system have been linked to **prions**, or proteinaceous infectious particles. Unlike all other infectious agents, prions appear to lack DNA or RNA and to consist only of protein; their presence in the body does not trigger an immune response. Prions have an abnormal shape and form deposits in the brain. They may spread by triggering normal proteins to change their structure to the abnormal and damaging form.

Prions are associated with a class of diseases known as *transmissible spongiform encephalopathies (TSEs)*, which are characterized by spongelike holes in the brain; symptoms of TSEs include loss of coordination, weakness, dementia, and death. Known prion diseases include Creutzfeldt-Jakob disease (CJD) in humans; bovine spongiform encephalopathy (BSE), or mad cow disease, in cattle; and scrapie in sheep. Some prion diseases are inherited or the result of spontaneous genetic mutations, whereas others are the result of eating infected tissue or being exposed to prions during medical procedures, such as organ transplants. A variant form of CJD referred to as vCJD occurs in humans who are infected by eating beef from cows with BSE.

As of 2006, 200 cases of vCJD had been reported worldwide, with 164 of those cases occurring in the United Kingdom. The first indigenous Canadian BSE case was identified in 2003 (the first case in Canada was found in 1993 in a cow originally imported from Britain, as discussed in Chapter 5). Steps have been taken or proposed to reduce the number of BSE-infected cows and the likelihood of meat from an infected animal entering the human food supply. These include increasing surveillance, limiting or banning the use of cattle products in feed for other cattle, prohibiting meat imports from countries with BSE-infected cattle, restricting certain people from giving blood, and banning the use of downer (nonambulatory) cattle for food for human consumption. Prions present special challenges because they are resistant to heat, radiation, and chemicals that kill other pathogens and because the diseases they cause have a long incubation period. In fact, experts say BSE can take 50 years to incubate. Authorities are now concerned that many more people may harbour BSE than estimated, leading to an epidemic of vCJD in coming decades. Scientists are working to develop new tests that would detect low levels of dangerous prions in asymptomatic cattle.

Emerging Infectious Diseases

Emerging infectious diseases are those infections whose incidence in humans has increased or threatens to increase in the near future. They include both known diseases that have experienced a resurgence, such as tuberculosis and cholera, and diseases that were previously unknown or confined to specific areas, such as the Ebola and West Nile viruses.

Selected Infections of Concern   Although the chances of the average Canadian contracting an exotic infection are very low, emerging infections are a concern to public health officials and represent a challenge to all nations in the future.

WEST NILE VIRUS A mini-outbreak of encephalitis in North America in 1999 led to the identification of West Nile virus, which had previously been restricted to Africa, the Middle East, and parts of Europe. In Canada, more than 2000 cases were confirmed in 2007 and only 36 cases in 2008. West Nile virus is carried by birds and then passed to humans when mosquitoes bite first an infected bird and then a person. Most people who are bitten have few or no symptoms, but the virus can cause permanent brain damage or death in some. Vaccines are being developed for West Nile virus, but it is important to protect yourself from mosquito bites.

SEVERE ACUTE RESPIRATORY SYNDROME (SARS) In February 2003, SARS appeared in southern China and quickly spread to more than 15 countries; it is a form of pneumonia that is fatal in about 5%–15% of cases. SARS is caused by a new type of coronavirus found in wildlife that may have crossed the species barrier when certain wildlife species were consumed as delicacies. By 2004 SARS had been responsible for more than 8000 illnesses and 800 deaths. No new cases have been reported since 2004.

ROTAVIRUS The leading viral cause of gastroenteritis, an intestinal inflammation that results in vomiting and diarrhea, rotavirus infects almost every child at one time or another. Worldwide, the virus kills about 600,000 children each year, mostly in developing countries. Left untreated, rotavirus-induced diarrhea can become severe and lead to dehydration, which can be fatal. Rotavirus spreads through poor hygiene and sanitation practices.

ESCHERICHIA COLI O157:H7 This potentially deadly strain of *E. coli*, transmitted in contaminated food, can cause

Insecticides, repellents, protective clothing, and screens are helpful in reducing mosquito bites. In developing countries, nets are a first line of defence against mosquitoes.

THINKING ABOUT THE ENVIRONMENT
Many environmental factors contribute to the spread of infectious diseases. Here are a few examples:

- In poverty-stricken regions, many people become ill as a result of unsanitary conditions and a lack of clean drinking water.

- Unsustainable development practices, such as clearing forests and draining wetlands, disturb the ecosystem and force many disease-carrying vectors (such as vermin and insects) out of their natural habitats and into contact with people.

- A shift in rainfall patterns (perhaps caused by global warming) may allow mosquito-borne diseases, such as malaria, to spread from the tropics into the temperate zones. Since many species of mosquito in North America can carry malaria, such changes could someday make malaria a widespread health threat to Canada.

For more information on the environment and environmental health, see Chapter 21.

bloody diarrhea and kidney damage. In 2000, more than 2000 people in Walkerton, Ontario, became ill, 68 were hospitalized, and 7 died from drinking well water contaminated by cattle fecal matter following heavy rains. Other outbreaks have been linked to spinach, lettuce, alfalfa sprouts, unpasteurized juice, petting zoos, and contaminated public swimming pools.

HANTAVIRUS Since first being recognized in 1993, 50 cases of hantavirus pulmonary syndrome (HPS) have been reported in Canada. HPS is caused by the rodent-borne Sin Nombre virus (SNV) and is spread primarily through airborne viral particles from rodent urine, droppings, or saliva. It is characterized by a dangerous fluid buildup in the lungs and is fatal in about 45% of cases.

EBOLA Human outbreaks of the often fatal Ebola hemorrhagic fever (EHF) have occurred only in Africa. The Ebola virus is transmitted by contact with infected blood or other body secretions, and many cases of EHF have been linked to unsanitary conditions in medical facilities. Because symptoms appear quickly and 70% of victims die, usually within a few days, the virus tends not to spread widely.

Factors Contributing to Emerging Infections What's behind this rising tide of infectious diseases? Contributing factors are complex and interrelated.

DRUG RESISTANCE New or increasing drug resistance has been found in organisms that cause malaria, tuberculosis, gonorrhea, influenza, AIDS, and pneumococcal and staphylococcal infections. Infections caused by drug-resistant organisms prolong illness, and—if not treated in time with more effective, expensive drugs—they can cause death. Some bacterial strains now appear to be resistant to all available antibiotics.

POVERTY More than 1 billion people live in extreme poverty, and half the world's population have no regular access to essential drugs. Population growth, urbanization, overcrowding, and migration (including the movement of refugees) also spread infectious diseases.

BREAKDOWN OF PUBLIC HEALTH MEASURES A poor public health infrastructure is often associated with poverty and social upheaval, but other problems, such as contaminated water supplies, can occur even in industrial countries. Inadequate vaccination has led to the reemergence of some diseases, such as diphtheria and pertussis. Natural disasters, such as floods and hurricanes, also disrupt the public health infrastructure, leaving survivors with contaminated water and food supplies and no shelter from disease-carrying insects.

TRAVEL AND COMMERCE More than 500 million travellers cross national borders each year, and international tourism and trade open the world to infectious agents. SARS was quickly spread throughout the world by infected air travellers. The reintroduction of cholera into the western hemisphere is thought to have occurred through the discharge of bilge water from a Chinese freighter into the waters off Peru.

MASS FOOD PRODUCTION AND DISTRIBUTION Food now travels long distances to our table, and microbes are transmitted along with it. Mass production of food increases the likelihood that a chance contamination can lead to mass illness.

HUMAN BEHAVIOURS Changes in patterns of human behaviour also influence the spread of infectious diseases. The widespread use of injectable drugs rapidly transmits HIV infection and hepatitis. Changes in sexual behaviour over the past 30 years have led to a proliferation of old and new STIs. The use of day care facilities for children has led to increases in the incidence of several infections that cause diarrhea.

BIOTERRORISM The deliberate release of deadly infectious agents is an ongoing concern, although Canadians' experience has, to date, been one of witness to what has happened to our southern neighbours. In 2001, infectious anthrax spores sent through the mail sickened 11 and killed 5 people in the United States. Potential bioterrorism agents that have been categorized as a highest concern are those that can be easily disseminated or transmitted from person to person and that have a high mortality rate and the potential for a major public health impact; these include anthrax, smallpox, plague, botulism, and viral hemorrhagic fevers, such as Ebola.

Other Immune Disorders: Cancer and Autoimmune Diseases

The immune system has evolved to protect the body from invasion by foreign microorganisms. Sometimes, as in the case of cancer, the body comes under attack by its own cells. As explained in Chapter 8, cancer cells cease to cooperate normally with the rest of the body and multiply uncontrollably. The immune system can often detect cells that have recently become cancerous and then destroy them just as it would a foreign microorganism. But if the immune system breaks down, as it may when people get older, when they have certain immune disorders (including HIV infection), or when they are receiving chemotherapy for other diseases, the cancer cells may multiply out of control before the immune system recognizes the danger. By the time the immune system gears up to destroy the cancerous cells, it may be too late.

Another immune disorder occurs when the body confuses its own cells with foreign organisms. As described earlier, the immune system must recognize many thousands of antigens as foreign and then be able to recognize the same antigens again and again. Our own tissue cells also are antigenic; that is, they would be recognized by another person's immune system as foreign. A delicate balance must be maintained to ensure that our immune system recognizes only truly foreign antigens as enemies; erroneous recognition of our own cells as foreign produces havoc.

This is what happens in autoimmune diseases, such as rheumatoid arthritis and systemic lupus erythematosus. In this type of malady, the immune system seems to be a bit too sensitive and begins to misapprehend itself as nonself. For reasons not well understood, these conditions are much more common in women than in men (see the box "Women and Autoimmune Diseases" on p. 304).

> **Nearly all** major bacterial infections are becoming resistant to common antibiotics.
>
> —CDC, 2007
>
> QUICK STATS

QUESTIONS FOR CRITICAL THINKING AND REFLECTION
Have you ever had any of the illnesses described in the preceding section? How were you exposed to the disease? Could you have taken any precautions to avoid it?

GENDER MATTERS

Women and Autoimmune Diseases

Although the immune systems of men and women are essentially the same, women have much higher rates of many autoimmune diseases. The reason gender is a determinant of autoimmune diseases is somewhat of a mystery. One clue may come from pregnancy: To conceive and carry a baby to term, a woman's body must temporarily suppress its immune response so it doesn't attack the sperm or the fetus. Another factor seems to be related to estrogen. Estrogen receptors have been found on suppressor T cells, pointing to a possible link between the glands controlling immunity and those controlling sex hormones. Women also appear to have somewhat enhanced immunity compared with men, a factor that could be linked to both longer lifespans and higher rates of autoimmune disorders.

Systemic lupus erythematosus is an autoimmune disease in which the immune system attacks the body's normal tissue, causing inflammation of the joints, blood vessels, heart, lungs, brain, and kidneys. Its symptoms include painful swollen joints, a rash on the nose and cheeks, sensitivity to sunlight, chest pain, fatigue, and dizziness. Tens of thousands of Canadians have lupus, 80% of them are women; the disorder is especially common among Aboriginal

peoples and black women. Lupus usually begins before menopause and may flare up during pregnancy; for some women, symptoms also increase in severity during menstruation or with the use of oral contraceptives. A link between these exacerbating factors is increased levels of estrogen, but this connection is not well understood. Researchers have also

identified genetic mutations that may be associated with lupus.

In rheumatoid arthritis, the body's immune system attacks the membranes lining the joints, causing pain and swelling. Among the estimated 300,000 Canadians with rheumatoid arthritis, women outnumber men three to one. The causes of the disease are not well understood. Researchers have hypothesized that an as-yet-unidentified virus may stimulate the immune system and trigger the disease. When the disease is present in younger women, symptoms often improve during pregnancy, when estrogen levels are higher, the opposite of what is seen in the case of lupus. Therefore, although estrogen levels may play a role in these disorders, its effects appear to be influenced by many other factors.

Other autoimmune disorders more common among women than men include multiple sclerosis, a neurological disease caused by the destruction of the protective coating around nerves; scleroderma, a connective tissue disease characterized by thickening, hardening, and tightening of the skin; and Graves' disease, characterized by an increase in the production of thyroid hormone, which affects metabolism and many body systems.

SUPPORTING YOUR IMMUNE SYSTEM

Pathogens threaten everyone's wellness, but you can take steps to prevent them from compromising your health. Here are some general guidelines for keeping pathogens at bay:

- Eat a balanced diet and maintain a healthy weight, as discussed in Chapters 4 and 5.

- Get enough sleep. Most people need six to eight hours every night. Sleep helps your body replenish itself and encourages the production of immune system cells. Lack of sleep can actually increase your chances of getting sick.

- Exercise, but not when you're sick. Exercise helps you stay healthy, as discussed in Chapter 6. It also staves off stress, which can weaken your immune system. For more information, see the box "Immunity and Stress."

- Don't smoke. Smoking decreases the levels of some immune cells (see Chapter 16).

- If you drink alcohol, do so only in moderation (see Chapter 14). Excessive drinking can interfere with normal immune system functioning.

Immunity and Stress

Studies have shown that rates of illness are higher for weeks or even months in people who have experienced the severe emotional trauma of divorce or the death of a loved one. But can commonplace anxieties and stresses also cause measurable changes in the immune system? And can common stress-management techniques boost the immune system? The answer to these questions appears to be yes. Consider the following research findings:

• Medical students taking final exams showed a much weaker immune response to a hepatitis vaccination than unstressed students. In other studies, stress was associated with lower T-cell responses and antibody levels following influenza vaccinations.

• People with higher levels of stress and who had a negative or pessimistic outlook developed more colds during a yearlong study than did individuals with lower levels of stress and a more positive outlook.

• In a study of caregivers, relaxation sessions were associated with increased secretion of cytokines in minor wounds, thus speeding healing. Relaxation and imagery have been shown to increase T-cell levels in some people.

• A study comparing parents of children with cancer (who presumably had high stress levels) with parents of healthy children found that stress appears to interfere with the body's ability to shut down the inflammatory response after it gets started. Continuing high levels of cytokines and inflammation could harm health. The same study found that social support is a determinant of improved immune response.

In seeking to explain these effects, researchers are looking at the connections among stress, hormones, and immunity. Some hormones, such as cortisol, appear to impair the ability of immune cells to multiply and function. Others, such as prolactin, seem to give immune cells a boost. By matching stress levels and

hormonal changes to the ups and downs of immune function, researchers hope to gain a better grasp of the shifting chemistry of mind and immunity.

• Wash your hands frequently, as advised throughout this chapter. Antibacterial soap has not been proven to reduce the risk of infection any better than regular soap, especially if you wash properly. Use hand sanitizer when soap and water aren't available; make sure the product is at least 60% alcohol.

• Avoid contact with people who are contagious with an infectious disease.

• Make sure you drink water only from clean sources. Unpurified water from lakes and streams can carry pathogens, even if it seems pristine.

• Avoid contact with disease carriers, such as rodents, mosquitoes, and ticks. Never touch or feed wild animals or rodents.

• Practise safer sex (as described in Chapter 13).

• Do not use injectable drugs of any kind (see Chapter 14).

• Make sure you have received all your recommended vaccinations, and keep them up-to-date. Your physician can tell you exactly what immunizations you need and when you should have them.

McGraw Hill connect™

Practise and learn online with Connect. Connect allows you to practise important skills at your own pace and on your own schedule, with 24/7 online access to an eBook, practice quizzes, interactivities, videos, study tools, additional resources, and more.

SUMMARY

• The step-by-step process by which infections are transmitted from one person to another involves the pathogen, its reservoir, a portal of exit, a means of transmission, a portal of entry, and a new host.

• Infection can be prevented by breaking the chain at any point. Strategies include public health measures, such as treatment of drinking water, and individual actions, such as handwashing.

• Physical and chemical barriers to microorganisms include skin, mucous membranes, and the cilia lining the respiratory tract.

• The immune response is carried out by white blood cells that are continuously produced in the bone marrow. These include neutrophils, macrophages, dendritic cells, natural killer cells, and lymphocytes.

• The immune response has four stages: recognition of the invading pathogen; rapid replication of killer T cells and B cells; attack by killer T cells and macrophages; and suppression of the immune response.

• Immunization is based on the body's ability to remember previously encountered organisms and retain its strength against them.

• Allergic reactions occur when the immune system responds to harmless substances as if they were dangerous antigens.

• Bacteria are single-celled organisms; some cause disease in humans. Bacterial infections include pneumonia, meningitis, strep throat, toxic shock syndrome, tuberculosis, Lyme disease, and ulcers.

• Most antibiotics work by interrupting the production of new bacteria; they do *not* work against viruses. Bacteria can become resistant to antibiotics.

• Viruses cannot grow or reproduce themselves; different viruses cause the common cold, influenza, measles, mumps, rubella, chicken pox, cold sores, mononucleosis, encephalitis, hepatitis, polio, and warts.

• Other diseases are caused by certain types of fungi, protozoa, parasitic worms, and prions.

• Autoimmune diseases occur when the body identifies its own cells as foreign.

• The immune system needs little help other than adequate nutrition and rest, a moderate lifestyle, and protection from excessive stress. Vaccinations also help protect against disease.

FOR MORE INFORMATION

BOOKS

Barry, J. 2005. *The Great Influenza: The Epic Story of the Deadliest Plague in History.* New York: Penguin. A compelling account of the medical, social, and political aspects of the Influenza epidemic of 1918–1919.

Bollet, A. J. 2004. *Plagues and Poxes: The Impact of Human History on Epidemic Disease.* New York: Demos Medical. Describes how human activity affects diseases.

Roitt, I. M., et al. 2006. *Roitt's Essential Immunology,* 11th ed. London: Blackwell. A highly readable introduction to the science of immunology.

Siegel, M. 2006. *Bird Flu: Everything You Need to Know About the Next Pandemic.* New York: Wiley. A practising physician and teacher examines the potential threat of an avian flu outbreak and explains the measures we can take to protect ourselves.

Sompayrac, L. M. 2008. *How the Immune System Works,* 3rd ed. Malden, Mass.: Blackwell Science. A highly readable overview of basic concepts of immunity.

ORGANIZATIONS, HOTLINES, AND WEB SITES

The Internet addresses listed here were accurate at the time of publication.

Alliance for the Prudent Use of Antibiotics. Provides information on the proper use of antibiotics and tips for avoiding infections.
    http://www.tufts.edu/med/apua

Canadian Cancer Society: The Human Papillomavirus and Cervical Cancer. Provides information about HPV.
    http://www.cancer.ca/Canada-wide/Prevention/Viruses%20and%20bacteria/Human%20papillomavirus%20HPV.aspx?sc_lang=en

Cells Alive! Includes micrographs of immune cells and pathogens at work.

http://www.cellsalive.com

Health Canada: Hepatitis. Provides information about hepatitis in Canada.

http://www.hc-sc.gc.ca/hc-ps/dc-ma/hep-eng.php

Health Canada: STI—Sexually Transmitted Infections. Provides information and resources about sexual health and STIs in Canada.

http://www.phac-aspc.gc.ca/publicat/std-mts/index-eng.php

Lupus Canada. Provides information and resources about lupus in Canada.

http://www.lupuscanada.org

Public Health Agency of Canada: Infectious Diseases. Provides information about infectious diseases.

http://www.phac-aspc.gc.ca/id-mi/index-eng.php

Public Health Agency of Canada: Immunization Schedules. Provides information about recommended immunizations for Canadian children and adults.

http://www.phac-aspc.gc.ca/im/is-vc-eng.php

Public Health Agency of Canada: Travel Health. Provides travel health information, including advisories, notices, and travel-related diseases.

http://www.phac-aspc.gc.ca/tmp-pmv/index-eng.php

Public Health Agency of Canada: Condoms, Sexually Transmitted Infections, Safer Sex and You. Provides tips on safer sex.

http://www.phac-aspc.gc.ca/publicat/epiu-aepi/std-mts/condom-eng.php

U.S. National Foundation for Infectious Diseases. Provides information about a variety of diseases and disease issues.

http://www.nfid.org

U.S. National Institute of Allergy and Infectious Diseases. Includes fact sheets about many topics relating to allergies and infectious diseases, including tuberculosis and STIs.

http://www.niaid.nih.gov

World Health Organization: Infectious Diseases. Provides fact sheets about many emerging and tropical diseases as well as information about current outbreaks.

http://www.who.int/topics/infectious_diseases/en/

See also the listings in Chapters 5 and 13.

SELECTED BIBLIOGRAPHY

Andries, K., et al. 2005. A diarylquinoline drug active on the ATP synthetase of *Mycobacterium tuberculosis*. *Science* 307(5707): 223–227.

Arbes, S. J., et al. 2005. Prevalences of positive skin test responses to 10 common allergens in the US population: Results from the third National Health and Nutrition Examination Survey. *Journal of Allergy and Clinical Immunology* 116(2): 377–383.

Cashman, N. R., and B. Caughey. 2004. Prion diseases—Close to an effective therapy? *Nature Reviews: Drug Discovery* 3(12): 874–884.

Canadian Institutes of Health Research. 2009. *About the Antibiotic Resistance Initiatives* (http://www.cihr-irsc.gc.ca/e/40485.html; retrieved April 14, 2011).

Centers for Disease Control and Prevention. 2007. *Healthcare-Associated Methicillin Resistant Staphylococcus Aureus (HA-MRSA)* (http://www.cdc.gov/ncidod/dhqp/ar-mrsa.html; retrieved February 16, 2009).

Cieslak, P. R., K. Hedberg, and L. E. Lee. 2004. Chickenpox outbreak in a highly vaccinated school population: In reply. *Pediatrics* 114(4): 1131.

Fairweather, D., and N. R. Rose. 2004. Women and autoimmune diseases. *Emerging Infectious Diseases* 10(11): 2005–2011.

Fauci, A. S. 2004. Emerging infectious diseases: A clear and present danger to humanity. *Journal of the American Medical Association* 292(15): 1887–1888.

Gupta, R. S., et al. 2006. The widening black/white gap in asthma hospitalizations and mortality. *Journal of Allergy and Clinical Immunology* 117(2): 351–358.

Immunization Safety Review Committee. 2004. *Immunization Safety Review: Vaccines and Autism.* Washington, D.C.: National Academy Press.

Keene, W. E., A. C. Markum, and M. Samadpour. 2004. Outbreak of *Pseudomonas aeruginosa* infections caused by commercial piercing of upper ear cartilage. *Journal of the American Medical Association* 291(8): 981–985.

Larson, E. L., et al. 2004. Effect of antibacterial home cleaning and handwashing products on infectious disease symptoms: A randomized, double-blind trial. *Annals of Internal Medicine* 140(5): 321–329.

Lee, G. M., et al. 2005. Illness transmission in the home: A possible role for alcohol-based hand gels. *Pediatrics* 115(4): 852–860.

Levy, S. B., and B. Marshall. 2004. Antibacterial resistance worldwide: Causes, challenges, and responses. *Nature Medicine* 10(12 Suppl.): S122–S129.

National Immunization Program. 2005. *Epidemiology and Prevention of Vaccine-Preventable Diseases,* 8th rev. ed. Waldorf, Md.: Public Health Foundation.

Orent, W. 2005. Worrying about killer flu. *Discover,* February.

Parker, S. K., et al. 2004. Thimerosal-containing vaccines and autistic spectrum disorder: A critical review of published original data. *Pediatrics* 114(3): 793–804.

Prusiner, S. B. 2004. Detecting mad cow disease. *Scientific American,* July.

Public Health Agency of Canada. 2008. *Hepatitis C Information for Health Professionals* (http://www.phac-aspc.gc.ca/hepc/pubs/ihp-ips/index-eng.php; retrieved April 15, 2011).

Public Health Agency of Canada. 2010. *Information on Seniors and the Flu Virus (Seasonal Flu and H1N1 Flu)* (http://www.phac-aspc.gc.ca/alert-alerte/h1n1/fs-fi-seniors-aines-eng.php; retrieved April 15, 2011).

Samandari, T., B. P. Bell, and G. L. Armstrong. 2004. Quantifying the impact of hepatitis A immunization in the United States, 1995–2001. *Vaccine* 22(31–32): 4342–4350.

Smeeth, L., et al. 2004. MMR vaccination and pervasive developmental disorders: A case-control study. *Lancet* 364(9438): 963–969.

Snow, R. W., et al. 2005. The global distribution of clinical episodes of *Plasmodium falciparum* malaria. *Nature* 434: 214–217.

Statistics Canada. 2010. *Leading Causes of Death, by Sex (Both Sexes)* (http://www40.statcan.gc.ca/l01/cst01/hlth36a-eng.htm; retrieved April 15, 2011).

Vazquez, M., et al. 2004. Effectiveness over time of varicella vaccine. *Journal of the American Medical Association* 291(7): 851–855.

World Health Organization. 2004. *WHO Guidelines for the Global Surveillance of Severe Acute Respiratory Syndrome (SARS), Updated Recommendations.* Geneva: World Health Organization.

World Health Organization. 2005. *Vaccine-Preventable Diseases* (http://www.who.int/mediacentre/events/2006/g8summit/vaccines/en/; retrieved April 15, 2011).

World Health Organization. 2007. *The World Health Report 2007.* Geneva: World Health Organization.

World Health Organization. 2010. *Poliomyelitis: Fact Sheet N°114* (http://www.who.int/mediacentre/factsheets/fs114/en/index.html; retrieved April 16, 2011).

Zoutman D. E., and B. D. Ford. 2008. A comparison of infection control program resources, activities, and antibiotic resistant organism rates in Canadian acute care hospitals in 1999 and 2005: pre- and post-severe acute respiratory syndrome. *American Journal of Infection Control* 36(10): 711–717.

McGraw Hill **connect**™

Practise and learn online with Connect.

HEALTHY RELATIONSHIPS AND COMMUNICATION

LOOKING AHEAD>>>>>

AFTER READING THIS CHAPTER, YOU SHOULD BE ABLE TO

- Explain the qualities that help people develop intimate relationships
- Describe different types of love relationships and the stages they often go through
- Identify common challenges of forming and maintaining intimate relationships
- Explain some elements of healthy and productive communication
- List some characteristics of successful families and some problems families may face

TEST YOUR KNOWLEDGE

ANSWERS

1. **What percentage of North Americans report having no one they want to confide in?**
   a. 10%
   b. 15%
   c. 25%

2. **In a typical long-term intimate relationship, commitment tends to increase over time.**
   True or false?

3. **Jealousy is a good indicator of what?**
   a. Love
   b. Insecurity
   c. Passion

4. **What percentage of Canadian children live in a single-parent home?**
   a. 2.5%
   b. 5%
   c. 25.8%

1. **C.** Nearly one-quarter of North Americans say they don't have a friend with whom they share intimate thoughts. The average person's circle of close friends has steadily shrunk over the last two decades.

2. **TRUE.** Although passion and physical attraction tend to decline over time, most couples become increasingly committed to their relationship as time goes by.

3. **B.** Some people think that the existence of jealousy proves the existence of love, but jealousy is actually a more accurate yardstick for measuring insecurity or possessiveness. Jealousy can destroy a relationship.

4. **C.** More than one-quarter of Canadian families with children are single-parent families. About 21% of those children live with their mother, while about 5% live with their father.

Human beings need social relationships; we cannot thrive as solitary creatures. Nor could the human species survive if adults didn't cherish and support each other, if we didn't form strong mutual attachments with our infants, and if we didn't create families in which to raise children. Simply put, people need people.

Although people are held together in relationships by a variety of factors, the foundation of many relationships is the ability to both give and receive love. Love in its many forms—romantic, passionate, platonic, parental—is the wellspring from which much of life's meaning and delight flows. In our culture, it binds us together as partners, parents, children, and friends.

Just as important is developing a healthy relationship with ourselves, which includes the ability to self-soothe, to regulate our emotions, and to be alone with ourselves at times.

DEVELOPING CLOSE RELATIONSHIPS

People who develop successful close, often called intimate, relationships believe in themselves and in the people around them. They are willing to give of themselves—to share their ideas, feelings, time, needs—and to accept what others want to give them.

Self-Concept and Self-Esteem

The principal element that we all bring to our relationships is our *selves*. To have successful relationships, we must first accept and feel good about ourselves. A positive self-concept and a healthy level of self-esteem help us love and respect others.

As discussed in Chapter 2, the roots of our identity and sense of self can be found in childhood, in the relationships we had with our parents and other family members. As adults, we probably have a sense that we're basically lovable, worthwhile people and that we can trust others if, as babies and children, we experienced the following:

- We felt loved, valued, and respected.
- Adults responded to our needs in a reasonably appropriate way.
- Adults gave us the freedom to explore and develop a sense of being separate individuals.

Gender Role Another thing we learn in early childhood is our *gender role*—the activities, abilities, and characteristics our culture deems appropriate for us based on whether we're male or female. In our society, men have traditionally been expected to work and provide for their families; to be aggressive, competitive, and power oriented; and to use thinking and logic to solve problems. Women have been expected to take care of the home and children; to be cooperative, supportive, and nurturing; and to approach life emotionally and intuitively. Although much more egalitarian gender roles are emerging in our society, the stereotypes we absorb in childhood tend to be deeply ingrained.

Attachment Our ways of relating to others may also be rooted in childhood. Although our ways of being with people can be affected by a variety of factors, some researchers, known as attachment theorists, have suggested that our adult styles of loving may be based on the style of **attachment** we established in infancy with our mother, father, siblings, or other primary caregiver. Much work has been done on attachment theory, and as a general overview, people who are *secure* in their intimate relationships probably had a secure, trusting, mutually satisfying attachment to their mother, father, or other parenting figure. As adults, they may find it relatively easy to get close to others. They don't worry about being abandoned or having someone get too close to them. They feel that other people like them and are generally well intentioned.

People who are clinging and dependent in their relationships may have had an *anxious/ambivalent* attachment, in which a parent's inconsistent responses made them unsure that their needs would be met. As adults, they may worry about whether their partners really love them and will stay with them. They tend to feel that others don't want to get as close as they do. They may want to merge completely with another person, which sometimes scares others away.

People who seem to run from relationships may have had an *anxious/avoidant* attachment, in which a parent's inappropriate responses made them want to escape from his or her sphere of influence. As adults, they feel uncomfortable being close to others. They may be distrustful and fearful of becoming dependent. Their partners usually want more intimacy than they do.

Even if people's earliest experiences and relationships were less than ideal, however, they can still establish satisfying relationships in adulthood. In fact, relationships in adolescence and adulthood give us an excellent opportunity to work on and through unresolved issues and conflicts from the past. After all, very few people have perfect parents and perfect siblings, and no one grows up without experiencing some sort of personal pain and conflict.

People can be resilient and flexible. They have the capacity to change their ideas, beliefs, and behaviour patterns. They can learn ways to raise their self-esteem; they can become more trusting, accepting, and appreciative of others; and they can acquire the communication and conflict-resolution skills required for maintaining successful relationships. Although it helps to have a good start in life, it may be even more important to begin again, right from where you are. Most important is to be accepting of and kind to ourselves as we are in the present and to do our best to grow and develop emotionally.

TERMS

attachment The emotional tie between an infant and his or her caregiver or between two people in a close relationship.

Friendship

The first relationships we form outside the family are friendships. The friendships we form in childhood are important in our development; through them we learn about tolerance, sharing, and trust. Friendships usually include most or all of the following characteristics:

- *Companionship.* Friends are usually relaxed and happy in each other's company. They typically have common values and interests and make plans to spend time together. But real friends are also able to be tense and unhappy with each other. Unlike fair-weather friends, we need to be able to support others as we would want support from them, even on bad days.

- *Respect.* Friends have a basic respect for each other's humanity and individuality. Good friends respect each other's feelings and opinions and work to resolve their differences without demeaning or insulting each other. They also show their respect by being honest with each other (see "Being a Good Friend" in the ▦ connect Library).

- *Acceptance.* Friends accept each other, flaws and all. They feel free to be themselves and express their feelings without fear of ridicule or criticism.

- *Help.* Sharing time, energy, and even material goods is important to friendship. Friends know they can rely on each other in times of need.

- *Trust.* Friends are secure in the knowledge that they will not intentionally hurt each other. They feel safe confiding in each other.

- *Loyalty.* Friends can count on each other. They stand up for each other in both word and deed.

- *Mutuality.* Friends retain their individual identities, but close friendships are characterized by a sense of mutuality: "What affects you affects me." Friends share the ups and downs in each other's lives.

- *Reciprocity.* Friendships are reciprocal. There is give-and-take between friends and the feeling that both share joys and burdens more or less equally over time.

Intimate romantic partnerships are like friendships in many ways, but they have additional characteristics. These relationships usually include sexual desire and expression, a greater demand for exclusiveness, and deeper levels of caring. Friendships are usually considered both more stable and longer lasting than intimate partnerships. Friends are often more accepting and less critical than lovers, probably because their expectations are different. Like love relationships, friendships bind society together, providing people with emotional support and buffering them from stress.

As important as friendships are, however, the average North American's social circle is shrinking—to the point that nearly 25% say they have no one they want to confide in. In 2006, sociological researchers released details of a study confirming the issue. According to the study, people have fewer close friends than ever before. Most have only two friends they consider close enough to discuss problems with. (In 1985, the average was three confidants per person.) That being said, in a recent Canadian study of more than 1700 university students, researchers found students to be more satisfied with their social health, including their connections with friends, family members, and romantic partners, than with any other aspect of their health. The value of having close friends and confidants is important for both emotional and physical health. In fact, a Canadian study published in the journal *Canadian Family Physician* found that the lack of a confidant was associated with not having a regular doctor.

Love, Sex, and Intimacy

Love is one of the most basic and profound human emotions. It is a powerful force in all our intimate relationships. Love encompasses opposites: affection and anger, excitement and boredom, stability and change, bonds and freedom. Love does not give us perfect happiness, but it does give our lives meaning.

In many kinds of adult relationships, love is closely intertwined with sexuality. In the past, marriage was considered the only acceptable context for sexual activities, but for many people today, sex is legitimized by love. Many couples, heterosexual and gay or lesbian, live together in committed relationships. We now use personal standards rather than social norms to make decisions about sex. Many people, however, worry about this trend toward personal responsibility and the bypassing of traditional norms and values. They fear that the prevailing attitude about sexuality has resulted in a greater emphasis on sex over love and a permissiveness that has undermined the commitment needed to make a true loving relationship work. This casual attitude toward sex may also make it easier for people to sexualize their dependency needs.

15%–18% of married people will have an affair during their marriage.

—**National Opinion Research Center, 2006**

QUICK STATS

For most people, love, sex, and commitment are closely linked ideals in intimate relationships. Love reflects the positive factors that draw people together and sustain them in a relationship. It includes trust, caring, respect, loyalty, interest in the other, and concern for the other's well-being. Sex brings excitement and passion to the relationship. It intensifies the relationship and adds fascination and pleasure.

Commitment, the determination to continue, reflects the stable factors that help maintain the relationship. Responsibility, reliability, and faithfulness are characteristics of commitment. Although love, sex, and commitment are related, they are not necessarily connected. One can exist without the others. Despite the various faces of love, sex, and commitment, most of us long for a special relationship that contains them all.

Other elements can be identified as features of love, such as euphoria, preoccupation with the loved one, idealization or devaluation of the loved one, and so on, but these tend to be temporary. These characteristics may include **infatuation**, which will fade or deepen into something more substantial. As relationships progress, the central aspects of love and commitment take on more importance.

Men and women tend to have different views of the relationship between love (or intimacy) and sex (or passion). Numerous studies have found that men can separate love from sex rather easily, although many men find that their most erotic sexual experiences occur in the context of a love relationship. Women generally view sex from the point of view of a relationship. Some people believe you can have satisfying sex without love—with friends, acquaintances, or strangers. Although sex with love is an important norm in our culture, it is frequently disregarded in practice, as the high incidence of extra-relational affairs attests.

The Pleasure and Pain of Love   The experience of intense love has confused and tormented lovers throughout history. They live in a tumultuous state of excitement, subject to wildly fluctuating feelings of joy and despair. They lose their appetite, can't sleep, and can think of nothing but the loved one. Is this happiness? Misery? Or both?

The contradictory nature of passionate love can be understood by recognizing that human emotions have two components: physiological arousal and an emotional explanation for the arousal. Love is just one of many emotions accompanied by physiological arousal; numerous unpleasant ones can also generate arousal, such as fear, rejection, frustration, and challenge. Although some experiences, such as attraction and sexual desire, are pleasant, extreme excitement is similar to fear and is unpleasant. For this reason, passionate love may be too intense to enjoy. Over time, the physical intensity and excitement tend to diminish. When this happens, pleasure may actually increase.

The Transformation of Love   All human relationships change over time, and love relationships are no exception. At first, love is likely to be characterized by high levels of passion and rapidly increasing intimacy. After a while, passion decreases as we become habituated to it and to the person. The diminishing of romance or passionate love is often experienced as a crisis in a relationship. If a more lasting love fails to emerge, the relationship will likely break up.

Unlike passion, however, commitment does not necessarily diminish over time. When intensity diminishes, partners often discover a more enduring love. They can now

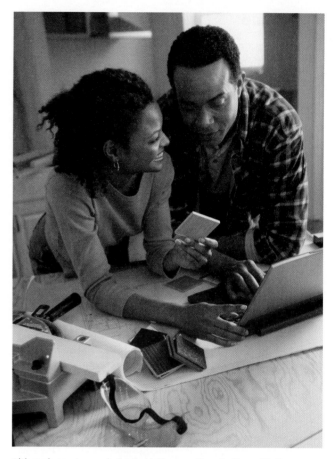

Although passion and physical intimacy often decline with time, other aspects of a relationship—such as commitment—tend to grow as the relationship matures.

move from absorption in each other to a relationship that includes external goals and projects, friends, and family. In this kind of intimate, more secure love, satisfaction comes not just from the relationship itself but also from achieving other creative goals, such as work or child rearing. The key to successful relationships is in transforming passion into an intimate love, based on closeness, caring, and the promise of a shared future.

Challenges in Relationships

Many people believe that love naturally makes an intimate relationship easy to begin and maintain, but in fact, obstacles arise and challenges occur. Even in the best of circumstances, a loving relationship will be tested. Individuals bring to a relationship diverse needs and wants, some of which emerge only at times of change or stress. Common relationship challenges relate to self-disclosure, commitment, expectations, competitiveness, and jealousy.

Is There Hidden Treasure in Our Relationships?   Obviously, we have relationships for fun, companionship, children, and support. But is that all there is to it? Is there hidden meaning to be found in our intimate relationships?

infatuation   An idealizing, obsessive attraction, characterized by a high degree of physical arousal.

Do they repeat issues and conflicts from our past *as well as* offer a way to heal and grow beyond these early-life difficulties? Some experts contend that, as adults, we unconsciously re-create relationships with others that play out the dramas of childhood. In doing so, they say, we attempt to work through and master problems from the past.

At various points in our lives, we may unconsciously play the part of our younger selves—or the part of another person (such as a parent or a sibling)—with the new emotional figure in our lives. We play these roles in the hope of getting emotionally what we didn't get as children or of giving back what we did get.

Quite often, conflicts in our later-life relationships have to do with our feelings and needs. We tend to expect too much, offer too little, or simply feel confused when it comes to our and the other's emotions. Problems in relationships are not always reflective of incompatibility and may sometimes indicate issues that are just very emotionally difficult because of past frustrations or hurt.

The good news is that our problems in relationships are the potential path to our growth as individuals as well as a couple. A man who feels he doesn't receive enough love from his partner (and didn't from his parents) may benefit from cultivating additional platonic relationships rather than hoping for complete satisfaction from one person. A woman who feels the need for more independence in a relationship (which she didn't have growing up) may grow from learning to stay with her discomfort around intimacy and see if she is gradually able to tolerate more closeness without becoming frightened or pulling back.

Ultimately, it seems that the best relationships are those in which we can be both securely connected and then separate and be on our own at times. Developmental psychology suggests that the healthiest infants are able to feel comforted by their mother without being engulfed and can be apart from her without feeling abandoned. Most important seems to be the mother's ability to be empathically attuned to the child to know when to comfort and when to let go.

Relationships in which we can be open, expressive, and understood offer us the greatest chance to grow, develop our potential, and awaken to as much life as possible. Perhaps the larger, hidden meaning of relationships is to help us cultivate the intimacy and freedom that may have been in short supply while we were growing up. We can help ourselves and others to heal and grow by offering and asking for love and compassion. We can free ourselves from the limits imposed on us from the past by challenging ourselves to see where we are afraid to go in our relationships and then going there with our partners.

Honesty and Openness Everyone looks for honesty and openness in an intimate relationship. However, especially at the beginning of a relationship, partners may engage in a certain amount of pretence in an effort to present themselves in the best possible manner. Although obvious when considering what is important in a relationship, for people in the excitement of a new relationship, it may be easy to forget that it is usually best to be yourself from the start to give both you and your potential partner a chance to find out if you are comfortable with each other's beliefs, interests, and lifestyles.

Getting close to another person by sharing thoughts and feelings may feel emotionally risky, but it is necessary for a relationship to deepen. In general, it is a good idea to take your time, and self-disclose at a slow but steady rate—one that doesn't make you feel too vulnerable or your partner too uncomfortable. Over time, you and your partner will learn more about each other and feel more comfortable sharing. In fact, intimate familiarity with your partner's life is a key characteristic of successful long-term relationships.

Unequal or Premature Commitment Sometimes one person in an intimate partnership becomes more serious about the relationship than the other partner. In this situation, it can be very difficult to maintain a friendship without hurting the other person. Sometimes a couple makes a premature commitment, and then one of the partners has second thoughts and wants to break off the relationship. Sometimes both partners begin to realize that something is wrong, but each is afraid to tell the other. Most such problems can be dealt with only by honest and sensitive communication.

Unrealistic Expectations Each partner brings hopes and expectations to a relationship, some of which may be unrealistic, unfair, and, ultimately, very damaging to the relationship (see the box "Are You Emotionally Intelligent?" on p. 314). For example, if you believe that love will eliminate all your problems, you may start to blame your partner for anything that goes wrong in your life. Other unrealistic expectations include the following:

- *Expecting your partner to change.* There are probably some things about your partner that you like more than other things. It's OK to discuss them with your partner; however, it's unfair to demand that your partner change to meet all of your expectations. Accept the differences between your ideal and reality.

- *Assuming that your partner has all the same opinions, priorities, interests, and goals as you.* Don't assume that you think the same about everything—or that you must if the relationship is to succeed. Agreement on key issues is important, but differences can enhance a relationship as long as partners understand and respect each other's points of view.

Are You Emotionally Intelligent?

Emotional intelligence (also known as E.Q. or E.I.Q.) can be defined as the degree to which we can skilfully and adaptively deal with our emotions and those of others.

More specifically, this involves the following:

1. Recognizing feelings as they occur

2. Responding to feelings with neither impulsive, aggressive reactivity, nor suppression, denial, distraction, or avoidance

3. Being able to tolerate and contain strong emotions and soothe yourself in the presence of powerful feelings

4. Being able to use the energy of strong emotions to motivate yourself and respond skilfully to the situation at hand

5. Being able to perceive the content of feelings to connect the emotion to its source and understand why you are feeling a particular emotion

6. Being able to recognize and bear the feelings of others without needing to distance yourself or dissuade the other person from having their feelings

7. Being able to persist in the face of fear or frustration and cultivate resilience

8. Being able to delay gratification

9. Being able to be curious and stay open to feelings rather than close down, tighten up, or turn away from emotions

10. Being able to express a wide range of emotions in a way that is natural and to a degree that is appropriate to the particular situation

How do you cultivate emotional intelligence? The key lies in the ability to develop the overarching skill of *mindfulness*—the ability to dispassionately observe thoughts and feelings as they occur and while they're occurring. This skill is aided by cultivating a *witness* or a *watcher* in your mind and noting the arising of strong reactions with a certain detachment. By holding our reactions in a larger mental space we can make more measured, wise, and skilful responses to the situation at hand.

Mindfulness can be cultivated by simply paying more attention to the operation of our minds, slowing down our lives enough to make more detailed observations, and staying in the moment so as to maximize awareness of ourselves and others. Although we often have a limited ability to control external events, it turns out that we have a great deal of ability to discipline, focus, and train our minds. With practice, we not only can become more emotionally intelligent but also may be able to cultivate an ongoing peace of mind that many people find so elusive.

- *Believing that a relationship will fulfil all of your personal, financial, intellectual, and social needs.* Expecting a relationship to fulfil all your needs places too much pressure on your partner and on your relationship, and it will inevitably lead to disappointment. For your own well-being, it's important to maintain some degree of autonomy and self-sufficiency.

Competitiveness   Games and competitive sports add flavour to the bonding process—as long as the focus is on fun. If one partner always feels the strong need to compete and win, it can detract from the sense of connectedness, interdependence, equality, and mutuality between partners. The same can be said for a perfectionistic need to be right in every instance—to win every argument.

If competitiveness is a problem for you, ask yourself if your need to win is more important than your partner's feelings or the future of your relationship. Try noncompetitive activities or an activity where you are a beginner and your partner excels. Accept that your partner's views may be just as valid and important to your partner as your own views are to you.

Balancing Time Spent Together and Apart   You may enjoy time together with your partner, but you may also want to spend time alone or with other friends. If you or your partner interprets time apart as rejection or lack of commitment, it can damage a relationship. Talk with your partner about what time apart means and share your feelings about what you expect from the relationship in terms of time together. Consider your partner's feelings carefully, and try to reach a compromise that satisfies both of you.

Differences in expectations about time spent together can mirror differences in ideas about emotional closeness. Any romantic relationship involves giving up some degree of autonomy in order to develop an identity as a couple. But remember that every person is unique and has different needs for distance and closeness in a relationship.

Jealousy   Jealousy is the angry, painful response to a partner's real, imagined, or likely involvement with a third person. Some people think that the existence of jealousy proves the existence of love, but jealousy is actually a sign of insecurity or possessiveness.

Strategies for Enhancing Support in Relationships

• *Be aware of the importance of support.* Time and energy spent on support will help both you and your partner deal with stress and create a positive atmosphere that will help when differences or conflicts do occur.

• *Learn to ask for help from your partner.* Try different ways of asking for help and support from your partner and make note of which approaches work best for your relationship.

• *Help your partner the way she or he would like to be helped.* Some people prefer empathy and emotional support, whereas others like more practical help with problems.

• *Avoid negativity, especially when being asked for help.* Asking for help puts a person in a vulnerable position. If your partner asks for your aid, be gracious and supportive; don't use phrases like "I told you so" or "You should have just. . . ." Otherwise, your partner may learn not to ask for your help or support at all.

• *Make positive attributions.* If you're unsure about the reasons for your partner's behaviour, give her or him the benefit of the doubt. For example, if your partner arrives for a date 30 minutes late and in a bad mood, assume it's because she or he had a bad day rather than attributing it to a character flaw or relationship problem. Offer appropriate support.

• *Help yourself.* Develop coping strategies for times your partner won't be available. These might include things you can do for yourself, such as going for a walk, or other people you can turn to for support.

• *Keep relationship problems separate.* Avoid bringing up relationship problems when you are offering or asking for help.

• *Avoid giving advice.* Immediately offering advice when asked for help implies that you are smarter or more capable than your partner at solving your partner's difficulty. Begin by providing emotional support and validating your partner's feelings. Then, if asked, help brainstorm solutions.

Source: Plante, T., and K. Sullivan. 2000. *Getting Together and Staying Together: The Stanford Course on Intimate Relationships.* Bloomington, Ind.: 1st Books Library. Reprinted with permission of the author.

In its irrational and extreme forms, jealousy can destroy a relationship by its insistent demands and attempts at control. Jealousy is a factor in precipitating violence in dating relationships among both high school and university students, and abusive spouses often use jealousy to justify their violence. (Problems with control and violence in relationships are discussed in Chapter 20.)

People with a healthy level of self-esteem are less likely to feel jealous. When jealousy occurs in a relationship, it's important for the partners to communicate clearly with each other about their feelings.

Supportiveness   Another key to successful relationships is the ability to ask for and give support. Partners need to know that they can count on each other during difficult times. If you are having trouble getting or giving the support that you or your partner needs, try some of the suggestions in the box "Strategies for Enhancing Support in Relationships" above.

Unhealthy Relationships

Everyone should be able to recognize when a relationship is unhealthy. Relatively extreme examples of unhealthy relationships are those that involve codependency or that are physically or emotionally abusive; strategies for addressing these problems are presented in Chapters 14 and 20, respectively.

Even relationships that are not abusive or codependent can still be unhealthy. If your relationship lacks love and respect and places little value on the time you and your partner or friend have spent together, it may be time to

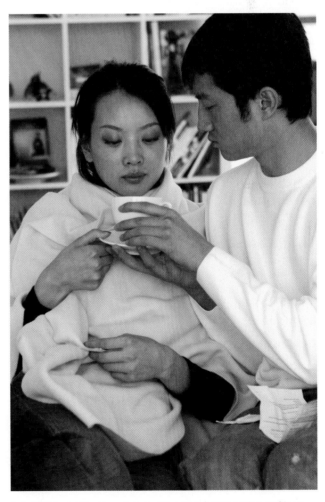

Supportiveness is a sign of commitment and compassion and is an important part of any healthy relationship.

get professional help or to end the partnership (partnerships can refer to both romantic relationships and platonic friendships). Further, if your relationship is characterized by communication styles that include criticism, contempt, defensiveness, and withdrawal—despite real efforts to repair these destructive patterns—the relationship may not be salvageable. Consider these questions:

- Do you and your partner have more negative than positive experiences and interactions?
- Are there old hurts that you or your partner cannot forgive?
- Do you feel disrespected or unloved?
- Do you find it hard to feel positive feelings of affection for your partner?
- Does it feel as if your relationship has been a waste of time?

Spiritual leaders suggest that relationships are unhealthy when you feel that your sense of spontaneity, your potential for inner growth and joy, and your connection to your spiritual life is deadened. Being in an unhappy relationship has negative physical and mental consequences of; although breaking up is painful and difficult, it is ultimately better than living in a toxic relationship.

Ending a Relationship

Even when a couple starts out with the best of intentions, an intimate relationship may not last. Some breakups occur quickly following direct action by one or both partners, but many others occur over an extended period as the couple goes through a cycle of separating and reconciling.

QUICK STATS

As much as **65%** of communication is nonverbal.

—**Ray Birdwhistell, Anthropologist, 1970**

Ending an intimate relationship is usually difficult and painful. Both partners may feel attacked and abandoned, but feelings of distress are likely to be more acute for the rejected partner. If you are involved in a breakup, the following suggestions may help make the ending easier:

- *Give the relationship a fair chance before breaking up.* If it's still not working, you'll know you did everything you could.
- *Be fair and honest.* If you're initiating the breakup, don't try to make your partner feel responsible.
- *Be tactful and compassionate.* You can leave the relationship without deliberately damaging your partner's self-esteem. Emphasize your mutual incompatibility, and admit your own contributions to the problem.
- *If you are the rejected person, give yourself time to resolve your anger and pain.* Mobilize your coping resources,

QUESTIONS FOR CRITICAL THINKING AND REFLECTION

Have you ever ended an intimate relationship? If so, how did you handle it? How did you feel after the breakup? How did the breakup affect your former partner? Did the experience help you in other relationships? If so, in what way did it help?

including social support and other stress-management techniques. You may go through a process of mourning the relationship, experiencing disbelief, anger, sadness, and finally acceptance. Remember that there are actually many people with whom you can potentially have an intimate relationship.

- *Recognize the value in the experience.* You honour the feelings that you shared with your partner by validating the relationship as a worthwhile experience. Ending a close relationship can teach you valuable lessons about your needs, preferences, strengths, and weaknesses. Use your insights to increase your chance of success in your next relationship.

Use the recovery period following a breakup for self-renewal. Redirect more of your attention to yourself, and reconnect with people and areas of your life that may have been neglected as a result of the relationship. Time will help heal the pain of the loss of the relationship.

COMMUNICATION

The key to developing and maintaining any type of intimate relationship is good communication. Most of the time, we don't actually think about communicating; we simply talk and behave naturally. But when problems arise—when we feel others don't understand us or when someone accuses us of not listening—we become aware of our limitations or, more commonly, what we think are other people's limitations. Miscommunication creates frustration and distances us from our friends and partners.

Nonverbal Communication

Even when we're silent, we're communicating. We send messages when we look at someone or look away, lean forward or sit back, smile or frown. Especially important forms of nonverbal communication are touch, eye contact, and proximity. If someone we're talking to touches our hand or arm, looks into our eyes, and leans toward us when we talk, we get the message that the person is interested in us and cares about what we're saying. If a person keeps looking around the room while we're talking or takes a step backward, we get the impression the person is uninterested or wants to end the conversation.

The ability to interpret nonverbal messages correctly is important to the success of relationships. It's also important, when sending messages, to make sure our body language agrees with our words. When our verbal and nonverbal messages don't correspond, we send a mixed message.

Communication Skills

Three keys to good communication in relationships are self-disclosure, listening, and feedback.

• *Self-disclosure* involves revealing personal information that we ordinarily wouldn't reveal because of the risk involved. It usually increases feelings of closeness and moves the relationship to a deeper level of intimacy. Friends often disclose the most to each other, sharing feelings, experiences, hopes, and disappointments; married couples sometimes share less because they think they already know everything there is to know about each other.

• *Listening*, the second key of good communication, is a rare skill. Good listening skills require that we spend more time and energy trying to fully understand another person's story and less time judging, evaluating, blaming, advising, analyzing, or trying to control. Empathy, warmth, respect, and genuineness are qualities of skilful listeners. Attentive listening encourages friends or partners to share more and, in turn, to be attentive listeners. To connect with other people and develop real emotional intimacy, listening is essential.

• *Feedback*, a constructive response to another's self-disclosure, is the third key to good communication. Giving positive feedback means acknowledging that the friend's or partner's feelings are valid—no matter how upsetting or troubling—and offering self-disclosure in response. If, for example, your partner discloses unhappiness about your relationship, it is more constructive to say that you're concerned or saddened by that and want to hear more about it than to get angry, to blame, to try to inflict pain, or to withdraw. Self-disclosure and feedback can open the door to change, whereas other responses block communication and change. (For tips on improving your skills, see the box "Guidelines for Effective Communication" on p. 318.)

Gender and Communication

Some of the difficulties people encounter in relationships can be traced to common gender differences in communication. Many authorities believe that, because of the way they've been raised, men and women generally approach conversation and communication differently. According to this view, men may be more inclined to use conversation in a *competitive* way, perhaps hoping to establish dominance in relationships. When male conversations are over, men may find themselves in a one-up or a one-down position. Women may be more inclined to use conversation in a more *affiliative* way, perhaps hoping to establish friendships. They negotiate various degrees of closeness,

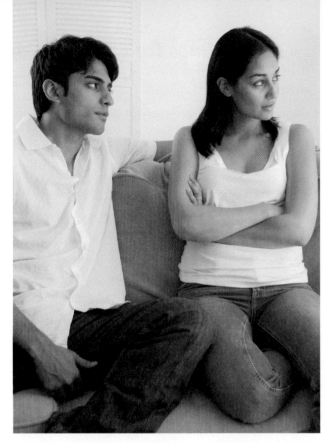

Conflict is an inevitable part of any intimate relationship. Couples need to develop constructive ways of resolving conflicts in order to maintain a healthy relationship.

seeking to give and receive support. Men may talk more—though without disclosing more—and listen less. Women may be more inclined to use good listening skills, such as eye contact, frequent nodding, focused attention, and asking relevant questions.

Although these are generalized patterns, they can translate into problems in specific conversations. Even when a man and a woman are talking about the same subject, their unconscious goals may be very different. The woman may be looking for understanding and closeness, while the man may be trying to demonstrate his competence by giving advice and solving problems. Both styles are valid; the problem comes when differences in style result in poor communication and misunderstanding. See the box "Gender and Communication" on p. 319 for more information.

Sometimes communication is not the problem in a relationship—the partners understand each other all too well. The problem is that they're unable or unwilling to change or compromise. Although good communication can't salvage a bad relationship, it does enable couples to see their differences and make more informed decisions.

Conflict and Conflict Resolution

Conflict is natural in intimate relationships. No matter how close two people become, they still remain separate individuals with their own needs, desires, past experiences,

Guidelines for Effective Communication

TAKE CHARGE

Getting Started

• When you want to have a serious discussion with your partner, find an appropriate time and place. Choose a block of time when you will not be interrupted or rushed and a place that is private.

• Face your partner and maintain eye contact. Use nonverbal feedback to show that you are interested and involved in the communication process.

Being an Effective Speaker

• State your concern or issue as clearly as you can.

• Use "I" statements—statements about how *you* feel—rather than statements beginning with "You," which tell another person how you think he or she feels. When you use "I" statements, you are taking responsibility for your feelings. "You" statements are often blaming or accusatory and will probably get a defensive or resentful response. The statement "I feel unloved," for example, sends a clearer, less blaming message than the statement "You don't love me."

• Focus on a specific behaviour rather than on the whole person. Be specific about the behaviour you like or don't like. Avoid generalizations beginning with "You always" or "You never." Such statements make people feel defensive.

• Make constructive requests. Opening your request with "I would like" keeps the focus on your needs rather than your partner's supposed deficiencies.

• Avoid blaming, accusing, and belittling. Even if you are right, you have little to gain by putting your partner down. Studies have shown that when people feel criticized or attacked, they are less able to think rationally or solve problems constructively.

• Ask for action ahead of time, not after the fact. Tell your partner what you would like to have happen in the future; don't wait for him or her to blow it and then express anger or disappointment.

Being an Effective Listener

• Provide appropriate nonverbal feedback (nodding, smiling, making eye contact, and so on).

• Don't interrupt.

• Develop the skill of reflective listening. Don't judge, evaluate, analyze, or offer solutions (unless asked to do so). Your partner may just need to have you there to sort out some feelings. By jumping in right away to fix the problem, you may actually be cutting off communication.

• Don't give unsolicited advice. Giving advice implies that you know more about what a person needs to do than he or she does; therefore, it often evokes anger or resentment.

• Clarify your understanding of what your partner is saying by restating it in your own words and asking if your understanding is correct. "I think you're saying that you would feel uncomfortable having dinner with my parents and that you'd prefer to meet them in a more casual setting. Is that right?" This type of specific feedback prevents misunderstandings and helps validate the speaker's feelings and message.

• Be sure you are really listening, not off somewhere in your mind rehearsing your reply. Try to tune in to your partner's feelings as well as the words.

• Let your partner know that you value what he or she is saying and want to understand. Respect for the other person is the cornerstone of effective communication.

---

and ways of seeing the world. In fact, the closer the relationship, the more differences and the more opportunities for conflict there will be.

Conflict itself isn't dangerous to a relationship; in fact, it may indicate that the relationship is growing. But if it isn't handled in a constructive way, conflict can damage—and ultimately destroy—the relationship. Consider the following guidelines, but remember that different couples communicate in different ways around conflict.

Conflict is often accompanied by anger—a natural emotion, but one that can be difficult to handle. If we express anger aggressively, we run the risk of creating distrust, fear, and distance; if we act it out without thinking things through, we can cause the conflict to escalate; if we suppress anger, it turns into resentment and hostility. The best way to handle anger in a relationship is to recognize it as a symptom of something that requires attention and needs to be changed. When angry, partners should exercise restraint so as not to become abusive. It is important to express anger skilfully and not in a way that is out of proportion to the issue at hand.

The sources of conflict for couples change over time but primarily revolve around the basic tasks of living together: dividing the housework, handling money, spending time together, and so on. Sexual interaction is also a source of disagreement for many couples.

Although there are numerous theories on and approaches to conflict resolution, the following strategies can be helpful when negotiating with a partner:

1. *Clarify the issue.* Take responsibility for thinking through your feelings and discovering what's really bothering you. Agree that one partner will speak first and have the chance to speak fully while the other listens. Then reverse the roles. Try to understand your partner's position fully by repeating what you've heard and asking questions to clarify or elicit more information. Agree to talk only about the topic at hand and not get distracted by other issues. Sum up what your partner has said.

318   PART IV   UNDERSTANDING SEXUALITY

Gender and Communication

From an early age, parents, teachers, and society send different messages to girls and boys regarding emotion; that is, researchers have found that males and females are socialized to communicate in different ways. Boys tend to learn to suppress and bury their feelings, especially fear and other emotions that make them feel vulnerable. Girls are generally encouraged to express and talk about their feelings.

These differences are further reinforced by peer groups. Gender segregation is already apparent in preschool and increases throughout middle childhood for most children. Boys and girls spend most of their time with peers of the same gender, and their communication styles are very different. For example, when conflict arises, girls tend to care more about preserving their relationships, and boys care more about maintaining the game they were playing.

Research also shows that men have a more intense physiological response to certain emotions. In discussions around conflict, a man's blood pressure and heart rate rise higher and remain elevated longer. Part of the reason may be that a man's internal dialogue repeats upsetting thoughts (for example, "How could she say that? I can't take this!"). When anyone is physiologically or emotionally overwhelmed ("flooded"), productive communication is impossible.

A common pattern that can arise between men and women is called "confront-withdraw." A woman often approaches her male partner because she is upset and wants to talk about it. The man tries to calm her down, provides solutions he sees as rational, and withdraws. This response may make his partner even more upset and demanding, which causes the man to further shut down. Given what we know about gender differences, we might understand the man's response as one of self-protection, because he is entering territory that is both unknown and physically unpleasant.

To enjoy intimacy, men and women must work to better understand each other and develop a more compatible communication style. Insufficient research exists currently to identify typical patterns in same-sex relationships. It may be advisable for sex-same partners to see which (if either) common pattern is more relevant for themselves and their partner.

Advice for Men

• When your partner raises an emotional topic, be aware of uncomfortable feelings and the desire to retreat.

• Do not run away (physically or emotionally)! Telling her to "calm down" will likely create the opposite response.

• Find a way to stay connected. This is the only way to deescalate the conflict.

• Empathize: Listen to what she is saying, and even if you disagree, communicate to her that you understand how she is feeling and where she is coming from. Often when a person feels genuinely heard, that is enough.

• Try not to think of her comments as personal attacks; instead, continue to empathize.

• You may need to calm yourself. Try taking long deep breaths, telling yourself that your partner needs to air her feelings, and remembering that she, too, wants the conflict to end.

• In some cases, a 20-minute break—during which you soothe yourself rather than think upsetting thoughts—can be helpful.

Advice for Women

• Try to be calm when approaching conflict; practise similar relaxation techniques to those described in "Advice for Men."

• Try to speak in ways that will not provoke defensiveness; complain rather than criticize, be specific, and use "I" statements.

• Try not to be critical of your partner's responses or his attempts to communicate.

• Be aware if he is withdrawing, and, if appropriate, help him to relax by using methods you have discussed previously.

Source: Gottman, J. 1994. *Why Marriages Succeed or Fail … and How You Can Make Yours Last.* New York: Simon & Schuster.

2. *Find out what each person wants.* Ask your partner to express his or her desires. Don't assume you know what your partner wants and don't speak for him or her.

3. *Determine how you both can get what you want.* Brainstorm to generate a variety of options.

4. *Decide how to negotiate.* Work out a plan for change; for example, one partner will do one task and the other will do another task, or one partner will do a

task in exchange for something he or she wants. Be willing to compromise, and avoid trying to win.

5. *Solidify the agreements.* Go over the plan verbally and write it down, if necessary, to ensure that you both understand and agree to it.

6. *Review and renegotiate.* Decide on a time frame for trying out your plan, and set a time to discuss how it's working. Make adjustments as needed.

To resolve conflicts, partners have to feel safe in voicing disagreements. They have to trust that the discussion won't get out of control, that they won't be abandoned by the other, and that the partner won't take advantage of their vulnerability. Partners should follow some basic ground rules when they argue, such as avoiding ultimatums, resisting the urge to give the silent treatment, refusing to "hit below the belt," and not using sex to smooth over disagreements.

When you argue, maintain a spirit of goodwill and avoid being harshly critical or contemptuous. Remember—you care about your partner and want things to work out. See the disagreement as a difficulty that the two of you have together rather than as something your partner does to you. Finish serious discussions on a positive note by expressing your respect and affection for your partner and your appreciation for having been listened to. If you and your partner find that you argue repeatedly over the same issue, it may be better to stop trying to resolve that problem and instead come to accept the differences between you.

PAIRING AND SINGLEHOOD

Although most people eventually marry or commit to a partner, everyone spends some time as a single person, and nearly all make some attempt, consciously or unconsciously, to find a partner. Intimate relationships are as important for singles as for couples.

Choosing a Partner

Most men and women select partners for long-term relationships through a fairly predictable process, although they may not be consciously aware of it. First attraction is based on easily observable characteristics: looks, dress, social status, and reciprocated interest. Most people pair with someone who lives in the same geographic area, is from a similar ethnic and socioeconomic background, has similar educational attainment, lives a similar lifestyle, and is like them in terms of physical attraction.

Once the euphoria of romantic love winds down, personality traits and behaviours become more significant factors in how the partners view each other. The emphasis shifts to basic values and future aspirations regarding career, family, and children. At some point, they decide whether the relationship feels viable and is worthy of their continued commitment.

Perhaps the most important question for potential mates to ask is, "How much do we have in common?" Although differences add interest to a relationship, similarities increase the chances of a relationship's success. Areas in which differences can affect a relationship include values, religion, ethnicity, attitudes toward sexuality and gender roles, socioeconomic status, familiarity with each other's culture, and interactions with the extended family (see the box "Interfaith and Intrafaith Partnerships"). Acceptance and communication skills go a long way toward making a relationship work, no matter how different the partners.

QUESTIONS FOR CRITICAL THINKING AND REFLECTION
How do you handle conflict in your relationships? Do you fight intensely and then make up? Discuss, negotiate, and compromise? Avoid conflict altogether? Whatever your pattern of conflict resolution (or avoidance), where do you think you learned it? How effective is it for you? If it isn't working well, what ideas do you have for improvement?

Dating

Every culture has certain rituals for pairing and finding mates. Parent-arranged marriages, still the norm in many cultures, are often very stable and permanent. Although the Canadian cultural norm is personal choice in courtship and mate selection, the popularity of dating services and online matchmaking suggests that many people want help finding a suitable partner (see the box "Online Relationships" on p. 322).

Most Canadians find romantic partners through some form of dating. They narrow the field through a process of getting to know each other. Dating often revolves around a mutually enjoyable activity, such as seeing a movie or having dinner. Traditionally, in the male-female dating pattern, the man took the lead, initiating the date, while the woman waited to be called. In this pattern, casual dating might evolve into steady or exclusive dating, then engagement, and finally marriage.

For many young people today, traditional dating has given way to a more casual form of getting together in groups. Greater equality between the sexes is at the root of this change. People go out in groups, rather than strictly

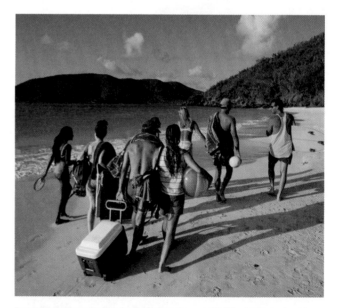

For many university students today, group activities have replaced dating as a way to meet and get to know potential partners.

Interfaith and Intrafaith Partnerships

Culture can be a determinant of partnership choices, but this is not always the case. Interfaith marriage is becoming more common among Canadians; in 2001, 19% of couples were in an interfaith marriage, up from 15% in 1981. There are many types of interfaith partnerships, including partners from (1) two completely different religions, (2) two religions with similar roots, (3) two divisions of the same religion, or (4) two denominations from the same religious division. The latter two are often called intrafaith partnerships.

Marrying someone of a different faith can broaden the partners' worldview and enrich their lives; however, it can also be a potential stressor and a challenge to a relationship.

The impact of being an interfaith couple depends on how religious the partners are. There is no specifically correct way to address religious diversity in a partnership, but the following are some potential approaches.

Withdrawal: In some couples, both partners withdraw from their respective religions. Religious differences may be minimized, but the withdrawal may not last. If a partner was observant before the relationship, it is likely that she or he will want to become actively involved again. This often occurs with a significant life event, such as the birth of a child or death of a parent.

Conversion: In many intrafaith couples, one partner converts to the religion of the other. Religious differences are decreased, but problems can occur if the partner who converts develops resentment, has difficulties with her or his family of origin, misses the old religion, or experiences feelings of guilt or betrayal.

Compromise: Some couples convert together to a new religion, possibly to a religion or denomination at a midpoint between their two religions. The couple may find a happy medium that is satisfying to both. However, both may experience the problems associated with conversion.

Multifaith: Some couples join both religions—formally or informally. They may alternate places of worship weekly or make other creative arrangements. The advantage of this pattern is that both partners maintain their religions and learn more about each other. Problems may arise if the religions have conflicting values or practices.

Ecumenical: In some relationships, partners merge their religions. They may combine the best of each or observe only the areas in which the religions intersect. They may get the best of both worlds or discover that their religions have more in common than they thought. In some cases, however, the original religious institutions may condemn compromise.

Diversity: In some couples, each partner chooses to follow his or her own religion. If both partners are very religious, they do not then have to give up an important part of their lives. However, some partners consider this approach undesirable because it means more time spent apart.

Do nothing: Some couples find no need to address religious differences because neither partner is observant or committed to a religion to an extent that it is a relationship challenge. They address specific issues if and when they arise.

Couples often handle their religious differences without a problem until they marry or have children. Planning an interfaith wedding can be fraught with unique stressors, such as differing rituals and the expectations of guests from different faiths. When children arrive, decisions may need to be made about many issues, such as baptism, circumcision, and religious upbringing.

To maintain a successful partnership, couples should communicate about religious issues before getting married and having children. Discuss the importance of your religions and religious needs. Consider ways that you can honour each other's religious traditions. Learn to discuss issues relating to religion and spirituality in ways that bring you closer together.

Sources: Statistics Canada. 2006. Study: Interreligious unions. *The Daily*, October 3 (http://www.statcan.gc.ca/daily-quotidien/061003/dq061003b-eng.htm; retrieved April 17, 2011); Robinson, B. A. 2007. *Inter-Faith Marriages* (http://www.religioustolerance.org/ifm_menu.htm; retrieved January 24, 2009); Robinson, B. A. 1999. *How Inter-Faith and Intra-Faith Couples Handle Religious Differences* (http://www.religioustolerance.org/ifm_diff.htm; retrieved January 24, 2009).

as couples, and each person pays his or her way. A man and woman may begin to spend more time together but often in the group context. If sexual involvement develops, it is more likely to be based on friendship, respect, and common interests than on expectations related to gender roles. In this model, mate selection may progress from getting together to living together to marriage.

Living Together

About 70% of adults Canadians are in opposite-sex marriages and 16% are in common law relationships. Nearly 76,000 Canadians are in same-sex common law partnerships, and approximately 15,000 are in same-sex marriages (representing 0.1% of all married couples in Canada).

Online Relationships

Worldwide, tens of millions of people use the World Wide Web to network and to find friends and partners. Social networking Web sites, such as Facebook, MySpace, and Friendster, offer places for profiles, photos, blogs, music, videos, and email to vast numbers of people, mostly teens and young adults, seeking to connect online.

Online dating sites and forums, such as Match.com or Lavalife, are also popular, especially among those recently out of university who are seeking an intimate partner or an expanded circle of friends. In fact, nearly 1.2 million Canadians have visited an online dating service.

Connecting with people online has its advantages and its drawbacks. It allows people to communicate in a relaxed way, to try out different personas, and to share things they might not share with family or friends face to face. Many find that it offers a sense of privacy, safety, and comfort. It is easy to put yourself out there without too much investment—you can get to know someone from the comfort of your own home, set your own pace, and start and end the relationships at any time. With millions of singles using dating forums that allow them to outline exactly what they are seeking, the Internet can increase a person's chance of finding a good match.

Meeting people online has drawbacks, however. People often misrepresent themselves, pretending to be very different— older or younger or even of a different sex—than they really are. Investing time and emotional resources in such relationships can be painful. In some instances, online romances have become dangerous or even deadly (see Chapter 20 for information on cyberstalking).

Because people have greater freedom to reveal only what they want to, users should also be aware of a greater tendency to idealize online partners—setting themselves up for later disappointment. If you find that your online friend seems perfect, consider that a warning sign. Looking for partners online can become like shopping: The choices available may increase your tendency to search for perfection or find fault quickly, thereby keeping you from giving people a chance. Remember what is most important to you and keep your expectations realistic.

When looking for friends and partners online, you are also missing important and powerful sources of information: chemistry and in-person intuition. Much of our communication is transmitted through body language and tone, which are not available online and cannot be fully captured even by Web cams. Trust your feelings regarding the process of the relationship. Are you revealing more than the other person? Is

there a balance in the amount of time spent talking by each of you? Is the other person respecting your boundaries? Just as in real-life dating, online relationships require you to use common sense and to trust your instincts.

If you decide to pursue an online relationship, here are some strategies that can help you have a positive experience and stay safe:

- To improve your chances of meeting people interested in you as a person, avoid sexually oriented Web sites.

- Know what you are looking for as well as what you have to offer someone else. If you are looking for a relationship, make that fact clear. About 80% of Canadian users of online dating services are single. Find out the other person's situation and intentions.

- Many Web sites let users upload photos. Know, however, that your photo can be downloaded by anyone, distributed to other individuals or sites, and even altered. Don't post photos unless you are completely comfortable with the potential consequences.

- Don't give out personal information, including your real full name, school, or place of employment, until you feel sure that you are giving the information to someone who is trustworthy. Do not give anyone your address or phone number over the Internet.

- Consider setting up a second email account for sending and receiving dating-related emails.

- If someone does not respond to a message, try not to take it personally. There are many reasons why a person may not pursue the connection. Do not send multiple messages to an unresponsive person; doing so could lead to an accusation of stalking. If someone stops responding to your messages, drop the interaction completely.

- Before deciding whether to meet an online friend in person, arrange to talk over the phone a few times.

- Don't agree to meet someone face to face unless you feel completely comfortable about it. Always meet initially in a very public place: a museum, a coffee shop, or a restaurant, not in private, and especially not at your home. Bring along a friend to further increase your safety, let a friend know where you will be, or plan to have a friend call you during the date.

If you pursue online relationships, don't let them interfere with your other interpersonal relationships and social activities. Online dating can have an addictive element that can become unhealthy. To maximize your emotional and interpersonal wellness, use the Internet to widen your circle of friends, not shrink it.

The decision to live together in a **common law** or **cohabitating relationship** is one of the most rapid and dramatic social changes that has ever occurred in our society (Figure 10.1). It seems to be gaining acceptance as part of the normal mate-selection process. By age 30, about half of all men and women will have cohabited. Several factors are involved in this change, including greater acceptance of premarital sex, increased availability of contraceptives, the tendency for people to wait longer before getting married, and a larger pool of single and divorced individuals.

Cohabitation is more popular among younger people than older, although a significant number of older couples live together without marrying as well. Living together provides many of the benefits of marriage: companionship; a setting for an enjoyable and meaningful relationship; the opportunity to develop greater intimacy through learning, compromising, and sharing; a satisfying sex life; and a way to save on living costs.

Living together has certain advantages over marriage. For one thing, it can give the partners a greater sense of

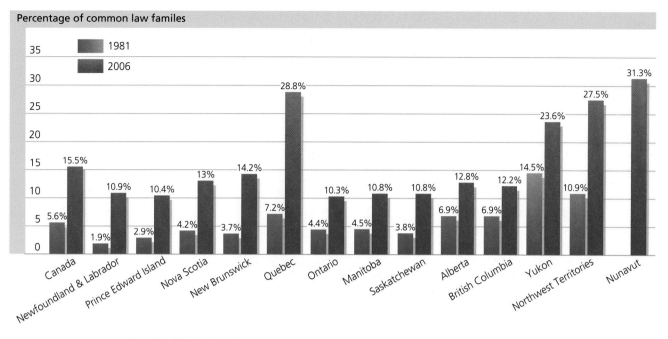

FIGURE 10.1 Common law families in Canada.

Note: For 1981, the Northwest Territories includes Nunavut. In 2006, same-sex couples are included.

Source: Human Resources and Skills Development Canada. 2011. *Canadians in Context—Households and Families* (http://www4.hrsdc.gc.ca/.3ndic.1t.4r@-eng.jsp?iid=37; retrieved April 17, 2011).

autonomy. Not bound by the social rules and expectations that are part of the institution of marriage, partners may find it easier to keep their identity and more of their independence. Cohabitation doesn't incur the same obligations as marriage. If things don't work out, the partners may find it easier to leave a relationship that hasn't been legally sanctioned.

But living together has some liabilities, too. In some cases, the legal protections of marriage are absent, such as health benefits and property and inheritance rights. These considerations can be particularly serious if the couple has children, from either former relationships or the current one. Couples may feel social or family pressure to marry or otherwise change their living arrangements, especially if they have young children. The general trend, however, is toward legitimizing nonmarital partnerships; for example, employers, communities, and provinces and territories now typically extend benefits to unmarried domestic partners.

Although many people choose cohabitation as a kind of trial marriage, unmarried partnerships tend to be less stable than marriages. In a survey of women ages 15–44 who had cohabited, fewer than half were still living—married (37%) or unmarried (10%)—with their first live-in partner, 34% had dissolved the relationship before marriage, and 21% had married and then divorced their partner. There is little evidence that cohabitation before marriage leads to happier or longer-lasting marriages; in fact, some studies have found slightly less marital satisfaction and slightly higher divorce rates among couples who had previously cohabited.

Same-Sex Partnerships

Regardless of **sexual orientation**, most people look for love in a close, satisfying, committed relationship. A person whose sexual orientation is **lesbian**, **gay**, or bisexual (LGB) may be involved in a same-sex relationship. Same-sex couples have many similarities with **heterosexual** couples (those who seek members of the other sex). According to one study, most gay men and lesbians have experienced at least one long-term relationship with a

common law or cohabiting relationship Living together in a sexual relationship without being married.

sexual orientation A consistent pattern of emotional and sexual attraction based on biological sex; it exists along a continuum that ranges from being exclusively heterosexual (attracted to people of the other sex) through being bisexual (attracted to people of both sexes) to being exclusively gay or lesbian (attracted to people of your own sex).

gay or lesbian Emotional and sexual attraction to people of your own sex.

heterosexual Emotional and sexual attraction to people of the other sex.

TERMS

Same-Sex Marriage and Civil Unions

Marriage is often viewed primarily as a social or religious institution, but it is in fact an institution defined by governmental statutes that confer legal and economic rights and responsibilities. Many laws include a distinction based on marriage. Marital status affects tax status, inheritance, medical decision making, and many other aspects of life.

The push for legal recognition of same-sex partnerships began decades ago, but it was brought to the forefront of public debate beginning in the 1990s. Supporters of same-sex marriage rights, however, met with stiff opposition at provincial, territorial, and federal levels.

In 2000, the Canadian Parliament enacted the Modernization of Benefits and Obligations Act, which extended benefits and obligations to common law couples, whether of opposite sexes or the same sex. Furthermore, the definition of "spouse" was changed to include any two persons who have lived together in a "marriage-like" relationship for at least two years. In 2001, the Netherlands became the first country to legalize same-sex marriage and was followed by Belgium in 2003 and Spain in 2005. In Canada, British Columbia and Ontario legalized same-sex marriage in 2003, and five other provinces and territories followed suit in 2004. In 2005, same-sex marriage was legalized nationwide.

Across Canada, same-sex couples are permitted to legally marry. This was safeguarded in legislation when the Civil Marriage Act, which was passed by Parliament, came into force on July 20, 2005. Before passage of the Civil Marriage Act, courts in nine jurisdictions, representing 89% of Canada's population, had already

extended equal civil marriage to same-sex couples.

Following the Civil Marriage Act ruling of 2005, members of Parliament were asked to re-open the equal marriage debate. The motion was rejected on December 7, 2006, and same-sex marriage in Canada seems to no longer be an issue for legal debate.

The court ruling to recognize same-sex marriages in Canada was based on the finding that excluding same-sex couples from civil marriage is unjustifiable discrimination, which violates section 15 of the Canadian Charter of Rights and Freedoms.

What cases are made for and against civil union and same-sex marriage? Opponents put forth numerous arguments, including that the purpose of marriage is to procreate, that the Bible forbids same-sex unions, that gay people are seeking special rights, that it's bad for children and families, and that the

majority of the population opposes such unions. The primary argument, however, is that same-sex marriage undermines the sanctity and validity of marriage as it is traditionally understood and thus undermines society. Rules and restrictions on who can marry preserve the value of the institution of marriage, according to this view. The underlying assumption of this position is that gay men and lesbians make a choice and that people can change their orientation, though the process may be difficult.

Proponents of civil unions and same-sex marriage believe that sexual orientation is outside the control of the individual and results from genetic and environmental factors that create an unchangeable orientation. The issue of same-sex union is then seen as one of basic civil rights, in which a group is being denied rights—to publicly express their commitment to one another, to provide security for their children, and to receive the legal and economic benefits afforded to married heterosexual couples—on the basis of something as unalterable as skin colour. Both opponents and proponents of same-sex marriage point out that marriage is healthy for both men and women and is the main social institution promoting family values; both sides see this assertion as supportive of their position.

Sources: Ambert, A. 2005. Same-sex couples and same-sex-parent families: Relationships, parenting, and issues of marriage. *Contemporary Family Trends* (http://www.vifamily.ca/media/node/476/attachments/samesex_05.pdf; retrieve April 17, 2011); Canadians for Equal Marriage. 2006. *Harper's Motion to Re-open Equal Marriage Defeated!* (http://www.equal-marriage.ca; retrieved November 16, 2009).

single partner. Like any intimate relationship, same-sex partnerships provide intimacy, passion, and security.

One difference between heterosexual and same-sex couples is that same-sex partnerships may be more egalitarian (equal) and less organized around traditional gender roles. Same-sex couples may put greater emphasis on partnership than on role assignment. Domestic tasks may be shared or split, and both partners often support themselves financially.

Another difference between heterosexual and same-sex relationships is that same-sex partners often have to deal with societal hostility or ambivalence toward their relationship, in contrast to the societal approval and rights given

to heterosexual couples (see the box "Same-Sex Marriage and Civil Unions" above). *Homophobia*, fear or hatred of gay people, can be obvious, as in the case of violence or discrimination, or more subtle, as in the way same-sex couples are portrayed in the media. Additional stress on a same-sex partnership may occur if an LGB individual is a member of a family or ethnic group that is not entirely accepting of her or his sexual orientation.

Bisexual individuals involved in heterosexual relationships may feel shame or guilt around the acceptance and privileges afforded to them by their heterosexual relationship. Because of the impact of societal disapproval, commu-

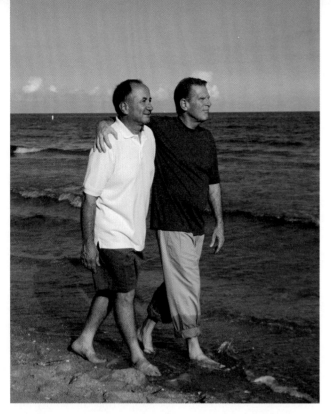

Greater openness has made gay men and lesbians more visible than they used to be, although they still constitute a minority of the population. Most gay people have experienced at least one long-term relationship with one partner.

nity resources and support may be more important for same-sex couples as a source of identity and social support than they are for heterosexuals. Many communities offer support groups for same-sex partners and families to help them build social networks and a sense of pride and acceptance.

Although many challenges for same-sex partnerships are common to all relationships, some issues are unique to LGB partnerships. Because men may not be socialized to communicate about interpersonal and emotional issues, communication problems may be particularly common or acute in gay relationships. Some researchers suggest that the process of female socialization, with its emphasis on creating and maintaining intimacy, makes lesbian relationships more likely to be characterized by fusion, enmeshment, and a blurring of boundaries. Problems may also arise when one member of a same-sex relationship has come out, or publicly identified as LGB, earlier than the other; consequently, the more experienced individual may wonder and worry whether the partner's sexual orientation is transient. The less experienced member of the relationship may feel threatened by the partner's level of "outness" or involvement in the LGB community. If same-sex couples decide to seek counselling, it is important to find a therapist who is an ally of the LGB community and who has training and experience working with LGB couples.

See Chapter 11 for more information on sexual orientation, gender identity, and sexual behaviour.

Singlehood

Despite the prevalence and popularity of marriage, a significant and growing number of adults in our society are unmarried—for the first time in Canada, being single is more common than being married, with 51.5% of Canadians (aged 15+) being unmarried. The largest group of unmarried adults have never been married (Figure 10.2).

Several factors contribute to the growing number of single people. One is the changing view of singlehood, which is increasingly being viewed as a legitimate alternative to marriage. Education and careers are delaying the age at which young people are marrying. The median age for marriage in Canada is now 30 years for men and 28 years for women. More young people are living with their parents as they complete their education, seek jobs, or strive for financial independence. Many other single people live together without being married. High divorce rates mean more singles, and people who have experienced divorce in their families may have more negative attitudes about marriage and more positive attitudes about singlehood.

Being single doesn't mean not having close relationships, however. Single people date, enjoy active and fulfilling social lives, and have a variety of sexual experiences and relationships. Other advantages of being single include more opportunities for personal and career development without concern for family obligations and more freedom and control in making life choices. Disadvantages include loneliness and a lack of companionship, as well as economic hardships (mainly for single women). Single men and women alike experience some discrimination and often are pressured to get married.

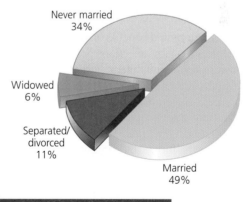

VITAL STATISTICS

FIGURE 10.2 Marital status of the Canadian population census 2001, ages 15+.

Source: Based on data from Statistics Canada. 2010. *Legal Marital Status (6), Age Groups (19) and Sex (3) for Population, for Canada, Provinces, Territories, Census Metropolitan Areas and Census Agglomerations, 1996 and 2001 Censuses—100% Data* (http://www12.statcan.ca/english/census01/products/standard/themes/RetrieveProductTable.cfm?Temporal=2001&PID=55523&GID=431515&METH=1&APATH=3&PTYPE=55440&THEME=38&AID=0&FREE=0&FOCUS=0&VID=0&VNAMEE=&VNAMEF=&GC=0&GK=0&SC=1&SR=1&RL=0&CPP=99&RPP=9999&d1=0&d2=0; retrieved June 6, 2011).

Nearly everyone has at least one episode of being single in adult life, whether before marriage, between marriages, following divorce or the death of a spouse, or for his or her entire life. How enjoyable and valuable this single time is depends on several factors, including how deliberately the person has chosen it; how satisfied the person is with his or her social relationships, standard of living, and job; how comfortable the person feels when alone; and how resourceful and energetic the person is about creating an interesting and fulfilling life.

MARRIAGE

The majority of Canadians marry at some time in their life. Marriage continues to remain popular because it satisfies several basic needs. Marriage has many important social, moral, economic, and political aspects, all of which have changed over the years. In the past, people married mainly for practical reasons, such as raising children or forming an economic unit. Today, people marry more for personal and emotional reasons.

Benefits of Marriage

The primary functions and benefits of marriage are those of any intimate relationship: affection, personal affirmation, companionship, sexual fulfillment, and emotional growth. Marriage also provides a setting in which to raise children, although an increasing number of couples choose to remain without children, and people can also choose to raise children without being married. Marriage is also important for providing for the future. By committing themselves to the relationship, people establish themselves with lifelong companions as well as some insurance for their later years.

Good marriages have been shown to have myriad positive effects on individuals' health (see the box "Are Intimate Relationships Good for Your Health?").

Issues in Marriage

Although we might like to believe otherwise, love is not enough to make a successful marriage. Couples have to be strong and successful in their relationship before getting married, because relationship problems will be magnified rather than solved by marriage. The following relation-

ship characteristics appear to be the best predictors of a happy marriage:

- The partners have realistic expectations about their relationship.
- Each feels good about the personality of the other.
- They communicate well.
- They have effective ways of resolving conflicts.
- They agree on religious and ethical values.
- They have an egalitarian role relationship.
- They have a good balance of individual versus joint interests and leisure activities.

Once married, couples must provide each other with emotional support, negotiate and establish marital roles, establish domestic and career priorities, handle their finances, make sexual adjustments, manage boundaries and relationships with their extended family, and participate in the larger community.

Marital roles and responsibilities have undergone profound changes in recent years. Many couples no longer accept traditional role assumptions, such as that the husband is solely responsible for supporting the family and the wife is solely responsible for domestic work. Today, many husbands share domestic tasks, and many wives work outside the home. In fact, more than 50% of married women are in the labour force, including women with babies less than one year of age. Although women still take most of the responsibility for home and children even when they work and although men still suffer more job-related stress and health problems than women do, the trend is toward an equalization of responsibilities.

The Role of Commitment

Coping with all these challenges requires that couples be committed to remaining in the relationship through its inevitable ups and downs. They need to be tolerant of each other's imperfections and keep their perspective and sense of humour. Commitment is based on conscious choice rather than on feelings, which, by their very nature, are transitory. Commitment is a promise of a shared future, a promise to be together, come what may. Committed partners put effort and energy into the relationship, no matter how they feel. They take time to attend to their partner, give compliments, and deal with conflict when necessary.

Commitment has become an important concept in recent years. To many people, commitment is a more important goal than living together or marriage.

Separation and Divorce

Canadians marrying today have a 35% chance of divorcing. The high rate of divorce in Canada reflects our extremely high expectations for emotional fulfillment and satisfaction in marriage (Figure 10.3). It also indicates that we no longer believe in the permanence of marriage.

MIND/BODY/SPIRIT

Findings suggest that marriage has intrinsic benefits. Married people, on average, live longer than unmarried people—whether single, divorced, or widowed—and they score higher on measures of mental health. They have a lower prevalence of headaches, low-back pain, inactivity, and psychological distress. Married people consistently report being happier than unmarried people.

The benefits of intimate relationships have been demonstrated for a range of conditions: People with strong social support are less likely to catch colds. They recover better from heart attacks, live longer with heart disease, and have higher survival rates for certain cancers. Among men with prostate cancer, those who are married live significantly longer than those who are single, divorced, or widowed. Women in satisfying marriages are less likely to develop risk factors associated with cardiovascular diseases than unmarried women or women in unhappy marriages. A 2006 study found that people who never marry have a higher chance of dying prematurely than people who have been divorced, separated, or widowed.

What is it about social relationships that supports wellness? Some studies suggest that friends and partners may encourage and reinforce healthy habits,

such as exercising, eating right, and seeing a physician when needed. In times of illness, a loving partner can provide both practical help (sometimes financial) and emotional support. Feeling loved, esteemed, and valued brings comfort at a time of vulnerability, reduces anxiety, and mitigates the damaging effects of stress and risks of social isolation.

Although good relationships may help the sick get better, bad relation-

ships may have the opposite effect. The impact of relationship quality on the course of illness may be partly explained by effects of the immune system: A study of married couples whose fighting went beyond normal conflict and into criticism and name-calling found them to have weaker immune responses than couples whose arguments were more civil. Hostile couples need more time for injuries to heal; their systems tend to contain higher levels of inflammatory agents, which have been linked to long-term illness. New research shows that high marital stress is linked with risky lifestyle choices and behaviours and nonadherence to medical regimens. Similarly, unhappy marriages are associated with risk factors for heart disease, such as depression, hostility, and anger.

Marriage, of course, isn't the only support system available. Whether married, in a committed partnership, or single, if you have supportive people in your life, you are likely to enjoy better physical and emotional health than if you feel isolated and alone. So when you start planning lifestyle changes to improve your health and well-being, don't forget to nurture your relationships with family and friends. Relationships are powerful medicine.

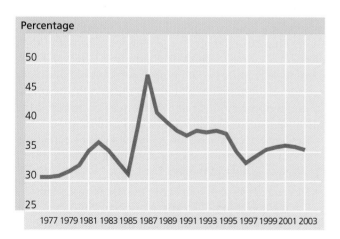

FIGURE 10.3 Percentage of divorces expected to end before the 25th year of marriage.

Note: "Divorces, expected" measures the percentage of married couples (existing in a certain year) that can expect to experience divorce before their 25th anniversary. This is a projection, which differs from the actual number of divorces occurring in a year (crude divorce rate).

Source: Statistics Canada. 2011. *Family Life—Divorce* (http://www4. hrsdc.gc.ca/.3ndic.1t.4r@-eng.jsp?iid=76; retrieved April 17, 2011).

The process of divorce usually begins with an emotional separation. Often one partner is unhappy and looks beyond the relationship for other forms of validation. Dissatisfaction increases until the unhappy partner decides he or she can no longer stay. Physical separation follows, although it may take some time for the relationship to be over emotionally.

Except for the death of a spouse or family member, divorce is the greatest stress-producing event in life. Research shows that divorced women are more likely to develop heart disease than married, remarried, or widowed women. Both men and women experience turmoil, depression, and lowered self-esteem during and after divorce. People experience separation distress and loneliness for about a year and then begin a recovery

74% of Canadians consider extramarital affairs to be immoral.

—Leger Marketing, 2006

QUICK STATS

period of one to three years. During this time they gradually construct a post-divorce identity, along with a new pattern of life. Most people are surprised by how long it takes to recover from divorce.

Children are especially vulnerable to the trauma of divorce, and sometimes counselling is appropriate to help them adjust to the changes in their lives. However, recent research has found that children who spend substantial time with both parents are usually better adjusted than those in sole custody arrangements and as well adjusted as their peers from intact families.

Despite the distress of separation and divorce, the negative effects are usually balanced sooner or later by the possibility of finding a more suitable partner, constructing a new life, and developing new aspects of the self. About 75% of all people who divorce remarry, often within five years. More Canadian men than women want to remarry following divorce. One result of the high divorce and remarriage rate is a growing number of stepfamilies (discussed in the next section).

FAMILY LIFE

Canadian families are very different today from what they were even a few decades ago. Currently, about half of all families are based on a first marriage; almost 26% are headed by a single parent; the remainder are remarriages or involve some other arrangement. Despite the tremendous variation apparent in Canadian families, certain patterns can still be discerned.

Becoming a Parent

Few new parents have any preparation for the job of parenting, yet they have to assume that role literally overnight. They have to learn quickly how to hold a baby, how to change it, how to feed it, how to interpret its cries. No wonder the birth of the first child is one of the most stressful transitions for any couple.

Even couples with an egalitarian relationship before their first child is born find that their marital roles become more traditional with the arrival of the new baby. The father becomes the primary provider and protector, and the mother becomes the primary nurturer. Most research indicates that mothers have to make greater changes in

their lives than fathers do. Although men today spend more time caring for their infants than ever before, women typically still take the ultimate responsibility for the baby. In addition, women are usually the ones who make job changes; they may quit working or reduce their hours to stay home with the baby for several months or more, or they may try to juggle the multiple roles of mother, homemaker, and employer/employee and feel guilty that they never have enough time to do justice to any of these roles.

Not surprisingly, marital satisfaction often declines after the birth of the first child. The wife who has stopped working may feel she is cut off from the world; the wife who is trying to fulfil duties both at home and on the job may feel overburdened and resentful. The husband may have a hard time adjusting to having to share his wife's love and attention with the baby.

But marital dissatisfaction after the baby is born is not inevitable. Couples who successfully weather the stresses of a new baby seem to have these three characteristics in common:

1. They had developed a strong relationship before the baby was born.

2. They had planned to have the child and want it very much.

3. They communicate well about their feelings and expectations.

Parenting

Sometimes being a parent is a source of unparalleled pleasure and pride: the first smile (at you), the first word, the first home run. But at other times parenting can seem like an overwhelming responsibility.

Parenting Styles   Most parents worry about their ability to raise a healthy, responsible, and well-adjusted child. Parents may wonder about the long-term impact of each decision they make on their child's well-being and personality. According to parenting experts, no one action or decision (within limits) will determine a child's personality or development; instead, what is most important is the *parenting style*, or overall approach to parenting.

Research has revealed four general styles of parenting. The four styles vary primarily according to the levels of two characteristics of the parents:

- *Demandingness* encompasses the use of discipline and supervision, the expectation that children act responsibly and maturely, and the direct response to disobedience.

- *Responsiveness* refers to a parent's warmth and his or her intent to facilitate independence and self-confidence in a child by being supportive, connected, and understanding of the child's needs.

Most parents use a blend of the four general styles but tend toward one style.

Setting clear boundaries, holding children to high expectations, and responding with warmth to children's needs are all positive parenting strategies.

AUTHORITARIAN Authoritarian parents are high in demandingness and low in responsiveness. They give orders and expect them to be obeyed, giving very little warmth or consideration to their children's special needs. They maintain a structured environment where the rules are explicit and set without input or discussion with the child. Children of authoritarian parents rate low on social competence, self-esteem, intellectual curiosity, spontaneity, and initiative. They perform fairly well in school and do not exhibit a lot of problem behaviour; however, they have higher levels of depression.

AUTHORITATIVE *Authoritative* parents are high in both demandingness and responsiveness. They set clear boundaries and expectations, but they are also loving, supportive, and attuned to their children's needs. They are firm in their decisions but allow for a give-and-take in discussions with the intent of fostering independent thinking.

Both authoritarian and authoritative parents hold their children to high expectations. The difference is that authoritarian parents expect their children to follow their commands without question or comment and authoritative parents are more likely to explain their reasoning and allow children to express themselves. Research consistently shows that children of authoritative parents are the best adjusted and rate particularly high in social competence.

PERMISSIVE (OR INDULGENT) *Permissive* parents are high in responsiveness and low in demandingness. They do not expect their children to act maturely but instead allow them to follow their own impulses. They are very warm, patient, and accepting, and they are focused on not stifling their child's innate creativity. They use little discipline and are often nontraditional. Children of permissive parents have difficulty with impulse control, are immature, perform more poorly in school, have more problem behaviours, and take less responsibility for their actions. They also have higher self-esteem, better social skills, and lower levels of depression.

UNINVOLVED *Uninvolved* parents are low in both demandingness and responsiveness. They require little from their children and respond with little attention, frequency, or effort. In extreme cases, this style might reach the level of child neglect. Research has found that children of uninvolved parents perform worse in all areas measured compared with children of parents who use the other styles.

Children's Temperaments Every child has a tendency toward certain moods and a style of reacting—a temperament—that is apparent from infancy and often lasts into adulthood. Research has identified three basic temperament types; most children show aspects of different temperaments but tend toward one.

- *Easy children* are happy, content, and have regular sleeping and eating habits. They are adaptable and not easily upset.

- *Difficult children* are fussy, fearful in new situations or with strangers, and have irregular sleeping and feeding habits. They are easily upset and often hard to soothe.

- *Slow-to-warm-up children* are somewhat fussy and tend to react negatively or fearfully to new people or situations; however, they slowly warm up and adapt positively.

A match between parental style and child temperament is ideal. Difficulties tend to arise when a mismatch occurs in temperaments and styles and the parent is not versed in parenting skills. For example, a parent who expects quick action in response to a command may not be a good match for a slow-to-respond child. Parents should be attuned to their child's distinct style and do their best to support the child.

According to psychologists, "optimal attunement" of the parent to the child involves allowing the child to feel close and connected without feeling engulfed or impinged on, while also allowing for separation and aloneness without the child feeling abandoned or rejected. *Attachment parenting* advocates believe that if children are consistently held, attended to, and not allowed to be unhappy for any length of time, they will internalize the parents' consistent care and support and grow up more able to provide this for themselves and others.

Parenting and the Family Life Cycle Parenting that is responsive and demanding is the most beneficial for children. Providing a balance of firm limits and clear structure along with high levels of warmth, nurturance, and respect for the child's own special needs and temperament as well as her or his growing independence is the best predictor for raising a healthy child. The important thing is to keep seeking ways to promote satisfaction for all family members—including the parents! It is also important for parents to develop and maintain confidence in their parenting skills, their common sense—and, above all, their love for their children.

At each stage of the family life cycle, the relationship between parents and children changes. And with those changes come new challenges. The parents' primary responsibility to a small, helpless baby is to ensure its physical well-being around the clock. As babies grow into toddlers and begin to crawl and walk and talk, they begin to be able to take care of some of their own physical needs. For parents, the challenge at this stage is to strike a balance between giving children the freedom to explore and setting limits that will keep the children safe and secure. As children grow toward adolescence, parents need to give them increasing independence and gradually be willing to let them risk success or failure on their own.

Marital satisfaction for most couples tends to decline somewhat while the children are in school. Reasons include the financial and emotional pressures of a growing family and the increased job and community responsibilities of parents in their thirties, forties, and fifties. Once the last child has left home, marital satisfaction usually increases because the couple have time to enjoy each other once more.

Single Parents

Today the family life cycle for many women is marriage, motherhood, divorce, single parenthood, remarriage, and widowhood.

In some single-parent families, the traditional family life cycle is reversed and the baby comes before the marriage. In some of these families, the single parent is a teenage mother; she may be of a lower socioeconomic status, and she may never get married or may not marry for several years. The number of Canadian women with children who are single and have never been married is also increasing. These lone parents of today tend to be older, on average, than their counterparts were in the past. In 2001, 30% of these lone parents were ages 35–44, up from 15% in 1981.

Economic difficulties are the primary problem for single mothers, especially for unmarried mothers who have not finished high school and have difficulty finding work. Divorced mothers usually experience a sharp drop in income the first few years on their own, but if they have job skills or education they usually can eventually support themselves and their children adequately. Other problems for single mothers are the often-conflicting demands of playing both father and mother and the difficulty of satisfying their own needs for adult companionship and affection.

Financial pressures are also a complaint of single fathers, but they do not experience them to the extent that single mothers do. Because they are likely to have less practice than mothers in juggling parental and professional roles, they may worry that they do not spend enough time with their children. Because single fatherhood is not as common as single motherhood, however, the men who choose it are likely to be stable, established, and strongly motivated to be with their children.

Research about the effect on children of growing up in a single-parent family is inconclusive. Evidence seems to indicate that these children tend to have less success in school and in their careers than children from two-parent families, but these effects may be associated more strongly with low educational attainment of the single parent than with the absence of the second parent. Two-parent families are not necessarily better if one of the parents spends little time relating to the children or is physically or emotionally abusive.

Stepfamilies

Single parenthood is usually a transitional stage: About three out of four divorced women and about four out of five divorced men will ultimately remarry. Rates are lower for widowed men and women, but overall, many of the marriages in North America are remarriages for the husband, the wife, or both. If either partner brings children from a previous marriage into the new family unit, a stepfamily (or blended family) is formed.

Stepfamilies are significantly different from primary families and should not be expected to duplicate the emotions and relationships of a primary family. Research has shown that healthy stepfamilies are less cohesive and more adaptable than healthy primary families; they have a greater capacity to allow for individual differences and accept that biologically related family members will have emotionally closer relationships. Stepfamilies gradually gain more of a sense of being a family as they build a history of shared daily experiences and major life events.

Successful Families

Family life can be extremely challenging. A strong family is not a family without problems; it's a family that copes successfully with stress and crisis (see "Strategies of Strong Families" in the ▤connect Library). Successful families are intentionally connected—members share experiences and meanings.

An excellent way to build strong family ties is to develop family rituals and routines: organized, repeated activities that have meaning for family members. Families with regular routines and rituals have healthier children, more satisfying marriages, and stronger family relationships. Some of the most common routines identified in research studies are dinnertime, a regular bedtime, and household chores; common rituals include birthdays, religious and other holidays, and Sunday activities. Family routines may even serve as protective factors, balancing out potential risk factors associated with single-parent families and families with divorce and remarriage. You may want to consider incorporating a regular family mealtime into your family routine, as it allows parents and children to develop closer relationships and leads to better parenting, healthier children, and better school performance.

Although Canadian families have tremendous variation, researchers have proposed that six major qualities or themes appear in strong families:

1. *Commitment.* The family is very important to its members; sexual fidelity between partners is included in commitment.

2. *Appreciation.* Family members care about one another and express their appreciation. The home is a positive place for family members.

3. *Communication.* Family members spend time listening to one another and enjoying one another's company. They talk about disagreements and attempt to solve problems.

4. *Time together.* Family members do things together, often simple activities that don't cost money.

5. *Spiritual wellness.* The family promotes sharing, love, and compassion for other human beings.

6. *Coping with stress and crisis.* When faced with illness, death, marital conflict, or other crises, family members pull together, seek help, and use other coping strategies to meet the challenge.

It may surprise some people that members of strong families are often seen at counselling centres. They know that the smartest thing to do in some situations is to get help. Many resources are available for individuals and families seeking counselling; people can turn to physicians, clergy, marriage and family counsellors, psychologists, or other trained professionals.

THINKING ABOUT THE ENVIRONMENT

Parents can instil a lifelong sense of environmental stewardship in their children by teaching them these simple habits:

- Recycle waste as much as possible.

- Purchase environmentally friendly products that are manufactured from recyclable materials.

- Turn off lights and appliances when they are not needed.

- Shop for locally grown foods that are raised through environmentally sustainable practices.

For more information on the environment, see Chapter 21.

QUESTIONS FOR CRITICAL THINKING AND REFLECTION

Do you think of your own family as a successful family? Why or why not? Either way, what could you do to make your relationships in your family more successful? Are you comfortable talking to your family about these issues?

Practise and learn online with Connect. Connect allows you to practise important skills at your own pace and on your own schedule, with 24/7 online access to an eBook, practice quizzes, interactivities, videos, study tools, additional resources, and more.

SUMMARY

• Healthy intimate relationships are an important component of the well-being of both individuals and society. Many intimate relationships are held together by love.

• Successful relationships begin with a positive sense of self and reasonably high self-esteem. Personal identity, gender roles, and styles of attachment are all rooted in childhood experiences.

• The characteristics of friendship include companionship, respect, acceptance, help, trust, loyalty, and reciprocity.

• Love, sex, and commitment are closely linked ideals in intimate relationships. Love includes trust, caring, respect, and loyalty. Sex brings excitement, fascination, and passion to the relationship.

• Common challenges in relationships relate to issues of self-disclosure, commitment, expectations, competitiveness, balancing time spent together and apart, and jealousy. Partners in successful relationships have strong communication skills and support each other in difficult times.

• The keys to good communication in relationships are self-disclosure, listening, and feedback.

• Conflict is inevitable in intimate relationships; partners need to have constructive ways to negotiate their differences.

• People usually choose partners like themselves. If partners are very different, acceptance and good communication skills are necessary to maintain the relationship.

• Most Canadians find partners through dating or getting together in groups. Cohabitation is a growing social pattern that allows partners to get to know each other intimately without being married.

• Gay and lesbian partnerships are similar to heterosexual partnerships, with some differences. Partners often don't conform to traditional gender roles, and they may experience hostility or ambivalence rather than approval toward their partnership from society.

• Singlehood is a growing option in our society. Advantages include greater variety in sex partners and more freedom in making life decisions; disadvantages include loneliness and possible economic hardship, especially for single women.

• Marriage fulfils many functions for individuals and society. It can provide people with affection, affirmation, and sexual fulfillment; a context for child rearing; and the promise of lifelong companionship.

• Love isn't enough to ensure a successful marriage. Partners have to be realistic, feel good about each other, have communication and conflict-resolution skills, share values, and have a balance of individual and joint interests.

• When problems can't be worked out, people often separate and divorce. Divorce is traumatic for all involved, especially children, but the negative effects are usually balanced in time by positive ones.

• Four general parenting styles are authoritarian, authoritative, permissive, and uninvolved; the authoritative style is usually associated with the best outcomes.

• At each stage of the family life cycle, relationships change. Marital satisfaction may be lower during the child-rearing years and higher later.

• Many families today are single-parent families. Problems for single parents include economic difficulties, conflicting demands, and time pressures.

• Stepfamilies are formed when single, divorced, or widowed people remarry and create new family units. Stepfamilies gradually gain more of a sense of being a family as they build a history of shared experiences.

• Important qualities of successful families include commitment to the family, appreciation of family members, communication, time spent together, spiritual wellness, and effective methods of dealing with stress.

For resources in your area, check your campus directory for a counselling centre or peer counselling program, or check the agencies listed in the Mental Health section of the phone book.

BOOKS

Brooks, J. B. 2008. *The Process of Parenting*, 7th ed. New York: McGraw-Hill. Demonstrates how parents and caregivers can translate their love and concern for children into effective parenting behaviour.

DeGenova, M. K., and F. P. Rice. 2006. *Intimate Relationships, Marriages, and Families,* 7th ed. New York: McGraw-Hill. A comprehensive introduction to relationships.

McKay, M., P. Fanning, and K. Paleg. 2007. *Couple Skills: Making Your Relationship Work,* 2nd rev. ed. New York: New Harbinger. A comprehensive guide to improving communication, resolving conflict, and developing greater intimacy and commitment in relationships.

Miller, R., D. Perlman, and S. S. Brehm. 2008. *Intimate Relationships,* 5th ed. New York: McGraw-Hill. A balanced presentation of both the positive and the problematic aspects of intimate relationships.

Olson, D., and J. DeFrain. 2007. *Marriages and Families: Intimacy, Diversity, and Strengths,* 6th ed. New York: McGraw-Hill. A comprehensive introduction to relationships and families.

ORGANIZATIONS AND WEB SITES

The Internet addresses listed here were accurate at the time of publication.

Association for Couples in Marriage Enrichment. An organization that promotes activities to strengthen marriage; a resource for books, tapes, and other materials.

http://www.bettermarriages.org

Canadians for Equal Marriage. A nationwide, bilingual campaign made up of individuals and organizations from all walks of Canadian life committed to upholding equal marriage rights for couples of any sexual orientation.

http://www.equal-marriage.ca

Charity Village Nonprofit Neighbourhood. A Web site and search engine that contains many links to information and support for lesbian, gay, bisexual, and transgendered (LGBT) people.

http://www.charityvillage.com/cv/nonpr/nonpr27.html

Conflict Resolution Information Source. Provides links to a broad range of Internet resources on conflict resolution. Information covers interpersonal, marriage, family, and other types of conflicts.

http://www.crinfo.org

Family Education Network. Provides information about education, safety, health, and other family-related issues.

http://www.familyeducation.com

Gottman Institute. Includes tips and suggestions for relationships and parenting, including an online relationships quiz.

http://www.gottman.com

Life Innovations. Provides materials for premarital counselling and marital enrichment.

http://www.prepare-enrich.com

Parents Without Partners. Provides educational programs, literature, and support groups for single parents and their children. Search the online directory for a referral to a local chapter.

http://www.parentswithoutpartners.org

Registry of Marriage and Family Therapists in Canada. Provides information about the profession, resources, and links to therapists in different area of Canada.

http://www.marriageandfamily.ca

Vanier Institute of the Family. Provides research, resources, consultation, and policy development regarding the importance of families to Canadian society.

http://www.vifamily.ca

See also the listings for Chapters 2 and 12.

SELECTED BIBLIOGRAPHY

Beaupré, P. 2008. I do… Take two? Changes in intentions to remarry among divorced Canadians during the past 20 years. *Matter of Fact* 5 (http://dsp-psd.tpsgc.gc.ca/collection_2008/statcan/89-630-X/89-630-XIE2008005.pdf; retrieved April 17, 2011).

Bookwala, J. 2005. The role of marital quality in physical health during the mature years. *Journal of Aging and Health* 17(1): 85–104.

Christakis, N. A., et al. 2006. Mortality after hospitalization of a spouse. *New England Journal of Medicine* 354(7): 719–730.

Holt-Lunstad, J., W. Birmingham, and B. Q. Jones. 2008. Is there something unique about marriage? *Annals of Behavioral Medicine* 35(2): 239–244.

Human Resources and Skills Development Canada. 2011. *Canadians in Context—Households and Families* (http://www4.hrsdc.gc.ca/.3ndic.1t.4r@-eng.jsp?iid=37; retrieved April 17, 2011).

Leger Marketing. 2006. *Morality Barometer* (http://www.legermarketing.com/documents/spclm/060612ENG.pdf; retrieved April 17, 2011).

Lichter, D. T., R. N. Turner, and S. Sassler. 2010. National estimates of the rise in serial cohabitation. *Social Science Research* 39(5): 754–765.

McPherson, M., L. Smith-Lovin, and M. Brashears. 2006. Social isolation in America: Changes in core discussion networks over two decades. *American Sociological Review* 71: 353–375.

Medical memo: Marital stress and the heart. 2004. *Harvard Men's Health Watch,* May.

Mookadam, F., and H. M. Arthur. 2004. Social support and its relationship to morbidity and mortality after acute myocardial infarction: Systematic overview. *Archives of Internal Medicine* 164(14): 1514–1518.

Najib, A., et al. 2004. Regional brain activity in women grieving a romantic relationship breakup. *American Journal of Psychiatry* 161(12): 2245–2256.

National Conference of State Legislatures. 2008 Update. *Same Sex Marriage, Civil Unions and Domestic Partnerships* (http://www.ncsl.org/programs/cyf/samesex.htm; retrieved January 21, 2009).

Pleis, J. R., and M. Lethbridge-Cejku. 2007. Summary health statistics for U.S. adults: National Health Interview Survey, 2006. *Vital and Health Statistics* 10(235): 1–153.

Roisman, G. I., et al. 2008. Adult romantic relationships as contexts of human development: A multimethod comparison of same-sex couples with opposite-sex dating, engaged, and married dyads. *Developmental Psychology* 44(1): 91–101.

Statistics Canada. 2005. *Women in Canada: A Gender-Based Statistical Report,* 5th ed. (http://www.statcan.gc.ca/pub/89-503-x/89-503-x2005001-eng.pdf; retrieved April 17, 2011).

Schoen, R., et al. 2007. Family transitions in young adulthood. *Demography* 44(4): 807–820.

Strong, B., et al. 2005. *Human Sexuality: Diversity in Contemporary America,* 5th ed. New York: McGraw-Hill.

Talbot, Y., et al. 2001. Canadians without regular medical doctors. Who are they? *Canadian Family Physician* 47(1), 58–64.

Tucker, P. and J. Irwin. 2009. University Students' Satisfaction With, Interest in Improving, and receptivity to Attending Programs Aimed at Health and Well-Being. *Health Promotion Practice.* [Published online before print February 5, 2009, doi: 10.1177/1524839908330814; http://hpp.sagepub.com/content/early/2009/02/05/1524839908330814.abstract]

Wainright, J. L., S. T. Russell, and C. J. Patterson. 2004. Psychosocial adjustment, school outcomes, and romantic relationships of adolescents with same-sex parents. *Child Development* 75(6): 1886–1898.

Whisman, M. A., L. A. Uebelacker, and L. M. Weinstock. 2004. Psychopathology and marital satisfaction: The importance of evaluating both partners. *Journal of Consulting and Clinical Psychology* 72(5): 830–838.

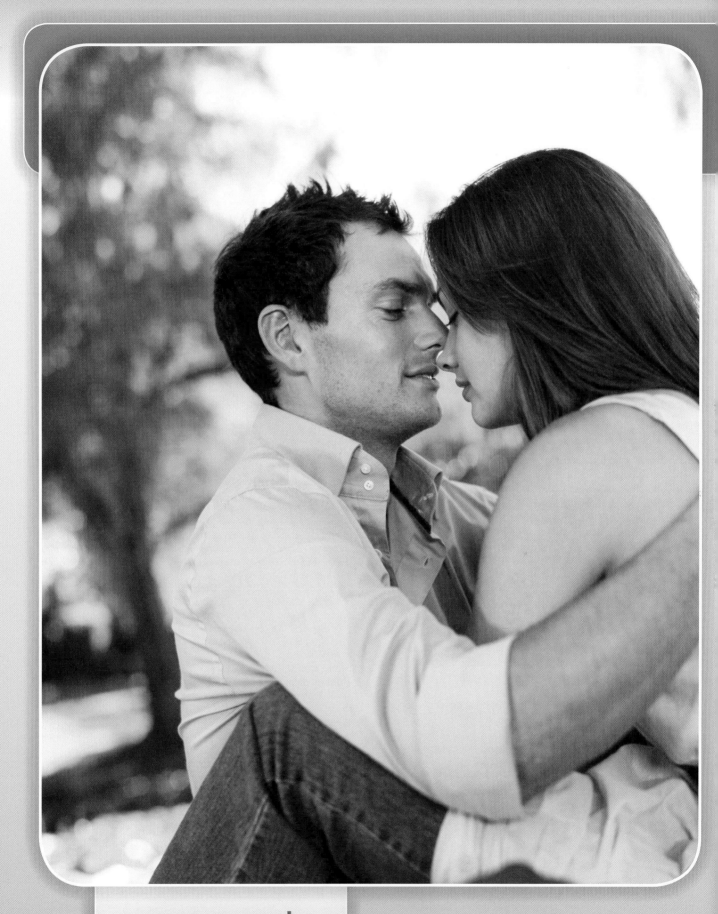

HEALTHY SEXUALITY

LOOKING AHEAD>>>>>

AFTER READING THIS CHAPTER, YOU SHOULD BE ABLE TO

- Describe the structure and function of the female and male sex organs
- Explain the changes in sexual functioning that occur during a person's life
- Describe how the sex organs function during sexual activity
- Identify common causes of sexual problems
- Outline the factors that influence sexual behaviour and the various ways human sexuality can be expressed
- Describe guidelines for safe, responsible sexual behaviour
- Identify the advantages, disadvantages, and level of effectiveness of commonly used reversible contraceptive methods
- Understand the different types of abortion procedures

TEST YOUR KNOWLEDGE

1. **Although testosterone is the primary male hormone, it is also produced in women.**
   True or false?

2. **Which of the following is a risk factor for erectile dysfunction (impotence)?**
   a. smoking
   b. overweight
   c. physical inactivity

3. **Calcium supplements may reduce symptoms of premenstrual syndrome (PMS) in some women.**
   True or false?

4. **Alcohol consumption by young people is associated with unplanned, unprotected sexual activity and higher rates of sexually transmitted infections (STIs).**
   True or false?

5. **Sperm can survive only about 24 hours inside a woman's body.**
   True or false?

6. **Abortion is illegal in some parts of Canada.**
   True of false?

ANSWERS

1. **TRUE.** Testosterone is produced in small amounts by a woman's ovaries.

2. **ALL THREE.** 70%–80% of cases of erectile dysfunction are thought to involve physical factors.

3. **TRUE.** Other self-help strategies for PMS include exercise, stress reduction, and a diet low in fat and rich in complex carbohydrates.

4. **TRUE.** Studies have shown that raising the drinking age and increasing the price of beer (through taxes) leads to a decrease in STI rates among young adults.

5. **FALSE.** Sperm usually live about 72 hours inside the woman's body but can live up to six or seven days.

6. **FALSE.** Abortion is legal throughout every province and territory in Canada.

Humans are sexual beings. Sexual activity is the source of our most intense physical pleasures, a central ingredient in many of our intimate emotional relationships, and the key to reproduction.

Sexuality is more than just sexual behaviour. It is a complex, interacting group of inborn, biological characteristics and acquired behaviours people learn in the course of growing up in a particular family, community, and society. Sexuality includes biological sex (being biologically male or female), gender (masculine and feminine behaviours), sexual anatomy and physiology, sexual functioning and practices, and social and sexual interactions with others. Our individual sense of identity is powerfully influenced by our sexuality. We think of ourselves in fundamental ways as male or female; as heterosexual, gay, or lesbian; as single, attached, married, or divorced.

Because it can arouse intense feelings, sexuality can be an emotionally charged topic. In many communities, sexual expression is regulated with restrictions and taboos, specifying which functions and behaviours are acceptable and "normal" and which are unacceptable and "abnormal." Young people in Canada are bombarded with conflicting messages about sex. The mass media suggest that the average person is a sexual athlete who continually jumps in and out of bed without using contraception, producing offspring, or contracting disease. Although parents, educators, and other responsible adults may try to present a more balanced picture, they often convey their own hidden messages as well. Ignorance, confusion, and fear are frequently the result.

Basic information about the body, sexual functioning, and sexual behaviour is vital to healthy adult life. Once we understand the facts, we have a better basis for evaluating the messages we get and for making informed, responsible choices about our sexual activities. If you have questions about some aspects of your physical sexuality, this chapter will provide you with answers.

SEXUAL ANATOMY

In spite of their different appearances, the sex organs of men and women arise from the same structures and fulfil similar functions. Each person has a pair of **gonads**; ovaries are the female gonads, and testes are the male gonads. The gonads produce **germ cells** and sex hormones. The germ cells are **ova** (eggs) in females and **sperm** in males. Ova and sperm are the basic units of reproduction; their union results in the creation of a new life.

Female Sex Organs

The external sex organs, or genitals, of the female are called the **vulva** (Figure 11.1). The mons pubis, a rounded mass of fatty tissue over the pubic bone, becomes covered with hair during puberty (biological maturation). Below it are two paired folds of skin called the labia majora (major lips) and the labia minora (minor lips). Enclosed within these folds are the clitoris, the opening of the urethra, and the opening of the vagina.

The **clitoris** is highly sensitive to touch and plays an important role in female sexual arousal and orgasm. The clitoris consists of a shaft, glans, and spongy tissue that fills with blood during sexual excitement. The glans is the most sensitive part of the clitoris and is covered by the clitoral hood, or **prepuce**, which is formed from the upper portion of the labia minora.

The female **urethra** is a duct that leads directly from the urinary bladder to its opening between the clitoris and the opening of the vagina; it conducts urine from the bladder to the outside of the body. The female urethra is independent of the genitals.

The vaginal opening is partially covered by a membrane called the **hymen**. This membrane can be stretched or torn during athletic activity or when a woman has sexual intercourse for the first time. (The idea that an intact hymen

FIGURE 11.1 The female sex organs.

Fallopian tube
Ovary
Uterus
Bladder
Pubic bone
Mons pubis
Urethra
Clitoris
Urethral opening
Labia majora

Cervix
Rectum
Vagina
Anus
Perinium
Vaginal opening
Labia minora

FIGURE 11.2   The male sex organs.

Bladder

Pubic bone

Vas deferens

Corpus
spongiosum

Penis

Urethra

Glans

Opening of
urethra

Seminal vesicle

Rectum

Prostate

Cowper's gland

Anus

Epididymis

Testis

Scrotum

is the sign of virginity is a myth.) The **vagina** is the passage that leads to the internal reproductive organs. It is the female structure for heterosexual sexual intercourse and also serves as the birth canal.

Projecting into the upper part of the vagina is the **cervix**, which is the opening of the **uterus**—or *womb*—where a fertilized egg is implanted and grows into a *fetus*.

A pair of **fallopian tubes** (or *oviducts*) extends from the top of the uterus. The end of each oviduct surrounds an **ovary** and guides the mature ovum down into the uterus after the egg exits the ovary.

Male Sex Organs

A man's external sex organs, or genitals, are the penis and the scrotum (Figure 11.2).

The **penis** consists of spongy tissue that becomes engorged with blood during sexual excitement, causing the organ to enlarge and become erect.

The **scrotum** is a pouch that contains a pair of sperm-producing male gonads, called **testes**. The scrotum maintains the testes at a temperature approximately 3°C below that of the rest of the body—that is, at about 34°C. The process of sperm production is extremely heat sensitive. In hot temperatures the muscles in the scrotum relax, and the testes move away from the heat of the body. This ability to regulate the temperature of the testes is important because elevated testicular temperature can interfere with normal sperm production.

Through the entire length of the penis runs the urethra, which can carry both urine and *semen*, the sperm-carrying fluid, to the opening at the tip of the penis. Although urine and semen share a common passage, they are prevented from mixing together by muscles that control their entry into the urethra.

TERMS

sexuality   A dimension of personality shaped by biological, psychosocial, and cultural forces and concerning all aspects of sexual behaviour.

gonads   The primary reproductive organs that produce germ cells and sex hormones; the ovaries and testes.

germ cells   Sperm and ova.

ovum (ova, plural)   A germ cell produced by a female, which combines with a male germ cell (sperm) to create a fetus; also called an *egg*.

sperm   A germ cell produced by a male, which combines with a female germ cell (ovum) to create a fetus.

vulva   The external female genitals or sex organs.

clitoris   The highly sensitive female genital structure.

prepuce   The foreskin of the clitoris or penis.

urethra   The duct that carries urine from the bladder to the outside of the body.

hymen   A membrane that partially covers the vaginal opening.

vagina   The passage leading from the female genitals to the internal reproductive organs; the birth canal.

cervix   The end of the uterus opening toward the vagina.

uterus   The hollow, thick-walled, muscular organ in which the fertilized egg develops; the womb.

fallopian tube   A duct that guides a mature ovum from the ovary to the uterus; also called an *oviduct*.

ovary   One of two female reproductive glands that produce ova and sex hormones; ovaries are the female gonads.

penis   The male genital structure consisting of spongy tissue that becomes engorged with blood during sexual excitement.

scrotum   The loose sac of skin and muscle fibres that contains the testes.

testis (testes, plural)   One of two male gonads, the site of sperm production; also called a *testicle*.

During its brief lifetime, a sperm takes the following route:

1. Sperm are produced inside a maze of tiny, tightly packed tubules within the testes. As they begin to mature, sperm flow into a single storage tube called the **epididymis**, which lies on the surface of each testis.

2. Sperm move from each epididymis into another tube called the **vas deferens**, which carries them upward into the abdominal cavity and through an organ called the **prostate gland**. This gland produces some of the fluid in semen, which helps transport and nourish the sperm.

3. The two *vasa deferentia* eventually merge into a pair of **seminal vesicles**, whose secretions provide nutrients for the semen.

4. On the final stage of their journey, sperm flow into the **ejaculatory ducts**, which join the urethra.

The **Cowper's glands** are two small structures flanking the urethra. During sexual arousal, these glands secrete a clear, mucuslike fluid that appears at the tip of the penis. The exact purpose of preejaculatory fluid is not known, but it is thought to help lubricate the urethra to facilitate the passage of sperm. In some men, preejaculatory fluid may contain sperm, so withdrawal of the penis before ejaculation is not a reliable form of contraception.

Circumcision The smooth, rounded tip of the penis is the highly sensitive **glans**, an important component in sexual arousal (Figure 11.3). The glans is partially covered by the foreskin, or prepuce, a retractable fold of skin that is removed by **circumcision** in about 9% of newborn males in Canada. Circumcision is performed for cultural, religious, and hygienic reasons, and rates of circumcision vary widely among different groups. Worldwide, the rate is about 30%. Most Europeans, Asians, South and Central Americans, and Africans do not perform circumcision; Jews and Muslims are the major groups who circumcise for religious reasons.

The pros and cons of this simple procedure have been widely debated. Citing research findings, proponents argue that it promotes cleanliness and reduces the risk of urinary tract infections in newborns and the risk of sexually transmitted infections (STIs), including HIV, later in life. STI education and the practice of abstinence or low-risk sexual behaviours have a far greater impact on the transmission of STIs than does circumcision. However, where safer sex practices are not adhered to, circumcision can have a protective effect. Recent studies in countries with high rates of HIV infection and AIDS have shown that circumcision can reduce the risk of acquiring HIV through heterosexual contact in men by as much as 60%.

In 2007, an expert panel from the World Health Organization (WHO) recognized that male circumcision is an effective intervention for decreasing the spread of HIV but stressed that circumcision provides only partial protection and must be combined with other preventive strategies, such as condom use and limiting the number of sexual partners.

Opponents of circumcision state that it is an unnecessary surgical procedure that causes pain and puts a baby at risk for complications. They also argue that, by removing the foreskin, circumcision exposes the glans of the penis to constant irritation by clothing, thereby reducing its sensitivity; research into this issue has been inconclusive.

The Canadian Paediatric Association (CPS) takes the position (opposed by some physicians) that although circumcision has potential medical benefits, the research is not sufficient to recommend the procedure routinely. The CPS issued a statement that "circumcision of newborns should *not* be routinely performed." All provincial health insurance plans have now removed non-therapeutic circumcision from the list of procedures covered, because of the lack of health benefits.

QUESTIONS FOR CRITICAL THINKING AND REFLECTION

What are your personal views on circumcision? Who or what has influenced those opinions? Are the bases of your views primarily cultural, moral, or medical?

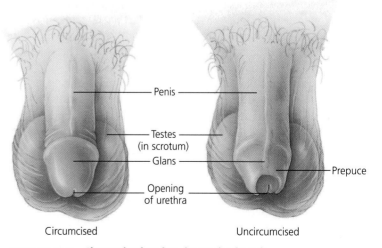

Penis

Testes (in scrotum)

Glans

Opening of urethra

Prepuce

Circumcised   Uncircumcised

FIGURE 11.3 Circumcised and uncircumcised penis.

HORMONES AND THE REPRODUCTIVE LIFE CYCLE

Many cultural and personal factors help shape the expression of your sexuality, but biology also plays an important role. The sex hormones produced by the ovaries or testes have a major influence on the development and function of the reproductive system throughout life.

The sex hormones made by the testes are called **androgens**, the most important of which is *testosterone*. The female sex hormones, produced by the ovaries, belong to two groups: **estrogens** and **progestins**, the most important of which is *progesterone*. The ovaries also produce a small amount of testosterone. The cortex of the **adrenal glands** also produces androgens in both males and females.

The hormones produced by the testes, the ovaries, and the adrenal glands are regulated by the hormones of the **pituitary gland**, located at the base of the brain. This gland in turn is controlled by hormones produced by the **hypothalamus** in the brain.

Differentiation of the Embryo

The biological sex of an individual is determined by the fertilizing sperm at the time of conception. All human cells normally contain 23 pairs of chromosomes. In 22 of the pairs, the two partner chromosomes match. But in the twenty-third pair, the **sex chromosomes**, two configurations are possible. Individuals with two matching X chromosomes are female, and individuals with one X and one

Y chromosome are male. Thus, at the time of conception, the genetic sex is established: Females are XX and males are XY (see the box "Sexual Differentiation, Hormones, and the Brain" on p. 340).

Genetic sex dictates whether the undifferentiated gonads become ovaries or testes. If a Y chromosome is present, the gonads become testes; the testes will produce the male hormone **testosterone**. Testosterone circulates throughout the body and causes the undifferentiated reproductive structures to develop into male sex organs (penis, scrotum, and so on). If a Y chromosome is not present, there is no testosterone and the gonads become ovaries and the reproductive structures develop into female sex organs (clitoris, labia, and so on).

TERMS

epididymis   A storage duct for maturing sperm, located on the surface of each testis.

vas deferens (vasa deferentia, plural**)**   A tube that carries sperm from the epididymis through the prostate gland to the seminal vesicles.

prostate gland   An organ in the male reproductive system; produces some of the fluid in semen, which helps transport and nourish sperm.

seminal vesicle   A tube leading from the vas deferens to the ejaculatory duct; secretes nutrients for the semen.

ejaculatory duct   A tube that carries mature sperm to the urethra so they can exit the body on ejaculation.

Cowper's gland   In the male reproductive system, a small organ that produces preejaculatory fluid.

glans   The rounded head of the penis or the clitoris.

circumcision   Surgical removal of the foreskin of the penis.

androgens   Male sex hormones produced by the testes in males and by the adrenal glands in both sexes.

estrogens   A class of female sex hormones, produced by the ovaries, that bring about sexual maturation at puberty and maintain reproductive functions.

progestins   A class of female sex hormones, produced by the ovaries, that sustain reproductive functions.

adrenal glands   Endocrine glands, located over the kidneys, that produce androgens (among other hormones).

pituitary gland   An endocrine gland at the base of the brain that produces follicle-stimulating hormone (FSH) and luteinizing hormone (LH), among others.

hypothalamus   A region of the brain above the pituitary gland whose hormones control the secretions of the pituitary; also involved in the nervous control of sexual functions.

sex chromosomes   The X and Y chromosomes, which determine an individual's biological sex.

testosterone   The most important androgen (male sex hormone); stimulates an embryo to develop into a male and induces the development of male secondary sex characteristics during puberty.

Sexual Differentiation, Hormones, and the Brain

Males and females are different from each other in many ways, but we are also very similar. We develop from the same embryonic tissue. The presence or absence of androgens determines how the sex organs develop. The entire process is known as *sexual differentiation*.

As described in the chapter, each male and female reproductive structure develops from the same undifferentiated tissue, so every structure in one sex has its counterpart in the other. For example, the tissue that gives rise to the clitoris in females becomes the penis in males, and the tissue that gives rise to the labia majora in females becomes the scrotum in males. The appearance of the genitals is sometimes called *gonadal sex*.

Exposure to hormones affects more than just the reproductive organs; it also influences development of the brain. It has been demonstrated many times that males tend to perform better than females at tasks requiring spatial skills and females perform better than males on tests of verbal skills. If androgens are involved in this gender difference, we would expect genetic females exposed to androgens to do better at spatial skills and genetic males deprived of androgens to do worse—and this is exactly what we find.

In a condition known as androgen insensitivity syndrome, genetic males do not have cell receptors for male hormones and they develop physically as females—and their spatial skills are more like those of females than males. The converse occurs when genetic females are exposed before birth to excess male hormones. In a fascinating study of twins, it was found that in opposite-sex

pairs, female twins had a more masculine pattern of skills and behaviour compared with same-sex female twins. In opposite-sex twins, the female twin is exposed in utero to some of the androgens produced by her male twin, and these androgens influence her brain organization and thus her spatial skills.

Each person is the product of biological events that act on the cells in the body, including the brain. However, the physical and social environment then shapes this biological foundation to produce unique individuals. Some researchers point to the human past as a way to explain sex differences in language and visual-spatial skills. For example, the early division of labour with men as hunters and women as food gatherers, camp organizers, and child raisers may have selected for different skills based on gender, including visual-spatial skills in men and communication skills in women.

Sources: Cohen-Bendahan, C., et al. 2004. Prenatal exposure to testosterone and functional lateralization: A study in same-sex and opposite-sex twin girls. *Psychoneuroendocrinology* 29(7): 911–916; Sinisi, A., et al. 2003. Sexual differentiation. *Journal of Endocrinological Investigation* 26(3 Suppl.): 23–28; Joseph, R. 2000. The evolution of sex differences in language, sexuality, and visual-spatial skills. *Archives of Sexual Behavior* 29(1): 35–66.

Female Sexual Maturation

Although humans are fully sexually differentiated at birth, the differences between males and females are accentuated at **puberty**, the period during which the reproductive system matures, secondary sex characteristics develop, and the bodies of males and females begin to appear more distinctive. The changes of puberty are induced by testosterone in the male and estrogen and **progesterone** in the female.

Physical Changes The first sign of puberty in girls is breast development, followed by a rounding of the hips and buttocks. As the breasts develop, hair appears in the pubic region and later in the underarms. Shortly after the onset of breast development, girls show an increase in growth rate. Breast development usually begins between ages 8 and 13, and the time of rapid body growth occurs between ages 9 and 15.

The Menstrual Cycle A major landmark of puberty for young women is the onset of the **menstrual cycle**, the monthly ovarian cycle that leads to menstruation (loss of blood and tissue lining the uterus) in the absence of pregnancy. The timing of **menarche** (the first *menstrual period*) varies with several factors, including ethnicity, genetics, and nutritional status. The "normal" range for the onset of menstruation is wide; some girls experience menarche as young as 9 or 10, and others when they are 16 or 17 years old. The current average age of menarche in Canada is around 12.5 years of age. Two hundred years ago, the average age of menarche was closer to 17 years. The earlier onset of menarche is probably due in large part to nutritional factors. When age at menarche is examined worldwide, menarche tends to come later to girls who live in relative poverty with diets lacking in protein and calories. Obesity is strongly correlated with earlier menarche, which may explain the current trend for earlier menarche in Canada and many

other countries. Some experts worry that exposure to estrogen-like chemicals in the environment may also be contributing to earlier menarche.

The day of the onset of bleeding is day 1 of the menstrual cycle. For the purposes of our discussion, a cycle of 28 days will be used; however, normal cycles vary in length from 21 to 35 days. The menstrual cycle consists of the following four phases (Figure 11.4):

1. Menses   During **menses**, characterized by the menstrual flow, blood levels of hormones from the ovaries and the pituitary gland are relatively low. This phase of the cycle usually lasts from day one to about day five.

2. Estrogenic Phase   The estrogenic phase begins when the menstrual flow ceases and the pituitary gland begins to produce increasing amounts of follicle-stimulating hormone (FSH) and luteinizing hormone (LH). Under the influence of FSH, an egg-containing ovarian **follicle** begins to mature, producing increasingly higher amounts of estrogens. Stimulated by estrogen, the **endometrium**, the uterine lining, thickens with large numbers of blood vessels and uterine glands.

3. Ovulation   A surge of a potent estrogen called *estradiol* from the follicle causes the pituitary to release a large burst of LH and a smaller amount of FSH. The high concentration of LH stimulates the developing follicle to release its ovum. This event is known as **ovulation**. After ovulation, the follicle is transformed into the **corpus luteum**, which produces progesterone and estrogen. Ovulation usually occurs about 14 days before the onset of menstrual flow,

Once they reach puberty, these adolescents are biologically adults, but it will take several more years for them to become adults in social and psychological terms.

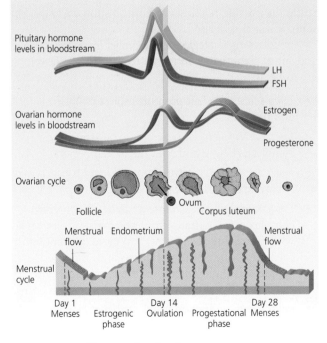

FIGURE 11.4   The menstrual cycle.

a fact that can be used to predict the most fertile time during the menstrual cycle, useful in both fertility treatment and natural family planning methods.

4. Progestational Phase During the progestational phase of the cycle, the amount of progesterone secreted from the corpus luteum increases and remains high until the onset of the next menses. Under the influence of estrogen and progesterone, the endometrium continues to develop, readying itself to receive and nourish a fertilized ovum. When pregnancy occurs, the fertilized egg produces the hormone human chorionic gonadotropin (HCG), which maintains the corpus luteum. Thus, levels of ovarian hormones remain high and the uterine lining is preserved, preventing menses.

If pregnancy does not occur, the corpus luteum degenerates, and estrogen and progesterone levels gradually fall. Below certain hormonal levels, the endometrium can no longer be maintained, and it begins to slough off, initiating menses. As the levels of ovarian hormones fall, a slight rise in LH and FSH occurs, and a new menstrual cycle begins.

MENSTRUAL PROBLEMS Menstruation is a normal biological process, but it may cause physical or psychological problems. **Dysmenorrhea** is characterized by cramps in the lower abdomen, backache, vomiting, nausea, a bloated feeling, diarrhea, and loss of appetite. Some of these symptoms can be attributed to uterine muscular contractions caused by chemicals called *prostaglandins*. Any drug that blocks the effects of prostaglandins, such as Aspirin or ibuprofen, will usually alleviate some of the symptoms of dysmenorrhea.

Many women experience transient physical and emotional symptoms before the onset of their menstrual flow. Depending on their severity, these symptoms may be categorized along a continuum from **premenstrual tension** through **premenstrual syndrome (PMS)** to **premenstrual dysphoric disorder (PMDD)**. Premenstrual tension symptoms are mild and may include negative mood changes and physical symptoms, such as abdominal cramping and backache. More severe symptoms are classified as PMS; very severe symptoms that cause impairment in social functioning and work-related activities are classified as PMDD. All three conditions share a definite pattern: Symptoms appear before the onset of menses and disappear within a few days after the start of menstruation.

Symptoms associated with PMS and PMDD include physical changes, such as breast tenderness, water retention (bloating), headache, and fatigue; insomnia or excessive sleep; appetite changes and food cravings; irritability, anger, and increased interpersonal conflict; mood swings; depression and sadness; anxiety and tearfulness; inability to concentrate; social withdrawal; and the sense that one is out of control or overwhelmed. The key to diagnosing PMS and PMDD is to keep a daily diary of symptoms over several menstrual cycles. PMDD is distinguished from PMS by the severity of symptoms, which in PMDD interfere significantly with work or school and with usual social activities and relationships.

Despite many research studies, the causes of PMS and PMDD are still unknown, and it is unclear why some women are more vulnerable than others. Research has focused on a variety of substances in the body that may fluctuate with the menstrual cycle. Most researchers feel that PMS is probably caused by a combination of hormonal, nutritional, and psychological factors.

Selective serotonin reuptake inhibitors (SSRIs), including Zoloft, Paxil, and Celexa, are the first-line treatment for PMDD. Until recently, women using SSRIs took the medication throughout the entire menstrual cycle, but it has now been shown that taking the medication during just the progestational phase of the cycle is similarly effective. Progestational phase use reduces the exposure to the drug and its associated side effects. Antianxiety medications and progesterone have also been tested for progestational phase administration but show little positive effect in easing symptoms.

Other drug treatments include estrogen, certain oral contraceptives, diuretics to minimize water retention, and drugs, such as Aspirin, ibuprofen, and more potent prescription prostaglandin inhibitors, that block the effects of prostaglandins. In 2009, the Yaz birth control pill was approved by Health Canada. In addition to birth control, Yaz can help to reduce PMDD. Yaz, and a similar oral contraceptive, Yasmin, contain drospirenone, a synthetic progestin that is similar to natural progesterone and has a diuretic effect that seems to counteract some premenstrual symptoms. Yaz can also reduce moderate acne in women who want an oral contraceptive for birth control. A number of vitamins, minerals, and other dietary supplements have also been studied for PMS relief. Only one supplement, calcium, has been shown in rigorous clinical studies to provide relief; several others show promise, but more research is needed.

The following strategies provide relief for many women, and all of them can contribute to a healthy lifestyle at any time:

- *Limit salt intake.* Salt promotes water retention and bloating.

- *Exercise.* Women who exercise experience fewer symptoms before and after menstrual periods.

- *Don't use alcohol or tobacco.* Alcohol and tobacco may aggravate certain symptoms of PMS and PMDD.

- *Eat a nutritious diet.* Choose a low-fat diet rich in complex carbohydrates from vegetables, fruits, and whole grain breads, cereals, and pasta. Get enough calcium from calcium-rich foods and, if needed, supplements. Minimize your intake of sugar and caffeine, and avoid chocolate, which is rich in both.

- *Relax.* Stress reduction is always beneficial, and stressful events can trigger PMS symptoms. Try relaxation techniques during the premenstrual time.

If symptoms persist, keep a daily diary to track both the types of symptoms you experience and their severity. See your physician for an evaluation and to learn more about treatments that are available only with a prescription.

Male Sexual Maturation

Reproductive maturation of boys occurs about two years later than that of girls; it usually begins at about age 10 or 11.

Testicular growth is usually the first obvious sign of sexual maturity in boys. The penis also grows at this time, reaching adult size by about age 18. Pubic hair begins to develop after the genitals begin to increase in size, with underarm and facial hair gradually appearing. Hair on the chest, back, and abdomen increases later in development. The voice deepens as a result of the lengthening and thickening of the vocal chords. A small amount of breast development occurs in many boys during puberty. This is called *gynecomastia*, and it usually decreases after puberty. Excessive breast growth can occur in some boys, especially if they are overweight. Boys grow taller for about six years after the first signs of puberty, with a very rapid period of growth about two years after puberty starts.

Acne A not-so-welcome aspect of puberty for many boys and girls is the development of acne, technically called *acne vulgaris*. During adolescence, acne is typically worse in males; in adulthood, women tend to have more acne than men. The production of male hormones in puberty is the initial trigger for acne in most boys and girls. Acne is caused by multiple factors, including hormones, excess oil production, plugging of hair follicles (pores), infection with the bacterium *Propionibacterium acnes*, and inflammation. Fortunately, many treatments for acne exist, making control of this skin disease possible in nearly all cases.

Aging and Human Sexuality

Changes in hormone production and sexual functioning occur as we age. As a woman approaches age 50, her ovaries gradually cease to function and she enters **menopause**, the cessation of menstruation. For some women, the associated drop in hormone production causes symptoms that are troublesome. The most common physical symptom of menopause is hot flashes, sensations of warmth rising to the face from the upper chest, with or without perspiration and chills. Other symptoms include headaches, dizziness, palpitations, and joint pains. Osteoporosis—decreasing bone density—can develop, making older women more vulnerable to fractures. Some menopausal women become moody, even markedly depressed, and they may also experience fatigue, irritability, and forgetfulness.

To alleviate the symptoms of menopause and reduce the risk of heart disease and osteoporosis, millions of women have been prescribed hormone therapy (HT), a regimen of hormones that includes estrogen and progesterone. In 2002, an ongoing study of HT involving more than 16,000 women was halted because the women in the study who had been taking HT for long periods had more strokes, heart attacks, and blood clots and had a higher incidence of breast cancer than women in the study taking a placebo. The risks for such health problems were small but significant enough to halt the study. The positive findings from this study were a reduction in hip fractures and a reduced risk of colon cancer among the women taking HT. Many women who were taking HT stopped and many more never started as a result of the publicity surrounding the 2002 study. In 2007, analysis of data on breast cancer in Canada showed a decline in 2003 and 2004, possibly because fewer women took HT (although other factors may also be responsible for the decline in breast cancer). At around the same time, scientists reanalyzed the original 2002 data on HT and found that women who started HT close to the time of menopause tended to have a reduced risk of cardiovascular disease, while women who took HT several years after going through menopause had a higher risk of heart disease. As a result of these findings, women taking HT were advised to consult their health care providers about their personal risks and benefits. (See Chapters 5, 7, 8, and 17 for more information on osteoporosis, heart disease, breast cancer, and HT.)

As a result of decreased estrogen production during menopause, the vaginal walls become thin, and lubrication in response to sexual arousal diminishes; sexual intercourse may become painful. Hormonal treatment or the use of lubricants during intercourse can minimize these problems.

TERMS

dysmenorrhea   Painful or problematic menstruation.

premenstrual tension   Mild physical and emotional changes associated with the time before the onset of menses; symptoms can include abdominal cramping and backache.

premenstrual syndrome (PMS)   A disorder characterized by physical discomfort, psychological distress, and behavioural changes that begin after ovulation and cease when menstruation begins.

premenstrual dysphoric disorder (PMDD)   Severe form of PMS, characterized by symptoms serious enough to interfere with work or school or with social activities and relationships.

menopause   The cessation of menstruation, occurring gradually around age 50.

Although sexual physiology changes as people get older, many men and women readily adjust to these alterations.

QUESTIONS FOR CRITICAL THINKING AND REFLECTION
Think about your own experience as you matured sexually during puberty and adolescence. In what ways did these changes affect your life? How did they contribute to the person you are today?

combine medication with a testosterone gel applied to the skin; see the section on sexual dysfunction later in the chapter for more information.

Unlike women, who are born with all the eggs they will ever have and stop being fertile at menopause, men continue to produce sperm throughout their lives and can sometimes father children when they are well into their eighties and even nineties. Starting at about age 30, however, men become gradually less fertile. Regardless of the age of their female partners, couples in which the male is over age 35 have a 50% lower pregnancy rate than couples in which the man is 30 years old or younger. Men who are over age 40 are more likely to produce children with health problems, such as autism, schizophrenia, and Down syndrome.

As women and men age, sexual activity can continue to be a source of pleasure and satisfaction for them. A recent study of sexuality in older adults found that three-fourths of those 57–64 years old were sexually active (defined as having at least one sexual partner in the last year). Half of those 65–74 years old, and about one-fourth of those 75–85, remained sexually active.

SEXUAL FUNCTIONING

In this section, we discuss sexual physiology—how the sex organs function during sexual activity—and problems that can occur with sexual functioning. Sexual activity is based on stimulus and response. Erotic stimulation leads to sexual arousal (excitement), which may culminate in the intensely pleasurable experience of orgasm. But sexual activity should not be thought of only in terms of the sex organs. Responses to sexual stimulation involve not just the genitals but the entire body—and the mind as well.

Sexual Stimulation

Sexual excitement can come from many sources, both physical and psychological. Although physical stimuli have an obvious and direct effect, some people believe psychological stimuli—thoughts, fantasies, desires, perceptions—are even more powerfully erotic. Regardless of the source of erotic stimuli, all stimulation has a physical basis, which is given meaning by the brain.

Between the ages of 35 and 65, men experience a gradual decline in testosterone production resulting in the aging male syndrome, sometimes referred to as *male menopause* or *andropause*. Experts generally prefer the term *aging male syndrome* because the process is much more gradual than female menopause. Symptoms vary widely among men, but most men experience at least some of the following symptoms as they age: loss of muscle mass, increased fat mass, decreased sex drive, erectile problems, depressed mood, irritability, difficulties with concentration, increased urination, loss of bone mineral density, and sleep difficulties. In some cases, treatment with testosterone can help. Although taking testosterone can be very harmful in young healthy men, older men with low testosterone levels may benefit from carefully prescribed testosterone treatment.

As men get older, they depend more on direct physical stimulation for sexual arousal. They take longer to achieve an erection and find it more difficult to maintain one; orgasmic contractions are less intense. Older men with erectile dysfunction are often prescribed medications, such as Viagra, or even more successful therapies that

Physical Stimulation Physical stimulation comes through the senses: We are aroused by things we see, hear, taste, smell, and feel. Most often, sexual stimuli come from other people, but they may also come from books, photographs, paintings, songs, films, or other sources.

The most obvious and effective physical stimulation is touching. Even though culturally defined practices vary and individual people have different preferences, most sexual encounters eventually involve some form of touching with hands, lips, and body surfaces. Kissing, caressing, fondling, and hugging are as much a part of sexual encounters as they are of expressing affection.

The most intense form of stimulation by touching involves the genitals. The clitoris and the glans of the penis are particularly sensitive to such stimulation. Other highly responsive areas include the vaginal opening, the nipples, the breasts, the insides of the thighs, the buttocks, the anal region, the scrotum, the lips, and the earlobes. Such sexually sensitive areas, or **erogenous zones**, are especially susceptible to sexual arousal for most people, most of the time. Often, though, what determines the response is not *what* is touched but how, for how long, and by whom. Under the right circumstances, touching any part of the body can cause sexual arousal.

Psychological Stimulation Sexual arousal also has an important psychological component, regardless of the nature of the physical stimulation. Fantasies, ideas, memories of past experiences, and mood can all generate sexual excitement. Erotic thoughts may be linked to an imagined person or situation or to a sexual experience from the past. Fantasies may involve activities a person doesn't actually want to experience in reality, usually because they're dangerous, frightening, or forbidden.

Arousal is also powerfully influenced by emotions. How you feel about a person and how the person feels about you matter tremendously in how sexually responsive you are likely to be. Even the most direct forms of physical stimulation carry emotional overtones. Kissing, caressing, and fondling express affection and caring. The emotional charge they give to a sexual interaction is at least as significant to sexual arousal as the purely physical stimulation achieved by touching.

The Sexual Response Cycle

Men and women respond physiologically with a predictable set of reactions, regardless of the nature of the stimulation.

Two physiological mechanisms explain most genital and bodily reactions during sexual arousal and orgasm. These mechanisms are vasocongestion and muscular tension. **Vasocongestion** is the engorgement of tissues that results when more blood flows into an organ than is flowing out. Thus, the penis becomes erect on the same principle that makes a garden hose become stiff when the water is turned on. Increased muscular tension culminates in rhythmical muscular contractions during orgasm.

In the late 1960s, Masters and Johnson first identified the four phases that characterize the sexual response cycle, and these four phases are still known to be accurate today:

1. In the *excitement phase*, the penis becomes erect as its tissues become engorged with blood. The testes expand and are pulled upward within the scrotum. In women, the clitoris, labia, and vaginal walls are similarly engorged with blood. Tension increases in the vaginal muscles, and the vaginal walls become moist with lubricating fluid.

2. The *plateau phase* is an extension of the excitement phase. Reactions become more marked. In men, the penis becomes harder, and the testes become larger. In women, the lower part of the vagina swells, as its upper end expands and vaginal lubrication increases.

3. In the *orgasmic phase*, or **orgasm**, rhythmic contractions occur along the man's penis, urethra, prostate gland, seminal vesicles, and muscles in the pelvic and anal regions. These involuntary muscular contractions lead to the ejaculation of **semen**, which consists of sperm cells from the testes and secretions from the prostate gland and seminal vesicles. In women, contractions occur in the lower part of the vagina and in the uterus, as well as in the pelvic region and the anus.

4. In the *resolution phase*, all the changes initiated during the excitement phase are reversed. Excess blood drains from tissues, the muscles in the region relax, and the genital structures return to their unstimulated state.

More general physical reactions accompany the genital changes in both men and women. Beginning with the excitement phase, nipples become erect, the woman's breasts begin to swell, and in both sexes the skin of the chest becomes flushed; these changes are more marked in women. The heart rate doubles by the plateau phase, and respiration becomes faster. During orgasm, breathing becomes irregular and the person may moan or cry out. A feeling of warmth leads to increased sweating during the resolution phase. Deep relaxation and a sense of well-being pervade the body and the mind.

---

erogenous zone Any region of the body highly responsive to sexual stimulation.

vasocongestion The accumulation of blood in tissues and organs.

orgasm The discharge of accumulated sexual tension with characteristic genital and bodily manifestations and a subjective sensation of intense pleasure.

semen Seminal fluid, consisting of sperm cells and secretions from the prostate gland and seminal vesicles.

Male and female reactions during the sexual response cycle differ somewhat. Generally, the male pattern is more uniform, whereas the female pattern is more varied. For instance, the female excitement phase may lead directly to orgasm, or orgasmic and plateau phases may be fused.

Male orgasm is marked by the ejaculation of semen. After ejaculation, men enter a *refractory period*, during which they cannot be restimulated to orgasm. Women do not have a refractory period, and immediate restimulation to orgasm is possible for some women.

Sexual Problems

Both physical and psychological factors can interfere with sexual functioning. Disturbances in sexual desire, performance, or satisfaction are referred to as **sexual dysfunctions**.

Common Sexual Health Problems Some problems with sexual functioning are due to treatable or preventable infections or other sexual health problems. Conditions that affect women include the following:

• *Vaginitis*, inflammation of the vagina, is caused by a variety of organisms: *Candida* (yeast infection), *Trichomonas* (trichomoniasis), and the overgrowth of a variety of bacteria (bacterial vaginosis). Symptoms include vaginal discharge, vaginal irritation, and pain during intercourse. (See Chapters 9 and 13 for more information.)

• *Endometriosis* is the growth of endometrial tissue (tissue normally found lining the uterus) outside the uterus. It occurs most often in women of childbearing age, and pain in the lower abdomen and pelvis is the most common symptom. Pain with premenstrual intercourse may occur. Endometriosis can cause serious problems if left untreated because the endometrial tissue can scar and partially or completely block the oviducts, causing infertility (difficulty conceiving) or sterility (the inability to conceive). Endometriosis is treated with hormone therapy or surgery.

• *Pelvic inflammatory disease (PID)* is an infection of the uterus, oviducts, or ovaries caused when microorganisms spread to these areas from the vagina. Approximately 50%–75% of PID cases are caused by sexually transmitted

organisms associated with diseases, such as gonorrhea and chlamydia. PID can cause scarring of the oviducts, resulting in infertility or sterility. Symptoms include pain in the abdomen and pelvis, fever, and possibly pain during intercourse. Sexually transmitted infections are discussed in detail in Chapter 13.

Sexual health problems that affect men include the following:

• *Prostatitis* is inflammation or infection of the prostate gland. Prostatitis can be acute (sudden) or chronic (gradual and long-lasting). The symptoms of *acute bacterial prostatitis* usually appear suddenly and may include fever, chills, flulike symptoms, pain in the lower back or groin, problems with urination, and painful ejaculation. Acute prostatitis is treated with antibiotics. It is potentially serious, so any man with these symptoms needs to seek immediate medical attention.

• *Chronic prostatitis* is more common in men over age 40. It can be caused by infection or inflammation of the prostate and is sometimes difficult to diagnose and treat.

• *Testicular cancer* occurs most commonly in men in their twenties and thirties. A rare cancer, it has a very high cure rate if detected early. Every man should perform testicular self-exams regularly (see Chapter 8).

Sexual Dysfunctions The term *sexual dysfunction* encompasses disturbances in sexual desire, performance, or satisfaction. A wide variety of physical conditions and drugs may interfere with sexual functioning; psychological causes and problems in intimate relationships can be important factors in many cases.

COMMON SEXUAL DYSFUNCTIONS Common sexual dysfunctions in men include **erectile dysfunction** (previously called *impotence*), the inability to have or maintain an erection sufficient for sexual intercourse; **premature ejaculation**, ejaculation before or just on penetration of the vagina or anus; and **retarded ejaculation**, the inability to ejaculate once an erection is achieved. Many men experience occasional difficulty achieving an erection or ejaculating because of excessive alcohol consumption, fatigue, or stress.

Female sexual problems generally involve either a lack of desire to have sex, the failure to become physically aroused even when sex is desired, the failure to have an orgasm (**orgasmic dysfunction**), or pain during sexual contact. All of these problems can have physical and psychological components. Many medical problems can influence a woman's desire and ability to respond sexually. Hormonal factors, especially menopause, also have a major influence. Psychological and social issues, such as relationship difficulties, family stresses, depression, and past sexual trauma, are all frequent causes of sexual dysfunction.

Orgasmic dysfunction has been the subject of a great deal of discussion over the years, as people debated the nature of the female orgasm and what constitutes dysfunction in

TERMS

sexual dysfunction A disturbance in sexual desire, performance, or satisfaction.

erectile dysfunction The inability to have or maintain an erection.

premature ejaculation Involuntary orgasm before or shortly after the penis enters the vagina or anus; ejaculation that takes place sooner than desired.

retarded ejaculation The inability to ejaculate when desired during intercourse.

orgasmic dysfunction The inability to experience orgasm.

women. Many women experience orgasm but not during intercourse, or they experience orgasm during intercourse only if the clitoris is directly stimulated at the same time. In general, the inability to experience orgasm under certain circumstances is a problem only if the woman considers it so.

TREATING SEXUAL DYSFUNCTION   Most forms of sexual dysfunction are treatable. The first step is to have a physical examination to find a possible medical cause. Heart disease and diabetes, for example, may cause erectile dysfunction; in fact, erectile dysfunction is often the first sign of a serious medical condition. This is one reason men who buy drugs online to treat their erectile dysfunction without first getting a good medical evaluation may be missing out on the opportunity to diagnose and treat a potentially life-threatening disease. Up to 80% of all erectile problems are thought to be due to physical factors, particularly vascular problems involving restriction of blood flow. Smoking affects blood flow in the penis and is an independent risk factor for erectile dysfunction.

Alcohol and many prescription and nonprescription drugs can inhibit sexual response. In particular, antidepressant drugs (especially the widely used SSRIs, such as Prozac) are believed to cause sexual dysfunction in up to half the people who take them. Switching to a different antidepressant often helps, and sometimes other drugs, such as Viagra, are used to counteract the side effects of antidepressants.

Other common medications that can inhibit sexual response include certain drugs that treat high blood pressure. Patients are sometimes reluctant to tell their physician that they are having sexual problems and may even stop taking their blood pressure medication for this reason. Letting the doctor know about sexual and other side effects is crucial because most of the time the problem can be solved by switching to a different medication. Newer antihypertensive drugs are highly effective and do not usually have sexual side effects.

Many treatments are available, particularly for erectile dysfunction. In 1999, Viagra (sildenafil citrate), the first-ever prescription pill for erectile dysfunction, was approved for use by Health Canada. Since then, two other oral medications with actions similar to Viagra, Cialis (tadalafil) and Levitra (vardenafil), have been approved. All three work by enhancing the effects of nitric oxide, a chemical that relaxes smooth muscles in the penis. This increases the amount of blood flow and allows a natural erection to occur in response to sexual stimulation. The medications are generally safe for healthy men, but they should not be used by men who have a high risk of heart attack or stroke. They are effective in about 70% of users, but they have potential side effects, including headaches, indigestion, facial flushing, back pain, visual and hearing disturbances, and changes in blood pressure. Viagra, Cialis, and Levitra should never be taken by anyone who takes nitrate medication (usually prescribed for heart problems). Also, the

recreational drugs amyl nitrate or nitrite (sometimes called "poppers") should never be combined with drugs for erectile dysfunction. The combination of nitrates and Viagra-like drugs can cause a sudden potentially lethal drop in blood pressure.

Viagra use by men between the ages of 18 and 45 has risen dramatically—possibly because use of the drug for recreational purposes (see Figure 11.5). The drug may cut the refractory period in men who do not have erectile dysfunction; younger men may also be using it to cope with performance anxiety or the effects of other drugs, such as antidepressants.

Although Viagra is not approved for use by women, a growing number of women are trying the drug. Research findings are mixed as to whether Viagra can increase sex drive and satisfaction levels in women. Recent studies have shown, however, that the drug can help women with sexual dysfunction caused by their use of antidepressant drugs.

Other treatments for erectile dysfunction in men are available. Medications, with the active ingredient alprostadil, can be administered with a fine needle into the penis or placed into the tip of the penis as a tiny suppository about the size of a grain of rice; it works by relaxing the smooth

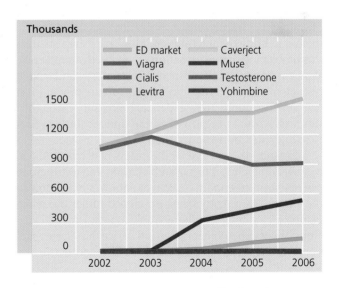

FIGURE 11.5   Prescription trends in medications for erectile dysfunction.

Source: Prescription trends (Canadian Pharmacists Association—*Guide to Drugs Canada*). As cited in IMS Health, Canada, CompuScript and Canadian Disease and Therapeutic Index. © 2006 IMS Health Canada (www.imsbrogan.com).

muscles lining the blood vessels in the penis. A topical cream can also be applied to the penis to improve erectile function. For a small number of men with testosterone deficiency, hormone replacement therapy is an option. There are also vacuum devices that pull blood into the penis, and in cases where other treatments are unsuccessful, penile implants can be used. Exercise may also help improve erectile function, especially exercises that target the muscles of the pelvic floor.

Even when sexual dysfunction has a physical cause, emotional and social factors frequently compound the problem. Many people with no obvious physical disorder have sexual problems because of psychological and social issues. Too often, sexual difficulties are treated with drugs when nondrug strategies may be more appropriate. Psychosocial causes of dysfunction include troubled relationships, a lack of sexual skills, irrational attitudes and beliefs, anxiety, and psychosexual trauma, such as sexual abuse or rape. Many of these problems can be addressed by sex therapy. A therapist may recommend books or films to help counter sexual myths and teach sexual skills. A therapist can also promote open discussion between partners and suggest specific techniques.

Women who seek treatment for orgasmic dysfunction often have not learned what types of stimulation will excite them and bring them to orgasm. Most sex therapists treat this problem with **masturbation** (genital self-stimulation). Women are taught about their own anatomy and sexual responses and then are encouraged to experiment with masturbation until they experience orgasm. Once they can masturbate to orgasm, they can transfer this learning to sexual intercourse with a partner.

Substances being tested for the treatment of female sexual dysfunction include prostaglandin creams and testosterone patches. A prostaglandin cream that improves blood flow to the clitoris is currently being developed under the name Femprox, and may soon be available to treat female sexual arousal disorder. Another option is a device that creates suction over the clitoris to increase blood flow and sensitivity.

SEXUAL BEHAVIOUR

Many behaviours stem from sexual impulses, and sexual expression takes a variety of forms. Probably the most basic aspect of sexuality is reproduction. But sexual excitement and satisfaction are aspects of sexual behaviour separate from reproduction. The intensely pleasurable sensations of arousal and orgasm are probably the strongest motivators for human sexual behaviour. People are infinitely varied in the ways they seek to experience erotic pleasure.

The Development of Sexual Behaviour

Sexual behaviour is a product of many factors, including genetics, physiology, psychology, and social and cultural influences. Our behaviour is shaped by the interplay of our biological predispositions and our life experiences.

Gender Roles and Gender Identity   As mentioned in Chapters 3 and 10, your *gender role* is everything you do in your daily life that expresses your maleness or femaleness to others, including dress, speech patterns, and mannerisms. Your **gender identity** is your personal, inner sense of being male or female.

Biological sex, gender role, and gender identity are usually in agreement, but some people experience conflict among them. For example, a male who feels trapped in the body of a male and who wants to be a female appears to others as a male, but his gender identity is that of a female. The umbrella term *transgender* is often used to describe any individual whose appearance, personal characteristics, or behaviour differs from the social and cultural norms for males and females. Transgender individuals include the following:

- *Transsexual* men and women, who feel their biological sex does not match their gender identity. Transsexuals may seek sex reassignment, which involves surgery to change the appearance of the genitals and hormonal treatments to induce secondary sex characteristics, such as breasts or facial hair.

- *Transvestites*, who enjoy wearing clothing identified with the other gender. Cross-dressing covers a broad range of behaviours, from wearing one article of clothing of the other sex in a private location to wearing an entire outfit in public.

- *Intersexed individuals*, who were born with ambiguous genitals—neither fully female nor fully male—because of genetic or hormonal abnormalities. Intersexed individuals may or may not have undergone surgery as infants to assign them to a particular sex.

- Men or women, regardless of sexual orientation, whose appearance, characteristics, or behaviour is perceived as gender atypical in their society or culture.

BIOLOGICAL AND CULTURAL INFLUENCES   Some gender characteristics are determined biologically, such as the genitals a person is born with and the secondary sex characteristics that develop at puberty. Others are defined by society and learned in the course of growing up. From birth, children are encouraged to behave in ways their culture

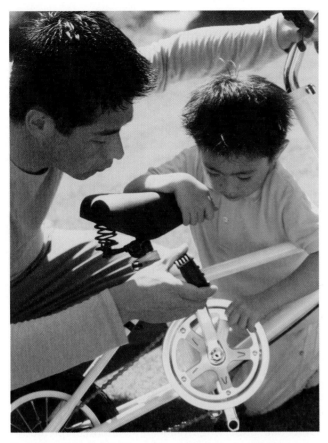
Our sense of gender identity and many of our gender-role behaviours are overwhelmingly influenced by cultural factors. This young boy is learning gender-specific behaviours by imitating his father.

deems appropriate for one sex or the other. In Canadian society, parents usually give children gender-specific names, clothes, and toys, and children may model their own behaviour after their same-sex parent. Family and friends create an environment that teaches the child how to act appropriately as a girl or a boy. Teachers, television, books, and even strangers model these gender roles.

Gender roles vary from one society to another and from one time to another. In Canada today, for example, many women shave their legs and wear makeup; in some Muslim countries, women wear robes and veils that conceal their face and body. Each set of behaviours expresses some learned aspect of the female gender role in that society, and each set may be inappropriate in the other society. Standards of sexual attractiveness also vary from one culture to another.

An extreme example of how cultural traditions can affect gender roles and sexual activity is female genital mutilation, or "female circumcision." Each year in 28 African countries, parts of Asia and the Middle East, and immigrant communities elsewhere, 3 million female children undergo this procedure. In some cases, only the hood of the clitoris is removed. In others, the entire clitoris, the labia minora, and parts of the labia majora are removed.

The sides of the labia majora may be sewn together, leaving only a small opening for the passage of urine and menstrual blood. The effects of these painful procedures can include bleeding, infection, the inability to enjoy sex, and infertility. Women who have endured genital mutilation commonly have difficulty during labour and childbirth. Children of such women are at far greater risk of dying during or after childbirth.

The practice probably developed as a way of controlling women's sexuality and ensuring that a woman would be a virgin when she married. After marriage, her husband reopens the labia to allow intercourse and childbirth.

Many countries now have laws against female genital mutilation. The WHO and other groups are trying to educate people about the negative medical consequences of this practice.

GENDER-ROLE FLEXIBILITY Historically, gender roles have tended to emphasize the differences between males and females, but new gender roles are emerging in our society that reflect more of a mix of male and female characteristics and behaviours. This tendency toward **androgyny** greatly broadens the range of experiences available to both males and females. Androgynous adults are less stereotyped in their thinking; in how they look, dress, and act; in how they divide work in the home; in how they think about jobs and careers; and in how they express themselves sexually. Women in our society today are able, and even expected, to be much more assertive, competitive, ambitious, and powerful than they were allowed to be in the past; likewise, men can be more sensitive, articulate, nurturing, and emotionally expressive.

Gender, Sexuality, and the Mass Media Many of our ideas about sexuality and gender roles are shaped by the mass media. Media images of sexuality are often more influential than the family in shaping the sexual attitudes and behaviours of adolescents and university students. Yet these images are usually unrealistic and help perpetuate stereotypes of women and men in our

TERMS

masturbation   Self-stimulation for the purpose of sexual arousal and orgasm.

gender identity   A person's personal, internal sense of maleness or femaleness.

androgyny   The state of being neither overtly male nor female.

society. The mass media rarely portray people negotiating safer sex or communicating seriously about other sexual issues.

Childhood Sexual Behaviour   The capacity to respond sexually is present at birth. Ultrasound studies suggest that boys experience erections in the uterus. After birth, both sexes have the capacity for orgasm, though many babies may not experience it. As people grow, many discover this capacity through self-exploration. Sexual behaviours gradually emerge in childhood; self-exploration and touching the genitals are common forms of play, observed among infants as young as six months. They gradually lead to more deliberate forms of masturbation, with or without orgasm.

Children often engage in sexual play with playmates by exploring each other's genitals. These activities are often part of games like "playing house" or "playing doctor." By age 12, 40% of boys have engaged in sex play; the peak exploration age for girls is 9, by which time 14% have had such experiences.

Adolescent Sexuality   A person who has experienced puberty is biologically an adult. But in psychological and social terms, people take five to ten more years to attain full adult status. This discrepancy between biological and social maturity creates considerable confusion over what constitutes appropriate sexual behaviour during adolescence.

Sexual fantasies and dreams become more common and explicit in adolescence than at earlier ages, often as an accompaniment to masturbation. Research has shown that about 80% of teenage boys and 55% of teenage girls masturbate more or less regularly. Once puberty is reached, orgasm in boys is accompanied by ejaculation. Teenage boys also experience **nocturnal emissions** ("wet dreams"). Some girls also have orgasmic dreams.

Sexual interaction during adolescence usually takes place between peers in the context of dating. Sexual intimacy is usually expressed in such relationships through petting and necking, which may involve kissing, caressing, and stimulating the breasts and genitals. These activities lead to arousal but may not culminate in orgasm.

Many Canadian teenagers also engage in premarital sexual relations. Recent surveys indicate that the average age of first sexual intercourse in Canada is about 16.5 years old. Twenty-eight percent of 15–19-year-olds in Canada have had sex at least once. Rates for premarital sex vary considerably from one group to another, however, based on ethnic, educational, socioeconomic, religious, geographic, and other factors. First-time intercourse is affected by these same factors, plus psychological readiness, fear of consequences, being in love, going steady, peer pressure, and the need to act like an adult, gain popularity, or rebel. A mother's relationship with her daughter influences the timing of first intercourse. Girls who perceive that their mother disapproves of their having sex are more likely to delay first intercourse.

Adolescent sexual behaviours are not confined to heterosexual relationships. Beginning in childhood, sex play involves members of one's own sex as well as of the other sex. Same-sex attractions, with or without sexual encounters, are common in adolescence. For many these are youthful experiments and don't mean that participants will ultimately be gay or lesbian. For some, they may be a factor in adult sexual orientation. Most adult gay men and women trace their orientation to childhood.

Adult Sexuality   Early adulthood is a time when people make important life choices—a time of increasing responsibility in terms of interpersonal relationships and family life (see the box "Sexual Decision Making"). In recent years, there has been a trend toward marriage at a later age than in past decades. And before marriage, more young adults are driven by a need to become sexually knowledgeable (see the box "Sexual Activity Among Postsecondary Students" on p. 352). Today, more people in their twenties believe that becoming sexually experienced rather than preserving virginity is an important prelude to selecting a mate. Take the quiz in the box "Your Sexual Attitudes" (on p. 353) to explore your own beliefs and opinions about sex.

Individual motivations for engaging in sexual activities change with age. Younger men state that they engage in sex for physical reasons, whereas women of the same age state that they engage in sex for emotional reasons. As men and women get older, their motives change; men more often engage in sex for emotional reasons, and women more often for physical reasons. In the oldest age groups, women's and men's motives for sex are actually the reverse of those of the earliest age groups. In addition to age, other factors, such as ethnicity, educational attainment, and living arrangements, also influence adult choices about sexuality.

Sexuality in Illness and Disability   Any disease or disability that affects mobility, well-being, self-esteem, or body image has the potential to affect sexual expression. People with chronic diseases or disabilities often have special needs regarding their sexual behaviour. They may also confront the perception that they are asexual. Sexuality is integral to all of us, regardless of our physical status.

The diagnosis of a chronic illness or the onset of a disability usually requires major adjustments in many areas of life, including sexuality. At first, sexual activity may take a low priority because of fear and the loss of self-esteem. Individuals and couples can learn to become creative about sexual expression and develop new approaches based on the limitations of the disability.

nocturnal emissions   Orgasm and ejaculation (wet dream) during sleep.

Sexual Decision Making

Choosing to have sex can change a relationship and a person's life. In making decisions about sexual activity, you owe it to yourself and your partner to think and talk honestly about your choices. Consider the following issues:

• *Your background, beliefs, and goals.* What are your religious, moral, or personal values regarding relationships and sex? What are your priorities at this time, and how will a sexual relationship fit into your goals and plans for the future? Are you physically, emotionally, and financially ready to accept the potential consequences of the choices you make?

• *Your relationship with your partner.* How do you feel about your partner and your relationship? Do you respect and trust each other? Do you feel comfortable talking about sexual issues, and

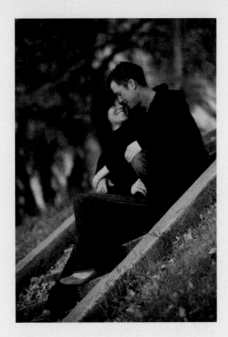

have you discussed contraception, pregnancy, and safer sex? How do you think having sex will affect your relationship and how you feel about yourself and your partner? What does having sex mean to each of you?

• *Your reasons for having sex.* What reasons do you have for moving into a sexual relationship? Are you being honest with yourself and your partner about this?

Personal decisions about sex should always be respected. You have the right to make your own choices and to do only what you feel comfortable with. When you make choices about sex based on self-respect, along with physical, emotional, and spiritual considerations, you'll be more likely to feel good about your decisions—now and in the future.

Developing a positive body image is often a particularly important, and difficult, adjustment for people with physical illness or limitations.

Sexual Orientation

Sexual orientation is a consistent pattern of emotional and sexual attraction based on biological sex. It exists along a continuum that ranges from being exclusively heterosexual (attracted to people of the other sex) through being bisexual (attracted to people of both sexes) to being exclusively gay or lesbian (attracted to people of your own sex). The term *straight* is often used to refer to heterosexuals and the preferred terms in the gay community are *gay men* (for men), *gay people* (for both men and women), and *lesbians* (for women). The terms *homosexual* and *homosexuality* are outdated and offensive to many gay people.

Sexual orientation involves feelings and self-concept, and individuals may or may not express their sexual orientation in their behaviour. In national surveys, about 2%–6% of men identify themselves as gay and about 1.5% of women identify themselves as lesbians. It is difficult to gauge the accuracy of these estimates because people may not tell the truth in surveys that probe very sensitive and private aspects of their lives.

Heterosexuality The great majority of people are heterosexual. The heterosexual lifestyle usually includes all the behaviour and relationship patterns described in Chapter 10: dating, engagement or living together, and marriage.

Same-Sex Attraction Same-sex attraction exists in almost all cultures. The major difference between heterosexuals and gay people is in their sex partners. Gay people are as varied and different from one another as are heterosexuals. Just like heterosexuals, lesbians and gay men may be in long-term, committed relationships or they may date different people.

Bisexuality Some bisexual individuals are involved with partners of both sexes at the same time, whereas others may alternate between same-sex partners and partners of the other sex ("serial bisexuality"). The largest group of bisexuals consists of married men who have secret sexual involvements with men but who rarely have female sexual contacts outside marriage.

The Origins of Sexual Orientation Many theories try to account for the development of sexual orientation. At this time, most experts agree that sexual orientation results from multiple genetic, biological, cultural, social, and psychological factors.

Scientists are now looking for genetic markers associated with sexual orientation in males. This study, funded by the National Institutes of Health, will examine the DNA of 1000 pairs of gay brothers and their families. Twin studies are another way of looking at the genetic contribution to sexual identity. Identical twins share the same DNA, so if sexual orientation were entirely genetically determined, we would expect that if one identical twin was gay or lesbian, the other would be as well. But studies

Sexual Activity Among Postsecondary Students

The popular perception of university and college students is that they are young, attractive, and highly sexually active. But how close are these stereotypes to reality? In a 2006 survey of nearly 95,000 students, about one-third of the respondents said they had never had a sexual partner or were currently not sexually active. Of those students who reported having sex with a partner, the vast majority said they had only one partner. Only a small group—about 1 in 10 students—reported having had three or more sexual partners in the last year.

Students tend to grossly overestimate the sexual activity level of their peers, mirroring the popular perception of university and college students. In the survey, students guessed that their peers had more than twice as many sex partners as they actually did.

Slightly more than half of all students said they had not had sexual intercourse in the past 30 days. When asked what types of intercourse they engaged in, most sexually active students reported participating in either vaginal or oral intercourse. Anal intercourse was relatively rare, with only about 1 in 20 stu-

dents reporting having had anal sex one or more times in the last month. Once again, students wildly overestimated the frequency of all types of intercourse among their fellow students; more than half of the students who were polled guessed that the typical student at their institution was participating in anal sex, while in reality only a small minority of students reported having had anal sex.

Judging from the results of this large survey, condom use among students is far from consistent. Only about 18% of students reported using a condom every time they had vaginal intercourse in the last month. Birth control pills were the most popular contraceptive, with condoms a close second. The vast majority of students do not use condoms when they engage in oral sex. When asked about condom use during anal sex—which is among the riskiest of all sexual behaviours in terms of acquiring a sexually transmitted infection—the majority of students who reported this activity did not use a condom the last time they had anal sex.

Among the men polled in this study, 93% described themselves as hetero-

sexual, as did 95% of women. About 4% of men identified themselves as gay and 1% of women identified themselves as lesbian. Another 2% of university men and 3% of women classified themselves as bisexual. Less than 1% of students described themselves as transgender.

---

of many identical twins (both gay men and lesbians) show that the odds are between 30% and 50% that both twins will have the same sexual orientation. These studies provide evidence that our genes make an important but limited contribution to our sexual orientation.

Exposure to hormones before birth also has a major impact on sexual orientation. Experiments with mice show that exposure to sex hormones early in development determines whether they will ultimately be sexually attracted to male or female mice. The situation is much more complicated in humans, but most researchers believe that the hormonal environment in the womb probably has an important influence on sexual orientation.

Researchers have also compared the brain structure of gay and heterosexual men. Although some differences have been found, they are not consistent across all studies. Also, even if brain structure differences exist, it is unclear whether they are the cause or an effect of differences in sexual orientation.

Several studies have shown that the more older brothers a boy has, the more likely he will grow up to be gay. The odds of being gay go up 33% with each older brother. There are numerous theories to explain this phenomenon.

One intriguing, but unproven, theory suggests that mothers with multiple biological sons may develop antibodies against proteins produced by male fetuses. The immune response by the mother may affect the fetal development of later sons, resulting in an increased chance of being gay.

Many psychological theories have also been proposed. Researchers have looked at how much contact children have with members of the two sexes, at the types of relationships children have with their parents, and at family dynamics. Early negative experiences with heterosexuality or positive experiences with same-sex attraction have also been proposed as possible influences. The significant growth of single-parent families over the past 40 years has not been accompanied by large shifts in sexual orientation among Canadians, so it is unlikely that family dynamics or early learning experiences are strong factors in determining sexual orientation. In addition, parents' sexual orientation seems to have little impact on children's sexual orientation. Studies of children raised by gay or lesbian parents show that these children's ultimate sexual orientation is similar to that of children raised by heterosexual parents.

So far, most studies on the origin of sexual orientation have focused on males. The factors that determine sexual

Your Sexual Attitudes

For each statement, circle the response that most closely reflects your position:

	AGREE	NOT SURE	DISAGREE
1. Sex education encourages young people to have sex.	3	2	1
2. Same-sex attraction is a healthy, normal expression of sexuality.	3	2	1
3. Members of the other sex will think more highly of you if you remain mysterious.	3	2	1
4. It's better to wait until marriage to have sex.	3	2	1
5. Abortion should be a personal, private choice for a woman.	3	2	1
6. It's natural for men to have more sexual freedom than women.	3	2	1
7. Condoms should not be made available to teenagers.	3	2	1
8. Access to pornography should not be restricted for adults.	3	2	1
9. A woman who is raped usually does something to provoke it.	3	2	1
10. Contraception is the woman's responsibility.	3	2	1
11. Feminism has had a positive influence on society.	3	2	1
12. Masturbation is a healthy expression of sexuality.	3	2	1
13. I have many friends of the other sex.	3	2	1
14. Prostitution should be legalized.	3	2	1
15. Women use sex for love; men use love for sex.	3	2	1
16. Our society is too sexually permissive.	3	2	1
17. The man should be the undisputed head of the household.	3	2	1
18. Having sex just for pleasure is OK.	3	2	1

Scoring

1–18: Traditional attitude about sexuality

19–36: Ambivalent attitude about sexuality

37–54: Open, progressive attitude about sexuality

orientation in women may be even more complex. Perhaps the most important message is that sexual orientation is most likely the result of the complex interaction of biological, psychological, and social factors, possibly different ones in each individual.

Varieties of Human Sexual Behaviour

Some sexual behaviours are aimed at self-stimulation only, whereas other practices involve interaction with a partner. Some people choose not to express their sexuality at all.

Celibacy Continuous abstention from sexual activities, termed **celibacy**, can be a conscious and deliberate choice, or it can be necessitated by circumstances. Health considerations and religious and moral beliefs may lead some people to celibacy, particularly until marriage or until an acceptable partner appears.

Many people use the related term *abstinence* to refer to avoidance of just one sexual activity—intercourse. Abstinence can also be chosen as a method to prevent pregnancy and sexually transmitted infections.

Autoeroticism and Masturbation The most common form of **autoeroticism** is **erotic fantasy**, creating imaginary experiences that range from fleeting thoughts to elaborate scenarios.

Masturbation involves manually stimulating the genitals, rubbing them against objects, or using stimulating devices, such as vibrators. Although commonly associated

celibacy Continuous abstention from sexual activity.

autoeroticism Behaviour aimed at sexual self-stimulation.

erotic fantasy Sexually arousing thoughts and daydreams.

TERMS

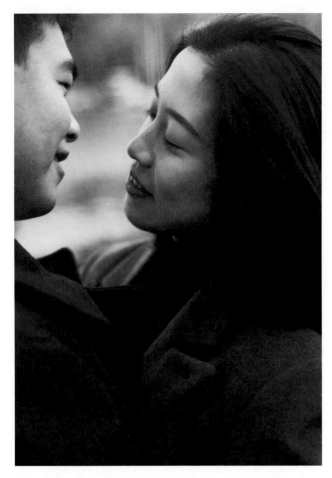

This couple's physical experiences together will be powerfully affected by their emotions, ideas, and values and by the quality of their relationship.

Oral-Genital Stimulation   **Cunnilingus** (the stimulation of the female genitals with the lips and tongue) and **fellatio** (the stimulation of the penis with the mouth) are common practices. Oral sex may be practised either as part of foreplay or as a sex act culminating in orgasm. Although prevalence varies in different populations, 90% of men, 88% of women, and more than 50% of teens report that they have engaged in oral sex. A recent study showed that more teens ages 15–19 had engaged in oral sex than in vaginal intercourse. The most common reasons given for postponing vaginal sex were avoidance of pregnancy and the desire to remain technically a virgin.

Like all acts of sexual expression between two people, oral sex requires the cooperation and consent of both partners. If they disagree about its acceptability, they need to discuss their feelings and try to reach a mutually pleasing solution.

Anal Intercourse   About 10% of heterosexuals and 50% of gay males regularly practise anal stimulation and penetration by the penis or a finger. The receiver does not usually reach orgasm from anal intercourse, though men usually experience orgasm while penetrating.

Because the anus is composed of delicate tissues that tear easily under such pressure, anal intercourse is one of the riskiest of sexual behaviours associated with the transmission of HIV and all other sexually transmitted infections. Anal intercourse is also associated with increased risk of anal cancer, hemorrhoids, anal fissures, prolapsed rectum, and fecal incontinence. The use of condoms is highly recommended for anyone engaging in anal sex. Special care and precaution should be exercised if anal sex is practised—cleanliness, lubrication, and gentle entry at the very least. Anything that is inserted into the anus should not subsequently be put into the vagina unless it has been thoroughly washed. Bacteria normally present in the anus can cause vaginal infections.

Sexual Intercourse   For most adults, most of the time, **sexual intercourse** (*coitus*) is the ultimate sexual experience. Men and women engage in vaginal intercourse to fulfil both sexual and psychological needs. In a 2006 study, 87% of men ages 15–44 and 98% of women in the same age group reported having had vaginal intercourse. The most common heterosexual practice is the man inserting his erect penis into the woman's dilated and lubricated vagina after sufficient arousal.

Much has been written on how to enhance pleasure through various coital techniques, positions, and practices. For a woman, the key factor in physical readiness for coitus is adequate vaginal lubrication, and in psychological readiness, being aroused and receptive. For a man, the setting and the partner must arouse him to attain and maintain an erection. Psychological factors and the quality of the relationship are more important to overall sexual satisfaction than sophisticated or exotic sexual techniques.

with adolescence, masturbation is practised by many throughout adult life. It may be used as a substitute for sexual intercourse or as part of sexual activity with a partner. Masturbation gives a person control over the pace, time, and method of sexual release and pleasure.

Touching and Foreplay   Touching is integral to sexual experiences, whether in the form of massage, kissing, fondling, or holding. Our entire body surface is a sensory organ, and touching almost anywhere can enhance intimacy and sexual arousal. Touching can convey a variety of messages, including affection, comfort, and a desire for further sexual contact.

During arousal, many men and women manually and orally stimulate each other by touching, stroking, and caressing their partner's genitals. Men and women vary greatly in their preferences for the type, pacing, and vigour of such **foreplay**. Working out the details to accommodate each other's pleasure is a key to enjoying these activities. Direct communication about preferences can enhance sexual pleasure and protect both partners from physical and psychological discomfort.

Atypical and Problematic Sexual Behaviours

In Canadian culture, many kinds of sexual behaviour are accepted. However, some types of sexual expression are considered harmful; they may be illegal, classified as mental disorders, or both. Because sexual behaviour occurs on a continuum, it is sometimes difficult to differentiate a behaviour that is simply atypical from one that is harmful. When attempting to evaluate an unusual sexual behaviour, experts consider the issues of consent between partners and whether physical or psychological harm is done to the individual or to others.

The term *paraphilia* is used to describe certain sexual behaviours that are atypical and cause harm to the self or others. Clinically, the term may be used for a sexual behaviour that causes significant distress to the individual involved or to other people. Paraphilias of clinical concern are characterized by recurring, intense sexual fantasies and urges that involve nonhuman objects, the suffering or humiliation of oneself or a partner, or children or nonconsenting individuals. Examples are peeping into strangers' homes, making obscene phone calls, and having sexual contact with children. The effects of paraphilic behaviour on others range from minor upset to serious physical and long-term psychological harm. Paraphilias are considered mental disorders according to the *Diagnostic and Statistical Manual of Mental Disorders*, the guidebook used by mental health care professionals in Canada and many other countries.

The use of force and coercion in sexual relationships is one of the most serious problems in human interactions. The most extreme manifestation of **sexual coercion**—forcing a person to submit to another's sexual desires—is rape, but sexual coercion occurs in many subtler forms, such as sexual harassment. Sexual coercion—including rape, the sexual abuse of children, and sexual harassment—is discussed in detail in Chapter 20.

Responsible Sexual Behaviour

Healthy sexuality is an important part of adult life. It can be a source of pleasurable experiences and emotions and an important part of intimate partnerships. But sexual behaviour also carries many responsibilities, as well as potential consequences, such as pregnancy, STIs, and emotional changes in the relationship. Every sexually active person should be aware of these consequences and accept responsibility for them.

Open, Honest Communication   Each partner needs to clearly indicate what sexual involvement means to him or her. Does it mean love, fun, a permanent commitment, or something else? The intentions of both partners should be clear. For strategies on talking about sexual issues with your partner, see the box "Communicating About Sexuality" (on p. 356).

Responsible sexual behaviour includes discussing potential consequences openly and honestly.

Agreed-On Sexual Activities   No one should pressure or coerce a partner. Sexual behaviours should be consistent with the sexual values, preferences, and comfort level of both partners. Everyone has the right to refuse sexual activity at any time.

Sexual Privacy   Intimate relationships involving sexual activity are based on trust, and that trust can be violated if partners reveal private information about the relationship to others. Sexual privacy also involves respecting other people—not engaging in activities in the presence of others that would make them uncomfortable. The question of how to handle bringing a partner back to a shared residence room is something that many university students must address. Roommates should be respectful of one another and discuss the situation in advance to avoid embarrassing encounters.

Using Contraception   If pregnancy is not desired, contraception should be used during sexual intercourse. Both partners need to take responsibility for protecting against

---

foreplay   Kissing, touching, and any form of oral or genital contact that stimulates people toward intercourse.

cunnilingus   Oral stimulation of the female genitals.

fellatio   Oral stimulation of the penis.

sexual intercourse   Sexual relations involving genital union; also called *coitus* and also known as *making love*.

sexual coercion   The use of physical or psychological force or intimidation to make a person submit to sexual demands.

TERMS

Communicating About Sexuality

TAKE CHARGE

To talk with your partner about sexuality, follow the general suggestions for effective communication given in Chapter 10. Getting started may be the most difficult part. Some people feel more comfortable if they begin by talking about talking— that is, initiating a discussion about why people are so uncomfortable talking about sexuality. Talking about sexual histories—how partners first learned about sex or how family and cultural background influenced sexual values and attitudes— is another way to get started. Reading about sex can also be a good beginning: Partners can read an article or a book and then discuss their reactions.

Be honest about what you feel and what you want from your partner. Cultural and personal obstacles to discussing sexual subjects can be difficult to overcome, but self-disclosure is important for successful relationships. Research indicates that when one partner openly discusses attitudes and feelings, the other partner is more likely to do the same. If your partner seems hesitant to open up, try asking open-ended or either/or questions: "Where do you like to be touched?" or "Would you like to talk about this now or wait until later?"

If something is bothering you about your sexual relationship, choose a good time to initiate a discussion with your partner. Be specific and direct but also tactful. Focus on what you actually observe, rather than on what you think the behaviour means.

"You didn't touch or hug me when your friends were around" is an observation. "You're ashamed of me around your friends" is an inference about your partner's feelings. Try focusing on a specific behaviour that concerns you rather than on the person as a whole—your partner can change behaviours but not his or her entire personality. For example, you could say "I'd like you to take a few minutes away from studying to kiss me" instead of "You're so caught up in your work, you never have time for me."

If you are going to make a statement that your partner may interpret as criticism, try mixing it with something positive: "I love spending time with you, but I feel annoyed when you . . ." Similarly, if your partner says something that upsets you, don't lash out. An aggressive response may make you feel better in the short run, but it will not help the communication process or the quality of the relationship.

If you want to say no to some sexual activity, say no unequivocally. Don't send mixed messages. If you are afraid of hurting your partner's feelings, offer an alternative if it's appropriate: "I am uncomfortable with that. How about . . .?"

If you're in love, you may think that the sexual aspects of a relationship will work out magically without discussion. However, partners who never talk about sex deny themselves the opportunity to increase their closeness and improve their relationship.

---

unwanted pregnancy. Partners should discuss contraception before sexual involvement begins. (Contraception is discussed in the next section of this chapter.)

Safer Sex Both partners should be aware of and practise safer sex to guard against sexually transmitted infections (STIs). Canada faces a significant challenge to the sexual health of its people because of the high numbers of STIs. Many sexual behaviours carry the risk of STIs, including HIV infection. Partners should be honest about their health and any medical conditions and work out a plan for protection. (For more information on STIs and safer sex practices, see Chapter 13.)

Sober Sex The use of alcohol or drugs in sexual situations increases the risk of unplanned, unprotected sexual activity. This is particularly true of young adults, many of

whom engage in episodes of binge drinking during social events. The link between intoxication and unsafe sex is illustrated by a recent study that found that areas with higher drinking ages and higher beer taxes have lower rates of STIs. Alcohol and drugs impair judgment and should not be used in association with sexual activity.

Aside from the dangers of mixing alcohol and sex, alcohol has a negative impact on sexual performance in both men and women. Although alcohol may lower sexual inhibition and make people more likely to attempt a sexual encounter, too much alcohol makes it difficult for a man to achieve or keep an erection, decreases vaginal lubrication in women, and makes orgasm more difficult to achieve in both sexes. Chronic overuse of alcohol reduces testosterone in men, ultimately causing erectile dysfunction, infertility, and body changes, such as enlarged breasts. Women who overuse alcohol often experience menstrual abnormalities and decreased sexual function. Similarly, cigarette smoking has a powerful negative effect on sexual function, primarily because it decreases blood flow to the genitals.

QUESTIONS FOR CRITICAL THINKING AND REFLECTION

If you are sexually active or plan to become active soon, how open have you been about communicating with your partner? Are you aware of your partner's feelings about sex and his or her comfort level with certain activities? Do you and your partner share the same views on contraception, STI prevention, and ethical issues about sex?

CONTRACEPTION

People have always had a compelling interest in managing fertility and preventing unwanted pregnancies, a practice commonly known as **birth control**. Records dating to the fourth century BC describe the use of foods, herbs, drugs, douches, and sponges to prevent **conception**, which is the fusion of an ovum and a sperm that creates a fertilized egg. Early attempts at **contraception** (blocking conception through the use of a device, substance, or method) were based on the same principle as many modern birth control methods.

Today, women and men can choose from many different types of **contraceptives** to avoid unwanted pregnancies. Modern contraceptives take a wide variety of forms and work in different ways. Modern contraceptive methods are much more predictable and effective than in the past, and people in developed countries now have many options when it comes to making decisions about their sexual and contraceptive behaviour.

Worldwide, however, the situation is quite different. People in many countries have little access to contraceptive information and supplies. The World Health Organization estimates that 80 million women worldwide have unintended or unwanted pregnancies every year and 500,000 women die from complications of pregnancy and childbirth.

Principles of Contraception

There are a variety of effective approaches to contraception, including the following:

- **Barrier methods** work by physically blocking the sperm from reaching the egg. Diaphragms, condoms, and several other methods are based on this principle.

- **Hormonal methods**, such as oral contraceptives (birth control pills), alter the biochemistry of the woman's body, preventing ovulation (the release of the egg) and producing changes that make it more difficult for the sperm to reach the egg if ovulation does occur.

- **Natural methods** of contraception are based on the fact that egg and sperm have to be present at the same time if fertilization is to occur.

- **Surgical methods**—female (**tubal sterilization** or **tubal ligation**, or **hysterectomy**) and male (**vasectomy**) **sterilization**—more or less permanently prevent transport of the sperm or eggs to the site of conception.

QUESTIONS FOR CRITICAL THINKING AND REFLECTION

Before reading this section, how familiar were you with the principles of contraception? Did you know as much as you thought? Does this kind of information make you feel as though you should be more or less directly responsible for the contraceptive choices in your life?

All contraceptive methods have advantages and disadvantages that make them appropriate for some people but not for others or the best choice at one period of life but not at another. Factors that affect the choice of method include effectiveness, convenience, cost, reversibility, side effects and risks, and protection against STIs. (See the box "Myths About Contraception on p. 358" to make sure you're not basing your current choices on common misinformation.)

REVERSIBLE CONTRACEPTION

Reversibility is an extremely important consideration for young adults when they choose a contraceptive method, because most people either plan to have children or at least want to keep their options open until they're older.

Oral Contraceptives: The Pill

About a century ago, a researcher noted that ovulation does not occur during pregnancy. Further research revealed the hormonal mechanism: During pregnancy, the corpus luteum secretes progesterone and estrogen in amounts

birth control The practice of managing fertility and preventing unwanted pregnancies.

conception The fusion of ovum and sperm, resulting in a fertilized egg, or zygote.

contraception The prevention of conception through the use of a device, substance, or method.

contraceptive Any agent or method that can prevent conception.

barrier methods A contraceptive that acts as a physical barrier, blocking the sperm from reaching the egg.

hormonal method A contraceptive that alters the biochemistry of the woman's body, preventing ovulation and making it more difficult for the sperm to reach the egg if ovulation does occur.

natural method An approach to contraception that does not use drugs or devices; requires avoiding intercourse during the time in a woman's menstrual cycle when an egg is likely to be present at the site of conception and the risk of pregnancy is greatest.

surgical methods Sterilization of a male or female to permanently prevent the transport of sperm or eggs to the site of conception.

sterilization Surgically altering the reproductive system to prevent pregnancy.

tubal sterilization Severing or blocking the oviducts to prevent eggs from reaching the uterus; also called *tubal ligation*.

hysterectomy Surgical removal of the uterus.

vasectomy The surgical severing of the ducts that carry sperm to the ejaculatory duct.

TERMS

Myths About Contraception

IN FOCUS

Myth Taking birth control pills for a few days before having sex gives reliable protection against pregnancy.

Fact Instructions for taking birth control pills must be followed carefully to provide effective contraception. With most pills, this means starting them with a menstrual period and then taking one every day.

Myth Pregnancy never occurs when unprotected intercourse takes place just before or just after a menstrual period.

Fact Menstrual cycles may be irregular, and ovulation may be unpredictable.

Myth During sexual relations, sperm enter the vagina only during ejaculation and never before.

Fact The small amount of fluid secreted before ejaculation may contain sperm. This is why withdrawing the penis from the vagina just before ejaculation is not an effective method of contraception.

Myth If semen is deposited just outside the vaginal entrance, pregnancy cannot occur.

Fact Although sperm usually live about 72 hours within the woman's body, they can live up to six or seven days and are capable of travelling through the vagina and up into the uterus and oviducts.

Myth Douching immediately after sexual relations can prevent sperm from reaching and fertilizing an egg.

Fact During ejaculation (within the vagina), some sperm begin to enter the cervix and uterus. Because these sperm are no longer in the vagina, it is impossible to remove them by douching after sexual relations. Douching may actually push the sperm up farther.

Myth A woman who is breastfeeding does not have to use any contraceptive method to prevent pregnancy.

Fact Frequent and regular breastfeeding may at times prevent ovulation, but not

consistently and reliably. Ovulation and pregnancy may occur before the first period after delivering a baby.

Myth Women can't become pregnant the first time they have intercourse.

Fact Any time intercourse without protection takes place, pregnancy may result. There is nothing unique about first intercourse that prevents this.

Myth Taking a break from the pill periodically is necessary for safety.

Fact Taking a prolonged break from oral contraceptive use has no known medical benefits; the risks and benefits of ongoing pill use should be evaluated for each individual. Pregnancy commonly occurs when one method of contraception is stopped and not immediately replaced by another method.

Myth Pregnancy is impossible if partners have sex while standing up.

Fact Sperm can travel and reach the egg regardless of body position.

high enough to suppress ovulation. **Oral contraceptives (OCs)**, or *birth control pills*, prevent ovulation by mimicking the hormonal activity of the corpus luteum. The active ingredients in OCs are estrogen and progestins, laboratory-made compounds that are closely related to progesterone. Today, OCs are the most widely used form of contraception among unmarried women and are second only to sterilization among married women.

In addition to preventing ovulation, the birth control pill has other backup contraceptive effects. It inhibits the movement of sperm by thickening the cervical mucus, alters the rate of ovum transport by means of its hormonal effects on the oviducts, and may prevent implantation by changing the lining of the uterus, in the unlikely event that a fertilized ovum reaches that area.

The most common type of OC is the *combination pill*. Each one-month packet contains a three-week supply of pills that combine varying types and amounts of estrogen and progestin. Most packets also include a one-week supply of inactive pills to be taken following the hormone pills; others simply instruct the woman to take no pills at all for one week before starting the next cycle. During the week in which no hormones are taken, a light menstrual period occurs. Many different types of combination pills are available.

Advantages Oral contraceptives are very effective in preventing pregnancy. Nearly all unplanned pregnancies

result because the pills were not taken as directed. The pill is relatively simple to use and does not hinder sexual spontaneity. Most women also enjoy the predictable regularity of periods, as well as the decrease in cramps and blood loss. For young women, the reversibility of the pill is especially important; **fertility**—the ability to reproduce—returns after the pill is discontinued (although not always immediately).

Medical advantages include a decreased incidence of benign breast disease, iron-deficiency anemia, pelvic inflammatory disease (PID), ectopic pregnancy, colon and rectal cancer, endometrial cancer (in the lining of the uterus), and ovarian cancer. Women who have never used the pill are twice as likely to develop endometrial or ovarian cancer as those who have taken it for at least five years.

Disadvantages Although oral contraceptives lower the risk of PID, they do not protect against HIV infection or other STIs in the lower reproductive tract. OCs have been associated with increased cervical chlamydia. Regular condom use is recommended for an OC user, unless she is in a long-term, mutually monogamous relationship with an uninfected partner.

The hormones in birth control pills influence all tissues of the body and can lead to a variety of disturbances. Symptoms of early pregnancy—morning nausea and swollen breasts, for example—may appear during the first few months of OC use. They usually disappear by the fourth cycle. Other side effects include depression, nervousness, changes in sex drive, dizziness, generalized headaches, migraine, bleeding between periods, and changes in the lining of the walls of the vagina, with an increase in clear or white vaginal discharge. Melasma, or "mask of pregnancy," sometimes occurs, causing brown pigmentation to appear on the face. Acne may develop or worsen but, in most women, using the pill causes acne to clear up, and it is sometimes prescribed for that purpose.

Serious side effects have been reported in a small number of women. These include blood clots, stroke, and heart attack, concentrated mostly in older women who smoke or have a history of circulatory disease. Recent studies have shown no increased risk of stroke or heart attack for healthy, young, nonsmoking women on lower-dosage pills. OC users may be slightly more prone to high blood pressure, blood clots in the legs and arms, and benign liver tumours that may rupture and bleed.

OC use is associated with little, if any, increase in breast cancer and a slight increase in cervical cancer; however, earlier detection and other variables, such as number of sexual partners, may account for much of this increase. The link between OC use and cervical cancer appears to pertain primarily to women infected with human papillomavirus, an STI.

Birth control pills are not recommended for women with a history of blood clots (or a close family member with unexplained blood clots at an early age), heart disease or stroke, migraines with changes in vision, any form of cancer or liver tumour, or impaired liver function. Women with certain other health conditions or behaviours, including migraines without changes in vision, high blood pressure, cigarette smoking, and sickle-cell disease, require close monitoring.

Effectiveness   Oral contraceptive effectiveness varies substantially because it depends so much on individual factors. If taken exactly as directed, the failure rate is extremely low (0.3%). However, among average users, lapses, such as forgetting to take a pill, do occur, and a typical first-year failure rate is 8.7%. The continuation rate for OCs also varies; the average rate is 68% after one year.

Contraceptive Skin Patch

The contraceptive skin patch, Ortho Evra, is a thin, 4.5 centimetre by 4.5 centimetre patch that slowly releases an estrogen and a progestin into the bloodstream. The contraceptive patch prevents pregnancy in the same way as combination OCs, following a similar schedule. Each patch is worn continuously for one week and is replaced on the same day of the week for three consecutive weeks. The fourth week is patch free, allowing a woman to have her menstrual period.

The patch can be worn on the upper outer arm, abdomen, buttocks, or upper torso (excluding the breasts); it

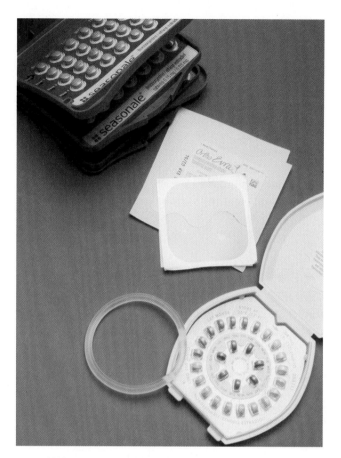

Reversible hormonal contraceptives are available in several forms. Shown here are the patch, the ring, and birth control pills.

is designed to stick to skin even during bathing or swimming. If a patch should fall off for more than a day, it is advisable to start a new four-week cycle of patches and use a backup method of contraception for the first week. Patches should be discarded according to the manufacturer's directions to avoid leakage of hormones into the environment.

Advantages   With both perfect and typical use, the patch is as effective as OCs in preventing pregnancy. Compliance seems to be higher with the patch than with OCs, probably because the patch requires weekly instead of daily action. Medical benefits are likely to be comparable to those of OCs.

Disadvantages   With patch use, additional measures must be taken to protect against STIs. Minor side effects are similar to those of OCs, although breast discomfort

oral contraceptive (OC)   Any of various hormone compounds (estrogen and progestins) in pill form that prevent conception by preventing ovulation.

fertility   The ability to reproduce.

TERMS

may be more common in patch users. Some women also experience skin irritation around the patch. More serious complications are thought to be similar to those of OCs, including an increased risk of side effects among women who smoke. However, because Ortho Evra exposes users to higher doses of estrogen than most OCs, patch use may further increase the risk of blood clots and other adverse effects.

Effectiveness With perfect use, the patch's failure rate is very low (0.3%) in the first year of use. The typical failure rate is assumed to be lower than the pill's 8.7%, because consistent use is better among patch users. The product appears to be less effective when used by women weighing more than 90 kilograms.

Vaginal Contraceptive Ring

The NuvaRing is a vaginal ring that is moulded with a mixture of progestin and estrogen. The five-centimetre ring slowly releases hormones and maintains blood hormone levels comparable to those found with OC use; it prevents pregnancy in the same way as OCs. A woman inserts the ring anytime during the first five days of her menstrual period and leaves it in place for three weeks. During the fourth week, which is ring-free, her next menstrual period occurs. A new ring is then inserted. Rings should be discarded according to the manufacturer's directions to avoid leakage of hormones into the environment.

Backup contraception must be used for the first seven days of the first ring use or if the ring has been removed for more than three hours during use. A diaphragm is not recommended as a backup contraceptive with the NuvaRing because the ring may interfere with the placement of a diaphragm. Diaphragm use is discussed on page 364.

Advantages The NuvaRing offers one month of protection with no daily or weekly action required. It does not require a fitting by a clinician, and exact placement in the vagina is not critical as it is with a diaphragm. Medical benefits are probably similar to those of OCs.

Disadvantages The NuvaRing gives no protection against STIs. Side effects are roughly comparable to those seen with OC use, except for a lower incidence of nausea and vomiting. Other side effects may include vaginal discharge, vaginitis, and vaginal irritation. Medical risks also are similar to those found with OC use.

Effectiveness As with the pill and patch, the perfect use failure rate is around 0.3% and the typical use failure rate is likely to be lower than the pill's 8.7%.

Contraceptive Implant

Contraceptive implants are placed under the skin of the upper arm and deliver a small but steady dose of progestin (a synthetic progesterone) over a period of years.

Only trained health professionals can insert a contraceptive implant.

The progestins in implants have several contraceptive effects. They cause hormonal shifts that may inhibit ovulation and affect development of the uterine lining. The hormones also thicken the cervical mucus, inhibiting the movement of sperm. Finally, they may slow the transport of the egg through the fallopian tubes. Contraceptive implants are best suited for women who want continuous and long-term protection against pregnancy.

Advantages Contraceptive implants are highly effective. After insertion of the implants, no further action is required; contraceptive effects are quickly reversed on removal. Because implants, unlike the combination pill, contain no estrogen, they carry a lower risk of certain side effects, such as blood clots and other cardiovascular complications. In addition, the progestin is released at a steady rate, in smaller quantities than are found in oral contraceptives. The thickened cervical mucus resulting from implant use has a protective effect against PID.

Disadvantages Like the pill, an implant provides no protection against HIV infection and STIs in the lower reproductive tract. Although the implants are barely visible, their appearance may bother some women. Only specially trained practitioners can insert or remove the implants, and removal is sometimes difficult.

The most common side effects of contraceptive implants are menstrual irregularities, including longer menstrual periods, spotting between periods, or no bleeding at all. The menstrual cycle usually becomes more regular after one year of use. Less common side effects include headaches, weight gain, breast tenderness, nausea, acne, and mood swings. Cautions and more serious health concerns are similar to those associated with oral contraceptives but are less common.

Effectiveness The overall failure rate is estimated at about 0.1%.

Injectable Contraceptives

Hormonal contraceptive injections were developed in the 1960s and are currently being used in at least 80 countries throughout the world. The first injectable contraceptive approved for use in Canada was Depo-Provera, which uses long-acting progestins. Injected into the arm or buttocks, Depo-Provera is usually given every 12 weeks, although it actually provides effective contraception for a few weeks beyond that. As another progestin-only contraceptive, it prevents pregnancy in the same ways as implants.

Advantages   Injectable contraceptives are highly effective and require little action on the part of the user. Because the injections leave no trace and involve no ongoing supplies, injectables allow women almost total privacy in their decision to use contraception. Depo-Provera has no estrogen-related side effects; it requires only periodic injections rather than the minor surgical procedures of implant insertion and removal.

Disadvantages   Injectable contraceptives provide no protection against HIV infection and STIs in the lower reproductive tract. A woman must visit a health care facility every three months to receive the injections. The side effects of Depo-Provera are similar to those of implants; menstrual irregularities are the most common, and after one year of using Depo-Provera many women have no menstrual bleeding at all. Weight gain is a common side effect. After discontinuing the use of Depo-Provera, women may experience temporary infertility for up to 12 months.

Reasons for not using Depo-Provera are similar to those for not using implants. Extended use of Depo-Provera is associated with decreased bone density, a risk factor for osteoporosis (see Chapter 5); women who use Depo-Provera are advised to do weight-bearing exercise and take 1000 milligrams of calcium daily. Women are advised to use Depo-Provera as a long-term contraceptive (longer than two years, for example) only if other methods are inadequate. Studies have found that bone density rebounds when use of Depo-Provera stops.

Effectiveness   The perfect use failure rate is 0.3% for Depo-Provera. With typical use, the failure rate increases to 6.7% in the first year of use. The one-year continuation rate for Depo-Provera is about 56%.

Emergency Contraception

Emergency contraception refers to postcoital methods—those used after unprotected sexual intercourse. An emergency contraceptive may be appropriate if a regularly used method has failed (for example, if a condom breaks) or if unprotected sex has occurred. Sometimes called the "morning-after pill," emergency contraceptives are designed only for emergency use and should not be relied on as a regular birth control method.

Until recently the most frequently used emergency contraceptive was a two-dose regimen of certain oral contraceptives. Researchers are still uncertain precisely how OCs work as emergency contraceptives. Opponents of their use argue that if they act by preventing implantation of a fertilized egg, they may actually be **abortifacients**; however, recent evidence indicates that prevention of implantation is not their primary mode of action. Postcoital pills appear to work primarily by inhibiting or delaying ovulation and by altering the transport of sperm or eggs; they do not affect a fertilized egg already implanted in the uterus.

Plan B is a newer product specifically designed for emergency contraception. It is available over the counter in Canada and contains two progestin-only pills. The first pill should be taken as soon as possible (no more than 120 hours) after inadequately protected sex. The second pill should be taken 12 hours after the first. Both pills may be taken together in a single dose with little change in effectiveness or side effects. If taken within 24 hours after intercourse, Plan B may prevent as many as 95% of expected pregnancies. Overall, Plan B reduces pregnancy risk by about 89%. It is most effective if initiated in the first 12 hours. Possible side effects are similar to those associated with the OC regimen and can include nausea, stomach pain, headache, dizziness, and breast tenderness.

Easy access to emergency contraception is important because the sooner the drug is taken, the more effective it is. Some clinicians advise women to keep a package of emergency contraception on hand in case their regular contraception method fails. Research has found that ready access to emergency contraception does not lead to an increase in unprotected intercourse, unintended pregnancies, or STIs.

Intrauterine devices, discussed in the next section, can also be used for emergency contraception: If inserted within five days of unprotected intercourse, they are even more effective than OCs. However, because their use is more complicated, they are not used nearly as frequently.

The Intrauterine Device (IUD)

The **intrauterine device (IUD)** is a small device placed in the uterus as a contraceptive. There are two types of IUDs in Canada, and they are effective for about five years.

Researchers do not know exactly how IUDs prevent pregnancy. Current evidence suggests that they work primarily by preventing fertilization. IUDs may cause

emergency contraception   A birth control method used after unprotected sexual intercourse has occurred.

abortifacient   An agent or a substance that induces abortion.

intrauterine device (IUD)   A plastic device inserted into the uterus as a contraceptive.

TERMS

biochemical changes in the uterus and affect the movement of sperm and eggs; although less likely, they may also interfere with implantation of fertilized eggs. Some IUDs slowly release very small amounts of hormones, which impede fertilization or implantation.

An IUD must be inserted and removed by a trained professional. It can be inserted at any time during the menstrual cycle, as long as the woman is not pregnant. The device is threaded into a sterile inserter, which is introduced through the cervix; a plunger pushes the IUD into the uterus. The threads protruding from the cervix are trimmed so that only 2.5–4 centimetres remain in the upper vagina.

Advantages   Intrauterine devices are highly reliable and are simple and convenient to use, requiring no attention except for a periodic check of the string position. They do not require the woman to anticipate or interrupt sexual activity. According to researchers, IUD use reduces the risk of developing endometrial cancer by as much as 40%. Usually IUDs have only localized side effects, and in the absence of complications they are considered a fully reversible contraceptive. In most cases, fertility is restored as soon as the IUD is removed. The risks of ectopic pregnancy and uterine cancer are both decreased with IUD use.

Disadvantages   Most side effects of IUD use are limited to the genital tract. Heavy menstrual flow and bleeding and spotting between periods may occur, although with some IUDs menstrual periods tend to become shorter and lighter over time. Another side effect is pain, particularly uterine cramps and backache, which seem to occur most often in women who have never been pregnant. Spontaneous expulsion of the IUD happens to 5%–6% of women within the first year, most commonly during the first months after insertion. The older the woman is and the more children she has had, the less likely she is to expel the device. In about 1 of 1000 insertions, the IUD punctures the wall of the uterus and may migrate into the abdominal cavity.

A serious but rare complication of IUD use is pelvic inflammatory disease (PID). Most pelvic infections among IUD users occur shortly after insertion, are relatively mild, and can be treated successfully with antibiotics. However, early and adequate treatment is critical—a lingering infection can lead to tubal scarring and subsequent infertility.

Some physicians advise against the use of IUDs by young women who have never been pregnant because of the increased incidence of side effects in this group and the risk of infection with the possibility of subsequent infertility.

IUDs are not recommended for women of any age who are at high risk for STIs. They are also unsuitable for women with suspected pregnancy, large tumours of the uterus or other anatomical abnormalities, irregular or unexplained bleeding, or rheumatic heart disease. No evidence has been found linking IUD use to an increased risk of cancer. IUDs offer no protection against STIs.

Early IUD danger signals are abdominal pain, fever, chills, foul-smelling vaginal discharge, irregular menstrual periods, and other unusual vaginal bleeding. A change in string length should also be noted. An annual checkup is important and should include a Pap test and a blood check for anemia if menstrual flow has increased.

Effectiveness   The typical failure rate of IUDs during the first year of use is 0.1%–0.6%. Effectiveness can be increased by periodically checking to see that the device is in place and by using a backup method for the first few months after IUD insertion. If pregnancy occurs, the IUD should be removed to safeguard the health of the woman and to maintain the pregnancy. The continuation rate of IUDs is about 80% after one year of use.

Male Condoms

The **male condom** is a thin sheath designed to cover the penis during sexual intercourse. Most brands available in Canada are made of latex, although condoms made of polyurethane are also now available. Condoms prevent sperm from entering the vagina and provide protection against disease. Condoms are the most widely used barrier method and the third most popular of all contraceptive methods used in North America, after the pill and female sterilization.

Condom sales have increased dramatically in recent years, primarily because they are the only method that provides substantial protection against HIV infection as well as some protection against other STIs. At least one-third of all male condoms are bought by women.

Advantages   Condoms are easy to purchase and are available without prescription or medical supervision. In addition to being free of medical side effects (other than occasional allergic reactions), latex condoms help protect against STIs. A recent study determined that condoms may also protect women from human papilloma virus (HPV), which causes cervical cancer. Condoms made of polyurethane are appropriate for people who are allergic to latex. However, they are more likely to slip or break than latex condoms and therefore may give less protection against STIs and pregnancy. (Lambskin condoms permit the passage of HIV and other disease-causing organisms, so they can be used only for pregnancy prevention, not the prevention of STIs.) Except for abstinence, correct and consistent use of latex male condoms offers the most reliable available protection against the transmission of HIV. (See Figure 11.6 for the proper way to use a condom.)

Disadvantages   The two most common complaints about condoms are that they diminish sensation and interfere with spontaneity. Although some people find these drawbacks serious, others consider them only minor disadvantages. Many couples learn to creatively integrate

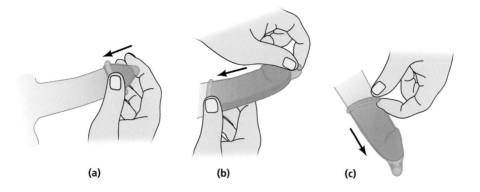

(a)   (b)   (c)

FIGURE 11.6   The male condom properly used.   (a) Check the expiration date and check to see that the package is intact. Put the condom on before any genital contact. If uncircumcised, pull back the foreskin. Cover the head of the penis with the condom. Leave some space at the tip for ejaculate, but gently press out any air. This will reduce the risk of breakage. **(b)** Unroll the condom so that the entire erect penis is covered all the way to the base. If needed, you may generously apply a water-based or silicone lubricant to the outside of the condom before penetration. Do not use oil-based lubricants. To prevent slippage, hold the condom at the base of the penis when withdrawing. **(c)** After ejaculation occurs, withdraw the penis before it gets soft. Hold onto the condom to prevent slippage. Throw the condom away.

Source: McKinley Health Center, University of Illinois at Urbana-Champaign. 2008. *How to Use a Condom and Spermicidal Jelly for Intercourse* (http://www.mckinley.illinois.edu/handouts/condom_spermicidal_jelly/condom_spermicidal_jelly.html; retrieved April 20, 2011).

condom use into their sexual practices. Indeed, it can be a way to improve communication and share responsibility in a relationship.

Effectiveness   In actual use, the failure rate of condoms varies considerably. First-year rates among typical users average about 17.4%. With perfect use, the first-year failure rate is about 2%. At least some pregnancies happen because the condom is carelessly removed after ejaculation. Some may also occur because of breakage or slippage, which may happen 1–2 times in every 100 instances of use for latex condoms and up to 10 times in every 100 instances for polyurethane condoms. Breakage is more common among inexperienced users. Other contributing factors include poorly fitting condoms, insufficient lubrication, excessively vigorous sex, and improper storage (because heat destroys rubber, latex condoms should not be stored for long periods in a wallet or a car's glove compartment). To help ensure quality, condoms should not be used past their expiration date or more than five years past their date of manufacture (two years for those with spermicide).

If a condom breaks or is carelessly removed, the risk of pregnancy can be reduced somewhat by the immediate use of a vaginal spermicide. Some clinicians recommend keeping emergency contraceptive pills on hand. If the emergency contraceptive Plan B is taken within one hour of inadequately protected sex, the failure rate is only about 0.14%. The most common cause of pregnancy with condom users is "taking a chance"—that is, occasionally not using a condom at all—or waiting to use it until after preejaculate fluid (which may contain some sperm) has already entered the vagina.

Female Condoms

A female condom is a latex or polyurethane pouch that can be inserted into a woman's vagina. Although the female condom is preferred in certain situations because it requires less participation on the part of the male partner, its overall popularity remains far below that of the male condom.

The female condom currently available is a disposable device that comes in one size and consists of a soft, loose-fitting polyurethane sheath with two flexible rings (Figure 11.7 on p. 364). The ring at the closed end is inserted into the vagina and placed at the cervix, much like a diaphragm. The ring at the open end remains outside the vagina. The walls of the condom protect the inside of the vagina.

The directions that accompany the condom should be followed closely. It can be inserted up to eight hours before intercourse and should be used with the supplied lubricant or a spermicide to prevent penile irritation. As with male condoms, users need to take care not to tear the condom during insertion or removal. Following intercourse, the woman should remove the condom immediately, before standing up. By twisting and squeezing the outer ring, she can prevent the spilling of semen. A new condom should be used for each act of sexual intercourse. A female condom should not be used with a male condom because when the two are used together slippage is more likely to occur.

Advantages   For many women, the greatest advantage of the female condom is the control it gives them over contraception and STI prevention. (Partner cooperation is still important, however.) Female condoms can be inserted

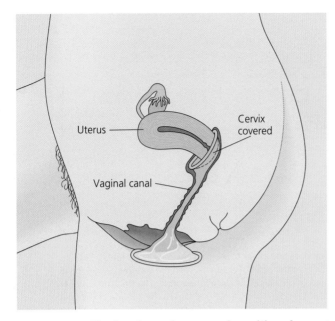

FIGURE 11.7 **The female condom properly positioned.**

Labels within the figure: Uterus, Cervix covered, Vaginal canal

before sexual activity and are thus less disruptive than male condoms. Because the outer part of the condom covers the area around the vaginal opening as well as the base of the penis during intercourse, it offers potentially better protection against genital warts or herpes. The polyurethane pouch can be used by people who are allergic to latex. And because polyurethane is thin and pliable, little loss of sensation occurs.

When used correctly, the female condom should theoretically provide protection against HIV transmission and STIs comparable to that of the latex male condom. However, in research involving typical users, the female condom was less effective in preventing both pregnancy and STIs. With careful instruction and practice, effectiveness can be improved.

Disadvantages   As with the traditional condom, interference with spontaneity is likely to be a common complaint. The outer ring, which hangs visibly outside the vagina, may be bothersome during foreplay; if so, couples may choose to put the device in just before intercourse. During coitus, both partners must take care that the penis is inserted into the pouch, not outside it, and that the device does not slip inside the vagina. Female condoms, like male condoms, are made for one-time use. A single female condom costs about four times as much as a single male condom.

Effectiveness   The typical first-year failure rate of the female condom is 27%. For women who follow instructions carefully and consistently, the failure rate is considerably lower—about 5%. Although the female condom rarely breaks during use, slippage occurs in nearly one in ten users. The risk of being exposed to semen is higher if

the relationship is new or short-term, if intercourse is very active, and if there is a large disparity between vagina and penis sizes. Having Plan B available as a backup contraceptive is recommended.

The Diaphragm with Spermicide

Before oral contraceptives were introduced, about 25% of all North American couples who used any form of contraception relied on the **diaphragm**. Many diaphragm users switched to the pill or IUDs, but the diaphragm offers advantages that are important to some couples.

The diaphragm is a dome-shaped cup of thin rubber stretched over a collapsible metal ring. When correctly used with spermicidal cream or jelly, the diaphragm covers the cervix, blocking sperm from entering the uterus.

Diaphragms are available only by prescription. Because of individual anatomical differences among women, a diaphragm must be carefully fitted by a trained clinician to ensure both comfort and effectiveness. The fitting should be checked with each routine annual medical examination, as well as after childbirth, abortion, or a weight change of more than 4.5 kilograms.

The woman spreads spermicidal jelly or cream on the diaphragm before inserting it and checking its placement (Figure 11.8). If more than six hours elapse between the time of insertion and the time of intercourse, additional spermicide must be applied. The diaphragm must be left in place for at least six hours after the last act of coitus to give the spermicide enough time to kill all the sperm. With repeated intercourse, a condom should be used for additional protection.

To remove the diaphragm, the woman simply hooks the front rim down from the pubic bone with one finger and pulls it out. She should wash it with mild soap and water, rinse it, pat it dry, and then examine it for holes or cracks. Defects would most likely develop near the rim and can be spotted by looking at the diaphragm in front of a bright light. After inspecting the diaphragm, she should store it in its case.

Advantages   Diaphragm use is less intrusive than male condom use because a diaphragm can be inserted up to six hours before intercourse. Its use can be limited to times of sexual activity only, and it allows for immediate and total reversibility. The diaphragm is free of medical side effects (other than rare allergic reactions).

When used along with spermicidal jelly or cream, it offers significant protection against gonorrhea and possibly chlamydia, STIs that are transmitted only by semen and for which the cervix is the sole site of entry. Diaphragm use can also protect the cervix from semen infected with the human papillomavirus, which causes cervical cancer. However, the diaphragm is unlikely to protect against STIs that can be transmitted through vaginal or vulvar surfaces (in addition to the cervix), including HIV infection, genital herpes, and syphilis.

(a)

(b)

(c)

FIGURE 11.8 Use of the diaphragm. Wash your hands with soap and water before inserting the diaphragm. It can be inserted while squatting, lying down, or standing with one foot raised. **(a)** Place about 15 millilitres (a tablespoon) of spermicidal jelly or cream in the concave side of the diaphragm, and spread it around the inside of the diaphragm and around the rim. **(b)** Squeeze the diaphragm into a long, narrow shape between the thumb and forefinger. Insert it into the vagina, and push it up along the back wall of the vagina as far as it will go. **(c)** Check its position to make sure the cervix is completely covered and that the front rim of the diaphragm is tucked behind the pubic bone.

Disadvantages Diaphragms must always be used with a spermicide, so a woman must keep both of these somewhat bulky supplies with her whenever she anticipates sexual activity. Diaphragms require extra attention, since they must be cleaned and stored with care to preserve their effectiveness. Some women cannot wear a diaphragm because of their vaginal or uterine anatomy. In other women, diaphragm use can cause an increase in bladder infections and may need to be discontinued if repeated infections occur.

Diaphragms have also been associated with a slightly increased risk of **toxic shock syndrome (TSS)**, an occasionally fatal bacterial infection. To reduce the risk of TSS, a woman should wash her hands carefully with soap and water before inserting or removing the diaphragm, should not use the diaphragm during menstruation or when abnormal vaginal discharge is present, and should never leave the device in place for more than 24 hours.

Effectiveness The diaphragm's effectiveness depends mainly on whether it is used properly. In actual practice, women rarely use it correctly every time they have intercourse. With perfect use, the failure rate is about 6%. Typical failure rates are 16% during the first year of use. The main causes of failure are incorrect insertion, inconsistent use, and inaccurate fitting. Sometimes, too, the vaginal walls expand during sexual stimulation, causing the diaphragm to be dislodged. If a diaphragm slips during intercourse, a woman may choose to use emergency contraception.

Lea's Shield

Lea's Shield is a one-size-fits-all diaphragm-like device, available by prescription. Made of silicone rubber, it can be used by women who are allergic to latex, and it is not damaged by petroleum-based products. The shield has a

diaphragm A contraceptive device consisting of a flexible, dome-shaped cup that covers the cervix and prevents sperm from entering the uterus.

toxic shock syndrome (TSS) A bacterial disease usually associated with tampon use; can also occur in men; symptoms include weakness, cold and clammy hands, fever, nausea, and headache. TSS can progress to life-threatening complications, including very low blood pressure (shock) and kidney and liver failure.

TERMS

valve that allows the flow of air and fluids from the cervix as well as a loop that aids in insertion and removal. The device may be inserted at any time before intercourse, but should be left in place for eight hours after last intercourse; it can be worn for up to 48 hours. Like the diaphragm, it must be used with spermicide. Studies completed thus far have reported advantages, disadvantages, and failure rates similar to those of the diaphragm.

FemCap

FemCap, another barrier device, is a small flexible cup that fits snugly over the cervix and is held in place by suction. This cervical cap is a clear silicone cup with a brim around the dome to hold spermicide and trap sperm and a removal strap over the dome. It comes in three sizes and must be fitted by a trained clinician. It is used like a diaphragm, with a small amount of spermicide placed in the cup and on the brim before insertion.

Advantages   Advantages of the cervical cap are similar to those associated with diaphragm use and include partial STI protection. It is an alternative for women who cannot use a diaphragm because of anatomical reasons or recurrent urinary tract infections. Because the cap fits tightly, it does not require backup condom use with repeated intercourse. It may be left in place for up to 48 hours.

Disadvantages   Along with most of the disadvantages associated with the diaphragm, difficulty with insertion and removal is more common for cervical cap users. Because there may be a slightly increased risk of TSS with prolonged use, the cap should not be left in place for more than 48 hours.

Effectiveness   Studies indicate that the average failure rate for the cervical cap is 16% for women who have never had a child and 32% for women who have had a child. Failure rates drop significantly with perfect use.

The Contraceptive Sponge

The **sponge** is a round, absorbent device about five centimetres in diameter with a polyester loop on one side (for removal) and a concave dimple on the other side, which helps it fit snugly over the cervix. The sponge is made of polyurethane and is presaturated with the same spermicide that is used in contraceptive creams and foams. The spermicide is activated when moistened with a small amount of water just before insertion. The sponge, which can be used only once, acts as a barrier, as a spermicide, and as a seminal fluid absorbent.

Advantages   The sponge offers advantages similar to those of the diaphragm and cervical cap, including partial protection against some STIs. In addition, sponges can be obtained without a prescription or professional fitting, and they may be safely left in place for 24 hours without the addition of spermicide for repeated intercourse.

Disadvantages   Reported disadvantages include difficulty with removal and an unpleasant odour if the sponge is left in place for more than 18 hours. Allergic reactions, such as irritation of the vagina, are more common with the sponge than with other spermicide products, probably because the overall dose contained in each sponge is significantly higher than that used with other methods. (A sponge contains one gram of spermicide compared with the 60–100 milligrams present in one application of other spermicidal products.) If irritation of the vaginal lining occurs, the risk of yeast infections and STIs (including HIV) may increase.

Because the sponge has also been associated with toxic shock syndrome, the same precautions must be taken as described for diaphragm use. A sponge user should be especially alert for symptoms of TSS when the sponge has been difficult to remove or was not removed intact.

Effectiveness   The typical effectiveness of the sponge is the same as the diaphragm (16% failure rate during the first year of use) for women who have never experienced childbirth. For women who have had a child, however, sponges are significantly less effective than diaphragms. One possible explanation is that the sponge's size may be insufficient to adequately cover the cervix after childbirth. To ensure effectiveness, the user should carefully check the expiration date on each sponge, as shelf life is limited.

Vaginal Spermicides

Spermicidal compounds developed for use with a diaphragm have been adapted for use without a diaphragm by combining them with a bulky base. Foams, creams, jellies, suppositories, and films are all available. Foam is sold in an aerosol bottle or a metal container with an applicator that fits on the nozzle. Creams and jellies are sold in tubes with an applicator that can be screwed onto the opening of the tube.

Foams, creams, and jellies must be placed deep in the vagina near the cervical entrance and must be inserted no more than 60 minutes before intercourse. After an hour, their effectiveness is drastically reduced, and a new dose must be inserted. Another application is also required before each repeated act of coitus. If the woman wants to **douche**, she should wait for at least six hours after the last intercourse to make sure that there has been time for the spermicide to kill all the sperm; douching is not recommended, however, because it can irritate vaginal tissue and increase the risk of various infections.

The spermicidal suppository is small and easily inserted like a tampon. Because body heat is needed to dissolve and activate the suppository, it is important to wait at least

15 minutes after insertion before having intercourse. The suppository's spermicidal effects are limited in time, and coitus should take place within one hour of insertion. A new suppository is required for every act of intercourse.

The Vaginal Contraceptive Film (VCF) is a paper-thin five centimetre by five centimetre film that contains spermicide. It is folded over one or two fingers and placed high in the vagina, as close to the cervix as possible. In about 15 minutes the film dissolves into a spermicidal gel that is effective for up to one hour. A new film must be inserted for each act of intercourse.

Advantages The use of vaginal spermicides is relatively simple and can be limited to times of sexual activity. They are readily available in most drugstores and do not require a prescription or a pelvic examination. Spermicides allow for complete and immediate reversibility, and the only medical side effects are occasional allergic reactions. Vaginal spermicides may provide limited protection against some STIs but should never be used instead of condoms for reliable protection.

Disadvantages When used alone, vaginal spermicides must be inserted shortly before intercourse, so their use may be seen as an annoying disruption. Some women find the slight increase in vaginal fluids after spermicide use unpleasant. Spermicides can alter the balance of bacteria in the vagina. Because this may increase the occurrence of yeast infections and urinary tract infections, women who are especially prone to these infections may want to avoid spermicides. Also, this method does not protect against gonorrhea, chlamydia, or HIV. Overuse of spermicides can irritate vaginal tissues; if this occurs, the risk of HIV transmission may increase.

Effectiveness The effectiveness rates of vaginal spermicides vary widely, depending partly on how consistently and carefully instructions are followed. The typical failure rate is about 29% during the first year of use. Foam is probably the most effective form of spermicide, because its effervescent mass forms a denser and more evenly distributed barrier to the cervical opening. Creams and jellies provide only minimal protection unless used with a diaphragm or cervical cap.

Spermicide is generally recommended only in combination with other barrier methods or as a backup to other contraceptives. Plan B provides a better backup than spermicides, however.

Whatever your needs, circumstances, or beliefs, *do* make a choice about contraception. Not choosing anything is the one method known *not* to work. This is an area in which taking charge of your health has immediate and profound implications for your future. The method you choose today won't necessarily be the one you'll want to use your whole life or even next year. But it should be one that works for you right now.

Even with the vast array of contraceptive options available to Canadians, unwanted pregnancies do occur for various reasons. When this happens, abortion may need to be considered.

ABORTION

Few issues are as complex and emotionally charged as abortion. In Canada, public attention has focused on the legal definition of abortion and the issue of restricting its practice. These far-reaching questions are important, but the most difficult aspects of abortion are personal—especially for women who must decide whether to have an abortion.

Because most women who undergo abortions are young, many university and college students have personal experience with unintended pregnancy and abortion. Therefore, students are in a good position not just to debate the larger issues surrounding abortion, but also to address the complex human factors involved in preventing pregnancy and dealing with unintended pregnancy.

Abortion is legal in throughout Canada; the number of abortions by province and territory from 1970 to 2004 are shown in Table 11.1 (on p. 368).

The word **abortion**, by strict definition, means the expulsion of an embryo or a fetus from the uterus before it is sufficiently developed to survive outside the uterus. As commonly used, however, the term *abortion* refers only to those expulsions that are artificially induced by mechanical means or drugs.

FemCap A small flexible cup that fits over the cervix, to be used with spermicide.

sponge A contraceptive device about five centimetres in diameter that fits over the cervix and acts as a barrier, spermicide, and seminal fluid absorbent.

douche To apply a stream of water or other solutions to a body part or cavity, such as the vagina; not a contraceptive technique.

abortion The artificially induced expulsion of an embryo or a fetus from the uterus.

Table 11.1	Total Induced Abortions by Province and Territory, 1970–2004	
Province	**Number of Abortions**	
Newfoundland and Labrador	19,065	
Prince Edward Island (1970–1982)	470	
Nova Scotia	60,941	
New Brunswick	20,596	
Quebec	636,733	
Ontario	1,146,255	
Manitoba	88,720	
Saskatchewan	48,602	
Alberta	256,362	
British Columbia	437,461	
Yukon Territory	3,753	
Northwest Territories (including Nunavut, 1974–1988)	4,454	
Northwest Territories (1999–2004)	1,569	
Nunavut (1999–2004)	288	
Total induced abortions	2,725,269	

Source: AbortionInCanada.ca. 2008. *Total Induced Abortions by Province, 1970–2004* (http://www.abortionincanada.ca/stats/total_abortions_province.html; retrieved April 21, 2011).

METHODS OF ABORTION

Abortion methods can be divided into two categories: surgical and medical. Surgical abortion is by far the most common.

Suction Curettage

First developed in China in 1958, **suction curettage** (commonly known as *dilation and curettage*, or D&C) is the most common method for abortions performed from the 6th to the 12th week of pregnancy. The procedure can be done quickly, usually on an outpatient basis, and the risk of complications is small.

A sedative may be given, along with a local anaesthetic. A speculum is inserted into the vagina, and the cervix is cleansed with a surgical solution. The cervix is dilated and a suction curette, a specially designed tube, is then inserted into the uterus (Figure 11.9). The curette is attached to the rubber tubing of an electric pump, and suction is applied. In 20–30 seconds, the uterus is emptied. Moderate cramping is common during evacuation. To ensure that no fragments of tissue are left in the uterus, the doctor usually scrapes the uterine lining with a metal curette, an instrument with a spoonlike tip. The entire suction curettage procedure takes five to ten minutes.

After a few hours in a recovery area, the woman can return home. She is usually instructed not to have intercourse or use tampons for several weeks after the abortion and to return for a postabortion examination. This follow-up exam is important to verify that the abortion was complete and that no signs of infection are present.

Manual Vacuum Aspiration

For more than 30 years, gynecologists have used **manual vacuum aspiration (MVA)** to manage incomplete abortions, for endometrial sampling in nonpregnant women, and for elective abortion. During this procedure, as in suction curettage, the woman receives a local anaesthetic and her cervix is dilated. A plastic tube attached to a handheld syringe is inserted through the cervix and into the uterus. The syringe provides gentle suction, which empties the uterus.

MVA has several advantages over the traditional D&C. Manual vacuum aspiration may be used earlier in pregnancy, can be performed in the office, and does not require an electric pump or additional equipment. It is also significantly cheaper than suction curettage, does not require electricity, and can be performed by mid-level providers, such as midwives and nurses. For these reasons, MVA is ideal for low-resource settings. A number of recent studies have shown that the two techniques have equivalent safety profiles and low rates of complications when done up to 10 weeks of gestation.

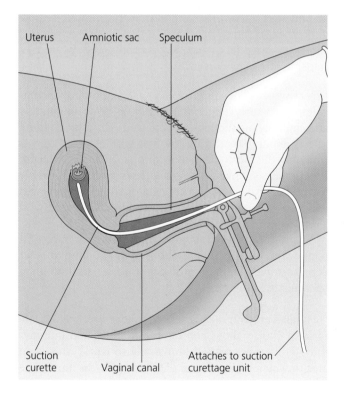

FIGURE 11.9 Suction curettage. This procedure takes five to ten minutes and can be performed up to the 12th week of pregnancy.

Medical Abortion

Medical abortion is generally used in very early pregnancy, within 49 days of the last menstrual period. The combination of drugs that is given causes the embryo and products of conception to be passed out through the vagina, as in a natural miscarriage. An ultrasound may be performed before giving the medication to make sure that the pregnancy dates are accurate, because complication rates for medical abortion are higher if the pregnancy is more advanced.

Advantages and Disadvantages of Medical Abortion

Medical abortion is generally safer than surgical abortion because it involves no anaesthesia or surgical risks. Some women feel that medical abortion allows them to take more control of the procedure and gives them more privacy than a surgical abortion would. Medical abortion can also be done very early in pregnancy.

The major disadvantages of medical abortion are that the process takes days or even weeks to complete (early surgical abortion generally takes less than an hour and can be done under sedation) and that bleeding after the procedure is often heavier and lasts longer than with surgical abortion. Medical abortion also generally requires more clinic visits than surgical abortion.

Possible Psychological Effects

After an exhaustive review completed in 1988, it was concluded that the available evidence failed to demonstrate either a negative or a positive long-term impact of abortion on mental health. More recent research has resulted in the same general conclusion. The frequency of any psychiatric diagnoses in women who have undergone an abortion procedure is no higher than in women with no such history.

The psychological side effects of abortion, however, are less clearly defined than the physical ones. Responses vary and depend on the individual woman's psychological makeup, family background, current personal and social relationships, cultural attitudes, and many other factors. A woman who has specific goals with a somewhat structured life may be able to incorporate her decision to have an abortion as the unequivocally best and most acceptable course more easily than a woman who feels uncertain about her future.

Although many women experience great relief after an abortion and virtually no negative feelings, some go through a period of ambivalence. Along with relief, they often feel a mixture of other responses, such as guilt, regret, loss, sadness, and anger. When a woman feels she was pressured into sexual intercourse or into the abortion, she may feel bitter. If she had strongly believed abortion to be immoral, she may wonder if she is still a good person. Many of these feelings are strongest immediately after the abortion, when hormonal shifts are occurring; such feelings often pass quite rapidly. Others take time to resolve and fade only slowly. It is important for a woman to realize that a mixture of feelings is natural. The decision-making process and feelings about abortion can be very complex for some women.

For a woman who experiences psychological or emotional effects after an abortion, talking with a close friend or family member can be very helpful. Supportive people can help her feel positive about herself and her decision. Although a legal and relatively common procedure in Canada, abortion is still treated very secretively in most of our society, so it is easy for a woman to feel isolated and alone. Many clinical centres that offer abortions make peer counselling available. Other women find they can identify with case histories in books written on abortion, which can help them deal with their own reactions. Unresolved emotions may persist, and a woman should seek professional counselling.

QUESTIONS FOR CRITICAL THINKING AND REFLECTION

What is your stand on the issue of late-term abortion? Do you feel it is never acceptable, or is it acceptable under certain circumstances? If so, what are those circumstances?

suction curettage   Removal of the embryo or fetus by means of suction; also called *dilation and curettage (D&C)*.

manual vacuum aspiration (MVA)   The vacuum aspiration of uterine contents shortly after a missed period by using a handheld syringe.

Mc Graw Hill connect™

Practise and learn online with Connect. Connect allows you to practise important skills at your own pace and on your own schedule, with 24/7 online access to an eBook, practice quizzes, interactivities, videos, study tools, additional resources, and more.

SUMMARY

• The female external sex organs are called the vulva; the clitoris plays an important role in sexual arousal and orgasm.

• The vagina leads to the internal sex organs, including the uterus, oviducts, and ovaries.

• The male external sex organs are the penis and the scrotum; the glans of the penis is an important site of sexual arousal.

• Internal sexual structures include the testes, vasa deferentia, seminal vesicles, and prostate gland.

• The fertilizing sperm determines the sex of the individual. Specialized genes on the Y chromosome initiate the process of male sexual differentiation in the embryo.

• Hormones initiate the changes that occur during puberty: The reproductive system matures, secondary sex characteristics develop, and the bodies of males and females become more distinctive.

• The menstrual cycle consists of four phases: menses, the estrogenic phase, ovulation, and the progestational phase.

• The ovaries gradually cease to function as women approach age 50 and enter menopause. The pattern of male sexual responses changes with age, and testosterone production gradually decreases.

• Sexual activity is based on stimulus and response. Stimulation may be physical or psychological.

• Vasocongestion and muscle tension are the primary physiological mechanisms of sexual arousal.

• The sexual response cycle has four stages: excitement, plateau, orgasm, and resolution.

• Physical and psychological problems can both interfere with sexual functioning.

• A treatment for sexual dysfunction first addresses any underlying medical conditions and then looks at psychosocial problems.

• Some gender characteristics are determined biologically, and others are defined by society. Children learn traits and behaviours traditionally deemed appropriate for one sex or the other.

• The ability to respond sexually is present at birth. Sexual behaviours emerging in childhood include self-exploration, perhaps leading to masturbation.

• Although puberty defines biological adulthood, people take five to ten more years to reach social maturity.

• Sexual fantasies and dreams and nocturnal emissions characterize adolescent sexuality.

• A person's sexual orientation can be heterosexual, gay or lesbian, or bisexual. Possible influences include genetics, hormonal factors, and early childhood experiences.

• Human sexual behaviours include celibacy, erotic fantasy, masturbation, touching, cunnilingus, fellatio, anal intercourse, and coitus.

• To evaluate whether an atypical sexual behaviour is problematic, experts consider the issues of consent between partners and whether the behaviour results in physical or psychological harm.

• Responsible sexuality includes open, honest communication; agreed-on sexual activities; sexual privacy; the use of contraception; safer sex practices; sober sex; and the taking of responsibility for consequences.

• Barrier methods of contraception physically prevent sperm from reaching the egg; hormonal methods are designed to prevent ovulation, fertilization, or implantation; and surgical methods permanently block the movement of sperm or eggs to the site of conception.

• The choice of contraceptive method depends on effectiveness, convenience, cost, reversibility, side effects and risk factors, and protection against STIs. Measures of effectiveness include failure rate and continuation rate.

• Hormonal methods of contraception include a combination of estrogen and progestins or progesterone alone. Hormones may be delivered via pills, patch, vaginal ring, implants, or injections.

- Hormonal methods of contraception prevent ovulation, inhibit the movement of sperm, and affect the uterine lining so that implantation is prevented.

- The most commonly used emergency contraceptives are two-dose regimens of oral contraceptives and Plan B, which is now available without a prescription to women 18 and older.

- How IUDs work is not clearly understood; they may cause biochemical changes in the uterus, affect movement of sperm and eggs, or interfere with the implantation of the egg in the uterus.

- Male condoms are simple to use, immediately reversible, and provide STI protection; female condoms are available but are more difficult to use.

- The diaphragm, Lea's Shield, cervical cap, and contraceptive sponge cover the cervix and block sperm from entering; all are used with or contain spermicide.

- Vaginal spermicides come in the form of foams, creams, jellies, suppositories, and film.

- Abortion is legal in Canada, and the procedure can be either surgical or medical.

- Psychological effects may be experienced by some women who undergo abortion; having a supportive friend, partner, or family is important to help with these challenges. Professional counselling may also be advised.

FOR MORE INFORMATION

BOOKS

Carlson, K. J., S. A. Eisenstat, and T. Ziporyn. 2004. *The New Harvard Guide to Women's Health.* Cambridge, Mass.: Belknap Press; Simon, H. B. 2004. *The Harvard Medical School Guide to Men's Health: Lessons from the Harvard Men's Health Studies.* New York: Free Press. These books provide research-based information about a wide variety of health issues, including sexuality, contraception, and sexually transmitted diseases.

Halbreich, U. 2003. New advances in premenstrual syndromes (PMS/PMDD). *Psychoneuroendocrinology* [Special Issue] 28(3 Suppl.). An entire issue devoted to all aspects of PMS and PMDD, including symptoms, treatments, and possible causes.

Kelly, G. F. 2007. *Sexuality Today,* 9th ed. New York: McGraw-Hill. An accessible approach that highlights cross-cultural examples, popular topics and issues, and case studies featuring college- and university-age individuals.

Marcus, E. 2005. *Is It a Choice? Answers to 300 of the Most Frequently Asked Questions About Gay and Lesbian People,* 3rd ed. San Francisco: Harper. Candid and informative information on coming out, family roles, and politics.

Omoto, A. M., and H. S. Kurtzman, eds. 2006. *Sexual Orientation and Mental Health: Examining Identity and Development in Lesbian, Gay, and Bisexual People.* Washington, D.C.: American Psychological Association. Covers topics in mental health as well as sexual

behaviour, work satisfaction, and the well-being of children of same-sex couples.

Strong, B., et al. 2008. *Human Sexuality: Diversity in Contemporary America,* 6th ed. New York: McGraw-Hill. A comprehensive introduction to human sexuality.

Taverner, W. J. 2006. *Taking Sides: Clashing Views on Controversial Issues in Human Sexuality,* 9th ed. New York: McGraw-Hill. Includes pro and con position statements on sexuality issues relating to biology, behaviour, and legal and social issues.

ORGANIZATIONS, HOTLINES, AND WEB SITES

The Internet addresses listed here were accurate at the time of publication.

Center for Young Women's Health. Includes information about many topics, such as menstruation, gynecological exams, eating disorders, body piercing, and sexual health.
   http://www.youngwomenshealth.org
International Planned Parenthood Federation. A global service provider and a leading advocate of sexual and reproductive health and rights for all
   http://www.ippf.org
The Kinsey Institute for Research in Sex, Gender, and Reproduction. One of the oldest and most respected institutions doing research on sexuality.
   http://www.kinseyinstitute.org
Public Health Agency of Canada. A list of frequently asked questions about contraception and their answers.
   http://www.phac-aspc.gc.ca/publicat/epiu-aepi/std-mts/
   contraceptives-eng.php
Sexuality and U. Administered by the Society of Obstetricians and Gynaecologists of Canada, this Web site provides credible and up-to-date information and education on sexual health.
   http://www.sexualityandu.ca
Sex Information and Education Council of Canada. Fosters professional education and public knowledge about sexuality and sexual health.
   http://www.sieccan.org
Sexuality Information and Education Council of the United States. Provides information on many aspects of sexuality and has an extensive library and numerous publications.
   http://www.siecus.org
Talking with Kids. Provides advice for parents about talking with children about difficult issues, including sex, relationships, and STIs.
   http://www.talkingwithkids.org
World Association for Sexual Health. Works to promote sexual health for all.
   http://www.worldsexualhealth.org

See also the listings for Chapters 10, 12, and 13.

SELECTED BIBLIOGRAPHY

Advance provision of emergency contraception for pregnancy prevention (full review). 2007. *Cochrane Database of Systematic Reviews* (2): CD005497.

Anawalt, B. D. 2007. Update on the development of male hormonal contraceptives. *Current Opinion in Investigational Drugs* 8(4): 318–323.

Ashok, P. W., et al. 2005. Patient preference in a randomized study comparing medical and surgical abortion at 10–13 weeks gestation. *Contraception* 71(2): 143–148.

Agot, K. E., et al. 2004. Risk of HIV-1 in rural Kenya: A comparison of circumcised and uncircumcised men. *Epidemiology* 15(2): 157–163.

Beckman, L. J., et al. 2006. Women's acceptance of the diaphragm: The role of relationship factors. *Journal of Sex Research* 43(4): 297–306.

Beksinska, M. E., et al. 2007. Bone mineral density in adolescents using norethisterone enanthate, depot-medroxyprogesterone acetate or combined oral contraceptives for contraception. *Contraception* 75(6): 438–443.

Bogaert, A. F. 2006. Biological versus nonbiological older brothers and men's sexual orientation. *Proceedings of the National Academy of Sciences* 103(28): 10771–10774.

Brohet, R. M., et al. 2007. Oral contraceptives and breast cancer risk in the international BRCA 1/2 carrier cohort study: A report from EMBRACE, GENEPSO, GEO-HEBON, and the IBCCS Collaborating Group. *Journal of Clinical Oncology* 25(25): 3831–3836.

Burkman, R. T. 2007. Transdermal hormonal contraception: Benefits and risks. *American Journal of Obstetrics and Gynecology* 197(2): 134.e1–134.e6.

Canadian Cancer Society/National Cancer Institute of Canada. 2009. *Canadian Cancer Statistics 2009* (http://www.cancer.ca/canada-wide/about%20cancer/cancer%20statistics/~/media/CCS/Canada%20wide/Files%20List/English%20files%20heading/pdf%20not%20in%20publications%20section/Stats%202009E%20Cdn%20Cancer.ashx; retrieved April 21, 2011).

Chamley, L. W., and G. N. Clarke. 2007. Antisperm antibodies and conception. *Seminars in Immunopathology* 29(2): 169–184.

Coffee, A. L., et al. 2007. Long-term assessment of symptomatology and satisfaction of an extended oral contraceptive regimen. *Contraception* 75(6): 444–449.

Consumer Reports On Health. 2009. *Healthy Sex: His and Hers* (http://www.consumerreports.org/health/conditions-and-treatments/sex-health/overview/sexual-health-ov.htm; retrieved June 21, 2011).

Curtis, K. M., et al. 2007. Neoplasia with use of intrauterine devices. *Contraception* 75(6 Suppl.): S60–S69.

Dailar, Cynthia. 2006. *Guttmacher Policy Review* (http://www.guttmacher.org/pubs/gpr/09/3/gpr090312.html; retrieved January 27, 2009).

Fazio, L., and G. Brock. 2004. Erectile dysfunction: management update. *Canadian Medical Association Journal* 170(9): 1429–1437.

Frye, C. A. 2006. An overview of oral contraceptives: Mechanism of action and clinical use. *Neurology* 66(6 Suppl.): S29–S36.

Gades, N. M., et al. 2005. Association between smoking and erectile dysfunction: A population-based study. *American Journal of Epidemiology* 161(4): 346–351.

Gilliam, M., et al. 2007. Factors associated with willingness to use the contraceptive vaginal ring. *Contraception* 76(1): 30–34.

Gordon, L., et al. 2007. Clinical inquiries. What hormonal contraception is most effective for obese women? *Journal of Family Practice* 56(6): 471–473.

Harris, M. A., J. C. Prior, and M. Koehoorn. 2008. Age at menarche in the Canadian population: Secular trends and relationship to adulthood BMI. *Journal of Adolescent Health* 43(6): 548–554.

Health Canada. 2006. *It's Your Health: Seniors and Aging—Sexual Activity* (http://www.hc-sc.gc.ca/hl-vs/iyh-vsv/life-vie/seniors-aines-eng.php; retrieved April 21, 2011).

Hershberger, S. L., and N. L. Segal. 2004. The cognitive, behavioral, and personality profiles of male monozygotic triplet set discordant for sexual orientation. *Archives of Sexual Behavior* 33(5): 497–514.

Hijazi, R. A., and G. R. Cunningham. 2004. Andropause: Is androgen replacement therapy indicated for the aging male? *Annual Review of Medicine* 56: 117–137.

Hutcheson, J. C. 2004. Male neonatal circumcision: Indications, controversies and complications. *Urologic Clinics of North America* 31(3): 461–471.

Isley, M. M., and A. Edelman. 2007. Contraceptive implants: An overview and update. *Obstetrics and Gynecology Clinics of North America* 34(1): 73–90.

Jick, S., et al. 2007. Further results on the risk of nonfatal venous thromboembolism in users of the contraceptive transdermal patch compared to users of oral contraceptives containing norgestimate and 35 micrograms of ethinyl estradiol. *Contraception* 76(1): 4–7.

Kalmuss, D., and C. Tatum. 2007. Patterns of men's use of sexual and reproductive health services. *Perspectives on Sexual and Reproductive Health* 39(2): 74–81.

Laumann, E. O., et al. 2005. Sexual problems among women and men aged 40–80 y: Prevalence and correlates identified in the Global Study of Sexual Attitudes and Behaviors. *International Journal of Impotence Research* 17(1): 39–57.

Lee, J. M., et al. 2007. Weight status in young girls and the onset of puberty. *Pediatrics* 119(3): 624–630.

Lewis, B. H., et al. 2006. Medical implications of the male biological clock. *Journal of the American Medical Association* 296(19): 2369–2371.

Lurie, G., et al. 2007. Association of estrogen and progestin potency of oral contraceptives with ovarian carcinoma risk. *Obstetrics and Gynecology* 109(3): 597–607.

Macaluso, M., et al. 2007. Efficacy of the male latex condom and of the female polyurethane condom as barriers to semen during intercourse: A randomized clinical trial. *American Journal of Epidemiology* 166(1): 88–96.

MacIsaac, L., and E. Espey. 2007. Intrauterine contraception: The pendulum swings back. *Obstetrics and Gynecology Clinics of North America* 34(1): 91–111.

Margolis, K. L., et al. 2007. A prospective study of oral contraceptive use and risk of myocardial infarction among Swedish women. *Fertility and Sterility* 88(2): 310–316.

Meirik, O., and T. M. Farley. 2007. Risk of cancer and the oral contraceptive pill. *British Medical Journal* 335(7621): 621–622.

Moreau, C., et al. 2007. Oral contraceptive tolerance: Does the type of pill matter? *Obstetrics and Gynecology* 109(6): 1277–1285.

National Institutes of Health. 2007. *Decrease in Breast Cancer Rates Related to Reduction in Use of Hormone Replacement Therapy* (http://www.nih.gov/news/pr/apr2007/nci-18a.htm; retrieved January 27, 2009).

Nettleman, M. D., et al. 2007. Reasons for unprotected intercourse: Analysis of the PRAMS survey. *Contraception* 75(5): 361–366.

Padian, N. S., et al. 2007. Diaphragm and lubricant gel for prevention of HIV acquisition in southern African women: A randomized controlled trial. *Lancet* 370(9583): 251–261.

Pills for erectile dysfunction: Now there are three. 2004. *Harvard Men's Health Watch*, April.

Rates of circumcision slashed in past 30 years. 2006. *The Gazette*. March 23: A13 (http://www.cirp.org/news/2006-03-23montrealgazette/; retrieved April 21, 2011).

Rossouw, J. E., et al. 2007. Postmenopausal hormone therapy and risk of cardiovascular disease by age and years since menopause. *Journal of the American Medical Association* 297(13): 1465–1477.

Prine, L. 2007. Emergency contraception, myths and facts. *Obstetrics and Gynecology Clinics of North American* 34(1): 127–136.

Roumen, F. J. 2007. The contraceptive vaginal ring compared with the combined oral contraceptive pill: A comprehensive review of randomized controlled trials. *Contraception* 75(6): 420–429.

Sulak, P. J., et al. 2006. Impact of an adolescent sex education program that was implemented by an academic medical center. *American Journal of Obstetrics and Gynecology* 195(1): 78–84.

Sanderson, C. A., and D. J. Yopyk. 2007. Improving condom use intentions and behavior by changing perceived partner norms: An evaluation of condom promotion videos for college students. *Health Psychology* 26(4): 481–487.

Shtarkshall, R. A., et al. 2007. Sex education and sexual socialization: Roles for educators and parents. *Perspectives on Sexual and Reproductive Health* 39(2): 116–119.

Swica, Y. 2007. The transdermal patch and the vaginal ring: Two novel methods of combined hormonal contraception. *Obstetrics and Gynecology Clinics of North America* 34(1): 31–42.

Wang, L., et al. 2004. Stress and dysmenorrhoea: A population based prospective study. *Occupational and Environmental Medicine* 61(12): 1021–1026.

WebMD. 2007. *Acne vulgaris* (http://www.emedicine.com/derm/topic2.htm; retrieved January 27, 2009).

Westhoff, C., et al. 2007. Initiation of oral contraceptives using a quick start compared with a conventional start: A randomized controlled trial. *Obstetrics and Gynecology* 109(6): 1270–1276.

Witte, S. S., et al. 2006. Promoting female condom use to heterosexual couples: Findings from a randomized clinical trial. *Perspectives on Sexual and Reproductive Health* 38(3): 148–154.

World Health Organization. 2007. *WHO and UNAIDS Announce Recommendations from Expert Consultation on Male Circumcision for HIV Prevention* (http://www.who.int/hiv/mediacentre/news68/en/print.html; retrieved January 27, 2009).

World Health Organization. 2008. *Female Genital Mutilation.* (http://www.who.int/gb/ebwha/pdf_files/EB122/B122_R13-en.pdf; retrieved January 27, 2009).

Zurawin, R. K., and L. Ayensu-Coker. 2007. Innovations in contraception: A review. *Clinical Obstetrics and Gynecology* 50(2): 425–439.

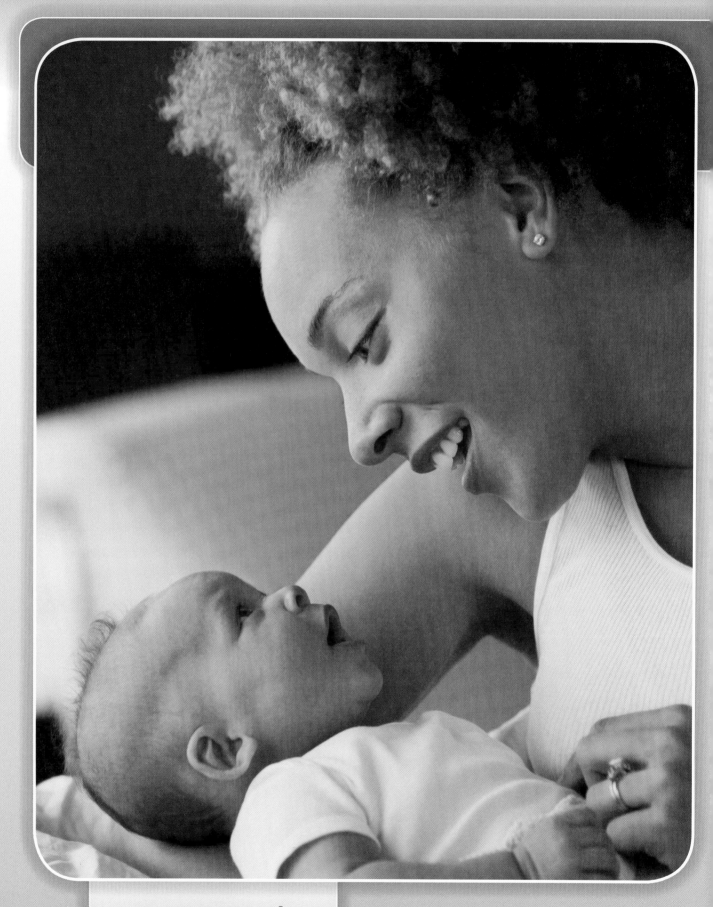

PREGNANCY AND CHILDBIRTH

12

LOOKING AHEAD>>>>>

AFTER READING THIS CHAPTER, YOU SHOULD BE ABLE TO

- List key issues to consider when deciding about parenthood
- Explain the process of conception, and describe the most common causes of and treatments for infertility
- Describe the physical and emotional changes a pregnant woman typically experiences
- Discuss the stages of fetal development
- List the important components of good prenatal care
- Describe the process of labour and delivery

TEST YOUR KNOWLEDGE

1. **What is the approximate cost of raising one child to the age of 18 in Canada?**
   a. $50,000–$100,000
   b. $100,000–$150,000
   c. $150,000–$200,000

2. **What is the leading cause of female infertility?**
   a. growths in the uterus
   b. exposure to radiation
   c. tubal factors, such as blockages and previous infection

3. **Before conception and in the early weeks of pregnancy, adequate intake of which of the following nutrients can reduce the risk of spina bifida and other neural tube defects?**
   a. iron
   b. folic acid
   c. calcium

4. **Cigarette smoking before or during pregnancy is linked to which of the following?**
   a. congenital anomalies
   b. low birth weight
   c. miscarriage
   d. central nervous system defects

ANSWERS

1. **C.** According to Manitoba Agriculture, the average cost of raising a daughter to the age of 18 was $166,549 in 2004. For a son, the cost was $166,972 (the difference was due to extra food costs).

2. **C.** If left untreated, the sexually transmitted infections (STIs) gonorrhea and chlamydia can lead to tubal scarring and blockage.

3. **B.** It is recommended that all reproductive-age women consume 400 micrograms of folic acid from fortified foods and supplements each day to reduce the risk of spina bifida and other neural tube defects.

4. **ALL FOUR.** Maternal smoking during pregnancy is associated with many types of birth defects and low birth weight. Lower measured intelligence levels and increased frequencies of behavioural and psychological abnormalities have been reported in children and adults whose mothers smoked cigarettes during pregnancy. Also, the risk of having a miscarriage is 20%–80% higher among women who smoke cigarettes during pregnancy than it is in nonsmokers.

Deciding whether to become a parent is one of the most important choices a person can ever make. Yet many people approach this decision with only a vague notion of what is involved in pregnancy and childbirth. This may help explain why about half of the pregnancies in Canada are unintentional.

Previous generations of Canadians assumed that virtually every married couple would have children. Today, however, with changing cultural expectations and more sophisticated contraceptive technology, you can choose whether and when to have a child. As a result of these changes, the average age of first-time mothers in Canada has steadily increased over the past 30 years. From 1975 to 2005, the average age of first-time mothers increased by 2.5 years to 29.2 years. Figure 12.1 illustrates these trends. The more you know about conception and pregnancy, fetal development and prenatal care, childbirth and parenting, the more capable you will be of making intelligent, informed decisions about them. This chapter presents information you can use both now and later in life to make the choices about pregnancy and childbirth that are right for you.

PREPARATION FOR PARENTHOOD

Before you decide whether or when to become a parent, you should consider your suitability and readiness. If you elect to have a child, you can take some actions before the pregnancy begins to help ensure a healthy outcome.

Deciding to Become a Parent

Many factors must be taken into account when you are considering parenthood. Some issues are relevant to both men and women; others apply only to women.

Health and Age   Generally speaking, healthier women tend to have more trouble-free pregnancies and healthier babies. Women who are considering motherhood should see their doctor for a complete medical checkup to catch problems that might interfere with pregnancy or childbirth. For example, high blood pressure and diabetes may require ongoing attention; if uncontrolled, these health problems can pose life-threatening dangers to mother or child.

A mother's age can also be a factor in pregnancy and childbirth. Teenagers and women over age 35 have a higher incidence of certain problems that can affect the health of

QUICK STATS

In 2007, approximately **3%** of babies were born to mothers ages 40 and older in Canada.

—Statistics Canada, 2009

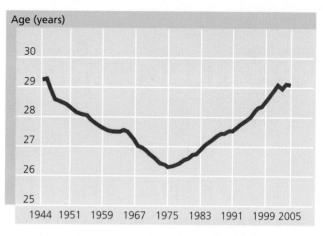

FIGURE 12.1   Average age of mother at childbirth.

Source: Human Resources and Skills Development Canada. 2010. *Indicators of Wellbeing in Canada: Age of Mother at Childbirth* (http://www4.hrsdc.gc.ca/.3ndic.1t.4r@-eng.jsp?iid=75; retrieved April 26, 2010).

both mother and baby. In fact, most experts automatically classify a pregnancy as high-risk if the mother is over age 35, especially if it is her first pregnancy.

Emotional Preparedness   Just as they need to be physically prepared, parents also need to be emotionally ready to have a child. A new baby is helpless and relies on adults for everything. For parents, this means being strong and stable enough to handle the responsibility and being mature enough to give up certain freedoms to care for a child.

Financial Circumstances   Parenthood is financially draining, even for families with steady incomes. As noted, the average cost of raising a child to the age of 18 in Canada was more than $166,000 in 2004.

If you are planning to have a child, try to make sure you are prepared financially—especially during the first few years, when the costs of diapers, furniture, and other necessities quickly add up. It makes good sense for all expecting parents to consult with a financial planner, regardless of income level. A qualified financial planner can help new parents see their larger financial picture and focus on important issues, such as taxes, insurance needs, and saving for long-term goals and emergencies. A good rule of thumb is to prepare to spend approximately $10,000 per year per child.

Relationships   The stress and expense of child rearing can strain any relationship, even a healthy one, which is why it is important for couples to plan for parenting. Through open, honest discussion, partners should make sure they are both ready to take the step of having a child. Both should be equally committed to parenthood and agree on matters of child care, housework, and other day-to-day responsibilities. Couples with relationship problems should work together to resolve their issues—with professional help, if necessary—before adding a child to the mix.

New parents also need a strong support network of friends and family members who can lend a hand when things get tough. Many first-time parents count on their own parents and siblings for aid with child care or household chores. It can be easy, however, to alienate family and friends with too many requests for assistance. To avoid this problem, parents-to-be should include members of their support network in the planning process, to figure out who will be able to help, in what ways, and at what times.

Future Plans   Having a child can put other life plans on hold, especially if the pregnancy is unintended. Anyone considering parenthood should make sure that it will fit with other goals. Otherwise, it may be necessary to postpone or cancel educational or career plans.

An important aspect of this planning is child care. New parents should figure out whether they will need child care services (such as a day care centre or a private caregiver) in order to work or attend school. The cost and availability of such services can be a deciding factor in determining whether parents can pursue their future plans. Canadian child care costs range from approximately $25 to $100 per day depending on the type of child care service; however, lower rates are often available for those in need of financial assistance.

Attitude and Aptitude   Before having a child, it's important for parents to recognize whether they have the right attitude about child rearing. If one parent is devoted to a child but the other views parenting as a burden, the partnership and the child will suffer. Before deciding to become a parent, it's a good idea to spend time with young children and see how you respond to them. It is also wise to talk to people who have raised children, and see if their experiences strike a positive chord in you.

Parents-to-be should also ask themselves how much they know about caring for a child and seek help according to their needs. Certain skills—such as diaper changing, bathing, and feeding—are essential but easy to learn and quickly become routine with a little practice. Other important parenting attributes, such as patience and the ability to stay calm in a crisis, aren't easily acquired if you don't already have them.

Luckily, many good sources of information are available for first-time parents. The best place to start is a family physician or pediatrician. Many hospitals and health units offer free or low-cost classes on labour, delivery, breastfeeding, and basic child care for expecting parents.

Preconception Care

The birth of a healthy baby depends in part on the mother's overall wellness before conception. The Society of Obstetricians and Gynaecologists of Canada (SOGC) recommends that all women receive health care to help them prepare for pregnancy. **Preconception care** should include an assessment of health risks, the promotion of healthy lifestyle behaviours, and any treatments necessary to reduce risk. The following are some of the issues, tests, and treatments involved during preconception care:

- *Preexisting conditions.* Medical conditions, such as diabetes, epilepsy, asthma, high blood pressure, and anemia, can cause problems during pregnancy. These conditions should be treated and monitored closely throughout pregnancy.

- *Medications.* Some medications and dietary supplements harm the **fetus** (the unborn baby from the ninth week after conception to the moment of birth), so a pregnant woman may need to change or stop taking certain drugs.

- *Prior pregnancies.* Problems with previous pregnancies or deliveries—such as miscarriage, premature birth, or delivery complications—may be due to a treatable physical condition.

- *Age.* As mentioned earlier, a woman's age may place her at risk for certain problems during pregnancy. A pregnant teenager, for example, may require special nutrition to meet her own growing body's needs and those of her baby. A woman over age 35 may need genetic testing because of the increased risk of her baby developing Down syndrome.

- *Tobacco, alcohol, and caffeine use.* These substances can harm a developing fetus. Women who smoke, drink, or consume caffeine should stop before becoming pregnant. (See Chapters 14–16 for more information on these and other substances.)

- *Infections.* A woman who has any type of infection should be treated for the infection before getting pregnant, if possible. This is good advice for men, too, to avoid transmitting an infection to their partner. A woman may need to be vaccinated against hepatitis B, rubella (German measles), varicella (chicken pox), and other communicable diseases if she is at risk for them. Testing for tuberculosis and some STIs can ensure treatment before pregnancy. (See Chapters 9 and 13 for more on infectious diseases and STIs.)

preconception care   Health care in preparation for pregnancy.

fetus   The developmental stage of a human from the ninth week after conception to the moment of birth.

TERMS

- *HIV.* Any woman who is at risk of HIV infection should be tested before getting pregnant; her partner should be tested as well. (See Chapter 13 for more on HIV and AIDS.)

- *Diet.* Good nutrition is essential to a healthy pregnancy. Nutritional counselling can help a woman create a plan for healthy eating before and during pregnancy. Diet is especially important for any woman with special nutritional needs or an eating disorder, or who is overweight or obese. Physicians commonly prescribe prenatal vitamin supplements to pregnant women. The SOGC recommends that all women of childbearing age take extra folic acid to reduce the risk of neural tube defects that can arise in the fetus. (See Chapter 5 for more information on nutrition.)

- *Multiple births.* If twins or multiple births run in a woman's family, she is more likely to have multiple births, too. Multiple births are also more prevalent in mothers who are obese, over 40, or using certain reproductive technologies to get pregnant.

- *Genetic diseases.* If either partner has a family history of any genetic disease, then genetic counselling may be in order before pregnancy. Genetic testing can determine whether the mother or father is a carrier for a specific disease. With counselling, a couple can decide how best to deal with the possibility of transferring a disease to a child. Members of some ethnic groups are at higher risk for genetic disorders; for more information on these disorders, see the box "Ethnicity and Genetic Diseases" on p. 380.

Additional tests or changes in behaviour may be recommended for prospective parents who have recently travelled outside Canada; who work with chemicals, radiation, or toxic substances; who participate in physically demanding or hazardous activities or occupations; or who face significant psychosocial risks, including homelessness, an unsafe home environment, or mental illness.

UNDERSTANDING FERTILITY

Conceiving a child is a highly complex process. Although many couples conceive readily, others can testify to the difficulties that can be encountered.

Conception

The process of conception involves the **fertilization** of an ovum (egg) from a woman by a sperm from a man (Figure 12.2). Every month during a woman's fertile years, her body prepares itself for conception and pregnancy. In one of her ovaries an egg matures and is released from its follicle. The egg, about the size of a pinpoint, travels through an oviduct, or fallopian tube, to the uterus in three to four days. The endometrium, or lining of

QUESTIONS FOR CRITICAL THINKING AND REFLECTION

If you don't have children now, do you plan to have them someday? Have you given any thought to the skills and qualities that make a good parent? Given what you know about yourself today, do you think you will make a good parent? What skills or qualities do you think you need to develop?

the uterus, has already thickened for the implantation of a **fertilized egg**, or *zygote*. If the egg is not fertilized, it lasts about 24 hours and then disintegrates. It is expelled along with the uterine lining during menstruation.

Sperm cells are produced in the man's testes and ejaculated from his penis into the woman's vagina during sexual intercourse (except in cases of artificial insemination or assisted reproduction; see p. 382). Sperm cells are much smaller than eggs. The typical ejaculate contains millions of sperm, but only a few complete the journey through the uterus and up the fallopian tube to the egg. Many sperm cells do not survive the acidic environment of the vagina.

Once through the cervix and into the uterus, many sperm cells are diverted to the wrong oviduct or get stuck along the way. Of those that reach the egg, only one will penetrate its hard outer layer. As sperm approach the egg, they release enzymes that soften this outer layer. Enzymes from hundreds of sperm must be released for the egg's outer layer to soften enough to allow one sperm cell to penetrate. The first sperm cell that bumps into a spot that is soft enough can swim into the egg cell. It then merges with the nucleus of the egg, and fertilization occurs. The sperm's tail, its means of locomotion, gets stuck in the outer membrane and drops off, leaving the sperm head inside the egg. The egg then releases a chemical that makes it impenetrable by other sperm.

The ovum carries the hereditary characteristics of the mother and her ancestors; sperm cells carry the hereditary characteristics of the father and his ancestors. Each parent cell—egg or sperm—contains 23 chromosomes, each of which contains genes, packages of chemical instructions for the developing baby. Genes provide the blueprint for a unique individual (see the box "Creating a Family Health Tree" on p. 381).

As soon as fertilization occurs, the zygote starts to undergo the cell division that begins the growth process. It continues to divide as it travels through the oviduct to the uterus. On reaching the uterus, the cluster of cells, now called a *blastocyst*, becomes implanted in the endometrium.

The usual course of events is that one egg and one sperm unite to produce one fertilized egg and one baby. But if the ovaries release two (or more) eggs during ovulation and if both eggs are fertilized, twins will develop. These twins will be no more alike than siblings from different pregnancies, because each will have come from a

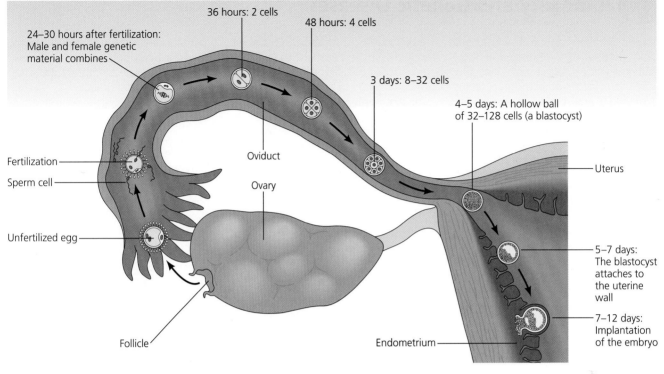

24–30 hours after fertilization: Male and female genetic material combines

36 hours: 2 cells

48 hours: 4 cells

3 days: 8–32 cells

4–5 days: A hollow ball of 32–128 cells (a blastocyst)

Oviduct

Ovary

Uterus

Fertilization

Sperm cell

Unfertilized egg

5–7 days: The blastocyst attaches to the uterine wall

7–12 days: Implantation of the embryo

Follicle

Endometrium

FIGURE 12.2   Fertilization and early development of the embryo.

different fertilized egg. Twins who develop this way are referred to as **fraternal twins**; they may be the same sex or different sexes. About 70% of twins are fraternal. Twins can also develop from the division of a single fertilized egg into two cells that develop separately. Because these babies share all genetic material, they are **identical twins**. The most serious complication of multiple births is preterm delivery (delivery before the fetuses are adequately mature). Studies show that the more fetuses a woman carries simultaneously, the shorter the gestational period will be. In 1934, the Dionne quintuplets were born in a northern Ontario farmhouse. This was Canada's most famous multiple birth because these quintuplets were the first in the world to be conceived and born naturally (before the advent of fertility medications) and to survive through infancy.

Infertility

Millions of couples have difficulty conceiving. **Infertility** is defined as the inability to conceive after trying for a year or more. It affects about 15% of the reproductive-age population of Canada. Many couples seek treatment for infertility each year. Although the focus is often on women (where the cause of infertility is found in 40% of cases), 20% of the factors contributing to infertility are male, and in 30% of infertile couples, both partners have problems. Therefore, it is important that each individual be evaluated.

Female Infertility   Female infertility usually results from one of two key causes—tubal blockage (40%) or failure to ovulate (40%). An additional 10% of cases of infertility are due to anatomical abnormalities, benign growths in the uterus, thyroid disease, and other uncommon conditions; the remaining 10% of cases are unexplained. Unexplained infertility implies that a cause for the infertility has not been found after completing all relevant investigations. This is often very frustrating for the couple involved.

Blocked fallopian tubes are most commonly the result of *pelvic inflammatory disease (PID)*, a serious complication of several sexually transmitted infections. Most cases of PID are associated with untreated cases of chlamydia or gonorrhea.

TERMS

fertilization   The initiation of biological reproduction: the union of the nucleus of an egg cell with the nucleus of a sperm cell.

fertilized egg   The egg after penetration by a sperm; a zygote.

fraternal twins   Twins who develop from separate fertilized eggs; not genetically identical.

identical twins   Twins who develop from the division of a single zygote; genetically identical.

infertility   The inability to conceive after trying for a year or more.

Ethnicity and Genetic Diseases

Genes carry the chemical instructions that determine the development of hundreds of individual traits, including disease risks, in every human being. Many traits and conditions involve multiple genes and environmental influences. Some diseases, however, can be traced to a mutation in a single gene.

Children inherit one set of genes from each parent. If only one copy of an abnormal gene is necessary to produce a disease, then it is called a *dominant* gene. Diseases caused by dominant genes seldom skip a generation; anyone who carries the gene will probably get the disease.

If two copies of an abnormal gene (one from each parent) are necessary for a disease to occur, then the gene is called *recessive*. Many diseases caused by recessive genes occur disproportionately in certain ethnic groups. Prospective parents who come from the same ethnic group can be tested for any recessive diseases that are known to occur in that group. If both parents are carriers, each of their children will have about a 25% chance of developing the disease.

The following list describes a few common conditions with proven genetic links in certain ethnic populations. If there is a history of any of these conditions in your family and you plan to have children, genetic tests and counselling can help assess the risk to your prospective offspring.

• *Sickle-cell disease* is common in the African-descended population of North America. It affects millions of people worldwide, primarily those whose ancestors come from sub-Saharan Africa, South America, Cuba, Central America, Saudi Arabia, India, and Mediterranean countries (Turkey, Greece, and Italy). In this disease,

red blood cells, which carry oxygen to the body's tissues, change shape; the normally disc-shaped cells become sickle shaped. The altered cells carry less oxygen and can block small blood vessels. People who inherit one gene for sickle-cell disease experience only mild symptoms; those with two genes become severely, often fatally, ill.

If you are at risk for sickle-cell disease, you should take care to reduce stress and respond to minor infections because red blood cells become sickle-shaped when the body is under stress. You should also have regular checkups and appropriate treatment, if required.

• *Hemochromatosis* (iron overload) affects about 1 in 200 people. At highest risk are people of Northern European (especially Irish), Mediterranean, and Hispanic descent. In hemochromatosis, the body absorbs and stores up to ten times the normal amount of iron. Iron deposits form in the joints, liver, heart, and pancreas. If untreated, the disease can cause organ failure and death.

Early symptoms are often vague and include weakness, lethargy, darkening of the skin, and joint pain. Early detection and treatment are necessary to prevent damage. Treatment involves reducing iron stores by removing blood from the body (a process known as phlebotomy or "bloodletting"). Sometimes, if the person is eligible, donating blood on a regular basis can serve as the treatment.

• *Tay-Sachs disease*, another recessive disorder, occurs in about 1 in 3000 Jewish people of Eastern European ancestry. People with Tay-Sachs disease cannot properly metabolize fat. As a result, the brain and other nerve tissues deteriorate. Affected children show weakness in their movements and eventually develop blindness (by age 12–18 months) and seizures. This disease is fatal, and death usually occurs by age six. No effective treatment is currently available.

• *Cystic fibrosis* occurs in 1 in 2500–3000 Caucasians; about 1 in 29 carries one copy of the cystic fibrosis gene. Because essential enzymes of the pancreas are deficient, the body cannot properly absorb nutrients. Thick mucus impairs functioning in the lungs and intestinal tracts of people with this disease. Cystic fibrosis is often fatal in early childhood,

but treatments are increasingly effective in reducing symptoms and prolonging life. In some cases, symptoms do not appear until early adulthood.

• *Thalassemia* is a blood disease found most often among Italians, Greeks, and to a lesser extent people of African and Asian descent. When inherited from one parent, this form of anemia is mild; when two genes are present, the disease is severe and can cause fetal death.

Children with this condition require repeated blood transfusions, eventually resulting in a damaging iron build-up. New interventions, such as genetic engineering, bone marrow transplants, and chemicals that bind with excess iron and remove it from the body, offer promise. Transplantation of stem cells from the umbilical cord blood of an unaffected sibling or donor is already being used in some cases.

If you are at risk of carrying thalassemia, you should get regular checkups and monitor your health for symptoms, and learn ways to manage symptoms if they start to occur.

• *Lactose intolerance*, or intolerance to lactose-containing foods (primarily dairy products), is a common problem that often has a genetic component. Clinical symptoms of lactose intolerance include diarrhea, abdominal pain, and flatulence after ingestion of milk or milk-containing products. These symptoms result from low intestinal lactase levels, which are commonly caused by the reduced genetic expression of the enzyme lactase-phlorizin hydrolase. Genetically regulated reduction of lactase activity determined by racial or ethnic factors is the underlying mechanism of lactose malabsorption in healthy individuals.

If you suspect lactose intolerance, see your doctor for a lactose absorption test. In the absence of a correctable underlying disease, lactose malabsorption is treated by reducing lactose intake, finding alternatives to foods containing lactose, taking an enzyme substitute, and maintaining calcium and vitamin D intake.

Other health problems that have a hereditary component and that disproportionately affect certain ethnic groups include diabetes, osteoporosis, high blood pressure, alcoholism, and certain cancers. Other chapters in this text discuss many of these links.

Creating a Family Health Tree

The genetic inheritance that each of us receives from our parents—and that our children receive from us—contains more than just physical characteristics, such as eye and hair colour. Heredity also contributes to our risk of developing certain diseases and disorders. For certain uncommon illnesses, such as hemophilia and sickle-cell disease, heredity is the primary cause; if your parents pass on the necessary genes, you'll get the disease. But heredity plays a subtler role in many other diseases, which are caused at least in part by environmental influences, such as infection, cancer-causing chemicals, and physical inactivity. Although your genes alone will not produce those diseases, they can determine how susceptible you are. Researchers have found a genetic influence in many common disorders, including heart disease, diabetes, depression, asthma, alcoholism, and certain forms of cancer.

Knowing that a specific disease runs in your family can save your life. It allows you to watch for early warning signs and get screening tests more often than you otherwise would. Changing health habits, too, can be valuable for people with a family history of certain diseases. An individual with a family history of high cholesterol and early heart disease can increase physical activity and pay special attention to diet.

In general, the more relatives with a genetically transmitted disease and the closer they are to you, the greater your risk. However, nongenetic factors—such as health habits—can also play a role. Signs of strong hereditary influence include early onset of the disease, appearance of the disease largely or exclusively on one side of the family, onset of the same disease at the same age in more than one relative, and developing the disease despite good health habits.

You can put together a simple family health tree by compiling a few key facts on your primary relatives: siblings, parents, aunts and uncles, and grandparents. Those facts include the date of birth, major diseases, health-related conditions and habits, and, for deceased relatives, the age at death as well as the cause. Because certain diseases are more common in particular ethnic groups, also record the ethnic background of each grandparent. Next, create a tree, using the example below as a guide. Then show your tree to a physician or genetic counsellor, who can help you target the health behaviours and screening tests that are most important for you and help you determine whether genetic testing might be appropriate.

A Sample Family Health Tree and What It Means

The 55-year-old woman who prepared this family tree has a strong family history of osteoporosis on her mother's side. She also has several close relatives on her father's side of the family who had high cholesterol levels and had heart attacks at an early age. These risk factors significantly increase her chance of having a heart attack.

The woman has two aunts who died of breast cancer, but there are several reasons not to be overly concerned. Aunts are second-degree relatives, more distantly related to her than her mother or sister (first-degree relatives). In addition, they came from different sides of the family, and they developed the disease quite late in life. Given these factors, it is likely that these cases of breast cancer did not have a significant genetic origin. Looking at her family history can help this woman make important decisions about behaviours, such as moderate alcohol consumption, which may lower the risk of heart attack but which may also slightly increase the risk of breast cancer. Based on her family history, her physician may recommend bone density testing to determine her risk of dangerous fractures and recommend medication and a heart-healthy diet to reduce her unhealthy cholesterol level and overall heart attack risk.

Sources: From "Prepare for the Future: Know Your Ancestors" and "Creating a Family Health Tree" © 1999 by Consumers Union of U.S., Inc. Yonkers, NY 10703-1057, a nonprofit organization. Reprinted with permission from the September 1999 issue of *Consumer Reports on Health*® for educational purposes only. No commercial use or reproduction permitted. www.ConsumerReports.org.

The Public Health Agency of Canada reports that there are approximately 100,000 cases of symptomatic PID per year in Canada; however, since PID is often asymptomatic and is not reportable, up to two-thirds of cases go unrecognized. It is estimated that 10%–15% of reproductive-age females have had PID. One episode of PID can result in infertility in 13% of patients. With a second infection, the risk increases to 36% and to 75% with a third infection. Tubal blockages can also be caused by prior surgery or by *endometriosis*, a condition in which endometrial (uterine) tissue grows outside of the uterus. This tissue responds to hormones and can cause pelvic pain, bleeding, scarring, and adhesions. Endometriosis is typically treated with hormonal therapy and surgery.

Age affects fertility; beginning at around age 30, a woman's fertility naturally begins to decline. Age is probably the main factor in ovulation failure. Exposure to toxic chemicals or radiation also appears to reduce fertility, as does cigarette smoking.

Male Infertility   Male factor infertility accounts for about 20% of infertile couples. The leading causes of male infertility can be divided into four main categories: hypothalamic pituitary disease or congenital disorders, testicular disease, disorders of sperm transport, and unexplained. Some acquired disorders of the testes can lead to infertility, such as damage from the following causes:

- Drug use (large doses of marijuana, for example, cause lower sperm counts and suppress certain reproductive hormones)
- Radiation
- Infection (such as having had mumps as a child)
- Environmental toxins
- Hyperthermia
- Smoking

Studies have identified a link between infertility and overweight and obesity in men, although the mechanism responsible for the relationship is not clear.

Treating Infertility   The cause of infertility can be determined for about 85% of infertile couples. Most cases of infertility are treated with conventional medical therapies. Surgery can repair oviducts, clear up endometriosis, and correct anatomical problems in both men and women. Fertility drugs can help women ovulate, although they may cause multiple births. If these conventional treatments don't work, couples can turn to **assisted reproductive technology (ART)** techniques, as described in the following sections.

Most infertility treatments are expensive and emotionally draining, however, and their success is hard to predict. Some infertile couples choose not to try to have children; others turn to adoption. One measure you can take now to avoid infertility is to protect yourself against STIs and to treat promptly and completely any disease you do

contract. Also, couples who are ready should consider trying to conceive before the woman's late 30s to decrease the probability of age-related infertility.

INTRAUTERINE INSEMINATION   Male infertility can sometimes be overcome by collecting and concentrating the man's sperm and introducing it by syringe into a woman's vagina or uterus, a procedure known as **artificial (intrauterine) insemination**. To increase the probability of success, the woman is often given fertility drugs to induce ovulation before the insemination procedure. The sperm can be provided by the woman's partner or, if there are severe problems with his sperm or he carries a serious genetic disorder, by a donor. Donor sperm are also used by single women and lesbian couples who want to conceive by using artificial insemination. The success rate is about 60%–70%.

IVF, GIFT, AND ZIFT   Three related techniques for overcoming infertility involve removing mature eggs from a woman's ovary.

- In **in vitro fertilization (IVF)**, the harvested eggs are mixed with sperm in a laboratory dish. If eggs are successfully fertilized, one or more of the resulting embryos are inserted into the woman's uterus. IVF is often used by women with blocked oviducts.
- In **gamete intrafallopian transfer (GIFT)**, eggs and sperm are surgically placed into the fallopian tubes before fertilization.
- In **zygote intrafallopian transfer (ZIFT)**, eggs are fertilized outside the woman's body and surgically introduced into the oviducts after they begin to divide.

GIFT and ZIFT can be used by women who have at least one open fallopian tube. Variations on these three techniques are also becoming available (see the box "Reproductive Technology").

THINKING ABOUT THE ENVIRONMENT

Global studies indicate that sperm counts have dropped by as much as 50% in the past 30 years. Many researchers believe that exposure to toxic substances (such as lead, chemical pollutants, and radiation) may be the cause.

- Of special interest is a class of chemicals called *endocrine disrupters*—substances found widely in the environment that mimic or interfere with the body's hormones. Endocrine disrupters may cause problems with reproduction, development, and fertility in humans; tests have linked these chemicals to reproductive problems in animals.

- Endocrine disrupters may be found in plastics, detergents, food, toys, cosmetics, pesticides, and other everyday products. The Government of Canada is taking national and international measures to investigate the effects of endocrine disruptors.

For more information on the environment and health, see Chapter 21.

Reproductive Technology

Research into the areas of genetics and cloning promise more breakthroughs for ART treatments. Below are a few of the most advanced techniques currently in use and under study.

Use of donor eggs, donor sperm, and donor embryos is fairly common in ART treatments. The use of donor eggs and embryos has allowed women in their fifties to complete pregnancy and deliver a baby. The resulting offspring is no more genetically related to the woman than an adopted child would be. Use of ART in women of this age is controversial.

Intracytoplasmic sperm injection (ICSI), in which a single sperm is injected into a mature egg, was originally developed to overcome cases of severe male infertility; it is now used for a broader range of conditions. Some studies have linked ICSI to an increase in genetic and birth defects in offspring. In addition, ICSI allows men who are infertile because of Y chromosome defects to have children, even though any sons they have will inherit the defect and also be infertile.

Cryopreservation of ovarian tissue and unfertilized eggs has been studied as a possible means of preserving fertility in women undergoing cancer therapy. In 2004, the first woman gave birth after having ovarian tissue removed and frozen before cancer chemotherapy and then reimplanted. This technique could potentially be used in women who choose to delay childbearing.

Freezing embryos is common in ART because multiple eggs are usually harvested and fertilized during IVF. If the initial IVF cycle is unsuccessful, the backup embryos can be used for additional attempts.

Preimplantation genetic diagnosis, in which embryos created through IVF undergo genetic analysis before implantation in the womb, was originally developed to help couples at risk for genetic diseases. According to the Assisted Human Reproduction Act, sex selection is prohibited in Canada, but outside Canada, some physicians now offer this technology for sex selection in couples who have no fertility problems.

Injection of cytoplasm (the material in a cell that surrounds the nucleus) from a younger woman's egg into an older woman's egg can be used as a possible means of reducing genetic errors in the older woman's egg. These errors occur in so-called mitochondrial DNA, genetic material in the cytoplasm of the cell that is passed along unchanged to offspring.

Nuclear transfer, a technique related to cytoplasm injection, uses cloning technology—the transfer of the nucleus from an older woman's egg into an egg from a younger woman from which the nucleus has been removed. In cytoplasm injection and nuclear transfer, the offspring carry DNA from two women—nuclear DNA from one woman and mitochondrial DNA from a second woman—and so have three genetic "parents."

Cloning is different from the techniques discussed here because it is a form of asexual reproduction. A clone carries the genes of only one person, not two. However, as described above, the cloning technique of nuclear transfer could potentially be used in the treatment of infertility. Nuclear transfer could theoretically also be used to create a child that is the genetic offspring of two people of the same sex. However, under the Assisted Human Reproduction Act, any form of human cloning is illegal in Canada.

IVF, GIFT, and ZIFT have drawbacks. Success rates vary from about 27% to 51%. They cost between $5000 and $13,000 per procedure and may require five or more cycles to produce one live birth. They also increase the chance of multiple births, which in turn increases the risk of premature birth and maternal complications, including pregnancy-related hypertension and diabetes.

SURROGATE MOTHERHOOD Surrogate motherhood involves a contract between an infertile couple and a fertile woman who agrees to carry a fetus. The surrogate mother agrees to be artificially inseminated by the father's sperm or to undergo IVF with the couple's embryo to carry the baby to term, and to give it to the couple at birth. In many areas of the world, the couple pays the surrogate mother for her services; however, in 2004, the Assisted Human Reproduction Act was passed in Canada, which prohibits payment to a surrogate mother, unless it is to reimburse her for expenses, such as medications, travel, and clothing.

Emotional Responses to Infertility Couples who seek treatment for infertility have often already confronted the possibility of not being able to become biological parents.

TERMS

assisted reproductive technology (ART) Advanced medical techniques used to treat infertility.

artificial (intrauterine) insemination The introduction of semen into the vagina by artificial means, usually by syringe.

in vitro fertilization (IVF) Combining egg and sperm outside the body and inserting the fertilized egg into the uterus.

gamete intrafallopian transfer (GIFT) Surgically introducing eggs and sperm into the fallopian tube before fertilization.

zygote intrafallopian transfer (ZIFT) Surgically introducing a fertilized egg into the fallopian tube.

cloning Asexual reproduction in which offspring are genetically identical to one parent.

Many infertile couples feel they have lost control over a major area of their lives. They may lose perspective on the rest of their lives as they focus more and more on the reasons for their infertility and on treatment. Infertile couples may need to set their own limits on how much treatment they are willing to undergo.

Support groups for infertile couples can provide help in this difficult situation, but there are few easy answers to infertility. If treatment is unsuccessful, couples must mourn the loss of the children they will never bear. They will need to make some kind of decision about their future—whether to pursue plans for adoption or another treatment or to adjust to childlessness and go on with their lives.

QUICK STATS

Only **15%** of couples affected by infertility can afford IVF treatment in Canada.

—Canadian Agency for Drugs and Technology in Health, 2009

PREGNANCY

Pregnancy is usually discussed in terms of **trimesters**—three periods of about three months (or 13 weeks) each. During the first trimester, the mother experiences a few physical changes and some fairly common symptoms. During the second trimester, often the most peaceful time of pregnancy, the mother gains weight, looks noticeably pregnant, and may experience a general sense of well-being if she is happy about having a child. The third trimester is the hardest for the mother because she must breathe, digest, excrete, and circulate blood for herself and the growing fetus. The weight of the fetus, the pressure of its body on her organs, and its increased demands on her system can cause discomfort and fatigue and may make the mother increasingly impatient to give birth.

QUICK STATS

377,703 babies were born in Canada between July 2008 and June 2009.

—Statistics Canada, 2010

Pregnancy Tests

The earliest tests for pregnancy are chemical tests designed to detect the presence of **human chorionic gonadotropin (HCG)**, a hormone produced by the implanted fertilized egg. These tests may be performed as early as two weeks after fertilization.

Home pregnancy test kits, which are sold in drugstores without a prescription, include a small sample of red blood cells coated with HCG antibodies, to which the woman adds a small amount of her urine. If the concentration of HCG is great enough, it will clump together with the HCG antibodies, indicating that the woman is pregnant. Home pregnancy tests can be very reliable, but the instructions must be followed carefully. If a home test done at the time of a missed menstrual period is negative, retesting after another week is recommended. In the first day or two following a missed period, the concentration of HCG may be too low to be detected by the test.

Changes in the Woman's Body

Hormonal changes begin as soon as the egg is fertilized, and for the next nine months the woman's body nourishes the fetus and adjusts to its growth. Let's take a closer look at the changes of early, middle, and late pregnancy (Figure 12.3).

Early Signs and Symptoms   Early recognition of pregnancy is important, especially for women with physical problems and nutritional deficiencies. The following symptoms are not absolute indications of pregnancy, but they are reasons to visit a health care provider:

- *A missed menstrual period.* If an egg has been fertilized and implanted in the uterine wall, the endometrium is retained to nourish the embryo. A woman who misses a period after having intercourse may be pregnant.

- *Slight bleeding.* Slight bleeding follows implantation of the fertilized egg in about 14% of pregnant women. Because this happens about the time a period is expected, the bleeding is sometimes mistaken for menstrual flow. It usually lasts only a few days.

- *Nausea.* About two-thirds of pregnant women feel nauseated, probably as a reaction to increased levels of progesterone and other hormones. Although this nausea is often called *morning sickness*, some women have it all day long. It frequently begins during the 6th week and disappears by the 12th week. In some cases, it lasts throughout the pregnancy.

- *Breast tenderness.* Some women experience breast tenderness, swelling, and tingling, usually described as different from the tenderness experienced before menstruation.

- *Increased urination.* Increased frequency of urination can occur soon after the missed period.

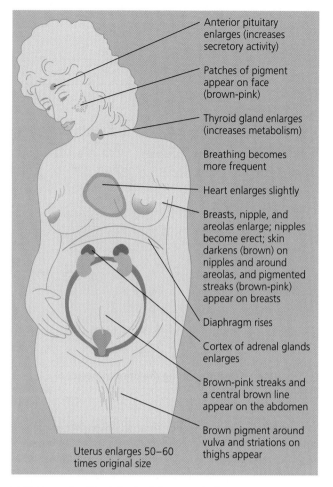

FIGURE 12.3 **Physiological changes during pregnancy.**

Labels in figure:
- Anterior pituitary enlarges (increases secretory activity)
- Patches of pigment appear on face (brown-pink)
- Thyroid gland enlarges (increases metabolism)
- Breathing becomes more frequent
- Heart enlarges slightly
- Breasts, nipple, and areolas enlarge; nipples become erect; skin darkens (brown) on nipples and around areolas, and pigmented streaks (brown-pink) appear on breasts
- Diaphragm rises
- Cortex of adrenal glands enlarges
- Brown-pink streaks and a central brown line appear on the abdomen
- Brown pigment around vulva and striations on thighs appear
- Uterus enlarges 50–60 times original size

- *Sleepiness, fatigue, and emotional upset.* These symptoms result from hormonal changes. Fatigue can be surprisingly overwhelming in the first trimester but usually improves significantly around the third month of pregnancy.

The first reliable physical signs of pregnancy can be distinguished about four weeks after a woman misses her menstrual period. A softening of the uterus just above the cervix, called *Hegar's sign*, and other changes in the cervix and pelvis are apparent during a pelvic examination. The labia minora and the cervix may take on a purple colour rather than their usual pink hue.

Four weeks after a woman misses her menstrual period, she would be considered to be about eight weeks pregnant because pregnancy is calculated from the time of a woman's last menstrual period rather than from the time of actual fertilization. (The timing of ovulation and fertilization is often difficult to determine.) Although a woman should see her physician to determine her due date, due dates can be approximated by subtracting three months from the date of the last menstrual period and then adding seven days. For example, a woman whose last menstrual period began on September 20 would have a due date of about June 27.

Continuing Changes in the Woman's Body The most obvious changes during pregnancy occur in the reproductive organs. During the first three months, the uterus enlarges to about three times its nonpregnant size, but it still cannot be felt in the abdomen. By the fourth month, it is large enough to make the abdomen protrude. By the seventh or eighth month, the uterus pushes up into the rib cage, which makes breathing slightly more difficult. The breasts enlarge and are sensitive; by week eight, they may tingle or throb. The pigmented area around the nipple, the areola, darkens and broadens.

Other changes are going on as well. Early in pregnancy, the muscles and ligaments attached to bones begin to soften and stretch. The joints between the pelvic bones loosen and spread, making it easier to have a baby but harder to walk. The circulatory system becomes more efficient to accommodate the blood volume, which increases by 50%, and the heart pumps it more rapidly. Much of the increased blood flow goes to the uterus and placenta (the organ that exchanges nutrients and waste between mother and fetus). The mother's lungs also become more efficient, and her rib cage widens to permit her to inhale up to 40% more air. Much of the oxygen goes to the fetus. The kidneys become highly efficient, removing waste products from fetal circulation and producing large amounts of urine by midpregnancy.

The average weight gain during a healthy pregnancy is 12.5 kilograms, although actual weight change depends on the individual. Table 12.1 on p. 386 shows the weight gains recommended by Health Canada, based on a woman's pre-pregnancy weight status. About 60% of the weight gain is directly related to the baby (such as the fetus and placenta); the rest accumulates over the woman's body as fluid and fat.

As the woman's skin stretches, small breaks may occur in the elastic fibres of the lower layer of skin, producing *stretch marks* on her abdomen, hips, breasts, or thighs. Increased pigment production darkens the skin in 90% of pregnant women, especially in places that have stretched.

Changes During the Later Stages of Pregnancy By the end of the sixth month, the increased needs of the fetus place a burden on the mother's lungs, heart, and kidneys. Her back may ache from the pressure of the baby's weight and from having to throw her shoulders back to keep her balance while standing (Figure 12.4 on p. 386). Her body retains more water, perhaps up to three extra litres of fluid. Her legs, hands, ankles, or feet may swell, and she may be bothered by leg cramps, heartburn, or constipation. Despite discomfort, both her digestion and her metabolism are working at top efficiency.

trimester One of the three, three-month periods of pregnancy.

human chorionic gonadotropin (HCG) A hormone produced by the fertilized egg that can be detected in the urine or blood of the mother within a few weeks of conception.

TERMS

Table 12.1	Recommended Weight Gain During Pregnancy				
Prepregnancy BMI Category	Mean* Rate of Weight Gain in the 2nd and 3rd Trimester		Recommended† Range of Total Weight Gain		
	kg/week	lb/week	kg	lb	
BMI < 18.5 Underweight	0.5	1.0	12.5–18	28–40	
BMI 18.5–24.9 Normal weight	0.4	1.0	11.5–16	25–35	
BMI 25.0–29.9 Overweight	0.3	0.6	7–11.5	15–25	
BMI ≥ 30‡ Obese	0.2	0.5	5–9	11–20	

* Rounded values.
† Calculations assume a total of 0.5–2 kg (1.1–4.4 lb) weight gain in the first trimester.
‡ A narrower range of weight gain may be advised for women with a prepregnancy BMI of 35 or greater. Individualized advice is recommended for these women.

Source: Health Canada: *Food and Nutrition: Canadian Gestational Weight Gain Recommendations.* Adapted from Institute of Medicine 2009 (http://www.hc-sc.gc.ca/fn-an/nutrition/prenatal/qa-gest-gros-qr-eng.php; retrieved April 26, 2010). © Her Majesty the Queen in Right of Canada.

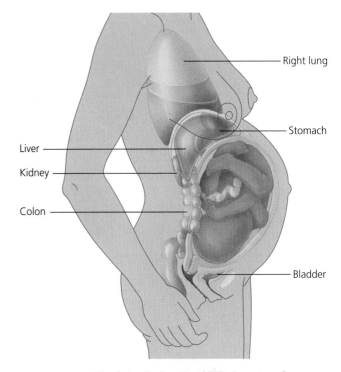

FIGURE 12.4   The fetus during the third trimester of pregnancy.

The uterus prepares for childbirth with preliminary contractions, called *Braxton Hicks contractions.* Unlike true labour contractions, these are usually short, irregular, and painless. The mother may only be aware that at times her abdomen is hard to the touch. These contractions become more frequent and intense as the delivery date approaches.

In the ninth month, the baby settles into the pelvic bones, usually head down, fitting snugly. This process, called **lightening**, allows the uterus to sink down about five centimetres, producing a visible change in the mother's profile. Pelvic pressure increases, and pressure on the diaphragm lightens. Breathing becomes easier; urination becomes more frequent. Sometimes, after a first pregnancy, the baby doesn't settle down into the pelvis until labour begins.

Emotional Responses to Pregnancy

Rapid changes in hormone levels can cause a pregnant woman to experience unpredictable emotions. A large part of pregnancy is beyond the woman's control—her changing appearance, her energy level, her variable moods—and some women need extra support and reassurance. Hormonal changes can also make women feel exhilarated and euphoric, although for some women such moods are temporary.

Like the physical changes that accompany pregnancy, emotional responses also change as the pregnancy develops. During the first trimester, the pregnant woman may fear that she may miscarry or that the child will not be normal. Education about pregnancy and childbirth and support from her partner, friends, relatives, and health care professionals are important antidotes to these fears (see the box "Pregnancy Tasks for Fathers").

During the second trimester, the pregnant woman can feel the fetus move within her, and worries about miscarriages usually begin to diminish. She may look and feel happy and be delighted as her pregnancy begins to show. However, she may also worry that her increasing size makes her unattractive. Reassurance from her partner can ease these fears.

The third trimester is the time of greatest physical stress during the pregnancy. A woman may find that her physical abilities are limited by her size. Because some women feel physically awkward and sexually unattractive, they may experience periods of depression. But many also feel a great deal of happy excitement and anticipation. The fetus may already be looked on as a member of the family, and both parents may begin talking to the fetus and interacting with it by patting the mother's belly. The upcoming birth will probably be a focus for both the woman and her partner.

Fetal Development

Now that we've seen what happens to the mother's body during pregnancy, let's consider the development of the fetus (Figure 12.5 on p. 388).

Pregnancy Tasks for Fathers

Before the Pregnancy

• *Consider your lifestyle and health habits.* A healthy lifestyle can help boost fertility and improve pregnancy outcome. Being too thin or too heavy may lower a man's sperm count, as may marijuana use. Men who smoke and drink have a lower concentration of sperm and a lower percentage of active sperm. Exposure to chemicals on the job may also affect pregnancy.

• *Check your budget and financial situation.* Make sure your finances are in order and that you have as much life, health, and disability insurance as you may need. See a financial planner for advice. Try putting away extra money every month now—both to practise living on a tighter budget and to save.

• *Get any necessary health checks and genetic counselling.* See the discussion of potential health concerns in the section "Preconception Care."

During the Pregnancy

• *Help your partner stay healthy during the pregnancy.* If you smoke, quit; second-hand smoke is dangerous for the developing fetus. Support your partner by making other lifestyle changes or joining her in any changes she's making; for example, drink non-alcoholic beverages, take walks with her, and get extra sleep.

• *Help around the home and with planning for the baby.* Help shop for necessities, and help get your home

ready for a baby. Pregnancy is hard work, so providing extra help with household chores and errands can be an important element of support. For example, because of the risk of infection by toxoplasmosis, pregnant women should avoid handling cat litter; if you and your partner have a cat, emptying the litter box should be your job.

• *Be involved.* Go to all the prenatal visits, birth preparation or education classes, hospital tours, and so on. Learn more about pregnancy, childbirth, and parenting by reading books, visiting Internet sites, and talking with other parents.

After the Baby Arrives

• *Help meet your baby's needs.* If your job allows, take parental leave to help with the new baby. Support the new mother by helping with baby care (feeding, diaper changes), laundry, shopping, and other chores. Take turns or join the mother when the baby needs care or feeding during the night; one survey found that more than half of fathers continue to sleep or pretend to be asleep when their babies cry during the night.

• *Support your partner, and ask others for help.* It is normal for a new mother to be tired and to experience mood changes, and some men also experience anxiety about their new role. Good communication between partners and help from supportive relatives and friends can help new parents adjust.

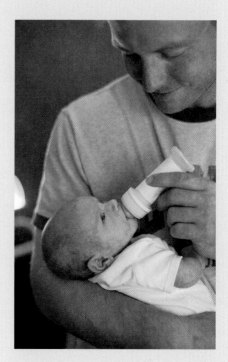

• *Give your partner some time off.* A new mother needs time to recover from childbirth, even after she leaves the hospital or birthing centre. This is especially true if the delivery was difficult, if a Caesarean section was performed, or if an episiotomy was required. Aside from doing the daily chores, the father can help the mother's recuperation by taking the baby for a few hours at a time. If the baby is being bottle-fed, take charge for a morning, an afternoon, or even the entire day.

The First Trimester About 30 hours after the egg is fertilized, the cell divides, and this process of cell division repeats many times. As the cluster of cells drifts down the oviduct, several different kinds of cells emerge. The entire set of genetic instructions is passed to every cell, but each cell follows only certain instructions; if this were not the case, we would not have different organs or body parts. For example, all cells carry genes for hair colour and eye colour, but only the cells of the hair follicles and irises (of the eye) respond to that information.

Around the fourth day after fertilization, the cluster, now about 32–128 cells and hollow, arrives in the uterus; this is a **blastocyst**. On about the sixth or seventh day, the blastocyst attaches to the uterine wall, usually along the upper curve; over the next few days, it becomes firmly implanted and begins to draw nourishment from the endometrium, the uterine lining.

The blastocyst becomes an **embryo** by about the end of the second week after fertilization. The inner cells of the blastocyst separate into three layers. One layer becomes inner body parts, the digestive and respiratory systems; the middle layer becomes muscle, bone, blood, kidneys, and sex glands; and the third layer becomes the skin, hair, and nervous tissue.

lightening A process in which the uterus sinks down because the baby's head settles into the mother's pelvic area.

blastocyst A stage of development, days 6–14, before the cell cluster becomes the embryo and placenta.

embryo The stage of development between blastocyst and fetus; about weeks two to eight.

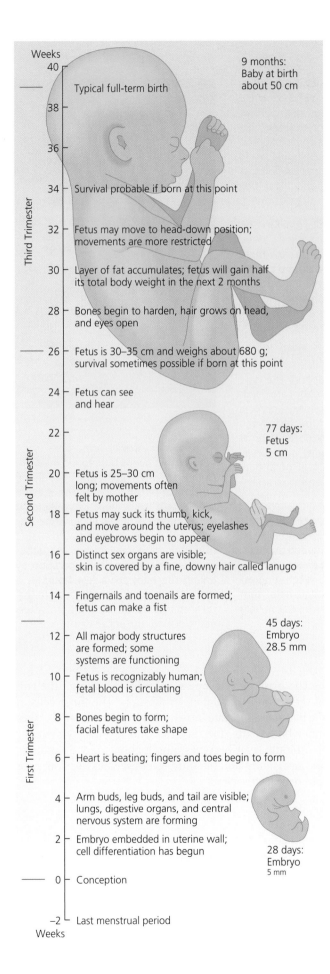

Weeks
40 ┤ Typical full-term birth

9 months:
Baby at birth
about 50 cm

38 ┤

36 ┤

Third Trimester

34 ┤ Survival probable if born at this point

32 ┤ Fetus may move to head-down position;
movements are more restricted

30 ┤ Layer of fat accumulates; fetus will gain half
its total body weight in the next 2 months

28 ┤ Bones begin to harden, hair grows on head,
and eyes open

26 ┤ Fetus is 30–35 cm and weighs about 680 g;
survival sometimes possible if born at this point

24 ┤ Fetus can see
and hear

22 ┤

77 days:
Fetus
5 cm

Second Trimester

20 ┤ Fetus is 25–30 cm
long; movements often
felt by mother

18 ┤ Fetus may suck its thumb, kick,
and move around the uterus; eyelashes
and eyebrows begin to appear

16 ┤ Distinct sex organs are visible;
skin is covered by a fine, downy hair called lanugo

14 ┤ Fingernails and toenails are formed;
fetus can make a fist

12 ┤ All major body structures
are formed; some
systems are functioning

45 days:
Embryo
28.5 mm

10 ┤ Fetus is recognizably human;
fetal blood is circulating

First Trimester

8 ┤ Bones begin to form;
facial features take shape

6 ┤ Heart is beating; fingers and toes begin to form

4 ┤ Arm buds, leg buds, and tail are visible;
lungs, digestive organs, and central
nervous system are forming

2 ┤ Embryo embedded in uterine wall;
cell differentiation has begun

28 days:
Embryo
5 mm

0 ┤ Conception

−2 ┘ Last menstrual period
Weeks

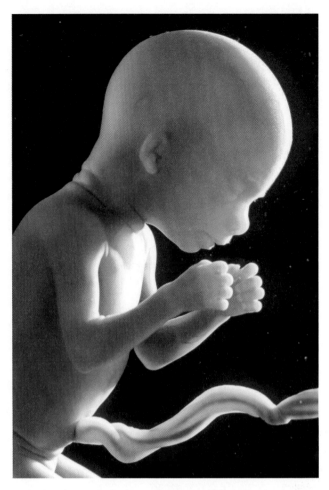

By the fourth month, the fetus is growing rapidly and is about
25 centimetres long. Weighing about 170 grams, it moves vigorously
in the uterus and can suck its thumb, frown, and turn its head.

The outermost shell of cells becomes the **placenta**, **umbilical cord**, and **amniotic sac** (Figure 12.6). A network of blood vessels called *chorionic villi* eventually forms the placenta. The human placenta allows a two-way exchange of nutrients and waste materials between the mother and the fetus. The placenta brings oxygen and nutrients to the fetus and transports waste products out. The placenta does not provide a perfect barrier between the fetal circulation and the maternal circulation, however. Some blood cells are exchanged and certain substances, such as alcohol, pass freely from the maternal circulation through the placenta to the fetus.

The period between weeks two and nine is a time of rapid differentiation and change. All the major body structures are formed during this time, including the heart, brain, liver, lungs, and sex organs; the eyes, nose, ears, arms, and legs also appear. Some organs begin to function—the heart begins to beat, and the liver starts producing blood cells. Because body structures are forming, the developing

FIGURE 12.5   A chronology of milestones in prenatal development.

Labels (left diagram, clockwise):
- Lining of uterus (endometrium)
- Muscle layer of uterine wall
- Umbilical cord
- Umbilical vein
- Amniotic sac filled with amniotic fluid
- Placenta
- Mucus plug
- Cervix
- Umbilical arteries
- Vagina (birth canal)

Labels (right diagram):
- Chorionic villi
- Placenta
- Maternal blood collects
- Maternal endometrial arteries
- Maternal endometrial vein

FIGURE 12.6   A cross-sectional view of the fetus in the uterus and an enlargement of the placenta.

organism is vulnerable to damage from environmental influences, such as drugs and infections (discussed in detail in sections that follow).

By the end of the second month, the brain sends out impulses that coordinate the functioning of other organs. The embryo is now a fetus, and most further changes will be in the size and refinement of working body parts. In the third month, the fetus begins to be quite active. By the end of the first trimester, the fetus is about 2.5 centimetres long and weighs less than 30 grams.

The Second Trimester   To grow during the second trimester, to about 35 centimetres and 680 grams, the fetus must have large amounts of food, oxygen, and water, which come from the mother through the placenta. All body systems are operating, and the fetal heartbeat can be heard with a stethoscope. The mother can detect fetal movements beginning in the fourth or fifth month. Against great odds, a fetus born prematurely at the end of the second trimester might survive.

The Third Trimester   The fetus gains most of its birth weight during the last three months. Some of the weight is fatty tissue under the skin that insulates the fetus and supplies food. The fetus needs a great deal of calcium, iron, and nitrogen from the food the mother eats. Some 85% of the calcium and iron she consumes goes into the fetal bloodstream.

Although the fetus may live if it is born during the seventh month, it needs the fat layer acquired in the eighth month and time for the organs, especially the respiratory

and digestive organs, to develop. It also needs the immunity supplied by the antibodies in the mother's blood during the final three months. The antibodies protect the fetus against many of the diseases to which the mother has acquired immunity. Breast milk can help the baby further resist infections because it also contains maternal antibodies.

Diagnosing Fetal Abnormalities   About 3% of babies are born with a major birth defect. Information about the health and sex of a fetus can be obtained before birth through prenatal testing.

Ultrasonography (also called *ultrasound*) uses high-frequency sound waves to create a **sonogram**, or visual image, of the fetus in the uterus. Sonograms show the position of the fetus, its size and gestational age, and the presence of certain anatomical problems. Sonograms can

placenta   The organ through which the fetus receives nourishment and empties waste via the mother's circulatory system; after birth, the placenta is expelled from the uterus.

umbilical cord   The cord connecting the placenta and fetus, through which nutrients pass.

amniotic sac   A membranous pouch enclosing and protecting the fetus; also holds amniotic fluid.

ultrasonography   The use of high-frequency sound waves to view the fetus in the uterus; also known as *ultrasound*.

sonogram   The visual image of the fetus produced by ultrasonography.

TERMS

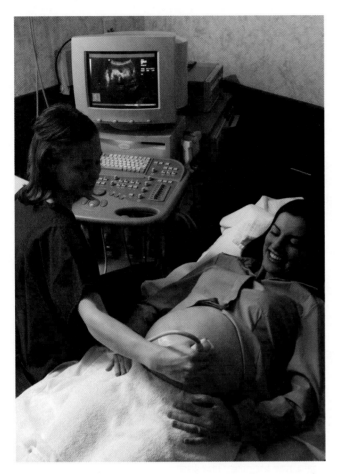

Ultrasonography provides information about the position, size, and physical condition of a fetus in the uterus.

sometimes be used to determine the sex of the fetus. Sonograms are considered safe for a pregnant woman and the fetus, but both the SOGC and Health Canada advise against "keepsake" sonograms performed for no medical purpose.

Amniocentesis involves the removal of fluid from the uterus with a long, thin needle inserted through the abdominal wall. It is usually performed between 15 and 18 weeks into the pregnancy, although earlier amniocentesis is available. A genetic analysis of the fetal cells in the fluid can reveal the presence of chromosomal disorders, such as Down syndrome, and some genetic diseases, including Tay-Sachs disease. The sex of the fetus can also be determined. Most amniocentesis tests are performed on pregnant women over age 35, who have a greater risk of chromosomal abnormalities, or in cases where the fetus is known to be at risk for a particular chromosomal or genetic defect. Amniocentesis carries a slight risk (a 0.3%–0.7% chance of miscarriage).

Another prenatal test is **chorionic villus sampling (CVS)**, which can be performed earlier in pregnancy than amniocentesis, between weeks 10 and 12. This procedure involves removal through the cervix (by catheter) or abdomen (by needle) of a tiny section of chorionic villi, which contain fetal cells that then can be analyzed. When CVS first became available, it was associated with a higher risk of miscarriage than amniocentesis, but by 2003 the two procedures were found to be equally safe.

Integrated prenatal screening (IPS) can be used to help identify fetuses with neural tube defects, Down syndrome, and other anomalies. IPS combines ultrasound evaluation of nuchal translucency (the thickness of the back of the fetus's neck) with two separate maternal blood tests done between the 11th and 14th week and the 15th and 18th week of pregnancy. The blood is analyzed for four hormone levels: human chorionic gonadotropin (HCG), unconjugated estriol, alpha-fetoprotein (AFP), and pregnancy associated plasma protein-A (PAPP-A). The hormone levels and ultrasound measurements are compared with appropriate standards, and the results are used to estimate the probability that the fetus has particular anomalies. IPS is a screening test rather than a diagnostic test and it has a false positive rate of about 2%–4%. In the case of abnormal IPS results, parents may choose further testing, such as amniocentesis or CVS. The SOGC recommends that amniocentesis or CVS be performed only in women with an abnormal IPS result or in pregnant woman over 40 years of age.

Genetic counsellors explain the results of the different tests so that parents can understand their implications. If a fetus is found to have a defect, it may be carried to term, aborted, or, in rare instances, treated while still in the uterus. Results of most current screening tests are not available until after week 12 of pregnancy; consequently, if abortion is chosen, it is likely to involve one of the more medically complex and physically difficult methods (see Chapter 11). Researchers are searching for new fetal screening techniques that are less invasive and that can be done earlier in pregnancy.

Fetal Programming Amniocentesis, CVS, and IPS look for chromosomal, genetic, and other anomalies that typically cause immediate problems. A new area of study known as *fetal programming theory* focuses on how conditions in the womb may influence the risk of adult diseases. For example, researchers have linked low birth weight to an increased risk of heart disease, high blood pressure, obesity, diabetes, and schizophrenia; high birth weight in female infants, however, has been linked to an increased risk of breast cancer in later life.

How might conditions during gestation affect the risk of adult diseases? A number of studies have looked at groups of people born in areas of poverty or at times of famine, when pregnant women were unable to eat properly. The poor prenatal conditions that stunt the growth of a developing fetus and lead to low birth weight may also affect specific organs. For example, if energy is limited, resources may be directed toward the developing fetal brain and away

Stress and Pregnancy

High levels of stress can have the same adverse effects on a pregnant woman as they do on anyone else (see Chapter 3). However, recent research suggests that stress can also affect the course of pregnancy and the health of the fetus.

Researchers have linked high levels of stress to miscarriage, preterm labour, and low birth weight. In one study, women who reported high levels of job stress were found to have a risk of miscarriage two to three times as high as that of less-stressed women. Other studies have found that pregnant women who experience major life changes, traumatic experiences, or high levels of pregnancy-related anxiety are at greater risk for preterm labour and for having a low-birth-weight infant.

Stress hormones may constrict blood flow to the placenta, depriving the fetus of the oxygen and nutrients needed for growth and development. Stress hormones also play a role in triggering labour, so high hormone levels may also increase the risk of preterm labour.

Stress may also affect the behaviour of a pregnant woman; negative coping techniques, such as use of tobacco, alcohol, and other drugs, can adversely affect a developing fetus. On the flip side, social support during pregnancy has been linked to improved fetal growth and healthy birth weight.

The time in pregnancy in which stress is experienced may be important in determining its effects. A study of earthquake survivors found that women who were in their first trimester when the earthquake occurred were at increased risk for preterm labour; women further along in their pregnancies experienced no such increase in risk. Researchers hypothesize that hormones produced in the later stages of pregnancy may protect both mother and fetus from the effects of stress.

High levels of stress have also been linked to birth defects. Although the overall risk of birth defects is very low, women who experience severe emotional trauma around the time of conception or during the first trimester are more likely to have an infant with defects of the skull, spine, palate, or limbs. The relationship between stress and birth defects has been found to be significantly greater in women with lower levels of education, suggesting that chronic stressors and behaviours that go along with low educational attainment and low income may increase the impact of stressful life events on fetal development.

Researchers have studied the long-term effects of stress by looking at children of pregnant Dutch women who experienced high levels of physical and emotional stress during the "Hunger

Winter" of 1944–1945, when the Nazis blockaded the western Netherlands. Fetuses exposed to the famine early in development were found to be at increased risk of central nervous system defects and, as adults, obesity and schizophrenia.

Although most women in North America do not experience such extreme stressors during pregnancy, these studies reinforce the importance of adequate prenatal care, including stress management and social support.

from other organs, including the liver and kidneys. Later in life, a small liver may be unable to clear cholesterol from the bloodstream, thereby increasing cholesterol levels and raising the risk of heart disease; undersized kidneys may be less able to regulate blood pressure. The fetus may also respond to limited resources by developing a permanently thrifty metabolism that triggers increased appetite and fat storage—leading to a greater risk of adult obesity and diabetes. Stress, both physical and emotional, increases maternal levels of the hormone cortisol, which in turn may permanently affect an infant's system of blood pressure regulation (see the box "Stress and Pregnancy," above).

Hormones may also be involved in the link between high birth weight and increased risk of breast cancer. Growth factors that contribute to high birth weight include leptin, insulin, and estrogen. Exposure to high levels of these in the womb may alter developing breast tissue in such a way that, when exposed to estrogen later in life, breast cells may be more likely to become malignant.

Although fetal programming theory is not yet embraced by all scientists, these studies emphasize that everything that occurs during pregnancy can have an impact on the developing fetus. In the future, people may be able to use information about their birth weight and other indicators of gestational conditions just as they can now use family history and genetic information—to alert them to special health risks and to help them improve their health.

amniocentesis A process in which amniotic fluid is removed and analyzed to detect possible birth defects.

chorionic villus sampling (CVS) Surgical removal of a tiny section of chorionic villi to be analyzed for genetic defects.

integrated prenatal screen (IPS) A combination of an ultrasound and two blood tests, used to assess the risk of fetal abnormalities.

TERMS

The Importance of Prenatal Care

Adequate prenatal care—as described in the following sections—is essential to the health of both mother and baby. All physicians recommend that women start getting regular prenatal checkups as soon as they become pregnant. Typically, this means one checkup every four weeks during the first 30 weeks, checkups every second week until the 36th week, then weekly checkups until delivery.

Regular Checkups   In the woman's first visit to her health care provider, she will be asked for a detailed medical history of herself and her family. The physician or midwife will note any hereditary conditions that may assume increased significance during pregnancy. The tendency to develop gestational diabetes (diabetes during pregnancy only), for example, can be inherited; appropriate treatment during pregnancy reduces the risk of serious harm.

The woman is given a complete physical exam and is informed about appropriate diet. She returns for regular checkups throughout the pregnancy, during which her blood pressure and weight gain are measured, her urine is analyzed, and the size and position of the fetus are monitored. Regular prenatal visits also give the mother a chance to discuss her concerns and assure herself that everything is proceeding normally. Physicians, midwives, health educators, and teachers of prenatal and childbirth classes can provide the mother with invaluable information.

Blood Tests   A blood sample is taken during the initial prenatal visit to determine blood type and detect possible anemia or Rh incompatibilities. The **Rh factor** is a blood protein. If an Rh-positive father and an Rh-negative mother conceive an Rh-positive baby, the baby's blood will be incompatible with the mother's. If some of the baby's blood enters the mother's bloodstream during delivery, she will develop antibodies to it just as she would toward a virus. If she has subsequent Rh-positive babies, the antibodies in the mother's blood, passing through the placenta, will destroy the fetus's red blood cells, possibly leading to jaundice, anemia, mental retardation, or death. This condition is completely treatable with a serum called Rh-immune globulin, which destroys Rh-positive cells as they enter the mother's body and prevents her from forming antibodies to them. Rh-immune globulin is given to Rh-negative mothers in the third trimester and again after the birth if the baby is found to be Rh-positive.

Blood may also be tested for evidence of hepatitis B, syphilis, rubella and varicella immunity, thyroid problems, and, with the mother's permission, HIV infection.

Prenatal Nutrition   A nutritious diet throughout pregnancy is essential for both the fetus and the mother. Not only does the baby get all its nutrients from the mother, but it also competes with her for nutrients not sufficiently available to meet both their needs. When a woman's diet is low in iron or calcium, the fetus receives most of it, and

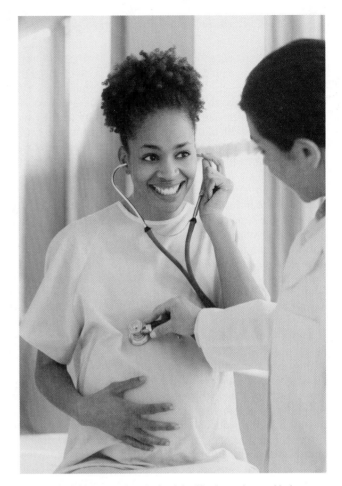

Prenatal care is essential to the health of both mother and baby.

the mother may become deficient in the mineral. To meet the increased nutritional demands of her body, a pregnant woman shouldn't just eat more; she should make sure that her diet is nutritionally adequate (see the box "Healthy Eating During Pregnancy").

Avoiding Drugs and Other Environmental Hazards   In addition to the food the mother eats, the drugs she takes and the chemicals she is exposed to affect the fetus. Everything the mother ingests may eventually reach the fetus in some proportion. Some drugs harm the fetus but not the mother because the fetus is in the process of developing and because the proper dose for the mother is a massive dose for the fetus.

During the first trimester, when the major body structures are rapidly forming, the fetus is extremely vulnerable to environmental factors, such as viral infections, radiation, drugs, and other **teratogens**, any of which can cause **congenital malformations**, or birth defects. The most susceptible body parts are those growing most rapidly at the time of exposure. The rubella (German measles) virus, for example, can cause a congenital malformation of a delicate system, such as the eyes or ears, leading to blindness or deafness, if exposure occurs during the first trimester, but it does no damage later in the pregnancy. Similarly,

Healthy Eating During Pregnancy

To maintain her own health and help the fetus grow, a woman needs to consume about 250–500 extra calories per day during pregnancy. Breastfeeding an infant requires even more energy—about 500 or more extra calories per day.

Healthy Choices

To ensure a balanced intake of key nutrients, pregnant women should follow *Eating Well with Canada's Food Guide*, which is based on four basic food groups. Pregnant women should and include two to three extra servings per day from one of the food groups. For women of childbearing age, the daily recommended intake from each group is as follows:

- Vegetables and fruit: seven to eight servings; choose dark green and brightly coloured vegetables and fruit.

- Grain products: six to seven servings; choose whole grain breads, rice, and pasta.

- Meat and alternatives: two servings; choose lean meats and meat alternatives.

- Milk and alternatives: two servings; choose low-fat varieties of milk, yogourt, and cheese.

A copy of *Eating Well with Canada's Food Guide* and recommendations for pregnant women can be found on Health Canada's Web site (listed in For More Information at the end of the chapter). See Chapter 5 for a more detailed discussion of *Eating Well with Canada's Food Guide*.

Supplements

Some physicians may prescribe vitamin and mineral supplements for women who are pregnant or lactating or who are trying to get pregnant. Adequate vitamin and mineral intake is important for many reasons. For example, women with low levels of vitamin D are more likely to have low-birth-weight babies.

Adequate intake of the B vitamin folate before conception and during pregnancy has been shown to decrease the risk of neural tube defects, including spina bifida. Any woman capable of becoming pregnant should consume at least 400 micrograms (0.4 milligrams) of folic acid (the synthetic form of folate) daily from fortified foods or supplements, in addition to folate from a varied diet. Pregnant women should have 400–1000 micrograms every day. Women who have already had a pregnancy involving a fetus with a neural tube defect should consult with a physician about taking a much larger amount of folic acid (4 milligrams), starting one month before conception and continuing through the first trimester. Folate is found naturally in leafy green vegetables, legumes, citrus fruits, and most berries. In 1998, it became mandatory for enriched grain products to be fortified with folic acid. This adds approximately 100 micrograms of folic acid to an average woman's daily diet.

It is important that a pregnant woman not supplement beyond her physician's advice because some vitamins and minerals are harmful if taken in excess. It is also important not to take herbal dietary supplements without consulting a physician; few dietary supplements have been tested for safety during pregnancy, but some have been shown to be dangerous.

Food Safety

Pregnant women should pay special attention to food safety because food-borne pathogens can be particularly dangerous during pregnancy. Two such pathogens are *Listeria monocytogenes* and *Toxoplasma gondii*. *Listeria* is a bacterium most often found in undercooked or ready-to-eat meat, poultry, or seafood; soft cheeses; products made with unpasteurized milk; and unpasteurized juice. Listeriosis causes flulike symptoms in pregnant women; if the fetus is infected, the result can be miscarriage, premature birth, or birth defects.

T. gondii, a parasite carried by cats, can also contaminate food or soil. Toxoplasmosis is typically caused by eating undercooked meat or poultry or unwashed fruits and vegetables, cleaning a litter box, or handling contaminated soil. Toxoplasmosis causes few symptoms in pregnant women, but if passed to the fetus it may cause miscarriage or mental impairment.

One further food safety recommendation for pregnant women relates to fish. Most types of fish are good choices for a healthy diet, but a few types can be contaminated with mercury or industrial pollutants. Health Canada recommends that pregnant women consume two food guide servings of fish per week (one serving is 75 grams). Fish contains important fats that are necessary for the development of a baby's brain, nerves, and eyes. Health Canada suggests consumption of the following fish as they have low levels of contaminants: salmon, trout, herring, haddock, canned light tuna, pollock (Boston bluefish), sole, flounder, anchovy, char, hake, mullet, smelt, Atlantic mackerel, and lake white fish. Certain types of fish should be limited or avoided during pregnancy including tuna (fresh, frozen, and canned albacore), shark, swordfish, marlin, orange roughy, and escolar. Health Canada recommends that pregnant women check with their provincial or territorial authority before consuming any fish caught in local waters.

For detailed information on food safety, see Chapter 5.

---

the drug thalidomide taken early in pregnancy prevents the formation of arms and legs in fetuses, but taken later, when limbs are already formed, it causes no damage. Other drugs can cause damage throughout prenatal development.

ALCOHOL Alcohol is a potent teratogen. Getting drunk just one time during pregnancy may be enough to cause brain damage in a fetus. Alcohol consumption during pregnancy can be associated with miscarriages, stillbirths, and, in live

Rh factor A protein found in blood; Rh incompatibility between a mother and fetus can jeopardize the fetus's health.

teratogen An agent or influence that causes physical defects in a developing fetus.

congenital malformation A physical defect existing at the time of birth, either inherited or caused during gestation.

TERMS

babies, **fetal alcohol spectrum disorder (FASD)**. FASD includes several alcohol-related diagnoses, such as alcohol-related birth defects (ARBD), alcohol-related neurodevelopmental disorder (ARND), partial fetal alcohol syndrome (pFAS), and the most severe disease, fetal alcohol syndrome (FAS). Babies with FASD many have a wide range of disabilities, including physical, social, cognitive, and emotional problems. These children may have difficulties with learning, behaviour, and social situations. They may also have a small head and body size, unusual facial characteristics, congenital heart defects, defective joints, impaired vision, mental impairment, and abnormal behaviour patterns. According to the Public Health Agency of Canada, there is no safe amount of alcohol and no safe time to drink alcohol during pregnancy (see Chapter 15).

TOBACCO According to Health Canada, in 2009, almost 9% of women reported smoking regularly during their pregnancy. Pregnant women who smoke should quit, and nonsmoking pregnant women should avoid places where people smoke. Smoking during pregnancy increases the risk of miscarriage, low birth weight, immune system impairment, and infant death; it may also cause genetic damage or physical deformations. If nicotine levels in a mother's bloodstream are high, fetal breathing rate and movement become more rapid; the fetus may also metabolize cancer-causing by-products of tobacco.

Infants of women who smoke during pregnancy have poorer lung function at birth, and exposure to second-hand smoke after birth increases a baby's susceptibility to pneumonia and bronchitis. If a mother who smokes also breastfeeds, her infant will be exposed to tobacco chemicals through breast milk. See Chapter 16 for more on the effects of smoking.

CAFFEINE Caffeine, a powerful stimulant, puts both mother and fetus under stress by raising the level of the hormone epinephrine. Caffeine also reduces the blood supply to the uterus. One study found that consuming the amount of caffeine in five or more cups of coffee a day doubled the risk of miscarriage. Coffee, colas, strong black tea, and chocolate are high in caffeine, as are some over-the-counter medications. A pregnant woman should limit her caffeine intake to no more than 300 milligrams per day, which is the equivalent of about two cups of coffee.

TERMS

fetal alcohol spectrum disorder (FASD) A combination of birth defects caused by alcohol consumption by the mother during pregnancy.

DRUGS Some prescription drugs, including some blood pressure medications, can harm the fetus, so they should be used only under medical supervision. Additionally, some babies born to women who use antidepressants during pregnancy suffer withdrawal symptoms after birth. Accutane, an anti-acne drug, may have caused more than 1000 cases of severe birth defects in the 1980s. Over-the-counter drugs should be used only under a physician's direction. Large doses of vitamin A, for example, can cause birth defects.

Recreational drugs, such as cocaine, are thought to increase the risk of major birth defects. Marijuana use may also interfere with fertility treatments, and methamphetamine use is associated with underweight babies.

STIS AND OTHER INFECTIONS Infections, including those that are sexually transmitted, are another serious problem for the fetus. The most common cause of life-threatening infections in newborns is Group B streptococcus (GBS), a type of bacterium that can cause pneumonia, meningitis, and blood infections. About 25% of all pregnant women carry GBS but do not become ill, so routine screening close to the time of delivery is recommended. A woman who carries GBS or who develops a fever during labour will be given intravenous antibiotics at the time of labour to reduce the risk of passing GBS to her baby.

Syphilis can infect and kill a fetus; if the baby is born alive, it will have syphilis. Penicillin taken by the mother during pregnancy cures syphilis in both mother and fetus. Gonorrhea can infect the baby during delivery and cause blindness. Because gonorrhea is often asymptomatic, in Canada the eyes of newborns are routinely treated with erythromycin ointment to destroy gonorrheal bacteria. All pregnant women should be tested for hepatitis B, a virus that can pass from the mother to the infant at birth. Infants of infected mothers can be immunized shortly after birth.

Herpes simplex can damage the baby's eyes and brain and cause death, and no cure has yet been discovered for it. Genital herpes can be transmitted to the baby during delivery if the mother's infection is in the active phase. If this is the case, the baby may be delivered by Caesarean section. An initial outbreak of herpes can be dangerous if it occurs during pregnancy because the virus may pass through the placenta to the fetus. For this reason, it is important to know if the pregnant woman or her partner has a history of herpes.

The human immunodeficiency virus (HIV), which causes AIDS, can be passed to the fetus by an HIV-infected mother during pregnancy, labour and delivery, or breastfeeding. According to the Public Health Agency of Canada, there were 242 reported AIDS cases in children under 15 years old in Canada between 1979 and 2007. Perinatal (mother-to-child) transmission was the cause in 176 of these cases. The babies most at risk are those whose mothers inject drugs or are the sex partners of men who inject drugs. HIV testing is critical for any woman at risk for HIV, and

Table 12.2 — Selected Environmental Factors Associated with Problems in a Fetus or an Infant

Agent or Condition	Potential Effects
Accutane (acne medication)	Small head, mental impairment, deformed or absent ears, heart defects, cleft lip and palate
Alcohol	Unusual facial characteristics, small head, heart defects, mental impairment, defective joints
Chlamydia	Eye infections, pneumonia
Cigarette smoking	Miscarriage, stillbirth, low birth weight, respiratory problems, sudden infant death
Cocaine	Miscarriage, stillbirth, low birth weight, small head, defects of genital and urinary tracts
Cytomegalovirus (CMV)	Small head, mental impairment, blindness
Diabetes (insulin-dependent)	Malformations of the brain, spine, and heart
Gonorrhea	Eye infection leading to blindness if untreated
Herpes	Brain damage, death
HIV infection	Impaired immunity, death
Lead	Reduced IQ, learning disorders
Marijuana	Impaired fetal growth, increase in alcohol-related fetal damage
Mercury	Brain damage
Propecia (hair loss medication)	Abnormalities of the male sex organs
Radiation (high dose)	Small head, growth and mental impairment, multiple birth defects
Rubella (German measles)	Malformation of eyes or ears causing deafness or blindness; small head; mental impairment
Syphilis	Fetal death and miscarriage, prematurity, physical deformities
Tetracycline	Pigmentation of teeth, underdevelopment of enamel
Vitamin A (excess)	Miscarriage; defects of the head, brain, spine, and urinary tract

some physicians recommend routine testing for all pregnant women. Antiviral drugs, given to a mother infected with HIV during pregnancy and delivery and to her newborn immediately following birth, reduce the rate of HIV transmission from mother to infant from 25% to 5% or less. Of course, women should also take all the necessary precautions against HIV infection during pregnancy. (See Chapter 13 for more on HIV and other STIs.)

Environmental factors affecting fetal or infant development are summarized in Table 12.2, above.

Prenatal Activity and Exercise   Physical activity during pregnancy contributes to mental and physical wellness. Women can continue working at their jobs until late in their pregnancy, provided the work isn't so physically demanding that it jeopardizes their health. At the same time, pregnant women need more rest and sleep to maintain their own well-being and that of the fetus.

A moderate exercise program during pregnancy does not adversely affect pregnancy or birth; in fact, regular exercise appears to improve a woman's chance of an on-time delivery and may reduce the risk of pregnancy-related diabetes. The amniotic sac protects the fetus, and normal activities will not harm it. A woman who exercised before becoming pregnant can often continue her program, with appropriate modifications to maintain her comfort and safety. A pregnant woman who hasn't been exercising and wants to start should first consult a physician.

The SOGC recommends that all pregnant women engage in aerobic and strength conditioning exercises, unless they have a contraindication to exercise, and provided they are not embarking on a physical activity regime for the first time. Walking, swimming, and stationary cycling are all good choices; more strenuous activities that could result in a fall are best delayed until after the birth.

Kegel exercises, to strengthen the pelvic floor muscles, are recommended for pregnant women. These exercises are performed by alternately contracting and releasing the muscles used to stop the flow of urine. Each contraction should be held for about five seconds. Kegel exercises should be done several times a day, for a total of about 50 repetitions daily.

Prenatal exercise classes are valuable because they teach exercises that tone the body muscles involved in birth, especially those of the abdomen, back, and legs. Toned-up muscles aid delivery and help the body regain its non-pregnant shape afterward.

Preparing for Birth   Childbirth (also called *prenatal*) classes are almost a routine part of the prenatal experience for both mothers and fathers these days. These classes typically teach the details of the birth process as well as relaxation techniques to help deal with the discomfort of labour and delivery. The mother learns and practises a variety of techniques so she will be able to choose what works best for her during labour when the time comes. The father typically acts as a coach, supporting his partner emotionally and helping her with her breathing and relaxing. He can remain with her throughout labour and delivery, even when a Caesarean section is performed.

Complications of Pregnancy and Pregnancy Loss

About 31% of mothers-to-be have complications during pregnancy. Some complications may prevent full-term development of the fetus or affect the health of the infant at birth. As discussed earlier in the chapter, exposure to harmful substances, such as alcohol or drugs, can harm the fetus. Other complications are caused by physiological problems or genetic abnormalities.

Ectopic Pregnancy   In an **ectopic pregnancy**, the fertilized egg implants and begins to develop outside of the uterus, usually in an oviduct (Figure 12.7). The incidence of ectopic pregnancy is about 2% in the general population. Ectopic pregnancies account for about 4% of the annual pregnancy-related deaths in Canada.

Ectopic pregnancies usually occur because the fallopian tube is blocked, most often as a result of pelvic inflammatory disease; smoking also increases a woman's risk for ectopic pregnancy. The embryo may spontaneously abort, or the embryo and placenta may continue to expand until they rupture the oviduct. Sharp pain on one side of the abdomen or in the lower back, usually in about the seventh or eighth week, may signal an ectopic pregnancy, and a woman may have irregular bleeding. If bleeding from a rupture is severe, the woman may go into shock, characterized by low blood pressure, a fast pulse, weakness, and fainting.

Surgical removal of the embryo and the oviduct may be necessary to save the mother's life, although microsurgery can sometimes be used to repair the damaged oviduct. If diagnosed early, before the oviduct ruptures, ectopic pregnancy can often be successfully treated without surgery. The incidence of ectopic pregnancy has more than quadrupled in the past 25 years.

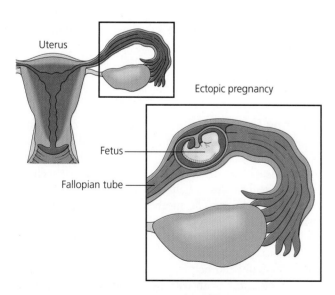

FIGURE 12.7   Ectopic pregnancy in a fallopian tube.

Spontaneous Abortion   A spontaneous abortion, or miscarriage, is the termination of pregnancy before the 20th week. About 15%–20% of all clinically diagnosed pregnancies end in miscarriage, and many women have miscarriages without knowing they were pregnant. About 30% of miscarriages occur before the 12th week of pregnancy. Most—about 60%—are due to chromosomal abnormalities in the fetus. Certain occupations that involve exposure to chemicals may increase the likelihood of a spontaneous abortion.

Vaginal bleeding (spotting) is usually the first sign that a pregnant woman may miscarry. She may also develop pelvic cramps, and her symptoms of pregnancy may disappear. (Note: Mild cramping is common in pregnancy and is usually not associated with miscarriage.)

One miscarriage doesn't mean that later pregnancies will be unsuccessful, and 70%–90% of women who miscarry eventually become pregnant again. About 1% of women suffer three or more miscarriages, possibly because of anatomical, hormonal, genetic, or immunological factors.

Stillbirth   The terms *fetal death, fetal demise, stillbirth,* and *stillborn* all refer to the delivery of a fetus that shows no signs of life. Each year, more than 3 million stillbirths occur worldwide. In Canada, the stillbirth rate is a little more than 6 in 1000. Risk factors for stillbirth include smoking, advanced maternal age, obesity, multiple gestations, and chronic disease. Race is also a factor; black women have twice as many stillbirths as white women.

Preeclampsia   A disease unique to human pregnancy, **preeclampsia**, is characterized by elevated blood pressure and the appearance of protein in the urine. Symptoms include headache, right upper-quadrant abdominal pain, vision changes (referred to as *scotomata*), and notable increased swelling and weight gain. If preeclampsia is untreated, patients can develop seizures, a condition called **eclampsia**. Other potential complications of preeclampsia are liver and kidney damage, bleeding, fetal growth restriction, and even fetal death.

The incidence of preeclampsia is commonly cited to be about 5%, but wide variations are reported. The incidence is related to race and ethnicity as well as to environmental factors and family history. It affects women at all reproductive ages. The incidence of preeclampsia in Canada is about 2.6%, and of these, 0.5% progress to eclampsia.

Women with mild preeclampsia may be monitored closely as outpatients and placed on home bed rest. More severe cases may require hospitalization for close medical management and early delivery.

Placenta Previa   In **placenta previa**, the placenta either completely or partially covers the cervical opening, preventing the mother from delivering the baby vaginally. As a result, the baby must be delivered by Caesarean section. This condition occurs in 1 in 250 live births. Risk factors include prior Caesarean delivery, multiple pregnancies, intrauterine surgery, smoking, multiple gestations, and advanced maternal age. Previas often present as painless bright red vaginal bleeding and may be associated with contractions. They account for 20% of bleeding in the third trimester.

Placental Abruption   In **placental abruption**, a normally implanted placenta prematurely separates from the uterine wall. Women experience abdominal pain, vaginal bleeding, and uterine tenderness. It account for 30% of all bleeding in the third trimester. The condition also increases the risk of fetal death. The risk factors for developing a placental abruption are maternal age, tobacco smoking, cocaine use, multiple gestation, trauma, preeclampsia, hypertension, and preterm premature rupture of membranes.

Gestational Diabetes   During gestation, about 4% of all pregnant women develop **gestational diabetes mellitus (GDM)**, in which the body loses its ability to use insulin properly. In these women, diabetes occurs only during pregnancy. The condition stems from placental secretion of certain hormones, including growth hormone, cortisol, placental lactogen, and progesterone. GDM arises when pancreatic function is not sufficient to overcome the insulin resistance created by these pregnancy-related hormones. Women diagnosed with GDM have an increased risk of developing type 2 diabetes later in life. It is important to accurately diagnose and treat GDM as it can lead to preeclampsia, polyhydramnios (increased levels of amniotic fluid), large fetuses, birth trauma, operative deliveries, perinatal mortality, and neonatal metabolic complications.

Preterm Labour   When a pregnant woman goes into labour before the 37th week of gestation, she is said to undergo *preterm labour*. Preterm labour is one of the most common reasons for hospitalizing pregnant women, but verifying true preterm labour can be difficult. About 30%–50% of preterm labours resolve themselves, with the pregnancy continuing to full term. In other cases, interventions may be required to delay labour and allow gestation to continue.

Labour Induction   If pregnancy continues well beyond the baby's due date, it may be necessary to induce labour artificially. This is one of the most common obstetrical procedures and is typically offered to pregnant women who have not delivered 7–14 days past their due date. Labour can be artificially induced in several ways.

Low Birth Weight and Premature Birth   A low-birth-weight (LBW) baby is one that weighs less than 2.5 kilograms at birth. LBW babies may be **premature** (born before the 37th week of pregnancy) or full-term. Babies who are born small even though they're full-term are referred to as *small-for-date* or *small-for-gestational-age* babies. Low birth weight affected about 6% of babies born in 2005 in Canada. About half of all cases are related to teenage pregnancy, cigarette smoking, poor nutrition, and poor maternal health. Other maternal factors include drug use, stress, depression, and anxiety. Adequate prenatal care is the best way to prevent LBW.

Full-term LBW babies tend to have fewer problems than premature infants. In Canada in 2006–2007, about 8% of babies were born prematurely. Many premature infants' organs are not sufficiently developed. Even mild prematurity increases an infant's risk of dying in the first month or year of life. Premature infants are subject to respiratory problems and infections. They may have difficulty eating because they may be too small to suck a breast or bottle and their swallowing mechanism may be underdeveloped. As they get older, premature infants may have problems, such as learning difficulties, behaviour problems, poor hearing and vision, and physical awkwardness.

Infant Mortality   The Canadian rate of **infant mortality**, the death of a child of less than one year of age, is near its lowest point ever; however, it remains far higher than that of most of the developed world. Canada ranks low among the world's developed countries for infant mortality, with 6 deaths for every 1000 live births. Many experts agree that it is difficult to make international comparisons because birth registration and reporting procedures are not standardized across the globe. Figure 12.8 on p. 398 shows the infant mortality rate across Canada in 2007, with the lowest rate in Nova Scotia and the highest in Nunavut. Infant mortality rates are higher among Aboriginal peoples in Canada; poverty and inadequate health care are key causes.

Other causes of infant death are congenital problems, infectious diseases, and injuries. According to Statistics Canada, congenital abnormalities and preterm births were the two leading causes of infant mortality in Canada from 2000 to 2004.

ectopic pregnancy   A pregnancy in which the embryo develops outside of the uterus, usually in the fallopian tube.

preeclampsia   A condition of pregnancy characterized by high blood pressure and protein in the urine.

eclampsia   A severe, potentially life-threatening form of preeclampsia, characterized by seizures.

placenta previa   A complication of pregnancy in which the placenta covers the cervical opening, preventing the mother from delivering the baby vaginally.

placental abruption   A complication of pregnancy in which a normally implanted placenta prematurely separates from the uterine wall.

gestational diabetes mellitus (GDM)   A form of diabetes that occurs during pregnancy.

low birth weight (LBW)   Weighing less than 2.5 kilograms at birth, often the result of prematurity.

premature   Born before the 37th week of pregnancy.

infant mortality   The death of a child less than one year of age.

TERMS

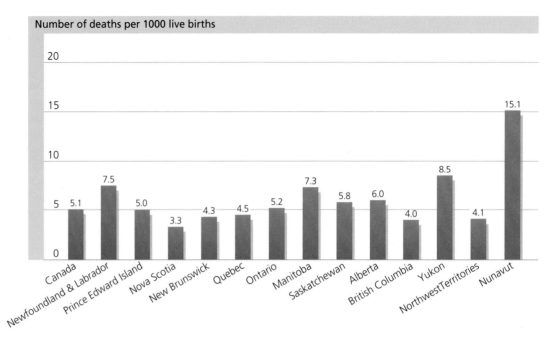

FIGURE 12.8
Infant mortality rates, by province and territory, 2007.

Note: The infant mortality rate is calculated as the number of deaths of children less than one year of age per 1000 live births in the same year.

Source: Human Resources and Skills Development Canada. 2010. *Indicators of Well-Being in Canada. Health: Infant Mortality* (http://www4.hrsdc.gc.ca/.3indic.1t.4r@-eng.jsp?iid=2; retrieved April 26, 2010). © Her Majesty the Queen in Right of Canada.

Number of deaths per 1000 live births

Canada	5.1
Newfoundland & Labrador	7.5
Prince Edward Island	5.0
Nova Scotia	3.3
New Brunswick	4.3
Quebec	4.5
Ontario	5.2
Manitoba	7.3
Saskatchewan	5.8
Alberta	6.0
British Columbia	4.0
Yukon	8.5
Northwest Territories	4.1
Nunavut	15.1

In **sudden infant death syndrome (SIDS)**, an apparently healthy infant dies suddenly while sleeping. The number of SIDS deaths has decreased since 1992, when the Back to Sleep campaign was instituted to make people aware that putting babies to bed on their backs rather than on their stomachs significantly reduces the risk of SIDS. Research suggests that abnormalities in the brainstem, the part of the brain that regulates breathing, heart rate, and other basic functions, underlie the risk for SIDS. Risk is greatly increased for infants with these innate differences if they are exposed to environmental risks, such as sleeping face down; being exposed to tobacco smoke, alcohol, or other drugs; or sleeping on a soft mattress or with fluffy bedding, pillows, or stuffed toys. Overbundling a baby or keeping a baby's room too warm also increases the risk of SIDS; because of this, SIDS deaths are more common in the colder months. Exposure to nitrous dioxide air pollution is also under investigation as a possible contributing factor. Several studies have found that the use of a pacifier significantly reduces the risk of SIDS.

QUICK STATS

In Canada, about **1** infant death per **1400** live births is due to SIDS.

—Health Canada, 2005

Coping with Loss Parents form a deep attachment to their children even before birth, and those who lose an infant before or during birth usually experience deep grief. Initial feelings of shocked disbelief and numbness may give way to sadness, anger, crying spells, and preoccupation with the loss. Physical sensations, such as tightness in the chest or stomach, loss of appetite, and sleeplessness, may also occur.

For the mother, physical exhaustion and hormone imbalances can compound the emotional and physical stress.

Experiencing the pain of loss is part of the healing process. A support group or professional counselling is also often helpful. Planning the next pregnancy, with a physician's input, can be an important step toward recovery, as long as the mind and body are given time to heal.

CHILDBIRTH

By the end of the ninth month of pregnancy, most women are tired of being pregnant; both parents are eager to start a new phase of their lives. Most couples find the actual process of birth to be an exciting and positive experience.

Choices in Childbirth

Many couples today can choose the type of practitioner and the environment they want for the birth of their child. A high-risk pregnancy is probably best handled by a specialist physician in a hospital with a nursery, but for low-risk births, many options are available.

Most babies in Canada are born in hospital. In 2003, more than 85% of women in Ontario gave birth in large community or teaching hospitals. During this time, more

QUESTIONS FOR CRITICAL THINKING AND REFLECTION

Do you know anyone who has lost a child to miscarriage, stillbirth, or a birth defect? If so, how did he or she cope with the loss? What would you do to help someone in this situation?

than 80% of women used an obstetrician, 11% used a family physician, 3.5% used a midwife in the hospital, and the remaining births took place at home with a midwife or another provider. Parents can choose to have their baby delivered by a physician (an obstetrician or family practitioner) or by a registered midwife. In Canada, most babies are delivered by an obstetrician. The number of babies delivered by family physicians is decreasing, while the number delivered by midwives is increasing. In Ontario, the number of deliveries by family physicians decreased by 50% between 1995 and 2004, and although the number of deliveries by midwives is less overall, it increased 400% over this same time period.

Midwives are health care providers who care for women and their babies during pregnancy, labour, delivery, and the postpartum period. Midwifery is regulated in Canada by provincial and territorial authorities. Midwives who are registered with these authorities use the title registered midwife (RM) or *sage-femme* (SF), and they are legally allowed to practise midwifery.

Some mothers-to-be are accompanied in the delivery room by a labour companion, called a *doula*. A doula is a woman who has either been through childbirth or has extensive experience with birth. She stays with the labouring woman continuously and provides emotional and tangible support, information, and advocacy. Supportive labour companions may improve labour progress by reducing maternal anxiety. Studies show that the presence of a knowledgeable doula can shorten the duration of labour, increase the rate of spontaneous vaginal birth, and reduce the use of narcotic painkillers, forceps delivery, and Caesarean birth.

It's important for prospective parents to discuss all aspects of labour and delivery with their physician or midwife beforehand so they can learn what to expect and can state their preferences. For more information, see the box "Making a Birth Plan" on p. 401.

Labour and Delivery

The birth process occurs in three stages (Figure 12.9 on p. 400). **Labour** begins when hormonal changes in both the mother and the baby cause strong, rhythmic uterine **contractions** to begin. These contractions exert pressure on the cervix and cause the lengthwise muscles of the uterus to pull on the circular muscles around the cervix, creating effacement (thinning) and dilation (opening) of the cervix. The contractions also pressure the baby to descend into the mother's pelvis, if it hasn't already. The entire process of labour and delivery usually takes between 2 and 36 hours, depending on the size of the baby, the baby's position in the uterus, the size of the mother's pelvis, the strength of the uterine contractions, the number of prior deliveries, and other factors. The length of labour is generally shorter for second and subsequent births.

The First Stage of Labour The first stage of labour averages 13 hours for a first birth, although wide variation exists among women. It begins with cervical effacement and dilation and continues until the cervix is completely dilated (10 centimetres). Contractions usually last about 30 seconds and occur every 15–20 minutes at first, more often later. The prepared mother relaxes as much as possible during these contractions to allow labour to proceed without being blocked by tension. Early in the first stage, a small amount of bleeding may occur as a plug of slightly bloody mucus that blocked the opening of the cervix during pregnancy is expelled. In some women, the amniotic sac ruptures and the fluid rushes out; this is sometimes referred to as the "water breaking."

The last part of the first stage of labour, called **transition**, is characterized by strong and frequent contractions, much more intense than in the early stages of labour. Contractions may last 60–90 seconds and occur every 1–3 minutes. During transition the cervix opens completely, to a diameter of about 10 centimetres. The head of the fetus usually measures 9–10 centimetres; thus once the cervix has dilated completely, the head can pass through. Many women report that transition, which normally lasts about 30–60 minutes, is the most difficult part of labour.

The Second Stage of Labour The second stage of labour begins with complete cervical dilation and ends with the delivery of the baby. The baby is slowly pushed down, through the bones of the pelvic ring, past the cervix, and into the vagina, which it stretches open. The mother bears down with the contractions to help push the baby down and out. Some women find this the most difficult part of labour; others find that the contractions and bearing down bring a sense of relief. The baby's back bends, the head turns to fit through the narrowest parts of the passageway, and the soft bones of the baby's skull move together and overlap as it is squeezed through the pelvis. When the top of the head appears at the vaginal opening, the baby is said to be crowning.

As the head of the baby emerges, the physician or midwife will remove any mucus from the mouth and nose, wipe the baby's face, and check to ensure that the umbilical cord is not around the neck. With a few more contractions, the baby's shoulders and body emerge. As the baby is squeezed through the pelvis, cervix, and vagina, the fluid in the

(a)

(b)

(c)

FIGURE 12.9   Birth: labour and delivery.   (a) The first stage of labour; **(b)** the second stage of labour: delivery of the baby; **(c)** the third stage of labour: expulsion of the placenta.

lungs is forced out by the pressure on the baby's chest. Once this pressure is released as the baby emerges from the vagina, the chest expands and the lungs fill with air for the first time. The baby will still be connected to the mother via the umbilical cord, which is not cut until it stops pulsating. The baby will appear wet and often is covered with a cheeselike substance. The baby's head may be oddly shaped at first, because of the moulding of the soft plates of bone during birth, but it usually takes on a more rounded appearance within 24 hours.

The Third Stage of Labour   In the third stage of labour, the uterus continues to contract until the placenta is expelled. This stage usually takes 5–30 minutes. It is important that the entire placenta be expelled; if part remains in the uterus, it may cause infection or bleeding. Breastfeeding soon after delivery helps control uterine bleeding because it stimulates the secretion of a hormone that makes the uterus contract.

The baby's physical condition is assessed with the **Apgar score**, a formalized system for assessing the baby's need for medical assistance. Heart rate, respiration, colour, reflexes, and muscle tone are individually rated with a score of 0–2, and a total score between 0 and 10 is given at one and five minutes after birth. A score of 7–10 at five minutes is considered normal. Most newborns are also tested for at least 30 rare disorders that can be treated early, decreasing future health problems for the child. In Canada, many newborns are screened for such disorders, but the specific disorders screened for varies across provinces and territories.

Pain Relief During Labour and Delivery   Women vary in how much pain they experience in childbirth. First babies are typically the most challenging to deliver, as the birth canal has never stretched to this extent before. It is recommended that women and their partners learn about labour and what kinds of choices are available for pain relief. Childbirth preparation courses are a good place to start, and communicating with the obstetrician or midwife is essential to assess the approaches that will be available. Breathing and relaxation techniques, such as Lamaze or Bradley, have been used effectively, and they are often modified by the labouring women to be even more effective. Forms of hypnosis can also be used.

The most commonly employed medical intervention for pain relief is the epidural. This procedure involves placing a thin plastic catheter between the vertebrae in the lower back. Medication that reduces the transmission of pain signals to the brain is given through this catheter. Local anaesthetic drugs are given in low concentration to minimize weakening of the leg muscles so that the mother can effectively push during the birth. The amount of medication given is quite low and does not accumulate in the baby or interfere with the baby's transition after birth. The mother is awake and is an active participant in the birth.

Women can also elect to have narcotics, such as morphine or demerol, given for pain relief during labour, but

Making a Birth Plan

A variety of birth situations can have positive physical and psychological outcomes. Parents should choose what is appropriate for their medical circumstances and what feels most comfortable to them. Prospective parents should discuss their preferences in the following areas with their physician or midwife:

1. Who will be present at the birth? The father? Friends? Children and other relatives? Will young siblings be allowed to visit the mother and new baby? What are the hospital/centre policies in terms of visitors and number of people present at the birth?

2. What type of room will the mother be in during labour, delivery, and recovery?

3. What types of tables, beds, or birthing chairs are available? What type of environment can be created for the birth? Can specific music be played?

4. Will the mother receive any routine preparation, such as an enema, intravenous feeding, or shaving of the pubic area?

5. What is the policy regarding food and drink during labour? Will the mother have the option of walking around or taking a shower or bath during labour?

6. Under what circumstances does the physician or midwife administer drugs to induce or augment labour? The use of these drugs tends to change the course of labour and carries a small risk.

7. How is the fetus monitored during labour? According to the SOGC, it is best to monitor the baby at regular intervals during labour; however, some circumstances require continuous monitoring.

8. Under what circumstances will an episiotomy, an incision at the base of the vaginal opening, be performed? Are any steps taken to avoid it? According to the SOGC, there is no reason to perform routine episiotomies.

9. Under what circumstances will forceps or vacuum extraction be used? In some cases of fetal distress, the use of forceps or vacuum extraction may be necessary to save the infant's life, but some authorities believe these techniques are overused.

10. What types of medications are typically used during labour and delivery? Some form of anaesthetic is usually administered during most hospital deliveries, as are hormones that intensify the contractions and shrink the uterus after delivery. Different types of anaesthetics, including short-acting narcotics, regional nerve blocks, and local anaesthetics, may be available; each has different effects on the mother and the fetus.

11. Under what conditions or circumstances does the physician perform a Caesarean section?

12. Who will "catch" the baby as she or he is born? Who will cut the umbilical cord?

13. What will be done to the baby immediately after birth? What kinds of tests and procedures will be done on the baby, and when?

14. How often will the baby be brought to the mother while they remain in the hospital or birthing centre? Can the baby stay in the mother's room rather than in a nursery? This practice is known as **rooming-in**. Research shows that rooming-in is best for babies and mothers. It gives the mother and baby an opportunity to bond, and the risk of infection is decreased for babies who room-in with their mother when compared with babies who stay in a nursery.

15. How will the baby be fed—by breast or bottle? Will feeding be on a schedule or on demand? Is there someone with breastfeeding expertise available to answer questions if necessary?

these medications usually provide less pain relief than the epidural and, if given shortly before the birth, can cause the baby to be less vigorous at birth. Local anaesthesia is available for repair of any tear or **episiotomy** if the mother has not used an epidural for the labour.

Caesarean Deliveries In a **Caesarean section**, the baby is removed through a surgical incision in the abdominal wall and uterus. Caesarean sections are necessary when a baby cannot be delivered vaginally—for example, if the baby's head is bigger than the mother's pelvic girdle or if the baby is in an unusual position. If the mother has a serious health condition, such as high blood pressure, a Caesarean may be safer for her than labour and a vaginal delivery. Caesareans are more common among women who are overweight or have diabetes. Other reasons for Caesarean delivery include abnormal or difficult labour, fetal distress, and the presence of a dangerous infection,

such as herpes, that can be passed to the baby during delivery. A growing number of Caesareans are performed on low-risk mothers; researchers hope further analysis will help determine if the trend is due to patient choice, physician choice, or a combination of the two.

Apgar score A formalized system for assessing a newborn's need for medical assistance.

rooming-in The practice of allowing the mother and baby to remain together in the hospital or birth centre after delivery.

episiotomy An incision made to widen the vaginal opening to facilitate birth and prevent uncontrolled tearing during delivery.

Caesarean section A surgical incision through the abdominal wall and uterus, performed to deliver a fetus.

TERMS

CRITICAL CONSUMER

According to Statistics Canada, the Caesarean delivery rate in Canada is the highest it has ever been, increasing from 5% of deliveries in the 1960s to 20% in the 1980s to more than 25% today (Figure 12.10). Like any major surgery, Caesarean sections carry some risk and should be performed only for valid medical reasons rather than for convenience. The SOGC encourages deliveries without interventions, such as Caesarean sections, unless medically necessary. Women who have Caesarean sections can remain conscious during the operation if they are given a regional anaesthetic, and the father or another person the mother chooses may be present.

Repeat Caesarean deliveries are also very common. In 2007–2008, about 82% of Canadian women who had had one child by Caesarean had subsequent children delivered the same way—an increase of 9% from 73% in 2001–2002. Although the risk of complications associated with a vaginal delivery after a previous Caesarean delivery is low, there is a small (1%) risk of serious complication to the mother and baby if the previous uterine scar opens during labour (uterine rupture). For this reason, women and their doctors may choose to deliver by elective repeat Caesarean.

The Postpartum Period

The **postpartum period**, a stage of about three months following childbirth, is a time of critical family adjustments. Parenthood begins literally overnight, and the transition can cause considerable stress.

Following a vaginal delivery, mothers usually leave the hospital within one to three days (after a Caesarean section, they usually stay three to five days). Uterine contractions will occur from time to time for several days after delivery, especially during nursing, as the uterus begins to return to its prebirth size. It usually takes six to eight weeks for a woman's reproductive organs to return to their prebirth condition. She will have a bloody discharge called *lochia* for three to six weeks after the birth.

Within the first few days after birth, a baby will undergo newborn screening for certain rare disorders as noted above. The baby's head—if somewhat pointed following a vaginal delivery—will become more rounded within a few days. It takes about a week for the umbilical cord stump to shrivel and fall off. Regular infant checkups for health screenings and immunizations usually begin when the infant is only a few weeks old.

Breastfeeding   In 2005, about 87% of Canadian mothers who had babies in the previous five years breastfed their infants after delivery. Across Canada, the rate of breastfeeding increased from east to west, with 62.3%

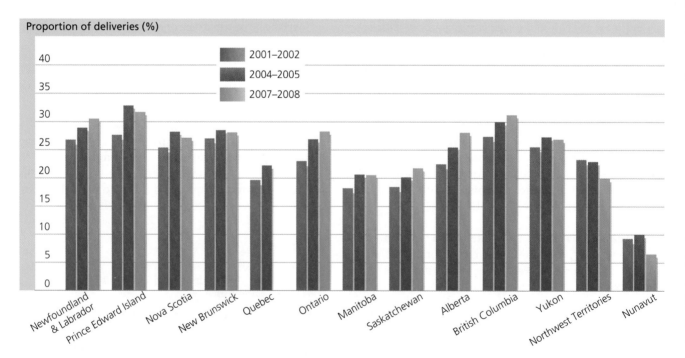

FIGURE 12.10   Caesarean section rates by province and territory.

Note: Data from Quebec for 2007–2008 were not available at time of publication.

Source: Canadian Institute for Health Information, *Health Indicators 2009* (Ottawa, Ontario: CIHI, 2009). Hospital Morbidity Database and Discharge: Abstract Database. Canadian Institute for Health Information.

of mothers breastfeeding in Newfoundland and Labrador and 98.8% in Yukon. **Lactation**, the production of milk, begins about three days after childbirth. before that time (sometimes as early as the second trimester), **colostrum** is secreted by the nipples. Colostrum contains antibodies that help protect the newborn from infectious diseases and is also high in protein.

Health Canada and the Canadian Paediatric Society recommend breastfeeding exclusively for six months, then in combination with solid food up to two years of age, and then for as long after that as a mother and baby desire. In 2005, only 16.4% of infants in Canada were exclusively breastfed for six months. Human milk is perfectly suited to the baby's nutritional needs and digestive capabilities, and it supplies the baby with antibodies. Breastfeeding decreases the incidence of infant ear infections, allergies, anemia, diarrhea, and bacterial meningitis. Preschoolers who were breastfed as babies are less likely to be overweight, and school-age children who were breastfed are less anxious and better able to cope with stress. Breastfeeding even has a beneficial effect on blood pressure and cholesterol levels later in life.

Breastfeeding is beneficial to the mother, as well. It stimulates contractions that help the uterus return to normal more rapidly, contributes to postpregnancy weight loss, and may reduce the risk of ovarian cancer, breast cancer, and postmenopausal hip fracture. Nursing also provides a sense of closeness and emotional well-being for mother and child. For women who want to breastfeed but who have problems, help is available from support groups, books, or a lactation consultant.

Breastfeeding can enhance the bond between mother and child. Health Canada and the Canadian Paediatric Society recommend breastfeeding exclusively for six months and then in combination with solid food up to two years of age and beyond.

For some women, physical problems, such as tenderness or infection of the nipples, can make breastfeeding difficult. If a woman has an illness or requires drug treatment, she may have to bottle-feed her baby because drugs and infectious agents may show up in breast milk. Breastfeeding can be restrictive, making it especially difficult for working mothers. Employers rarely provide nursing breaks, so bottle-feeding or the use of a breast pump (to express milk for use while the mother is away from her infant) may be the only practical alternatives. Bottle-feeding also allows the father or other caregiver to share in the nurturing process. Both breastfeeding and bottle-feeding can be part of loving, secure parent-child relationships.

When a mother doesn't nurse, menstruation usually begins within about 10 weeks. Breastfeeding can prevent the return of menstruation for six months or longer because the hormone prolactin, which aids milk production, suppresses hormones vital to the development of mature eggs. However, ovulation—and pregnancy—can occur before menstruation returns, so breastfeeding is not a reliable contraceptive method; if a woman wants to avoid pregnancy, she should use a more reliable method. If the mother becomes pregnant while still nursing, she needs to make sure that she is receiving adequate nutrition, because the energy requirement for both breastfeeding and gestating is immense. With proper counselling, breastfeeding can continue until near delivery.

Postpartum Depression Many women experience fluctuating emotions during the postpartum period as hormone levels change. The physical stress of labour, as well as dehydration, blood loss, and other physical factors, lowers the woman's stamina. About 50%–80% of new mothers experience "baby blues," characterized by episodes of sadness, weeping, anxiety, headache, sleep disturbances, and irritability. A mother may feel lonely and anxious about caring for her infant. About 5%–9% of new mothers experience **postpartum depression**, a more disabling syndrome characterized by despondency, mood swings, guilt, and occasional hostility. Rest, sharing feelings and concerns with others, and relying on supportive relatives and friends for assistance are usually helpful in dealing with mild cases of the baby blues or postpartum depression, which generally lasts only a few weeks. If the depression is serious, professional treatment may be needed. Some

postpartum period The period of about three months after delivering a baby.

lactation The production of milk.

colostrum A yellowish fluid secreted by the mammary glands around the time of childbirth until milk comes in, about the third day.

postpartum depression An emotional low that may be experienced by the mother following childbirth.

TERMS

men also seem to get a form of postpartum depression, characterized by anxiety about their changing role and feelings of inadequacy. Both mothers and fathers need time to adjust to their new roles as parents.

Attachment   Another feature of the postpartum period is the development of attachment—the strong emotional tie that grows between the baby and the adult who cares for the baby. Parents can foster secure attachment relationships in the early weeks and months by responding sensitively to the baby's needs. Parents who respond appropriately to the baby's signals of gazing, looking away, smiling, and crying establish feelings of trust in their child. They feed the baby when she's hungry, for example; respond when she cries; interact with her when she gazes, smiles, or babbles; and stop stimulating her when she frowns or looks away. A secure attachment relationship helps the child develop and function well socially, emotionally, and mentally.

QUESTIONS FOR CRITICAL THINKING AND REFLECTION

If you are a woman, what are your views on labour and delivery options? if you have a child in the future, which facility, delivery, and pain management options do you think you would prefer? If you are a man, what are your views on participating in delivery? What role would you want to play?

For most people, the arrival of a child provides a deep sense of joy and accomplishment. However, adjusting to parenthood requires effort and energy. Talking with friends and relatives about their experiences during the first few weeks or months with a baby can help prepare new parents for the period when the baby's needs may require all the energy that both parents have to expend. But the pleasures of nurturing a new baby are substantial, and many parents look back on this time as one of the most significant and joyful of their lives.

SUMMARY

• Factors to consider when deciding if and when to have a child include physical health and age; financial circumstances; relationship with your partner; educational, career, and child care plans; emotional readiness for parenthood; social support system; personal qualities, attitudes toward children, and aptitude for parenting; and philosophical or religious beliefs.

• Preconception care examines many factors, such as preexisting medical conditions, current medications, age of the mother, lifestyle behaviours, infections, nutritional status, and family history of genetic disease.

• Fertilization is a complex process culminating when a sperm penetrates the membrane of the egg released from the woman's ovary.

• The leading causes of infertility in women are blocked oviducts and ovulation disorders. Exposure to toxins, injury to the testicles, and infection can cause infertility in men.

• Early signs and symptoms of pregnancy include a missed menstrual period; slight bleeding; nausea; breast tenderness; increased urination; fatigue and emotional upset; and a softening of the uterus just above the cervix.

• During pregnancy, the uterus enlarges until it pushes up into the rib cage; the breasts enlarge and may secrete colostrum; the muscles and ligaments soften and stretch; and the circulatory system, lungs, and kidneys become more efficient.

• The fetal anatomy is almost completely formed in the first trimester and is refined in the second; during the third trimester, the fetus grows and gains most of its weight, storing nutrients in fatty tissues.

• Prenatal tests include ultrasound, amniocentesis, chorionic villus sampling, and integrated prenatal screening.

• Health care during pregnancy includes a complete history and physical at the beginning, followed by regular checkups and monitoring of blood pressure, weight gain, and size and position of the fetus.

• Important elements of prenatal care include good nutrition; avoidance of drugs, alcohol, tobacco, infections, and other harmful environmental agents or conditions; regular physical activity; and childbirth or prenatal classes.

• Pregnancy usually proceeds without major complications. Problems that can occur include ectopic pregnancy, spontaneous abortion, preeclampsia, and low birth weight. The loss of a fetus or an infant is deeply felt by most parents, who need time to grieve and heal.

• Couples preparing for childbirth may have many options to choose from, including type of practitioner and facility.

• The first stage of labour begins with contractions that exert pressure on the cervix, causing effacement and dilation. The second stage begins with complete cervical dilation and ends when the baby emerges. The third stage of labour is expulsion of the placenta.

• During the postpartum period, the mother's body begins to return to its prepregnancy state, and she may begin to breastfeed. Both mother and father must adjust to their new roles as parents, as they develop a strong emotional tie to their baby.

FOR MORE INFORMATION

BOOKS

Beer, A. E., J. Kantecki, and L. Reed. 2006. *Is Your Body Baby-Friendly? Unexplained Infertility, Miscarriage, and IVF Failure Explained and Treated.* Chicago: AJR Publishing. Covers many issues facing women and couples who are trying to overcome infertility.

Lees, C., K. Reynolds, and G. McCarten. 2007. *Pregnancy and Birth: Your Questions Answered.* London: Dorling Kindersley. Answers hundreds of common questions about conception, pregnancy, and delivery.

Lichtman, R., L. Simpson, and A. Rosenfield. 2005. *Dr. Guttmacher's Pregnancy, Birth & Family Planning,* updated ed. New York: New American Library. A complete guide to contraception, conception, pregnancy, and childbirth.

Riley, L. 2006. *Healthy Eating During Pregnancy.* New York: Meredith Books. Provides up-to-date dietary information and meal-planning guides for pregnant women.

Schuurmans, N., V. Senikas, and A. B. Lalonde. 2009. *Healthy Beginnings: Giving Your Baby the Best Start from Preconception to Birth*, 4th ed. Toronto: John Wiley and Sons Canada. A step-by-step guide to pregnancy and childbirth.

Wynbrandt, J. 2007. *Encyclopedia of Genetic Disorders and Birth Defects*. New York: Facts on File. A detailed overview of many types of birth defects, both inherited and noninherited.

ORGANIZATIONS AND WEB SITES

The Internet addresses listed here were accurate at the time of publication.

Assisted Human Reproduction Canada. Provides publications, reports, and brochures relating to assisted reproduction in Canada.
    http://www.ahrc-pac.gc.ca
Canadian Agency for Drugs and Technologies in Health. Provides information relating to many health technologies, including those related to assisted reproduction.
    http://www.cadth.ca
Canadian Association of Midwives. Provides information about midwifery in Canada.
    http://www.canadianmidwives.org
Caring for Kids. A Web site developed by the Canadian Paediatric Society to provide information regarding health of babies and children, including safe sleep and reducing the risk of sudden infant death syndrome.
    http://www.caringforkids.cps.ca
Childbirth.Org. Contains medical information and personal stories about all phases of pregnancy and birth.
    http://www.childbirth.org
Health Canada. Provides publications and other resources on many health issues including assisted human reproduction (AHR), healthy diet and pregnancy, and healthy babies.
    http://www.hc-sc.gc.ca
Health Canada: Women of Childbearing Age and Eating Well with Canada's Food Guide. Provides information on proper nutrition before and during pregnancy.
    http://www.hc-sc.gc.ca/fn-an/food-guide-aliment/choose-choix/
    advice-conseil/women-femmes-eng.php
International Council on Infertility Information Dissemination. Includes information on current research and treatments for infertility.
    http://www.inciid.org
La Leche League International. Provides advice and support for breastfeeding mothers.
    http://www.llli.org/
March of Dimes. Provides public education materials on many pregnancy-related topics, including preconception care, genetic screening, diet and exercise, and the effects of smoking and drinking during pregnancy.
    http://www.marchofdimes.com
Motherisk. Provides information about pregnancy and breastfeeding, with counsellors available by phone. Run by the Hospital for Sick Children in Toronto, Ontario.
    http://www.motherisk.org
Public Health Agency of Canada: The Sensible Guide to a Healthy Pregnancy. Reviews lifestyle choices to ensure a healthy pregnancy.
    http://www.phac-aspc.gc.ca/hp-gs/guide-eng.php
Society of Obstetricians and Gynaecologists of Canada. Provides up-to-date information on women's health topics including infertility, pregnancy, and childbirth.
    http://www.sogc.org

SELECTED BIBLIOGRAPHY

American Academy of Pediatrics Section on Breastfeeding. 2005. Breastfeeding and the use of human milk. *Pediatrics* 115(2): 496–506.

American Academy of Pediatrics Task Force on Sudden Infant Death Syndrome. 2005. The changing concept of sudden infant death syndrome. *Pediatrics* 116(5): 1245–1255.

Canadian Agency for Drugs and Technology in Health. 2009. *Health Technology Update 10: Assisted Reproductive Technologies in Canada* (http://www.cadth.ca/index.php/en/hta/reports-publications/health-technology-update/issue-10-september-2008/assisted-reproductive; retrieved April 26, 2010).

Canadian Council on Social Development. 2006. *Stats and Facts: Canadian Families—The Costs of Raising Children* (http://www.ccsd.ca/factsheets/family/index.htm; retrieved April 26, 2010).

Canadian Institute for Health Information. 2009. *Executive Summary.* (http://secure.cihi.ca/cihiweb/dispPage.jsp?cw_page=AR1106_2009 summary_e; retrieved April 26, 2010).

Canadian Institute for Health Information. 2009. *Health Indicators 2009.* (http://www.cihi.ca/cihiweb/products/Healthindicators2009_en.pdf; retrieved April 26, 2010).

Case, A. M. 2003. Infertility evaluation and management. Strategies for family physicians. *Canadian Family Physician* 49(11): 1465–1472.

Centers for Disease Control and Prevention. 2006. *Preconception Health and Care, 2006* (http://www.cdc.gov/ncbddd/preconception/documents/Ata-glance-4-11-06.pdf; retrieved January 29, 2006).

Central Intelligence Agency. 2009. *The World Factbook: Rank Order—Infant Mortality Rate* (https://www.cia.gov/cia/publications/factbook/rank order/2091rank.html; retrieved January 29, 2009).

de la Chica, R. A., et al. 2005. Chromosomal instability in amniocytes from fetuses of mothers who smoke. *Journal of the American Medical Association* 293(10): 1212–1222.

Davies, G. A. L., et al. 2003. *Exercise in Pregnancy and the Postpartum Period. Joint SOGC/CSEP Clinical Practice Guideline 129* (http://www.sogc.org/guidelines/public/129E-JCPG-June2003.pdf; retrieved April 26, 2010).

Does caffeine in pregnancy cause birth defects? 2006. *Child Health Alert* 24: 2.

Department of Justice of Canada. 2010. *Assisted Human Reproduction Act 2004.* (http://laws.justice.gc.ca/en/A-13.4/FullText.html; retrieved April 26, 2010).

De Sutter, P. 2006. Rational diagnosis and treatment of infertility. *Best Practice & Research: Clinical Obstetrics and Gynaecology* 20: 647–664.

Duncombe, D., et al. 2006. Vigorous exercise and birth outcomes in a sample of recreational exercisers: A prospective study across pregnancy. *The Australian & New Zealand Journal of Obstetrics & Gynaecology* 46(4): 288–292.

Gorman, C. 2006. What alcohol does to a child. *Time,* 5 June.

Harrison, E. C., and J. S. Taylor. 2006. IVF therapy for unexplained infertility. *American Family Physician* 73(1): 63–65.

Health Canada. 2005. *Sudden Infant Death: The Back to Sleep Campaign* (http://hc-sc.gc.ca/ahc-asc/activit/marketsoc/camp/sids-eng.php; retrieved April 26, 2010).

Health Canada. 2007. *Pregnancy: Smoking and Your Body* (http://www.hc-sc.gc.ca/hc-ps/tobac-tabac/body-corps/preg-gros-eng.php; retrieved April 26, 2010).

Health Canada. 2009. *Food and Nutrition: Canadian Gestational Weight gain recommendations* (http://www.hc-sc.gc.ca/fn-an/nutrition/prenatal/qa-gest-gros-qr-eng.php; retrieved April 26, 2010).

Health Canada. 2009. *Food and Nutrition: Prenatal Nutrition Guidelines for Health Professionals—Fish and Omega-3 Fatty Acids* (http://www.hc-sc.gc.ca/fn-an/pubs/nutrition/omega3-eng.php; retrieved April 26, 2010).

HealthyOntario. 2009. *Conditions: Preeclampsia.* (http://www.healthyontario.com/ConditionDetails.aspx?disease_id=107; retrieved April 26, 2010).

Human Resources and Skills Development Canada. 2010. *Indicators of Well Being in Canada: Age of Mother at Childbirth* (http://www4.hrsdc.gc.ca/.3ndic.1t.4r@-eng.jsp?iid=75; retrieved April 26, 2010).

Human Resources and Skills Development Canada. 2010. *Indicators of Well Being in Canada. Health: Infant Mortality* (http://www4.hrsdc.gc.ca/.3ndic.1t.4r@-eng.jsp?iid=2; retrieved April 26, 2010).

Human Resources and Skills Development Canada. 2010. *Indicators of Well Being in Canada. Health: Low Birth Weight* (http://www4.hrsdc.gc.ca/.3ndic.1t.4r@-eng.jsp?iid=4; retrieved April 26, 2010).

Jimenez-Chillaron, J. C., et al. 2005. Beta-cell secretory dysfunction in the pathogenesis of low birth weight–associated diabetes. *Diabetes* 54(3): 702–711.

Lavender, T., et al. 2006. Caesarean section for non-medical reasons at term. *Cochrane Database of Systematic Reviews* 19(3) (http://www2.cochrane.org/reviews/en/ab004660.html; retrieved April 25, 2011).

Leguizamon, G. F., and N. P. Zeff. 2006. Hypertension and the pregnancy complicated by diabetes. *Current Diabetes Reports* 6(4): 297–304.

Levine, R. J., et al. 2005. Urinary placental growth factor and risk of pre-eclampsia. *Journal of the American Medical Association* 293(1): 77–85.

Macfarlane, A., and D. Tuffnell. 2006. Diabetes and pregnancy. *British Medical Journal* 333(7560): 157–158.

March of Dimes. 2009. *Pregnancy Complications: Depression* (http://www.marchofdimes.com/complications_depression.html; retrieved April 25, 2011).

Mannion, C. A., et al. 2006. Association of low intake of milk and vitamin D during pregnancy with decreased birth weight. *Canadian Medical Association Journal* 174(9): 1273–1277.

McCormack, V. A., et al. 2005. Birth characteristics and adult cancer incidence: Swedish cohort of over 11,000 men and women. *International Journal of Cancer* 115: 611–617.

Murray, H., et al. 2005. Diagnosis and treatment of ectopic pregnancy. *Canadian Medical Association Journal* 173(8) (http://www.cmaj.ca/cgi/content/full/173/8/905; retrieved April 26, 2010).

Ontario Medical Association. 2008. *Policy on Maternal and Newborn Care in Ontario* (http://www.oma.org/Health/IPC/MaternalandNewbornCare2008.pdf; retrieved April 26, 2010).

Pattenden, S., et al. 2006. Parental smoking and children's respiratory health: Independent effects of prenatal and postnatal exposure. *Tobacco Control* 15(4): 294–301.

Public Health Agency of Canada. 2004. *Fetal Alcohol Spectrum Disorder: Frequently Asked Questions* (http://www.phac-aspc.gc.ca/fasd-etcaf/faq-eng.php#7; retrieved April 26, 2010).

Public Health Agency of Canada. 2007. *Canadian Guidelines on Sexually Transmitted Infections 2006: Pelvic Inflammatory Disease—Updated 2007* (http://www.phac-aspc.gc.ca/std-mts/sti_2006/pdf/pid06_e.pdf; retrieved April 26, 2010).

Public Health Agency of Canada. 2008. *Canadian Perinatal Health Report, 2008 Edition* (http://www.phac-aspc.gc.ca/publicat/2008/cphr-rspc/pdf/cphr-rspc08-eng.pdf; retrieved April 26, 2010).

Public Health Agency of Canada. 2008. *HIV and AIDS in Canada Surveillance Report to December 31, 2007* (http://www.phac-aspc.gc.ca/aids-sida/publication/survreport/pdf/survrep1207.pdf; retrieved April 26, 2010).

Public Health Agency of Canada. 2008. *The Sensible Guide to a Healthy Pregnancy* (http://www.phac-aspc.gc.ca/hp-gs/pdf/hpguide-eng.pdf; retrieved April 26, 2010).

Schuurmans, N., V. Senikas, and A. B. Lalonde. 2009. *Healthy Beginnings: Giving Your Baby the Best Start from Preconception to Birth,* 4th ed. Toronto: John Wiley and Sons Canada.

Scollan-Koliopoulos, M., et al. 2006. Gestational diabetes management: Guidelines to a healthy pregnancy. *Nurse Practitioner* 31(6): 14–23.

Statistics Canada. 2009. *Births 2007* (http://www.statcan.gc.ca/pub/84f0210x/84f0210x2007000-eng.pdf; retrieved April 26, 2010).

Statistics Canada. 2009. *Overview of the 10 Leading Causes of Infant Death in Canada* (http://www.statcan.gc.ca/pub/84-215-x/2008000/ana-eng.htm#f; retrieved April 26, 2010).

Statistics Canada. 2010. *Births and Birth Rate by Province and Territory* (http://www40.statcan.gc.ca/l01/cst01/demo04a-eng.htm; retrieved April 26, 2010).

Statistics Canada. 2010. *Infant Mortality Rates by Province and Territory* (http://www40.statcan.gc.ca/l01/cst01/health21a-eng.htm; retrieved January 2, 2011).

Summers, A. M., et al. 2007. Prenatal screening for fetal aneuploidy. *SOGC Clinical Practice Guideline 187* (http://www.sogc.org/guidelines/documents/187E-CPG-February2007.pdf; retrieved April 26, 2010).

UNICEF. 2009. *The State of the World's Children: Basic Indicators* (http://www.unicef.org/rightsite/sowc/statistics.php; retrieved April 26, 2010).

Voelker, R. 2005. The business of baby pictures: Controversy brews over "keepsake" fetal ultrasounds. *Journal of the American Medication Association* 293(1): 25–27.

World Health Organization. 2010. Genomic *Resource Centre: Genes and Human Disease* (http://www.who.int/genomics/public/geneticdiseases/en/index2.html; retrieved April 26, 2010).

SEXUALLY TRANSMITTED INFECTIONS (STIs)

13

LOOKING AHEAD >>>>>

AFTER READING THIS CHAPTER, YOU SHOULD BE ABLE TO

- Discuss the symptoms of, risks for, and treatments for the major sexually transmitted infections (STIs)

- Explain how HIV infection affects the body and how it is transmitted, diagnosed, and treated

- List strategies for protecting yourself from STIs

TEST YOUR KNOWLEDGE

1. **If you have a sexually transmitted infection (STI), you will know it.**
   True or false?

2. **Of the developed countries, which one has the highest rate of STIs?**
   a. Germany
   b. Canada
   c. United States
   d. France

3. **A man with an STI is more likely to transmit the infection to a female partner than vice versa.**
   True or false?

4. **After you have had an STI once, you become immune to that disease and cannot get it again.**
   True or false?

5. **Worldwide, HIV infection is spread primarily via which of the following?**
   a. injection drug use
   b. sex between men
   c. mother-to-child transmission
   d. heterosexual sex

ANSWERS

1. **FALSE.** Many people with STIs have no symptoms and do not know they are infected; however, they can still pass an infection to any partner.

2. **C.** The United States has the highest rate of STIs of any developed nation. If current trends continue, 50% of Americans will contract a sexually transmitted infection by age 25.

3. **TRUE.** For many STIs, infected men are at least twice as likely as infected women to transmit an STI to a partner.

4. **FALSE.** Reinfection with STIs is very common. For example, if you are treated for and cured of chlamydia and then you have sex with your untreated partner, the chances are very good that you will be infected again.

5. **D.** The vast majority of HIV infection cases worldwide result from heterosexual contact, and nearly two-thirds of all new cases occur in teenage girls and young women.

Considering the intimate nature of sexual activity, it is not surprising that many infections can be transmitted from one person to another through sexual contact. Of course, colds, influenza, and many other infections can spread from one sexual partner to another, but sexual contact is not the primary means of transmission for these illnesses. **Sexually transmitted infections (STIs)**—previously referred to as sexually transmitted diseases (STDs)—spread from person to person mainly through sexual activity.

STIs are a particularly insidious group of illnesses because a person can be infected and able to transmit the disease yet not look or feel sick; this is why the term *sexually transmitted infection (STI)* has replaced the term *sexually transmitted disease* in Canada. Everyone should have a clear understanding of what STIs are, how they are transmitted, and how they can be prevented. Many STIs can also be cured if treated early and properly. This chapter introduces the major forms of sexually transmitted infections; it also provides information about healthy, safer sexual behaviour to help you understand how to reduce the further spread of these infections.

THE MAJOR STIs

The following seven STIs pose a major health threat:

- Chlamydia
- Gonorrhea
- Syphilis
- Human papillomavirus (HPV)
- Genital herpes (HSV 1 and HSV 2)
- HIV/AIDS
- Hepatitis B (HBV)

These diseases are considered major threats because they are serious in themselves, cause serious complications if left untreated, and pose risks to a fetus or newborn. STIs can result in serious long-term consequences, including chronic pain, infertility, stillbirths, genital cancers, and death.

All these diseases have a relatively high incidence among Canadians (Table 13.1). In fact, a 2010 report from the Public Health Agency of Canada shows that many of the most common STIs are on the rise in Canada. To assess your current level of responsibility for STI prevention, complete the quiz in the box "Do Your Attitudes and Behaviours Put You at Risk for STIs?" on p. 412.

Chlamydia

STIs are caused by more than 30 different organisms, including viruses, bacteria, fungi, and protozoa. *Chlamydia trachomatis* causes **chlamydia**, the most prevalent bacterial STI in Canada. According to Health Canada, rates of chlamydia infection in Canada have been increasing steadily since 1997, with more than 65,000 cases reported in 2006. Many experts believe, however, that chlamydia is vastly underreported because it is often symptomless, and they estimate that as many as 40,000 new cases of the disease occur each year. The highest rates of infection occur in single people ages 15–24. In 2007, reported chlamydia rates were highest in Nunavut, the Northwest Territories, and Yukon. (Table 13.2 on p. 412 shows rates of common STIs in all provinces and territories). Both men and women are susceptible to chlamydia, but, as with most STIs, women bear the greater burden because of possible complications and consequences of the disease (see the box "Women Are Hit Hard by STIs" on p. 413). *C. trachomatis* can be transmitted by oral sex as well as by other forms of sexual intercourse.

In most women, chlamydia produces no early symptoms. If left untreated, it can lead to pelvic inflammatory disease (PID), which is discussed later in this chapter. Chlamydia also greatly increases a woman's risk for infertility and ectopic (tubal) pregnancy. Because rates of infection are high and most women with chlamydia have no symptoms, many physicians screen sexually active women at the time of their routine pelvic exam. Chlamydia can also lead to infertility in men, although not as often as in women. In men under age 35, chlamydia is the most common cause of **epididymitis**, inflammation of the sperm-carrying ducts. And up to half of all cases of **urethritis**, inflammation of the urethra, in men are caused by chlamydia. Despite these statistics, many infected men have no symptoms. The Public Health Agency of Canada currently recommends routine screening for all at-risk groups, including sexually active women and men 25 years old or younger.

Infants of infected mothers can acquire the infection through contact with the pathogen in the birth canal during delivery. The Canadian Paediatric Society recommends routine prenatal screening for chlamydia; testing pregnant women and treating those infected is a highly effective way to prevent infection of newborns.

Symptoms In men, chlamydia symptoms include painful urination, a slight watery discharge from the penis, and sometimes pain around the testicles. Although most women with chlamydia are asymptomatic, some notice increased vaginal discharge, burning with urination, pain or bleeding with intercourse, and lower abdominal pain. Less common symptoms in both men and women include arthritis, conjunctivitis, sore throat, and rectal inflammation and pain (in people who become infected during receptive anal intercourse). Symptoms in both men and women can begin within five days of infection. However,

Table 13.1	Epidemiology of STIs in Canada		
STI	**How Common in Clinical Practice?**	**Trends in Incidence**	**Groups Most Affected**
Chlamydia	• Most commonly diagnosed and reported bacterial STI • 82,919 cases reported in 2008	• Steadily increasing in Canada since 1997	• Young women ages 15–24 • Young men ages 20–29
Gonorrhea	• Second most commonly diagnosed and reported bacterial STI • 12,723 cases reported in 2008	• Steadily increasing in Canada since 1997 • Quinolone (antibiotic) resistance increased from <1% in early 1990s to 15.7% in 2005 (national rate)	• Males account for two-thirds of reported cases • Men who have sex with men • Young men ages 20–29 • Young women ages 15–24
Syphilis	• Previously rare in Canada • 1394 cases reported in 2008	• Dramatic national increases since 1997 • Related to regional outbreaks across Canada	• Men who have sex with men ages 30–39 • Sex workers and their clients • Acquisition in endemic regions
Human papillomavirus (HPV)	• Very common • 70% of the adult population will have had at least one genital HPV infection in their lifetime	• True incidence is not known as HPV is not a reportable STI	• Adolescent and young adult women and men (although it affects women and men of all ages)
Genital herpes (HSV 1 and HSV 2)	• Common	• True incidence is not known as HSV is not a reportable STI	• Very common in adolescent and adult men and women • Women are affected more often than men
HIV/AIDS	• Rare in general practice • 2623 new cases reported in Canada in 2008	• 7% rise in number of HIV-positive test reports from 2007–2008	• Men who have sex with men • Acquisition in endemic regions • People who inject drugs • Young women ages 15–19
Hepatitis B (HBV)	• Low to moderate in general practice and varies in different populations • Approximately 700 acute cases per year in Canada	• Acute HBV twice as high for men • Peak incidence rates are found in the 30–39 age group	• People who inject drugs and share equipment • People with multiple sexual partners • Acquisition in endemic regions • Sexual and household contacts of an acute or a chronic carrier • Infants born to hepatitis B surface antigen-positive (HbsAg+) mothers

Sources: Public Health Agency of Canada. 2008. *Canadian Guidelines on Sexually Transmitted Infections—2008 Edition* (http://www.phac-aspc.gc.ca/std-mts/sti-its/pdf/sti-its-eng. pdf; retrieved February 18, 2010); Public Health Agency of Canada. 2009. *HIV and AIDS in Canada. Surveillance Report to December 31, 2008.* (http://www.phac-aspc.gc.ca/ aids-sida/publication/survreport/2008/dec/index-eng.php#toc; retrieved March 4, 2010); Public Health Agency of Canada. 2005. National Microbiology Laboratory, unpublished data; Public Health Agency of Canada. 2010. *Primary Care and Sexually Transmitted Infections* (http://www.phac-aspc.gc.ca/std-mts/sti-its/pdf/secii-eng.pdf; retrieved January 22, 2011).

most people experience few or no symptoms, increasing the likelihood that they will inadvertently spread the infection to their partners.

Diagnosis Chlamydia is typically diagnosed through laboratory tests on a urine sample or a small amount of fluid from the urethra or cervix. The lab test may involve growing the organism in culture, using special dyes to detect bacterial proteins, or a process that quickly copies and detects genetic material from the bacteria. A home test is currently being studied.

Treatment Once chlamydia has been diagnosed, the infected person and his or her partner(s) are given antibiotics—usually doxycycline, erythromycin, or a newer drug,

azithromycin, which can cure infection in one dose. Treatment of partners is important because people who have been treated for chlamydia are susceptible to getting the

sexually transmitted infection (STI) An infection that can be transmitted by sexual contact; some can also be transmitted by other means.

chlamydia An STI transmitted by the pathogenic bacterium Chlamydia trachomatis.

epididymitis An inflammation of the small body of sperm-carrying ducts that rests on the testes.

urethritis An inflammation of the tube that carries urine from the bladder to the outside opening.

TERMS

Do Your Attitudes and Behaviours Put You at Risk for STIs?

To identify your STI risk factors, read the following statements and identify whether each one is true or false for you.

True or False

1. I have never been sexually active. (If false, continue. If true, you are not at risk; respond to the remaining statements based on how you realistically believe you would act.)

2. I am in a mutually monogamous relationship with an uninfected partner or am not currently sexually active. (If false, continue. If true, you are at minimal risk now; respond to the remaining statements according to your attitudes and past behaviours.)

3. I have only one sex partner.

4. I always use a condom for each act of intercourse, even if I am fairly certain my partner has no infections.

5. I do not use oil-based lubricants or other products with condoms.

6. I discuss STIs and prevention with new partners before having sex.

7. I do not use alcohol or other mood-altering drugs in sexual situations.

8. I would tell my partner if I thought I had been exposed to an STI.

9. I am familiar with the signs and symptoms of STIs.

10. I regularly perform genital self-examinations.

11. When I notice any sign or symptom of any STI or if I engage in risky sexual behaviour, I consult my physician immediately.

12. I obtain screening for HIV and STIs regularly. In addition (if female), I obtain yearly pelvic exams and Pap tests.

13. When diagnosed with an STI, I inform all recent partners.

14. When I have a sign or symptom of an STI that goes away on its own, I still consult my physician.

15. I do not use drugs prescribed for friends or partners or left over from other illnesses to treat STIs.

16. I do not share syringes or needles to inject drugs.

False answers indicate attitudes and behaviours that may put you at risk for contracting STIs or for suffering serious medical consequences from them. (For a more detailed self-assessment, take the quiz at http://www.thebody.com/surveys/sexsurvey.html.)

---

disease again if they have sexual contact with an infected person. Because the risk of repeat infection is so high, the Public Health Agency of Canada now recommends that all people who have been treated for chlamydia be retested six months after treatment is completed.

Gonorrhea

Almost 13,000 cases of **gonorrhea** were reported to Health Canada in 2008. Like chlamydia, however, gonorrhea is underreported because it is often symptomless, so the number of actual cases is likely much higher. The highest incidence is among Canadians under the age of 30. Like chlamydia, untreated gonorrhea can cause PID in women and urethritis and epididymitis in men. It can also cause arthritis, rashes, and eye infections, and it occasionally involves internal organs. Being infected with gonorrhea increases the likelihood that HIV will be transmitted. A woman who is infected during pregnancy is at risk for preterm delivery and for having a baby with life threatening

gonorrhea   A sexually transmitted bacterial infection that usually affects mucous membranes.

gonococcal conjunctivitis   An inflammation of the mucous membrane lining of the eyelids, caused by the gonococcus bacterium.

TERMS

Table 13.2	Rates of Common STIs by Province and Territory, 2007		
	Chlamydia	Gonorrhea	Syphilis
British Columbia	**233.3**	29.8	6.9
Alberta	**318.8**	**62.5**	7.1
Saskatchewan	**440.1**	**103.3**	1.0
Manitoba	**471.0**	**124.4**	2.3
Ontario	182.3	31.0	3.0
Quebec	173.7	8.3	2.9
New Brunswick	159.2	4.8	0.3
Nova Scotia	191.0	7.7	0.3
Prince Edward Island	124.5	2.2	0.7
Newfoundland and Labrador	99.3	3.6	0.4
Yukon	**669.1**	**46.0**	0.0
Northwest Territories	**1,727.3**	**507.6**	0.0
Nunavut	**3,486.3**	**476.8**	0.0

Source: Rates of Common STIs by Province/Territory: 2007. Public Health Agency of Canada. Reproduced with the permission of the Minister of Health, 2009.

Notes: Rates are per 100,000 population. Bolded numbers indicate rates above national average.

Women Are Hit Hard by STIs

Sexually transmitted infections cause suffering for all who are infected, but in many ways, women and girls are the hardest hit, for both biological and social reasons.

Male-to-female transmission of many infections is more likely to occur than female-to-male transmission. This is particularly true of HIV: Studies show that it is three to eight times easier for a man infected with HIV to transmit the virus to a woman than it is for a woman with HIV to infect a man. Researchers have also found that after one episode of sexual intercourse, a female has a 60%–90% chance of contracting gonorrhea from her infected male partner, whereas the risk of transmission from a woman to a man is 20%–30%.

Young women have been hit especially hard by STIs. A 2007 report from the Public Health Agency of Canada shows that the highest rates of STIs are among Canadian women ages 15–24 (for chlamydia and gonorrhea) and 25–29 (for syphilis). Young women are more vulnerable to STIs than older women because the less mature cervix is more susceptible to injury and infection. As a woman ages, the type of cells at the opening of the cervix gradually changes so that the tissue becomes more resistant to infection. Young women are also more vulnerable for social and emotional reasons: Lack of control in relationships, fear of discussing condom use, and an older sex partner are all linked to increased STI risk.

Once infected, women tend to suffer more consequences of STIs than men. For example, gonorrhea and chlamydia can cause PID and permanent damage to the oviducts in women, but these infections tend to have less serious effects in men. HPV infection causes nearly all cases of cervical cancer. HPV infection is also associated with penile cancer in men, but penile cancer is much less common

than cervical cancer. Women also have the added concern of the potential effects of STIs during pregnancy.

Worldwide, as many women as men now die from AIDS each year, and in the hardest-hit regions of Africa, nearly 60% of adults infected with HIV are women. Before 1994, the proportion of new cases of AIDS in women in Canada was 6.4%; by 2002, it was 16.5%. Women with HIV infection often face tremendous challenges when they are ill because they may be caring for family members who are also infected and ill. In addition, women may become sicker at lower viral loads than men do. Women and men with HIV do about equally well if they have similar access to treatment, but in many cases women are diagnosed later in the course of HIV infection, receive less treatment, and die sooner.

Worldwide, social and economic factors play a large role in the transmission and consequences of AIDS and other STIs for women. Sexual violence against women is spreading AIDS, as are such practices as very early marriage for women, often to much older men who have had many sexual partners. Cultural gender norms that promote premarital and extramarital relationships for men, combined with women's lack of power to negotiate safer sex, make HIV a risk even for women who are married and monogamous. In addition, lack of education and economic opportunities can force women into commercial sex work, placing them at high risk for all STIs.

In some parts of the world, the stigma of AIDS hits women harder. Men with HIV are typically cared for by female family members, without being questioned about the source of their infection. Women, in contrast, may be accused of having had extramarital sex and receive less help and support. It is women who

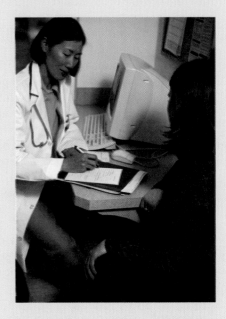

typically provide care to relatives with HIV as well as support the household financially when other earners are too ill to work. But if husbands die, women often do not inherit property and can be thrown deeper into poverty. Solutions to the STI crisis in women must include empowerment in the social sphere in addition to direct health care.

Sources: Dunkle, K. M., et al. 2004. Gender-based violence, relationship power, and risk of HIV infection in women attending antenatal clinics in South Africa. *Lancet* 363(9419): 1415–1421; Health Canada. 2003. *HIV and AIDS in Canada. Surveillance Report to June 30, 2003.* Ottawa: Surveillance and Risk Assessment Division, Centre for Infectious Disease Prevention and Control; Joint United Nations Programme on HIV/AIDS. 2004. *AIDS Epidemic Update, December 2004.* Geneva: UNAIDS; World Health Organization. 2003. *Gender and HIV/AIDS.* Geneva: World Health Organization; Wong, T., et al. 2004. Gender differences in bacterial STIs in Canada. *BMC Women's Health* 4(1 Suppl.): S26 (http://www.biomedcentral.com/1472-6874/4/S1/S26; retrieved March 2, 2010).

gonorrheal infection of the blood or joints. An infant passing through the birth canal of an infected mother may contract **gonococcal conjunctivitis**, an infection in the eyes that can cause blindness if not treated. In Canada, newborn babies are routinely treated with antimicrobial eyedrops to prevent eye infection.

Gonorrhea is caused by the bacterium *Neisseria gonorrhoeae*, which flourishes in mucous membranes. The microbe cannot thrive outside the human body and dies

within moments of exposure to light and air. Consequently, gonorrhea cannot be contracted from toilet seats, towels, or other objects.

Symptoms　In males, the incubation period for gonorrhea is brief, generally two to seven days. The first symptoms are due to urethritis, which causes urinary discomfort and a thick, yellowish-white or yellowish-green discharge from the penis. The lips of the urethral opening may become inflamed and swollen. In some cases, the lymph glands in the groin become enlarged and swollen. Up to half of males have minor symptoms or none at all.

Most females with gonorrhea are asymptomatic. Those who do have symptoms often experience pain with urination, increased vaginal discharge, and severe menstrual cramps. Up to 40% of women with untreated gonorrhea develop PID. Women may also develop painful abscesses in the Bartholin's glands, a pair of glands located on either side of the opening of the vagina.

Gonorrhea can also infect the throat or rectum of people who engage in oral or anal sex. Gonorrhea symptoms in the throat may be a sore throat or pus on the tonsils, and those in the rectum may be pus or blood in the feces or rectal pain and itching.

Diagnosis   Several tests—gram stain, detection of bacterial genes or DNA, or culture—may be performed; depending on the test, samples of urine or cervical, urethral, throat, or rectal fluids may be collected.

Treatment   Gonorrhea can be cured with antibiotics, but increasing drug resistance is a major concern. Today only one class of antibiotics, the cephalosporins, remains consistently effective against gonorrhea. People with gonorrhea often also have chlamydia, so additional antibiotics are typically given to treat chlamydia. Follow-up tests are sometimes performed to make sure the infection has been eradicated. If you have had gonorrhea and have been treated, you can still get the disease again if you have sexual contact with an infected partner.

Pelvic Inflammatory Disease

Pelvic inflammatory disease (PID) is a major complication in 10%–40% of women who have been infected with either gonorrhea or chlamydia and have not received adequate treatment. PID occurs when the initial infection with gonorrhea or chlamydia travels upward, often along with other bacteria, beyond the cervix into the uterus, oviducts, ovaries, and pelvic cavity. PID is often serious enough to require hospitalization and sometimes surgery. Even if the disease is treated successfully, about 25% of affected women will have long-term problems, such as a continuing susceptibility to infection, ectopic pregnancy, infertility, and chronic pelvic pain.

PID is the leading cause of infertility in young women, often going undetected until the inability to become pregnant leads to further evaluation. Infertility occurs in 8% of women after one episode of PID, 20% after two episodes, and 40% after three episodes. The risk of ectopic pregnancy increases significantly in women who have had PID.

Women under age 25 are much more likely to develop PID than are older women. As with all STIs, the more sex partners a woman has had, the greater her risk of PID. Smokers have twice the risk of PID as nonsmokers. Using intrauterine devices (IUDs) for contraception also increases the risk of PID. Research into whether the use of other contraceptives protects against PID has yielded mixed results; oral contraceptive use may reduce the severity of PID symptoms.

Symptoms   Symptoms of PID vary greatly. Some women, especially those with chlamydia, may be asymptomatic; others may feel very ill with abdominal pain, fever, chills, nausea, and vomiting. Early symptoms are essentially the same as those described earlier for chlamydia and gonorrhea. Symptoms often begin or worsen during or soon after a woman's menstrual period. Many women have abnormal vaginal bleeding—either bleeding between periods or heavy and painful menstrual bleeding.

Diagnosis   Diagnosis of PID is made on the basis of symptoms, physical examination, ultrasound, and laboratory tests. Laparoscopy may be used to confirm the diagnosis and obtain material for cultures. Cultures from the rectum or cervix may also be taken to help identify the specific organism. The symptoms of PID, ectopic pregnancy, and appendicitis can be quite similar, so careful evaluation is required to make the correct diagnosis.

Treatment   Starting treatment of PID as quickly as possible is important to minimize damage to the reproductive organs. Antibiotics are usually started immediately; in severe cases, the woman may be hospitalized and antibiotics given intravenously. It is especially important that an infected woman's partners be treated. As many as 60% of the male contacts of women with PID are infected with the bacteria that caused the infection but are asymptomatic.

Syphilis

Syphilis, a disease that once caused death and disability for millions, can now be effectively treated with antibiotics. In 2008, close to 1400 cases of syphilis were reported in Canada. The number of new cases hit an all-time low from 1994 to 2000, but has been on the rise since then. Recent outbreaks of syphilis have been reported in a number of locations across Canada, including Calgary, Edmonton, Vancouver, Winnipeg, Toronto, Ottawa, Montreal, Halifax, and Yukon. In British Columbia, Alberta, and Yukon, Aboriginal people are disproportionately affected by syphilis; although Aboriginal people compose about 4% of the Canadian population, they account for more than 25% of syphilis cases in these locations. A number of factors have contributed to this trend, including a wide array of social and health inequities.

The increase in syphilis has been greatest in gay and bisexual men, prompting health officials to call for increased education in safer sex practices among these groups. Studies have found an association between syphilis infection and the use of the Internet as a means to meet sex partners among men who have sex with men. Another recent trend is an increase in the proportion of cases of syphilis from oral sex. People with syphilis in the mouth may not have symptoms, or they may mistake the sores for another illness. The sores associated with syphilis, regardless of their location, dramatically increase the risk of acquiring HIV or transmitting it to someone else.

Syphilis is caused by a spirochete called *Treponema pallidum*, a thin, corkscrew-shaped bacterium. The disease is usually acquired through sexual contact, although infected pregnant women can transmit it to the fetus. The pathogen passes through any break or opening in the skin or mucous membranes and can be transmitted by kissing, vaginal or anal intercourse, or oral-genital contact. Although easy to treat, syphilis can be difficult to recognize, and if left untreated the disease can cause devastating damage to almost any system of the body.

Symptoms   Syphilis progresses through several stages. *Primary syphilis* is characterized by an ulcer called a **chancre** that appears within 3–90 days after exposure. The chancre is usually found at the site where the organism entered the body, such as the genital area, but it may also appear in other sites, such as the mouth, breasts, or fingers. Chancres contain large numbers of bacteria and make the disease highly contagious when present; they are often painless and typically heal on their own within a few weeks. If the disease is not treated during the primary stage, about a third of infected individuals progress to chronic stages of infections.

Secondary syphilis is usually marked by mild, flulike symptoms and a skin rash that appears three to six weeks after the chancre. The rash may cover the entire body or only a few areas, but the palms of the hands and soles of the feet are usually involved. Areas of skin affected by the rash are highly contagious but usually heal within several weeks or months.

If the disease remains untreated, the symptoms of secondary syphilis may recur over several years; affected individuals may then lapse into an asymptomatic *latent stage* in which they experience no further consequences of infection. However, in about a third of cases of untreated secondary syphilis, the individual develops *tertiary syphilis*. Tertiary syphilis can damage many organs of the body, possibly causing severe dementia, cardiovascular damage, blindness, and death.

In infected pregnant women, the syphilis bacterium can cross the placenta. If the mother is not treated, the probable result is stillbirth, prematurity, or congenital deformity. In many cases, the infant is also born infected (*congenital syphilis*) and requires treatment.

Diagnosis and Treatment   Syphilis is diagnosed by examination of infected tissues and with blood tests. All stages can be treated with antibiotics, but damage from tertiary syphilis can be permanent.

Human Papillomavirus Infection

Human papillomavirus (HPV) infection is estimated to be one of the most common STIs in Canada and around the world (see the box "STIs: A Growing Public Health Concern for All Canadians" on p. 416). HPV infection causes a variety of human diseases, including common warts, **genital warts**, and genital cancers. HPV is the cause of virtually all cervical cancer, but it also causes penile cancer and some forms of anal and oropharyngeal cancers. Genital HPV is usually spread from one person to another through sexual activity, including oral sex.

The Society of Obstetricians and Gynaecologists of Canada (SOGC) estimates that 10%–30% of Canadian adults are infected with HPV. It is also estimated that up to 70% of adults will have at least one HPV infection in their lifetime. Most people infected with HPV have no symptoms at all and are unaware that they are infected and contagious. The good news is that the immune system usually clears the virus, and the infection disappears without any treatment. But in some cases, the infection persists and causes genital warts or cancers.

HPV is especially common in young people, with some of the highest rates of infection among Canadians under the age of 25 (see the box "Postsecondary Students and STIs" on p. 417). Many young women contract HPV infection within three months of becoming sexually active; it is estimated that 2% of sexually active young women have genital warts.

Human papillomaviruses cause many types of human warts. There are more than 100 different strains of HPV, and different strains infect specific locations. More than 30 types are likely to cause genital infections, and five of these are often implicated in cervical cancer; other strains are linked to anal, penile, and other genital cancers. The HPV

pelvic inflammatory disease (PID)   An infection that progresses from the vagina and cervix to the uterus, oviducts, and pelvic cavity.

syphilis   A sexually transmitted bacterial infection caused by the spirochete *Treponema pallidum*.

chancre   The sore produced by syphilis in its earliest stage.

human papillomavirus (HPV)   The pathogen that causes human warts, including genital warts.

genital warts   A sexually transmitted viral infection characterized by growths on the genitals; also called *genital HPV infection* or *condyloma*.

TERMS

STIs: A Growing Public Health Concern for All Canadians

The most recent statistics show that chlamydia, gonorrhea, and syphilis—three nationally reportable STIs—are all on the rise in Canada. Although chlamydia and gonorrhea rates continue to be higher among younger adults, rates of all three STIs have increased dramatically among middle-aged adults (ages 40–59). For example, from 1997 to 2007, cases of gonorrhea among middle-aged Canadians increased by 210%. It is evident that STIs pose a major threat to the health and well-being of all Canadians. STIs are public health challenges for many reasons.

• *STIs are stealth diseases.* Many STIs, including chlamydia, genital herpes, trichomoniasis, HPV, and even early HIV infection often have few, if any, recognizable symptoms. The large number of disease carriers who are unaware of their infection makes these diseases extremely difficult to control. Experts believe that in most cases, HIV is transmitted very early in the disease, before people are aware of the infection. The fact that most people are symptom-free for the first several years of HIV infection highlights the need to frequently test people who are at risk.

• *Viral STIs are persistent and incurable.* Even if detected, most viral STIs—genital herpes, HPV infection, and HIV infec-

tion—are not curable with current therapies. This means that the number of people capable of infecting others continues to grow. The best hope for controlling viral STIs is the development and widespread use of effective vaccines.

• *Screening tests may be underutilized.* Many individuals are unaware of or too embarrassed to request STI screening. Testing more people for STIs could potentially bring STI rates down; it would at least provide an opportunity to counsel people about risky sexual behaviours. Also potentially helpful would be media messages about the benefits and availability of confidential STI screening services.

• *Young people are particularly vulnerable to STIs.* Some of the highest rates and increases in STIs are in Canadians ages 15–24. Young adults are more likely to be ignorant about STIs and safer sex, embarrassed to ask for information, and unaware of how to access appropriate STI testing and treatment services. Many young adults are sexually active by age 25, but young people are more likely to be unmarried, have more than one partner over time, and have a partner who has an STI. Young people need medically accurate information about abstinence, condoms, and other contraceptive methods—and open communication and encourage-

ment from family, friends, and the community to behave responsibly.

Until STIs are controllable with vaccines or effective screening and treatment, the only way to reduce your risk is to limit the number of sexual partners and to use condoms consistently. Those who choose abstinence or a mutually monogamous relationship with one uninfected partner have no risk of STIs.

---

strains that cause most visible genital warts are less likely to cause cancer than some of the other strains. A person can be infected with several different strains.

Genital HPV infection is quite contagious. Condoms and other barrier methods can help prevent the transmission of HPV, but HPV infection frequently occurs in areas where condoms are not fully protective. These areas are the labia in women, the base of the penis and the scrotum in men, and around the anus in both men and women. Still, a three-year study showed that women who always use condoms cut their risk of HPV infection by 70%.

Most people who carry HPV have no visible warts or any other symptoms and are not aware that they are infected and contagious to others. The strains of HPV that are linked with cancer are especially stealthy in that they generally do not cause warts or any obvious signs of their presence.

In 2006, Health Canada approved a vaccine for HPV in females (Gardasil). This vaccination protects against four types of HPV that together account for 90% of genital warts and 70% of cervical cancers; the drug has also been shown

to prevent cancers of the vagina and vulva. The vaccine is not a treatment for girls or women who are infected with HPV and is most effective when given before exposure to genital HPV. Vaccination is available for females ages 9–26. All provinces and territories now offer school-based immunization programs with Gardasil, in which girls (the age range varies depending on the province or territory) are vaccinated against HPV. In 2010, Gardasil was also approved as a vaccination to prevent genital warts in males ages 9–26.

Health Canada has recently approved a second HPV vaccine for females, called Cervarix. This vaccine is designed to offer protection against two specific types of HPV, but not against genital warts. Further research is needed to evaluate the effectiveness of this drug in comparison with Gardasil.

The use of the vaccine for HPV has been limited by political and moral considerations. Many parents have opted not to vaccinate their daughters at least in part because they want their daughters to choose abstinence and fear that giving the vaccine will be viewed as an endorsement for premarital sexual activity. Public health experts generally

Postsecondary Students and STIs

Why Do Postsecondary Students Have High Rates of STIs?

• Risky sexual behaviour is common. One study of university students found that fewer than half used condoms consistently and one-third had had 10 or more sex partners. Another study found that 19% of male students and 33% of female students had consented to sexual intercourse simply because they felt awkward refusing.

• University students underestimate their risk of STIs. Although students may have considerable knowledge about STIs, they often feel the risks do not apply to them—a dangerous assumption. One study of students with a history of STIs showed that more than half had unprotected sex while they were infected, and 25% of them continued to have sex without ever informing their partners.

• Many students are infected but don't know it. A 2006 study of asymptomatic college women revealed that nearly 10% were infected with chlamydia.

What Effect Does Alcohol or Drug Use Have on My Likelihood of Getting an STI?

• Between one-third and one-half of university students report participating in sexual activity as a direct result of being intoxicated. All too often, sexual activity while intoxicated leads to unprotected intercourse.

• Students who binge-drink are more likely to have multiple partners, use condoms inconsistently, and delay seeking treatment for STIs than students who drink little or no alcohol. Sexual assaults occur more frequently when either the perpetrator or the victim has been drinking.

What Can Students Do to Protect Themselves Against STIs?

• Limit the number of sex partners. Even people who are always in a monogamous relationship can end up with extensive potential exposure to STIs if, over the years, they have numerous relationships.

• Use condoms consistently, and don't assume it's safe to stop after you've been with a partner for several months. HIV infection, HPV infection, herpes, and chlamydia can be asymptomatic for months or years and can be transmitted at any time. If you haven't been using condoms with your current partner, start now.

• Enjoy sexuality on your own terms. Don't let the expectations of friends and partners cause you to ignore your own feelings. Let your own wellness be your first priority. If you choose to be sexually active, learn about safer sex practices.

• Get to know your partner, and talk to him or her before becoming intimate. Be honest about yourself, and encourage your partner to do the same. But practise safer sex no matter what.

---

believe that giving the vaccine has little effect on girls' sexual choices and that the vaccine offers the opportunity to prevent the majority of cases of cervical cancer.

Symptoms HPV-infected tissue often appears normal; it may also look like anything from a small bump on the skin to a large, warty growth. Depending on location and size, genital warts are sometimes painful. Untreated warts can grow together to form a cauliflower-like mass. In males, they appear on the penis and often involve the urethra, appearing first at the opening and then spreading inside. The growths may cause irritation and bleeding, leading to painful urination and a urethral discharge. Warts may also appear around the anus or within the rectum. In women, warts may appear on the labia or vulva and may spread to the perineum, the area between the vagina and the rectum. They may also appear on the cervix.

The incubation period ranges from one month to two years from the time of contact. People can be infected with the virus and be capable of transmitting it to their sex partners without having any symptoms at all. The vast majority of people with HPV infection have no visible warts or symptoms of any kind.

Genital warts sometimes grow very large during pregnancy and can occasionally be large enough to make vaginal

delivery difficult. However, most pregnant women with HPV infection can deliver vaginally. HPV infection is infrequently transmitted to an infant during delivery but can occasionally cause warts to form on the infant's vocal cords.

Diagnosis Genital warts are usually diagnosed based on the appearance of the lesions. Sometimes examination with a special magnifying instrument or biopsy is done to evaluate suspicious lesions. HPV infection of the cervix is often detected on routine Pap tests. Special tests are now available to detect the presence of HPV infection and to distinguish among the more common strains of HPV, including those that cause most cases of cervical cancer.

Treatment Treatment of genital HPV infection depends on whether the infection manifests as genital warts or as a cancerous or precancerous condition. Treatment of genital warts focuses on reducing the number and size of warts, although most warts eventually disappear, even without treatment. The currently available treatments do not eradicate HPV infection. Warts may be removed by cryosurgery (freezing), electrocautery (burning), or laser surgery. Direct applications of podophyllin or other cytotoxic acids may be used, and there are treatments that patients can use at home. The success rates of methods vary, and warts often recur despite initial improvement. Warts are more likely to persist and become severe in people with an impaired immune system.

Even after treatment and the disappearance of visible warts, the individual may continue to carry HPV in healthy-looking tissue and can probably still infect others. Anyone who has ever had HPV infection should inform all partners and use condoms, even though they do not provide total protection. Because of the relationship between HPV and cervical cancer, women who have had genital warts should have Pap tests at least every 12 months. Cervical HPV infection associated with precancerous changes is treated by destroying the abnormal tissue with laser, freezing, heat, or other surgical means. Women who have regular screening exams almost never develop full-blown cervical cancer.

Genital Herpes

Because herpes simplex virus (HSV) infection is not a reportable STI in Canada, the annual incidence of **genital herpes** is unknown. We do know, however, that most people with genital herpes do not know they are infected. Worldwide, genital herpes is extremely common and is a major factor in the transmission of HIV. Most people with HIV are also infected with HSV 2, and their herpes lesions contain large amounts of HIV, making it more likely that the virus will be transmitted. The presence of herpes lesions in an HIV-negative person increases the likelihood that she or he will be infected by a partner who is infected with HIV. Genital herpes may also interact with HPV infection to increase the risk of cervical cancer.

Two types of herpes simplex viruses, HSV 1 and HSV 2, cause genital herpes and oral-labial herpes (cold sores). Genital herpes is usually caused by HSV 2, and oral-labial herpes is usually caused by HSV 1, although both virus types can cause either genital or oral-labial lesions. Many people wrongly assume that they are unlikely to pick up an STI if they limit their sexual activity to oral sex, but this is not true, particularly in the case of genital herpes. HSV can also cause rectal lesions, usually transmitted through anal sex. Infection with HSV is generally lifelong; after infection, the virus lies dormant in nerve cells and can reactivate at any time.

HSV 1 infection is so common that an estimated 50% of Canadians have antibodies to HSV 1 (which indicates previous exposure to the virus); most were exposed during childhood. HSV 2 infection usually occurs between the ages of 18 and 25. In Canada, approximately 17% of women of childbearing age have antibodies to HSV 2.

HSV 2 is almost always sexually transmitted. The infection is more easily transmitted when people have active sores, but HSV 2 can be transmitted to a sex partner even when no obvious lesions are present. A recent study of women with HSV 2 showed the presence of the virus in genital secretions more than one-fourth of the time when the women were symptom free. Because new HSV 2 infec-

tions are asymptomatic in about 60% of people, the infection is often acquired from a person who does not know that he or she is infected. If you have ever had an outbreak of genital herpes, you should consider yourself always contagious and inform your partners. Avoid intimate contact when any sores are present, and use condoms during all sexual contact.

Newborns can occasionally be infected with HSV, usually during passage through the birth canal of an infected mother (or through an HSV infection acquired by the mother during the third trimester of pregnancy). Without treatment, 65% of newborns with HSV will die, and most who survive will have some degree of brain damage. The risk of mother-to-child HSV transmission during pregnancy and delivery is low (less than 1%) in women with long-standing herpes infection. New herpes blood tests to screen pregnant women and their sexual partners could substantially reduce neonatal herpes infections. If an uninfected pregnant woman's partner carries HSV, abstinence or the use of condoms could prevent infection during pregnancy.

Pregnant women who have been exposed to genital herpes should inform their health care providers so that appropriate precautions can be taken to protect the baby from infection. These precautions sometimes include a Caesarean section if active lesions are present at the time of delivery.

Symptoms   A large number of people who are infected with HSV have no symptoms. Those that do develop symptoms often first notice them within 2–20 days of having sex with an infected partner. (However, it is not unusual for the first outbreak to occur months or even years after initial exposure.) The first episode of genital herpes frequently causes flulike symptoms in addition to genital lesions. The lesions usually heal within three weeks, but the virus remains alive in an inactive state within nerve cells. A new outbreak of herpes can occur at any time.

On average, newly diagnosed people will experience five to eight outbreaks per year, with a decrease in the frequency of outbreaks over time. Recurrent episodes are usually less severe than the initial one, with fewer and less painful sores that heal more quickly. Outbreaks can be triggered by stress, illness, fatigue, sun exposure, sexual intercourse, and menstruation (see the box "Stress and Genital Herpes").

Diagnosis   Genital herpes is often diagnosed on the basis of symptoms; a sample of fluid from the lesions may also be sent to a laboratory for culture. This test is helpful if the specimen is obtained within about two days of the lesion's development. If the lesion has been around for longer than two days, the culture will often be negative even if the person has genital herpes.

Several blood tests can detect the presence of HSV antibodies. Older tests don't distinguish between HSV 1 and HSV 2. Because HSV 1 infection is extremely common, most people will test positive even if they have not had genital herpes. Newer tests can determine if a person is infected with HSV 1 or HSV 2 and may potentially alert many asymptomatic people to the fact that they are infected. This knowledge

Patients and health care workers alike have long suspected that stress and genital herpes outbreaks are related. Research into this potential link has yielded mixed results. A recent study of women with genital herpes found that persistent stressors (those lasting more than a week) and persistent high levels of anxiety were associated with increased outbreaks. Short-term stress, mood changes, and brief negative life experiences did not influence the rate of herpes outbreaks.

Experts suspect that stress has a negative impact on the immune system. Studies have shown that cell-mediated immune function and antibody levels may drop in response to psychological stress. Perhaps herpes viruses that are usually dormant in nervous system tissue become activated when immune function declines because of stress.

The next step is to investigate whether stress-reduction techniques, such as meditation or exercise, result in reduced rates of herpes outbreaks. Until such research becomes available, it makes sense for people who suffer recurrent genital herpes outbreaks to do what they can to reduce stress, especially long-term stress and anxiety (see Chapter 3).

If you have herpes, joining a support group may help reduce your stress and improve your ability to cope with this chronic disease. If you have several outbreaks a year, or if you have recently had your first episode of genital herpes, talk to your health care provider about suppressive antiviral medication, which can reduce outbreaks substantially. Keep in mind that regardless of stress level, genital herpes outbreaks naturally tend to become less and less frequent over time. Knowing that your outbreaks are likely to diminish can, in and of itself, help reduce your feelings of stress.

---

may help prevent transmission of HSV in couples where one partner is infected and the other is not (particularly important for uninfected women who are pregnant). The more accurate tests for HSV rely on the development of antibodies to the virus, which can take several weeks or months after exposure to the virus. For this reason, doctors often recommend that people wait for 12–16 weeks after possible exposure before having a blood test.

Anyone who has any STI should also be tested for HIV, but this is especially true for people who have HSV 2. Recent studies suggest that adults who are infected with HSV 2 are 15 times as likely as those without HSV 2 to be infected with HIV.

Treatment There is no cure for herpes. Once infected, a person carries the virus for life. Antiviral drugs, such as acyclovir, can be taken at the beginning of an outbreak to shorten the severity and duration of symptoms. People who have frequent outbreaks can take acyclovir or similar drugs daily to suppress outbreaks and decrease viral shedding between outbreaks. Anyone diagnosed with a first episode of genital herpes should talk with a health care provider about suppressive treatment.

A person on suppressive therapy can still transmit HSV to an uninfected partner, but the risk is probably reduced by about half. Using condoms consistently and taking suppressive medication is a reasonable way to reduce the risk of passing herpes to an uninfected sexual partner. It is always important to inform a sexual partner if you have genital herpes.

A herpes vaccine is currently undergoing testing, but results to date have been frustrating because the vaccine appears to be effective only for women who have not been exposed to HSV 1 or 2, and it is ineffective for men. Several microbicides are under development that may someday be available to help stop the transmission of HSV.

HIV Infection and AIDS

The **human immunodeficiency virus (HIV)** causes **acquired immune deficiency syndrome (AIDS)**, a disease that ultimately kills most of its victims, especially in parts of the world where adequate treatment is not available. AIDS originated in Africa sometime during the early twentieth century but was not recognized or named until 1981. The disease spread rapidly throughout the world and is now a leading cause of death globally.

An estimated 65 million people have been infected since the epidemic began—nearly 1% of the world's population—and tens of millions of those people have died (see the box "HIV/AIDS Around the World" on p. 420). Currently, about 33 million people are infected with HIV/AIDS worldwide (Table 13.3 on p. 420), and most of these people will die within the next 10 years.

For the first time in the history of the AIDS epidemic, the number of people worldwide that are living with HIV infection has begun to level off. Many experts believe that the global HIV epidemic peaked in the late 1990s, at about 3 million new infections per year, compared with an estimated 2.6 million new infections in 2009. Despite a slowing of the epidemic, however, AIDS remains the primary cause of death in Africa and continues to be a major cause of mortality around the world.

genital herpes A sexually transmitted infection caused by the herpes simplex virus.

human immunodeficiency virus (HIV) The virus that causes HIV infection and AIDS.

acquired immune deficiency syndrome (AIDS) A generally fatal, incurable, sexually transmitted viral infection.

TERMS

HIV/AIDS Around the World

In 2006, the world marked the 25th year since AIDS, a previously unknown disease, was diagnosed in five young gay men in Los Angeles. We now know that HIV originated in Africa about five decades earlier. HIV is now a worldwide scourge (see Figure 13.1), with approximately 65 million people infected and 25 million deaths since the epidemic began. Because of the many promising developments and efforts to address the epidemic, experts have suggested that the world has turned the corner in the fight against HIV. Worldwide, there has been a 19% decrease in new HIV infections since 1999, the year in which it is believed the HIV epidemic peaked.

The vast majority of HIV cases occur in developing countries, where heterosexual contact is the primary means of transmission and is responsible for 85% of all adult infections. In the developed world, HIV is increasingly becoming an infection that disproportionately affects the poor and ethnic minorities. Worldwide, women are the fastest-growing group of newly infected people; approximately half of adults living with HIV in 2009 were women. In addition, an estimated 2.5 million children are living with HIV infection and about 12 million children are AIDS orphans.

Sub-Saharan Africa remains the hardest hit of all areas of the world. Two-thirds of all adults and children with HIV live in this region, and close to three-quarters of all deaths from AIDS in 2009 occurred here. However, because the epidemic started about 10 years later in Asia than in Africa, experts expect an explosion of new cases in Asia. And because Asia accounts for more than 50% of the world's population, the pool of people at risk is much larger than in Africa. HIV is also spreading rapidly in Eastern Europe, and former Soviet countries have seen a fiftyfold increase in HIV infection in the last decade.

Globally, an increasing number of people living with HIV/AIDS have access to treatment, which has resulted in fewer AIDS-related deaths. However, efforts to combat HIV/AIDS are still complicated by political, economic, and cultural barriers.

Education and prevention programs are often hampered by resistance from social and religious institutions and by the taboo on openly discussing sexual issues. Condoms are not commonly used in many countries, and women in many societies do not have sufficient control over their lives to demand that men use condoms during sex. Prevention approaches that have had success include STI treatment and education, public education campaigns about safer sex, and syringe exchange programs for injection drug users.

In countries with a substantial imbalance in the social power of men and women, empowering women is a crucial priority in reducing the spread of HIV. In particular, reducing sexual violence against women, allowing women property and inheritance rights, and increasing women's access to education and employment are essential.

International efforts are under way to make condoms more available by lowering their price and to develop effective antiviral creams that women can use without the knowledge of their partners. Other potential strategies for fighting the spread of HIV include the widespread use of drugs to suppress genital herpes simplex, an extremely common STI that can dramatically increase transmission of HIV. Also, the practice of male circumcision might be useful in reducing the spread of HIV (and chlamydia, discussed earlier in this chapter). Recent research has shown a 60% reduction in HIV transmission among circumcised men compared with uncircumcised men, even when controlling for other factors.

In developed nations, such as Canada, new drugs are easing AIDS symptoms and lowering viral levels dramatically for some patients. In the past few years, a small but growing number of people in poor countries have gained access to antiviral drugs because of the introduction of inexpensive generic drugs and increasing international funding for HIV treatment. Still, the vast majority of people with HIV remain untreated.

Table 13.3	HIV/AIDS Global Summary, 2009
People Living with HIV	
Adults	30.8 million
Adult women	15.9 million
Children (<15 years old)	2.5 million
Total	33.3 million
People Newly Infected with HIV	
Adults	2.2 million
Children (<15 years old)	370,000
Total	2.6 million
AIDS Deaths	
Adults	1.6 million
Children (<15 years old)	260,000
Total	1.8 million

Source: Data from Joint United Nations Programme on HIV/AIDS (UNAIDS). 2010. *Global Report: UNAIDS Report on the Global AIDS Epidemic 2010.* Geneva: Joint United Nationals Programme on HIV/AIDS (UNAIDS) (http://www.unaids.org/en/media/unaids/contentassets/documents/unaidspublication/2010/20101123_globalreport_en.pdf and http://www.unaids.org/documents/20101123_epislides_core_en.pdf; retrieved April 25, 2011). Copyright © 2010 Joint United Nations Programme on HIV/AIDS (UNAIDS). All rights reserved.

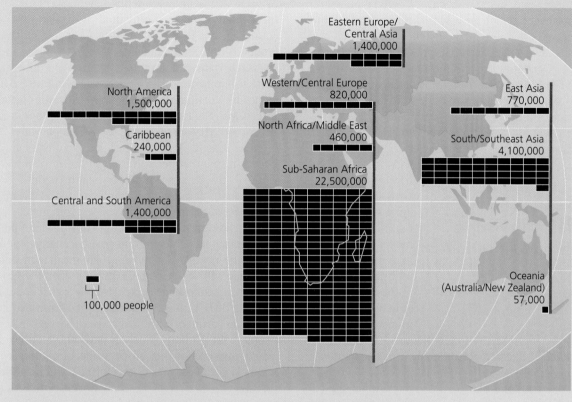

FIGURE 13.1 Approximate number of adults and children living with HIV in 2009.

Source: Data from Joint United Nations Programme on HIV/AIDS (UNAIDS). 2010. *Global Report: UNAIDS Report on the Global AIDS Epidemic 2010.* Geneva: Joint United Nationals Programme on HIV/AIDS (UNAIDS) (http://www.unaids.org/en/media/unaids/contentassets/documents/unaidspublication/2010/20101123_globalreport_en.pdf; retrieved April 25, 2011). Copyright © 2010 Joint United Nations Programme on HIV/AIDS (UNAIDS). All rights reserved.

Since 1985 (when HIV reporting began in Canada), more than 69,000 positive HIV tests have been reported. In Canada, the first death attributed to AIDS occurred in 1983; since then, approximately 21,000 Canadians have died from HIV or AIDS. In 2009, 2417 new HIV infections were reported, a decrease of 8.3% from the number of positive cases in Canada in 2008. But the number of Canadians living with HIV infection continues to rise; today, it is estimated that about 30% of HIV-infected Canadians are unaware of their condition.

HIV is thought to be a relatively new infection in humans. In 1998, researchers discovered a group of wild chimpanzees in west equatorial Africa that carry simian immunodeficiency virus (SIV), a virus very similar to the pandemic strain of HIV seen around the world in humans. Genetic evidence shows that SIV first spread from chimpanzees to humans in the 1930s, when the trapping and butchering of chimpanzees was common. SIV is fairly benign in chimps,

but when it made the jump to humans, it became more virulent and deadly. Poverty, the harsh environment, crowded living conditions, and unsound vaccination practices contributed to the disease's spread through local populations. Eventually, global travel allowed the disease to spread to the rest of the world.

What Is HIV/AIDS? **HIV infection** is a chronic disease that progressively damages the body's immune system, making an otherwise healthy person less able to resist a variety of infections and disorders. Normally, when a virus or other pathogen enters the body, it is targeted and destroyed

HIV infection A chronic, progressive viral infection that damages the immune system.

by the immune system. But HIV attacks the immune system itself, invading and taking over **CD4 T cells**, monocytes, and macrophages, which are essential elements of the immune system (Chapter 9). HIV enters a human cell and converts its own genetic material, RNA, into DNA. It then inserts this DNA into the chromosomes of the host cell. The viral DNA takes over the CD4 cell, causing it to produce new copies of HIV; it also makes the CD4 cell incapable of performing its immune functions.

Immediately following infection with HIV, billions of infectious particles are produced every day. For a time, the immune system keeps pace, also producing billions of new cells. Unlike the virus, however, the immune system cannot make new cells indefinitely; as long as the virus keeps replicating, it wins in the end. The destruction of the immune system is signalled by the loss of CD4 T cells (Figure 13.2). As CD4 cells decline, an infected person may begin to experience mild to moderately severe symptoms. In Canada, a person is diagnosed with full-blown AIDS when he or she (1)

receives a positive test result for HIV and (2) develops one or more of the illnesses defined as markers for AIDS. In the United States, an individual must also have a CD4 count that it is less than 200 cells per cubic millimetre of blood (200/μL) to be diagnosed with AIDS; this indicates a severely damaged immune system. AIDS represents the most severe form of HIV infection. People with AIDS are vulnerable to a number of serious **opportunistic (secondary) infections**. The infections that most often prove deadly for people with HIV are seldom serious in people with a healthy immune system. Opportunistic infections are usually caused by organisms that are common in the environment and generally do not cause illness in healthy people.

The first weeks after being infected with HIV are called the *primary/acute infection* phase. Most, but not all, infected people develop flulike symptoms during this time. During primary HIV infection, people have large amounts of HIV in the bloodstream, making them much more infectious than they will be several months later when they enter the chronic infection stages. Experts believe that about half of all cases of HIV infection are acquired from people who are in the primary infection stage. The vast majority of people with primary infection have no idea they are infected, and even if they suspect infection and get tested, the most commonly used tests for HIV will be negative in this stage. Special tests can detect primary infection, and

During the initial acute illness, CD4 levels fall sharply and HIV RNA levels increase; 60%–90% of infected people experience flulike symptoms during this period. Antibodies to HIV usually appear 2–12 weeks after the initial infection. During the asymptomatic phase that follows, CD4 levels gradually decline, and HIV RNA levels again increase. Because of declines in immunity, infected individuals eventually begin to experience symptoms; when CD4 levels drop very low, people become vulnerable to serious opportunistic infections characteristic of full-blown AIDS. Chronic or recurrent illnesses continue until the immune system fails and death results.

FIGURE 13.2 The general pattern of untreated HIV infection. The blue line represents the number of CD4 cells in the blood, a marker for the status of the immune system. The orange line shows the amount of HIV RNA in the blood.

Source: Adapted from A. S. Fauci and Giuseppe Pantaleo, 1996, "Immunopathogenic Mechanisms of HIV infection," *Annals of Internal Medicine* 124(7), 654–663, Figure 1. Reprinted with permission of the American College of Physicians.

experts believe that improved detection of primary infection could help reduce the spread of the virus.

The next phase of HIV infection is the *chronic **asymptomatic*** (symptom-free) stage. This period can last from 2–20 years, with an average of 11 years in untreated adults. During this time the virus progressively infects and destroys the cells of the immune system. People infected with HIV can transmit the infection to others, even if they are symptom free. Even if they receive treatment, they remain infectious to varying degrees throughout their lives.

The final phase of HIV infection before an individual may or may not progress from HIV to AIDS is the *chronic symptomatic stage*. This phase is characterized by a further depletion of CD4 cells and a severely damaged immune system. Loss of vision, unexplained fever, and encephalopathy are just a few of the many possible signs and symptoms of the chronic symptomatic stage of HIV infection.

Transmitting the Virus HIV lives only within cells and body fluids, not outside the body. It is transmitted by blood and blood products, semen, vaginal and cervical secretions, and breast milk. It cannot live in air, in water, or on objects or surfaces, such as toilet seats, eating utensils, or telephones. The three main routes of HIV transmission are from (1) specific kinds of sexual contact, (2) direct exposure to infected blood, and (3) an HIV-infected woman to her fetus during pregnancy or childbirth or to her infant during breastfeeding.

SEXUAL CONTACT HIV is more likely to be transmitted by unprotected anal or vaginal intercourse than by other sexual activities. During vaginal intercourse, male-to-female transmission is more likely to occur than female-to-male transmission. HIV has been found in preejaculatory fluid, so transmission can occur before ejaculation. Being the receptive partner during unprotected anal intercourse is the riskiest of all sexual activities. Oral-genital contact carries some risk of transmission, although less than anal or vaginal intercourse. HIV can be transmitted through tiny tears, traumatized points, or irritated areas in the lining of the vagina, cervix, penis, anus, mouth, and throat and through direct infection of cells in these areas. Sexual assault is an important factor in the transmission of HIV both in Canada and throughout the world. Protection is almost never used during sexual assault, and tissue trauma is generally greater than in unforced sexual activity.

The presence of lesions, blisters, or inflammation from other STIs in the genital, anal, or oral areas makes it two to nine times easier for the virus to be passed. Spermicides may also cause irritation and increase the risk of HIV transmission. Recent studies of the widely used spermicide nonoxynol-9 (N-9) found that frequent use may cause vaginal and rectal irritation, increasing the risk of transmission of HIV and other STIs. The World Health Organization (WHO) recommends that spermicides containing N-9 not be used for protection against HIV and STIs. Condoms or lubricants with N-9 should never be used during anal intercourse because N-9 damages the lining of the rectum, providing an entry point for HIV and other STIs.

The risk of HIV transmission during oral sex increases if a person has poor oral hygiene, has oral sores, or has brushed or flossed just before or after oral sex. Some evidence suggests that recent consumption of alcohol may make the cells that line the mouth more susceptible to infection with HIV.

Studies in developing nations with high rates of HIV infection have found that circumcised males have a lower risk of HIV infection than uncircumcised males. A study in South Africa showed a 60% reduction in new infections among men who were circumcised as part of the study, and another study in Kenya and Uganda showed an approximate halving of risk among men who were circumcised. Circumcision is uncommon in most parts of the world, but these findings are heightening interest in the practice. In Canada, where circumcision is fairly common and HIV infection rates are much lower, circumcision does not appear to offer any significant protection against HIV.

DIRECT CONTACT WITH INFECTED BLOOD Direct contact with the blood of an infected person is another major route of HIV transmission. Needles used to inject drugs (including heroin, cocaine, and anabolic steroids) are routinely contaminated by the blood of the user. If needles are shared, small amounts of one person's blood are directly injected into another person's bloodstream. HIV may be transmitted through subcutaneous and intramuscular injection as well, from needles or blades used in acupuncture, tattooing, ritual scarring, and piercing of the earlobes, nose, lip, nipple, navel, or other body part.

In 2009, 21.6% of all new Canadian cases of HIV were caused, directly or indirectly, by sharing drug injection equipment contaminated with HIV. Drug users, their sex partners, and their children are all at extremely high risk for HIV infection. Most experts agree that syringe exchange programs combined with increased substance abuse treatment and prevention could significantly reduce the spread of HIV. One example of such a program is Insite, North America's first legal and medically supervised drug injection facility. Insite opened in Vancouver, British Columbia, in 2003 and has been described as a safe and sterile "health-focused place" where individuals do not have to abstain from drug use. Insite clients can inject pre-obtained illicit drugs under the supervision of nurses, and they also have access to a wide range of community resources and services,

---

CD4 T cell A type of white blood cell that helps coordinate the activity of the immune system; the primary target for HIV infection; a decrease in the number of these cells correlates with the risk and severity of HIV-related illness.

opportunistic (secondary) infection An infection caused when organisms take the opportunity presented by a primary (initial) infection to multiply and cause a new, different infection.

asymptomatic Showing no signs or symptoms of a disease.

such as addiction counselling and treatment. A considerable number of research studies have reported that Insite is associated with several positive and important outcomes for its clients and the surrounding community, including lower levels of public injecting; reduced HIV-risk behaviours, such as syringe sharing; and greater enrolment in addiction treatment services among the facility's users.

HIV has also been transmitted in blood and blood products used in the medical treatment of injuries and illnesses. In Canada, blood donors have been screened for HIV infection since 1985. Since then, the estimated risk of infection through blood transfusion has been reduced substantially, from about 1 in 16,000 units of blood in 1985 to 1 in more than 1 million units of blood currently. Unfortunately, the blood supply is much less safe in the rest of the world. In the developing world in particular, blood is often not adequately tested and blood donors are not always appropriately screened. In these countries, the risk of contracting HIV or another serious infection from a blood transfusion is very high. The WHO estimates that about 5% of all cases of HIV infection worldwide have resulted from the transfusion of infected blood and blood products.

A small number of health care workers have acquired HIV on the job; most of these cases involve needle sticks, in which a health care worker is accidentally stuck with a needle used on an infected patient. The likelihood of a patient acquiring HIV infection from a health care worker is almost negligible; the risk to health care workers from infected patients is much greater.

What about contact with other body fluids? Trace amounts of HIV have been found in the saliva and tears of some infected people. However, researchers believe that these fluids do not carry enough of the virus to infect another person. (In the rare cases of HIV infection linked to deep kissing or biting, the virus is thought to have been transmitted in blood from oral sores rather than in saliva.) Contact with the urine or feces of an infected person may carry some risk, but contact with sweat is not believed to carry any risk. There is no evidence that HIV can be spread by insects, such as mosquitoes.

MOTHER-TO-CHILD TRANSMISSION The final major route of HIV transmission is mother-to-child, also called *vertical*, or *perinatal, transmission*, which can occur during pregnancy, childbirth, or breastfeeding. About one in four infants born to untreated HIV-infected mothers is also infected with the virus; testing and treatment can reduce this infection rate to as low as 1% or 1 in 100 infants. Worldwide, about two-thirds of vertical transmission occurs during pregnancy and childbirth and one-third through breastfeeding.

HIV-infected children rarely appear ill at birth, but they begin to develop health problems over the first months and years of life. About 20% of infected children become very ill and progress to AIDS or death by age four; the remaining 80% develop problems more slowly. In many developed countries, new treatments to reduce vertical transmission are in use, and in Canada, the use of these treatments by pregnant women with HIV infection is increasing.

NOT THROUGH CASUAL CONTACT A person is not at risk of getting HIV infection by being in the same classroom, dining room, or even household with someone who is infected. Before this was generally known, many people with HIV infection, including children, were the targets of ostracism, hysteria, and outright violence. Today, it is an acknowledged responsibility of everyone to treat people with HIV infection with respect and compassion, regardless of their age or how they became infected.

Populations of Special Concern for HIV Infection

Among Canadians with AIDS, the most common means of HIV exposure is sexual activity between men; heterosexual contact and injection drug use (IDU) are the next most common (Figure 13.3). Although HIV transmission occurs through specific individual behaviours, disproportionately high rates of infection in certain groups are tied to social, cultural, and economic factors. HIV in Canada is increasingly becoming a disease that affects ethnic minorities, women, and poor people. Women, especially Aboriginal women, make up an increasingly large proportion of all Canadian AIDS cases. In 2006, the Public Health Agency

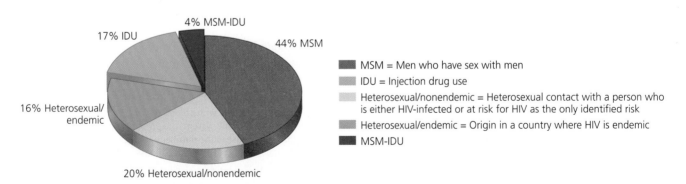

FIGURE 13.3 Routes of HIV transmission among Canadians.

Source: Estimated Prevalence by Transmission Category, 2008 Chart. *HIV/AIDS Epi Updates 2007.* Public Health Agency of Canada. Reproduced with the permission of the Minister of Health, 2008.

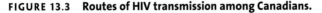

of Canada estimated that approximately 28% of Canadians infected with HIV were women. Overall, Aboriginal people made up almost one-quarter of the reported AIDS cases, with half the cases occurring in Aboriginal women. See the box "HIV/AIDS: Canada's At-Risk Populations" on p. 426 for more on these trends.

Another group of people at increased risk for HIV infection are young men who have sex with men. HIV infection has increased in recent years among this group, primarily because more young men are engaging in unsafe sexual practices, such as unprotected anal intercourse. There are probably several factors underlying this trend. Young gay men are less likely than older men to have seen friends die from AIDS and thus are more removed from the reality of the disease. They may be less afraid of acquiring HIV because of advances in treatment and a false belief that a cure is just around the corner. Drug use, especially use of crystal methamphetamine or club drugs, and the practice of meeting sex partners over the Internet are also associated with increased rates of unsafe sex and HIV infection among men who have sex with men.

There also appears to be a growing number of cases among men who acquire HIV through sex with other men but who do not identify themselves as gay. Some men who have sex with men also have sex with women, and they identify themselves as heterosexual, not as gay or bisexual. Men who have sex with men and still identify themselves as heterosexual are just as likely to be infected with HIV as are gay and bisexual men who are out, but they are much less likely to know their HIV status and so may be more likely to transmit HIV to a male or female partner. Public health efforts directed toward gay men may not reach men in this group, and negative cultural attitudes toward same-sex attraction may make it difficult for gay and bisexual men to be honest with their partners. This trend endangers not only the men but also their partners, both male and female.

These patterns of HIV infection reflect complex social, economic, and behavioural factors. Reducing the rates of HIV transmission and AIDS death in minorities, women, and other groups at risk will require dealing with the difficult problems of drug abuse, poverty, and discrimination. HIV prevention programs must be tailored to meet the special needs of minority communities.

Increased testing is one of the most important aspects of HIV prevention, but knowledge of HIV status may not be enough to change behaviour. Studies show that up to one-third of people who have been diagnosed with HIV continue to have unprotected sex. Testing must be coupled with strategies not only to encourage individuals with HIV to take the steps necessary to avoid infecting others but also to encourage all individuals to consistently practise safer sex.

Symptoms of HIV Infection

Within a few days or weeks of infection with HIV, some people will develop symptoms of primary/acute HIV infection. These can include fever, fatigue, rashes, headache, swollen lymph nodes, body aches, night sweats, sore throat, nausea, and diarrhea. Because the symptoms of primary HIV infection are similar to those of many common viral illnesses, the condition often goes undiagnosed, even if an infected individual sees a physician.

Diagnosis of HIV at this very early stage of infection, although uncommon, is extremely beneficial. Immediate treatment is sometimes given to help preserve immune function, slow the progress of the disease, and reduce transmission of HIV to others. It is critical for people who have engaged in behaviour that places them at risk for HIV infection and who then experience symptoms of primary HIV infection to immediately inform their physician of their risk status.

Other than the initial flulike symptoms associated with primary/acute HIV infection, most people in the first months or years of HIV infection have few if any symptoms. As the immune system weakens, however, a variety of symptoms can develop: persistent swollen lymph nodes; lumps, rashes, sores, or other growths on or under the skin or on the mucous membranes of the eyes, mouth, anus, or nasal passages; persistent yeast infections; unexplained weight loss; fever and drenching night sweats; dry cough and shortness of breath; persistent diarrhea; easy bruising and unexplained bleeding; profound fatigue; memory loss; difficulty with balance; tremors or seizures; changes in vision, hearing, taste, or smell; difficulty in swallowing; changes in mood and other psychological symptoms; and persistent or recurrent pain. Obviously, many of these symptoms can also occur with a variety of other illnesses. Because the immune system is weakened, people with HIV infection are also highly susceptible to a number of opportunistic infections, both common and uncommon.

Diagnosing HIV Infection

The most common HIV tests check for antibodies to the virus. HIV infection primarily disrupts T-cell immunity; B cells are still able to produce antibodies to HIV, which show up in tests. These antibodies, however, do not protect against the spread of the virus. For most other diseases, the presence of an antibody to a particular pathogen may indicate protective immunity. In the case of HIV, however, the presence of the antibody indicates an active case of the disease. **HIV antibody tests** are used because they are accurate and relatively inexpensive (see the box "Getting an HIV Test" on p. 429).

HIV antibody test   A blood test to determine whether a person has been infected by HIV; becomes positive within weeks or months of exposure.

TERMS

HIV/AIDS: Canada's At-Risk Populations

HIV does not discriminate; it affects males and females of all ages, religions, education and income levels, and ethnicities. However, the reality is that in Canada, specific populations are disproportionately affected by HIV and AIDS.

• *Aboriginal peoples.* Individuals who identify themselves as Aboriginal (including First Nations, Inuit, and Metis) represent a growing percentage of reported HIV-positive and AIDS cases in Canada (see Figure 13.4). Injection drug use is a primary mode of HIV transmission in the Aboriginal community. Aboriginal peoples also test positive for HIV at a younger age than non-Aboriginals.

• *Canadians of African ancestry.* Black Canadians make up a growing percentage of positive HIV reports and reported AIDS cases (see Figure 13.4). Heterosexual exposure accounts for more than 80% of positive HIV test reports in Canadians of African ancestry. About half of the positive HIV test reports in this group are in women.

• *Injection drug users (IDU) and men who have sex with men (MSM).* As was shown in Figure 13.3, men who have sex with men represent the largest category of positive HIV test reports in Canada. Interestingly, although injection drug use represents a large exposure category in Canada, the number of HIV infections in this group appears to be decreasing. The overall heterosexual exposure category (including individuals from HIV-endemic and nonendemic countries) now represents a growing number of positive HIV tests, surpassing injection drug use as the second-largest exposure category.

• *Prison inmates.* Rates of HIV infection in Canadian prisons appear to be considerably higher than in the general population. In federal prisons, the prevalence of HIV among women is higher than among men. It is probable that some offenders

FIGURE 13.4   Distribution of positive HIV test reports in Canada, by ethnic status.

Note: Ethnic status is available only for provinces and territories that submitted ethnicity data (Ontario, Quebec, and the Northwest Territories did not).

Source: HIV and AIDS in Canada: Surveillance Report to December 31, 2008. Public Health Agency of Canada. Reproduced with the permission of the Minister of Health, 2008.

infected with HIV engaged in risky behaviours before going to prison; however, some inmates also engage in high-risk behaviours while in prison, including needle-sharing, tattooing, and unprotected sex. The potential for HIV transmission is great in penitentiaries, with possible infection of spouses and partners once inmates are released.

Not everyone with HIV infection will test positive on antibody tests. Antibodies may not appear in the blood for weeks or months after infection, so people who are newly infected are likely to have a negative antibody test. If an individual is tested during this window and the result is negative, he or she will have to be retested later to confirm a negative diagnosis.

If a person is diagnosed as **HIV positive**, the next step is to determine the disease's severity to plan appropriate treatment. The immune system's status can be gauged by measuring CD4 T cells every few months. The infection itself can be monitored by tracking the viral load (the amount of virus in the body); this helps physicians evaluate the effects of treatment and can also help predict the likelihood of long-term survival in a person infected with HIV.

Many people are not aware that rapid HIV tests are now available in Canada. These tests must be performed by a health care professional in a setting where HIV counselling is available. Results are typically obtained within 15 minutes. Whereas a negative test result is considered accurate (and no further testing is necessary), an initially positive (or

"initially reactive") test result requires another test at an approved HIV-testing laboratory for confirmation.

The Public Health Agency of Canada recommends that anyone who engages in risky behaviour should be tested (refer to the box "Getting an HIV Test" on p. 429 for a list of risky behaviours). Since it takes the body three to six months to produce enough HIV antibodies to be detectable by a blood test, individuals should get tested approximately three months after the last time they engaged in such behaviour(s). In the meantime, it is important for individuals to practise safer sex (or to abstain) and to not share needles or other injecting equipment. It should be noted that being tested once is not enough. Periodic routine testing is the best way for anyone to find out if he or she has HIV, and early detection is important to minimize the disease's effects and reduce the risks to others.

Reporting   In Canada, all diagnosed cases of HIV or AIDS must be reported to public health authorities. In addition, the patient (or a health care professional) must notify all of his or her sexual partners and other contacts that may

- *Youth.* Approximately one-quarter of the positive HIV cases in 2006 were among youth ages 20–29. In comparison with other age groups, the proportion of HIV tests attributed to females is highest among youth, with approximately 41% of positive test reports being for females ages 15–29.

- *Women.* Women represent an increasing proportion of reported HIV and AIDS cases in Canada. Approximately 28% of the positive HIV test reports in 2006 were in women, compared with less than 10% before 1995. Heterosexual exposure and injection drug use are the two main risk behaviours for HIV infection in women.

- *People from countries where HIV is endemic.* In 2006, about 8% of new HIV test reports were among individuals who were from countries where HIV is endemic. Women from countries were HIV is endemic represented more than half of the HIV-positive test reports and approximately 42% of the AIDS cases in this category between 1998 and 2006.

New approaches to prevention and treatment will likely be needed to combat the high incidence of HIV/AIDS among the populations discussed above. HIV prevention messages need to communicate effectively with the populations most at risk. Programs stressing ethnic and gender pride have been effective for some groups. For those who are already HIV positive, other resources, such as peer networks, legal assistance, and on-site child care at clinics, may help improve treatment access and success.

In January 2005, the Government of Canada launched the Federal Initiative to Address HIV/AIDS in Canada, a joint initiative of the Public Health Agency of Canada, Health Canada, the Canadian Institutes of Health Research, and Correctional Service Canada. In addition to increased HIV/AIDS funding and several other areas of action, this initiative focuses on some of the populations discussed above. The use of population-specific approaches is considered essential to developing culturally appropriate strategies that can address the factors that contribute to infection in these at-risk groups.

Some of the factors contributing to disparities in HIV incidence include the following:

- *Poverty, drug use, and associated problems:* Low income is linked to lack of information about safer sex and HIV testing and treatment, higher rates of injection drug use, and limited access to health care. Women who are poor and unemployed are more likely to be financially dependent on a male partner and less likely to use condoms; they are more likely to trade sex for money or drugs. Higher rates of incarceration among members of some minority groups also contribute to the spread of HIV.

- *Social, economic, and behavioural factors:* Poverty, substance use, previous and current sexually transmitted infections, and limited access to health services all contribute to an increase in vulnerability to HIV infection in certain at-risk populations in Canada.

- *Social patterns and perception of risk:* High prevalence of infection in a group, combined with a low perception of risk, contributes to the spread of HIV as people are more likely to encounter an infected sex partner if they choose partners from a group with a high prevalence.

Sources: Health Canada. 2007. *Health Concerns: Federal Initiative to Address HIV/AIDS in Canada* (http://www.hc-sc.gc.ca/hc-ps/dc-ma/int_aids-sida_fed-eng.php; retrieved February 24, 2010); Public Health Agency of Canada. 2007. *Populations at Risk—Federal Initiative to Address HIV/AIDS in Canada* (http://www.phac-aspc.gc.ca/aids-sida/populations-eng.php; retrieved February 21, 2010); Public Health Agency of Canada. 2008. *Canadian Guidelines on Sexually Transmitted Infections* (http://www.phac-aspc.gc.ca/std-mts/sti-its/index-eng.php; retrieved February 10, 2010).

have been exposed in the past. Partner notification is a prevention process through which at-risk individuals are identified, located, assessed, and treated if necessary.

Tracking the Canadian HIV epidemic has been particularly difficult for several reasons. Before 2003, HIV infection was not reported in all provinces and territories. All positive HIV test reports and AIDS cases now are legally reportable everywhere in Canada. Despite efforts to safeguard confidentiality and prohibit discrimination, mandatory reporting of HIV infection remains controversial. If people believe they are risking their jobs, friends, or social acceptability, they may be less likely to be tested. At the same time, it is essential that enough information be disclosed to monitor the epidemic. Although anonymous testing may encourage more people to get tested for HIV, it is not available in all provinces and territories.

Treatment Although HIV infection has no cure yet, medications can significantly alter the course of the disease and extend life. The drop in the number of deaths in Canada from AIDS since 1996 is in large part due to the increasing use of combinations of new drugs. However, this progress is irrelevant to the vast majority of people with AIDS worldwide, who can't afford treatment.

ANTIVIRAL DRUGS Antiviral drugs in current use to combat HIV fall into several categories based on how they block HIV replication. HIV uses the enzyme reverse transcriptase to integrate its genetic material into human cells. Drugs that inhibit this process (see Figure 13.5 on p. 428) were the first approved for treatment of HIV.

Having many drugs that work against HIV in different stages of its life cycle is crucial to keeping the virus at bay. HIV is an incredibly agile virus that constantly changes, mutates, and adapts to its environment. The virus can easily become resistant to any given drug, but when an HIV-

HIV positive A diagnosis resulting from the presence of HIV in the bloodstream; also referred to as *seropositive*.

TERMS

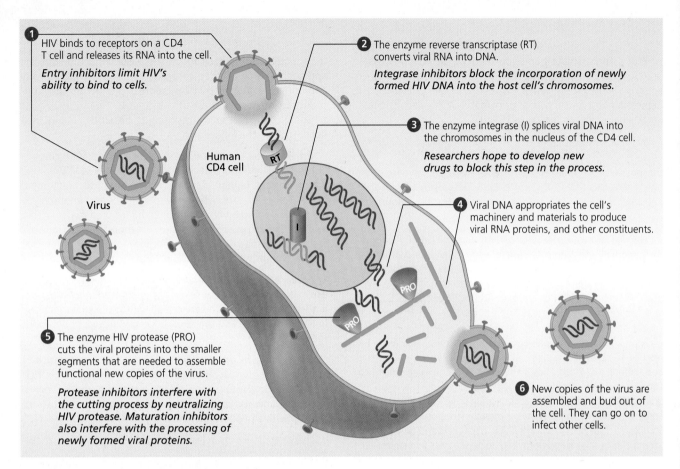

The life cycle of HIV: How antiviral drugs work.

① HIV binds to receptors on a CD4 T cell and releases its RNA into the cell.

Entry inhibitors limit HIV's ability to bind to cells.

Virus

Human CD4 cell

② The enzyme reverse transcriptase (RT) converts viral RNA into DNA.

Integrase inhibitors block the incorporation of newly formed HIV DNA into the host cell's chromosomes.

③ The enzyme integrase (I) splices viral DNA into the chromosomes in the nucleus of the CD4 cell.

Researchers hope to develop new drugs to block this step in the process.

④ Viral DNA appropriates the cell's machinery and materials to produce viral RNA proteins, and other constituents.

⑤ The enzyme HIV protease (PRO) cuts the viral proteins into the smaller segments that are needed to assemble functional new copies of the virus.

Protease inhibitors interfere with the cutting process by neutralizing HIV protease. Maturation inhibitors also interfere with the processing of newly formed viral proteins.

⑥ New copies of the virus are assembled and bud out of the cell. They can go on to infect other cells.

FIGURE 13.5 **The life cycle of HIV: How antiviral drugs work.** Different classes of drugs block the replication of HIV at different points in the virus's life cycle.

Sources: A virus in action. 2001. *Scientific American*, November; Dickinson, G., et al. 1998. The latest recommendations for antiretroviral therapy. *Patient Care*, 15 August.

infected person takes several types of drugs that attack the virus at different stages of its life, the virus is much less likely to develop resistance.

Treatment with combinations of drugs, referred to as *highly active antiretroviral therapy*, or HAART, can reduce HIV in the blood to undetectable levels in many people. However, research indicates that the latent virus is still present in the body and that HIV-infected people on HAART carry potentially transmissible HIV in their body fluids. Even people who respond well to HIV treatment may still be able to infect others, although successful treatment greatly reduces the risk.

HIV/AIDS treatment is becoming increasingly complex. More than 20 drugs have been approved specifically for use against HIV/AIDS, and many others are being developed. One way to simplify treatment is by combining medicines.

For example, in October 2007, Health Canada approved Atripla, the first once-a-day tablet for HIV patients that combines three medicines into one.

TREATMENTS FOR OPPORTUNISTIC INFECTIONS In addition to antiviral drugs, most patients with low CD4 T-cell counts also take a variety of antibiotics to help prevent opportunistic infections, such as pneumonia and tuberculosis. A person with advanced HIV infection may need to take 20 or more pills every day. Medication side effects can become severe when so many drugs are used in combination.

What About a Vaccine? If an effective, safe, affordable vaccine against HIV could be developed, it might be possible to stop the worldwide HIV epidemic. Unfortunately, making a vaccine against HIV is proving to be exceedingly difficult. Methods that have been used to produce vaccines against other diseases are often ineffective or unsafe when used against HIV. Adding to the challenge is the fact that HIV comes in numerous subtypes, mutates rapidly, and destroys the very cells that normally protect the body against infectious diseases. Vaccines are being tested in humans, but experts are discouraged by recent vaccine trial failures.

Getting an HIV Test

You should strongly consider being tested for HIV if any of the following apply to you or any past or current sexual partners:

• You have had unprotected sex (vaginal, anal, or oral) with more than one partner or with a partner who was not in a mutually monogamous relationship with you.

• You have had sex while under the influence of alcohol or drugs (you might not have used protection).

• You have used or shared needles, syringes, or other paraphernalia for injecting drugs (including steroids).

• You have had tattooing, piercing, or acupuncture with unsterilized equipment.

• You received a transfusion of blood or blood products before November 1986.

• You have ever been diagnosed with an STI.

Physician or Clinic Testing

Your physician, student health clinic, public health department, or local AIDS association can arrange your HIV test. Before you take the test, a nurse or counsellor will ask you why you want to take the test, when and how you think you were exposed to HIV, and whether you have any questions. This is also a good time to obtain accurate information about HIV and AIDS and to talk about the implications of the test result, especially if it is positive. It is your choice to get tested, and you must give your consent in writing.

The standard test involves drawing a sample of blood from your arm. The sample is then sent to a laboratory for analysis; if the first stage of testing is positive, the test is repeated. If the results from the second stage of testing are positive, a final (and different) test is done to confirm the result. A positive test means that you have tested positive for the virus. If the result of the confirmatory test is indeterminate you will need to be tested again, usually about one month later.

In Canada, HIV testing is not automatically anonymous. *Anonymous testing* is available, but you will need to find a clinic that offers this service. Having an anonymous test means that only you will know you took the test and what the result was. The only identification is a code or name that is assigned by clinic staff. Although your name is not revealed, the result of your test may be reported to public health units in some jurisdictions.

If you give your name when having an HIV test, the test and results are confidential, not anonymous. Confidential tests may be *nominal* or *non-nominal*. Having a nominal test means that your name will appear on the test form and test result. The test result will be made available to your physician or health care provider and entered in your medical record. In some places, the test result may also be reported to the public health authorities. For non-nominal tests, a code is used instead of your name. Only you and your physician will know to whom the code refers.

Home Testing

Using an HIV home test kit requires an individual to prick his or her finger with a supplied lancet, blot a few drops of blood onto

blotting paper, and mail it to a laboratory. In a few days, the test result is retrieved over the telephone. Anyone who tests positive is connected to a trained counsellor, who can provide emotional and medical support. These results are anonymous.

While home test kits have been available in the United States since 1996, these kits have not been approved for use in Canada. Both Canadian and U.S. governments have warned individuals about the dangers of purchasing unapproved HIV home test kits sold over the Internet. In June 2009, Health Canada advised consumers not to use HIV home test kits as they have not been authorized for home use and may provide false results.

Understanding the Results

A negative test result means that no antibodies were found in your sample. However, it usually takes at least three months after exposure to HIV (and possibly as long as six months in some people) for antibodies to appear. Therefore, an infected person may receive a false-negative result. In patients with a negative HIV test result and a high risk of infection, repeat testing is recommended.

A positive result means that you are infected with HIV—it does not mean that you have AIDS. It is important to seek medical care and counselling immediately. You need to know more about your medical options; the possible psychological, social, and financial repercussions, and how to avoid spreading the disease. Rapid progress is being made in treating HIV, and treatments are potentially much more successful when begun early.

For more information about HIV testing and a list of AIDS service organizations in your region, visit the Canadian AIDS Society Web site (http://www.cdnaids.ca). You can also find a testing centre in your area (including anonymous test sites) by calling your provincial or territorial HIV/AIDS hotline. These numbers are listed on the Public Health Agency of Canada's Web site (http://www.phac-aspc.gc.ca/aids-sida/info/4-eng.php#find).

A licensed AIDS vaccine is now estimated to be at least a decade away, and some experts think that a fully effective AIDS vaccine may never be developed. Vaccines are also being tested as therapy for people already infected with HIV.

Researchers are making relatively rapid progress in producing a **microbicide** that could be used to prevent HIV and other STIs. A microbicide in the form of a cream, gel, sponge, ring, or suppository that could be inserted into the vagina or rectum could function as a kind of chemical condom. A microbicide could fill the urgent need for a prevention method that can be used by a woman without requiring cooperation from her partner. Several microbicides are currently undergoing human testing for safety and effectiveness.

The female condom may someday play a larger role in HIV prevention. Female condoms are more expensive than male condoms and aren't widely available in developing countries, but they offer the advantage that women can initiate their use. Scientists are developing a cheaper, easier-to-use female condom and are evaluating whether diaphragms (in combination with microbicides) protect against HIV.

Another approach is the use of preexposure treatment as prevention. Individuals who are not infected with HIV but are at a high risk for infection would take an anti-HIV medication before an activity that might expose them to HIV. This approach is controversial but might be effective in stopping the spread of HIV in highly vulnerable populations, such as sex workers. Unlike a vaccine, this form of prevention could be tested and put into practice in a relatively short time, especially if an existing HIV drug is used.

How Can You Protect Yourself? Although AIDS is currently incurable, it is preventable. You can protect yourself by avoiding behaviours that may bring you into contact with HIV. This means making careful choices about sexual activity and not sharing needles if you inject drugs.

MAKE CAREFUL CHOICES ABOUT SEXUAL ACTIVITY In a sexual relationship, the current and past behaviours of you and your partner determine the amount of risk involved. If you are uninfected and in a mutually monogamous relationship with another uninfected person, you are not at risk for HIV. Of course, it is often hard to know for sure whether your partner is completely faithful and is truly uninfected. Having a series of monogamous relationships is not a safe prevention strategy.

QUICK STATS

40% of individuals infected with HIV do not tell their sexual partners.

—Allen et al., 2008

For anyone not involved in a long-term, mutually monogamous relationship, abstinence from any sexual activity that involves the exchange of body fluids is the only sure way to prevent HIV infection (Figure 13.6).

High Risk

Unprotected anal sex is the riskiest sexual behaviour, especially for the receptive partner.

Unprotected vaginal intercourse is the next riskiest, especially for women, who are much more likely to be infected by an infected male partner than vice versa.

Oral sex is probably considerably less risky than anal and vaginal intercourse but can still result in HIV transmission.

Sharing of sex toys can be risky because they can carry blood, semen, or vaginal fluid.

Use of a condom reduces risk considerably but not completely for any type of intercourse. Anal sex with a condom is riskier than vaginal sex with a condom; oral sex with a condom is less risky, especially if the man does not ejaculate.

Hand-genital contact and deep kissing are less risky but could still theoretically transmit HIV; the presence of cuts or sores increases risk.

Sex with only one uninfected and totally faithful partner is without risk, but effective only if both partners are uninfected and completely monogamous.

Activities that don't involve the exchange of body fluids carry no risk: hugging, massage, closed-mouth kissing, masturbation, phone sex, and fantasy.

Abstinence is completely without risk. For many people, it can be an effective and reasonable method of avoiding HIV infection and other STIs during certain periods of life.

No Risk

FIGURE 13.6   What's risky and what's not: The approximate relative risk of HIV transmission of various sexual activities.

Anal and vaginal intercourse are the sexual activities associated with the highest risk of HIV infection. If you have intercourse, always use a condom. Use of a lubricated condom reduces the risk of transmitting HIV during all forms of intercourse. Condoms are not perfect, and they do not provide risk-free sex; however, when used properly, a condom provides a high level of protection against HIV. Experts also suggest the use of latex squares and dental dams, rubber devices that can be used as barriers during oral-genital or oral-anal sexual contact. As mentioned already, avoid using nonoxynol-9 lubricants because of the risk of tissue irritation, which can make STI transmission more likely.

Like condom use, many of the same steps you can take to avoid an unintended pregnancy can help you prevent STI and HIV infection. These methods are discussed in detail in Chapter 11 and are covered again later in this chapter.

DON'T SHARE DRUG NEEDLES People who inject drugs should avoid sharing needles, syringes, or anything that might have blood on it. Any injectable drug, legal or illegal, can be associated with HIV transmission. Needles can be decontaminated with a solution of bleach and water, but it is not a foolproof procedure, and HIV can survive in a syringe for a month or longer. (Boiling needles and syringes does not necessarily destroy HIV either.) As described in Chapter 14, obtaining sterile syringes through a syringe exchange program is much more effective than attempting to sterilize used syringes. Many prominent health organizations, including the Joint United Nations Programme on HIV/AIDS (UN-AIDS) and the Canadian Public Health Association, support syringe exchange programs, but these programs are unavailable or illegal in many other parts of the world.

If you are an injection drug user, your best protection is to obtain treatment and refrain from using drugs.

PARTICIPATE IN AN HIV EDUCATION PROGRAM   Many schools, universities, and colleges have peer education programs about preventing the transmission of HIV. These programs give you a chance to practise communicating with potential sex partners and negotiating safer sex, to engage in role playing to build self-confidence, and to learn how to use condoms. Studies show that educational programs in which students learn from their peers and then try out what they've learned through role playing are more likely to result in real behaviour change.

Many young people still believe that they are invulnerable to most kinds of harm and persist in thinking of themselves as not being at risk for HIV. The attitude of "it won't happen to me" is pervasive among high school and postsecondary students and is a major stumbling block to HIV/AIDS prevention. Until an effective vaccine and a cure are found, HIV infection will remain one of the biggest challenges of this generation. Education and individual responsibility can lead the way to controlling this devastating epidemic (see the box "Preventing HIV Infection and Other STIs on p. 432").

Hepatitis B

Hepatitis (inflammation of the liver) can cause serious and sometimes permanent damage to the liver, which can result in death in severe cases. One of the many types of hepatitis is caused by hepatitis B virus (HBV). HBV is somewhat similar to HIV; it is found in most body fluids, and it can be transmitted sexually, by injection drug use, and during pregnancy and delivery. However, HBV is much more contagious than HIV, and it can also be spread through nonsexual close contact. Health care workers who are exposed to blood are frequently infected, as are people who live in close contact with one another, such as prisoners and residents of mental health care facilities.

Hepatitis B is a potentially fatal disease with no cure, but an effective vaccine is available. In Canada, a universal HBV immunization program includes school-based vaccinations for children ages 9–13. An infant vaccination program is also offered in some provinces and territories. The number of cases of acute hepatitis B in Canada has decreased in all age groups, coinciding with the increasing use of the vaccine. In addition, mother-to-child transmission has been greatly reduced because of routine HBV screening

Accurate information about HIV/AIDS, including where to go for testing and treatment, is available from many sources, including health professionals, community-based organizations, and national hotlines.

of pregnant women. Vaccination is recommended for all individuals at increased risk for hepatitis B, including men who have sex with men, those who inject illegal drugs, people with a recent history of STIs or multiple sexual partners, prison inmates, household and sexual contacts of people infected with HBV, and health care workers who are exposed to blood and body fluids.

Other forms of viral hepatitis can also be sexually transmitted. Hepatitis A is of particular concern for people who engage in anal sex; a vaccine is available and is recommended for all people at risk. Less commonly, hepatitis C can be transmitted sexually. Experts believe that traumatic sexual activity that causes tissue damage is most likely to transmit HCV. See Chapter 9 for more on these forms of hepatitis.

Transmission   HBV is found in all body fluids, including blood and blood products, semen, saliva, urine, and vaginal secretions. It is easily transmitted through any sexual activity that involves the exchange of body fluids, the use of contaminated needles, and any blood-to-blood contact, including the use of contaminated razor blades, toothbrushes, and eating utensils. The primary risk factors for acquiring HBV are sexual exposure and injection drug use; having multiple partners greatly increases risk. As mentioned, a pregnant woman can transmit HBV to her unborn child.

Symptoms   Many people infected with HBV never develop symptoms; they have what are known as silent infections. The normal incubation period is 30–180 days. Mild cases of hepatitis cause flulike symptoms, such as

microbicide   An agent that destroys microorganisms; also known as an *antiseptic*.

TERMS

Preventing HIV Infection and Other STIs

For those who aren't in a long-term monogamous relationship with an uninfected partner, abstinence is the only truly safe option for avoiding STIs. Remember that it's OK to say no to sex and drugs.

Safer sexual activities that allow close person-to-person contact with almost no risk of contracting STIs or HIV include fantasy, hugging, massage, rubbing clothed bodies together, self-stimulation by both partners, and kissing with lips closed. If you choose to be sexually active, talk with potential partners about HIV, safer sex, and the use of condoms before you begin a sexual relationship. The following behaviours will help lower your risk of exposure to STIs during sexual activities:

• Don't drink alcohol or use drugs in sexual situations. Mood-altering drugs can affect your judgment and make you more likely to take risks. Having sex when intoxicated significantly increases the risk of STIs.

• Limit the number of partners. Avoid sexual contact with people who have HIV or an STI or who have engaged in risky behaviours in the past, including unprotected sex and injection drug use.

• Use condoms during every act of intercourse and oral sex. Condoms do not provide perfect protection, but they greatly reduce your risk of contracting an infection. Multiple studies show that regular condom use can reduce the risk of several diseases, including HIV, chlamydia, and genital herpes.

• Use condoms properly to obtain maximum protection (see Chapter 11). Use a water-based lubricant; don't use oil-based lubricants, such as petroleum jelly or baby oil, or any vaginal product containing mineral or vegetable oil. Avoid using lubricants or condoms containing nonoxynol-9, particularly for anal intercourse. Unroll condoms gently to avoid tearing them, and smooth out any air bubbles. If you accidentally put a condom on the wrong way, remove it and throw it away; do not flip it over and try again.

• Avoid sexual contact that could cause cuts or tears in the skin or tissue. Using extra lubricant (water-based) can help prevent damage to delicate tissues.

• Get periodic screening tests for STIs and HIV. Young women need yearly pelvic exams and Pap tests.

• Get vaccinated for hepatitis B. Young women and men should also consider getting vaccinated against HPV.

• Get prompt treatment for any STIs you contract.

If you inject drugs of any kind, don't share needles, syringes, or anything that might have blood on it. If your community has a syringe exchange program, use it. Seek treatment; stop using injectable drugs.

If you are at risk for HIV infection, don't donate blood, sperm, or body organs. Don't have unprotected sex or share needles or syringes. Get tested for HIV soon, and get treated. People infected with HIV who get early treatment generally feel better and live longer than those who delay treatment.

---

fever, body aches, chills, and loss of appetite. As the illness progresses, people may experience nausea, vomiting, dark-coloured urine, abdominal pain, and jaundice. Some people with hepatitis also develop a skin rash and joint pain or arthritis. Acute hepatitis B can sometimes be severe, resulting in prolonged illness or even death.

Most adults who have acute hepatitis B recover completely within a few weeks or months. But a small number of adults who are infected with HBV become chronic carriers of the virus, capable of infecting others for the rest of their life. The prevalence of chronic carriers varies in different populations. For example, it is estimated that 7.4% of immigrants to Canada and 0.3% of First Nations are chronic carriers. Some chronic carriers remain asymptomatic, while others develop chronic liver disease. Chronic hepatitis can cause cirrhosis of the liver, liver failure, and a deadly form of liver cancer. Hepatitis B kills about 100 Canadians each year; worldwide, the annual death toll exceeds 600,000.

Diagnosis and Treatment Blood tests can diagnose hepatitis by analyzing liver function and detecting the infecting organism. Hepatitis B has no cure and no specific treatment for acute infections; antiviral drugs and immune system modulators may be used for cases of chronic HBV infection. For people exposed to HBV, treat-ment with hepatitis B immunoglobulin can provide protection against the virus.

Prevention Preventive measures for hepatitis B are similar to those for HIV infection: Avoid sexual contact that involves sharing body fluids, including saliva; use condoms during sexual intercourse; and don't share needles. If you have tattooing or body piercing done, make sure all needles and equipment are sterile. The vaccine for hepatitis B is safe and highly effective.

Other STIs

A few other infections are transmitted sexually and require responsible sexual behaviour.

Trichomoniasis (often called *trich*) is one of the most curable STIs among young women. The single-celled organism that causes trich, *Trichomonas vaginalis*, thrives in warm, moist conditions, making women particularly susceptible to these infections in the vagina. Women who become symptomatic with trich develop a greenish, foul-smelling vaginal discharge and severe itching and pain in the vagina. Prompt treatment with metronidazole is important because studies suggest that trich may increase the risk of HIV transmission and, in pregnant women, premature delivery.

THINKING ABOUT THE ENVIRONMENT

In some parts of the world, the human environment is far more responsible than the natural one for the spread of STIs.

As has been mentioned in this chapter, people in remote and poverty-stricken areas typically have little access to health care resources, information on safer sex practices, and barrier devices, such as condoms. Without access to medical testing and treatment, whole populations have little means for preventing or dealing with STIs of any kind.

Making matters worse is the harsh male-dominated sexual environments found in some regions. Whether these circumstances are based on local religious or social mores, they often place women (and children, in some cases) at risk of exploitation and greatly increase the risks of STIs. For example, some cultures allow or even encourage male infidelity. In many parts of the world, women have little or no say in their sexual relationships, meaning they may not be able to use protective measures against STIs. Often, the cultures that prevent women from protecting themselves shun or punish women who become infected with a sexually transmitted infection.

See Chapter 21 for more information on the environment and environmental health.

Bacterial vaginosis (BV) is the most common cause of abnormal vaginal discharge in women of reproductive age. BV occurs when healthy bacteria that normally inhabit the vagina become displaced by unhealthy species. BV is clearly associated with sexual activity and often occurs after a change in partners. Douching has been correlated with an increased risk of BV, especially in women who douche more than once a month. Symptoms of BV include vaginal discharge with a fishy odour and sometimes vaginal irritation. BV is treated with topical and oral antibiotics.

Pubic lice (commonly known as *crabs*) and **scabies** are highly contagious parasitic infections. Treatment is generally easy, although lice infestation can require repeated applications of medications.

WHAT YOU CAN DO

You can take responsibility for your health and contribute to a general reduction in the incidence of STIs in three major areas: education, diagnosis and treatment, and prevention.

Education

Since the AIDS epidemic began, public and private agencies have grown more serious about educating the public and increasing their awareness of all STIs. This campaign may already be paying off in changing attitudes and sexual behaviours, at least among certain segments of the population. For example, in comparison with previous years,

QUESTIONS FOR CRITICAL THINKING AND REFLECTION

Have you ever had sex and regretted it later? If so, what were the circumstances, and what influenced you to act the way you did? Were there any negative consequences? What preventive strategies can you use in the future to make sure it doesn't happen again?

---

data from 2005 show that the percentage of Canadian women ages 15–19 who reported engaging in sexual intercourse had decreased, while the use of condoms among these women had increased. But some groups seem to be growing weary of messages about safer sex. Many younger gay men are participating in high-risk behaviours, and a second wave of the AIDS epidemic among gay men can be expected if younger men fail to use preventive measures. Also discouraging is the fact that the number of cases of HIV infection among harder-to-reach groups, such as injection drug users and their partners and children, is still increasing. In particular, more educational efforts are needed among Canadian ethnic minority groups.

Education efforts targeted at increasing public awareness about AIDS through the media have included public service announcements, dramatic presentations, and support from well-known public figures. Universities and colleges offer courses in health and human sexuality. Free pamphlets and other literature are available from public health departments, health clinics, physicians' offices, and student health centres, and easy-to-understand books are available in libraries and bookstores. Several national hotlines have been set up to provide free, confidential information and referral services to callers anywhere in the country.

Learning about STIs is still up to every person individually. You must assume responsibility for learning about the causes and nature of STIs and their potential effects on you, those with whom you have sexual relationships, and the children you may have. Once you know about STIs—their symptoms, how they're transmitted, and how they can be prevented—you are in a position to educate others. Providing information to your friends and partners, whether in casual conversation or in more serious decision-making discussions, is an important way that you can make a difference in both your own wellness and that of others.

---

trichomoniasis A protozoal infection caused by *Trichomonas vaginalis*, transmitted sexually and externally.

bacterial vaginosis (BV) A condition linked to sexual activity; caused by an overgrowth of certain bacteria inhabiting the vagina.

pubic lice Parasites that infest the hair of the pubic region, commonly called *crabs*.

scabies A contagious skin disease caused by a type of burrowing parasitic mite.

Diagnosis and Treatment

Early diagnosis and treatment of STIs can help you and your sex partner(s) avoid unnecessary complications and help prevent the spread of STIs.

Get Vaccinated   Every young, sexually active person should be vaccinated for hepatitis B; vaccines are available for all age groups. Men who have sex with men should be vaccinated for hepatitis A, and girls and women ages 9–26 should be vaccinated for HPV.

Be Alert for Symptoms   If you are sexually active, be alert for any sign or symptom of infection, such as a rash, a discharge, sores, or unusual pain, and don't hesitate to have a professional examination if you notice such a symptom. Although only a physician can make a proper diagnosis of an STI, you can perform *genital self-examinations* between checkups to look for early warning signs of infection. Women should examine the entire genital area, including the area covered by pubic hair, the outer and inner lips of the vagina, the clitoris, and the area around the urinary and vaginal openings. Men should look at the entire head, shaft, and base of the penis and the scrotum. A mirror may be helpful for checking difficult-to-see areas.

Throughout the exam, look for bumps, sores, blisters, or warts on the skin. Bumps or blisters may be red or light coloured; they may look like pimples, or they may develop into open sores. Genital warts may appear as very small bumpy spots, or they may have a fleshy, cauliflower-like appearance. Also stay alert for other signs of STIs, including pain or burning on urination, itchiness in the genital area, abnormal discharge from the vagina or penis, pelvic pain, and, in women, bleeding between menstrual periods. Be alert for these signs or symptoms in your partner, too.

Get Tested   Remember that almost all STIs—including HIV infection—can be completely asymptomatic for a long time. If you are sexually active, be sure to get periodic STI checks, even if you have no symptoms. If you have a risky sexual encounter, see a physician as soon as possible (see the box "Don't Wait—Early Treatment of STIs Really Matters").

Sexually active young women should have pelvic exams and Pap tests at least once a year, with chlamydia and gonorrhea screening in most cases. Sexually active men, especially if they have had more than one partner, should have periodic STI screenings.

Men who have sex with men are at especially high risk for HIV and other STIs. Sexually active men who have sex with men should be tested regularly for HIV, chlamydia (anal and urethral), syphilis, and gonorrhea (anal, urethral, and pharyngeal). Men who have multiple anonymous partners or who are injection drug users should also be screened frequently. All sexually active gay and bisexual men should be vaccinated for hepatitis A and B.

Testing for STIs is done through private physicians, public health clinics, community health agencies, and most student health services.

Inform Your Partners   Telling a partner that you have exposed him or her to an STI isn't easy. You may be afraid your partner will be angry or resentful, or you may worry that your partner will think less of you or reject you. At the same time, you may be feeling afraid, ashamed, embarrassed, or angry yourself. Despite the awkwardness and difficulty, it is crucial that your sex partner(s) be informed and urged to seek testing and treatment as quickly as possible.

You can get help telling your partner if you need it. Public health departments will notify sex partners of their possible exposure while maintaining your confidentiality and anonymity. Peer counselling and student health programs often help students with practice in role-playing in these circumstances, and health care personnel can provide assistance.

As emphasized throughout this chapter, undetected and untreated STIs can lead to serious medical complications and even death. In asymptomatic cases, the only way infected people can find out they have a disease is by being tested. Uninformed, untested partners can go on to spread the disease, contributing to anguish for others as well as spiralling public health problems.

Get Treated   Generally speaking, treatments for STIs are safe and (with the exception of AIDS treatments) fairly inexpensive. Many Canadians have access to insurance coverage, through public or private insurance plans, for STI treatments. If you are being treated, follow instructions carefully and take all the medication as prescribed. Don't stop taking the medication just because you feel better or your symptoms have disappeared. Above all, don't give any of your medication to anyone else, including your partner. If you have an STI, your partner needs to be tested and, if necessary, treated. Taking a few of your pills is unlikely to cure your partner, and may make your treatment incomplete, leaving you both at risk for reinfection.

Being cured of an STI does not mean that you will not get it again, and exposure does not confer lasting immunity, nor does it prevent you from getting any other STI—all the more reason to be informed, to inform your partner(s), and to practise safer sex.

Prevention   STIs *are* preventable. As discussed earlier, the only sure way to avoid exposure to STIs is to abstain from sexual activity. But if you choose to be sexually active, the key is to think about prevention *before* you have a sexual encounter or find yourself in the heat of the moment. Find out what your partner thinks before you become sexually involved. Remember, you can become infected with an STI from just one unprotected encounter.

All your good intentions are likely to fly out the window if you enter into a sexual situation when you are intoxicated. If you or your partner (or both of you) is drunk,

Don't Wait—Early Treatment of STIs Really Matters

If you have had a recent risky sexual encounter, visit your physician, student health centre, or local STI clinic and ask for testing. Don't wait for symptoms to develop—you may never have any. Permanent damage from STIs, including infertility, can occur even if you have no symptoms. Treating some STIs, such as chlamydia and gonorrhea, within a few days of infection is very likely to prevent complications, such as PID and infertility. You will also be much less likely to pass the infection on to anyone else.

Unsafe sex with a person who is infected with HIV meets the criteria for postexposure prophylaxis (PEP) treatment, which involves taking antiviral medication as soon as possible. If you are treated within 72 hours of possible exposure, PEP will significantly reduce your risk of HIV infection. If you develop flulike symptoms in the days or weeks following risky sexual or drug-taking behaviour, see your physician immediately. If HIV treatment is begun within the first weeks of the infection, there is still a good chance that damage to the immune system can be reduced or even prevented. Many physicians will not think of primary HIV infection when you describe flulike symptoms, so be sure to speak up about your recent risky activities and your concerns about HIV.

If tests come back positive for a particular STI, you need to be tested for others, including HIV infection. Infection with any STI means that you are at higher risk for all others. Women should also have a pelvic exam and a Pap test. If you are given medication to treat an STI, take all of it as directed. Incomplete treatment can result in an incomplete cure, thereby contributing to the development of drug-resistant organisms.

Do not have sexual intercourse until your treatment—and your partner's treatment—is complete. If your partner still carries the infection, you are likely to be reinfected when you resume sexual activity. If you have an incurable STI, such as herpes or HPV infection, always use a condom and make sure your partner is fully informed of the potential risks of being intimate with you, even if you are using condoms.

The use of condoms declined as more advanced methods of contraception, such as birth control pills and IUDs, became available. But condoms are once again gaining in popularity because of the protection they provide against STIs.

you are likely to be less cautious about sex than you would be if you were sober. Many people use alcohol and drugs as a way to deal with their anxiety in social and sexual situations. However, being intoxicated leaves you vulnerable to sexual assault and greatly increases your risk of acquiring a serious STI.

Most people don't want to think, talk, or ask questions about STIs for a variety of reasons. They may think it detracts from the appeal and excitement of the moment, that it takes away from the spontaneity of the experience, or that it will be perceived as a personal insult. For others, simply not knowing how to talk about STIs and safer sex may prevent them from bringing up the issue with a partner. (For advice on communicating with potential sex partners, see the box "Talking About Condoms and Safer Sex" on p. 436.)

Find out about your partner's sexual history and practices. Be honest, and ask your partner to do the same, but don't stake your health and life on assumptions about your partner's honesty. Even if your partner's past seems low risk, still insist on using a condom every time you have sex. Any sexual activity exposes partners to everyone from their partner's sexual past and everyone from those people's pasts. In one recent study, researchers mapped the sexual relationships of a group of high school students and found a chain of 288 one-to-one sexual relationships, meaning the teen at the end of the chain may have had direct sexual contact with only 1 person, but was indirectly exposed to 286 others.

You may find that your partner is just as concerned as you are. By thinking and talking about responsible sexual behaviour, you are expressing a sense of caring for yourself, your potential partner, and your future children. Taking STIs seriously is practical, courageous, and loving; it means giving yourself the respect you deserve.

QUESTIONS FOR CRITICAL THINKING AND REFLECTION

If you are sexually active, have you talked seriously with your partner about STIs and safer sex practices? If not, why? How would you react if your partner started such a discussion?

Talking About Condoms and Safer Sex

The only sure way to prevent STIs, including HIV infection, is to abstain from sexual activity. If you choose to be sexually active, you should do everything possible to protect yourself from STIs. This includes good communication with your sex partner(s).

The time to talk about safer sex is before you begin a sexual relationship. However, even if you've been having unprotected sex with your partner, it is still worth it to start practising safer sex now. If you're nervous about initiating a conversation about safer sex, rehearse what you will say first.

There are many ways to bring up the subject of safer sex and condom use with your partner. Be honest about your concerns and stress that protection against STIs means that you care about yourself and your partner. Here are a few suggestions:

- "I heard on the news that more and more people are using condoms. I think it shows that people are being more responsible about sex. What do you think?"

- "I'm worried about the diseases we can get from having sex because so many don't have symptoms. I want to protect both of us by using condoms whenever we have sex."

- "I've been thinking about making love with you. But first we need to talk about how to have safer sex and be protected."

You may find that your partner shares your concerns and also wants to use condoms. He or she may be happy and relieved that you have brought up the subject of safer sex. However, if he or she resists the idea of using condoms, you may need to negotiate. Stress that you both deserve to be protected and that sex will be more enjoyable when you aren't worrying about STIs (see the suggestions that follow). If you and your partner haven't used condoms before, buy some and familiarize yourselves with how to use them. Once you feel more comfortable handling condoms, you'll be able to use them correctly and incorporate them into your sexual activity in fun ways. Consider trying the female condom.

If your partner still won't agree to use condoms, think carefully about whether you want to have a sexual relationship with him or her. Safer sex is part of a responsible, caring sexual relationship, and it's smart to say no to a partner who won't use a condom. It's up to you to protect yourself.

If your partner says ...	Try saying ...
"They're not romantic."	"Worrying about AIDS isn't romantic, and with condoms we won't have to worry." OR "If we put one on together, a condom could be fun."
"You don't trust me."	"I do trust you, but how can I trust your former partners or mine?" OR "It's important to me that we're both protected."
"I don't have any diseases. I've been tested."	"I'm glad you've been tested, but tests aren't foolproof for all diseases. To be safe, I always use condoms."
"I forgot to bring a condom. But it's OK to skip it just this once."	"I'd really like to make love with you, but I never have sex without a condom. Let's go get some."
"I don't like the way they feel."	"They might feel different, but let's try." OR "Sex won't feel good if we're worrying about diseases." OR "How about trying the female condom?"
"I don't use condoms."	"I use condoms every time." OR "I don't have sex without condoms."
"But I love you."	"Being in love can't protect us from diseases." OR "I love you, too. We still need to use condoms."
"But we've been having sex without condoms."	"I want to start using condoms now so we won't be at any more risk." OR "We can still prevent infection or reinfection."

Source: Dialogue from San Francisco AIDS Foundation. 1998. *Condoms for Couples* (IMPACT AIDS, 3692 18th Street, San Francisco, CA 94110). Copyright © 1998 San Francisco AIDS Foundation. All rights reserved. Used with permission.

Mc Graw Hill connect™

Practise and learn online with Connect. Connect allows you to practise important skills at your own pace and on your own schedule, with 24/7 online access to an eBook, practice quizzes, interactivities, videos, study tools, additional resources, and more.

SUMMARY

- Chlamydia causes epididymitis and urethritis in men; in women, it can lead to pelvic inflammatory disease (PID) and infertility if untreated.

- Untreated gonorrhea can cause PID in women and epididymitis in men, leading to infertility. In infants, untreated gonorrhea can cause blindness.

- PID, a complication of untreated gonorrhea or chlamydia, is an infection of the uterus and oviducts that may extend to the ovaries and pelvic cavity. It can lead to infertility, ectopic pregnancy, and chronic pelvic pain.

- Syphilis is a highly contagious bacterial infection that can be treated with antibiotics. If left untreated, it can lead to deterioration of the central nervous system and death.

- Human papillomavirus (HPV) causes genital warts and cervical cancer. Treatment does not eradicate the virus, which can be passed on by asymptomatic people.

- Genital herpes is a common incurable infection that can be fatal to newborns. After an initial infection, outbreaks may recur at any time.

- HIV affects the immune system, making an otherwise healthy person less able to resist a variety of infections.

- HIV is carried in blood and blood products, semen, vaginal and cervical secretions, and breast milk. HIV is transmitted through the exchange of these fluids.

- There is currently no cure or vaccine for HIV infection. Drugs have been developed to slow the course of the disease and to prevent or treat certain secondary infections.

- HIV infection can be prevented by making careful choices about sexual activity, not sharing drug needles, and learning how to protect yourself from HIV.

- Hepatitis B is a viral infection of the liver transmitted through sexual and nonsexual contact. Following an initial infection, most people recover; but some become carriers and may develop serious complications.

- Other infections that can be transmitted sexually or are linked to sexual activity include trichomoniasis, bacterial vaginosis, pubic lice, and scabies. Any STI that causes sores or inflammation can increase the risk of HIV transmission.

- Successful diagnosis and treatment of STIs involve being alert for symptoms, getting tested, informing partners, and following treatment instructions carefully.

- All STIs are preventable; the key is practising responsible sexual behaviours. Those who are sexually active are safest with one mutually monogamous, uninfected partner. Using a condom properly with every act of sexual intercourse helps protect against STIs.

FOR MORE INFORMATION

BOOKS

Engel, J. 2007. *The Epidemic: A Global History of AIDS*. New York: Collins. A historical, social, and cultural perspective on the AIDS epidemic, from its beginning in 1981 to the present day, from a medical historian.

Hyde, J. S., and J. D. DeLamater. 2008. *Understanding Human Sexuality*, 10th ed. New York: McGraw-Hill. A comprehensive, multidisciplinary introduction to human sexuality; includes material on STIs.

Klausner, J. D., and E. W. Hook. 2007. *Current Diagnosis and Treatment of Sexually Transmitted Diseases*. New York: McGraw-Hill. Written for the clinician; provides an easy-to-use reference of the latest diagnostic and treatment information available on STIs.

Marr, L. 2007. *Sexually Transmitted Diseases: A Physician Tells You What You Need to Know*. Baltimore, Md.: Johns Hopkins University Press. Practical information on the diagnosis, treatment, and prevention of sexually transmitted infections of all types.

McIlvenna, T. 2005. *The Complete Guide to Safer Sex*. Fort Lee, N.J.: Barricade Books. Provides practical advice for STI prevention.

Moore, E. A. 2008. *Encyclopedia of Sexually Transmitted Diseases*, Illustrated ed. Jefferson, N.C.: McFarland. Includes a variety of information about STIs in an easy-to-use format.

ORGANIZATIONS, HOTLINES, AND WEB SITES

The Internet addresses listed here were accurate at the time of publication.

Aboriginal Canada Portal. Provides resources, up-to-date information (including health and social services information), and government programs in Canada for First Nations, Inuit, and Metis.

http://www.aboriginalcanada.gc.ca

Canadian AIDS Society. Provides information about a variety of topics, including AIDS-related events, HIV and poverty, and harm reduction, as well as other resources (including links, hotline information, and online discussion groups).

http://www.cdnaids.ca

Canadian AIDS Treatment Information Exchange. Provides free, confidential information about all aspects of HIV, including prevention, medications, nutrition, supplements, side effects, and complementary therapies.

http://www.catie.ca

Canadian Federation for Sexual Health. Promotes sexual and reproductive health and rights in Canada and internationally. Provides information pertaining to STIs, pregnancy, and contraception.

http://www.cfsh.ca

Canadian Foundation for Women's Health. Provides information about research and resources related to women's sexual and reproductive health. Founded by the Society of Obstetricians and Gynaecologists of Canada.

http://www.cfwh.org

Canadian Public Health Association. Provides information and resources related to public health issues in Canada, with links to provincial and territorial public health associations.

http://www.cpha.ca

Federal Initiative to Address HIV/AIDS in Canada. Provides information on HIV/AIDS funding and the use of population-specific approaches to develop culturally appropriate strategies to reduce HIV/AIDS transmission in at-risk groups.

http://www.phac-aspc.gc.ca/aids-sida/fi-if/

Health Canada: Sexually Transmitted Infections. Offers information on prevention and control of STIs, along with links to resources statistics, educational materials, and support programs.

http://www.hc-sc.gc.ca/hc-ps/dc-ma/sti-its-eng.php

Joint United Nations Programme on HIV/AIDS (UNAIDS). Provides statistics and information on the international HIV/AIDS situation.

http://www.unaids.org

NAMES Project Foundation AIDS Memorial Quilt. Includes the story behind the quilt, images of quilt panels, and information and links relating to HIV infection.

http://www.aidsquilt.org

Public Health Agency of Canada: Sexual Health and Sexually Transmitted Infections. Provides a wealth of credible and up-to-date information on sexual health and sexually transmitted infections.

http://www.phac-aspc.gc.ca/std-mts/index-eng.php

SexualityandU. Provides information and education on sexual health for teens, adults, parents, teachers, and health professionals. Administered by the Society of Obstetricians and Gynaecologists of Canada.

http://www.sexualityandu.ca

Society of Obstetricians and Gynaecologists of Canada. Provides information, research, and resources related to women's health issues and clinical practice guidelines.

http://www.sogc.org

Vancouver Coastal Health Supervised Injection Site. Contains information and research (including user statistics) related to Insite, North America's first legal supervised injection facility.

http://supervisedinjection.vch.ca/home/

WHO: Sexually Transmitted Infections. Provides information on international statistics and prevention efforts.

http://www.who.int/topics/sexually_transmitted_infections/en

See also the listings for Chapters 9 and 11.

SELECTED BIBLIOGRAPHY

Agot, K. E., et al. 2004. Risk of HIV-1 in rural Kenya: A comparison of circumcised and uncircumcised men. *Epidemiology* 15(2): 157–163.

Alary, M. 1997. Gonorrhea: Epidemiology and control strategies. *Canadian Journal of Human Sexuality* 6(2): 151–159.

Allen, M., et al. 2008. Persons living with HIV: Disclosure to sexual partners. *Communication Research Reports* 25(3): 192–199.

AVERT. 2009. *The Origin of AIDS and HIV and The First Cases of AIDS* (http://www.avert.org/origins.htm; retrieved February 17, 2009).

Baeten, J. M., et al. 2005. Female-to-male infectivity of HIV-1 among circumcised and uncircumcised Kenyan men. *Journal of Infectious Diseases* 191(4): 546–553.

British Columbia Centre for Excellence in HIV/AIDS, Urban Health Research Initiative. 2009. *Findings from the Evaluation of Vancouver's Pilot Medically Supervised Safer Injecting Facility: Insite.* (http://uhri.cfenet.ubc.ca/images/Documents/insite_report-eng.pdf; retrieved January 21, 2011).

Brown, D. R., et al. 2005. A longitudinal study of genital human papillomavirus infection in a cohort of closely followed adolescent women. *Journal of Infectious Diseases* 191(2): 182–192.

Canadian AIDS Society, Centre for Infectious Disease Prevention and Control, and Health Canada. 2002. *A Guide to HIV/AIDS Epidemiological and Surveillance Terms* (http://www.phac-aspc.gc.ca/publicat/haest-tesvs/pdf/hiv_glossary_e.pdf; retrieved February 20, 2010).

Canadian Public Health Association. 2005. *Leading Together: Canada Takes Action on HIV/AIDS (2005–2010)* (http://www.leadingtogether.ca/pdf/Leading_Together.pdf; retrieved March 1, 2010).

Centers for Disease Control and Prevention. 2006. Trends in HIV-related risk behaviors among high school students—United States, 1991–2005. *Morbidity and Mortality Weekly Report* 55(31): 851–854.

Cohen, M. 2004. HIV and sexually transmitted diseases: A lethal synergy. *Topics in HIV Medicine* 12(4):104–107.

Crosby, R., and R. J. DiClemente. 2004. Use of recreational Viagra among men having sex with men. *Sexually Transmitted Infections* 80(6): 466–468.

Erbelding, E. J., and J. M. Zenilman. 2005. Toward better control of sexually transmitted diseases. *New England Journal of Medicine* 352(7): 720–721.

Gupta, R., et al. 2004. Valacyclovir and acyclovir for suppression of shedding of herpes simplex virus in the genital tract. *Journal of Infectious Diseases* 190(8): 1374–1381.

Health Canada. 2009. *Health Canada Is Warning Canadians Not to Use Clean Testing HIV Home Test Kit, or Any Home HIV Test Kit* (http://www.hc-sc.gc.ca/ahc-asc/media/advisories-avis/_2009/2009_97-eng.php; retrieved February 19, 2010).

Hampton, T. 2006. High prevalence of lesser-known STDs. *Journal of the American Medical Association* 295(21): 2467.

Huppert, J. S. 2006. New detection methods for trichomoniasis may help curb more serious STIs. *Patient Care for the Nurse Practitioner* 40(5): 32–36.

Joint United Nations Programme on HIV/AIDS (UNAIDS). 2010. *UNAIDS Report on the Global AIDS Epidemic 2010.* Geneva: UNAIDS (http://www.unaids.org/en/media/unaids/contentassets/documents/unaidspublication/2010/20101123_globalreport_en.pdf; April 27, 2011).

Kimberlin, D., and D. Rouse. 2004. Genital herpes. *New England Journal of Medicine* 350(19): 1970–1977.

Mathers, C. D., and Loncar, D. 2006. Projections of global mortality and burden of disease from 2002 to 2030. Public Library of Science, *Medicine* 3(11): 2011–2030.

Merson, M. 2006. The HIV-AIDS pandemic at 25—The global response. *New England Journal of Medicine* 354(23): 2414–2417.

Miller, W. C., et al. 2004. Prevalence of chlamydial and gonococcal infections among young adults in the United States. *Journal of the American Medical Association* 291(18): 2229–2236.

Money, D., and M. Steben. 2008. Genital herpes: Gynaecological aspects. *Journal of Obstetrics and Gynaecology Canada* 30(4): 347–353.

National Institutes of Allergy and Infectious Diseases. 2009. *HIV Infection in Women* (http://www.niaid.nih.gov/topics/HIVAIDS/Understanding/Population%20Specific%20Information/Pages/womenHiv.aspx; retrieved February 17, 2009).

Ness, R. B., et al. 2005. Douching, pelvic inflammatory disease, and incident gonococcal and chlamydial genital infection in a cohort of high-risk women. *American Journal of Epidemiology* 61(2): 186–195.

Public Health Agency of Canada. 2003. *HIV and AIDS in Canada. Surveillance Report to June 30, 2003* (http://www.phac-aspc.gc.ca/publicat/aids-sida/haic-vsac0604/pdf/haic-vsac0604.pdf; retrieved April 27, 2011).

Public Health Agency of Canada. 2008. *Canadian Guidelines on Sexually Transmitted Infections—2008 Edition* (http://www.phac-aspc.gc.ca/std-mts/sti-its/pdf/sti-its-eng.pdf; retrieved February 18, 2010).

Public Health Agency of Canada. 2009. *Brief Report on Sexually Transmitted Infections in Canada: 2007* (http://www.phac-aspc.gc.ca/publicat/2009/sti-its/index-eng.php#toc; retrieved March 2, 2010).

Public Health Agency of Canada. 2009. *Summary: Estimates of HIV Prevalence and Incidence in Canada, 2008* (http://www.phac-aspc.gc.ca/aids-sida/publication/survreport/pdf/estimat08-eng.pdf; retrieved February 26, 2010).

Public Health Agency of Canada. 2010. *HIV and AIDS in Canada. Surveillance Report to December 31, 2009* (http://www.phac-aspc.gc.ca/aids-sida/publication/survreport/2009/dec/pdf/2009-Report-Rapport.pdf; retrieved January 22, 2011).

Public Health Agency of Canada. 2010. *Primary Care and Sexually Transmitted Infections* (http://www.phac-aspc.gc.ca/std-mts/sti-its/pdf/secii-eng.pdf; retrieved January 22, 2011).

Remis, R. S., et al. 2003. *Report on HIV/AIDS in Ontario 2002.* Toronto: Ontario Ministry of Health and Long-Term Care.

Rodriguez, B., et al. Predictive value of plasma HIV RNA level on rate of CD4 T-cell decline in untreated HIV infection. *Journal of the American Medical Association* 296(12): 1498–1506.

Sanders, G. D., et al. 2005. Cost-effectiveness of screening for HIV in the era of highly active antiretroviral therapy. *New England Journal of Medicine* 352(6): 570–585.

Sepkowitz, K. 2006. One disease, two epidemics—AIDS at 25. *New England Journal of Medicine* 354(23): 2411–2414.

Wang, C., et al. 2004. Mortality in HIV-seropositive versus -seronegative persons in the era of highly active antiretroviral therapy: Implications for when to initiate therapy. *Journal of Infectious Diseases* 190(6): 1046–1054.

Weinstock, H., S. Berman, and W. Cates. 2004. Sexually transmitted diseases among American youth: Incidence and prevalence estimates, 2000. *Perspectives on Sexual and Reproductive Health* 36(1): 6–10.

World Health Organization. 2007. *Post-exposure Prophylaxis to Prevent HIV Infection: Joint WHO/ILO Guidelines on Post-exposure Prophylaxis (PEP) to Prevent HIV Infection* (http://whqlibdoc.who.int/publications/2007/9789241596374_eng.pdf; retrieved March 1, 2010).

Yeni, P. G., et al. 2004. Treatment for adult HIV infection. *Journal of the American Medical Association* 292(2): 251–265.

Mc Graw Hill connect™   Practise and learn online with Connect.

THE USE AND ABUSE OF PSYCHOACTIVE DRUGS

LOOKING AHEAD >>>>>

AFTER READING THIS CHAPTER, YOU SHOULD BE ABLE TO

- Define and discuss the concepts of addictive behaviour, substance abuse, and substance dependence
- Explain factors contributing to drug use and dependence
- List the major categories of psychoactive drugs and describe their effects, methods of use, and potential for abuse and dependence
- Discuss social issues related to psychoactive drug use and its prevention and treatment
- Evaluate the role of drugs and other addictive behaviours in your life and identify your risk factors for abuse or dependence

TEST YOUR KNOWLEDGE

1. **Addictions always involve drugs that cause physical withdrawal symptoms when the person stops taking them.**
   True or false?

2. **Which of the following is the most widely used illegal drug among Canadian university students?**
   a. cocaine
   b. hallucinogens
   c. marijuana
   d. opioids

3. **Caffeine use can produce physical dependence.**
   True or false?

4. **Which of the following drugs is most addictive?**
   a. marijuana
   b. nicotine
   c. LSD

5. **About what percentage of street drugs contain the promised primary ingredient?**
   a. 50%
   b. 66%
   c. 75%

ANSWERS

1. **FALSE.** Both assertions in this statement are wrong. Addiction does not always involve a drug, but even when it does, withdrawing from that drug may not result in physical symptoms.

2. **C.** Marijuana ranks first, followed by hallucinogens and opioids. Alcohol remains by far the most popular drug among postsecondary students.

3. **TRUE.** Regular users of caffeine develop physical tolerance, needing more caffeine to produce the same level of alertness. Many also experience withdrawal symptoms, such as headaches and irritability, when they decrease their intake.

4. **B.** Nicotine is believed to be the most highly addictive psychoactive drug.

5. **A.** This figure is even lower for drugs that are difficult to obtain or manufacture. Street drugs may be sold in unsafe dosages and are typically mixed ("cut") with cheaper and often more hazardous substances.

The use of **drugs** for both medical and social purposes is widespread in Canada (Table 14.1). Many people believe that every problem has or should have a chemical solution. For fatigue, many turn to caffeine; for insomnia, sleeping pills; for anxiety or boredom, alcohol or other recreational drugs. Advertisements, social pressures, and the human desire for quick solutions to life's difficult problems all contribute to the prevailing attitude that drugs can ease all pain. Unfortunately, using drugs can—and often does—have serious consequences.

The most serious consequences are abuse and addiction. The drugs most often associated with abuse are **psychoactive drugs**—those that alter a person's experiences or consciousness. In the short term, psychoactive drugs can cause **intoxication**, a state in which sometimes unpredictable physical and emotional changes occur. A person who is intoxicated may experience potentially serious changes in physical functioning. His or her emotions and judgment may be affected in ways that lead to uncharacteristic and unsafe behaviour. In the long term, recurrent drug use can have profound physical, emotional, and social effects.

This chapter introduces the concept of addictive behaviour, and then focuses on the major classes of psychoactive drugs, their effects, their potential for abuse and addiction, and other issues related to their use. Alcohol and nicotine—two of the most widely used and most harmful psychoactive drugs—are discussed in Chapters 15 and 16.

ADDICTIVE BEHAVIOUR

Although addiction is most often associated with drug use, many experts now extend the concept of addiction to other behaviours. **Addictive behaviours** are habits that have gotten out of control, with resulting negative effects on a person's health. Looking at the nature of addiction and a range of addictive behaviours can help us understand similar behaviours when they involve drugs.

What Is Addiction?

The word *addiction* tends to be a highly charged one for most people. Most of us think of true addiction as a habitual and uncontrollable behaviour, usually involving the use of a drug. Some people think of addiction as a moral flaw or a personal weakness. Others think addictions arise from certain personality traits, genetic factors, or socioeconomic influences. Views on the causes of addictions have an impact on our attitudes toward people with addictive disorders, as well as on the approaches to treatment.

Historically, the term *addiction* was applied only when the habitual use of a drug produced chemical changes in the user's body. One such change is physical tolerance, in which the body adapts to a drug so that the initial dose no longer produces the original emotional or psychological effects. This process, caused by chemical changes, means the user has to take larger and larger doses of the drug to

VITAL STATISTICS

Table 14.1 — Nonmedical Drug Use Among Canadians, 2009

	Percentage Using Substance in the Past Year	
	Young Adults (ages 15–24)	All Canadians (ages 15 and older)
Tobacco (cigarettes*)	36.0	18.0
Alcohol	75.5	76.5
Heavy drinker†	22.3	8.8
Cannabis (marijuana and hashish)	26.3	10.6
Cocaine/crack	3.0	1.2
Methamphetamine/ crystal meth	N/A	0.1
Hallucinogens	4.4	0.9
Ecstasy	3.6	0.9
Speed	3.7‡	0.4
Nonmedical use of pharmaceuticals	1.7	0.6
Pain relievers	1.2	0.4
Sedatives	0.8‡	0.2
Stimulants	1.2‡	0.1

Sources: Health Canada. 2009. *Canadian Alcohol and Drug Use Monitoring Survey (CADUMS): Summary of Results for 2008* (http://www.hc-sc.gc.ca/hc-ps/drugs-drogues/stat/_2008/summary-sommaire-eng.php#intro; retrieved March 31, 2010); Health Canada. 2010. *Canadian Alcohol and Drug Use Monitoring Survey (CADUMS): Summary of Results for 2009* (http://www.hc-sc.gc.ca/hc-ps/drugs-drogues/stat/_2009/summary-sommaire-eng.php; retrieved February 5, 2011); Health Canada. 2010. *Canadian Tobacco Use Monitoring Survey (CTUMS) 2009: Summary of Annual Results for 2009* (http://www.statcan.gc.ca/daily-quotidien/100927/dq100927c-eng.htm; retrieved February 5, 2011).

* Percentage of Canadians who identified themselves as a "current smoker" in 2009.

† A person who usually consumes five or more drinks on each drinking occasion.

‡ Most recent data available are from 2008.

N/A = data not available

achieve the same high. (Tolerance is discussed in greater detail later in the chapter.) The concept of addiction as a disease process, one based in brain chemistry rather than a moral failing, has led to many advances in the understanding and treatment of drug addiction.

As scientists have learned about addictive behaviours, they have been able to distinguish between different levels of addiction. In particular, the concepts of drug **addiction** and drug **habituation** have been defined over the past few decades to help explain how drug use affects people's lives in different ways. These two terms are often differentiated as follows:

- *Drug addiction* is defined by four important characteristics: the compulsive desire for a drug, the need to increase the dosage associated with psychological and physical dependence, harmful effects to the individual, and harm to society.

- *Drug habituation* (or habit) is often considered to mean a lesser version of addiction. While sharing the same behavioural patterns with drug addiction, drug habituation is defined by the routine use of a drug but without reaching a level of compulsion or increased need for greater dosage associated with drug addiction. Further, drug habituation is accompanied by psychological but not physical dependence.

Distinguishing among different levels of drug addiction is important for developing and implementing successful prevention and treatment strategies for drug use. The definitions of drug addiction and drug habituation, however, are under continual debate.

Some scientists think that other behaviours may share some of the chemistry of drug addiction. They suggest that some activities, such as gambling, eating, exercising, and having sex, trigger the release of brain chemicals that cause a pleasurable rush in much the same way that psychoactive drugs do. The brain's own chemicals thus become the "drug" that can cause addiction. These theorists suggest that all addictions—whether to drugs or to pleasurable activities—have a common mechanism in the brain. In this view, addiction is partly the result of our own natural wiring.

The view that addiction is based in our brain chemistry does *not* imply that people are not responsible for their addictive behaviour. Many experts believe that it is inaccurate and counterproductive to think of all bad habits and excessive behaviours as diseases. They point to other factors, especially lifestyle and personality traits, that play key roles in the development of addictive behaviours.

Characteristics of Addictive Behaviour

It is often difficult to distinguish between a healthy habit and one that has become an addiction. Experts have identified some general characteristics typically associated with addictive behaviours:

- *Reinforcement.* Addictive behaviours are reinforcing. Some aspect of the behaviour produces pleasurable physical or emotional states or relieves negative ones.

- *Compulsion or craving.* The individual feels a strong compulsion—a compelling need—to engage in the behaviour, often accompanied by obsessive planning for the next opportunity to perform it.

- *Loss of control.* The individual loses control over the behaviour and cannot block the impulse to do it.

- *Escalation.* Addiction often involves a pattern of escalation, in which more and more of a particular substance or activity is required to produce its desired effects.

- *Negative consequences.* The behaviour continues despite serious negative consequences, such as problems with academic or job performance, personal relationships, and health; legal or financial troubles are also typical.

The Development of Addiction

We all engage in activities that are potentially addictive. Some of these activities can be good for you if they are done appropriately and in moderation. But if a behaviour starts to be excessive, it may become an addiction.

An addiction often starts when a person does something to bring pleasure or avoid pain. The activity may be drinking a beer, using the Internet, playing the lottery, or going shopping. If it works, the person is likely to repeat it. He or she becomes increasingly dependent on the behaviour, and tolerance may develop—that is, the person needs more of the behaviour to feel the same effect. Eventually, the behaviour becomes a central focus of the person's life, and there is a deterioration in other areas, such as academic or job performance or relationships. The behaviour no longer brings pleasure, but it is necessary to avoid the pain of going without it. What started as a seemingly innocent way of feeling good can become a prison.

Although many common behaviours are potentially addictive, most people who engage in them do not develop problems. The reason lies in the combination of factors that are involved in the development of addiction, including personality, lifestyle, heredity, the social and physical environment, and the nature of the substance or behaviour in question. For a behaviour to become an addiction, these diverse factors must come together in a certain way. For example, nicotine (the psychoactive drug in tobacco) has very high potential for physical addiction; but a person must submit to the temptation to start using tobacco—whether prompted by peer pressure, stress, or personality traits—to develop an addiction to it.

Characteristics of People with Addictions

The causes and course of an addiction are extremely varied, but people with addictions seem to share some characteristics. Many use a substance or an activity as a substitute for healthier coping strategies. People vary in their ability

drug   Any chemical other than food intended to affect the structure or function of the body.

psychoactive drug   A chemical that can alter a person's consciousness or experience.

intoxication   The state of being mentally affected by a chemical (literally, a state of being poisoned).

addictive behaviour   Any habit that has gotten out of control, resulting in a negative effect on a person's health.

addiction   Psychological or physical dependence on a substance or behaviour, characterized by a compulsive desire and increasing need for the substance or behaviour, and by harm to the individual or society.

habituation   Similar to addiction, involving the routine use of a substance, but without the level of compulsion or increasing need that characterizes addiction.

TERMS

to manage their lives, and those who have the most trouble dealing with stress and painful emotions may be more susceptible to addiction.

Some people may have a genetic predisposition to addiction to a particular substance; such predispositions may involve variations in brain chemistry. People with addictive disorders usually have a distinct preference for a particular addictive behaviour. They also often have problems with impulse control and self-regulation, and tend to be risk takers.

Examples of Addictive Behaviours

Some behaviours that are not related to drugs can become addictive for some people.

Compulsive or Pathological Gambling   Compulsive gamblers cannot control the urge to gamble, even in the face of financial and personal ruin. Most compulsive gamblers seek excitement even more than money. Increasingly larger bets are necessary to produce the desired level of excitement. When financial resources become strained, the person may lie or steal to pay off debts. The consequences of compulsive gambling are not just financial; the Canada Safety Council estimates that more than 200 compulsive gamblers take their own lives every year.

The American Psychiatric Association (APA), an organization composed of mental health professionals from around the world, recognizes pathological gambling as a mental disorder. The APA lists 10 characteristic behaviours associated with pathological gambling, including preoccupation with gambling, unsuccessful efforts to cut back or quit, using gambling to escape problems, and lying to family members to conceal the extent of involvement with gambling. Gambling is often linked to other risky behaviours, and many compulsive gamblers also have drug and alcohol abuse problems.

In Canada, it is estimated that 1% of adults are compulsive (pathological) gamblers, and another 5% develop gambling-related problems. In a 2004 survey of more than 6000 undergraduate students from 40 Canadian universities, 61.5% of students reported having gambled at least once since the beginning of the school year, and 7.9% were considered to be at risk for developing serious gambling problems.

Compulsive Exercising   When taken to a compulsive level, even healthy activities may develop into harmful addictions. For example, compulsive exercising has been

Many postsecondary students have gotten caught up in the poker craze. A 2006 survey of Ontarians revealed that approximately one-third of young adults ages 18–34 play poker for money.

widely studied and is now recognized as a serious departure from normal behaviour. Compulsive exercising is often accompanied by more severe psychiatric disorders, such as anorexia nervosa and bulimia (Chapter 4). Traits frequently associated with compulsive exercising include an excessive preoccupation and dissatisfaction with body image, the use of laxatives or vomiting to lose weight, and the development of other obsessive-compulsive symptoms.

Experts don't completely agree on what frequency and intensity of physical activity constitute compulsive exercising. Many compulsive exercisers, however, get involved in physical activities that cause bodily harm. For example, research has shown that professional bodybuilders, when compared with recreational exercisers engaged in weight lifting, are often dissatisfied with muscle size. Because of their preoccupation with muscle size, and because of the frequency and intensity of their workouts, some body builders face an increased risk of injuries through harmful weight-lifting practices.

Work Addiction   The term *workaholic* is often used to describe individuals with an excessive preoccupation with work and work-related activities. Work addiction, however, is actually based on a set of symptoms, including the following:

• An intense work schedule

• The inability to limit your own work schedule

• The inability to relax, even when away from work

• Failed attempts at curtailing the intensity of work (in some cases)

Many of these traits are also seen in other types of addiction, such as alcoholism—hence the popularity of the word *workaholism*.

Work addiction is a serious concern for various reasons. Someone suffering from this addiction is likely to neglect other areas of his or her life. For example, work addicts may tend to exercise less, spend less time with family and friends, and stay away from social activities.

Further, work addiction typically coincides with a well-known risk factor for cardiovascular disease—the type A personality (Chapter 7). Traits associated with type A personality include competitiveness, ambition, drive, time urgency, restlessness, and hyperalertness.

Many researchers see work addiction as a culture-bound disorder arising from a workplace that encourages these harmful behavioural patterns. The changing landscape of the modern workplace is likely to make work addiction a source of disability for a growing number of people.

Sex and Love Addiction   More controversial is the notion of addiction to sex or love. Some researchers believe that the initial rush of arousal and erotic or romantic chemistry produces an effect in the brain comparable to that of taking amphetamines or morphine. After a time, the brain becomes desensitized, and the addict must then seek his or her next rush by pursuing a new partner. According to this view, cheating on a partner, having many partners, and sexually victimizing others are behaviours parallel to drug-seeking behaviour. Behaviours associated with sex addiction include having an extreme preoccupation with sex, feeling a compulsion to have sex repeatedly within a short time, spending a great deal of time and energy looking for partners or engaging in sex, using sex as a means of relieving painful feelings, and suffering negative emotional, personal, and professional consequences as a result of sexual activities.

Some experts are reluctant to call compulsive sexual activity a true addiction. However, even therapists who challenge the concept of sex addiction recognize that some people become overly preoccupied with sex, cannot seem to control their sex drive, and act in potentially harmful ways to obtain satisfaction. This pattern of sexual behaviour seems to meet the criteria for addictive behaviours discussed earlier.

Compulsive Buying or Shopping   A compulsive buyer repeatedly gives in to the impulse to buy more than he or she needs or can afford. Compulsive spenders usually buy

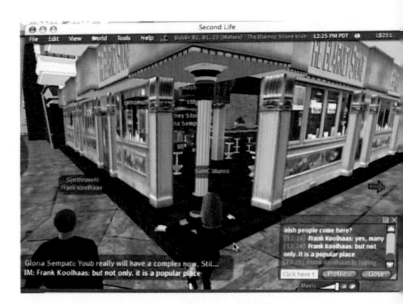

Because the Internet provides easy access to so many different kinds of content, many Canadians experience Internet addiction.

luxury items rather than daily necessities. Compulsive shoppers are usually distressed by their behaviour and its social, personal, and financial consequences. Some experts link compulsive shopping with neglect or abuse during childhood; it also seems to be associated with eating disorders, depression, and bipolar disorder.

Internet Addiction   In the years since the Internet became widely available, millions of Canadians have become compulsive Internet users. To spend more time online, Internet addicts skip important school, social, or recreational activities; compulsive Internet users often spend their work time online, a fact that has led many employers to adopt strict Internet usage policies. Despite negative financial, social, or academic consequences, compulsive Internet users don't feel able to stop. As with other addictive behaviours, online addicts may be using their behaviour to alleviate stress or avoid painful emotions.

Generally speaking, studies have shown that 5%–10% of Internet users may experience Internet addiction. One study showed that Internet addicts spent an average of 38 hours online every week. There is concern that the number of Internet addicts will continue growing as the Internet becomes more accessible.

Other behaviours that can become addictive include eating, watching TV, and playing video games. Any substance or activity that becomes the focus of a person's life at the expense of other needs and interests can be damaging to health.

DRUG USE, ABUSE, AND DEPENDENCE

The substances most commonly associated with addiction are psychoactive drugs. Drugs are chemicals other than food that are intended to affect the structure or function of the body. They include prescription medicines, such as antibiotics and antidepressants; nonprescription or over-the-counter (OTC) substances, such as alcohol, tobacco, and caffeine products; and illegal substances, such as LSD and heroin. The use of drugs is not new in society; drug use has a long history.

The Drug Tradition

Using drugs to alter consciousness is an ancient and universal pursuit. People have used alcohol for celebration and intoxication for thousands of years. People in all parts of the world have exploited the psychoactive properties of various local plants, such as the coca plant in South America and the opium poppy in the Far East.

In the nineteenth century, chemists began extracting the active chemicals from medicinal plants, such as morphine from the opium poppy and cocaine from the coca leaf. This was the beginning of modern **pharmacy**, the art of compounding drugs, and of **pharmacology**, the science and study of drugs. From this point on, a variety of drugs began to be produced, including codeine, LSD, methamphetamine, and heroin.

For generations, the manufacture and sale of these new drugs were not regulated. Pure morphine or cocaine could be purchased by mail order, and the makers of patent medicines and tonics included potentially addictive drugs in their products without informing consumers of either the ingredients or the dangers. The earliest version of the soft drink Coca-Cola contained cocaine, for example, which accounted for the lift it provided.

Drug addiction among middle-class Europeans and North Americans was more common by 1900 than at any time before or since. Concerns about drug addiction and the need to regulate drug sales and manufacture led in the early 1900s to the passage of harsh federal drug laws in Canada. Middle-class use of regulated drugs dropped, and drug use became increasingly identified with criminal subcultures.

Nonmedical (recreational) drug use expanded in Canada during the 1960s and 1970s and then declined until the early to mid-1990s, when drug use rates began to rise in certain high-risk segments of the Canadian population. According to Health Canada, illicit drug use among youth ages 12–17 has increased consistently since the late 1980s. In 2008, drug use among young adults ages 15–24 remained substantially higher than that reported by Canadians 25 years and older: four times as high for cannabis use and nine times as high for the use of any other illicit drug.

Drug Abuse and Dependence

The APA's *Diagnostic and Statistical Manual of Mental Disorders* is used by Canadian mental health professionals and is the authoritative reference for defining all sorts of behavioural disorders, including those related to drugs. The APA

has chosen not to use the term addiction, in part because it is so broad and has so many connotations. Instead, the APA refers to two forms of substance (drug) disorders: substance abuse and substance dependence. Both are maladaptive patterns of substance use that lead to significant impairment or distress. Although the APA's definitions are more precise and more directly related to drug use, they clearly encompass the general characteristics of addictive behaviour described in the preceding section.

Abuse   As defined by the APA, **substance abuse** involves one or more of the following:

- Recurrent drug use, resulting in a failure to fulfil major responsibilities at work, school, or home
- Recurrent drug use in situations in which it is physically hazardous, such as before or while driving a car
- Recurrent drug-related legal problems
- Continued drug use despite persistent social or interpersonal problems caused or exacerbated by the effects of the drug

The pattern of use may be constant or intermittent, and **physical dependence** may or may not be present. For example, a person who smokes marijuana once a week and cuts classes because he or she is high is abusing marijuana, even though he or she is not physically dependent.

Dependence   Substance dependence is a more complex disorder and is what many people associate with the idea of addiction. The seven specific criteria the APA uses to diagnose substance dependence are listed below. The first two are associated with physical dependence; the final five are associated with compulsive use. To be considered dependent, a person must experience a cluster of three or more of these symptoms during a 12-month period.

1. Developing **tolerance** to the substance. When a person requires increased amounts of a substance to achieve the desired effect or notices a markedly diminished effect with continued use of the same amount, he or she has developed tolerance.

2. Experiencing **withdrawal**. In an individual who has maintained prolonged, heavy use of a substance, a drop in its concentration within the body can result in unpleasant physical and cognitive withdrawal symptoms. Withdrawal symptoms are different for different drugs. For example, nausea, vomiting, and tremors are common for alcohol, opioids, and sedatives. Some drugs have no significant withdrawal symptoms.

3. Taking the substance in larger amounts or over a longer period than was originally intended.

4. Expressing a persistent desire to cut down or regulate substance use.

5. Spending a great deal of time obtaining the substance, using the substance, or recovering from its effects.

6. Giving up or reducing important social, school, work, or recreational activities because of substance use.

7. Continuing to use the substance in spite of recognizing that it is contributing to a psychological or physical problem.

If a person who is drug dependent experiences either tolerance or withdrawal, he or she is considered physically dependent. However, not everyone who experiences tolerance or withdrawal is drug dependent. For example, a hospital patient who is prescribed therapeutic doses of morphine to relieve pain may develop a tolerance to the drug and experience withdrawal symptoms when the prescription is discontinued. But without showing any signs of compulsive use, this individual would not be considered dependent.

Conversely, dependence can occur without a physical component, based solely on compulsive use. For example, people with at least three symptoms of compulsive use of marijuana who show no signs of tolerance or withdrawal are suffering from substance dependence. In general, dependence problems that involve physical dependence carry a greater risk of immediate general medical problems and higher relapse rates.

Who Uses Drugs?

The use and abuse of drugs occur at all income and education levels, among all ethnic groups, and at all ages (see the box "Drug Use Among University Students" on p. 448). Society is concerned with the casual or recreational use of illegal drugs because it is not really possible to know when drug use will lead to abuse or dependence. Some casual users develop substance-related problems; others do not. Some psychoactive drugs are more likely than others to lead to dependence, but some users of even heroin or cocaine do not meet the APA's criteria for substance dependence.

It isn't possible to accurately predict which drug users will become abusers, but young people at a high risk of *trying* drugs share certain characteristics:

- *Being young.* People who start using drugs when they're very young have a greater risk of dependence and health consequences.

- *Being male.* Males are typically more likely than females to abuse illicit drugs (see the box "Gender Differences in Drug Use and Abuse" on p. 449).

- *Being a troubled adolescent.* Teens are more likely to try drugs if they have poor self-image or self-control, use tobacco, or suffer from certain mental or emotional problems.

- *Being a thrill-seeker.* A sense of invincibility is a factor in drug experimentation.

- *Being in a dysfunctional family.* A chaotic home life or parental abuse increases the risk of drug use. The same is true for children from a single-parent home or whose parents didn't complete high school.

- *Being in a peer group that accepts drug use.* Young people who are uninterested in school and earn poor grades are more likely to try drugs.

- *Being poor.* Young people who live in disadvantaged areas are more likely to be around drugs at a young age.

- *Dating young.* Adolescent girls who date boys two or more years older than themselves are more likely to use drugs.

What about people who *don't* use drugs? As a group, nonusers also share some characteristics. Not surprisingly, people who perceive drug use as risky and who disapprove of it are less likely to use drugs than those who believe otherwise. Drug use is also less common among people who have positive self-esteem and self-concept and who are assertive, independent thinkers who are not controlled by peer pressure. Self-control, social competence, optimism, academic achievement, and regular church attendance are also linked to lower rates of drug use (see the box "Spirituality and Drug Abuse" on p. 450).

Home environments are also influential: Coming from a strong family, one that has a clear policy on drug use, is another characteristic of people who don't use drugs. Young people who communicate openly with their parents and feel supported by them are also less likely to use drugs.

TERMS

pharmacy The art of compounding drugs from various substances.

pharmacology The science and study of drugs.

substance abuse A maladaptive pattern of using any substance that persists despite adverse social, psychological, or medical consequences. The pattern may be intermittent, with or without tolerance and physical dependence.

physical dependence The result of physiological adaptation that occurs in response to the frequent presence of a drug; typically associated with tolerance and withdrawal.

substance dependence A cluster of cognitive, behavioural, and physiological symptoms that occur in someone who continues to use a substance despite suffering significant substance-related problems, leading to considerable impairment or distress; also known as *addiction*.

tolerance Lower sensitivity to a drug so that a given dose no longer exerts the usual effect and larger doses are needed.

withdrawal Physical and psychological symptoms that follow the interrupted use of a drug on which a user is physically dependent; symptoms may be mild or life threatening.

Drug Use Among University Students

Drug use in university has long been recognized as a significant health problem that affects many students. According to the 2004 *Canadian Campus Survey* data from the Centre for Addiction and Mental Health, 16.7% of university undergraduates reported the use of cannabis (marijuana or hashish or both) in the past 30 days, while 2.2% reported using other illicit drugs. Overall, these numbers remained relatively stable from 1998 to 2004. The same survey shows that past-year alcohol use, heavy and frequent drinking, and hazardous and harmful drinking remained steady among Canadian undergraduates from 1998 to 2004, while cigarette smoking and past-year use of hallucinogens decreased.

The *Canadian Campus Survey* shows that recreational drug use is fairly common among university students. For example, 5.6% of university students reported using hallucinogens at least once in the past year, while another 5% reported using opioids and 2.5% reported using ecstasy. Finally, 2.1% said they had used cocaine at least once in the past year, and 2.6% reported using amphetamines.

Drug use on university campuses has been examined extensively, and many experts believe that no single factor can explain the widespread impact of this phenomenon. Family history, peer pressure, depression, anxiety, low self-esteem, and the dynamics of university life (for example, the drive to compete and distorted perceptions of drug use among peers) have been suggested as potential explanations for drug use among university students.

Excessive alcohol use often accompanies illicit drug use. In fact, the term *AOD* (alcohol and other drug) has been developed to refer to this type of substance use among university students. Further, AOD use and depression or anxiety are generally recognized as coexisting conditions that require a comprehensive approach to prevention and treatment. Despite the growing awareness among university counsellors and other health professionals who work with university students, it is not entirely clear whether anxiety and depression precede the onset of alcohol and drug use, or whether early exposure to alcohol and drug use before university exacerbates more serious psychiatric disorders by the time a student enters university. A third line of research suggests that AOD use, depression, and anxiety share common causes, such as genetic predisposition or family history. However, one aspect of drug use among university students remains clear: AOD use has dramatic consequences for the educational, family, and community life of students. Poor academic performance has been linked with AOD use. Further, driving while intoxicated remains one of the most dangerous outcomes associated with AOD use affecting families and communities. Fortunately, several AOD prevention programs are now under way at university campuses across Canada.

Source for data: Adlaf, E. M., et al. (eds.). 2005. *Canadian Campus Survey 2004.* Toronto: Centre for Addiction and Mental Health.

Why Do People Use Drugs?

Young people, especially those from middle-class backgrounds, are frequently drawn to drugs by the allure of the exciting and illegal. They may be curious, rebellious, or vulnerable to peer pressure. Young people may want to imitate adult models in their lives or in the movies. Most people who take illicit drugs do so experimentally, typically trying the drug one or more times but not continuing. The main factors in the initial choice of a drug are whether it is available and whether peers are using it.

Although some people use drugs because they have a desire to alter their mood or are seeking a spiritual experience, others are motivated primarily by a desire to escape boredom, anxiety, depression, feelings of worthlessness, or other distressing symptoms of psychological problems. They use drugs as a way to cope with the difficulties they are experiencing in life. The common practice in our society of seeking a drug solution to every problem is a factor in the widespread reliance on both illicit and prescription drugs.

For people living in poverty, many of these reasons for using drugs are magnified. The problems are more devastating, the need for escape more compelling. Furthermore, the buying and selling of drugs provide access to an unofficial, alternative economy that may seem like an opportunity for success.

Risk Factors for Dependence

Why do some people use psychoactive drugs without becoming dependent, whereas others aren't as lucky? The answer seems to be a combination of physical, psychological, and social factors. Research indicates that some people may be born with certain characteristics of brain chemistry or metabolism that make them more vulnerable to drug dependence. Other research suggests that people who were exposed to drugs while still in the womb may have an increased risk of abusing drugs themselves later in life.

Psychological risk factors for drug dependence include difficulty controlling impulses and a strong need for

Gender Differences in Drug Use and Abuse

Generally speaking, men are more likely than women to use, abuse, and be dependent on illicit drugs (see table). In Canada, men are also more likely than women to have problems associated with drug use, including harm to at least one of the following: physical health; friendships and social life; financial position; home life or marriage; work, studies, or employment opportunities; legal problems; difficulty learning; and housing problems.

Drug use among Canadian youth has increased consistently since the late 1980s. Gender differences in *why* and *how* young people use drugs are well known. Young males tend to use alcohol or drugs for sensation seeking or to enhance their social status, factors tied to culturally based gender roles. Young women tend to use drugs to improve mood, increase confidence, and reduce inhibitions. Boys are more likely to receive offers to use drugs in public settings, whereas girls are more likely to receive offers in a private place, such as a friend's residence.

Despite overall lower rates of drug use, females may have unique biological vulnerabilities to certain drugs, and they may move more quickly from use to abuse. Major life transitions, including the physical and emotional changes associated with puberty, increase the risk of drug use and abuse for girls more so than for

boys. Certain other drug abuse risk factors are also more common in female adolescents, including depression, low self-esteem, eating disorders, and a history of physical or sexual abuse.

Adolescent boys and girls share some protective factors relating to drug abuse, including positive family relationships and extracurricular activities; religious involvement is protective for both boys and girls but may be more protective for girls.

Among older men and women, marriage, children, and employment are associated with lower rates of drug abuse and dependence. Rates of drug abuse and dependence among married adults are less than half of those among unmarried adults. Similar patterns are seen when comparing adults who live with children versus those who do not live with children and adults who are employed versus those who are unemployed.

	National Survey Results, 2009: Percentage of Adults (Ages 15+) Reporting Usage in Past Year	
	Males	Females
Cannabis (marijuana and hashish)	14.2	7.2
Cocaine/crack	1.5	0.9
Speed	1.3†	0.8†
Hallucinogens	1.1	0.8
Ecstasy	1.1	0.7
Any pharmaceutical* used to get high	0.7	0.4
Drug-related harms to self	3.5†	1.8†

* Pharmaceuticals include prescription-type pain relievers, stimulants, and sedatives.
† Most recent data available are from 2008.

Sources: Health Canada. 2009. *Canadian Alcohol and Drug Use Monitoring Survey (CADUMS): Summary of Results for 2008* (http://www.hc-sc.gc.ca/hc-ps/drugs-drogues/stat/_2008/summary-sommaire-eng.php#drug; retrieved February 5, 2011); Health Canada. 2010. *Canadian Alcohol and Drug Use Monitoring Survey (CADUMS): Summary of Results for 2009* (http://www.hc-sc.gc.ca/hc-ps/drugs-drogues/stat/_2009/summary-sommaire-eng.php; retrieved February 5, 2011).

excitement, stimulation, and immediate gratification. Feelings of rejection, hostility, aggression, anxiety, or depression are also associated with drug dependence. People may turn to drugs to blot out their emotional pain.

People with mental health problems have a very high risk of substance dependence. Research shows that about one-third of people with psychological disorders also have a substance-dependence problem and about one-third of those have another mental disorder. People with two or more coexisting mental disorders are referred to as having **dual (co-occurring) disorders**. Diagnosis of psychological problems among people with substance dependence can be very difficult because drug intoxication and withdrawal can mimic the symptoms of a mental health problem.

Social factors that may influence drug dependence include growing up in a family in which a parent or sibling abused drugs, belonging to a peer group that emphasizes and encourages drug abuse, and living in poverty. Because they have easy access to drugs, health care professionals

are also at a higher risk. To determine whether you are at risk, take the quiz in the box "Do You Have a Problem with Drugs?" on p. 251.

Other Risks of Drug Use

Dependence is not the only serious potential consequence of drug use. In 2002, illnesses related to illegal drug use accounted for more than 350,000 days of acute care in Canadian hospitals.

Intoxication   People who are under the influence of drugs—intoxicated—may act in uncharacteristic and unsafe ways because both their physical and their mental func-

dual (co-occurring) disorder   The presence of two or more mental disorders, such as drug dependence and depression, simultaneously in the same person.

TERMS

Spirituality and Drug Abuse

Although religious viewpoints on drug use are diverse, many religions infer some link between psychoactive drugs and spirituality. Some religions use drugs in the quest for spiritual transcendence: for example, Polynesian, African, and other indigenous religions have used psychoactive drugs, such as peyote, khat, alcohol, and hashish, for expanding consciousness and developing personal spirituality. Other religions view psychoactive drugs as a threat to spirituality. In Islam, for example, the consumption of alcohol and certain other drugs is strictly forbidden.

Research with teens and adults has shown that spiritual or religious involvement is generally associated with a lower risk of trying psychoactive drugs and, for those who do use drugs, a lower risk of heavy use and dependence. The mechanism for this protective effect is unclear; possibilities include the adoption of a strict code of behaviour or set of principles that forbids drug use, the presence of a social support system for abstinence or moderation, and the promotion of values that include avoidance of drug use.

The relationship between religious faith and avoidance of drug use appears to be even stronger in teens than in adults. One study found that teens who felt they had a personal relationship with the divine or who belonged to a more fundamentalist religious denomination were less likely to engage in substance use and abuse than other teens. Teens who attend 25 or more religious services per year are about half as likely to use illicit drugs as teens who attend services less frequently. Overall, people who spend time regularly engaging in spiritual practices, such as prayer and transcendental meditation, have lower rates of drug abuse.

People with current substance-abuse problems tend to have lower rates of religious affiliation and involvement and lower levels of spiritual wellness, characterized by a lack of a sense of meaning in life. One of the hallmarks of drug dependence is spending increasing amounts of time and energy obtaining and using drugs; such a pattern of behaviour inevitably reduces the resources an individual puts toward developing physical, emotional, and spiritual wellness.

Among people in treatment for substance abuse, higher levels of religious faith and spirituality may contribute to the recovery process. A study of people recovering from alcohol or other drug abuse found that spirituality and religiousness were associated with better coping skills, greater optimism about life, greater resilience to stress, and greater perceived social support.

More research is needed to clarify the relationships among spirituality, religion, drug use, and recovery. One of the difficulties in conducting research in this area is the difficulty in defining and measuring spirituality and religious involvement. Spirituality is a complex part of human nature, involving behaviour, belief, and

experience. And although some behaviours, such as the spiritual practices of prayer or meditation, can be measured, it is more difficult to determine what such practices mean to an individual and her or his overall sense of self.

Sources: Brown, A. E., et al. 2006. Alcohol recovery and spirituality: Strangers, friends, or partners? *Southern Medical Journal* 99(6): 654–657; Substance Abuse and Mental Health Network. 2004. Religious beliefs and substance use among youths. *NSDUH Report*, January; Dunn, M. S. 2005. The relationship between religiosity, employment, and political beliefs on substance use among high school seniors. *Journal of Alcohol and Drug Education* 49(1): 73.

tioning are impaired. They are more likely to be injured from a variety of causes, including falls, drowning, and automobile crashes; to engage in unsafe sex, increasing their risk for sexually transmitted infections and unintended pregnancy; and to be involved in incidents of aggression and violence, including sexual assault.

Unexpected Side Effects Psychoactive drugs have many physical and psychological effects beyond the alteration of consciousness. These effects range from nausea and constipation to paranoia, depression, and heart failure. Some drugs also carry the risk of fatal overdose.

Unknown Drug Constituents There is no quality control in the illegal drug market, so the composition, dosage, and toxicity of street drugs is highly variable. Studies indicate that half of all street drugs don't contain their promised primary ingredient; in some cases, a drug may be present in unsafe dosages or mixed with other drugs to boost the effects. Careless manufacturing practices can result in the presence of toxic contaminants.

Risks Associated with Injection Drug Use Heroin and related substances are the most commonly injected drugs, but individuals can also inject cocaine, amphetamines, and other drugs. Many people who inject drugs share or reuse needles, syringes, and other injection equipment, which can easily become contaminated with the user's blood. Small amounts of blood can carry enough human immunodeficiency virus (HIV) and hepatitis C virus (HCV) to be infectious. In 2008, injection drug use (IDU) accounted for about 19% of all new HIV/AIDS cases in

Do You Have a Problem with Drugs?

Answer yes (Y) or no (N) to the following questions:

_____ 1. Do you take the drug regularly?

_____ 2. Have you been taking the drug for a long time?

_____ 3. Do you always take the drug in certain situations or when you're with certain people?

_____ 4. Do you find it difficult to stop using the drug? Do you feel powerless to quit?

_____ 5. Have you tried repeatedly to cut down or control your use of the drug?

_____ 6. Do you need to take a larger dose of the drug to get the same high you're used to?

_____ 7. Do you feel specific symptoms if you cut back or stop using the drug?

_____ 8. Do you frequently take another psychoactive substance to relieve withdrawal symptoms?

_____ 9. Do you take the drug to feel normal?

_____ 10. Do you go to extreme lengths or put yourself in dangerous situations to get the drug?

_____ 11. Do you hide your drug use from others? Have you ever lied about what you're using or how much you use?

_____ 12. Do people close to you ask you about your drug use?

_____ 13. Are you spending more and more time with people who use the same drug as you?

_____ 14. Do you think about the drug when you're not high, figuring out ways to get it?

_____ 15. If you stop taking the drug, do you feel bad until you can take it again?

_____ 16. Does the drug interfere with your ability to study, work, or socialize?

_____ 17. Do you skip important school, work, social, or recreational activities to obtain or use the drug?

_____ 18. Do you continue to use the drug despite a physical or mental disorder or despite a significant problem that you know is made worse by drug use?

_____ 19. Have you developed a mental or physical condition or disorder because of prolonged drug use?

_____ 20. Have you done something dangerous or that you regret while under the influence of the drug?

The more times you answer yes, the more likely it is that you are developing a dependence on the drug. If your answers suggest dependence, talk to someone at your school health clinic or to your physician about taking care of the problem before it gets worse.

Canada; many more were attributed to sexual contact with people who inject drugs. IDU also accounts for the majority of HCV infections.

Unsterile injection practices can cause skin and soft tissue infections, which can progress to gangrene and be fatal if untreated. Other risks include endocarditis (infection of the heart valves), tuberculosis, and tetanus.

The surest way to prevent diseases related to IDU is never to inject drugs. Those who inject drugs should use a new needle and syringe with each injection and should use sterile water and other equipment to prepare drugs. Bleach or boiling water may kill some viruses and bacteria, but they are not foolproof sterilization methods. Many viruses can survive in a syringe for a month or more.

Syringe exchange programs (SEPs)—where people who inject drugs can trade a used syringe for a new one—have been advocated to help slow the spread of HIV and reduce the rates and cost of other health problems associated with IDU. Opponents of SEPs argue that supplying injection drug users with syringes gives them the message that illegal drug use is acceptable and could thus exacerbate the nation's drug problem. However, studies have shown that well-implemented SEPs do not increase the use of drugs, and most offer AIDS counselling and provide referrals to drug treatment programs. Getting people off drugs is clearly the best solution, but there are far more people who inject drugs than treatment facilities can currently handle.

Legal Consequences Many psychoactive drugs are illegal, so using them can result in large fines or imprisonment. According to Statistics Canada, the rate of police-reported drug offences reached 305 incidents per 100,000 Canadians in 2007—the highest rate in 30 years. This peak is likely related to a number of factors, including police policies, charging practices, and available resources. For example, targeted

> QUICK STATS
>
> Between **75,000 and 125,000** Canadians inject heroin, cocaine, methamphetamine, Talwin and Ritalin, or steroids.
>
> —Canadian Centre on Substance Abuse, 2009

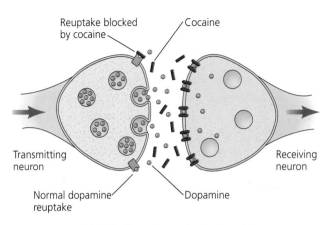

FIGURE 14.1 Effect of cocaine on brain chemistry.
Under normal circumstances, the amount of dopamine at a synapse is controlled in part by the reuptake of dopamine by the transmitting neuron. Cocaine blocks the removal of dopamine from a synapse; the resulting buildup of dopamine causes continuous stimulation of the receiving neurons.

initiatives to crack down on drugs may result in more incidents being identified by police, rather than more incidents actually occurring.

HOW DRUGS AFFECT THE BODY

The drugs discussed in this chapter have complex and variable effects, many of which can be traced to changes in brain chemistry. However, the same drug may affect different people differently or the same person in different ways under different circumstances. Beyond a fairly predictable general change in brain chemistry, the effects of a drug may vary depending on drug factors, individual factors, and social factors.

Changes in Brain Chemistry

Psychoactive drugs produce most of their key effects by acting on brain chemistry in a characteristic fashion. Before any changes in brain chemistry can occur, however, molecules of the drug have to be carried to the brain through the bloodstream via a particular route of administration. A drug that is taken by mouth has to dissolve in the stomach, be absorbed into the bloodstream through the lining of the small intestine, and then pass through the liver, heart, and lungs before returning to the heart to be carried via arteries to the brain. A drug that is already dissolved and is injected directly into the bloodstream will reach the brain in much less time, and drugs that are inhaled and absorbed by the lungs travel to the brain even more rapidly. The faster a drug reaches the brain, the more likely the user is to become dependent.

Once a psychoactive drug reaches the brain, it acts on one or more **neurotransmitters**, either increasing or decreasing the neurotransmitters' concentration and actions. Cocaine, for example, affects dopamine, a neurotransmitter thought to play a key role in the process of reinforcement—the brain's way of telling itself "That's good; do the same thing again." When a neurotransmitter is released by one neuron to signal another neuron, its level or concentration is controlled in part by the reuptake or resorption of the neurotransmitter by the releasing neuron. Cocaine inhibits the resorption of dopamine, thereby increasing the concentration of dopamine in the synapse and lengthening the time of its action (Figure 14.1). The euphoria produced

by cocaine is thought to be a result of its effect on dopamine. Heroin, nicotine, alcohol, and amphetamines also affect dopamine levels through their effects on the brain.

The duration of a drug's effect depends on many factors and may range from five minutes (crack cocaine) to 12 or more hours (LSD). As drugs circulate through the body, they are metabolized by the liver and eventually excreted by the kidneys in urine. Small amounts may also be eliminated in other ways, including in sweat, in breast milk, and via the lungs.

Drug Factors

When different drugs or dosages produce different effects, the differences are usually caused by one or more of five different drug factors:

1. The **pharmacological properties** of a drug are its overall effects on a person's body chemistry, behaviour, and psychology. The pharmacological properties also include the amount of a drug required to exert various effects, the time course of these effects, and other characteristics, such as a drug's chemical composition.

2. The **dose-response function** is the relationship between the amount of drug taken and the type and intensity of the resulting effect. Many psychological effects of drugs reach a plateau in the dose-response function and increasing the dose does not increase the effect any further. With LSD, for example, the maximum changes in perception occur at a certain dose, and no further changes in perception take place if higher doses are taken. However, all drugs have more than one effect, and the dose-response functions usually are different for different effects. This means that increasing the dose of any drug may begin to result in additional effects, which are likely to be increasingly unpleasant or dangerous at high doses.

The method of use (or route of administration) is one variable in the overall effect of a drug on the body.

Individual Factors

Certain physical and psychological characteristics also help determine how a person will respond to a drug. Body mass is one variable. The effects of a certain dose of a drug on a 50-kilogram person will be twice as great as on a 100-kilogram person. Other variables include general health and genetic factors. For example, some people have an inherited ability to rapidly metabolize a cough suppressant called dextromethorphan, which also has psychoactive properties. These people must take a higher-than-normal dose to get a given cough-suppressant effect.

If a person's biochemical state is already altered by another drug, this too can make a difference. Some drugs intensify the effects of other drugs, as is the case with alcohol and sedatives. Some drugs block the effects of other drugs, such as when a tranquilizer is used to relieve anxiety caused by cocaine. Interactions between drugs, including many prescription and OTC medications, can be unpredictable and dangerous.

One physical condition that requires special precautions is pregnancy. It can be risky for a woman to use any drugs at all during pregnancy, including alcohol and common OTC preparations like cough medicine. The risks are greatest during the first trimester, when the fetus's body is rapidly forming and even small biochemical alterations in the mother can have a devastating effect on fetal development. Even later, the fetus is more susceptible than the mother to the adverse effects of any drugs she takes. The fetus may even become physically dependent on a drug being taken by the mother and suffer withdrawal symptoms after birth.

Sometimes a person's response to a drug is strongly influenced by the individual's expectations about how he or she will react (the psychological set). With large doses, the drug's chemical properties seem to have the strongest effect on the individual's response. But with small doses, psychological (and social) factors are often more important. When people strongly believe that a given drug will affect them a certain way, they are likely to experience those effects regardless of the drug's pharmacological properties. In one study, regular users of marijuana reported a moderate level of intoxication (**high**) after using a cigarette that smelled and tasted like marijuana but contained no THC,

3. The **time-action function** is the relationship between the time elapsed since a drug was taken and the intensity of its effect. The effects of a drug are greatest when concentrations of the drug in body tissues are changing fastest, especially if they are increasing.

4. The person's drug use history may influence the effects of a drug. A given amount of alcohol, for example, will generally affect a habitual drinker less than an occasional drinker. Tolerance to some drugs, such as LSD, builds rapidly. To experience the same effect, a user has to abstain from the drug for a time before that dosage will again exert its original effects.

5. The method of use (or route of administration) has a direct effect on how strong a response a drug produces. Methods of use include ingestion, inhalation, injection, and absorption through the skin or tissue linings. Drugs are usually injected in one of three ways: intravenously (IV, or mainlining), intramuscularly (IM), or subcutaneously (SC, or skin popping).

TERMS

neurotransmitter   A brain chemical that transmits nerve impulses.

pharmacological properties   The overall effects of a drug on a person's behaviour, psychology, and chemistry.

dose-response function   The relationship between the amount of a drug taken and the intensity and type of the resulting effect.

time-action function   The relationship between the time elapsed since a drug was taken and the intensity of its effect.

high   The subjectively pleasing effects of a drug, usually felt quite soon after the drug is taken.

the active ingredient in marijuana. This is an example of the **placebo effect**: A person receives an inert substance yet responds as if it were an active drug. (The placebo effect is discussed in more detail in Chapter 19.) In other studies, subjects who smoked low doses of real marijuana that they believed to be a placebo experienced no effects from the drug. Clearly, the person's expectations had a greater effect on the smokers than the drug itself.

Social Factors

The *setting* is the physical and social environment surrounding the drug use. If a person uses marijuana at home with trusted friends and pleasant music, the effects are likely to be different from the effects if the same dose is taken in an austere experimental laboratory with an impassive research

placebo effect   A response to an inert or innocuous medication given in place of an active drug.

opioid   Any of several natural or synthetic drugs that relieve pain and cause drowsiness or euphoria; examples are opium, morphine, and heroin; also called a *narcotic*.

euphoria   An exaggerated feeling of well-being.

technician. Similarly, the dose of alcohol that produces mild euphoria and stimulation at a noisy, active cocktail party might induce sleepiness and slight depression when taken at home while alone.

REPRESENTATIVE PSYCHOACTIVE DRUGS

The following sections introduce six representative groups of psychoactive drugs (Figure 14.2 on p. 455): opioids, central nervous system (CNS) depressants, central nervous system stimulants, marijuana and other cannabis products, hallucinogens, and inhalants. Some of these drugs are classified according to how they affect the body; others— the opioids and the cannabis products—are classified according to their chemical makeup.

Opioids

Also called *narcotics*, **opioids** are natural or synthetic (laboratory-made) drugs, such as opium, morphine, heroin, methadone, codeine, hydrocodone, oxycodone, meperidine, and fentanyl. Opioids relieve pain, cause drowsiness, and induce **euphoria**. Especially in small doses, opioids have beneficial medical uses, including pain relief and cough suppression. Opioids tend to reduce anxiety and produce lethargy, apathy, and an inability to concentrate. People who use opioids become less active and less responsive to frustration, hunger, and sexual stimulation. These effects are more pronounced in novice users; with repeated use, many effects diminish.

Opioids are typically injected or absorbed into the body from the stomach, intestines, nasal membranes (from snorting or sniffing), or lungs (from smoking). Effects depend on the method of administration. If brain levels of the drug change rapidly, more immediate effects will result. Although the euphoria associated with opioids is an important factor in their abuse, many people experience a feeling of uneasiness when they first use these drugs. People who use opioids also often feel nauseated and vomit, and they may have other unpleasant sensations. Even so, the abuse of opioids often results in dependence. Tolerance can develop rapidly and be pronounced. Withdrawal symptoms include cramps, chills, sweating, nausea, tremors, irritability, and feelings of panic.

Rates of heroin use have always been low, but there are periodic episodes of increased use among some groups. In Canada, about twice as many males as females use heroin. Whereas first-time users are often young (typically in their teens or 20s), most people who use heroin regularly are over the age of 30. Heroin use among youth remains low but has increased in some locations, mostly through increased rates of sniffing or smoking the drug. Although these users avoid the special disease risks of injection drug use, including HIV infection, dependence can readily result from sniffing and smoking heroin. In

Category	Representative drugs	Street names	Appearance	Methods of use	Short-term effects
Opioids	Heroin	Dope, H, junk, brown sugar, smack	White/dark brown powder; dark tar or coal-like substance	Injected, smoked, snorted	Relief of anxiety and pain; euphoria; lethargy, apathy, drowsiness, confusion, inability to concentrate; nausea, constipation, respiratory depression
	Opium	Big O, black stuff, hop	Dark brown or black chunks	Swallowed, smoked	
	Morphine	M, Miss Emma, monkey, white stuff	White crystals, liquid solution	Injected, swallowed, smoked	
	Oxycodone, codeine, hydrocodone	Oxy, O.C., killer, Captain Cody, schoolboy, vike	Tablets, powder made from crushing tablets	Swallowed, injected, snorted	
Central nervous system depressants	Barbiturates	Barbs, reds, red birds, yellows, yellow jackets	Coloured capsules	Swallowed, injected	Reduced anxiety, mood changes, lowered inhibitions, impaired muscle coordination, reduced pulse rate, drowsiness, loss of consciousness, respiratory depression
	Benzodiazepines (e.g., Valium, Xanax, Rohypnol)	Candy, downers, tranks, roofies, forget-me pill	Tablets	Swallowed, injected	
	Methaqualone	Ludes, quad, quay	Tablets	Injected, swallowed	
	Gamma hydroxy-butyrate (GHB)	G, Georgia home boy, grievous bodily harm	Clear liquid, white powder	Swallowed	
Central nervous system stimulants	Amphetamine, methamphetamine	Bennies, speed, black beauties, uppers, chalk, crank, crystal, ice, meth	Tablets, capsules, white powder, white crystals	Injected, swallowed, smoked, snorted	Increased heart rate, blood pressure, metabolism; increased mental alertness and energy; nervousness, insomnia, impulsive behaviour; reduced appetite
	Cocaine, crack cocaine	Blow, C, candy, coke, flake, rock, toot	White powder, beige pellets or rocks	Injected, smoked, snorted	
	Ritalin	JIF, MPH, R-ball, Skippy	Tablets	Injected, swallowed, snorted	
Marijuana and other cannabis products	Marijuana	Dope, grass, joints, Mary Jane, reefer, skunk, weed	Dried leaves and stems	Smoked, swallowed	Euphoria, slowed thinking and reaction time, confusion, anxiety, impaired balance and coordination, increased heart rate
	Hashish	Hash, hemp, boom, gangster	Dark, resin-like compound formed into rocks or blocks	Smoked, swallowed	
Hallucinogens	LSD	Acid, boomers, blotter, yellow sunshines	Blotter paper, liquid, gelatin tabs, pills	Swallowed, absorbed through mouth tissues	Altered states of perception and feeling; nausea; increased heart rate, blood pressure; delirium; impaired motor function; numbness, weakness
	Mescaline (peyote)	Buttons, cactus, mesc	Brown buttons, liquid	Swallowed, smoked	
	Psilocybin	Magic mushrooms, shrooms, mushies, fungus delight	Mushrooms, light to dark brown; available fresh, dried, or powdered	Swallowed (eaten raw or cooked, or steeped in hot water)	
	Ketamine	K, special K, cat valium, vitamin K	Clear liquid, white or beige powder	Injected, snorted, smoked	
	PCP	Angel dust, hog, love boat, peace pill	White to brown powder, tablets	Injected, swallowed, smoked, snorted	
	MDMA (ecstasy)	X, peace, clarity, Adam	Tablets	Swallowed	
Inhalants	Solvents, aerosols, nitrites, anaesthetics	Laughing gas, poppers, snappers, whippets	Household products, sprays, glues, paint thinner, petroleum products	Inhaled through nose or mouth	Stimulation, loss of inhibition, slurred speech, loss of motor coordination, loss of consciousness

FIGURE 14.2   Commonly abused drugs and their effects.

Sources: Health Canada. 2010. *Health Concerns: Psilocybin (Magic Mushrooms)* (http://www.hc-sc.gc.ca/hc-ps/drugs-drogues/learn-renseigne/psilocybin-eng.php; retrieved April 19, 2010); The Partnership for a Drug-Free America. 2006. *Drug Guide by Name* (http://www.drugfree.org/portal/drug_guide; retrieved August 7, 2006); U.S. Drug Enforcement Agency. 2006. *Photo Library* (http://www.usdoj.gov/dea/photo_library.html; retrieved August 7, 2006); U.S. Drug Enforcement Agency. 2005. *Drug Information* (http://www.usdoj.gov/dea/concern.concern.htm; retrieved August 7, 2006); National Institute on Drug Abuse. 2004. *Commonly Abused Drugs* (http://www.drugabuse.gov/DrugPages/DrugsofAbuse.html; retrieved August 7, 2006).

addition, the potentially high but variable purity of street heroin poses a risk of unintentional overdose. Symptoms of overdose include respiratory depression, coma, and constriction of the pupils; death can also result.

Nonmedical use of prescription pain relievers that contain oxycodone and hydrocodone, including Oxycontin and Vicodin, has increased in recent years. When taken as prescribed in tablet form, these drugs treat moderate to severe chronic pain and do not typically lead to abuse. However, like other opioids, use of prescription painkillers can lead to abuse and dependence. Oxycodone and hydrocodone can be abused orally; the long-acting form of oxycodone is also sometimes crushed and snorted or dissolved and injected, providing a powerful heroin-like high. When taken in large doses or combined with other drugs, oxycodone and hydrocodone can cause fatal respiratory depression.

Central Nervous System Depressants

Central nervous system **depressants**, also known as **sedative-hypnotics**, slow down the overall activity of the **central nervous system (CNS)**. The result can range from mild **sedation** to death, depending on the various factors involved—which drug is used, how it's taken, how tolerant the individual who is using the drug is, and so on. CNS depressants include alcohol (Chapter 15), barbiturates, and other sedatives.

Types   The various types of barbiturates are similar in chemical composition and action, but they differ in how quickly and how long they act. People who use drugs call barbiturates "downers" or "downs" and refer to specific brands by names that describe the colour and design of the capsules. People usually take barbiturates in capsules, but they may also inject them.

TERMS

depressant or sedative-hypnotic   A drug that decreases nervous or muscular activity, causing drowsiness or sleep.

central nervous system (CNS)   The brain and spinal cord.

sedation   The induction of a calm, relaxed, often sleepy state.

tranquilizer   A CNS depressant that reduces tension and anxiety.

anaesthetic   A drug that produces a loss of sensation with or without a loss of consciousness.

stimulant   A drug that increases nervous or muscular activity.

Antianxiety agents, also called sedatives or **tranquilizers**, include the benzodiazepines, such as Xanax, Valium, Librium, clonazepam (Klonopin), and flunitrazepam (Rohypnol, also called *roofies*). Other CNS depressants include methaqualone (Quaalude), ethchlorvynol (Placidyl), chloral hydrate ("mickey"), and gamma hydroxy butyrate (GHB, or "liquid ecstasy").

Effects   CNS depressants reduce anxiety and cause mood changes, impaired muscular coordination, slurring of speech, and drowsiness or sleep. Mental functioning is also affected, but the degree varies from person to person and also depends on the kind of task the person is trying to do. Most people become drowsy with small doses, although a few become more active.

Medical Uses   Barbiturates, antianxiety agents, and other sedative-hypnotics are widely used to treat insomnia and anxiety disorders and to control seizures. Some CNS depressants are used for their calming properties in combination with **anaesthetics** before operations and other medical or dental procedures.

From Use to Abuse   People are usually introduced to CNS depressants either through a medical prescription or through peers who use drugs. The use of Rohypnol and GHB is often associated with dance clubs and raves (see the box "Club Drugs"). The abuse of CNS depressants by a medical patient may begin with repeated use for insomnia and progress to dependence through increasingly larger doses at night, coupled with a few capsules at stressful times during the day.

Most CNS depressants, including alcohol, can lead to classical physical dependence. Tolerance, sometimes for up to 15 times the usual dose, can develop with repeated use. Tranquilizers have been shown to produce physical dependence even at ordinary prescribed doses. Withdrawal symptoms can be more severe than those accompanying opioid dependence and are similar to the DTs of alcoholism (see Chapter 15). They may begin as anxiety, shaking, and weakness but may turn into convulsions and possibly cardiovascular collapse and death.

While intoxicated, people on depressants cannot function well. They are confused and are frequently obstinate, irritable, and abusive. Even prescription use of benzodiazepines has been associated with an increased risk of automobile crashes. After long-term use, depressants, such as alcohol, can lead to poor health and brain damage, with impaired ability to reason and make judgments.

Overdosing with CNS Depressants   Too much depression of the central nervous system slows respiration and may stop it entirely. CNS depressants are particularly dangerous in combination with another depressant, such as alcohol. People who combine depressants with alcohol account for numerous emergency room visits and overdose deaths each year. Rohypnol is 10 times as potent as Valium and can be fatal if combined with alcohol. GHB is

Club Drugs

Club drugs are part of the popular dance culture of clubs and raves—all-night dance parties held in fields or abandoned buildings. Some people refer to club drugs as soft drugs because they see them as recreational—for the casual, weekend user—rather than as addictive. But club drugs have many potential negative effects and are particularly potent and unpredictable when mixed with alcohol. Substitute drugs are often sold in place of club drugs, putting users at risk for taking dangerous combinations of unknown drugs.

MDMA (*ecstasy, E, X, XTC, Adam, hug drug, lover's speed*): Taken in pill form, MDMA (methylenedioxymethamphetamine) is a stimulant with mildly hallucinogenic and amphetamine-like effects. Users may experience euphoria, increased energy, and a heightened sense of belonging. In club settings, using MDMA

can produce a dangerously high body temperature and potentially fatal dehydration; some users experience confusion, depression, anxiety, paranoia, muscle tension, involuntary teeth clenching, blurred vision, nausea, and seizures. Even low doses can affect concentration, judgment, and driving ability. Tolerance can develop, leading users to take the drug more frequently, to use higher doses, or to combine MDMA with other drugs to enhance the drug's effects.

In addition to MDMA, many ecstasy tablets include other drugs, such as methamphetamine, ephedrine, or cocaine. At high doses or mixed with other drugs, MDMA is extremely dangerous; most deaths linked to MDMA have occurred as a result of multidrug toxicity or traumatic injuries.

MDMA increases the activity of three neurotransmitters: serotonin, dopamine, and norepinephrine. Increases in serotonin are likely the cause of the drug's mood-elevating effects, but use of MDMA can deplete the brain of serotonin and may cause an emotional letdown (sadness, irritability, etc.) in the days following use.

People who use MDMA perform worse than nonusers on complex cognitive tasks of memory, attention, and general intelligence. Long-term effects may include physical symptoms and psychological problems, such as confusion or paranoia. Research suggests that pregnant women who use MDMA are at increased risk for having a baby with congenital malformations and long-term impairment in memory and other cognitive functions.

LSD (*acid, boomers, yellow sunshines, red dragon*): A potent hallucinogen, LSD (lysergic acid diethylamide) is sold in tablets or capsules, in liquid form, or on small squares of paper called blotters. LSD

increases heart rate and body temperature and may cause nausea, tremors, sweating, numbness, and weakness.

Ketamine (*special K, vitamin K, K, cat valium, jet*): A veterinary anaesthetic that can be taken in powdered or liquid form, ketamine may cause hallucinations and impaired attention and memory. At higher doses, ketamine can cause delirium, amnesia, high blood pressure, and potentially fatal respiratory problems. Tolerance to ketamine develops rapidly.

GHB (*Georgia home boy, G, grievous bodily harm, liquid ecstasy*): GHB (gamma hydroxybutyrate) can be produced in clear liquid, white powder, tablet, and capsule form. GHB is a CNS depressant that in large doses or when taken in combination with alcohol or other depressants can cause sedation, loss of consciousness, respiratory arrest, and death. GHB may cause prolonged and potentially life-threatening withdrawal symptoms.

Rohypnol (*roofies, roche, forget-me pill*): Taken in tablet form, Rohypnol (flunitrazepam) is a sedative that is 10 times as potent as Valium. Its effects, which are magnified by alcohol, include reduced blood pressure, dizziness, confusion, gastrointestinal disturbances, and loss of consciousness. Users of Rohypnol may develop physical and psychological dependence on the drug.

Several club drugs are used as "date rape drugs" or to facilitate sexual assault. Because they can be added to beverages surreptitiously, these drugs may be unknowingly consumed by intended rape victims. In addition to depressant effects, some drugs also cause *anterograde amnesia*, the loss of memory of things occurring while under the influence of the drug.

---

often produced clandestinely, resulting in widely varying degrees of purity; it has been responsible for many poisonings and a number of deaths.

Central Nervous System Stimulants

CNS **stimulants** speed up the activity of the nervous or muscular system. Under their influence, the heart rate

accelerates, blood pressure rises, blood vessels constrict, the pupils of the eyes and the bronchial tubes dilate, and gastric and adrenal secretions increase. There is greater muscular tension and sometimes an increase in motor activity. Small doses usually make people feel more awake and alert, less fatigued and bored. The most common CNS stimulants are cocaine, amphetamines, nicotine (Chapter 16), ephedrine, and caffeine.

Cocaine Usually derived from the leaves of coca shrubs that grow high in the Andes in South America, cocaine is a potent CNS stimulant. For centuries, natives of the Andes have chewed coca leaves both for pleasure and to increase their endurance. For a short time during the nineteenth century, some physicians were enthusiastic about the use of cocaine to cure alcoholism and addiction to the pain-killer morphine. Enthusiasm waned after the drug's adverse side effects became apparent.

Cocaine—also known as *coke* or *snow*—quickly produces a feeling of euphoria, which makes it a popular recreational drug. Cocaine use surged in popularity during the early 1980s, when the drug's high price made it a status drug. The introduction of crack cocaine during the 1980s made the drug available in smaller quantities and at lower prices to more people. The typical recreational user shifted rapidly from wealthy professionals snorting powdered cocaine to poor inner-city smokers of crack cocaine. The 2008 prevalence of cocaine use among the general Canadian population was 1.6%; this percentage is comparable to the rates of use reported in 2004.

METHODS OF USE Cocaine is usually snorted and absorbed through the nasal mucosa or injected intravenously, providing rapid increases of the drug's concentration in the blood and therefore fast, intense effects. Another method of use involves processing cocaine with baking soda and water, yielding the ready-to-smoke form of cocaine known as crack. Crack is typically available as small beads or pellets smokable in glass pipes. The tiny but potent beads can be handled more easily than cocaine powder and marketed in smaller, less expensive doses.

EFFECTS The effects of cocaine are usually intense but short-lived. The euphoria lasts from 5 to 20 minutes and ends abruptly, to be replaced by irritability, anxiety, or slight depression. When cocaine is absorbed via the lungs, by either smoking or inhalation, it reaches the brain in about 10 seconds, and the effects are particularly intense. This is part of the appeal of smoking crack. The effects from IV injections occur almost as quickly—in about 20 seconds. Since the mucous membranes in the nose briefly slow absorption, the onset of effects from snorting takes two three minutes. Heavy users may inject cocaine intravenously every 10–20 minutes to maintain the effects.

The larger the cocaine dose and the more rapidly it is absorbed into the bloodstream, the greater the immediate—and sometimes lethal—effects. Sudden death from cocaine is most commonly the result of excessive CNS stimulation that causes convulsions and respiratory collapse, irregular heartbeat, extremely high blood pressure, blood clots, and possibly heart attack or stroke. Although rare, fatalities can occur in healthy young people; among people ages 18–59, people who use cocaine are seven times as likely as nonusers to have a heart attack. Chronic cocaine use produces inflammation of the nasal mucosa, which can lead to persistent bleeding and ulceration of the septum between the nostrils. The use of cocaine may also cause paranoia and aggressiveness.

ABUSE AND DEPENDENCE When steady cocaine users stop taking the drug, they experience a sudden crash characterized by depression, agitation, and fatigue, followed by a period of withdrawal. Their depression can be temporarily relieved by taking more cocaine, so its continued use is reinforced. A binge cocaine user may go for weeks or months without using any cocaine and then take large amounts repeatedly. Although not physically dependent, a binge cocaine user who misses work or school and risks serious health consequences is clearly abusing the drug.

COCAINE USE DURING PREGNANCY Cocaine rapidly passes from the mother's bloodstream into the placenta and can have serious effects on the fetus. A woman who uses cocaine during pregnancy is at higher risk for miscarriage, premature labour, and stillbirth. She is more likely to deliver a low-birth-weight baby who has a small head circumference. Her infant may be at increased risk for defects of the genito-urinary tract, cardiovascular system, central nervous system, and extremities. It is difficult to pinpoint the effects of cocaine because many women who use cocaine also use tobacco or alcohol or both.

Infants whose mothers use cocaine may also be born intoxicated. They are typically irritable and jittery and do not eat or sleep normally. These characteristics may affect their early social and emotional development because it may be more difficult for adults to interact with them. Cocaine also passes into breast milk and can intoxicate a breastfeeding infant.

Amphetamines Amphetamines (uppers) are a group of synthetic chemicals that are potent CNS stimulants. Some common drugs in this family are amphetamine (Benzedrine), dextroamphetamine (Dexedrine), and methamphetamine (Methedrine or "meth"). Meth is more addictive and dangerous than most forms of amphetamine because it is more toxic and its effects last longer. Once taken, the drug causes the brain to release high amounts of dopamine, a key neurotransmitter. Methamphetamine is highly addictive; many casual users rapidly become regular users. Crystal methamphetamine ("crystal meth" or "ice"), a smokable, high-potency form of methamphetamine, is popular in some cities across Canada. Easy to manufacture, crystal meth is cheaper than crack and produces a similar but longer-lasting euphoria. The use of crystal meth can quickly lead to dependence. Despite recent media attention given to methamphetamine and crystal methamphetamine use in various populations, a 30-year study of thousands of Ontario students in grades 7 to 12 revealed that as of 2009, past-year use of methamphetamine had significantly decreased since 1999.

EFFECTS Small doses of amphetamines usually make people feel more alert. Amphetamines generally increase motor activity but do not measurably alter a normal, rested person's ability to perform tasks calling for challenging motor skills or complex thinking. When amphetamines do improve performance, it is primarily by counteracting fatigue and boredom. Amphetamines in small doses also increase heart rate and blood pressure and change sleep patterns.

Amphetamines are sometimes used to curb appetite, but after a few weeks the user develops tolerance and higher doses are necessary. When people stop taking the drug, their appetite usually returns, and they gain back the weight they lost unless they have made permanent changes in their eating behaviour.

Short-term effects associated with methamphetamine use can include euphoria, rapid breathing, increased body temperature (hyperthermia), insomnia, tremors, anxiety, and convulsions. In the long term, methamphetamine's effects can be devastating. Severe weight loss, heart attack, stroke, hallucinations, violence, paranoia, and psychotic behaviour have all been linked to meth addiction. Meth use causes extensive tooth decay and tooth loss, a condition referred to as "meth mouth." The drug takes a severe toll on the heart, increasing heart rate and blood pressure, damaging blood vessels, and causing irregular heartbeat. Such damage can be fatal.

FROM USE TO ABUSE   Much amphetamine abuse begins as an attempt to cope with a temporary situation. A student cramming for an exam or an exhausted long-haul truck driver can go a little longer by taking amphetamines, but the results can be disastrous. The likelihood of making bad judgments significantly increases. The stimulating effects may also wear off suddenly, and the individual may precipitously feel exhausted or fall asleep (crash).

Another problem is **state dependence**, the phenomenon whereby information learned in a certain drug-induced state is difficult to recall when the person is not in that same physiological state. Test performance may deteriorate when students use drugs to study and then take tests in their normal, nondrug state. (Users of antihistamines may also experience state dependence.)

Methamphetamine intoxication leads to unsafe and uncharacteristic behaviour. It has been linked to high-risk sexual activity and increased rates of STIs, including HIV infection (Chapter 13).

DEPENDENCE   Repeated use of amphetamines, even in moderate doses, often leads to tolerance and the need for increasingly larger doses. The result can be severe disturbances in behaviour, including a temporary state of paranoid **psychosis**, with delusions of persecution and episodes of unprovoked violence. If injected in large doses, amphetamines produce a feeling of intense pleasure, followed by sensations of vigour and euphoria that last for several hours. As these feelings wear off, they are replaced by feelings of irritability and vague uneasiness. Long-term use of amphetamines at high doses can cause paranoia, hallucinations, delusions, and incoherence.

Methamphetamine users have signs of brain damage similar to those seen in individuals with Parkinson's disease that appear to persist even after drug use ceases, causing impaired memory and motor coordination. Withdrawal symptoms may include muscle aches and tremors, profound fatigue, deep depression, despair, and apathy. Chronic high-dose use is often associated with pronounced psychological cravings and obsessive drug-seeking behaviour.

Women who use amphetamines during pregnancy risk premature birth, stillbirth, low birth weight, and early infant death. Babies born to mothers who use amphetamines have a higher incidence of cleft palate, cleft lip, and deformed limbs. They may also experience symptoms of withdrawal from amphetamines.

Ritalin   A stimulant with amphetamine-like effects, Ritalin (methylphenidate) is used to treat attention deficit hyperactivity disorder (ADHD). When taken orally at prescribed levels, it has little potential for abuse. When injected or snorted, however, dependence and tolerance can rapidly result. There is growing concern that more and more young people are abusing these drugs for various reasons, including appetite suppression, alertness, increased concentration and focus, and euphoria.

Ephedrine   Although somewhat less potent than amphetamine, ephedrine does produce stimulant effects. Ephedrine has been linked to heart arrhythmia, stroke, psychotic reactions, seizures, and some deaths, and it may be particularly dangerous at high doses or when combined with another stimulant, such as caffeine. Health Canada has issued several warnings to consumers about the dangers of using unauthorized products containing ephedra or ephedrine, either alone or in combination with other stimulants, for weight loss, body building, or increased energy.

Caffeine   Caffeine is probably the most popular psychoactive drug and also one of the most ancient. It is found in coffee, tea, cocoa, soft drinks, headache remedies, and OTC preparations. (Table 14.2 on p. 460 lists typical levels of caffeine in several popular products.) In ordinary doses, caffeine produces greater alertness and a sense of well-being. It also decreases feelings of fatigue or boredom; using caffeine may enable a person to keep at physically tiring or

state dependence   A situation in which information learned in a drug-induced state is difficult to recall when the effect of the drug wears off.

psychosis   A severe mental disorder characterized by a distortion of reality; symptoms might include delusions or hallucinations.

TERMS

Table 14.2 Caffeine Content of Popular Products

	Serving Size	Typical Caffeine Level (mg)*
Coffee		
Regular coffee, brewed	237 mL (1 cup)	135
Regular coffee, instant	237 mL	76–106
Decaffeinated coffee, brewed	237 mL	5
Decaffeinated coffee, instant	237 mL	5
Tea		
Regular tea, brewed	237 mL	43
Decaffeinated tea, brewed	237 mL	2
Green tea	237 mL	30
Snapple Iced Tea	473 mL (1 bottle)	18
Nestea	355 mL (1 can)	17
SoBe Green Tea	355 mL	14
Lipton Brisk Iced Tea, Lemon	355 mL	10
Cola Beverages		
Diet Coke	355 mL (1 can)	47
Dr. Pepper, Diet Dr. Pepper	355 mL	41
Pepsi	355 mL	38
Coca-Cola Classic, Diet Pepsi	355 mL	35
A&W Crème Soda	355 mL	29
Barq's Root Beer	355 mL	23
Energy Drinks		
SoBe No Fear	473 mL	174
Monster Energy, Rockstar	473 mL	160
SoBe Adrenaline Rush	473 mL	152
AMP Energy Drink	473 mL	143
Red Bull	245 mL	76
Cocoa Products		
Chocolate milk	237 mL	8
Hot-cocoa mix, 1 envelope	237 mL	5
Candy, milk chocolate	28 g	7
Chocolate cake	80 g	36

Sources: Center for Science in the Public Interest. 2007. *Caffeine Content of Food & Drugs* (http://www.cspinet.org/new/cafchart.html; retrieved February 3, 2009); Health Canada. 2010. *Food and Nutrition: Caffeine in Food* (http://www.hc-sc.gc.ca/fn-an/securit/addit/caf/food-caf-aliments-eng.php; retrieved April 15, 2010); Mayo Clinic. 2007. *How Much Caffeine Is in Your Daily Habit?* (http://www.mayoclinic.com/health/caffeine/AN01211; retrieved February 3, 2009); U.S. Department of Agriculture, Agricultural Research Service. 2007. *USDA National Nutrient Database for Standard Reference, Release 20* (http://www.ars.usda.gov/ba/bhnrc/ndl; retrieved February 3, 2009); U.S. Department of Agriculture, Agricultural Research Service. 2007. *USDA National Nutrient Database for Standard Reference, Release 20* (http://www.ars.usda.gov/ba/bhnrc/ndl; retrieved February 3, 2009).

* Caffeine levels vary greatly by brand of product, manner of preparation, and amount consumed. The amounts shown here are averages based on tests conducted by a variety of organizations. To find the exact amount of caffeine in any product, check that product's label.

Caffeine mildly stimulates the heart and respiratory system, increases muscular tremor, and enhances gastric secretion. Higher doses may cause nervousness, anxiety, irritability, headache, disturbed sleep, and gastric irritation or peptic ulcers. In people with high blood pressure, caffeine can cause blood pressure to rise even further above normal; in people with type 2 diabetes, caffeine may cause glucose and insulin levels to rise after meals. Some people, especially children, are quite vulnerable to the adverse effects of caffeine. They become hyperactive and overly sensitive to any stimulation in their environment. In rare instances, the disturbance is so severe that they experience misperceptions of their surroundings—a toxic psychosis.

Drinks containing caffeine are rarely harmful for most people, but some tolerance develops, and withdrawal symptoms of irritability, headaches, and even mild depression do occur. Thus, although we don't usually think of caffeine as a dependence-producing drug, for some people it is. People can usually avoid problems by simply decreasing their daily intake of caffeine; if intake is decreased gradually, withdrawal symptoms can be reduced or avoided. For the general population of healthy adults, Health Canada advises an intake of no more than 400 milligrams of caffeine per day.

Marijuana and Other Cannabis Products

Marijuana is the most widely used illegal drug in Canada (hallucinogens are second). According to the 2008 *Canadian Alcohol and Drug Use Monitoring Survey*, more than 40% of Canadians have tried marijuana at least once in their lifetime; among 15–24-year-olds, more than 52% have tried marijuana. In 2004, 16.7% of Canadian university students reported using marijuana at least once within the past month.

Marijuana is a crude preparation of various parts of the Indian hemp plant *Cannabis sativa*, which grows in most parts of the world. THC (tetrahydrocannabinol) is the main active ingredient in marijuana. Based on THC content, the potency of marijuana preparations varies widely. Marijuana plants that grow wild often have less than 1% THC in their leaves. When selected strains are cultivated by separation of male and female plants (*sinsemilla*), the bud leaves from the flowering tops may contain 7%–8% THC. Hashish, a potent preparation made from the thick resin that exudes from the marijuana leaves, may contain up to 14% THC.

These various preparations have all been known and used for centuries, so the frequently heard claim that today's marijuana is more potent than the marijuana of the 1970s is not strictly true. However, a greater proportion of the marijuana sold today is the higher-potency (and more expensive) sinsemilla; hence, the average potency of street marijuana has increased.

Marijuana is usually smoked, but it can also be ingested. The classification of marijuana is a matter of some debate. For this reason, it is treated separately here.

repetitive tasks longer. Such use is usually followed, however, by a sudden letdown. Caffeine does not noticeably influence a person's ability to perform complex mental tasks unless fatigue, boredom, or other factors have already affected normal performance.

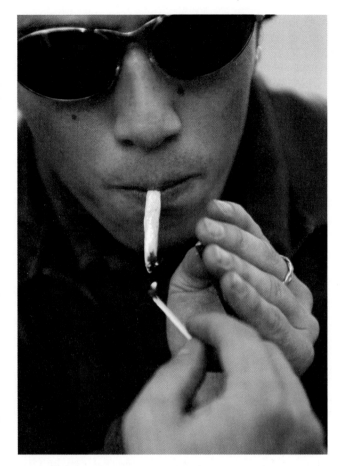
Marijuana is the most widely used illegal drug in Canada.

characteristic bloodshot eyes. Individuals who use marijuana may also feel less inclined toward physical exertion and may feel particularly hungry or thirsty. THC affects parts of the brain controlling balance, coordination, and reaction time; thus marijuana use impairs driving performance. The combination of alcohol and marijuana is even more dangerous: Even a low dose of marijuana, when combined with alcohol, significantly impairs driving performance and increases crash risk.

Some compounds in marijuana may have legitimate medical use. For example, marijuana has been shown to ease pain, reduce nausea, and increase appetite. These benefits led Health Canada to approve the use of "medical marijuana" by extremely ill patients, in situations where conventional treatments are not appropriate or do not provide adequate relief. Despite these benefits, Health Canada warns that the use of medical marijuana should not be confused with the legalization of marijuana in Canada. Marijuana remains an illegal and controlled substance; therefore, it is not legal to grow or possess marijuana except with permission from Health Canada. The ethical debates over medical marijuana use continue, as do court cases.

Short-Term Effects and Uses As is true with most psychoactive drugs, the effects of a low dose of marijuana are strongly influenced both by the individual's expectations and by past experiences. At low doses, people who use marijuana typically experience euphoria, a heightening of subjective sensory experiences, a slowing down of the perception of passing time, and a relaxed, laid-back attitude. These pleasant effects are the reason this drug is so widely used. With moderate doses, these effects become stronger, and the user can also expect to have impaired memory function, disturbed thought patterns, lapses of attention, and feelings of **depersonalization**, in which the mind seems to be separated from the body.

The effects of marijuana in higher doses are determined mostly by the drug itself rather than by the individual's expectations and setting. Very high doses produce feelings of depersonalization, as well as marked sensory distortion and changes in body image (such as a feeling that the body is very light). Inexperienced users sometimes think these sensations mean they are going crazy, and they become anxious or even panicky. Unexpected reactions are the leading reason for emergency room visits by users of marijuana or hashish.

Physiologically, marijuana increases heart rate and dilates certain blood vessels in the eyes, which creates the

Long-Term Effects The most probable long-term effect of smoking marijuana is respiratory damage, including impaired lung function and chronic bronchial irritation. Although no evidence links marijuana use to lung cancer, it may cause changes in lung tissue that promote cancer growth. Individuals who use marijuana may be at increased risk for emphysema and cancer of the head and neck; among people with chronic conditions, such as cancer and AIDS, marijuana use is associated with increased risk of fatal lung infections. Heavy users may experience learning problems, as well as subtle impairments of attention and memory that may or may not be reversible following long-term abstinence. Long-term use may also decrease testosterone levels and sperm counts and increase sperm abnormalities.

Heavy marijuana use during pregnancy may cause impaired fetal growth and development, low birth weight, and increased risk of ectopic pregnancy. Marijuana may act synergistically with alcohol to increase the damaging effects of alcohol on the fetus. THC rapidly enters breast milk and may impair an infant's early motor development.

depersonalization A state in which a person loses the sense of his or her reality or perceives his or her body as unreal.

TERMS

Dependence Regular users of marijuana can develop tolerance, and some develop dependence. In 2002, Statistics Canada estimated that 3.4% of Canadians were dependent on marijuana. Withdrawal symptoms may occur in the majority of dependent or heavy users; common symptoms include anger or aggression, irritability, nervousness or restlessness, sleep difficulties, and decreased appetite or weight loss.

Hallucinogens

Hallucinogens are a group of drugs whose predominant pharmacological effect is to alter perceptions, feelings, and thoughts. Hallucinogens include the following:

- LSD (lysergic acid diethylamide)
- Psilocybin
- STP (4-methyl-2,5-dimethoxyamphetamine)
- DMT (dimethyltryptamine)
- MDMA (3,4-methylenedioxymethamphetamine)
- Ketamine
- PCP (phencyclidine)

These drugs are most commonly ingested or smoked.

LSD LSD is one of the most powerful psychoactive drugs. Tiny doses will produce noticeable effects in most people, such as an altered sense of time, visual disturbances, an improved sense of hearing, mood changes, and distortions in how people perceive their bodies. Dilation of the pupils and slight dizziness, weakness, and nausea may also occur. With larger doses, individuals may experience a phenomenon known as **synaesthesia**, feelings of depersonalization, and other alterations in the perceived relationship between the self and external reality.

> **QUICK STATS**
>
> **10.2%** of Canadians ages 15–24 have tried hallucinogens at least once in the past year.
>
> —Health Canada, 2009

Many hallucinogens induce tolerance so quickly that after only one or two doses their effects decrease substantially. The user must then stop taking the drug for several days before his or her system can be receptive to it again. Typically, these drugs cause little drug-seeking behaviour and no physical dependence or withdrawal symptoms.

The immediate effects of low doses of hallucinogens are largely determined by expectations and setting. Many effects are hard to describe because they involve subjective and unusual dimensions of awareness—the **altered states of consciousness** for which these drugs are famous. For this reason, hallucinogens have acquired a certain aura not associated with other drugs. People have taken LSD in search of a religious or mystical experience or in the hope of exploring new worlds. During the 1960s, some psychiatrists gave LSD to their patients to help them talk about their repressed feelings.

A severe panic reaction, which can be terrifying in the extreme, can result from taking any dose of LSD. It is impossible to predict when a panic reaction will occur. Some LSD users report having had hundreds of pleasurable and ecstatic experiences before having a bad trip, or "bummer." If the user is already in a serene mood and feels no anger or hostility and if he or she is in secure surroundings with trusted companions, a bad trip may be less likely, but a tranquil experience is not guaranteed.

Even after the drug's chemical effects have worn off, spontaneous flashbacks and other psychological disturbances can occur. **Flashbacks** are perceptual distortions and bizarre thoughts that occur after the drug has been entirely eliminated from the body. Although they are relatively rare phenomena, flashbacks can be extremely distressing. They are often triggered by specific psychological cues associated with the drug-taking experience, such as certain mood states or even types of music.

Other Hallucinogens Most other hallucinogens have the same general effects as LSD, but there are some variations. For example, a DMT or ketamine high does not last as long as an LSD high; an STP high lasts longer. MDMA has both hallucinogenic and amphetamine-like properties. Tolerance to MDMA develops quickly, and high doses can cause anxiety, delusions, and paranoia. (Refer back to the box "Club Drugs" on p. 457 for more on MDMA.)

PCP reduces and distorts sensory input, especially proprioception, the sensation of body position and movement; it creates a state of sensory deprivation. PCP was initially used as an anaesthetic but was unsatisfactory because it caused agitation, confusion, and delirium (loss of contact with reality). Because it can be easily made, PCP is often available illegally and is sometimes used as an inexpensive replacement for other psychoactive drugs.

The effects of ketamine are similar to those of PCP—confusion, agitation, aggression, and lack of coordination—but they tend to be less predictable. Tolerance to either drug can develop rapidly.

Hallucinogenic effects can also be obtained from certain mushrooms (psilocybin, or "magic mushrooms"), certain morning glory seeds, nutmeg, jimsonweed, and other botanical products, but unpleasant side effects, such as dizziness, have limited the popularity of these products.

Inhalants

Inhaling certain chemicals can produce effects ranging from heightened pleasure to delirium and death. Inhalants fall into several major groups:

- Volatile solvents, which are found in many products, such as paint thinner, glue, and gasoline
- Aerosols, which are sprays that contain propellants and solvents

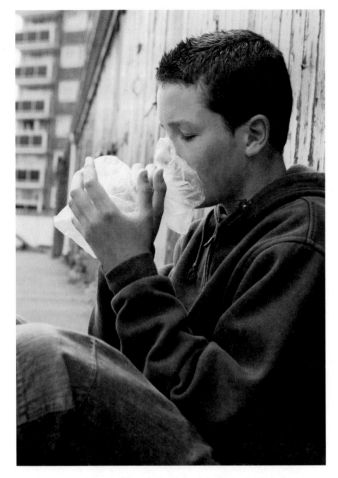
Inhalant use is difficult to monitor and control because inhalants are found in many inexpensive and legal products.

- Nitrites, such as butyl nitrite and amyl nitrite
- Anaesthetics, which include nitrous oxide, or laughing gas

Inhalant use tends to be highest among younger adolescents and declines with age. It is estimated that 3%–5% of Canadian adolescents have tried inhalants, although this statistic does not take into consideration the growing and rampant problem of inhalant use in some remote Inuit and First Nations communities across Canada.

Inhalant use is difficult to control because inhalants are easy to obtain. They are present in a variety of seemingly harmless products, from dessert-topping sprays to under-arm deodorants, that are both inexpensive and legal. Using the drugs also requires no illegal or suspicious paraphernalia. People who use inhalants get high by sniffing, snorting, "bagging" (inhaling fumes from a plastic bag), or "huffing" (placing an inhalant-soaked rag against the mouth).

Although different in makeup, nearly all inhalants produce effects similar to those of anaesthetics, which slow down body functions. Low doses may cause people to feel slightly stimulated; at higher doses, people may feel less inhibited and less in control. Sniffing high concentrations of the chemicals in solvents or aerosol sprays can cause a

loss of consciousness, heart failure, and death. High concentrations of any inhalant can also cause death from suffocation by displacing the oxygen in the lungs and central nervous system. Deliberately inhaling from a bag or in a closed area greatly increases the chances of suffocation. Other possible effects of the excessive or long-term use of inhalants include damage to the nervous system (impaired perception, reasoning, memory, and muscular coordination); hearing loss; increased risk of cancer; and damage to the liver, kidneys, and bone marrow.

DRUG USE: THE DECADES AHEAD

Drug research will undoubtedly provide new information, new treatments, and new chemical combinations in the decades ahead. New psychoactive drugs may present unexpected possibilities for therapy, social use, and abuse. Making honest and unbiased information about drugs available to everyone, however, may cut down on their abuse.

Although the use of some drugs, both legal and illegal, has declined dramatically since the 1970s, the use of others has held steady or increased. Mounting public concern has led to great debate and a wide range of opinions about what should be done. Efforts to combat the problem include workplace drug testing, tougher law enforcement and prosecution, and treatment and education.

In October 2007, the Government of Canada launched its National Anti-Drug Strategy, which consists of action plans to improve law enforcement, prevent drug abuse, and treat people who have drug addictions. Law enforcement measures include building and strengthening the capacities of police, investigation, and prosecution units, and enhancing border control. The action plan on drug abuse prevention includes a national awareness campaign

hallucinogen   Any of several drugs that alter perception, feelings, or thoughts; examples are LSD and PCP.

synaesthesia   A condition in which a stimulus evokes not only the sensation appropriate to it but also another sensation of a different character, such as when a colour evokes a specific smell.

altered states of consciousness   Profound changes in mood, thinking, and perception.

flashback   A perceptual distortion or bizarre thought that recurs after the chemical effects of a drug have worn off.

involving mass media, youth and their parents, and community-based projects on drug abuse prevention. The action plan on the treatment of people who are addicted to illicit drugs aims to enhance treatment and support for First Nations and Inuit, provide treatment programs for young offenders with drug-related problems, and support research on new treatment models. The Government allocated $102 million to law enforcement, $30 million to drug abuse prevention, and $100 million to the treatment of people with drug addiction, over five years. With drugs entering the country on a massive scale from a variety of countries and being distributed through tightly controlled drug-smuggling organizations and street gangs, it remains to be seen how effective any program will be.

Drugs, Society, and Families

The economic cost of drug abuse is staggering. According to the Canadian Centre on Substance Abuse, the justice-related cost to society of illicit drug use, including police, courts, and correctional services, is $2 billion annually. That figure expands substantially when combined with the costs of alcohol and tobacco use and when other expenses, such as health care costs and lost productivity, are taken into account. But the costs are more than just financial; they are also paid in human pain and suffering.

The relationship between drugs and crime is complex. The criminal justice system is inundated with people accused of crimes related to drug possession, sale, or use. In Canada, the overall rate of police-reported drug offences has been increasing since 1993. Many assaults and murders are committed when people try to acquire or protect drug territories, settle disputes about drugs, or steal from dealers. Violence and the use of guns are more common in neighbourhoods where drug trafficking is prevalent. People addicted to drugs commit more robberies and burglaries than criminals who are not on drugs. People under the influence of drugs, especially alcohol, are more likely to commit violent crimes, such as rape and murder, than are people who do not use drugs. Although often associated with poor inner-city areas and ethnic minorities, drug-related problems affect all groups and every area of the country.

Drug use is also a health care issue for society. In Canada, illegal drug use leads to more than 47,000 deaths and thousands more injuries and disabilities each year. Although it is in the best interest of society to treat people who want help, not nearly enough space is available in treatment facilities to help the vast number of Canadians who need immediate treatment. Individuals who are addicted to drugs and who want to quit, especially those among the urban poor, often have to wait a year or more for acceptance into a residential care or other treatment program.

Drug abuse also takes a toll on individuals and families. Children born to women who use drugs, such as alcohol, tobacco, or cocaine, may have long-term health problems. Drug use in families can become a vicious cycle. Observing adults around them using drugs, children assume it is an acceptable way to deal with problems. Problems, such as abuse, neglect, lack of opportunity, and unemployment, become contributing factors to drug use and serve to perpetuate the cycle.

Legalizing Drugs

Pointing out that many of the social problems associated with drugs are related to prohibition rather than to the effects of the drugs themselves, some people have argued for various forms of drug legalization or decriminalization. Proposals range from making some drugs, such as marijuana and heroin, available by prescription to allowing licensed dealers to sell some of these drugs to adults. Proponents argue that legalizing some currently illicit drugs—but putting controls on them similar to those used for alcohol, tobacco, and prescription drugs—could eliminate many of the problems related to drug use.

Opponents of drug legalization argue that allowing easier access to drugs would expose many more people to possible abuse and dependence. Drugs would be cheaper and easier to obtain, and drug use would be more socially acceptable. Legalizing drugs could cause an increase in drug use among children and teenagers. Opponents point out that alcohol and tobacco are major causes of disease and death in our society and that they should not be used as models for other practices.

Treatment for Drug Dependence

Treatment for drug dependence is sometimes characterized by discrete episodes of short-term abstinence and relapse. Regardless of the therapeutic approach used for drug dependence, many individuals undergoing treatment will often slide back into their drug habits. Often, this backsliding results in worsening of the original substance-abuse problem. For some substances, the period from abstinence to relapse occurs within one year after treatment.

Preventing relapse and maintaining long-term cessation of drug use is an exceedingly complex medical goal. Medical interventions based on pharmaceutical aids to enhance the individual's long-term commitment to change and stay drug-free remain an elusive goal. Relapse prevention research is instead increasingly focusing on the need to expand the behavioural repertoire of skills needed to decrease the risk of recidivism among individuals receiving drug-treatment services.

Choosing a Drug-Treatment Program

When evaluating different facilities or programs for drug treatment, consider the following issues:

• *What type of treatment or facility is most appropriate?* Intensive outpatient treatment is available through many community mental health centres, as well as through specialized drug-treatment facilities. Such programs typically require several sessions per week, combining individual therapy, group counselling, and attendance at 12-step meetings. Residential, or inpatient, facilities may be associated with a medical facility, such as a hospital, or they may be freestanding programs that focus solely on substance-abuse treatment. Some residential treatment programs last longer or cost more per week than some health insurance plans will cover.

• *How will treatment be paid for?* Many services are covered by provincial or territorial health insurance plans. However, additional fees may be incurred for services, which may be covered in part, or in full, by workplace extended health benefits plans or other private insurance health care plans.

• *Is there likely to be a need for medical support?* Chronic alcoholics or abusers of other CNS depressants may experience life-threatening seizures or other withdrawal symptoms during the first few days of detoxification. Malnutrition is common among substance abusers, and people who inject drugs may suffer from local infections and blood-borne diseases, such as hepatitis or HIV infection. Any medical problems, such as these, are best handled in an inpatient program with good medical support.

• *What is the level of professional training of the staff?* Is there a medical doctor on-site or making frequent visits? Are there trained nurses? Licensed psychologists or social workers? Many successful programs are staffed primarily by recovering alcoholics or drug users. Do those staff members have training and certification as addiction specialists or some other licence or certificate?

• *Does the program provide related services, such as family and job counselling and post-treatment follow-up?* These types of services are extremely important for the long-term success of drug-abuse treatment.

• *Can you visit the facility and speak with the staff and clients?* A prospective client and his or her family should be allowed to visit any treatment centre or program.

Medication-Assisted Treatment Medications are increasingly being used in addiction treatment—to reduce the craving for the abused drug or to block or oppose its effects. Perhaps the best-known medication for drug abuse is methadone, a synthetic drug used as a substitute for heroin. Use of methadone prevents withdrawal reactions and reduces the craving for heroin; it enables dependent people to function normally in social and vocational activities, although they remain dependent on methadone. The narcotic buprenorphine, approved by Health Canada in 2007 for treatment of opioid addiction, also reduces cravings. Many other medications are under study; drugs used specifically in the treatment of nicotine and alcohol dependence are discussed in Chapters 15 and 16.

Medication therapy is relatively simple and inexpensive and is therefore popular among patients and health care providers. However, the relapse rate is high. Combining drug therapy with psychological and social services improves success rates, underscoring the importance of psychological factors in drug dependence.

Treatment Centres Treatment centres offer a variety of short-term and long-term services, including hospitalization, detoxification, counselling, and other mental health services. The therapeutic community is a specific type of centre, a residential program run in a completely drug-free atmosphere. Administered by ex-addicts, these programs use confrontation, strict discipline, and unrelenting peer pressure to attempt to resocialize individuals with addictions with a different set of values. Halfway houses, transitional settings between a 24-hour-a-day program and independent living, are an important phase of treatment for some people. Strategies for evaluating programs are given in the box "Choosing a Drug-Treatment Program," above.

Self-Help Groups and Peer Counselling Self-help groups, such as Alcoholics Anonymous (AA) and Narcotics Anonymous (NA), have helped many people. People treated in drug-substitution programs or substance-abuse treatment centres are often urged or required to join a self-help group as part of their recovery. These groups follow a 12-step program. Group members' first step is to acknowledge that they have a problem over which they have no control. Peer support is a critical ingredient of these programs, and members usually meet at least once a week. Each member is paired with a sponsor to call on for advice and support if the temptation to relapse becomes overwhelming. With such support, thousands of substance-dependent people have been able to recover, remain abstinent, and reclaim their lives. Chapters of AA and NA meet on some university campuses; community-based chapters are typically listed in the phone book, online, and in local newspapers.

Many universities also have peer counselling programs, in which students are trained to help other students who have drug problems. A peer counsellor's role may be as limited as referring a student to a professional with expertise in substance dependence for an evaluation or as involved as helping arrange a leave of absence from school for participation in a drug-treatment program. Most peer counselling programs are founded on principles of strict confidentiality.

If Someone You Know Has a Drug Problem

Changes in behaviour and mood in someone you know may signal a growing dependence on drugs. Signs that a person's life is beginning to focus on drugs include the following:

- Sudden withdrawal or emotional distance

- Rebellious or unusually irritable behaviour

- A loss of interest in usual activities or hobbies

- A decline in school or work performance

- A sudden change in the chosen group of friends

- Changes in sleeping or eating habits

- Frequent borrowing of money or stealing

- Secretive behaviour about personal possessions, such as a backpack or the contents of a drawer

- Deterioration of physical appearance

If you believe a family member or friend has a drug problem, obtain information about resources for drug treatment available on your campus or in your community. Communicate your concern, provide him or her with information about treatment options, and offer your support during treatment. If the person continues to deny having a problem, you may want to talk with an experienced counsellor about setting up an intervention—a formal, structured confrontation designed to end denial by having family, friends, and other caring individuals present their concerns to the person using drugs. Participants in an intervention would indicate the ways in which the individual is hurting others as well as himself or herself. If your friend or family member agrees to treatment, encourage him or her to attend a support group, such as Narcotics Anonymous or Alcoholics Anonymous. And finally, examine your relationship with the individual who is using drugs for signs of codependency. If necessary, get help for yourself; friends and family of people who use drugs can often benefit from counselling.

Peer counsellors may also be able to help students who are concerned about a classmate or loved one with an apparent drug problem (see the box "If Someone You Know Has a Drug Problem," above). Information about peer counselling programs is usually available from the student health centre.

Harm-Reduction Strategies Recognizing that many attempts at treatment are at first unsuccessful and that a drug-free society may be an unobtainable goal, some experts advocate the use of harm-reduction strategies. The goal of harm reduction is to minimize the negative effects of drug use and abuse; a common example is the use of designated drivers to reduce alcohol-related motor vehicle crashes. In terms of illicit drugs, drug substitution programs, such as methadone maintenance, are one form of harm reduction; although participants remain drug dependent, the negative individual and social consequences of their drug use is reduced. Syringe exchange programs, designed to reduce transmission of HIV and hepatitis C, are another harm-reduction approach. Some experts have also suggested free testing of street drugs for purity and potency to help people who use drugs avoid unintentional toxicity or overdose.

Codependency Many treatment programs also offer counselling for those who are close to people who abuse drugs. Drug abuse takes a toll on friends and family members, and counselling can help people work through painful feelings of guilt and powerlessness. **Codependency**, in which a person close to the drug abuser is controlled by the abuser's behaviour, sometimes develops. Codependent people may come to believe that love, approval, and security are contingent on their taking care of the person who abuses drugs. People can become codependent naturally because they want to help when someone they love becomes dependent on a drug. They may assume that their good intentions will persuade the individual to stop using drugs.

Codependent people often engage in behaviours that remove or soften the effects of drug use on the user—so-called *enabling* behaviours. However, the habit of enabling can inhibit a drug-dependent person's recovery because the person never has to experience the consequences of his or her behaviour. Often, the enabler is dependent, too—on the patterns of interaction in the relationship. People who need to take care of people often marry people who need to be taken care of. Children in these families often develop the same behaviour pattern as one of their parents, by either becoming helpless or becoming a caregiver. For this reason, many treatment programs involve the whole family.

Have you ever been an enabler in a relationship? You may have, if you've ever done any of the following:

- Given someone one more chance to stop abusing drugs, then another, and another...

- Made excuses or lied for someone to his or her friends, teachers, or employer
- Joined someone in drug use and blamed others for your behaviour
- Loaned money to someone to continue drug use
- Stayed up late waiting for or gone out searching for someone who uses drugs
- Felt embarrassed or angry about the actions of someone who uses drugs
- Ignored the drug use because the person got defensive when you brought it up
- Not confronted a friend or relative who was obviously intoxicated or high on a drug

If you come from a codependent family or see yourself developing codependency relationships or engaging in enabling behaviours, consider acting now to make changes in your patterns of interaction. Remember, you cannot cause or cure drug dependence in another person.

Preventing Drug Abuse

Obviously, the best solution to drug abuse is prevention. Government attempts at controlling the drug problem often focus on stopping the production, importation, and distribution of illegal drugs. Creative effort also has to be put into stopping the demand for drugs. Developing persuasive antidrug educational programs offers the best hope for solving the drug problem in the future. Indirect approaches to prevention involve building young people's self-esteem, improving their academic skills, and increasing their recreational opportunities. Direct approaches involve giving information about the adverse effects of drugs and teaching tactics that help students resist peer pressure to use drugs in various situations. Developing strategies for resisting peer pressure is one of the more effective techniques.

Prevention efforts need to focus on the different motivations individuals have for using and abusing specific drugs at different ages. For example, grade-school children seem receptive to programs that involve their parents or well-known adults, such as professional athletes. Adolescents in high school are often more responsive to peer counsellors. Many young adults tend to be influenced by efforts that focus on health education. For all ages, it is important to provide nondrug alternatives—such as recreational facilities, counselling, greater opportunities for leisure activities, and places to socialize—that speak to the individual's or group's specific reasons for using drugs. Reminding young people that most people, no matter what age, are *not* users of illegal drugs, do *not* smoke cigarettes, and do *not* get drunk frequently is a critical part of preventing substance abuse.

The Role of Drugs in Your Life

Where do you fit into this complex picture of drug use and abuse? Chances are that you've had experience with OTC and prescription drugs, and you may or may not have had experience with one or more of the drugs described in this chapter. You probably know someone who has used or abused a psychoactive drug. Whatever your experience has been up to now, it's likely that you will encounter drugs at some point in your life. To make sure you'll have the inner resources to resist peer pressure and make your own decisions, cultivate a variety of activities you enjoy doing, realize that you are entitled to have your own opinion, and don't neglect your self-esteem.

Before you try a psychoactive drug, consider the following questions:

- *What are the risks involved?* Many drugs carry an immediate risk of injury or death. Most involve the longer-term risk of abuse and dependence.
- *Is using the drug compatible with your goals?* Consider how drug use will affect your education and career objectives, your relationships, your future happiness, and the happiness of those who love you.
- *What are your ethical beliefs about drug use?* Consider whether using a drug would cause you to go against your personal ethics, religious beliefs, social values, or family responsibilities.
- *What are the financial costs?* Many drugs are expensive, especially if you become dependent on them.
- *Are you trying to solve a deeper problem?* Drugs will not make emotional pain go away; in the long run, they will only make it worse. If you are feeling depressed or anxious, seek help from a mental health professional instead of self-medicating with drugs.

Like all aspects of health-related behaviour, making responsible decisions about drug use depends on information, knowledge, and insight into yourself. Many choices are possible; making the ones that are right for you is what counts.

QUESTIONS FOR CRITICAL THINKING AND REFLECTION
Do you know someone who may have a drug problem? What steps, if any, have you taken to help that person? If you were using drugs and felt that things were out of control, what would you want your friends to do for you?

Changing Your Drug Habits

This behaviour change strategy focuses on one of the most commonly used drugs: caffeine. If you are concerned about your use of a different drug or another type of addictive behaviour, you can devise your own plan based on this one and on the steps outlined in Chapter 1.

Because caffeine supports certain behaviours that are characteristic of our culture, such as sedentary, stressful work, you may find yourself relying on coffee (or tea, chocolate, or cola) to get through a busy schedule. Such habits often begin in university. Fortunately, it's easier to break a habit before it becomes entrenched as a lifelong dependency.

When you are studying for exams, the forced physical inactivity and the need to concentrate even when fatigued may lead you to overuse caffeine. But caffeine doesn't help unless you are already sleepy. And it does not relieve any underlying condition (you are just more tired when it wears off). How can you change this pattern?

Self-Monitoring

Keep a log of how much caffeine you eat or drink. Use a measuring cup to measure coffee or tea. Using Table 14.2 on p. 460, convert the amounts you drink into an estimate expressed in milligrams of caffeine. Be sure to include all forms, such as chocolate bars and OTC medications, as well as caffeine candy, colas, cocoa or hot chocolate, chocolate cake, tea, and coffee.

Self-Assessment

At the end of the week, add up your daily totals and divide by seven to get your daily

average in milligrams. How much is too much? At more than 250 milligrams per day, you may well be experiencing some adverse symptoms. If you are experiencing at least five of the following symptoms, you may want to cut down:

- Restlessness
- Nervousness
- Excitement
- Insomnia
- Flushed face
- Excessive sweating
- Gastrointestinal problems
- Muscle twitching
- Rambling thoughts and speech
- Irregular heartbeat
- Periods of inexhaustibility
- Excessive pacing or movement

Set Limits

Can you restrict your caffeine intake to a daily total and stick to this contract? If so, set a cutoff point, such as one cup of coffee. Pegging it to a specific time of day can be helpful, because then you won't confront a decision at any other point (and possibly fail). If you find you cannot stick to your limit, you may want to cut out caffeine altogether; abstinence can be easier than moderation for some people. If you experience caffeine withdrawal symptoms (headache, fatigue), you may want to cut your intake more gradually.

Find Other Ways to Keep Up Your Energy

If you are fatigued, it makes sense to get enough sleep or exercise more, rather than drowning the problem in coffee or tea. Different people need different amounts of sleep; you may also need more sleep at different times, such as during a personal crisis or an illness. Also, exercise raises your metabolic rate for hours afterward—a handy fact to exploit when you want to feel more awake and want to avoid an irritable caffeine jag. And if you've been compounding your fatigue by not eating properly, try filling up on complex carbohydrates, such as whole-grain bread or crackers, instead of candy bars.

Tips on Cutting Out Caffeine

Here are some more ways to decrease your consumption of caffeine:

- Keep some uncaffeinated drinks on hand, such as decaffeinated coffee, herbal teas, mineral water, bouillon, or hot water.
- Alternate between hot and very cold liquids.
- Fill your coffee cup only halfway.
- Avoid the office or school lunchroom or cafeteria and the chocolate sections of the grocery store. (Often people drink coffee or tea and eat chocolate simply because they're available.)
- Read labels of OTC medications to check for hidden sources of caffeine.

SUMMARY

- Addictive behaviours are reinforcing. People with addictions experience a strong compulsion for the behaviour and a loss of control over it; an escalating pattern of abuse with serious negative consequences may result.

- The sources or causes of addiction include heredity, personality, lifestyle, and environmental factors. People may use an addictive behaviour as a means of alleviating stress or painful emotions.

- Many common behaviours are potentially addictive, including gambling, shopping, sexual activity, Internet use, eating, and working.

- Drug abuse is a maladaptive pattern of drug use that persists despite adverse social, psychological, or medical consequences.

- Drug dependence involves taking a drug compulsively, which includes neglecting constructive activities because of it and continuing to use it despite experiencing adverse effects resulting from its use. Tolerance and withdrawal symptoms are often present.

- Reasons for using drugs include the lure of the illicit; curiosity; rebellion; peer pressure; and the desire to alter one's mood or escape boredom, anxiety, depression, or other psychological problems.

- Psychoactive drugs affect the mind and body by altering brain chemistry. The effect of a drug depends on the properties of the drug and how it's used (drug factors), the physical and psychological characteristics of the individual (individual factors), and the physical and social environment surrounding the drug use (social factors).

- Opioids relieve pain, cause drowsiness, and induce euphoria; they reduce anxiety and produce lethargy, apathy, and an inability to concentrate.

- CNS depressants slow down the overall activity of the nerves; they reduce anxiety and cause mood changes, impaired muscular coordination, slurring of speech, and drowsiness or sleep.

- CNS stimulants speed up the activity of the nerves, causing acceleration of the heart rate, a rise in blood pressure, dilation of the pupils and bronchial tubes, and an increase in gastric and adrenal secretions.

- Marijuana usually causes euphoria and a relaxed attitude at low doses; very high doses produce feelings of depersonalization and sensory distortion. The long-term effects may include chronic bronchitis and cancer; use during pregnancy may impair fetal growth.

- Hallucinogens alter perception, feelings, and thought and may cause an altered sense of time, visual disturbances, and mood changes.

- Inhalants are present in a variety of harmless products; they can cause delirium. Their use can lead to loss of consciousness, heart failure, suffocation, and death.

- Economic and social costs of drug abuse include the financial costs of law enforcement, treatment, and health care, and the social costs of crime, violence, and family problems. Drug testing and drug legalization have been proposed to address some of the problems related to drug abuse.

- Approaches to treatment include medication, treatment centres, self-help groups, and peer counselling; many programs also offer counselling to family members.

FOR MORE INFORMATION

BOOKS

Aue, P. W. 2006. *Teen Drug Abuse: Opposing Viewpoints.* San Diego: Greenhaven Press. Explores key issues relating to drug use and abuse by teenagers.

Drug Abuse and Society Series. Various authors and various years. New York: Rosen Publishing. A series of short books, each exploring a different type of drugs—from prescription medicine to club drugs—and their use and abuse.

Hanson, G. R., et al. 2008. *Drugs and Society,* 10th ed. Boston: Jones & Bartlett. Discusses the impact of drug abuse on individuals' lives and on the broader society.

Karch, S. B. 2006. *Drug Abuse Handbook,* 2nd ed. London: CRC Press. Explores drug abuse from a variety of perspectives, including clinical and criminological.

Ksir, C., C. L. Hart, and O. S. Ray. 2008. *Drugs, Society, and Human Behavior,* 12th ed. New York: McGraw-Hill. Examines drugs and behaviour from the behavioural, pharmacological, historical, social, legal, and clinical perspectives.

Lessa, N. R., et al. 2006. *Wiley Concise Guides to Mental Health: Substance Use Disorders.* New York: Wiley. A clearly written introduction to the diagnosis and treatment of various kinds of substance abuse.

Murphy, P. J. M., and M. Shlafer. 2006. *Over-the-Counter Drugs of Abuse.* New York: Chelsea House Publications. An up-to-date discussion of nonprescription medicines and their abuse.

ORGANIZATIONS, HOTLINES, AND WEBSITES

The Internet addresses listed here were accurate at the time of publication.

Aboriginal Canada Portal. Provides resources, information (including health and social services information), and a list of government programs for First Nations, Inuit, and Metis in Canada.
   http://www.aboriginalcanada.gc.ca
Canadian Centre on Substance Abuse. Provides information relating to substance-abuse issues; contains a number of links and resources.
   http://www.ccsa.ca
Center for Online Addiction. Contains information about Internet and cybersex addiction.
   http://netaddiction.com
Centre for Addiction and Mental Health. Provides information and resources pertaining to clinical care, research, education, policy development, and health promotion in relation to mental health and addiction.
   http://www.camh.net
ClubDrugs.Org. Provides information on drugs commonly classified as "club drugs."
   http://www.clubdrugs.org
Do It Now Foundation. Provides youth-oriented information about drugs.
   http://www.doitnow.org
Gamblers Anonymous. Includes questions to help diagnose gambling problems and provides resources for getting help.
   http://www.gamblersanonymous.org
Health Canada: Drug and Alcohol Statistics. Offers information and statistics on alcohol and drug use in Canada, including findings from the *Canadian Alcohol and Drug Use Monitoring Survey 2008,* the Not4Me Youth Drug Prevention Program.
   http://www.hc-sc.gc.ca/hc-ps/drugs-drogues/stat/index-eng.php
Higher Education Center for Alcohol, Drug Abuse, and Violence Prevention. Gives information about alcohol and drug abuse on campus and links to related sites.
   http://www.edc.org/hec
Narcotics Anonymous. Similar to Alcoholics Anonymous, NA sponsors 12-step meetings and provides other support services for drug abusers.
   http://www.na.org

There are also 12-step programs that focus on specific drugs:
Cocaine Anonymous
   http://www.ca.org
Marijuana Anonymous
   http://www.marijuana-anonymous.org

National Anti-Drug Strategy (Government of Canada). Offers information and news related to three identified priority areas: preventing illicit drug use, treating illicit drug dependency, and combating the production and distribution of illicit drugs. Also offers resources related to youth drug prevention for parents.
   http://www.nationalantidrugstrategy.gc.ca
Responsible Gambling Council. Creates awareness programs related to problem gambling prevention; provides information on problem gambling, treatment, and warning signs, as well as other resources, such as brochures and videos.
   http://www.responsiblegambling.org/en/index.cfm

See also the listings for Chapters 15 and 16.

SELECTED BIBLIOGRAPHY

Adams, G. R., et al. 2007. A study of differences in Canadian university students' gambling and proximity to a casino. *Journal of Gambling Issues* 19: 9–17 (http://www.camh.net/egambling/issue19/pdfs/adams.pdf; retrieved April 1, 2010).

Adlaf, E. M., et al. (eds.). 2005. *Canadian Campus Survey 2004.* Toronto: Centre for Addiction and Mental Health.

American Psychiatric Association. 2000. *Diagnostic and Statistical Manual of Mental Disorders,* 4th ed., text rev. Washington, D.C.: American Psychiatric Association.

Beers, M. H., et al. 2006. *The Merck Manual of Diagnosis and Therapy,* 18th ed. New York: Wiley.

Braine, N. 2004. Long-term effects of syringe exchange on risk behavior and HIV prevention. *AIDS Education and Prevention* 16(3): 264–275.

Budney, A. J., et al. 2004. Review of the validity and significance of cannabis withdrawal syndrome. *American Journal of Psychiatry* 161(11): 1967–1977.

Canada Safety Council. 2005. Canadian roulette. *Safety Canada* 49(1) (http://archive.safety-council.org/news/sc/2005/Eng-1-05.pdf; retrieved April 2, 2010).

Canadian Centre on Substance Abuse. 2009. *Injection Drug Users Overview* (http://www.ccsa.ca/Eng/Topics/Populations/IDU/Pages/InjectionDrug UsersOverview.aspx; retrieved April 19, 2010).

Canadian Psychological Association. 2009. *Gambling* (http://www.cpa.ca/publications/yourhealthpsychologyworksfactsheets/gambling/; retrieved April 4, 2010).

Dauvergne, M. 2009. Trends in police-reported drug offences in Canada. *Juristat,* May (http://www.statcan.gc.ca/pub/85-002-x/2009002/article/10847-eng.htm; retrieved April 19, 2010).

Delaney-Black, V., et al. 2004. Prenatal cocaine: Quantity of exposure and gender moderation. *Journal of Developmental and Behavioral Pediatrics* 25(4): 254–263.

Foreign Affairs and International Trade Canada. 2009. *Consular Activity in 2008: Incident Report for Canadians Abroad* (http://www.voyage.gc.ca/statistics_ statistiques/report-08-rapport-eng.asp#stats; retrieved April 19, 2010).

Government of Canada. 2009. *The National Anti-Drug Strategy* (http://www.nationalantidrugstrategy.gc.ca/nads-sna.html; retrieved April 19, 2010).

Grant, J. E., et al. 2006. Multicenter investigation of the opioid antagonist nalmefene in the treatment of pathological gambling. *American Journal of Psychiatry* 163(2): 303–312.

Health Canada. 2007. *Canadian Addiction Survey (CAS): A National Survey of Canadians' Use of Alcohol and Other Drugs: Substance Use by Canadian Youth* (www.hc-sc.gc.ca/hl-vs/alt_formats/hecs-sesc/pdf/pubs/adp-apd/cas-etc/youth-jeunes/youth-jeunes-eng.pdf (retrieved March 31, 2010).

Health Canada. 2008. *Health Canada Reminds Canadians Not to Use Ephedra/Ephedrine Products* (http://www.hc-sc.gc.ca/ahc-asc/media/advisories-avis/_2008/2008_41-eng.php; retrieved April 16, 2010).

Health Canada. 2009. *Canadian Alcohol and Drug Use Monitoring Survey (CADUMS): Summary of Results for 2008* (http://www.hc-sc.gc.ca/hc-ps/drugs-drogues/stat/_2008/summary-sommaire-eng.php#intro; retrieved March 31, 2010).

Health Canada. 2010. *Canadian Alcohol and Drug Use Monitoring Survey (CADUMS): Summary of Results for 2009* (http://www.hc-sc.gc.ca/hc-ps/drugs-drogues/stat/_2009/summary-sommaire-eng.php; retrieved February 5, 2011).

Health Canada. 2010. *Canadian Tobacco Use Monitoring Survey (CTUMS) 2009: Summary of Annual Results for 2009* (http://www.statcan.gc.ca/daily-quotidien/100927/dq100927c-eng.htm ; retrieved February 5, 2011).

Health Canada. 2010. *Food and Nutrition: Caffeine in Food* (http://www.hc-sc.gc.ca/fn-an/securit/addit/caf/food-caf-aliments-eng.php; retrieved April 15, 2010)

Health Canada. 2010. *Health Concerns: Psilocybin (Magic Mushrooms)* (http://www.hc-sc.gc.ca/hc-ps/drugs-drogues/learn-renseigne/psilocybin-eng.php; retrieved April 19, 2010)

Holmes, N., et al. 2008. Drug testing in the workplace. *Library of Parliament—Parliamentary Information and Research Service* (PRB 07-51E) (http://www.parl.gc.ca/Content/LOP/ResearchPublications/prb0751-e.pdf; retrieved April 19, 2010).

Hurd, Y. L., et al. 2005. Marijuana impairs growth in mid-gestation fetuses. *Neurotoxicology and Teratology* 27(2): 221–229.

Iannone, M., et al. 2006. Electrocortical effects of MDMA are potentiated by acoustic stimulation in rats. *BMC Neuroscience* 7: 13.

International Narcotics Control Board. 2010. *Report of the International Narcotics Control Board for 2009*. New York: United Nations (http://www.incb.org/pdf/annual-report/2009/en/AR_09_English.pdf; retrieved April 3, 2010).

Johnston, L. D., et al. 2008. *Monitoring the Future: National Results on Adolescent Drug Use: Overview of Key Findings, 2007*. Bethesda, Md.: National Institute on Drug Abuse.

Juliano, L. M., and R. R. Griffiths. 2004. A critical review of caffeine withdrawal: Empirical validation of symptoms and signs, incidence, severity, and associated features. *Psychopharmacology* 176(1): 1–29.

Kim, S. W., et al. 2006. Pathological gambling and mood disorders: Clinical associations and treatment implications. *Journal of Affective Disorders* 92(1): 109–116.

Lane, J. D., et al. 2004. Caffeine impairs glucose metabolism in type 2 diabetes. *Diabetes Care* 27(8): 2047–2048.

Lynch, W. J., P. K. Maciejewski, and M. N. Potenza. 2004. Psychiatric correlates of gambling in adolescents and young adults grouped by age at gambling onset. *Archives of General Psychiatry* 61(11): 1116–1122.

Mahowald, M. L., J. A. Singh, and P. Majeski. 2005. Opioid use by patients in an orthopedics spine clinic. *Arthritis and Rheumatology* 52(1): 312–321.

McBride, B. F., et al. 2004. Electrocardiographic and hemodynamic effects of a multicomponent dietary supplement containing ephedra and caffeine. *Journal of the American Medical Association* 291(4): 216–221.

McCusker, R. R., et al. 2006. Caffeine content of energy drinks, carbonated sodas, and other beverages. *Journal of Analytical Toxicology* 30(2): 112–114.

Messinis, L., et al. 2006. Neuropsychological deficits in long-term frequent cannabis users. *Neurology* 66(5): 737–739.

National Institute on Drug Abuse. 2008. *NIDA InfoFacts: Treatment Approaches for Drug Addiction* (http://www.drugabuse.gov/infofacts/treatmeth.html; retrieved February 3, 2009).

Opioid abuse. 2004. *Journal of the American Medical Association* 291(11): 1394.

Paglia-Boak, A., et al. 2009. *Drug Use Among Ontario Students, 1977–2009: OSDUHS Highlights* (CAMH Research Document Series No. 28). Toronto: Centre for Addiction and Mental Health (http://www.camh.net/Research/Areas_of_research/Population_Life_Course_Studies/OSDUS/Highlights_DrugReport_2009OSDUHS_Final_Web.pdf; retrieved April 15, 2010).

Parrott, A. C. 2005. Chronic tolerance to recreational MDMA (3,4-methyl-enedioxymethamphetamine) or ecstasy. *Journal of Psychopharmacology* 19(1): 71–83.

Public Health Agency of Canada. 2009. *HIV and AIDS in Canada. Surveillance Report to December 31, 2008* (http://www.phac-aspc.gc.ca/aids-sida/publication/survreport/2008/dec/index-eng.php#toc; retrieved March 4, 2010).

Ramaekers, J. G., et al. 2004. Dose-related risk of motor vehicle crashes after cannabis use. *Drug and Alcohol Dependence* 73(2): 109–119.

Rehm, J., et al. 2006. Global burden of disease from alcohol, illicit drugs and tobacco. *Drug and Alcohol Review* 25(6): 503–513.

Rehm, J., et al. 2006. The *Costs of Substance Abuse in Canada, 2002: Highlights*. Ottawa: Canadian Centre on Substance Abuse (www.ccsa.ca/2006 CCSA Documents/ccsa-011332-2006.pdf; retrieved April 1, 2010).

Ren, S., et al. 2006. Effect of long-term cocaine use on regional left ventricular function as determined by magnetic resonance imaging. *American Journal of Cardiology* 97(7): 1085–1088.

Responsible Gambling Council. 2009. *Gambling Facts & Stats* (http://www.responsiblegambling.org/en/media/stats.cfm; retrieved April 1, 2010).

Savoca, M. R., et al. 2005. Association of ambulatory blood pressure and dietary caffeine in adolescents. *American Journal of Hypertension* 18(1): 116–120.

Singer, L. T., et al. 2004. Cognitive outcomes of preschool children with prenatal cocaine exposure. *Journal of the American Medical Association* 291(20): 2448–2456.

Statistics Canada. 2009. *Perspectives on Labour and Income: Gambling* (http://www.statcan.gc.ca/pub/75-001-x/topics-sujets/pdf/topics-sujets/gambling-jeuxdehasard-2009-eng.pdf; retrieved April 1, 2010).

Substance Abuse and Mental Health Services Administration. 2005. Nonmedical oxycodone users: A comparison with heroin users. *The NSDUH Report*, January.

Tjepkema, M. 2004. Alcohol and illicit drug dependence. *Health Reports* (15 Suppl.) (http://www.statcan.gc.ca/pub/82-003-s/2004000/pdf/7447-eng.pdf; retrieved April 19, 2010).

Wareing, M., et al. 2005. Visuo-spatial working memory deficits in current and former users of MDMA ("ecstasy"). *Human Psychopharmacology* 20(2): 115–23.

Waska, R. 2006. Addictions and the quest to control the object. *American Journal of Psychoanalysis* 66(1): 43–62.

Weir, E. 2001. Inhalant use and addiction in Canada. *Canadian Medical Association Journal* 164(3): 397.

Zakzanis, K. K., and Z. Campbell. 2006. Memory impairment in now abstinent MDMA users and continued users: A longitudinal follow-up. *Neurology* 66(5): 740–741.

Practise and learn online with Connect.

THE RESPONSIBLE USE OF ALCOHOL

LOOKING AHEAD>>>>>

AFTER READING THIS CHAPTER, YOU SHOULD BE ABLE TO

- Explain how alcohol is absorbed and metabolized by the body
- Describe the immediate and long-term effects of drinking alcohol
- Define moderate alcohol consumption and discuss its possible benefits
- Describe the different forms of alcohol abuse and their consequences
- Evaluate the role of alcohol in your life, and list strategies for using it responsibly

TEST YOUR KNOWLEDGE

1. **"Moderate drinking" is having three or fewer drinks per day.**
   True or false?

2. **Approximately how many adults in Canada do not drink alcohol?**
   a. 56%
   b. 23%
   c. 4%

3. **If a man and a woman of the same weight drink the same amount of alcohol, the woman will become intoxicated more quickly than the man.**
   True or false?

4. **Drinking too much alcohol in too short a time can cause death from alcohol poisoning.**
   True or false?

5. **Drinking coffee will help you sober up.**
   True or false?

ANSWERS

1. **FALSE.** Moderate drinking is no more than one drink per day for women and no more than two drinks per day for men.

2. **B.** In 2008, approximately 10% of Canadian adults indicated that they were lifetime abstainers; another 13% indicated that they had abstained from alcohol in the past year, for a total of 23%. About 68% of Canadian adults drink lightly; a smaller number of Canadians (about 9%) identify themselves as heavy drinkers.

3. **TRUE.** Women are usually smaller than men, have a higher percentage of body fat, and have a less active form of a stomach enzyme that breaks down alcohol. These factors cause them to become intoxicated more quickly and to a greater degree.

4. **TRUE.** Consuming several drinks in a few hours is likely to cause intoxication, followed by a hangover; chugging the same amount in an hour or less can be lethal.

5. **FALSE.** Once alcohol has been absorbed by the body, nothing speeds its metabolism.

Throughout history, alcohol has been more popular than any other psychoactive drug in the Western world, despite numerous prohibitions against it. Alcohol has a somewhat contradictory role in human life. Used in moderation, alcohol can enhance social occasions by loosening inhibitions and creating a pleasant feeling of relaxation. But alcohol use can also be unhealthy. Like other drugs, alcohol has physiological effects on the body that can impair functioning in the short term and cause devastating damage in the long term. For some people, alcohol becomes an addiction, leading to a lifetime of recovery or, for a few, to debilitation and death. Many of our slang expressions for intoxication reflect its less positive aspects; we describe someone who is drunk as being "smashed," "bombed," or "wasted."

The use of alcohol is a complex issue, one that demands conscious thought and informed decisions. In our society, some people choose to drink in moderation while some choose not to drink at all. Still others realize too late that they've made an unwise choice—when they become dependent on alcohol, are involved in an alcohol-related car crash, or simply wake up to discover they've done something they regret.

This chapter discusses the complexities of alcohol use and provides information that will help you make choices that are right for you.

THE NATURE OF ALCOHOL

If you have ever been around people who are drinking, you probably noticed that alcohol seems to affect different people in different ways. One person may seem to get drunk after just a drink or two, while another appears to tolerate a great deal of alcohol without becoming intoxicated. These differences make alcohol's effects on the body seem mysterious and help explain why there are many misconceptions about alcohol use. The following sections describe how alcohol works in the body.

Alcoholic Beverages

Technically speaking, there are many kinds of **alcohol**, and each is an organic compound. In this book, however, the term *alcohol* refers only to ethyl alcohol (or ethanol, often abbreviated as ETOH). Several kinds of alcohol are similar to ethyl alcohol, such as methanol (wood alcohol) and isopropyl alcohol (rubbing alcohol), but they are highly toxic; if consumed, these forms of alcohol can cause serious illness, blindness, and even death.

Common Alcoholic Beverages   Alcoholic beverages come in several basic types; ethanol is the psychoactive ingredient in each of them:

- Beer is a mild intoxicant brewed from a mixture of grains. By volume, beer usually contains 3%–6% alcohol.

- Ales and malt liquors, which are similar to beer, typically contain 6%–8% alcohol by volume.
- Wines are made by fermenting the juices of grapes or other fruits. During *fermentation*, sugars from the fruit react with yeast to create ethanol and other by-products. In table wines, the concentration of alcohol is about 9%–14%. A more potent type of wine, called *fortified wine*, is so called because extra alcohol is added during its production. Fortified wines—such as sherry, port, and Madeira—contain about 20% alcohol.
- Hard liquor—such as gin, whiskey, rum, tequila, vodka, and liqueur—is made by *distilling* brewed or fermented grains or other plant products. Hard liquors usually contain 35%–50% alcohol but can be much stronger.

In Canada, any beverage containing 1.1% or more alcohol by volume is considered an alcoholic beverage. By law, all labels on alcoholic beverages must include the amount of alcohol in the product.

Standard Drinks Versus Actual Servings   When discussing alcohol consumption, the term **one drink** (or *a standard drink*) means the amount of a beverage that typically contains 13.6 grams of alcohol. Figure 15.1 shows the amounts of some popular beverages that are considered to be one standard drink, based on their alcohol content.

People don't always limit themselves to one drink. In fact, a typical serving of most alcoholic beverages is larger (sometimes significantly larger) than a single standard drink. This is particularly true of mixed drinks, which often include more than one type of hard liquor. Alcoholic beverages are usually purchased in packages that contain multiple servings, as shown in Table 15.1.

Caloric Content   Alcohol provides seven calories per gram, and the alcohol in one drink (14–17 grams) supplies about 100–120 calories. Most alcoholic beverages also

341 mL =
(12 oz.)
beer*
(5% alcohol)

142 mL =
(5 oz.)
wine
(12% alcohol)

85 mL =
(3 oz.)
fortified wine**
(16%–18%
alcohol)

43 mL =
(1.5 oz.)
liquor
(40% alcohol)

*Regular beers have an average alcohol content of 5%, but some have as much as 6% or 7%, making them stronger than a "standard" drink. "Light" beers have an average alcohol content of 4%.

**Such as sherry, port, or vermouth

FIGURE 15.1   One drink of various alcoholic beverages.

Source: Centre for Addiction and Mental Health. 2009. *Do You Know... Alcohol* (http://www.camh.net/About_Addiction_Mental_Health/Drug_and_Addiction_Information/alcohol_dyk.html; retrieved May 3, 2010).

Table 15.1	Serving Sizes Versus Standard Drinks of Common Alcoholic Beverages	
Beverage	**Serving/ Container Size**	**No. of Standard Drinks**
Beer	341 mL (12 oz.)	1
	473 mL (16 oz.)	1.3
Table wine	750 mL (25 oz.) bottle	5
Hard liquor	1 mixed drink	1 or more
	750 mL (25 oz.) bottle	17

Source: Based on Department of Health and Human Services. 2007. *The Surgeon General's Call to Action to Prevent and Reduce Underage Drinking.* Washington, D.C.: Department of Health and Human Services, Office of the Surgeon General.

contain some carbohydrate, so, for example, one beer provides about 150 total calories. The "light" in light beer refers to calories; a light beer typically has close to the same alcohol content as a regular beer and about 100 calories. A 145-millilitre glass of red wine has 100 calories; white wine has 96. An 85-millilitre margarita supplies 157 calories, a 175-millilitre cosmopolitan has 143 calories, and a 175-millilitre rum and Coke contains about 180 calories.

Absorption

When a person ingests alcohol, about 20% is rapidly absorbed from the stomach into the bloodstream. About 75% is absorbed through the upper part of the small intestine. Any remaining alcohol enters the bloodstream further along the gastrointestinal tract. Once in the bloodstream, alcohol produces feelings of intoxication. The rate of absorption is affected by a variety of factors. For example, the carbonation in a beverage like champagne increases the rate of alcohol absorption. Artificial sweeteners (commonly used in drink mixers) have been shown to have the same effect. Food in the stomach slows the rate of absorption, as does the drinking of highly concentrated alcoholic beverages, such as hard liquor. But remember: *All* alcohol a person consumes is eventually absorbed.

Metabolism and Excretion

Alcohol is quickly transported throughout the body by the blood. Because alcohol easily moves through most biological membranes, it is rapidly distributed throughout most body tissues. The main site of alcohol **metabolism** is the liver, though a small amount of alcohol is metabolized in the stomach. Alcohol can be metabolized by several processes. Most is converted first to acetaldehyde, then to acetate, which is ultimately burned for energy or converted to fat. The enzymes needed for this process vary slightly among individuals, creating differences in how people react to

alcohol. (See the box "Metabolizing Alcohol: Our Bodies Work Differently.")

About 2%–10% of ingested alcohol is not metabolized in the liver or other tissues but is excreted unchanged by the lungs, kidneys, and sweat glands. Excreted alcohol causes the telltale smell on a drinker's breath and is the basis of breath and urine analyses for alcohol levels. Although such analyses do not give precise measurements of alcohol concentrations in the blood, they provide a reasonable approximation if done correctly.

Alcohol readily enters the human brain, crossing the restrictive layer of cells that ordinarily shields that organ. There, alcohol affects neurotransmitters, the chemicals that carry messages between brain cells. The ability of brain cells to receive these messages is changed, and networks within the brain that connect different brain regions are disrupted. These changes are temporary, creating many of the immediate effects of drinking alcohol.

With chronic heavy usage, however, alcohol's effects become permanent, resulting in lasting disruption of brain function and changes in brain structure. Alcohol interferes with the production of new brain cells in unborn children, young children, adolescents, and young adults in whom the brain continues to develop until about age 21. Even in mature adults, new brain cells are produced to replace damaged ones, and alcohol is likely to affect that process as well.

Alcohol Intake and Blood Alcohol Concentration

Blood alcohol concentration (BAC), a measure of intoxication, is determined by the amount of alcohol consumed in a given amount of time and by individual factors:

- *Body weight:* In most cases, a smaller person develops a higher BAC than a larger person after drinking the same amount of alcohol (Figure 15.2 on p. 476). A smaller person has less overall body tissue into which alcohol can be distributed.

- *Percentage of body fat:* A person with a higher percentage of body fat will usually develop a higher BAC than a more muscular person of the same weight. Alcohol does not concentrate as much in fatty tissue as in muscle and most other tissues, in part because fat has fewer blood vessels.

alcohol The intoxicating ingredient in fermented or distilled beverages; a colourless, pungent liquid.

one drink The amount of a beverage that typically contains 13.6 grams of alcohol; also called a *standard drink.*

metabolism The chemical transformation of food and other substances in the body into energy and wastes.

blood alcohol concentration (BAC) The amount of alcohol in the blood in terms of weight per unit volume; used as a measure of intoxication.

TERMS

Metabolizing Alcohol: Our Bodies Work Differently

DIMENSIONS OF DIVERSITY

Do you notice that you react differently to alcohol than some of your friends do? If so, you may be seeing genetic differences in alcohol metabolism that are associated with ethnicity. Alcohol is metabolized mainly in the liver, where it is converted by an enzyme (alcohol dehydrogenase) to a toxic substance called acetaldehyde. Acetaldehyde is responsible for many of alcohol's noxious effects. Ideally, it is quickly broken down by another enzyme (acetaldehyde dehydrogenase).

But some people, primarily those of Asian descent, have inherited ineffective or inactive variations of the latter enzyme. Other people, including some of African descent and some Jewish population groups, have forms of alcohol dehydrogenase that metabolize alcohol to acet-aldehyde unusually quickly. In either case, the result is a buildup of acetaldehyde when these people drink alcohol. They experience a reaction called *flushing syndrome*. Their skin feels hot, their heart and respiration rates increase, and they may get a headache, vomit, or break out in hives. The severity of their reaction is affected by the inherited form of their alcohol-metabolizing enzymes. Drinking makes some people so uncomfortable that it's unlikely they could ever become addicted to alcohol.

How people behave in relation to alcohol is influenced in complex ways by many factors, including social and cultural ones. But in this case at least, individual choices and behaviour are strongly influenced by a specific genetic characteristic.

- *Sex:* Women metabolize less alcohol in the stomach than men do because the stomach enzyme that breaks down alcohol before it enters the bloodstream is four times as active in men as in women. This means that more unmetabolized alcohol is released into the bloodstream in women. Because women are also generally smaller than men and have a higher percentage of body fat, women will have a higher BAC than men after consuming the same amount of alcohol. Hormonal fluctuations may also affect the rate of alcohol metabolism, making a woman more susceptible to high BACs at certain times during her menstrual cycle (usually just before the onset of menstruation).

BAC also depends on the balance between the rate of alcohol absorption and the rate of alcohol metabolism. A man who weighs 69 kilograms and has normal liver function metabolizes 6.8 grams of alcohol per hour, the equivalent of about half a 341-millilitre bottle of beer or a 145-millilitre glass of wine.

The rate of alcohol metabolism varies among individuals and is largely determined by genetic factors and drinking behaviour. Chronic drinking activates enzymes that metabolize alcohol in the liver, so people who drink frequently metabolize alcohol more rapidly than nondrinkers do. Although the rate of alcohol absorption can be slowed by factors like food, the metabolic rate *cannot* be influenced

FIGURE 15.2 Approximate blood alcohol concentration and body weight. This chart illustrates the BAC an average person of a given weight would reach after drinking the specified number of drinks in the time shown. In Canada, it is a criminal offence to drive with a BAC of 0.08%, or 80 milligrams of alcohol in 100 millilitres of blood; for drivers in a graduated licensing system, most provinces have zero-tolerance laws that set BAC limits at 0%.

Table 15.2	The Effects of Alcohol	
BAC (%)	**Common Behavioural Effects**	**Hours Required to Metabolize Alcohol**
0.00–0.05	Slight change in feelings, usually relaxation and euphoria. Decreased alertness.	2–3
0.05–0.10	Emotional instability, with exaggerated feelings and behaviour. Reduced social inhibitions. Impairment of reaction time and fine motor coordination. Increasingly impaired during driving. Legally drunk at 0.08%.	3–6
0.10–0.15	Unsteadiness in standing and walking. Loss of peripheral vision. Driving is extremely dangerous.	6–10
0.15–0.30	Staggering gait. Slurred speech. Pain and other sensory perceptions greatly impaired.	10–24
More than 0.30	Stupor or unconsciousness. Anaesthesia. Death possible at 0.35% and above. Can result from rapid or binge drinking with few earlier effects.	More than 24

by exercising, breathing deeply, eating, drinking coffee, or taking other drugs. The rate of alcohol metabolism is the same whether a person is asleep or awake.

If a person absorbs slightly less alcohol each hour than he or she can metabolize in an hour, the BAC remains low. People can drink large amounts of alcohol this way over a long period without becoming noticeably intoxicated; however, they do run the risk of significant long-term health hazards (described later in the chapter). If a person drinks alcohol more quickly than it can be metabolized, the BAC will steadily increase, and he or she will become increasingly drunk (Table 15.2, above). Think of a quantity of alcohol drunk over two or three hours—enough to cause intoxication and a hangover the next day. Now, imagine chugging that same quantity in an hour or less. Drinking that much alcohol so quickly could be lethal.

ALCOHOL AND HEALTH

The effects of alcohol consumption on health depend on the individual, the circumstances, and the amount of alcohol consumed.

The Immediate Effects of Alcohol

BAC is a primary factor determining the effects of alcohol (see Table 15.2, above). At low concentrations, alcohol tends to make people feel relaxed and jovial, but at higher concentrations people are more likely to feel angry, sedated, or sleepy. Alcohol is a central nervous system depressant, and its effects vary because body systems are affected to different degrees at different BACs. At any given BAC, the effects of alcohol are more pronounced when the BAC is rapidly

increasing than when it is slowly increasing, steady, or decreasing. The effects of alcohol are more pronounced if a person drinks on an empty stomach, because alcohol is absorbed more quickly and the BAC rises more quickly.

Low Concentrations of Alcohol The effects of alcohol can first be felt at a BAC of about 0.03%–0.05%. These effects may include light-headedness, relaxation, and a release of inhibitions. Most drinkers experience mild euphoria and become more sociable. When people drink in social settings, alcohol often seems to act as a stimulant, enhancing conviviality or assertiveness. This apparent stimulation occurs because alcohol depresses inhibitory centres in the brain.

Higher Concentrations of Alcohol At higher concentrations, the pleasant effects tend to be replaced by more negative ones: interference with motor coordination, verbal performance, and intellectual functions. The drinker often becomes irritable and may be easily angered or given to crying. When the BAC reaches 0.1%, most sensory and motor functioning is reduced, and many people become sleepy. Vision, smell, taste, and hearing become less acute. At 0.2%, most drinkers are unable to function, either physically or psychologically, because of the pronounced depression of the central nervous system, muscles, and other body systems. Coma usually occurs at a BAC of 0.35%, and any higher level can be fatal.

Small doses of alcohol may improve sexual functioning for individuals who are especially anxious or self-conscious, but higher doses often have negative effects, such as reduced erectile response. (Chronic effects of heavy drinking include reduction of testosterone levels and impairment of sperm production.)

Alcohol causes blood vessels near the skin to dilate, so drinkers often feel warm; their skin flushes, and they may sweat more. Flushing and sweating contribute to heat loss, however, so the internal body temperature falls. High doses of alcohol may impair the body's ability to regulate temperature, causing it to drop sharply, especially if the surrounding temperature is low. Drinking alcoholic beverages to keep warm in cold weather does not work and can even be dangerous.

QUESTIONS FOR CRITICAL THINKING AND REFLECTION
Have you ever had a hangover or watched someone else suffer through one? Did the experience affect your attitude about drinking? In what way?

Since alcohol is a sedative, it induces sleepiness. But for those using alcohol as a sleep aid, its utility is short lived, because people quickly build up a tolerance to it. Moreover, large amounts of alcohol disturb normal sleep patterns. The sleep that follows drinking becomes poor quality after some hours, fitful and unrefreshing as the person dreams, awakens, and often stays wakeful. Alcohol can also cause or worsen sleep apnea, a breathing disorder in which the air passage at the back of the mouth narrows or closes during sleep. The condition, evidenced by loud snoring and gasping for breath, greatly reduces the restfulness of sleep. All these sleep disturbances adversely affect next-day performance and alertness. Performance is further impaired if total sleep time is inadequate. Fatigue and sleepiness compromise memory, response time, and ability to perform difficult tasks. These effects become cumulative if, over time, alcohol use and insufficient sleep become routine.

Alcohol Hangover Alcohol's effects wear off slowly, and anyone who has experienced a severe hangover knows they are no laughing matter. The symptoms include headache, shakiness, nausea, diarrhea, fatigue, and impaired mental functioning. Table 15.2 on p. 477 shows how much time is needed to metabolize alcohol. But even after sobering up, at high BACs the resulting hangover can continue to leave a person impaired.

A hangover is probably caused by a combination of the toxic products of alcohol breakdown, dehydration, and hormonal effects. During a hangover, heart rate and blood pressure increase, making some individuals more vulnerable to heart attacks. Electroencephalography or EEGs (brain wave measurement) shows diffuse slowing of brain waves for up to 16 hours after BAC drops to zero. Studies of pilots, drivers, and skiers all indicate that coordination and cognition are impaired in a person with a hangover, increasing the risk of injury.

The best treatment for hangover is prevention. Nearly all men can expect a hangover if they drink more than five or six drinks; for women, the number is three or four drinks. Drinking less, drinking at a slower pace, and consuming food and plenty of non-alcoholic liquids decrease the risk of hangover. If you get a hangover, remember that your ability to drive is definitely impaired, even after your BAC has returned to zero.

Alcohol Poisoning Acute alcohol poisoning occurs much more frequently than most people realize, and all too often it causes death. Drinking large amounts of alcohol in a short time can rapidly raise the BAC into the lethal range. Alcohol, either alone or in combination with other drugs, is responsible for more toxic overdose deaths than any other drug.

Death from alcohol poisoning may be caused either by central nervous system and respiratory depression or by inhaling fluid or vomit into the lungs. The amount of alcohol it takes to make a person unconscious is dangerously close to a fatal dose. Although passing out may prevent someone from drinking more, BAC can keep rising during unconsciousness, because the body continues absorbing ingested alcohol into the bloodstream. Special care should be taken to ensure the safety of anyone who has been drinking heavily, especially if the person becomes unconscious (see the box "Dealing with an Alcohol Emergency").

Using Alcohol with Other Drugs Alcohol-drug combinations are a leading cause of drug-related deaths. Using alcohol while taking a medication that can cause central nervous system depression increases the effects of both drugs, potentially leading to coma, respiratory depression, and death. Such drugs include barbiturates; Valium-like drugs; narcotics, such as codeine; and OTC antihistamines, such as Benadryl. For people who consume three or more drinks per day, use of OTC pain relievers, such as Aspirin, ibuprofen, or acetaminophen increases the risk of stomach bleeding or liver damage. Some antibiotics and diabetes medications can also interact dangerously with alcohol.

Many illegal drugs are especially dangerous when combined with alcohol. Life-threatening overdoses occur at much lower doses when heroin and other narcotics are combined with alcohol. When cocaine and alcohol are used together, a toxic substance called cocaethylene is formed; this substance is responsible for more than half of all cocaine-related deaths.

The safest strategy is to avoid combining alcohol with any other drug—prescription, OTC, or illegal. If in doubt, ask your pharmacist or physician before using any drug in combination with alcohol, or just don't do it.

Alcohol-Related Injuries and Violence The combination of impaired judgment, weakened sensory perception, reduced inhibitions, impaired motor coordination, and increased aggressiveness and hostility that characterizes alcohol intoxication can be dangerous. Through homicide, suicide, automobile crashes, and other traumatic incidents (and not taking into account deaths caused by alcohol-related health issues), alcohol use was linked to close to 3000 Canadian deaths in 2001. The majority of people who attempt suicide have been drinking. Among suicide-related deaths, alcohol use is common; a recent analysis of 5550 suicide deaths found that one-third involved alcohol. Alcohol use more than triples the chances of fatal injuries during leisure activities, such as swimming and boating, and more than half of all fatal falls and serious burns happen to people who have been drinking.

Alcohol and Aggression Worldwide, alcohol is associated with more acts of aggression and violence than any

TAKE CHARGE

Remember: Being very drunk is potentially life threatening. Helping a drunk friend could save a life.

• Be firm but calm. Don't engage the person in an argument or discuss his or her drinking behaviour while the person is intoxicated.

• Get the person out of harm's way—don't let him or her drive or wander outside. Don't let the person drink any more alcohol.

• If the person is unconscious, don't assume he or she is just "sleeping it off." Place your friend on his or her side with the knees up. This position will help prevent choking if the person vomits.

• Stay with the person—you need to be ready to help if he or she vomits or stops breathing.

• Don't try to give the person anything to eat or drink, including coffee or other drugs. Don't give cold showers or try to make your friend walk around. None of these things help anyone to sober up, and they can be dangerous.

Call 911 immediately in any of the following instances:

• You can't wake the person even with shouting or shaking.

• The person is taking fewer than eight breaths per minute or the breathing pattern seems shallow or irregular.

• You think the person took other drugs in addition to alcohol.

• The person has had an injury, especially a blow to the head.

• The person drank a large amount of alcohol within a short time and then became unconscious. Death caused by alcohol poisoning most often occurs when the blood alcohol level rises very quickly because of the rapid ingestion of alcohol.

If you aren't sure what to do, call 911. You may save a life.

---

other legal or illegal drug. In fact, alcohol use contributes to more than 50% of all murders, assaults, and rapes. Not surprisingly, alcohol is frequently found in the bloodstream of victims as well as perpetrators. One study of emergency room departments in Canada found that 42% of patients with violent injuries had a BAC of more than 0.08%. However, only some people become violent under alcohol's influence. These people are often predisposed to aggressive behaviour, are highly impulsive, and may have an underlying psychiatric condition called *antisocial personality disorder*. Their bad behaviour—repeated criminal acts, deceitfulness, impulsiveness, repeated fights or assaults, and disregard for the safety of others—worsens under alcohol's influence. They are also more likely to become alcohol dependent. Alcohol is an important component of gang life, affirming masculinity and male togetherness, and contributing to gang violence.

Alcohol abuse can wreak havoc on home life. Marital discord and domestic violence often exist in the presence of excess alcohol. Heavy drinking by parents is associated with abuse of their children, typically emotional or psychological abuse. Links between parental drinking and physical or sexual abuse are not found consistently, but when such mistreatment does take place, the damaging effect is often long lasting and associated with alcohol misuse in the grown child. (See the box "Growing Up with Alcoholism" on p. 480)

Alcohol and Sexual Decision Making Alcohol seriously affects a person's ability to make wise decisions about sex. A recent survey of university students revealed that frequent binge drinkers were five times as likely to engage in unplanned sexual activity and five-and-a-half times as likely to have unprotected sex as non-binge drinkers. Heavy drinkers are also more likely to have multiple sex partners and to engage in other forms of high-risk sexual behaviour. For all these reasons, rates of sexually transmitted infections (including HIV) and unwanted pregnancy are higher among people who drink heavily than among people who drink moderately or not at all.

Women who binge-drink are at increased risk for rape and other forms of nonconsensual sex. The laws regarding sexual consent are clear: A person who is very drunk or passed out cannot consent to sex. Having sex with a person who is drunk or unconscious is sexual assault.

Drinking and Driving

In Canada, drinking and driving remains the single largest criminal cause of death. According to Mothers Against Drunk Driving (MADD) Canada, more than 41% of the 3045 crash fatalities in 2007 were impairment related. Impaired driving is particularly problematic among young Canadians. In 2006, 16–25-year-olds represented only 13.2% of the population but were involved in 33.4% of Canada's alcohol-related traffic deaths. The highest rate of impaired driving deaths occurs at age 19. More than 73,000 Canadians were injured in alcohol-related car crashes in 2007—approximately 200 people per day. According to a 2009 survey conducted by the Traffic Injury Research Foundation, 5.6% of Canadians admitted to using alcohol before driving. Meanwhile, more than 79% of Canadians say they are "very" or "extremely" concerned about drinking and driving.

People who drink and drive are unable to drive safely because their judgment is impaired, their reaction time is slower, and their coordination is reduced. Some driving skills are affected at BACs of 0.02% and lower; at 0.05%, visual perception, reaction time, and certain steering tasks are all impaired. Any amount of alcohol impairs your ability to drive safely, and fatigue augments alcohol's effects.

Growing Up with Alcoholism

For a child growing up in a household where alcoholism exists, family life can take a painful toll. Whether the alcoholic is a parent, a sibling, or another relative living with the family, the dysfunctional environment's effects start in childhood and can last throughout adulthood. Children from households where there is alcoholism—particularly the children of alcoholics (COAs)—deal with constant stress, anxiety, and embarrassment. Many, feeling that the alcohol abuse was somehow their fault, carry a burden of guilt from early childhood on. Nevertheless, most COAs somehow escape the major damage to which dysfunctional family life contributes: mental health problems, alcohol dependence, and alcohol abuse.

In such households there is often neglect, with household activities revolving around the needs of the alcoholic. The child may witness or be the victim of verbal or physical abuse. The child may simply learn that drinking is an accepted approach to problem solving.

The presence of an alcoholic parent or close relative affects the health and well-being of all members of the household. Other family members are frequently the target of the alcoholic's verbal or physical abuse and all too often have their own problems with alcohol. Nondrinking female spouses of heavy drinkers experience high levels of psycho-

logical distress. A recent study found that both adults and children in the households of alcohol abusers had more medical problems than people from households without alcohol abusers and, not surprisingly, also incurred greater health care costs.

But children are most vulnerable, and an environment of alcoholism results in poor health early on. A very young child is almost completely dependent on the attention and reasonable actions of his caregivers, who may be unable to respond appropriately when the child gets sick. As the child gets older, the caregivers' inability to provide adequate supervision leaves the child vulnerable in other ways.

Yet, the outlook for COAs is not as grim as we might expect, given the hurdles they must overcome. Even though their risk of illness, alcohol dependence, and alcohol abuse is greater than for those without a history of family alcoholism, an impressive majority of COAs are not

alcohol abusers or alcoholics. In 2001–2002, the U.S. National Institute on Alcohol Abuse and Addiction undertook a comprehensive, in-depth survey on alcohol use, interviewing more than 43,000 adults ages 18 and older. The table below shows some of the survey's results.

Although adults with a family background of alcoholism were more likely to drink currently, and to drink more heavily, a sizable proportion had chosen to never drink, and even more had used alcohol in the past but had abstained for at least a year.

The likelihood of problematic alcohol use is also greater among adults with a family background of alcoholism; approximately 6% of these adults abused alcohol, and 7.4% were alcohol dependent. By comparison, 3.4% of respondents without such a family history abused alcohol, and 2.3% were alcohol dependent. Thus, about three times as many people with a family history of alcoholism became alcoholics.

Alcohol Status	No Family Alcoholism	Family History of Alcoholism
Current drinker (1 or more drinks in past 12 months)	61%	71%
Current heavy drinker (men: more than 2 drinks/day; women: more than 1 drink/day)	8%	14%
Former drinker (no drinks in past 12 months)	16%	20%
Lifetime abstainer	23%	9%

The *dose-response function* (see Chapter 14) is the relationship between the amount of alcohol or drug consumed and the type and intensity of the resulting effect. Higher doses of alcohol are associated with a much greater probability of automobile crashes (Figure 15.3). A person driving with a BAC of 0.14% is more than 40 times as likely to be involved in a crash as someone with no alcohol in his or her blood. For those with a BAC above 0.14%, the risk of a fatal crash is estimated to be 380 times as high. The risks for young drivers are even greater than indicated in Figure 15.3, even at very low BACs. Younger drivers have less experience with both driving and alcohol, which results in significant impairment with BACs as low as 0.02%.

In addition to an increased risk of injury and death, driving while intoxicated can have serious legal consequences. Drunk driving is against the law. Since 1969, the legal limit for driving a vehicle has been a BAC of 0.08%, or 80 milligrams of alcohol in 100 millilitres of blood, in all provinces and territories. There are stiff penalties for

drunk driving, including fines, loss of licence, confiscation of vehicle, and jail time. Drivers with lower BACs may also be punishable by law and are dealt with under provincial and territorial traffic acts. Researchers have found that drivers with a BAC of 0.05% may experience difficulties with vision, a reduced ability to perform simple motor tasks, slower reaction times, and less accurate responses—even if they don't appear to be intoxicated. All these problems negatively affect driving performance and lead to an increased risk of collision. For this reason, many provinces have implemented legal consequences, such as licence suspensions, for individuals who are caught driving with a BAC between 0.05% and 0.08% (known as the "warn range"). Additionally, under current zero-tolerance laws in most provinces, drivers with a graduated licence must maintain a 0% BAC while driving.

If you are out of your home and drinking, find alternative transportation or have a *designated driver* who doesn't drink and can provide safe transportation home. The responsibility

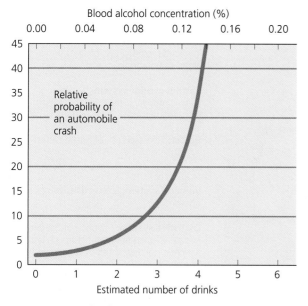

Blood alcohol concentration (%)

FIGURE 15.3   The dose-response relationship between BAC and automobile crashes.

can be rotated for different occasions. Remember, you risk more than your own life when you drink and drive. Causing serious injury or death results in lifelong feelings of sadness and guilt for the driver and grief for friends and families of victims.

It's more difficult to protect yourself against someone else who drinks and drives. Learn to be alert to the erratic driving that signals an impaired driver. Warning signs include making wide, abrupt, and illegal turns; straddling the centre line or lane marker; driving against traffic; driving on the shoulder; weaving, swerving, or nearly striking an object or another vehicle; following too closely; driving at erratic speeds; driving with the headlights off at night; and driving with the window down in very cold weather. If you see any of these signs, try the following strategies:

- If the driver is ahead of you, maintain a safe following distance. Don't try to pass.
- If the driver is behind you, turn right at the nearest intersection, and let the driver pass.
- If the driver is approaching your car, move to the shoulder and stop. Avoid a head-on collision by sounding your horn or flashing your lights.
- When approaching an intersection, slow down and stay alert for vehicles that don't appear to be slowing.
- Make sure your seat belt is fastened and children are in approved safety seats.
- Report suspected impaired drivers to the nearest police station by phone.

The Effects of Chronic Abuse

Because alcohol is distributed throughout most of the body, it can affect many different organs and tissues (Figure 15.4 on p. 482). Problems associated with chronic or habitual excessive use of alcohol include diseases of the digestive and cardiovascular systems and some cancers. Drinking during pregnancy risks the health of both the woman and the developing fetus.

The Digestive System   Even in the short term, alcohol can alter the functioning of the liver. Within just a few days of heavy alcohol consumption, fat begins to accumulate in liver cells, resulting in the development of "fatty liver." If drinking continues, inflammation of the liver can occur, resulting in alcoholic hepatitis, a frequent cause of hospitalization and death in alcoholics. Both fatty liver and alcoholic hepatitis are potentially reversible if the person stops drinking. With continued alcohol use, however, liver cells are progressively damaged and then permanently destroyed. The destroyed cells are replaced by fibrous scar tissue, a condition known as **cirrhosis**. As cirrhosis develops, a drinker may gradually lose his or her capacity to tolerate alcohol, because fewer and fewer healthy cells remain in the liver to metabolize it.

As with most health hazards, the risk of cirrhosis depends on an individual's susceptibility, largely genetically determined, and the amount of alcohol consumed over time. Some people show signs of cirrhosis after a few years of consuming three or four drinks per day. Women generally develop cirrhosis at lower levels of alcohol consumption than men. Heavy drinkers who also inject drugs place themselves at risk of acquiring infection with hepatitis C virus (HCV); the combination of alcohol abuse and HCV infection greatly increases the risk for cirrhosis and liver cancer.

Signs of cirrhosis can include jaundice (a yellowing of the skin and white part of the eyes) and the accumulation of fluid in the abdomen and lower extremities. Some people with cirrhosis have no obvious outward signs of the disease. Treatment for cirrhosis includes correcting nutrient deficiencies and complete abstinence from alcohol. People with cirrhosis who continue to drink have only a 50% chance of surviving five or more years.

Alcohol can inflame the pancreas, causing nausea, vomiting, abnormal digestion, and severe pain. Acute alcoholic pancreatitis generally occurs in binge drinkers. Unlike cirrhosis, which usually occurs after years of fairly heavy alcohol use, pancreatitis can occur after just

cirrhosis   A disease in which the liver is severely damaged by alcohol, other toxins, or infection.

TERMS

Central nervous system: Impaired reaction time and motor coordination; impaired judgment and sedation; coma and death at high BACs

Senses: Less acute vision, smell, taste, and hearing

Stomach: Nausea, inflammation, and bleeding

Skin: Flushing; sweating; heat loss and hypothermia; formation of broken capillaries

Sexual functioning: In men, reduced erection response

Brain: Damaged/destroyed brain cells; impaired memory; loss of sensation in limbs; brain atrophy

Cardiovascular system: Weakened cardiac muscle; elevated blood pressure; irregular heartbeat; increased risk of stroke

Breast: Increased risk of breast cancer

Immune system: Lowered resistance to disease

Digestive system: Cirrhosis of the liver; hepatitis; inflammation of stomach and pancreas; increased risk of cancers of the lip, mouth, larynx, esophagus, liver, rectum, stomach, and pancreas

Kidney: Kidney failure associated with end-stage liver disease

Nutrition: Nutrient deficiencies; obesity

Reproductive system: In women, menstrual irregularities and increased risk of having children with fetal alcohol syndrome (FAS); in men, impotence and impaired sperm production

Bone: Increased risk of osteoporosis; increased risk of fractures from frequent falls

FIGURE 15.4   The immediate and long-term effects of alcohol abuse.

one or two severe binge-drinking episodes. Acute pancreatitis is often fatal; in survivors it can develop into a chronic condition.

Overuse of alcohol is a common cause of bleeding in the gastrointestinal tract. Cirrhosis frequently results in development of enlarged, fragile esophageal and rectal veins, which can easily burst or tear with potentially fatal results. Enlarged esophageal veins are especially vulnerable when the drinker vomits after an alcoholic binge. Even a relatively small amount of alcohol can cause painful irritation of the lining of the stomach.

The Cardiovascular System   The effects of alcohol on the cardiovascular system depend on the amount of alcohol consumed. Moderate doses of alcohol—one drink or less a day for women and one to two drinks a day for men—may reduce the risk of heart disease and heart attack in some people. (The possible health benefits of alcohol are discussed later in this chapter.)

However, higher doses of alcohol have harmful effects on the cardiovascular system. In some people, more than two drinks a day will elevate blood pressure, making stroke and heart attack more likely. Some alcoholics show a weakening of the heart muscle, a condition known as **cardiac**

myopathy. Binge drinking can cause "holiday heart," a syndrome characterized by serious abnormal heart rhythms, which usually appear within 24 hours of a binge episode.

Cancer   Both the International Agency for Research on Cancer and the United States National Toxicology Program have identified alcohol as a known human carcinogen. The Canadian Cancer Society suggests that alcohol consumption is a risk factor for the development of cancers of the breast, colon, rectum, esophagus, larynx, liver, mouth, and pharynx. (Some of these cancers are also associated with use of tobacco, with which alcohol frequently acts as a cocarcinogen.) Five or six daily drinks, especially combined with smoking, increase risk of these cancers by a factor of 50 or more. Alcohol also is largely responsible for the most common form of liver cancer, and continued heavy drinking in people with hepatitis accelerates progression to this cancer. In all alcohol-related cancers, however, genetics and other biological factors play important roles and help explain why some chronic alcohol abusers do not get cancer.

As mentioned above, alcohol increases the risk of breast cancer, but the risks of light to moderate drinking are unclear and somewhat controversial. Recent studies show that breast cancer risk, although still small, begins to increase

at two to three drinks per day, and continues to rise with increasing numbers of daily drinks. The kind of alcohol does not seem to matter. Women at otherwise increased risk of breast cancer (for example, those with a family history of breast or ovarian cancer) should carefully weigh the risks of even moderate drinking.

Brain Damage Brain damage from chronic alcohol abuse is also tempered by an individual's physiology and genetics. Imaging studies document that many alcoholics experience brain shrinkage, with loss of both grey and white matter, reduced blood flow, and slowed metabolic rates in some brain regions. To some extent, brain shrinkage can be reversed over time with abstinence. Individuals who are dependent on alcohol often have cognitive impairments, ranging from mild to severe. These include memory loss, dementia, and compromised problem-solving and reasoning abilities. Even mild-to-moderate drinking can negatively affect certain mental activities that involve acquiring, storing, retrieving, and using information. Additionally, malnutrition, particularly thiamine deficiency, contributes to severe brain damage and the disabling condition known as Wernicke-Korsakoff syndrome.

Mortality Worldwide, alcohol causes 3.2% of all deaths each year. Excessive alcohol consumption is also a factor in several of the leading causes of death for Canadians. Average life expectancy among alcoholics is about 15 years less than among nonalcoholics. About half the deaths caused by alcohol are due to chronic conditions, such as cirrhosis and cancer; the other half are due to acute conditions or events, such as car crashes, falls, and suicide. Because many deaths from acute conditions occur in youths and young adults, alcohol is responsible for thousands of years of potential life lost each year. In 2001, close to 150,000 years of life were lost prematurely in Canada because of alcohol.

The Effects of Alcohol Use During Pregnancy

During pregnancy, alcohol and its metabolic product acetaldehyde readily cross the placenta, potentially harming the developing fetus. Damage to the fetus depends on the amount of alcohol consumed and the stage of the pregnancy. Early in pregnancy, heavy drinking can cause spontaneous abortion or miscarriage. Alcohol in early pregnancy can also cause a range of disabilities known as fetal alcohol spectrum disorder (FASD). The most severe diagnosis of FASD is **fetal alcohol syndrome (FAS)**. Children with FAS have a characteristic mixture of deformities that can include a small head, abnormal facial structure, heart defects, and other physical abnormalities. Their physical and mental growth is slower than normal, and most have a mental disability.

Because rapid brain development continues throughout pregnancy, the fetal brain stays vulnerable to alcohol use until delivery. Although effects of drinking later in preg-

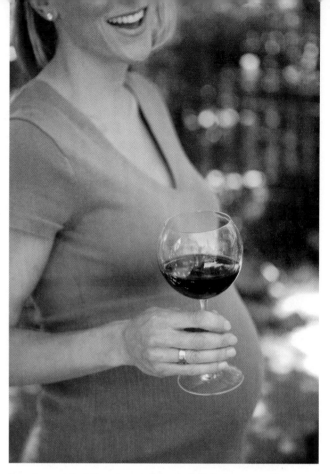

Experts warn that there is no safe level of alcohol consumption during pregnancy.

nancy do not typically cause the characteristic physical deformities of FAS, getting drunk just once during the final three months of pregnancy could damage fetal brain cells.

FASD is a permanent, incurable condition that causes lifelong disability; it is among the most common preventable causes of intellectual disability in the Western world. It is estimated that in Canada, more than 3000 babies are born with FASD each year. Research also suggests that rates of FASD are significantly higher in Aboriginal populations and in rural, remote, and Northern communities.

About three times as many babies are born with **alcohol-related neurodevelopmental disorder (ARND)**. Children with ARND appear physically normal but often have significant learning and behavioural disorders. As adults,

cardiac myopathy Weakening of the heart muscle through disease.

fetal alcohol syndrome (FAS) A characteristic group of birth defects caused by alcohol consumption by the mother, including facial deformities, heart defects, and physical and mental disabilities.

alcohol-related neurodevelopmental disorder (ARND) Cognitive and behavioural problems seen in people whose mothers drank alcohol during pregnancy.

TERMS

they are more likely to develop substance abuse problems and to have criminal records. No one is sure exactly how much alcohol causes FAS or ARND. Like other untoward effects of alcohol, genetics and individual differences in metabolism, along with environmental factors, such as diet, are thought to affect vulnerability. A 2002 study found that children born to mothers who drank as little as one and a half alcoholic drinks per week during their pregnancy weighed less and were shorter at age 14 than children of mothers who drank nothing during pregnancy. This is one of the first studies to show a significant difference between the children of nondrinkers and those of light drinkers. The children's smaller size may be a marker for subtle, persistent alcohol damage. Therefore, no amount of alcohol during pregnancy is considered safe.

Women who are trying to conceive, or who are sexually active without using effective contraception, should abstain from alcohol to avoid inadvertently harming their baby in the first few days or weeks of pregnancy, before they know they're expecting. Binge drinking among women of childbearing age is a particular concern. In the United States, labels on alcoholic beverages are required to carry a warning on the dangers of drinking during pregnancy. In Canada, only Yukon and the Northwest Territories have adopted the use of similar alcohol warning labels. Any alcohol consumed by a nursing mother quickly enters the breast milk. What impact this has on the child or on the mother's milk production is a matter of controversy. Dosage may again be the key issue. However, many physicians advise nursing mothers to abstain from drinking alcohol because of the belief that any amount may have negative effects on the baby's brain development.

Possible Health Benefits of Alcohol

Numerous studies have shown that, on average, light to moderate drinkers (no more than one drink per day for women, and one to two drinks per day for men) live longer than either abstainers or heavy drinkers.

The risks and benefits of drinking alcohol vary considerably with the age of the drinker. If you are 35 or younger, your odds of dying *increase* in direct proportion to the amount of alcohol you drink. Among people under age 35, even light drinkers have slightly higher mortality rates than nondrinkers. In other words, young adults who drink *any* amount of alcohol are more likely to die than nondrinkers of the same age. By contrast, alcohol consumption appears to confer health benefits primarily to older individuals.

The clearest evidence of benefit relates to coronary heart disease (CHD). The lowest rates of CHD deaths occur with moderate alcohol use, which in studies had a positive effect on both healthy people and individuals at risk for CHD. (CHD is discussed in detail in Chapter 7.) In a 2006 study of men ages 50 and over, those who drank moderately each day reduced their risk of CHD by about 40%, compared with men who never drank. The difference was not as great in women. Moderate drinking may improve heart health by raising blood levels of HDL (the beneficial form of cholesterol), by thinning the blood, and by reducing inflammation and the risk of dangerous blood clots, all of which can contribute to the risk of a heart attack. Individuals with heart disease or with strong risk factors should talk with their doctors about the possible health benefits of moderate drinking.

Some evidence also suggests that moderate drinkers may be less likely to develop or better able to manage a variety of other conditions, including diabetes, high blood pressure, strokes, arterial blockages in the legs, cognitive decline (including Alzheimer's disease), and benign prostate enlargement. A 2010 study of more than 1800 older adults who were followed for 20 years showed that moderate drinkers had a lower mortality risk than both abstainers and heavy drinkers. It is still unclear if these effects are due to the alcohol itself or to the nonalcoholic components of alcoholic drinks (the substances that give each different kind of beverage its distinctive character).

Research is under way to determine whether the apparent health benefits of wine are due to the alcohol or to some other substance found in wine. Some experts believe that the apparent benefit of wine may merely reflect the fact that wine drinkers tend to be more affluent and to have healthier lifestyles than those who don't drink wine.

ALCOHOL ABUSE AND DEPENDENCE

Abuse of and dependence on alcohol affect more than just the drinker. Friends, family members, co-workers, strangers that drinkers encounter on the road, and society as a whole pay the physical, emotional, and financial costs of the misuse of alcohol.

Statistics on Alcohol Use

According to the 2008 *Canadian Alcohol and Drug Use Monitoring Survey*, about 77% of Canadians ages 15 and older

drink alcohol, whether infrequently or routinely. Approximately 13% of Canadians are former drinkers, and 10% are lifetime abstainers. More than 9% of Canadians are classified as heavy alcohol users. Heavy drinkers account for more than half of all the alcohol consumed, as well as a disproportionate amount of the social costs of alcohol abuse (death, illness, and economic costs were estimated at $14.6 billion in 2002). In 2002, alcohol use was responsible for more than 8000 deaths in Canada, or 6.2% of deaths in people under the age of 70. The biggest contributing factors were motor vehicle crashes, liver cirrhosis, suicides, oesophageal cancer, and arrhythmias. Alcohol is among the top three risk factors contributing to the burden of disease, disability, and death in Canada (after tobacco and high blood pressure).

Abuse Versus Dependence

As explained in Chapter 14, the American Psychiatric Association's *Diagnostic and Statistical Manual of Mental Disorders* makes a distinction between substance abuse and substance dependence.

Alcohol abuse is recurrent alcohol use that has negative consequences, such as drinking in dangerous situations (before driving, for instance), or drinking patterns that result in academic, professional, interpersonal, or legal difficulties. A person does not have to be an alcoholic to have problems with alcohol. The person who drinks only once a month, perhaps after an exam, but then drives while intoxicated is an alcohol abuser.

Alcohol dependence, or **alcoholism**, involves more extensive problems with alcohol use, usually involving physical tolerance and withdrawal. Alcoholism is discussed in greater detail later in the chapter.

How can you tell if you or someone you know is becoming alcohol dependent? Look for the following warning signs:

- Drinking alone or secretively
- Using alcohol deliberately and repeatedly to perform or get through difficult situations
- Feeling uncomfortable on certain occasions when alcohol is not available
- Escalating alcohol consumption beyond an already established drinking pattern
- Consuming alcohol heavily in risky situations, such as before driving
- Getting drunk regularly or more frequently than in the past
- Drinking in the morning or at other unusual times

Binge Drinking

Although many different definitions can be found in the literature, **binge drinking** has recently been defined as a pattern of alcohol use that brings a person's BAC up to 0.08% or above (typically four drinks for men or three drinks for

VITAL STATISTICS		
Table 15.3	**The Effects of Binge Drinking on University Students**	

	Percentage of Students Experiencing Problems	
Alcohol-Related Problem	**Non-Binge Drinkers**	**Frequent Binge Drinkers**
Drove after drinking alcohol	18	58
Did something they regretted	17	62
Argued with friends	10	43
Engaged in unplanned sex	9	41
Missed a class	9	60
Got behind in schoolwork	9	42
Had unprotected sex	4	21
Got hurt or injured	4	28
Got into trouble with police	2	14
Had five or more of these problems since school year began	4	48

Source: Wechsler, H., and B. Wuethrich. 2003. *Dying to Drink: Confronting Binge Drinking on College Campuses*, reprint ed. Emmaus, Pa.: Rodale.

women), consumed within about two hours. Binge drinking is also referred to as *heavy drinking* or *heavy episodic drinking*. For example, Statistics Canada defines "heavy drinking" as having five or more drinks on one occasion, at least once a month over the past year; a 2008 survey estimated that almost 17% of Canadians (more than 4.5 million people) over the age of 12 were classified as heavy drinkers.

Among university- and college-aged Canadians, drinking often takes place in the form of a binge. In 2004–2005, almost 65% of 15–19-year-old drinkers and 76% of 20–24-year-old drinkers reported binge drinking (five or more drinks on one occasion) at least once in the past 12 months. Approximately half of these binge drinkers reported doing so at least 12 times in the past year.

Binge drinking has a profound effect on students' lives (see the box "Campus Binge Drinking" on p. 486). Frequent binge drinkers have been found to be three to seven times more likely than non-binge drinkers to engage in unplanned or unprotected sex, to drive after drinking, and to get hurt or injured (Table 15.3, above). Binge

alcohol abuse The use of alcohol to a degree that causes physical damage, impairs functioning, or results in behaviour harmful to others.

alcohol dependence A pathological use of alcohol or impairment in functioning caused by alcohol; characterized by tolerance and withdrawal symptoms; alcoholism.

alcoholism A chronic psychological disorder characterized by excessive and compulsive drinking.

binge drinking Periodically drinking alcohol to the point of severe intoxication.

Campus Binge Drinking

Binge drinking among postsecondary students, a serious problem for decades, has recently come under a harsh spotlight largely because of highly publicized alcohol-related tragedies on campuses across Canada and worldwide. Deaths from alcohol overdose, alcohol-related injuries (including motor vehicle crashes), violent crimes, student riots, and serious vandalism have all drawn attention to the epidemic of heavy drinking on university and college campuses.

To many people, heavy drinking is considered a normal and integral part of campus life. But research has shown that heavy drinking has had a devastating impact on far too many students—drinkers and nondrinkers alike—as well as on their families and communities.

Drinking on campus is pervasive. More than 80% of Canadian undergraduate students drink alcohol; that's more than use cigarettes, marijuana, and cocaine combined. Much of the current data on university drinking in Canada comes from the *Canadian Campus Survey*, conducted in 2004. This survey includes the responses of 6282 undergraduate students from 40 universities across Canada. Results show that almost half of students binge-drink; 41% of students reported consuming five or more drinks on a single occasion at least twice in the

past month. Furthermore, about 17% of students reported consuming eight or more drinks on a single occasion at least twice in the past month.

The consequences of campus drinking are serious. According to the *Canadian Campus Survey*, 32% of students reported hazardous or harmful patterns of drinking. Hazardous alcohol-related behaviours included unplanned sexual relations, driving after drinking too much, engaging in unsafe sex, and driving while drinking. The most common alcohol-related harms reported by students were experiencing a hangover, memory loss, and regrets, and missing classes because of a hangover. The negative effects associated with excessive alcohol consumption were also experienced by those around the drinker; secondary alcohol-related harms included study or sleep disruptions, serious arguments, being pushed or assaulted, and experiencing sexual harassment as a result of someone else's drinking.

Approximately 25% of students took advantage of low-priced promotions at bars on campus in the month before the survey. About 15% of students went to happy hours, 12.2% made use of special promotions by beer companies, and 7% attended events that included unlimited drinking for a cover charge. Canadian students who identified themselves as

frequent drinkers found their campus environment to be conducive to drinking, and heavy drinkers believed that the alcohol policies on their campus were not enforced.

Working together, students, faculty, administrators, parents, and the community are beginning to put an end to the destructive culture of heavy drinking on campuses. At some schools in the United States, for example, there is an effort to shift classes to Fridays and even Saturdays, after it was found that binge drinking increases when students don't have Friday classes. Increasingly, social events held during orientation week on many Canadian campuses are becoming "dry" or alcohol free. At some institutions, incoming students are required to take online classes about alcohol; peer health education programs are also being offered. And there is stricter punishment for underage drinking and public drunkenness on some campuses, with the likelihood of suspension for repeat offenders.

Source: Adlaf, E. M., et al. (eds.). 2005. *Canadian Campus Survey 2004.* Toronto: Centre for Addiction and Mental Health (http://www.camh.net/Research/Areas_of_research/Population_Life_Course_Studies/CCS_2004_report.pdf).

drinkers were also more likely to miss classes, get behind in schoolwork, and argue with friends. The more frequent the binges, the more problems the students encountered. Despite their experiences, fewer than 1% of the binge drinkers identified themselves as problem drinkers.

Alcoholism

As mentioned earlier, alcoholism, or alcohol dependence, is usually characterized by tolerance to alcohol and withdrawal symptoms. Everyone who drinks—even non-alcoholics—develops tolerance after repeated alcohol use.

Patterns and Prevalence Alcoholism occurs among people of all ethnic groups and at all socioeconomic levels. The stereotype of the homeless, impoverished alcoholic actually accounts for fewer than 5% of all alcohol-dependent people and usually represents the final stage of a drinking career that began years earlier. Alcohol dependence has different patterns, including these four common ones:

1. Regular daily intake of large amounts
2. Regular heavy drinking limited to weekends
3. Long periods of sobriety interspersed with binges of daily heavy drinking lasting for weeks or months
4. Heavy drinking limited to periods of stress

Once established, alcoholism often exhibits a pattern of exacerbations and remissions. The person may stop drinking and abstain from alcohol for days or months after a frightening problem develops. After a period of abstinence, an alcoholic often attempts controlled drinking, which almost inevitably leads to an escalation in drinking and more problems. Alcoholism is not hopeless, however; many alcoholics do achieve permanent abstinence.

Health Effects Tolerance and withdrawal can have a serious impact on health. As described in Chapter 14, *tolerance* means that a drinker needs more alcohol to achieve intoxication or the desired effect, that the effects of continued use of the same amount of alcohol are diminished, or

that the drinker can function adequately at doses or a BAC that would produce significant impairment in a casual user. Heavy users of alcohol may need to consume about 50% more than they originally needed to experience the same degree of intoxication.

When alcoholics stop drinking or sharply decrease their intake, they experience withdrawal. Symptoms include trembling hands (shakes, or jitters), a rapid pulse and accelerated breathing rate, insomnia, nightmares, anxiety, and gastrointestinal upset. These symptoms usually begin 5–10 hours after alcohol intake is decreased and improve after four to five days. After a week, most people feel much better, but occasionally anxiety, insomnia, and other symptoms persist for six months or more.

More severe withdrawal symptoms occur in about 5% of alcoholics. These include seizures (sometimes called *rum fits*), confusion, and **hallucinations**. Still less common is **delirium tremens** (the **DTs**), a medical emergency characterized by severe disorientation, confusion, epileptic-like seizures, and vivid hallucinations, often of vermin and small animals. The mortality rate from DTs can be as high as 15%, especially in very debilitated people with preexisting medical illnesses.

Alcoholics face all the physical health risks associated with intoxication and chronic drinking described earlier in the chapter. Some of the damage is compounded by nutritional deficiencies that often accompany alcoholism. A mental problem associated with alcohol use is profound memory gaps (commonly known as blackouts), which are sometimes filled by conscious or unconscious lying.

The specific health effects of alcoholism tend to vary from person to person. For example, one individual may suffer from problems with memory and central nervous system defects and have no liver or gastrointestinal problems. Another person with a similar drinking and nutritional history may have advanced liver disease but no memory gaps.

Social and Psychological Effects   Alcohol use causes more serious social and psychological problems than all other forms of drug abuse combined. For every person who is an alcoholic, another three or four people are directly affected. Alcohol is a major source of trouble in many families.

People with alcoholism frequently have mental disorders in addition to their substance dependence. They are also much more likely than nonalcoholics to experience clinical depression, panic disorder, schizophrenia, and antisocial personality disorders. People with anxiety or panic attacks may try to use alcohol to lessen their anxiety, even though alcohol often makes these disorders worse. Individuals with alcoholism also often have other substance-abuse problems.

Causes of Alcoholism   The precise causes of alcoholism are unknown, but many factors are probably involved. Studies of twins and adopted children clearly demonstrate the importance of genetics. If one of a pair of fraternal twins is alcoholic, then the other has about twice the chance of

becoming alcoholic. For the identical twin of an alcoholic, the risk of alcoholism is about four times that of the general population. These risks persist even when the twins have little contact with each other or their biological parents. Similarly, adoption studies show an increased risk among children of alcoholics, even if they were adopted at birth into nondrinking families. Alcoholism in adoptive parents, contrarily, doesn't make individuals more or less likely to become dependent on alcohol. Some studies suggest that as much as 50%–60% of a person's risk for alcoholism is determined by genetic factors.

Not all children of alcoholics become alcoholics, however, and it is clear that other factors are involved. A person's risk of developing alcoholism may be increased by certain personality disorders, having grown up in a violent or otherwise troubled household, and imitating the alcohol abuse of peers and other role models. People who begin drinking excessively in their teens are especially prone to binge drinking and alcoholism later in life. Common psychological features of individuals who abuse alcohol are denial ("I don't have a problem") and rationalization ("I drink because I need to socialize with my customers"). Certain social factors have also been linked with alcoholism, including urbanization, disappearance of the extended family, a general loosening of kinship ties, increased mobility, and changing values.

Treatment   Some alcoholics recover without professional help. How often this occurs is unknown, but possibly as many as one-third stop drinking on their own or reduce their drinking enough to eliminate problems. Often these spontaneous recoveries are linked to an alcohol-related

TERMS

hallucination   A false perception that does not correspond to external reality, such as seeing visions or hearing voices that are not there.

delirium tremens (DTs)   A state of confusion brought on by the reduction of alcohol intake in an alcohol-dependent person; other symptoms are sweating, trembling, anxiety, hallucinations, and seizures.

crisis, such as a blackout or alcohol-related automobile crash, a health problem, or the threat of being fired. Not all alcoholics must hit bottom before they are motivated to stop. People vary markedly in what induces them to change their behaviour.

Most alcoholics, however, require a treatment program of some kind to stop drinking. Many different kinds of programs exist. No single treatment works for everyone, so a person may have to try different programs before finding the right one.

Although treatment is not successful for all alcoholics, considerable optimism has replaced the older view that nothing could be done. Many alcoholics have patterns of drinking that fluctuate widely over time. These fluctuations indicate that their alcohol abuse is a response to environmental factors, such as life stressors or social pressures, and therefore may be influenced by treatment.

One of the oldest and best-known recovery programs is Alcoholics Anonymous (AA). AA consists of self-help groups that meet several times each week and follow a 12-step program. Important steps for people in these programs include recognizing that they are "powerless over alcohol" and must seek help from a "higher power" to regain control of their lives. By verbalizing these steps, the individual directly addresses the denial that is often prominent in alcoholism and other addictions. Many AA members have a sponsor of their choosing who is available by phone 24 hours a day for individual support and crisis intervention. AA convincingly shows the individual that abstinence can be achieved and also provides a sober peer group of people who share the same identity—that of recovering alcoholics. Many AA members find that it works best in combination with counselling and medical care.

Other recovery approaches are available. Some, like Rational Recovery and Women for Sobriety, deliberately avoid any emphasis on higher spiritual powers. A more controversial approach to problem drinking is offered by the group Moderation Management, which encourages people to manage their drinking behaviour by limiting intake or abstaining.

Al-Anon is a companion program to AA for families and friends of people with alcoholism. In Al-Anon, spouses and others explore how they enabled the alcoholic to drink by denying, rationalizing, or covering up his or her drinking and how they can change this codependent behaviour. Alateen is a part of Al-Anon dedicated to young people, typically teenagers, whose lives have been affected by another individual's drinking. Similar to Al-Anon groups, Alateen members meet regularly to share experiences and learn effective coping mechanisms. Employee assistance programs and school-based programs represent another approach to alcoholism treatment. These programs can deal directly with work and campus issues, often important sources of stress for the person who is abusing alcohol. They encourage effective coping responses for internal and external stressors.

Inpatient hospital rehabilitation is useful for some alcoholics, especially if they have serious medical or psycho-logical problems or if life stressors threaten to overwhelm them. When the person returns to the community, however, it is critical that there be some form of active, continuing, long-term treatment. Patients who return to a spouse or family often need to address issues involving those significant others, and to establish new routines and shared recreational activities that do not involve drinking.

Several medical treatments are available for alcoholism. All of these work best in combination with counselling or other nonpharmacological programs:

- *Naltrexone* (ReVia) binds to a brain pleasure centre that reduces the craving for alcohol and decreases its pleasant, reinforcing effects. When taken correctly, naltrexone usually does not make the user feel ill.
- *Acamprosate* (Campral) helps people maintain abstinence after they have stopped drinking. It is unclear how acamprosate works, but it appears to act on brain pathways related to alcohol abuse.

In people who abuse alcohol and have significant depression or anxiety, the use of antidepressant or anti-anxiety medication can improve both mental health and drinking behaviour. In addition, other drugs, such as diazepam (Valium), are sometimes prescribed to replace alcohol during initial stages of withdrawal. Such chemical substitutes are usually useful for only a week or so, because alcoholics are at particularly high risk for developing dependence on other drugs.

Alcohol-treatment programs are successful in achieving an extended period of sobriety for about half of those who participate. Success rates of conventional treatment programs are about the same for men and women and for people from different ethnic groups. Women, minority group members, and the poor often face major economic and social barriers to receiving treatment. Many inpatient treatment programs are financially out of reach for people of low income or those without insurance coverage. AA remains the mainstay of treatment for most people and is often a component of even the most expensive treatment programs. Special AA groups exist in many communities for young people, women, gay men and lesbians, people whose first language isn't English, and a variety of interest groups.

Gender, Setting, and Population Differences

People who abuse alcohol come from all socioeconomic levels and cultural groups, but notable differences exist in patterns of drinking between men and women, across provinces and territories, and among Canadian populations. Table 15.4 contains an overview of the rates of past-year alcohol use for males and females and across provinces.

Men In 2008, Canadian males reported significantly higher rates of heavy drinking than Canadian females. Among men, excessive drinking often begins in the teens

Table 15.4	Users of Alcohol in Canada, by Gender and Province, 2008	
		Past Year Prevalence (percentage)
Gender		
Men		81.4
Women		73.5
Province		
Newfoundland and Labrador		73.1
Prince Edward Island		73.7
Nova Scotia		71.6
New Brunswick		74.0
Quebec		80.9
Ontario		76.4
Manitoba		77.4
Saskatchewan		75.4
Alberta		76.7
British Columbia		77.0
Total Population		**77.3**

Source: Canadian Alcohol and Drug Use Monitoring Survey 2008. Summary of Results for 2008. Health Canada. Reproduced with the permission of the Minister of Health, 2008.

or twenties and progresses gradually through the thirties until the individual is clearly identifiable as an alcoholic by the time he is in his late thirties or early forties. Other men remain controlled drinkers until later in life, sometimes becoming alcoholic in association with retirement, the loss of friends and loved ones, boredom, illness, or psychological disorders. (See the box "Gender and Alcohol Use and Abuse" on p. 490.)

Women   Compared with men, more Canadian women abstain from alcohol completely or are light infrequent drinkers. The progression of alcoholism in women is usually different than it is in men. Women tend to become dependent on alcohol at a later age and with fewer years of heavy drinking. It is not unusual for women in their forties or fifties to become alcoholic after years of controlled drinking. Women who abuse alcohol develop cirrhosis and other medical complications somewhat more often than men; they may have more medical problems because they are less likely to seek early treatment. In addition, women who drink may have an inherently greater biological risk for such complications.

Provincial and Territorial Differences   According to the *Canadian Alcohol and Drug Use Monitoring Survey*, some notable differences in drinking patterns emerged across provinces in 2008. The overall rate of drinking in the year before the survey was about 77%, with Quebec having the highest rate in the country and Nova Scotia having the lowest rate (refer back to Table 15.4). In terms

of light frequent drinking, Quebec had the highest rate at 37.8%, and Newfoundland and Labrador had the lowest rate at 18.8%. Newfoundland and Labrador also had the highest rate of heavy frequent drinking in Canada. In contrast, Quebec had the lowest rate of heavy frequent drinking.

The prevalence of heavy drinking is much higher in the Northwest Territories than in the provinces. According to the 2004 *Northwest Territories Addiction Survey*, almost half of the respondents who indicated that they had consumed alcohol in the previous year reported that they had consumed five or more drinks on a single occasion at least once a month, and close to 15% stated that they had engaged in such heavy drinking at least once a week. Another 40% of drinkers said that they normally consumed five or more drinks on a typical drinking day. More than 40% of drinkers in the Northwest Territories indicated that they had engaged in hazardous drinking in the year before the survey. Similar to those in the rest of Canada, heavy drinkers in the Northwest Territories are more likely to be young males than females.

The legal drinking age is **19** in Canada, except in Alberta, Manitoba, and Quebec, where it is **18**.

—Canadian Centre on Substance Abuse, 2008

QUICK STATS

First Nations Communities   Alcohol abuse is a widespread and severe health problem in many First Nations communities, especially for adolescents and young adults. The 2002–2003 *First Nations Regional Longitudinal Health Survey* revealed that the overall frequency of alcohol use was actually lower among First Nations adults than it was for the general population. However, there was a greater proportion of heavy drinkers (defined as those who drink five or more alcoholic beverages on one occasion) among First Nations adults. The highest-risk group includes young males ages 18–29.

The Canadian Centre on Substance Abuse identified several issues, such as poverty, low education levels, unstable family lives, unemployment, physical and mental abuse, poor social support, and problems with the law, as factors that are related to alcohol abuse within First Nations communities. From a historical and cultural perspective, alcohol and substance abuse problems are (and have been) compounded by discrimination, the effects of residential schools, and barriers to health care. As a result, it has been suggested that treatment and prevention efforts in First Nations communities would be more effective if cultural and historical components are included. Many First Nations communities have succeeded in preventing or reducing alcohol and substance use problems among their people by applying community-based, culturally appropriate solutions to the issues noted above.

Gender and Alcohol Use and Abuse

GENDER MATTERS

Men are more likely than women to drink alcohol, to abuse alcohol, and to have alcohol dependency. In Canada, men account for the majority of alcohol-related deaths and injuries. Most alcohol-related deaths and injuries among men result from incidents involving intoxication, such as motor vehicle crashes, falls, drowning, suicide, and homicide.

A variety of factors contribute to the higher rates of alcohol use and abuse among men. Traditional or stereotypic gender roles and ideas regarding masculinity and drinking behaviour may promote excessive alcohol consumption among men. Young men in particular are also more likely to engage in all types of risky health behaviours. Men drive more kilometres, drive more dangerously, and are more likely to drive while intoxicated. They tend to have greater access to firearms, contributing to their increased rates of suicide and homicide. Men may also be more likely than women to use alcohol to cope with stress and other life challenges.

Generally speaking, alcohol use among Canadian women has decreased since 2004. However, women are not immune to alcohol problems. Whether a woman is a "social drinker," a binge drinker, or a heavy daily user, the impact of alcohol on her will be different from and generally greater than the impact of comparable use on a man. And because of the social stigma attached to problem drinking, particularly among women, women are less likely to seek early treatment.

Women become intoxicated at lower doses of alcohol than men, and they tend to experience the adverse physical effects of chronic drinking sooner and at lower levels of alcohol consumption than men. They develop alcohol liver disease and alcohol-related brain damage after a comparatively shorter period of heavy drinking and a lower level of drinking than men. Some alcohol-related health problems are unique to women, including an increased risk of breast cancer, menstrual disorders, infertility, and, in pregnant women, giving birth to a child with FASD.

Women from all walks of life and all ethnic groups can develop alcohol problems, but those who have never married or are divorced are more likely to drink heavily than married or widowed women. Women who have multiple life roles, such as parent, worker, and spouse, are less vulnerable to alcohol problems than women who have fewer roles.

Helping Someone with an Alcohol Problem

Helping a friend or relative with an alcohol problem requires skill and tact. Start by making sure you are not enabling someone to continue excessively using alcohol. Enabling takes many forms, such as making excuses for the person who is abusing alcohol—for example, saying "he has the flu" when it is really a hangover.

QUICK STATS

8.6% of Canadians ages **20–24** reported symptoms of alcohol dependence in 2002.

—*Canadian Community Health Survey, 2002*

Another important step is open, honest labelling: "I think you have a problem with alcohol." Such explicit statements usually elicit emotional rebuttals and may endanger a relationship. However, you are not helping your friends by allowing them to deny their problems with alcohol or other drugs. Taking action shows that you care.

Even when problems are acknowledged, people are usually reluctant to get help. You can't cure a friend's drinking problem, but you can guide him or her to appropriate help. Your best role might be to obtain information about the available resources and persistently encourage their use. Consider making an appointment for your friend at the student health centre and then go with him or her to the appointment. Most student health centres will be able to recommend local options for self-help groups and formal treatment. You can also check the phone book and the Internet for local chapters of AA and other groups (see For More Information at the end of the chapter). And don't underestimate the power of families to help. An honest phone call to your friend's parents could save a life if your friend is in serious trouble with alcohol.

QUESTIONS FOR CRITICAL THINKING AND REFLECTION

Do you know anyone with a serious alcohol problem? From what you have read in this chapter, would you say that person abuses alcohol or is dependent on it? What effects, if any, has this person's problem had on your life? Have you thought about getting support or help?

DRINKING BEHAVIOUR AND RESPONSIBILITY

The responsible use of alcohol means keeping your BAC low, so that your behaviour is always under your control. In addition to controlling your own drinking, you can promote responsible alcohol use in others.

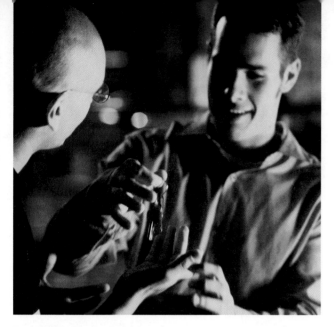

By choosing a designated driver, these men are ensuring a safe trip home.

Examine Your Drinking Behaviour

When you want to drink responsibly, it's helpful to know, first of all, why you drink. The following are common reasons given by university students:

- "It lets me go along with my friends."
- "It makes me less self-conscious and more social."
- "It makes me less inhibited."
- "It relieves depression, anxiety, tension, or worries."
- "It enables me to experience a different state of consciousness."

If you drink alcohol, what are your reasons for doing so?

After examining your reasons for drinking, take a closer look at your drinking behaviour. Is it moderate and responsible? Or do you frequently overindulge and suffer negative consequences? The Behaviour Change Strategy at the end of the chapter explains how to keep and analyze a record of your drinking. The CAGE screening test can help you determine whether you, or someone close to you, may have a drinking problem. Answer yes or no to the following questions:

- Have you ever felt you should
  Cut down on your drinking?
- Have people
  Annoyed you by criticizing your drinking?
- Have you ever felt bad or
  Guilty about your drinking?
- Have you ever had an
  Eye-opener (a drink first thing in the morning to steady your nerves or get rid of a hangover)?

One "yes" response suggests a possible alcohol problem; if you answered yes to more than one question, it is highly likely that a problem exists. For a more detailed evaluation of your drinking habits, complete the AUDIT question-

naire in the box "Do You Have a Problem with Alcohol?" on p. 492. If the results of either assessment test indicate a potential problem, get help right away.

Drink Moderately and Responsibly

Sometimes people lose control when they misjudge how much they can drink. At other times, they set out deliberately to get drunk. The following are some strategies for keeping your drinking and your behaviour under control:

- *Drink slowly.* Sip your drinks rather than gulp them. Do not drink alcoholic beverages to quench your thirst. Avoid drinks made with carbonated mixers, especially if you're thirsty; you'll be more likely to gulp them down.
- *Space your drinks.* Drink nonalcoholic drinks at parties, or alternate them with alcoholic drinks. Learn to refuse a round: "I've had enough for right now." Parties are easier for some people if they hold a glass of something nonalcoholic that has ice and a twist of lime floating in it so it looks like an alcoholic drink.
- *Eat before and while drinking.* Avoid drinking on an empty stomach. Food in your stomach will not prevent the alcohol from eventually being absorbed, but it will slow down the rate somewhat and lower the peak

Do You Have a Problem with Alcohol?

The Alcohol Use Disorders Test (AUDIT) is a screening tool for problem drinking. It can also be used for self-assessment. For each question, choose the answer that best describes your behaviour. Then total your scores.

Questions	Points					Your Score
	0	**1**	**2**	**3**	**4**	
1. How often do you have a drink containing alcohol?	Never	Monthly or less	2–4 times a month	2–3 times a week	4 or more times a week	_____
2. How many drinks containing alcohol do you have on a typical day when you are drinking?	1 or 2	3 or 4	5 or 6	7–9	10 or more	_____
3. How often do you have six or more drinks on one occasion?	Never	Less than monthly	Monthly	Weekly	Daily or almost daily	_____
4. How often during the past year have you found that you were not able to stop drinking once you had started?	Never	Less than monthly	Monthly	Weekly	Daily or almost daily	_____
5. How often during the past year have you failed to do what was normally expected because of drinking?	Never	Less than monthly	Monthly	Weekly	Daily or almost daily	_____
6. How often during the past year have you needed a first drink in the morning to get yourself going after a heavy drinking session?	Never	Less than monthly	Monthly	Weekly	Daily or almost daily	_____
7. How often during the past year have you had a feeling of guilt or remorse after drinking?	Never	Less than monthly	Monthly	Weekly	Daily or almost daily	_____
8. How often during the past year have you been unable to remember what happened the night before because you had been drinking?	Never	Less than monthly	Monthly	Weekly	Daily or almost daily	_____
9. Have you or someone else been injured as a result of your drinking?	No	Yes, but not in the past year (2 points)		Yes, during the past year (4 points)		_____
10. Has a relative, friend, doctor, or other health worker been concerned about your drinking or suggested you cut down?	No	Yes, but not in the past year (2 points)		Yes, during the past year (4 points)		_____
					Total	_____

A total score of 8 or more indicates a strong likelihood of hazardous or harmful alcohol consumption. Even if you score below 8, if you are encountering drinking-related problems with your academic performance, job, relationships, health, or the law, you should consider seeking help.

Source: Sanders, J. B. et al. 1993, *Development of the Alcohol Use Disorders Identification Test (AUDIT):* WHO collaborative project on early detection of persons with harmful alcohol consumption-II. *Addiction,* 88(6), Appendix, p. 803. Reprinted by permission of Blackwell Publishers.

BAC. In restaurants, order your food before you order a drink. Try to have something to eat before you go out to a party where alcohol will be served.

• *Know your limits and your drinks.* Learn how different BACs affect you. In a safe setting, such as your home, with your roommate, friend, or family member, see how a set (and reasonable) amount—say, two drinks in an hour—affects you. A good test is walking heel to toe in a straight line with your eyes closed or standing with your feet crossed and trying to touch your finger to your nose with your eyes closed.

Be aware that in different settings your performance, and especially your ability to judge your behaviour, may change. At a given BAC, you will perform less well when surrounded by activity and boisterous companions than you will in a quiet test setting with just one or two other people. This impairment results partially because alcohol reduces your ability to perform when your brain is bombarded by multiple stimuli.

Promote Responsible Drinking in Others

Although you cannot completely control the drinking behaviour of others, you can do things to help promote responsible drinking.

Encourage Responsible Attitudes Our society teaches us attitudes toward drinking that contribute to alcohol-related problems. Many of us have difficulty expressing disapproval about someone who has drunk too much, and we are amused by the antics of a funny drunk. We accept the alcohol industry's linkage of drinking with virility or

Alcohol Advertising

To be a careful and informed health consumer, you need to consider the effects that advertisements have on you.

In 2002, alcohol manufacturers spent approximately $160 million on advertising in Canada. They claim that the purpose of their advertising is to persuade adults who already drink to choose a certain brand. But in reality, ads cleverly engage young people and children—never overtly suggesting that young people should drink, but clearly linking alcohol and good times.

Alcohol ads are common during televised sporting events and other shows popular with young adults. Studies show that the more TV adolescents watch, the more likely they are to take up drinking in their teens. New alcoholic drinks geared to the tastes of young people are heavily promoted. "Hard lemonade" and other fruity or sweetened drinks ("alcopops" or "low-alcohol refreshers") have been described by teens as a way to get drunk without suffering the bitter taste of most alcoholic beverages. Though only recently introduced, these drinks have been tried by almost half of 14–18-year-olds.

Alcohol manufacturers also reach out to young people at youth-oriented activities, such as concerts and sporting events. Product logos are heavily marketed through sales of T-shirts, hats, and other items, and many universities allow alcohol manufacturers to advertise at campus events.

What is the message of all these advertisements? Think about the alcohol ads you've seen. Many give the impression that drinking alcohol is a normal part of everyday life and good times. This message seems to work well on the young, many of whom believe that heavy-duty drinking at parties is normal and fun. The use of famous musicians, athletes, or actors in commercials increases the appeal of alcohol by associating it with fame, wealth, sex, and popularity. Many beer advertisements, for example, portray beer drinking as a critical part of success in finding an attractive mate.

What ads don't show is the darker side of drinking. You never see hangovers, car crashes, slipping grades, or violence. Although some ads include a brief message, such as "know when to say when," the impact of such cautions is small compared with that of the image of happy, attractive young people having fun while drinking.

The next time you see an advertisement for alcohol, take a critical look. What is the message of the ad? What audience is being targeted, and what is the ad implying about alcohol use? Be aware of its effect on you.

---

sexuality (see the box "Alcohol Advertising"). And many people treat nondrinkers as nonconformists in social settings. Recognize that the choice to abstain is neither odd nor unusual. Close to one-quarter of Canadian adults do not drink at all or have not had an alcoholic beverage in the past year. Most adults are capable of enjoying their leisure time without alcohol or drugs. In hazardous situations, such as driving or operating machinery, abstinence is the only appropriate choice.

Be a Responsible Host   When you are the host, serve nonalcoholic beverages as well as alcohol. Have only enough alcohol on hand for each guest to have a moderate amount. Don't put out large kegs of beer, as these invite people to overindulge. For parties hosted by a dorm, fraternity or sorority, or other campus group, don't allow guests to have unlimited drinks for a single admission fee, as this also encourages binge drinking.

Always serve food along with alcohol, and stop serving alcohol an hour or more before people will leave. If possible, arrange carpools with designated nondrinking drivers in advance. Remind your guests with a graduated licence about the zero-tolerance laws—even a single drink can result in an illegal BAC. Insist that guests who drink too much take a taxi, ride with someone else, or stay overnight.

Plan social functions with no alcohol at all. Outdoor parties, hikes, and practically every other type of social occasion can be enjoyable without alcohol. If that doesn't seem possible to you, then examine your own drinking patterns and attitudes toward alcohol. If you can't have fun without drinking, you may have a problem with alcohol.

Hold the Drinker Responsible   The individual who consumes alcohol must take full responsibility for his or her behaviour. Pardoning unacceptable behaviour fosters the attitude that the behaviour is caused by the drug. The drinker is thereby excused from responsibility and learns to expect minimal adverse consequences for bad behaviour. The opposite approach—holding the individual fully accountable—is a more effective policy. For example, alcohol-impaired drivers who receive strict penalties have fewer subsequent rearrests than those who receive only mandatory treatment. Other people's drunkenness can impinge on your living or study environment. Speak up against this behaviour—and insist on your rights.

Take Community Action   Consider joining an action group, such as BACCHUS Canada. Through education, training, and the promotion of informed decision making regarding the responsible use of alcohol, BACCHUS Canada helps students avoid the dangers of drinking, impaired driving, and other destructive choices.

QUESTIONS FOR CRITICAL THINKING AND REFLECTION

Are you aware of the campus and community resources that can help someone overcome an alcohol problem? For example, does your college or university offer alternatives to keg parties or other events where alcohol is traditionally provided? Are there dorms, organizations, or clubs whose members agree to abstain from alcohol? Are counselling services readily available to students?

Developing Responsible Drinking Habits

How much do you drink? Is it the right amount for you? You may know the answer to this question already, or you may not have given it much thought. Many people learn through a single unpleasant experience how alcohol affects them. Others suffer ill effects but choose to ignore or deny them.

To make responsible and informed choices about using alcohol, consider, first, whether there is any history of alcohol abuse in your family. If someone in your family is dependent on alcohol, you have a higher-than-average likelihood of becoming dependent too. Second, consider whether you are dependent on other substances or behaviours. Do you smoke, drink strong coffee every day, or use other drugs regularly? Does some habit control your life? Some people have more of a tendency to become addicted than others, and a person with one addiction is often likely to have other addictions as well. If this is the case for you, again you may need to be more cautious with alcohol.

Keep a Record

Once you have answered these questions, find out more about your alcohol-related behaviour by keeping track of your drinking for two weeks in a health journal. Keep a daily alcohol behaviour record like the one illustrated in Chapter 1 for eating behaviour. Include information on the following:

■ *The drinking situation*, including type of drink, time of day, how fast you drank it, where you were, and what else you were doing.

■ *Your internal state*, including what made you want to drink and your feelings, thoughts, and concerns at the time. Note how others influenced you.

■ *The consequences of drinking*, including any changes in your feelings or behaviour while or after you were drinking, such as silliness, assertiveness, aggressiveness, or depression.

Analyze Your Record

Next, analyze your record to detect patterns of feelings and environmental cues. Do you always drink when you're at a cer-

tain place or with certain people? Do you sometimes drink just to be sociable, when you don't really want a drink and would be satisfied with a nonalcoholic beverage? Refer to the list of warning signs of alcohol abuse given in the text. Are any of them true for you? For example, do you feel uncomfortable in a social situation if alcohol is *not* available?

Set Goals

Now that you've analyzed your record, think about whether you want to change any of your behaviours. Would you do better academically if you drank less? Has drinking had a negative impact on any of your relationships? Have you risked infection and unplanned pregnancy by having unprotected sex while drunk? Do you depend on alcohol to have a good time? Have you been injured while drinking? If you drink and drive or if you feel you are becoming dependent on alcohol, it is time to change your drinking behaviour. Decide on goals that will give you the best health and safety returns, such as a beer or a glass of wine with dinner, one drink per hour at a party, or no alcohol at all.

Devise a Plan

Refer to your health journal to see what kinds of patterns your drinking falls into and where you can intervene to break the behaviour chain. If you have determined that your life would be improved if you changed your drinking habits, now is the time to make changes. For some people, simple changes in the environment, such as stocking the refrigerator with alternative beverages like juices or sparkling water, can be helpful. If you feel self-conscious about ordering a nonalcoholic drink when you're out with a group, try recruiting a friend to do the same. If it's too difficult to avoid drinking in some situations, such as at a bar or a beer party, you may decide to avoid those situations for a time.

Examine your friendships. If drinking is becoming a problem for you and some of your friends drink heavily, you may need to think about letting those relationships go. If you find support groups helpful, check with your campus health clinic;

most schools sponsor peer group activities for those who are working to change their drinking habits. Local chapters of AA and other organizations may have groups geared toward university-age people.

Instead of drinking, try other activities that produce the same effect. For example, if you drink to relieve anxiety or tension, try adding 20–30 minutes of exercise to your schedule to help manage stress. Or try doing a relaxation exercise or going for a brisk walk to help reduce anxiety before a party or date. If you drink to relieve depression or to stop worrying, consider finding a trustworthy person (perhaps a professional counsellor) to talk to. If you drink to feel more comfortable sexually, consider ways to improve communication with your partner so you can deal with sexual issues more openly. When these activities are successful, they will reinforce your responsible drinking decisions and make it more likely that you'll make the same decisions again in the future.

For other ways to monitor and control your drinking behaviour, see the suggestions in the section "Drinking Behaviour and Responsibility," which starts on p. 490.

Reward Yourself and Monitor Your Progress

If changing your drinking behaviour turns out to be difficult, it may be a clue that drinking is becoming a problem for you—all the more reason to get it under control now. Be sure to reward yourself as you learn to drink responsibly (or not at all). You may lose weight, look better, feel better, and have higher self-esteem as a result. Keep track of your progress in your health journal, and use the strategies described in Chapter 1 for maintaining your program. Remember, when you establish sensible drinking habits, you're planning not just for this week or month—but for your whole life.

Practise and learn online with Connect. Connect allows you to practise important skills at your own pace and on your own schedule, with 24/7 online access to an eBook, practice quizzes, interactivities, videos, study tools, additional resources, and more.

SUMMARY

- Although alcohol has long been a part of human celebrations, it is a psychoactive drug capable of causing addiction.

- After being absorbed into the bloodstream in the stomach and small intestine, alcohol is transported throughout the body. The liver metabolizes alcohol as blood circulates through it.

- If people drink more alcohol each hour than the body can metabolize, blood alcohol concentration (BAC) increases. The rate of alcohol metabolism depends on a variety of individual factors.

- Alcohol is a central nervous system depressant. At low doses, it tends to make people feel relaxed.

- At higher doses, alcohol interferes with motor and mental functioning; at very high doses, alcohol poisoning, coma, and death can occur. Effects may be increased if alcohol is combined with other drugs.

- Alcohol use increases the risk of injury and violence; drinking before driving is particularly dangerous, even at low doses.

- Continued alcohol use has negative effects on the digestive and cardiovascular systems and increases cancer risk and overall mortality.

- Pregnant women who drink risk giving birth to children with a cluster of birth defects known as fetal alcohol spectrum disorder (FASD). Even occasional drinking during pregnancy can cause brain injury in the fetus.

- Moderate drinking may decrease the risk of coronary heart disease in some people.

- Alcohol abuse involves drinking in dangerous situations or drinking to a degree that causes academic, professional, interpersonal, or legal difficulties.

- Alcohol dependence, or alcoholism, is characterized by more extensive problems with alcohol, usually involving tolerance and withdrawal.

- Binge drinking is a common form of alcohol abuse on university and college campuses that has negative effects on both drinking and nondrinking students.

- Physical consequences of alcoholism include the direct effects of tolerance and withdrawal, as well as all the problems associated with chronic drinking. Psychological problems include memory loss and additional mental disorders, such as depression.

- Treatment approaches include mutual support groups like AA, job- and school-based programs, inpatient hospital programs, and pharmacological treatments.

- Helping someone who abuses alcohol means avoiding being an enabler and obtaining information about available resources and persistently encouraging their use.

- Strategies for keeping drinking under control include examining attitudes about drinking and drinking behaviour, drinking slowly, spacing drinks, eating before and while drinking, and knowing your limits.

- Strategies for promoting responsible drinking in others include encouraging responsible attitudes, being a responsible host, holding the drinker responsible for his or her actions, learning about prevention programs, and taking community action.

FOR MORE INFORMATION

BOOKS

Auth, J. 2007. *Emmy's Questions.* St. Augustine, Fla.: Morningtide Press. A young girl's experience growing up in an alcoholic household; for children age 9–12.

Herrick, C. 2007. *100 Questions & Answers About Alcoholism & Drug Addiction.* Boston: Jones and Bartlett. Answers specific questions about alcohol abuse, dependence, and treatment options.

Kinney, J. 2007. *Loosening the Grip: A Handbook of Alcohol Information,* 9th ed. New York: McGraw-Hill. A fascinating book about alcohol, including information on physical effects, abuse, alcoholism, and cultural aspects of alcohol use.

Lu, K. 2006. *Media and College Binge-Drinking: Direct and Indirect Media Influences on Drinking Norm*. Ann Arbor: ProQuest/UMI. A quantitative review of the effect of the media on students' perceptions about drinking.

Seaman, B. 2006. *Binge: Campus Life in an Age of Disconnection and Excess*. New York: Wiley. An exploration of campus life at 12 residential colleges and universities, with discussions on the effects of student isolation, peer pressure, and drinking on students.

Wholey, D. 2007. *Why Do I Keep Doing That?* Deerfield Beach, Fla.: Health Communications. An optimistic approach to breaking self-destructive habits.

Zailckas, K. 2006. *Smashed: Story of a Drunken Girlhood,* reprint ed. New York: Penguin. A young woman writes about her experiences of drinking through high school and college; also includes information from surveys and research into the effects of alcohol use.

ORGANIZATIONS, HOTLINES, AND WEB SITES

The Internet addresses listed here were accurate at the time of publication.

Aboriginal Canada Portal. Provides resources, information (including health and social services information), and government programs for First Nations, Inuit, and Metis in Canada.
http://www.aboriginalcanada.gc.ca

Al-Anon Family Group Headquarters. Provides information and referrals to local Al-Anon and Alateen groups. The Web site includes a self-quiz to determine if you are affected by someone's drinking.
888-4AL-ANON
http://www.al-anon.alateen.org

Alcoholics Anonymous (AA) World Services. Provides general information on AA, literature on alcoholism, and information about AA meetings and related 12-step organizations.
http://www.aa.org

AlcoholScreening.Org. Provides information about alcohol and health, referrals for treatment and support groups, and a drinking self-assessment.
http://www.alcoholscreening.org

BACCHUS Canada. Focuses on alcohol-related issues on post-secondary campuses across Canada.
http://www.studentlifeeducation.com/BACCHUSCanada

Betty Ford Center. In addition to its residential treatment program, the centre offers symposia, newsletters, and programs for children of alcoholics.
http://www.bettyfordcenter.org

Canadian Centre on Substance Abuse. Provides information relating to substance abuse issues; contains a number of links and resources.
http://www.ccsa.ca

Centre for Addiction and Mental Health. Provides information and resources about clinical care, research, education, policy development, and health promotion in relation to mental health and addiction.
http://www.camh.net

Facts on Tap. Provides information about alcohol and postsecondary life, sex and alcohol, and children of alcoholics, as well as suggestions for students who have been negatively affected by other students' alcohol use.
http://www.factsontap.org

Higher Education Center for Alcohol, Drug Abuse, and Violence Prevention. Provides support for campus alcohol and illegal drug prevention efforts; gives information about alcohol and drug abuse on campus and links to related sites.
http://www.edc.org/hec

Moderation Management Network. Provides information on the controversial self-help program designed to help early problem drinkers limit their drinking; not intended for serious alcohol abusers or alcoholics.
http://www.moderation.org

Mothers Against Drunk Driving Canada. Supports efforts to develop solutions to the problems of drunk driving and underage drinking; provides news, information, and brochures about many topics, including a guide to understanding and avoiding alcohol liability when hosting a party.
http://www.madd.ca

Rational Recovery. A free self-help program that offers an alternative to 12-step programs; the emphasis is on learning the skill of abstinence.
http://www.rational.org

Student Life Education Company. Provides students and student advisers with materials, resources, and training pertaining to health-related issues, including the use or nonuse of alcohol.
http://www.studentlifeeducation.com

U.S. National Council on Alcoholism and Drug Dependence. Provides information and resources.
http://www.ncadd.org

See also the listings for Chapter 14.

SELECTED BIBLIOGRAPHY

Addolorato, G., et al. 2006. Baclofen: A new drug for the treatment of alcohol dependence. *International Journal of Clinical Practice* 60(8): 1003–1008.

Adlaf, E. M., et al. (eds.). 2005. *Canadian Campus Survey 2004*. Toronto: Centre for Addiction and Mental Health.

Anton, R. F., et al. 2006. Combined pharmacotherapies and behavioral interventions for alcohol dependence: The COMBINE study: A randomized controlled trial. *Journal of the American Medical Association* 295(17): 2003–2017.

Aronson, K. 2003. Alcohol: A recently identified risk factor for breast cancer. *Canadian Medical Association Journal* 168(9): 1147–1148 (http://ecmaj.ca/cgi/content/full/168/9/1147; retrieved May 5, 2010).

Austin, E. W., and S. J. T. 2005. Targeting adolescents? The content and frequency of alcoholic and nonalcoholic beverage ads in magazine and video formats November 1999–April 2000. *Journal of Health Communication* 10(8): 769–785.

Callahan, M. 2006. Cocktail confidential. *Health,* June, 169–171.

Canadian Cancer Society. 2009. *Alcohol* (http://www.cancer.ca/canada-wide/prevention/alcohol.aspx?sc_lang=en; retrieved February 13, 2011).

Canadian Centre on Substance Abuse. 2009. *First Nations, Inuit and Métis People Overview* (http://www.ccsa.ca/Eng/Topics/Populations/FirstNations_Inuit_MétisPeople/Pages/AboriginalPeoplesOverview.aspx; retrieved February 13, 2011).

Canadian Food Inspection Agency. 2009. *Guide to Food Labelling and Advertising: Chapter 10—Guide to the Labelling of Alcoholic Beverages* (http://www.inspection.gc.ca/english/fssa/labeti/guide/ch10e.shtml; retrieved May 3, 2010).

Centers for Disease Control and Prevention. 2004. Alcohol-attributable deaths and years of potential life lost, United States, 2001. *Morbidity and Mortality Weekly Report* 53(37): 866–870.

Clifasefi, S. L., et al. 2006. Blind drunk: The effects of alcohol on inattentional blindness. *Applied Cognitive Psychology* 20(5): 697–704.

College Drinking Prevention. 2007. *A Snapshot of Annual High-Risk College Drinking Consequences* (http://www.collegedrinkingprevention.gov/StatsSummaries/snapshot.aspx; retrieved February 4, 2009).

Collins, G. B., et al. 2006. Drug adjuncts for treating alcohol dependence. *Cleveland Clinic Journal of Medicine* 73(7): 641–644.

Costello, R. M. 2006. Long-term mortality from alcoholism: A descriptive analysis. *Journal of Studies on Alcohol* 67(5): 694–699.

Dawson, D. A., et al. 2005. Recovery from *DSM-IV* alcohol dependence: United States, 2001–2002. *Addiction* 100(3): 281–292.

Department of Health and Human Services. 2007. *The Surgeon General's Call to Action to Prevent and Reduce Underage Drinking.* Washington, D.C.: Department of Health and Human Services, Office of the Surgeon General.

First Nations Centre. 2005. *First Nations Regional Longitudinal Health Survey (RHS) 2002/03: Results for Adults, Youth and Children Living in First Nations Communities* (http://www.rhs-ers.ca/sites/default/files/ENpdf/RHS_2002/ rhs2002-03-technical_report.pdf; retrieved April 11, 2011).

Gruenewald, P. J., and L. Remer. 2006. Changes in outlet densities affect violence rates. Alcoholism: *Clinical and Experimental Research* 30(7): 1184–1193.

Health Canada. 2007. *Canadian Addiction Survey (CAS): A National Survey of Canadians' Use of Alcohol and Other Drugs: Substance Use by Canadian Youth* (http://www.hc-sc.gc.ca/hl-vs/alt_formats/hecs-sesc/pdf/pubs/adp-apd/cas-etc/youth-jeunes/youth-jeunes-eng.pdf; retrieved March 31, 2010).

Health Canada. 2009. *Canadian Alcohol and Drug Use Monitoring Survey 2008: Summary of Results for 2008* (http://www.hc-sc.gc.ca/hc-ps/drugs-drogues/stat/_2008/summary-sommaire-eng.php#intro; retrieved March 31, 2010).

Heilig, M., and M. Egli. 2006. Pharmacological treatment of alcohol dependence: Target symptoms and target mechanisms. *Pharmacology and Therapeutics* 111(3): 855–876.

Hingson, R., et al. 2005. Magnitude of alcohol-related mortality and morbidity among U.S. college students ages 18–24. *Annual Review of Public Health* 26: 259–279.

Hingson, R. W., et al. 2006. Age at drinking onset and alcohol dependence: Age at onset, duration, and severity. *Archives of Pediatrics and Adolescent Medicine* 160(7): 739–746.

Holahan, C. J., et al. 2010. Late-life alcohol consumption and 20-year mortality. *Alcohol: Clinical and Experimental Research* 34(11): 1961–1971.

Krampe, H., et al. 2006. Follow-up of 180 alcoholic patients for up to 7 years after outpatient treatment: Impact of alcohol deterrents on outcome. *Alcohol: Clinical and Experimental Research* 30(1): 86–95.

Mayo Clinic. 2006. Pain relievers and alcohol: A potentially risky combination. *Mayo Clinic Health Letter,* May.

McCaig, L. F., and E. N. Nawar. 2006. National Hospital Ambulatory Medical Care Survey: 2004 emergency department summary. Advance Data from *Vital and Health Statistics* No. 372. Hyattsville, Md.: National Center for Health Statistics.

Mercer, G. 2009. *Estimating the Presence of Alcohol and Drug Impairment in Traffic Crashes and Their Costs to Canadians: 1999 to 2006.* Vancouver: Applied Research and Evaluation Services.

Miller, T. R., et al. 2006. Societal costs of underage drinking. *Journal of Studies on Alcohol* 67(4): 519–528.

Monti, P. M., et al. 2005. Adolescence: Booze, brains, and behavior. *Alcoholism: Clinical and Experimental Research* 29(2): 207–220.

National Center for Health Statistics. 2008. Deaths: Preliminary data for 2006. *National Vital Statistics Reports* 56(16).

National Institute on Alcohol Abuse and Alcoholism. 2006. *Young Adult Drinking. Alcohol Alert No. 68.* Bethesda, Md.: National Institute on Alcohol Abuse and Alcoholism.

Nelson, T. F., et al. 2005. The state sets the rate: The relationship of college binge drinking rates and selected state alcohol control policies. *American Journal of Public Health* 95(3): 441–446.

Office of Applied Studies, Substance Abuse and Mental Health Services Administration. 2008. *Results from the 2007 National Survey on Drug Use and Health: National Findings* (http://www.drugabusestatistics.samhsa.gov; retrieved February 4, 2009).

Perreira, K. M., and K. E. Cortes. 2006. Explaining race/ethnicity and nativity differences in alcohol and tobacco use during pregnancy. *American Journal of Public Health,* 27 July [epub].

Public Health Agency of Canada. 2008. *Canadian Perinatal Health Report, 2008 edition* (http://www.phac-aspc.gc.ca/publicat/2008/cphr-rspc/pdf/cphr-rspc08-eng.pdf); retrieved May 5, 2010).

Rehm, J., J. Patra, and S. Popova. 2006. Alcohol-attributable mortality and potential years of life lost in Canada 2001: Implications for prevention and policy. *Addiction* 101(3): 373–384.

Rehm, J., et al. 2006. *The Costs of Substance Abuse in Canada 2002.* Ottawa: Canadian Centre on Substance Abuse.

Slutska, W. S. 2005. Alcohol use disorders among US college students and their non-college-attending peers. *Archives of General Psychiatry* 62(3): 321–327.

Statistics Canada. 2005. *Leading Causes of Death in Canada* (http://www.statcan. gc.ca/bsolc/olc-cel/olc-cel?catno=84-215-x&lang=eng; retrieved April 30, 2010).

Traffic Injury Research Foundation. 2009. *The Road Safety Monitor 2009: Drinking and Driving in Canada* (http://www.tirf.ca/publications/PDF_publications/rsm_2009_dd_nat_print.pdf; retrieved May 6, 2010).

Willford, J., et al. 2006. Moderate prenatal alcohol exposure and cognitive status of children at age 10. *Alcoholism: Clinical and Experimental Research* 30(6): 1051–1059.

TOWARD A TOBACCO-FREE SELF AND SOCIETY

16

LOOKING AHEAD >>>>>

AFTER READING THIS CHAPTER, YOU SHOULD BE ABLE TO

- List the reasons people start using tobacco and why they continue to use it

- Explain the short- and long-term health risks associated with tobacco use

- Discuss the effects of environmental tobacco smoke on nonsmokers

- Describe the social costs of tobacco, and list actions that have been taken to combat smoking in the public and private sectors

- Prepare plans to stop using tobacco and to avoid environmental tobacco smoke

TEST YOUR KNOWLEDGE

1. **"Light" or low-tar cigarettes are safer than regular cigarettes.**
   True or false?

2. **Which of the following substances is found in tobacco smoke?**
   a. acetone (nail polish remover)
   b. ammonia (cleaner)
   c. hexamine (lighter fluid)
   d. toluene (industrial solvent)

3. **Each year in Canada, the equivalent of the population of a small city dies from tobacco use.**
   True or false?

4. **Cigarette smoking increases the risk for which of the following conditions?**
   a. facial wrinkling
   b. miscarriage
   c. impotence

5. **A person who quits smoking now will reduce his or her risk of lung cancer within 10 years.**
   True or false?

ANSWERS

1. **FALSE.** Smokers who choose light or low-tar cigarettes do not reduce tar intake or smoking-related disease risks, nor is there any evidence that switching to light cigarettes helps smokers quit.

2. **ALL FOUR.** Tobacco contains thousands of chemical substances, including many that are poisonous or are linked to the development of cancer.

3. **TRUE.** Approximately 47,500 Canadians die each year from tobacco-related causes.

4. **ALL THREE.** Cigarette smoking reduces quality of life and is the leading preventable cause of death in Canada.

5. **TRUE.** The lung cancer risk of a former smoker is 50% of that of a continuing smoker within 10 years of quitting.

moking is the leading cause of preventable death in Canada. Each year, in fact, nearly 45,000 Canadians die prematurely from tobacco-related causes (Figure 16.1). Tobacco use accounts for nearly one of every five deaths in Canada.

Smoking affects the health of people at all stages of life and from all walks of life. On average, a male smoker loses about 6.5 years from his life; a female smoker loses nearly 9 years. Nonsmokers also suffer, especially the children of parents who smoke. Exposure to environmental tobacco smoke (ETS) kills thousands of nonsmokers every year.

In spite of these facts—and despite increasing public and private efforts to restrict smoking—approximately 5.1 million Canadians are smokers, with thousands more joining their ranks each year. This chapter discusses the reasons people use tobacco, the negative impact of smoking, and the measures being taken to stop this public health threat.

WHO USES TOBACCO?

According to the 2005 *Canadian Tobacco Use and Monitoring Survey* (CTUMS), 21% of the Canadian population, or nearly 5.1 million people, reported using a tobacco product at least once in the preceding month. Thirty percent of all university students described themselves as current smokers, meaning they smoke cigarettes every day or most days.

Smoking rates reported in such surveys are essentially unchanged from those reported in 2005, suggesting that a decades-long decline in smoking prevalence has stalled. Until 2005, smoking rates had dropped steadily from a high of roughly 49% in 1964, when the surgeon general's report linked smoking and lung cancer.

In 2009, 19% of men and almost 16% of women smoked cigarettes. Rates of smoking varied based on gender, age, ethnicity, and education level (see Table 16.1 and the box "Smoking Among Canadian Ethnic Populations"). By 2009, adults with less than a grade 12 education were much more likely to smoke cigarettes than those with a postsecondary education. The reverse is true for cigars; cigar smoking is most common among the affluent and those with high educational attainment.

For more than a decade, there has been a gradual increase in the number of "occasional smokers" (people who smoke on some days but not daily). Most such smokers are young adults ages 18–25 who say they smoke only at parties or when they are with friends who smoke. Health officials warn that occasional smokers are as vulnerable as other smokers to the health dangers of tobacco. Occasional smokers are also less likely to try to quit.

Most current smokers, however, seem to understand the risks of tobacco use. For example, more than 80% of adult smokers believe tobacco will shorten their life and would like to stop smoking. Each year, approximately 1 million smokers quit; however, 43% will relapse. It takes the average smoker 3.2 quit attempts before quitting successfully.

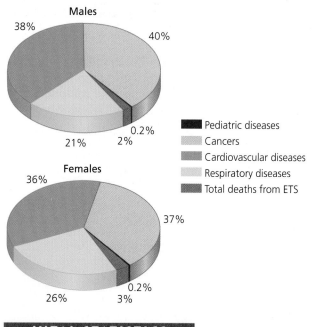

Males

38%
40%
0.2%
2%
21%

Females

36%
37%
0.2%
3%
26%

■ Pediatric diseases
■ Cancers
■ Cardiovascular diseases
■ Respiratory diseases
■ Total deaths from ETS

VITAL STATISTICS

FIGURE 16.1 **Proportion of deaths attributable to smoking in Canada, by sex.**

Source: Makomaski Illing, E. M., and M. J. Kaiserman. 2004. Mortality attributable to tobacco use in Canada and its regions, 1998. *Canadian Journal of Public Health* 95(1) (http://journal.cpha.ca/index.php/cjph/article/download/457/457; retrieved May 1, 2011). © Her Majesty the Queen in Right of Canada.

Table 16.1	Who Smokes?		
	Percentage of the Population Who Smoke		
	Men	Women	Total
Ethnic group (age 18+) in 2007			
Anglophones			25
Francophones			35
Inuit			70
First Nations on-reserve			60
Education and smoking prevalence (age 15+)	**2005**		**2009**
Less than high school	23	19	23
Finished high school	30	25	22
Some postsecondary	27	23	16
Postsecondary graduate	21	18	9

Sources: Data for ethnic groups from Centre for Addiction and Mental Health. 2007. *New Prevention Program to Address Smoking in Ethnic Francophone Communities* (http://www.camh.net/News_events/News_releases_and_media_advisories_and_backgrounders/francophone%20smoking/francophone%20smoking%20cessation.html; retrieved May 2, 2011); and Health Canada. 2007. *First Nations, Inuit and Aboriginal Health: Substance Use and Treatment of Addictions—Tobacco* (http://www.hc-sc.gc.ca/fniah-spnia/substan/tobac-tabac/index-eng.php#facts; retrieved May 2, 2011). Data for education level from Physicians for a Smoke-Free Canada. 2005. *Smoking in Canada: A Statistical Snapshot of Canadian Smokers* (http://www.smoke-free.ca/pdf_1/SmokinginCanada-2005.pdf; retrieved May 2, 2011); and Health Canada. 2010. *Canadian Tobacco Use Monitoring Survey, 2009: Table 8—Smoking and Education, Age 15+ Years, Canada 2009* (http://www.hc-sc.gc.ca/hc-ps/tobac-tabac/research-recherche/stat/_ctums-esutc_2009/ann-eng.php#t7; retrieve May 2, 2011).

Smoking Among Canadian Ethnic Populations

The overall rate of tobacco use among Canadians ages 12 and older was 21% in 2008; on average, any group of a dozen people is likely to include three or four who use tobacco. But averages include wide variations among populations, and ethnic differences appear in the earliest stages of tobacco use. Similar to a number of health-related issues, ethnicity and cultural background serve as determinants of tobacco use.

About 24% of all Canadian high school students described themselves as "current cigarette users" in 2008. Francophone students (35.6%) were more likely than Anglophone students (23%) to smoke in high school. However, far more First Nations students living on-reserve (60%) described themselves as smokers than did either Anglophone or Francophone students.

The use of smokeless tobacco products in high school is not nearly as prevalent as cigarette use. Only 1% of students age 15 and older reported using smokeless tobacco products.

Wide ethnic variations also exist among smokers over 18 years old. Almost 72% of Inuit and 52% of Metis adults are smokers, a rate that is almost double that of the general population.

Within broad ethnic categories, even greater variation occurs. Among people grouped under the broad category of Aboriginal people, which represents only 4.4% of the total population, 60% smoke. The health-related implications of such a high Aboriginal smoking rate results in an adjusted smoking attributable mortality

rate almost 1.5 times as high as in the general population. This means that approximately one in five adult deaths among Aboriginal people is tobacco related.

The staggering smoking rate of Aboriginal people is not restricted to adults: Smoking rates of Aboriginal youth are double that of the smoking rate of other Canadian youth.

The variations between and within ethnic populations reflect a complex interplay of social, environmental, and cultural factors. For example, tobacco is used in important Aboriginal spiritual ceremonies, specifically, sweat lodges, pipe ceremonies, and smudges. Tobacco is used in cleansing rituals to enable communication with spirits as a way of seeking the Creator.

The substantial tobacco use among Aboriginal people requires culturally sensitive quitting initiatives. Canada's Aboriginal culture gravitates toward a four-body approach when confronting health issues. The four-body approach encompasses the physical, mental, emotional, and spiritual aspects of the individual in relation with the health concern. As such, initiatives would need to address not only the physical addiction but also the other three components of the four-body approach. More specifically, cessation efforts may be more successful if they address the mental relationship of tobacco use in spiritual ceremonies as compared with that in tobacco misuse; the emotional aspect of dealing with smoking habits that are encouraged through role modelling; and the spiritual aspect of an individual for whom the misuse of tobacco can negatively affect the effectiveness of communicating with the spirits.

Sources: McKennit, D. 2007. A smoking prevention program for Aboriginal youth. *First Peoples Child and Family Review* 3(2): 52–55; Reading, J., and Y. Allard. 1999. *The Tobacco Report: Report of the FNIRHS.* Ottawa: First Nations and Inuit Health Survey National Steering Committee; Wardman, D., and N. Khan. 2004. Smoking-attributable mortality among British Columbia's First Nations populations. *International Journal on Circumpolar Health* 63: 81–92; Wardman, D., and N. Khan. 2005. Registered Indians and tobacco taxation: A culturally appropriate strategy? *Canadian Journal of Public Health* 96: 451–453.

Young People and Tobacco

Although all provinces and territories ban the sale of tobacco to anyone younger than 18 years of age, at least 50 million packs of cigarettes are consumed by minors each year. In one month, 30,000 teens under the age of 19 reported smoking tobacco.

Almost 20% of Canadian teens ages 12–19 smoke. Among high school students, about 23% of males and 21% of females are smokers. An estimated 1% of high school students use spit or smokeless tobacco. (The various types of tobacco products are described in detail later in this chapter.) In 2009, 30% of cigarettes smoked by high school students in Ontario and Quebec were contraband cigarettes. All of this is particularly worrisome given that one out of two lifetime smokers will die from tobacco use.

Tobacco and Other Drugs

Men and women with other drug abuse problems frequently use tobacco. For example, studies show that roughly 70% of alcoholics and more than 90% of heroin addicts are heavy smokers.

QUESTIONS FOR CRITICAL THINKING AND REFLECTION

Do any of your friends or family members smoke or use smokeless tobacco? What effect has it had on their health and relationships? Have you ever discussed their tobacco use with them? Why or why not?

Smoking also is two to four times as prevalent among people with mental health diagnoses, including major depression, social phobias, and generalized anxiety disorder, as it is in the general population. Such findings suggest that underlying psychological or physiological traits may predispose people to drug use, including tobacco.

WHY PEOPLE USE TOBACCO

Although people start smoking for a variety of reasons, they usually become long-term smokers after becoming addicted to nicotine—the key psychoactive ingredient in tobacco smoke.

Nicotine Addiction

The primary reason people continue to use **tobacco** is that they have become addicted to a powerful psychoactive drug: **nicotine**. Although the tobacco industry long maintained that nicotine had not been proven to be addictive, scientific evidence overwhelmingly shows that nicotine is highly addictive. Many researchers consider nicotine to be the most physically addictive of all the psychoactive drugs.

Some neurological studies indicate that nicotine acts on the brain in much the same way as cocaine and heroin. Nicotine reaches the brain via the bloodstream seconds after it is inhaled or, in the case of spit tobacco, absorbed through membranes of the mouth or nose. It triggers the release of powerful chemical messengers in the brain, including epinephrine, norepinephrine, and dopamine. But unlike street drugs, most of which are used to achieve a high, nicotine's primary attraction seems to lie in its ability to modulate everyday emotions.

At low doses, nicotine acts as a stimulant. It increases heart rate and blood pressure. In adults, nicotine can enhance alertness, concentration, rapid information processing, memory, and learning. The opposite effect occurs in teens who smoke, however; they show impairment in memory and other cognitive functions.

In some circumstances, nicotine acts as a mild sedative. Most commonly, nicotine relieves withdrawal symptoms, such as anxiety, irritability, and mild depression, in tobacco users who are trying to quit. Some studies have shown that high doses of nicotine and rapid smoking cause increases in levels of glucocorticoids and endorphins, chemicals that act in the brain to moderate moods and reduce stress. Tobacco users are able to fine-tune nicotine's effects and regulate their moods by increasing or decreasing their intake of the drug. Studies have shown that smokers experience milder mood variation than nonsmokers while performing long, boring tasks or while watching emotional movies, for example.

All tobacco products contain nicotine, and the use of any of them can lead to addiction (see the box "Nicotine Dependence: Are You Hooked?"). Nicotine addiction fulfils the criteria for substance dependence described in Chapter 14, including loss of control, tolerance, and withdrawal.

Loss of Control Half of all Canadian smokers would like to quit smoking. Canadian cessation programs are considered successful if 15% of smokers are able to quit. Of the people who try to quit smoking, 60% typically relapse in the first three months and 75% relapse within six months. This relapse rate is similar to rates for alcoholics and heroin addicts. Quitting may be even harder for smokeless users: In one study, only 1 of 14 spit tobacco users who participated in a tobacco-cessation clinic was able to stop for more than four hours.

Regular tobacco users live according to a rigid cycle of need and gratification. On average, they can go no more than 40 minutes between doses of nicotine; otherwise, they begin feeling edgy and irritable and have trouble concentrating. If ignored, nicotine cravings build until getting tobacco becomes a paramount concern, crowding out other thoughts. Tobacco users may plan their daily schedule around opportunities to satisfy their nicotine cravings; this loss of control and personal freedom can affect all the dimensions of wellness (see the box "Tobacco Use and Religion: Global Views" on p. 504).

Tobacco users become adept, therefore, at keeping a steady amount of nicotine circulating in the blood and going to the brain. In one experiment, smokers were given cigarettes that looked and tasted alike but varied in nicotine content. The subjects automatically adjusted their rate and depth of inhalation so that they absorbed their usual amount of nicotine. In other studies, heavy smokers were given nicotine without knowing it, and they cut down on their smoking without a conscious effort. Spit tobacco users maintain blood nicotine levels as high as those of cigarette smokers.

Tolerance and Withdrawal Using tobacco builds up tolerance. Where one cigarette may make a beginning smoker nauseated and dizzy, a long-term smoker may have to chain-smoke a pack or more to experience the same effects. For most regular tobacco users, sudden abstinence from nicotine produces predictable withdrawal symptoms as well. These symptoms, which come on several hours after the last dose of nicotine, can include severe cravings, insomnia, confusion, tremors, difficulty concentrating, fatigue, muscle pains, headache, nausea, irritability, anger, and depression. Users undergo measurable changes in brain waves, heart rate, and blood pressure, and they perform poorly on tasks requiring sustained attention. Although most of these symptoms of physical dependence pass in two or three days, the craving associated with addiction persists. Many ex-smokers report intermittent, intense urges to smoke for years after quitting.

Social and Psychological Factors

Why do tobacco users have such a hard time quitting even when they want to? Social and psychological forces

Nicotine Dependence: Are You Hooked?

Answer each question in the list below, giving yourself the appropriate number of points.

_____ 1. How soon after you wake up do you have your first cigarette?

    a. within 5 minutes (3)

    b. 6–30 minutes (2)

    c. 31–60 minutes (1)

    d. after 60 minutes (0)

_____ 2. Do you find it difficult to refrain from smoking in places where it is forbidden, such as the library, a theatre, or a doctor's office?

    a. yes (1)

    b. no (0)

_____ 3. Which cigarette would you most hate to give up?

    a. the first one in the morning (1)

    b. any other (0)

_____ 4. How many cigarettes a day do you smoke?

    a. 10 or less (0)

    b. 11–20 (1)

    c. 21–30 (2)

    d. 31 or more (3)

_____ 5. Do you smoke more frequently during the first hours after waking than during the rest of the day?

    a. yes (1)

    b. no (0)

_____ 6. Do you smoke if you are so ill that you are in bed most of the day?

    a. yes (1)

    b. no (0)

_____ TOTAL

A total score of 7 or more indicates that you are very dependent on nicotine and are likely to experience withdrawal symptoms when you stop smoking. A score of 6 or less indicates low to moderate dependence.

Source: Heatherton, T. F., et al. 1991. The Fagerstrom Test for Nicotine Dependence: A revision of the Fagerstrom Tolerance Questionnaire. *British Journal of Addictions* 86(9): 1119–1127.

---

combine with physiological addiction to maintain the tobacco habit. Many people, for example, have established habits of smoking while doing something else—while talking, working, drinking, and so on. The spit tobacco habit is also associated with certain situations—studying, drinking coffee, or playing sports. It is difficult for these people to break their habits because the activities they associate with tobacco use continue to trigger their urge. Such activities are called **secondary reinforcers**; they act together with the physiological addiction to keep the user dependent on tobacco.

Genetic Factors

Inherited characteristics play an important role in some aspects of tobacco use. Genetic factors may be more important than social and environmental factors in smoking initiation and in the development of nicotine dependence.

For example, a gene that influences the way in which nicotine is metabolized, or broken down in the body, helps regulate the activity of an enzyme called CYP2A6. When people with slow CYP2A6 metabolism use tobacco, the nicotine remains in their blood longer than in people who have the gene for a faster metabolizing form of the enzyme. The slow metabolizers are more likely to feel nausea or dizziness when they first use tobacco, are less likely to continue smoking if they try it, and find it easier to quit if they do become regular smokers.

Scientists have also shown that a gene called *DRD2* (associated with the brain chemical dopamine, which plays a key role in the pleasurable effects of nicotine) appears to influence the progression of smoking in adolescence. Among students in grade 10 who took one puff of a cigarette, those with one form of the gene were more than three times as likely as those with the other form to have become regular smokers when they finished grade 11.

QUICK STATS

12 years is the average age at which a Canadian starts smoking.

—**Smoke-Free Living, 2008**

TERMS

tobacco The leaves of cultivated tobacco plants prepared for smoking or chewing or for use as snuff.

nicotine A poisonous, addictive substance found in tobacco and responsible for many of the effects of tobacco.

secondary reinforcers Stimuli that are not necessarily pleasurable in themselves but that are associated with other stimuli that are pleasurable.

Tobacco Use and Religion: Global Views

SMOKING IS NOT ALLOWED IN THE CHURCH YARD

Religious traditions can best assist adult smokers by reminding them of two principles: one, the value of liberation from any form of slavery, and two, respect for life out of deference to their god.

Tobacco Use as a Violation of Religious Principles

All religions condemn tobacco use for its damaging effects on the body. Most religions regard the human body as the dwelling place of the spirit; as such, it deserves care and respect.

The Baha'i faith, for example, strongly discourages smoking as unclean and unhealthy. Some Protestant churches consider tobacco use a violation of the body. For Hindus, smoking goes against one of the primary spiritual practices, the care of the body. The Roman Catholic Church endorses the age-old adage "a sound mind in a sound body." For Muslims, one of the five essential principles on which religious law is based is protection of the integrity of the individual. In Judaism, people are urged to "choose life" and to choose whatever strengthens the capacity to live. Buddhists believe that the body doesn't belong to the person at all— even suicide is considered murder—and a person must do nothing to harm it.

Most religions also contend that dependence and addiction run counter to ideas of freedom, choice, and human dignity. Buddhism teaches a path of freedom—a way of life without dependence on anything. Hindus regard tobacco use as a dependence that is not necessary for the preservation of health. Protestant churches caution that any form of dependence is contrary to the notion of Christian freedom.

Another argument against tobacco use is the immorality of imposing secondhand smoke on nonsmokers, which is seen as inflicting harm on others. In Hinduism, harming others is sinful. In the Jewish tradition, those who force nonsmokers to breathe smoke jeopardize the lives of others, and to do so is to jeopardize the whole universe.

The Role of Individual Responsibility

Most religions focus on the role of individual responsibility in overcoming dependence on tobacco. In Buddhism, for example, people must assume responsibility for their habits; they practise introspection to understand the cause of problems within themselves and the effects of their actions on others. The principles of Islam are based on notions of responsibility and protection; you are responsible for your body and health.

Religion and Tobacco Control

Different religions share common views on how the problem of tobacco use should be approached. The Islamic view is that the campaign to control tobacco use must be based on awareness, responsibility, and justice. Developing awareness means providing information on the global problem. Fostering responsibility means helping people understand what they need to do to attain well-being. Emphasizing social and human justice means helping the farmers and societies that depend on tobacco cultivation to find alternative crops.

According to the Geneva Interreligious Platform (a project involving Hindus, Buddhists, Jews, Christians, Muslims, and Baha'is), the best approach is prevention. Here, the rights of nonsmokers clearly prevail over the freedom of smokers. In support of this position, the common religious exhortation not to do unto others what you would not have them do unto you can be invoked. Further, adequate information should be provided to counter the deceptive images projected by tobacco industry advertising, especially where minors are concerned. Protection of the weak and denunciation of dishonesty are underlying values of all religious traditions.

Why Start in the First Place?

By grade 4 students are thinking about smoking, and by grade 6, students are likely to start experimenting with smoking. Almost 85% of all smokers started smoking before they were 18 years old. Children—especially girls—are beginning to experiment with tobacco at ever-younger ages. The earlier people begin smoking, the more likely they are to become heavy smokers—and to die of tobacco-related disease.

Not all young people are equally vulnerable to the lure of tobacco. According to Health Canada's *Youth Smoking Survey*, fewer Canadian youth are starting to smoke and more are never smokers in recent years (Figure 16.2). Research suggests that the more of the following characteristics that apply to a child or adolescent, the more likely he or she is to use tobacco:

- A parent or sibling uses tobacco.
- Peers use tobacco.
- The child comes from a blue-collar family.
- The child comes from a low-income home.
- The family is headed by a single parent.
- The child performs poorly in school.
- The child drops out of school.
- The child has positive attitudes about tobacco use.

Young people start using tobacco for a variety of reasons. Some young, male athletes, for example, begin using spit

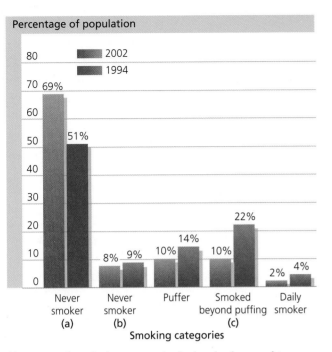

Percentage of population

■ 2002
■ 1994

- 80
- 70 — 69%
- 60
- 50 — 51%
- 40
- 30
- 20 — 22%
- 10 — 8% 9% 10% 14% 10% 2% 4%
- 0

Never smoker (a) | Never smoker (b) | Puffer | Smoked beyond puffing (c) | Daily smoker

Smoking categories

(a) Never smoker who has never seriously thought about smoking
(b) Never smoker who has seriously thought about smoking
(c) Smoked beyond puffing, not daily smoker
Percentages may not add to 100 because of rounding.

FIGURE 16.2   Comparison of smoking categories in youth, grades 5 to 9, by year in Canada.

Source: Health Canada. 2002. *Youth Smoking Survey: Technical Report*, Chapter 3, p. 45 (http://www.hc-sc.gc.ca/hc-ps/alt_formats/hecs-sesc/pdf/pubs/tobac-tabac/yss-etj-2002/yss-etj-2002-eng.pdf; retrieved May 1, 2011). © Her Majesty the Queen in Right of Canada.

Most adult smokers began as teenagers.

tobacco to emulate their favourite professional athletes. Young women commonly take up smoking because they think it will help them lose weight or stay thin. Most often, however, young people start smoking simply because their peers are already doing it; smoking gives them a way to fit in with a crowd or to look cool.

Rationalizing the Dangers   Making the decision to smoke requires minimizing or denying both the health risks of tobacco use and the tremendous pain, disability, emotional trauma, family stress, and financial expense involved in tobacco-related diseases, such as cancer and emphysema. A sense of invincibility, characteristic of many adolescents and young adults, also contributes to the decision to use tobacco. Young people may persuade themselves they are too intelligent, too lucky, or too healthy to be vulnerable to tobacco's dangers. "I'm not dumb enough to get hooked," they may argue. "I'll be able to quit before I do myself any real harm."

Many teenagers believe they will be able to stop smoking when they want. In fact, adolescents are more vulnerable to nicotine than are older tobacco users. Compared with older smokers, adolescents become heavy smokers and develop dependence after fewer cigarettes. Nicotine addiction can start within a few days of smoking and after just a few cigarettes. More than half of teenagers who try cigarettes progress to daily use, and about half of those who ever smoke daily progress to nicotine dependence. In surveys, about 70% of smoking teens state they wish they had never started. Another survey revealed that only 5% of high school smokers predicted they would definitely be smoking in five years; in fact, close to 75% were smoking seven to nine years later.

Emulating Smoking in the Media   Researchers have found that smoking in movies has increased significantly since 1990, to levels not seen since 1960. Between 1998 and 2000, smoking in PG-13 movies increased by 50%. Half the tobacco shots in the top movies from 2002 to 2003 were in G, PG, and PG-13 movies.

The portrayal of smoking in films does not reflect Canadian patterns of tobacco use. The prevalence of smoking among lead characters is three to four times that among comparable Canadians. Films typically show the smoker as white, male, well educated, successful, and attractive. In reality, smokers tend to be poor and to have less education. In the top-grossing films in the early 2000s, smoking was portrayed in more than 73% of the films, including 82% of PG-13 films; smoking was often shown positively as a means to relieve tension or as something to do while socializing. Negative consequences resulting from tobacco use were depicted for only 3% of the major characters who used tobacco. By showing smoking in an unrealistically positive light, films may be acting as advertisement (see the box "Tobacco Advertising" on p. 506).

CRITICAL CONSUMER

Tobacco Advertising

Advertising is a powerful influence. In 2003, the Canadian tobacco industry spent more than $388 million on advertising that portrayed users as confident, popular, fit, and sexually attractive. That same year approximately 45,000 people died from tobacco-related causes.

Youth Appeal

Young people were a prime target of tobacco ads because nicotine addiction can lead to a lifetime of purchasing tobacco. The tobacco industry also understood that young smokers are most likely to buy familiar brands. The most heavily advertised cigarettes were the choice of 90% of teen smokers. In the 1980s and 1990s, for example, R.J. Reynolds Tobacco Company's promotion of the Camel brand recruited millions of new smokers. In surveys, more than 90% of six-year-olds recognized the Camel character ("Joe Camel"), who became as familiar to children as Mickey Mouse.

Limits on Ads

In Canada, tobacco companies must adhere to the Canadian Tobacco Act (enacted in 1997), which regulates the manufac-

turing, sale, labelling, and promotion of tobacco products. The act specifically prohibits the following:

- Testimonials in favour of tobacco use

- Brand stretching to products and services associated with young people

- All forms of promotion except those explicitly stated in the act, which include the following:

  - A mailed publication addressed to an adult who is identified by name

  - A publication with an adult readership of not less than 85%

  - Signage in locations where young persons are not permitted by law

Regardless, the tobacco industry continues to spend millions of dollars annually to promote its product. Much of this money is spent on print ads and coupons, but a great deal is also given to retailers to help offset ever-increasing taxes levied on tobacco products by provinces and territories.

Does smoking on-screen affect real-life smoking habits? Studies of adolescents have consistently found a strong association between seeing tobacco use in films and trying cigarettes. Adolescents who see more smoking in films or whose favourite movie stars frequently use tobacco on-screen have more positive attitudes about smoking and are as much as three times as likely to have tried smoking as teens with less exposure to films. Teens may be particularly sensitive to on-screen portrayals of smoking because they are in the process of developing adult identities; during this period, they may try out different personas, including those of their favourite movie stars.

Some groups suggest an automatic R rating for any film that shows tobacco use, equating smoking with violence, strong language, sexuality, and nudity in determining a film's rating.

QUICK STATS

70% of Inuit people ages 18–45 years smoke—the highest rate among Canadian ethnicities.

—Health Canada, 2007

QUESTIONS FOR CRITICAL THINKING AND REFLECTION

What has influenced your decision to smoke, not to smoke, or to quit smoking? Have you ever felt that images or messages in the media were encouraging you to use tobacco? How do you react to such messages?

Although tobacco advertising has been severely restricted, smoking is still commonly portrayed in movies. In the 2009 movie *Avatar*, Dr. Grace Augustine (played by Sigourney Weaver) is seldom without a cigarette.

HEALTH HAZARDS

Tobacco adversely affects nearly every part of the body, including the brain, stomach, mouth, and reproductive organs.

Tobacco Smoke: A Toxic Mix

Tobacco smoke contains hundreds of damaging chemical substances, including acetone (nail polish remover), ammonia, hexamine (lighter fluid), and toluene (industrial solvent). Smoke from a typical unfiltered cigarette contains about 5 billion particles per cubic millimetre—50,000 times as many as are found in an equal volume of smoggy urban air. These particles, when condensed, form a brown, sticky mass called **cigarette tar**.

Carcinogens and Poisons   At least 43 chemicals in tobacco smoke are linked to the development of cancer. Some, such as benzo(a)pyrene and urethane, are **carcinogens**; that is, they directly cause cancer. Other chemicals, such as formaldehyde, are **cocarcinogens**; they do not themselves cause cancer but combine with other chemicals to stimulate the growth of certain cancers, at least in laboratory animals. Other substances in tobacco cause health problems because they damage the lining of the respiratory tract or decrease the lungs' ability to fight off infection.

Tobacco also contains poisonous substances, including arsenic and hydrogen cyanide. In addition to being an addictive psychoactive drug, nicotine is also a poison and can be fatal in high doses. Many cases of nicotine poisoning occur each year in toddlers and infants who pick up and eat cigarette butts they find at home or on the playground.

Cigarette smoke contains carbon monoxide, the deadly gas in automobile exhaust, in concentrations 400 times as high as is considered safe in industrial workplaces. Not surprisingly, smokers often complain of breathlessness when they require a burst of energy to climb stairs or lift something. Carbon monoxide displaces oxygen in red blood cells, depleting the body's supply of oxygen needed for extra work. Carbon monoxide also impairs visual acuity, especially at night.

Additives   Tobacco manufacturers use additives to manipulate the taste and effect of cigarettes and other tobacco products. Additives account for roughly 10%, by weight, of a cigarette, and include sugars and other flavouring agents, humectants (compounds that keep tobacco from drying out), and chemicals that enhance the addicting properties of nicotine.

Added sugars—including liquorice, cocoa, and honey—have a dual role. As flavour enhancers, sugars mask the harsh, bitter taste of tobacco, so smokers can inhale more smoke and absorb more nicotine. When sugars burn, they produce acetaldehyde, a chemical that enhances the addictive effect of nicotine and is a carcinogen.

Other flavour components, such as the obromine and glycyrrhizin, act as bronchodilators, opening the lungs'

airways and making it easier for nicotine to get into the bloodstream.

Ammonia plays a complex role in tobacco products, but its chief purpose is to boost the amount of addictive nicotine delivered by cigarettes. Ammonia reduces the acidity of tobacco smoke and releases nicotine in the form of a base (alkaline) rather than a salt (acid) bound to other acid components of smoke. As a free base, nicotine is more readily absorbed into the blood.

Some additives are intended to make **sidestream smoke** (the uninhaled smoke from a burning cigarette) less obvious and objectionable. For example, potassium citrate, aluminum, and clay are added to cigarette wrappers to convert particulate ash into an invisible gas with less irritating odour than would be given off by a conventional paper wrapper. These additives serve no purpose in making cigarettes more desirable and addicting to the smoker; instead, they are intended to reduce social pressures from nonsmokers.

QUICK STATS

Nicotine levels increased more than 1% per year in major cigarette brands from 1998 to 2005.

—Harvard School of Public Health, 2007

Nearly 600 chemicals, approved as safe when used as food additives, are used in manufacturing cigarettes. Canada is a world leader in cigarette testing. In 1998, British Columbia became the first jurisdiction to successfully demand disclosure of the chemicals in cigarette smoke from tobacco companies. Canadian tobacco manufacturers now must disclose all additives in their products.

The Results of Inhaling Tobacco Smoke   All smokers absorb some gases, tar, and nicotine from cigarette smoke, but smokers who inhale bring most of these substances into their bodies and keep them there. In one year, a typical pack-a-day smoker takes in 50,000 to 70,000 puffs. Smoke from a cigarette, pipe, or cigar directly assaults the mouth, throat, and respiratory tract. The nose, which normally filters about 75% of foreign matter we breathe, is completely bypassed.

In a cigarette, the unburned tobacco itself acts as a filter. As a cigarette burns down, there is less and less filter. Thus, more chemicals are absorbed into the body during the

TERMS

cigarette tar   A brown, sticky mass created when the chemical particles in tobacco smoke condense.

carcinogen   Any substance that causes cancer.

cocarcinogen   A substance that works with a carcinogen to cause cancer.

sidestream smoke   The uninhaled smoke from a burning cigarette.

Cigarette making is an elaborate process involving industrial machinery and chemistry. Dozens of compounds may be added to tobacco to produce a specific brand of cigarette.

last third of a cigarette than during the first. A smoker can cut down on the absorption of harmful chemicals by not smoking cigarettes down to short butts. Any gains, of course, will be offset by smoking more cigarettes, inhaling more deeply, or puffing more frequently.

"Light" and Low-Tar Cigarettes   Some smokers switch to low-tar, low-nicotine, or filtered cigarettes because they believe them to be healthier alternatives. But there is no such thing as a safe cigarette, and smoking behaviour is a more important factor in tar and nicotine intake than the type of cigarette smoked. Smokers who switch to a low-nicotine brand often compensate by smoking more cigarettes, inhaling more deeply, taking larger or more frequent puffs, or blocking ventilation holes with lips or fingers to offset the effects of filters.

Studies have found that people who smoke "light" cigarettes inhale up to eight times as much tar and nicotine as printed on the label. Studies also show that smokers of light cigarettes are less likely to quit than smokers of regular cigarettes, probably because of the misperception that light cigarettes are safer. Use of light and low-tar cigarettes does not reduce the risk of smoking-related illnesses.

Menthol Cigarettes   Concerns have also been raised about menthol cigarettes. Menthol is a bronchodilator; as mentioned earlier, bronchodilators open the lungs' airways and make it easier for nicotine to enter the bloodstream. Younger smokers are using more menthol cigarettes than are older smokers. Studies have found that 44% of current smokers, ages 12–17 years have tried menthol cigarettes, compared with 31% of smokers ages 18 and older. The anaesthetizing effect of menthol, which may allow smokers to inhale more deeply and hold smoke in their lungs for longer, may be partly responsible for these differences. Research is needed to determine the relationship between menthol cigarettes and illnesses, such as cancer and cardiovascular disease.

The Immediate Effects of Smoking

The beginning smoker often has symptoms of mild nicotine poisoning: dizziness; faintness; rapid pulse; cold, clammy skin; and sometimes nausea, vomiting, and diarrhea. The seasoned smoker occasionally suffers these effects of nicotine poisoning, particularly after quitting and then returning to a previous level of consumption. The effects of nicotine on smokers vary, depending greatly on the size of the nicotine dose and how much tolerance previous smoking has built up. Nicotine can either excite or tranquilize the nervous system, depending on dosage.

Nicotine has many other immediate effects (Figure 16.3). It stimulates the part of the brain called the **cerebral cortex**. It also stimulates the adrenal glands to discharge adrenaline. Nicotine inhibits the formation of urine; constricts the blood vessels, especially in the skin; accelerates the heart rate; and elevates blood pressure. Higher blood pressure, faster heart rate, and constricted blood vessels require the heart to pump more blood. In healthy people, the heart can usually meet this demand, but in people whose coronary arteries are damaged enough to interfere with the flow of blood, the heart muscle may be strained.

Smoking depresses hunger contractions and dulls the taste buds; smokers who quit often notice that food tastes much better. Smoking is not useful for weight loss, however. Smoking for decades may lessen or prevent age-associated weight gain for some smokers, but for people under 30, smoking is not associated with weight loss.

QUICK STATS

More than **4000** chemicals have been identified in tobacco smoke.

—Physicians for a Smoke-Free Canada, 2003

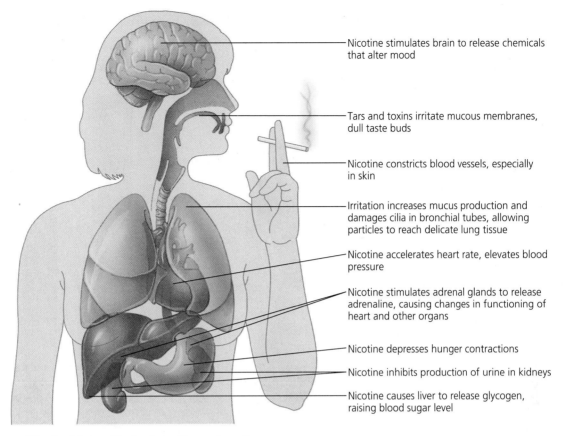

FIGURE 16.3   The short-term effects of smoking a cigarette.

The figure shows labels pointing to various parts of the body:

- Nicotine stimulates brain to release chemicals that alter mood
- Tars and toxins irritate mucous membranes, dull taste buds
- Nicotine constricts blood vessels, especially in skin
- Irritation increases mucus production and damages cilia in bronchial tubes, allowing particles to reach delicate lung tissue
- Nicotine accelerates heart rate, elevates blood pressure
- Nicotine stimulates adrenal glands to release adrenaline, causing changes in functioning of heart and other organs
- Nicotine depresses hunger contractions
- Nicotine inhibits production of urine in kidneys
- Nicotine causes liver to release glycogen, raising blood sugar level

The Long-Term Effects of Smoking

Smoking is linked to many deadly and disabling diseases. Research indicates that the total amount of tobacco smoke inhaled is a key factor contributing to disease. People who smoke more cigarettes per day, inhale deeply, puff frequently, smoke cigarettes down to the butts, or begin smoking at an early age run a greater risk of disease than do those who smoke more moderately or who do not smoke at all.

As more research is done, even more diseases associated with smoking are being uncovered. The costliest ones—to society as well as to the individual—are cardiovascular diseases; respiratory diseases, such as emphysema and lung cancer; and other cancers.

Cardiovascular Disease   Although lung cancer tends to receive the most publicity, one form of cardiovascular disease, coronary heart disease (CHD), is actually the most widespread single cause of death for cigarette smokers. CHD often results from atherosclerosis, a condition in which fatty deposits called plaques form on the inner walls of heart arteries, causing them to narrow and stiffen. Smoking and exposure to environmental tobacco smoke (ETS) permanently accelerate the rate of plaque accumulation in the coronary arteries—50% for smokers, 25% for ex-smokers, and 20% for people regularly exposed to ETS. The crushing chest pain of angina pectoris, a primary

symptom of CHD, results when the heart muscle, or myocardium, does not get enough oxygen. Sometimes a plaque forms at a narrow point in a main coronary artery. If the plaque completely blocks the flow of blood to a portion of the heart, that portion may die. This type of heart attack is called a **myocardial infarction**.

CHD can also interfere with the heart's electrical activity, resulting in disturbances of the normal heartbeat rhythm. Sudden and unexpected death is a common result of CHD, particularly among smokers. (See Chapter 7 for a more extensive discussion of cardiovascular disease.)

Smokers have a death rate from CHD that is 70% higher than that of nonsmokers. Deaths from CHD associated with cigarette smoking are most common in people age 40–50. (In contrast, deaths from lung cancer caused by smoking are most likely to occur in 60–70-year-olds.) Among people *under* age 40, smokers are five times as likely as nonsmokers to have a heart attack. Cigar and pipe smokers run a lower risk than cigarette smokers.

> **cerebral cortex**   The outer layer of the brain, which controls complex behaviour and mental activity.
>
> **myocardial infarction**   A heart attack caused by the complete blockage of a main coronary artery.

TERMS

We do not completely understand how cigarette smoking increases the risk of CHD, but researchers are beginning to shed light on the process. Smoking reduces the amount of good cholesterol (high-density lipoprotein, or HDL) in the blood, and creates lesions or roughness in arterial walls, which promote plaque deposit. Smoking may also increase tension in heart muscle walls, speeding up the rate of muscular contraction and accelerating the heart rate. The workload of the heart thus increases, as does its need for oxygen and other nutrients. Carbon monoxide produced by cigarette smoking combines with hemoglobin in the red blood cells, displacing oxygen and thus providing less oxygen to the heart. One study showed that the additional blood supply available to the heart during stress was 21% less in smokers than in nonsmokers. This reduced blood flow is an early indicator of future heart attacks or strokes.

The risks of CHD decrease rapidly when a person stops smoking; this is particularly true for younger smokers, whose coronary arteries have not yet been extensively damaged.

Lung Cancer and Other Cancers Cigarette smoking is the primary cause of lung cancer (Figure 16.4). A recent study identified the precise mechanism: Benzo(a)pyrene, a chemical found in tobacco smoke, causes genetic mutations in lung cells that are identical to those found in many patients with lung cancer. Those who smoke two or more packs of cigarettes a day have lung cancer death rates 12–25 times the rates of nonsmokers. The dramatic rise in lung cancer rates among women in the past 40 years clearly parallels the increase of smoking in this group; lung cancer now exceeds breast cancer as the leading cause of cancer deaths among women. The risk of developing lung cancer increases with the number of cigarettes smoked each day, the number of years of smoking, and the age at which the person started smoking.

Cigarette smoking has been linked to other cardiovascular diseases, including the following:

- *Stroke*, a sudden interference with the circulation of blood in a part of the brain, resulting in the destruction of brain cells
- *Aortic aneurysm*, a bulge in the aorta caused by a weakening in its walls
- *Pulmonary heart disease*, a disorder of the right side of the heart, caused by changes in the blood vessels of the lungs

Although cigar and pipe smokers have a higher risk of lung cancer than nonsmokers do, the risk is lower than that for cigarette smokers. Smoking filter-tipped cigarettes slightly reduces health hazards, unless the smoker compensates by smoking more, as is often the case.

QUICK STATS

85% of lung cancer deaths are attributable to smoking.

—Canadian Cancer Society, 2002

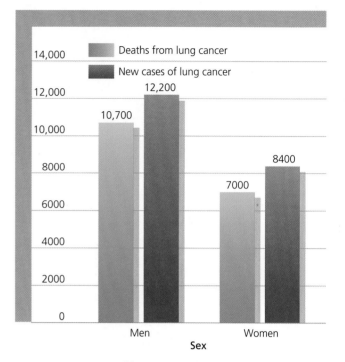

FIGURE 16.4 Annual lung cancer deaths and new cases of lung cancer, 2000.

Source: Data from Health Canada. 2000. *Lung Cancer* (http://www.hc-sc.gc.ca/hc-ps/tobac-tabac/body-corps/disease-maladie/lung-poumon_more-plus-eng.php; retrieved April 11, 2011). © Her Majesty the Queen in Right of Canada.

Evidence suggests that after one year without smoking, the risk of lung cancer decreases substantially. After 10 years, the risk of lung cancer among ex-smokers is 50% lower than that of continuing smokers.

Research has also linked smoking to cancers of the trachea, mouth, pharynx, esophagus, larynx, pancreas, bladder, kidney, breast, cervix, stomach, liver, colon, and skin. For more information on cancer, see Chapter 8.

Chronic Obstructive Pulmonary Disease The lungs of a smoker are constantly exposed to dangerous chemicals and irritants, and they must work harder to function adequately. The stresses placed on the lungs by smoking can permanently damage lung function and lead to *chronic obstructive pulmonary disease (COPD)*, also known as chronic obstructive lung disease (COLD), or chronic lower respiratory disease. COPD is the fourth leading cause of death in Canada. This progressive and disabling disorder consists of several different but related diseases; emphysema and chronic bronchitis are two of the most common.

Cigarette smokers are up to 18 times as likely as nonsmokers to die from emphysema and chronic bronchitis. (Pipe and cigar smokers are more likely to die from COPD than are nonsmokers, but they have a smaller risk than cigarette smokers.) A 2008 study estimated that 6% of the Canadian population has COPD. The risk rises with the number of cigarettes smoked and falls when smoking ceases. In 80%–90% of COPD cases in Canada, cigarette smoking is the main cause; however, air pollution also plays a role and exposure to both is more dangerous than exposure to either by itself.

EMPHYSEMA Smoking is the primary cause of **emphysema**, a disabling condition in which the walls of the lungs' air sacs lose their elasticity and are gradually destroyed. The lungs' ability to obtain oxygen and remove carbon dioxide is impaired. A person with emphysema is breathless, is constantly gasping for air, and has the feeling of drowning. The heart must pump harder and may become enlarged. People with emphysema often die from a damaged heart. There is no known way to reverse this disease. In its advanced stage, the person is bedridden and severely disabled.

CHRONIC BRONCHITIS Persistent, recurrent inflammation of the bronchial tubes characterizes **chronic bronchitis**. When the cell lining of the bronchial tubes is irritated, it secretes excess mucus. Bronchial congestion is followed by a chronic cough, which makes breathing more and more difficult. If smokers have chronic bronchitis, they face a greater risk of lung cancer, no matter how old they are or how many cigarettes they smoke. Chronic bronchitis seems to be a shortcut to lung cancer.

Other Respiratory Damage Even when the smoker shows no signs of lung impairment or disease, cigarette smoking damages the respiratory system. Normally the cells lining the bronchial tubes secrete mucus, a sticky fluid that collects particles of soot, dust, and other substances in inhaled air. Mucus is carried up to the mouth by the continuous motion of the cilia, hairlike structures that protrude from the inner surface of the bronchial tubes (Figure 16.5). If the cilia are destroyed or impaired, or if the pollution of inhaled air is more than the system can remove, the protection provided by cilia is lost.

Cigarette smoke first slows and then stops the action of the cilia. Eventually it destroys them, leaving delicate membranes exposed to injury from substances inhaled in cigarette smoke or from the polluted air in which the person lives or works. Special cells, called *macrophages*, a type of white blood cell, also work to remove foreign particles from the respiratory tract by engulfing them. Smoking appears to make macrophages work less efficiently. This interference with the functioning of the respiratory system often leads rapidly to the conditions known as smoker's throat and smoker's cough, as well as to shortness of breath. Even smokers of high school age show impaired respiratory function, compared with nonsmokers of the same age. Other respiratory effects of smoking include a worsening of allergy and asthma symptoms and an increase in the smoker's susceptibility to colds.

Although cigarette smoking can cause many respiratory disorders and diseases, the damage is not always permanent. Once a person stops smoking, steady improvement in overall lung function usually takes place. Chronic coughing subsides, mucus production returns to normal, and breathing becomes easier. The likelihood of lung disease drops sharply. People of all ages, even those who have been smoking for decades, improve after they stop smoking.

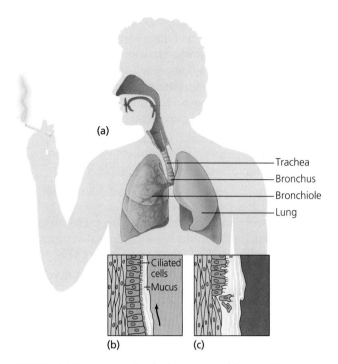

FIGURE 16.5 Damage to the lungs caused by smoking. **(a)** The respiratory system. **(b)** The inside of a bronchiole of a nonsmoker. **(c)** The inside of a bronchiole of a smoker.

Additional Health, Cosmetic, and Economic Concerns
Smoking has many effects and plays a role in the following health, aesthetic, and economic problems:

- *Ulcers.* People who smoke are more likely to develop peptic ulcers and are more likely to die from them (especially stomach ulcers), because smoking impairs the body's healing ability. Smoking also increases the risk of gastroesophageal reflux, which causes heartburn and can, if severe, raise the risk of esophageal cancer.

- *Impotence.* Smoking affects blood flow in the veins and arteries of the penis, and it is an independent risk factor for impotence. In one recent study, smokers were twice as likely as nonsmokers to experience erectile dysfunction (impotence).

emphysema A disease characterized by a loss of lung tissue elasticity and breakup of the air sacs, impairing the lungs' ability to obtain oxygen and remove carbon dioxide.

chronic bronchitis Recurrent, persistent inflammation of the bronchial tubes.

TERMS

- *Reproductive health problems.* Smoking is linked to reduced fertility in both men and women. A study of 18-year-old men who smoked found that they had a significantly higher proportion of abnormally shaped sperm and sperm with genetic defects than nonsmokers. In women, smoking can contribute to menstrual disorders, early menopause, and complications of pregnancy.
- *Dental diseases.* Smokers are at increased risk for tooth decay and gum and periodontal diseases, with symptoms appearing by the mid-20s.
- *Diminished physical senses.* Smoking dulls the senses of taste and smell. Over time, it increases the risk for hearing loss, and for macular degeneration and cataracts (both serious eye conditions that can result in partial or total blindness; see Chapter 17).
- *Injuries.* Smokers have higher rates of motor vehicle crashes, fire-related injuries, and back pain.
- *Cosmetic concerns.* Smoking can cause premature skin wrinkling, premature baldness, stained teeth, discoloured fingers, and a persistent tobacco odour in the smoker's clothes and hair.
- *Economic costs.* In 2009, the average per-pack price of cigarettes was between $10 and $13 dollars. A pack-a-day habit costs approximately $4200 each year for cigarettes alone.

In addition, smoking contributes to osteoporosis, increases the risk of complications from diabetes, and accelerates the course of multiple sclerosis. Further research may link tobacco use to still other disorders.

Cumulative Effects   The cumulative effects of tobacco use fall into two general categories. The first category is reduced life expectancy. A male who takes up smoking before age 15 and continues to smoke is only half as likely to live to age 75 as a male who never smokes. Females who have similar smoking habits also have a reduced life expectancy.

The second category involves quality of life. A long-term study shows that smokers take an average of eight additional sick days away from their jobs because of illness than nonsmokers. Female smokers spend 17% more days sick in bed than female nonsmokers. Lost workdays because of smoking number in the millions.

Both men and women smokers show a greater rate of acute and chronic disease than people who have never smoked (see the box "Gender and Tobacco Use"). Smokers become disabled at younger ages than nonsmokers and have more years of unhealthy life as well as a shorter life-span. In Canada, it is estimated 1 person in 20 has chronic bronchitis; smoking accounts for 90% of those cases.

Other Forms of Tobacco Use

Many smokers have switched from cigarettes to other forms of tobacco, such as spit (smokeless) tobacco, cigars, cigarillos, and pipes, and clove cigarettes and bidis. These alternatives,

Percentage of respondents

FIGURE 16.6   **Percentage of youth who have ever tried various tobacco products, grades 6–9, 2008–2009, and ages 15–19, 2009.**

Source: Reid, J. L., and D. Hammond. 2011. *Tobacco Use in Canada: Patterns and Trends*, 2011 ed. Waterloo, ON: Propel Centre for Population Health Impact, University of Waterloo (http://www.tobaccoreport.ca/tobacco%20Use%20in%20Canada_2011.pdf; retrieved April 11, 2011).

however, are far from safe. Among students and teenagers, cigarillos (little cigars) were the most popular tobacco product after cigarettes (Figure 16.6, above).

Spit (Smokeless) Tobacco   Spit tobacco use has increased in recent years and is especially common among Aboriginal and rural Canadians, adolescent males, and male athletes. Geographically, use of spit tobacco is higher in the Prairies than in parts of Canada. About 17% of Canadians will experiment with spit tobacco some time in their life.

Spit tobacco comes in two major forms: snuff and chewing tobacco (chew). In snuff, the tobacco leaf is processed into a coarse, moist powder and mixed with flavourings. Snuff is usually sold in small tins. Users place a "pinch," "dip," or "quid" between the lower lip or cheek and gum and suck on it. In chewing tobacco, the tobacco leaf may be shredded ("leaf"), pressed into bricks or cakes ("plugs"), or dried and twisted into ropelike strands ("twists"). Chew is usually sold in pouches. Users place a wad of tobacco in their mouth and then chew or suck it to release the nicotine. All types of smokeless tobacco cause an increase in saliva production, and the resulting tobacco juice is spit out or swallowed. A recent innovation in smokeless tobacco, called *snus*, comes in a tiny pouch that is placed between the lip and gum. Snus does not require the user to spit, as do other forms of smokeless tobacco.

Gender and Tobacco Use

Canadian men are currently more likely than women to smoke, but women younger than age 17 are becoming smokers at a faster rate than any other population segment. As the rate of smoking among women approaches that of men, so do rates of tobacco-related illness and death. More Canadians women now die each year from lung cancer than from breast cancer.

Although overall risks of tobacco-related illness are similar for women and men, sex appears to make a difference in some diseases. Women, for example, are more at risk for smoking-related blood clots and strokes than are men, and the risk is even greater for women who use oral contraceptives. Among men and women with the same smoking history, the odds for developing three major types of cancer, including lung cancer, is 1.2–1.7 times as high in women as in men. Women may also have a greater biological vulnerability to lung cancer.

For both men and women, tobacco use is associated with increased incidence of sex-specific health problems. Men who smoke increase their risk of erectile dysfunction and infertility because of reduced sperm density and motility. Women who smoke have higher rates of osteoporosis

(a bone-thinning disease that can lead to fractures), thyroid-related diseases, and depression.

Women who smoke also have risks associated with reproduction and the reproductive organs. Smoking is associated with greater menstrual bleeding, greater duration of painful menstrual cramps, and more variability in menstrual cycle length. Smokers have a more difficult time becoming pregnant, and they reach menopause on average a year or two earlier than nonsmokers. When female smokers become pregnant, they face increased chances of miscarriage or placental disorders that lead to bleeding and premature delivery; rates of ectopic pregnancy, preeclampsia, and stillbirth are also higher among women who smoke. Smoking is a risk factor for cervical cancer.

When women decide to try to stop smoking, they are more likely than men to join a support group. Overall, though, women are less successful than men in quitting. Women report more severe withdrawal symptoms when they stop smoking and are more likely than men to report cravings in response to social and behavioural cues associated with smoking.

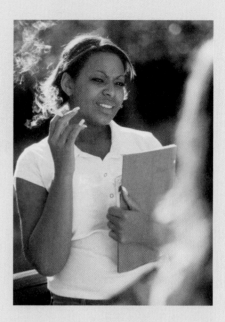

For men, relapse to smoking is often associated with work or social pressure; women are more likely to relapse when sad or depressed or concerned about weight gain. Women and men also respond differently to medications: Nicotine replacement therapy appears to work better for men, whereas the non-nicotine medication bupropion appears to work better for women.

The nicotine in spit tobacco—along with flavourings and additives—is absorbed through the gums and lining of the mouth. Holding an average-size dip in the mouth for 30 minutes delivers about the same amount of nicotine as two or three cigarettes. Because of its nicotine content, spit tobacco is highly addictive. Some users keep it in their mouth even while sleeping.

Although not as dangerous as smoking cigarettes, the use of spit tobacco carries many health risks. Changes can occur in the mouth after only a few weeks of use. Gums and lips become dried and irritated and may bleed. White or red patches may appear inside the mouth; this condition, known as *leukoplakia*, can lead to oral cancer. About 25% of regular spit tobacco users have *gingivitis* (inflammation), recession of the gums, and bone loss around the teeth, especially where the tobacco is usually placed. The senses of taste and smell are usually dulled. In addition, other people find the presence of wads of tobacco in the mouth, stained teeth, bad breath, and behaviours, such as frequent spitting, to be unpleasant.

One of the most serious effects of spit tobacco is an increased risk of oral cancer—cancers of the lip, tongue, cheek, throat, gums, roof and floor of the mouth, and larynx.

Spit tobacco contains at least 28 chemicals known to cause cancer, and long-term snuff use may increase the risk of oral cancer by as much as 50 times. Surgery to treat oral cancer is often disfiguring and may involve removing parts of the face, tongue, cheek, or lip.

Dipping and chewing tobacco produce blood levels of nicotine similar to those in cigarette smokers. Other chemicals in spit tobacco are believed to pose risks to developing fetuses.

Cigars and Pipes   After decades of decline, in 2007 cigar smoking rates were double those in the 1990s. The popularity of cigars is highest among white males ages 25–44 with higher-than-average income and education, but women are also smoking cigars in record numbers. Cigar use is also growing among young people: In government surveys, 4% of Canadians 15 years and older reported having smoked at least one cigar in the previous month. Less than 0.5% of Canadians, mostly males who also smoke cigarettes, are pipe smokers.

Cigars are made from rolled whole tobacco leaves; pipe tobacco is made from shredded leaves and often flavoured. Because cigar and pipe smoke are more alkaline than

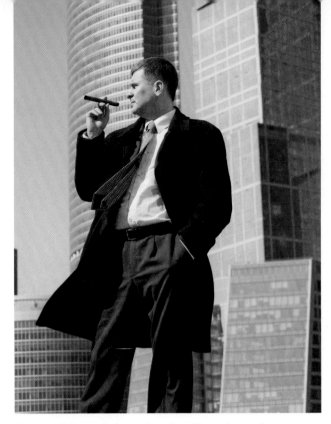

Cigars contain more tobacco than cigarettes and so produce more tar when smoked. Cigar smokers face an increased risk of cancer even if they don't inhale the smoke.

QUESTIONS FOR CRITICAL THINKING AND REFLECTION
Do you know anyone who has had an illness related to tobacco use? If so, what problems did that person face? What was the outcome? Did the experience have any effect on your views about using tobacco?

cigarette smoke, users of cigars and pipes do not need to inhale to ingest nicotine; instead, they absorb nicotine through the gums and lining of the mouth. Cigars contain more tobacco than cigarettes and so contain more nicotine and produce more tar when smoked. Large cigars may contain as much tobacco as a whole pack of cigarettes and take one to two hours to smoke.

The smoke from cigars contains many of the same toxins and carcinogens as the smoke from cigarettes, some in much higher quantities. The health risks of cigars depend on the number of cigars smoked and whether the smoker inhales. Because most cigar and pipe users do not inhale, they have a lower risk of cancer and cardiovascular and respiratory diseases than cigarette smokers. However, their risks are substantially higher than those of nonsmokers. For example, compared with nonsmokers, people who smoke one or two cigars per day without inhaling have six times the risk of cancer of the larynx. The risks are much higher for cigar smokers who inhale: They have 27 times the risk of oral cancer and 53 times the risk of cancer of the larynx compared with nonsmokers, and their risk of heart and lung diseases approaches that of cigarette smokers. Smoking a cigar immediately impairs the ability of blood vessels to dilate, reducing the amount of oxygen delivered to tissues, including the heart muscle, especially during times of stress. Pipe and cigar smoking are also risk factors for pancreatic cancer, which is almost always fatal.

Nicotine addiction is another concern. Most adults who smoke cigars do so only occasionally, and little evidence suggest that use of cigars by adults leads to addiction. The recent rise in cigar use among young adults has raised concerns, however, because nicotine addiction almost always develops in the teen or young adult years. More research is needed to determine if cigar use by teens will develop into nicotine addiction and frequent use of either cigarettes or spit tobacco. In July 2000 the Canadian government announced an agreement to put warning labels on cigar packages, 34 years after warning labels first appeared on cigarette packages.

Clove Cigarettes and Bidis Clove cigarettes, also called *kreteks* or *chicartas*, are made of tobacco mixed with chopped cloves; they are imported primarily from Indonesia and Pakistan. Clove cigarettes contain almost twice as much tar, nicotine, and carbon monoxide as conventional cigarettes and so have all the same health hazards. Some chemical constituents of cloves may also be dangerous. For example, eugenol, an anaesthetic compound found in cloves, may impair the respiratory system's ability to detect and defend against foreign particles. A number of serious respiratory injuries and deaths have resulted from the use of clove cigarettes.

Bidis, or *beadies*, are small cigarettes imported from India that contain species of tobacco different from those used by North American cigarette manufacturers. The tobacco in bidis is hand-rolled in Indian ebony leaves (tendu) and then often flavoured; clove, mint, chocolate, and fruit varieties are available. Bidis contain up to four times as much nicotine and twice as much tar as North American cigarettes. Use of bidis has been growing among teens, possibly because of the flavourings they contain or because they look and smell somewhat like marijuana cigarettes (*joints*); they do not produce the same effects as marijuana, however.

An estimated 4% of Canadians have tried clove cigarettes or bidis. Neither is a safe or healthy alternative to conventional tobacco cigarettes.

THE EFFECTS OF SMOKING ON THE NONSMOKER

Tobacco users aren't the only ones who suffer ill effects from their habits. Tens of thousands of nonsmokers die each year because of excess exposure to second-hand smoke. Further, the medical and societal costs of tobacco use are enormous.

Environmental Tobacco Smoke

Environmental tobacco smoke (ETS)—more commonly called second-hand smoke—has been designated a Class A carcinogen and is a known human carcinogen. These designations put ETS in the same category as such notorious cancer-causing agents as asbestos. No level of exposure to ETS is safe; even brief exposure can cause serious harm.

ETS consists of mainstream smoke and sidestream smoke. Smoke exhaled by smokers is referred to as **mainstream smoke**. Sidestream smoke enters the atmosphere from the burning end of a cigarette, cigar, or pipe. Nearly 85% of the smoke in a room where someone is smoking comes from sidestream smoke. Undiluted sidestream smoke, because it is not filtered through either a cigarette filter or a smoker's lungs, has twice as much tar and nicotine, three times as much benzo(a)pyrene, almost three times as much carbon monoxide, and three times as much ammonia.

In rooms where people are smoking, levels of carbon monoxide can exceed those deemed acceptable by the Canadian Environmental Protection Act for outside air. In a typical home with the windows closed, it takes about six hours for 95% of the airborne cigarette smoke particles to clear.

The carcinogens in the second-hand smoke from a single cigar exceed that of three cigarettes, and cigar smoke contains up to 30 times as much carbon monoxide.

ETS Effects   Nonsmokers subjected to ETS frequently develop coughs, headaches, nasal discomfort, and eye irritation. Other symptoms range from breathlessness to sinus problems. People with allergies tend to suffer the most (see the box "Avoiding ETS" on p. 516).

ETS causes 330 lung cancer deaths and about 2000 deaths from heart disease each year in people who do not smoke. As described earlier, exposure to ETS is associated with a 20% increase in the progression of atherosclerosis. ETS also aggravates asthma and increases the risk for breast and cervical cancers.

Scientists have been able to measure changes that contribute to lung tissue damage and potential tumour promotion in the bloodstreams of healthy young test subjects who spend just three hours in a smoke-filled room. After just 30 minutes of exposure to ETS, the function in the coronary arteries of healthy nonsmokers is reduced to the same level as that of smokers. And nonsmokers can still be affected by the harmful effects of ETS hours after they have left a smoky environment. Carbon monoxide, for example, lingers in the bloodstream five hours later.

Infants, Children, and ETS   Recent studies have found three times as many infants die from second-hand smoke related sudden infant death syndrome (SIDS) as from child abuse or homicide. Children under five whose primary caregiver smokes 10 or more cigarettes per day have measurable blood levels of nicotine and tobacco carcinogens. Chemicals in tobacco smoke also show up in breast milk, and breastfeeding may pass more chemicals to the infant of a smoking mother than direct exposure to ETS.

About 1.6 million Canadian infants and children are regularly exposed to environmental tobacco smoke.

ETS triggers approximately 115,000 cases of bronchitis, pneumonia, and other respiratory infections in Canadian children annually, resulting in more than 200,000 visits to physicians.

Older children suffer, too. ETS is a risk factor for asthma in children who have not previously displayed symptoms of the disease, and it aggravates the symptoms of children who already have asthma. ETS is also linked to reduced lung function and fluid buildup in the middle ear, a contributing factor in middle-ear infections, a leading reason for childhood surgery. Children and teens exposed to ETS score lower on tests of reading and reasoning. Later in life, people exposed to ETS as children are at increased risk for lung cancer, emphysema, and chronic bronchitis.

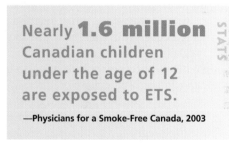

Nearly **1.6 million** Canadian children under the age of 12 are exposed to ETS.

—Physicians for a Smoke-Free Canada, 2003

QUICK STATS

Smoking and Pregnancy

Smoking almost doubles a pregnant woman's chance of having a miscarriage, and it significantly increases her risk of ectopic pregnancy. Maternal smoking causes an

environmental tobacco smoke (ETS)   Smoke that enters the atmosphere from the burning end of a cigarette, cigar, or pipe, as well as smoke that is exhaled by smokers; also called *second-hand smoke*.

mainstream smoke   Smoke that is inhaled by a smoker and then exhaled into the atmosphere.

TERMS

Avoiding ETS

Given the health risks of exposure to ETS, try these strategies to keep the air around you safe:

• *Speak up tactfully.* Smokers may not know the dangers they are causing or may not know it bothers you.

• *Display reminders.* Put up signs asking smokers to refrain in your home, work area, and car.

• *Don't allow smoking in your home or room.* Get rid of ashtrays and ask smokers to light up outside.

• *Open a window.* If you cannot avoid being in a room with a smoker, at least try to provide some ventilation.

• *Discuss quitting strategies.* Social pressure is a major factor in many former smokers' decisions to quit. Help the smokers in your life by sharing quitting strategies with them.

estimated 100 infant deaths in the Canada each year, primarily because of premature delivery and smoking-related problems with the placenta. Maternal smoking is a major factor in low birth weight, which puts newborns at high risk for infections and other serious problems. If a nonsmoking mother is regularly exposed to ETS, her infant is also at greater risk for low birth weight. Recent studies have also shown that babies whose mothers smoked during pregnancy had higher rates of colic, clubfoot, cleft lip and palate, and impaired lung function; they may also have genetic damage.

Babies born to mothers who smoke more than two packs a day perform poorly on developmental tests in the first hours after birth, compared with babies of nonsmoking mothers. Later in life, obesity, hyperactivity, short attention span, and lower scores on spelling and reading tests all occur more frequently in children whose mothers smoked during pregnancy than in those born to nonsmoking mothers. Prenatal tobacco exposure has also been associated with behavioural problems in children, including immaturity, emotional instability, physical aggression, and hyperactivity. Other research shows that teenagers whose mothers smoked during pregnancy have lower scores on tests of general intelligence and poorer performance on tasks requiring auditory memory than do children who were not exposed to cigarette smoke before birth. Males born to smoking mothers have higher rates of adolescent and adult criminal activity, suggesting that maternal smoking may cause brain damage that increases the risk of criminal behaviour. Nevertheless, in Canada, almost 9% of pregnant women reported smoking regularly during pregnancy in 2009.

The Cost of Tobacco Use to Society

The annual health-related costs of smoking in Canada exceed $24 billion. These costs far exceed the tax revenues that are collected on the sale of tobacco products, even though the average cigarette tax was 70% of the cost per pack in 2009.

Tobacco Legislation in Canada A major step in regulating tobacco in Canada occurred in 1999 when the National Strategy on Tobacco Control was adopted by both the federal and the provincial and territorial governments.

Since then, although the strategy's name has changed several times, the focus remains on protection, prevention, cessation, and harm reduction (see the box "Regulation of Tobacco").

The Tobacco Act, enacted in 1997, regulates the manufacture, sale, labelling, and promotion of tobacco in Canada through a variety of methods, including legislation and fines for noncompliance. For example, in Ontario, selling cigarettes to minors has a graduated penalty structure with fines up to $25,000 for infractions.

Canada is considered to be at the forefront of anti-smoking legislation, with bans on smoking in public places being enacted across all provinces and territories over the last decade:

• Prince Edward Island banned smoking in public places and workplaces in 2003.

• Manitoba banned smoking in any indoor location where children or youth where present in 2002 and subsequently banned smoking in public areas in 2004.

• New Brunswick banned smoking in public places in 2004.

• Nunavut and the Northwest Territories banned smoking in business and work sites in 2004.

• Saskatchewan banned smoking in bars, casinos, and restaurants in 2002 and in all public places in 2005.

• Newfoundland and Labrador amended the Smoke-Free Environment Act in 2005 to ban smoking in all public places.

• Alberta banned smoking in public places in 2006.

• Quebec made restaurants, bars, clubs, casinos, and shelters smoke-free in May 2006 and subsequently banned smoking in all public places in June 2006.

• In Halifax, Nova Scotia, smoking was restricted in 2009 in outdoor venues where children are present (i.e., parks, rinks, and sports fields).

• Ontario banned smoking in public places in various cities between 2001 and 2006, banned tobacco displays in 2008, and banned smoking in vehicles carrying children in 2009.

Regulation of Tobacco

Tobacco kills more Canadians annually than motor vehicle accidents, accidental falls, murders, suicides, and alcohol combined. Given the danger associated with tobacco, Canada has imposed regulations in an attempt to regulate tobacco products. The Tobacco Reporting Regulation was created to better control the tobacco industry. This regulation requires that Canadian tobacco companies and tobacco importers in Canada provide annual reports to the federal minster of health. The information that is required in the reports includes the following:

• Tobacco sales

• Ingredients in all tobacco products

• Toxic constituents (20 are identified that require reporting)

• Toxic emissions (40 are identified and require reporting)

• Research activities

• Promotional initiatives

The regulation further details the methods that must be used when analyzing and evaluating the ingredients in tobacco products and the toxic emissions for various types of smoke and tobacco. The Canadian government has clearly outlined sets of rules for mainstream smoke, sidestream smoke, and whole tobacco testing, along with specific guidelines for testing the various components of tobacco. For example, each ingredient in tobacco, including ammonia, carbon monoxide, mercury, tar, and nicotine, must be tested for and reported.

• British Columbia banned smoking in public places in 2008 and smoking in vehicles with minors in 2009.

• Yukon was the last jurisdiction to ban smoking in public places in 2009.

In 2009 Bill C-32, An Act to Amend the Tobacco Act, was passed in Canada, which bans flavours in cigarillos, cigarettes, and blunts (tobacco rolling papers). This bill also prohibits advertising of tobacco products in both newspapers and magazines. Bill C-32 came about as new research in tobacco use among youth in Canada from the *Youth Smoking Survey* (2006–2007) found high rates of cigarillo use by youth. With the removal of tobacco advertising in print resources, the Canadian government hopes to reduce youths' exposure to tobacco products and reduce their tobacco use.

Court Cases In 2009, the Ontario government launched a $50 billion lawsuit against big tobacco companies, seeking damages for both past and ongoing health care costs associated with tobacco-related illnesses from 1955 to 2009. As the attorney general in charge of prosecution stated, "the tax payers of the province of Ontario have paid a lot of money for health-care costs directly related to tobacco use over the decades."

The government recently passed the Tobacco Damages and Health Care Costs Recovery Act, which allows provinces to sue for the recovery of past, present, and continuing tobacco-related damages. This legislation is consistent with legislation in other parts of the world. The Imperial Tobacco Company, the largest manufacturer of tobacco in Canada, was named in the lawsuit, along with 14 other Canadian-, American-, and British-based tobacco companies.

The first successful lawsuit against tobacco companies concluded in 1999 in California. Patricia Henley, a woman diagnosed with inoperable lung cancer, was awarded $51.5 million from the Philip Morris tobacco company. Appeals, over seven years, reduced the award to $10.5 million. Henley died in 2009.

THINKING ABOUT THE ENVIRONMENT

The buildings in which you live, work, and learn are important parts of your environment, as are the skies and oceans. The health and safety of indoor air are threatened by second-hand smoke, just as the outside air is threatened by other forms of pollution.

Physicians for a Smoke-Free Canada estimate that anywhere from 1000 to 7500 nonsmokers die annually from exposure to tobacco smoke report the following facts:

■ Children exposed to second-hand smoke are more likely to die of sudden infant death syndrome and to develop severe infections.

■ Adults exposed to second-hand smoke experience immediate harmful effects to the cardiovascular system and increased risk of coronary heart disease and lung cancer.

■ No level of exposure to second-hand smoke is safe.

■ Completely eliminating indoor smoking is the only way to fully protect nonsmokers from exposure to second-hand smoke. Ventilating buildings or separating smokers from nonsmokers is not sufficient.

For more information on the environment and environmental health, see Chapter 21.

QUESTIONS FOR CRITICAL THINKING AND REFLECTION

What are your views on the government's role in regulating tobacco products? Is there currently enough regulation, or should the government go further in controlling the production and marketing of these products? What events or experiences have shaped your views on this issue?

WHAT CAN BE DONE?

Many things can be done to act against this public health threat.

Action at the Local Level

Since the 1980s, local government agencies—such as city councils, school boards, and county boards of commissioners—have been passing ordinances designed to discourage smoking in public places. Thousands of local ordinances across Canada now restrict or ban smoking in restaurants, stores, workplaces, and even public outdoor areas.

International Action

Many countries are restricting smoking. Smoking is now banned on many international air flights, as well as in many restaurants and hotels and on public transportation in some countries. The World Health Organization has taken the lead in international anti-tobacco efforts by sponsoring the Framework Convention on Tobacco Control. World No Tobacco Day (observed on May 31) encourages smokers to stop smoking for one day. A smoker who successfully takes the first step of quitting for a day may be encouraged enough to follow through on the commitment and become a permanent nonsmoker. With more than 1 billion smokers worldwide, addressing the global impact of tobacco use will require a massive coordinated effort.

Action in the Private Sector

The information available about the negative effects of second-hand smoke gave employers reason to worry about workers' compensation claims and lawsuits based on exposure to workplace smoke. Most provinces have enacted smoke-free workplaces legislation.

Individual Action

Such local, provincial and territorial, national, and international efforts represent progress, but health activists warn that tobacco industry influence remains strong. But nonsmokers have the right not only to breathe clean air but also to take action to help solve one of society's most serious public health threats. Here are just some of the many ways in which individuals can help support tobacco prevention and stop-smoking efforts:

Smokers can light up only in designated smoking areas, which are outdoors and a specified distance from building entrances.

- When a smoker violates a no-smoking designation, complain.
- If you see children buying tobacco, report this illegal activity to the facility manager or the police.
- Learn more about addiction and tobacco cessation so you can better support the tobacco users you know. (See the box "Helping a Friend or Partner Stop Using Tobacco" in the ▣connect Library.)
- Vote for candidates who support anti-tobacco measures; contact local, provincial or territorial, and national representatives to express your views.
- Cancel your subscriptions to magazines that carry tobacco advertising; send a letter to the publisher explaining your decision.
- Voice your opinion about other positive representations of tobacco use. (A recent study found that more than two-thirds of children's animated feature films depicted tobacco or alcohol use with no clear message that such practices were unhealthy.)
- Volunteer with the Canadian Lung Association, the Canadian Cancer Society, or the Heart and Stroke Foundation of Canada.

QUESTIONS FOR CRITICAL THINKING AND REFLECTION

What anti-smoking ordinances are in effect in your community? Does your school prohibit smoking on campus? Do you think these rules have been effective in reducing smoking or exposure to ETS? Do you support such regulations? Why or why not?

HOW A TOBACCO USER CAN QUIT

Giving up tobacco is a long-term, intricate process. Heavy smokers who say they have just stopped cold turkey often don't tell of the struggling and mental processes that contributed to their final victory over this powerful addiction.

Research shows that tobacco users move through predictable stages—from being uninterested in stopping, to thinking about change, to making a concerted effort to stop, to finally maintaining abstinence. But most attempt to quit several times before they finally succeed. Relapse is a normal part of the process.

The Benefits of Quitting

Giving up tobacco provides immediate health benefits to men and women of all ages (Table 16.2). People who quit smoking find that food tastes better. Their sense of smell is sharper. Circulation improves, heart rate and blood pressure drop, and lung function and heart efficiency increase. Ex-smokers can breathe more easily, and their capacity for exercise improves. Many ex-smokers report feeling more energetic and alert. They experience fewer headaches. Even their complexion may improve.

Quitting also has a positive effect on long-term disease risk. From the first day without tobacco, ex-smokers begin to decrease their risk of cancer of the lung, larynx, mouth, pancreas, bladder, cervix, and other sites. Risk of heart attack, stroke, and other cardiovascular diseases drops quickly, too.

The younger people are when they stop smoking, the more pronounced the health improvements. And these improvements gradually but invariably increase as the period of nonsmoking lengthens. It's never too late to quit, though. People who quit smoking, regardless of age, live longer than people who continue to smoke. Even smokers who have already developed chronic bronchitis or emphysema may show some improvement when they quit.

Options for Quitting

Half of tobacco users want to quit, and half of those who want to quit will make an attempt this year. What are their options? No single method works for everyone, but each does work for some people some of the time. Health Canada offers online resources to help smokers quit, as well as information on pharmacological interventions, including nicotine replacement therapy, which can serve as a valuable aid for some people. Health Canada's Web site also provides behavioural strategies to aid in cessation, along with a toll-free number for people who want more information.

Choosing to quit requires developing a strategy for success (see the box "Building Motivation to Quit Smoking" on p. 520). Some people quit cold turkey, whereas others taper off slowly. There are over-the-counter and prescription products that help many people (see the box "Smoking Cessation Products" on p. 521 for more on these options).

Table 16.2	Benefits of Quitting Smoking

Within 20 minutes of your last cigarette
- You stop polluting the air.
- Blood pressure drops to normal.
- Pulse rate drops to normal.
- Temperature of hands and feet increases to normal.

8 hours
- Carbon monoxide level in blood drops to normal.
- Oxygen level in blood increases to normal.

24 hours
- The chance of heart attack decreases.

48 hours
- Nerve endings start regrowing.
- Ability to smell and taste is enhanced.

2–3 months
- Circulation improves.
- Walking becomes easier.
- Lung function increases up to 30%.

1–9 months
- Coughing, sinus congestion, fatigue, and shortness of breath all decrease.

1 year
- Heart disease death risk is half that of a smoker.

5 years
- Stroke risk drops nearly to the risk for nonsmokers.

10 years
- Lung cancer death risk drops to 50% of that of a continuing smoker.
- Incidence of other cancers (mouth, throat, larynx, esophagus, bladder, kidney, and pancreas) decreases.
- Risk of ulcer decreases.

15 years
- Risk of lung cancer is about 25% of that of continuing smokers.
- Risks of heart disease and death are close to those for nonsmokers.

Sources: American Lung Association. 2002. *Benefits of Quitting* (http://www.lungusa.org/tobacco/quit_ben.html; retrieved August 18, 2006); American Cancer Society. 2000. *Quitting Smoking* (http://www.cancer.org/tobacco/quitting.html; retrieved August 18, 2006).

Behavioural factors that have been shown to increase the chances of a smoker's permanent smoking cessation are support from others and regular exercise. Support can come from friends and family or formal group programs sponsored by organizations, such as the Canadian Cancer Society and the Canadian Lung Association, or by your campus health centre or community hospital. Programs that combine group support with nicotine replacement therapy have rates of continued abstention as high as 35% after one year.

QUICK STATS

In 2008, **513,426** Canadians quit smoking without relapse.

—Physicians for a Smoke-Free Canada, 2008

Building Motivation to Quit Smoking

A common misconception among smokers is that a few cigarettes a day aren't enough to cause harm. Among postsecondary students who smoke, many describe themselves as casual smokers, smoking ten or fewer cigarettes a day. These smokers are ignoring the very real health risks of even one cigarette. One strategy to enhance motivation to quit is the 5Rs. If you are a smoker or are trying to help one, think about these areas of concern and see if they help develop a desire and readiness to make a real attempt at quitting.

Relevance: Think about the personal relevance of quitting tobacco use. What would the effects be on your family and friends? How would your daily life improve? What is the most important way that quitting would change your life?

Risks: Smokers face immediate risks, such as shortness of breath, infertility, and impotence, and long-term risks, including cancer, heart disease, and respiratory problems. Remember, smoking is harmful to you and you extend that risk to anyone exposed to your smoke.

Rewards: The list of the rewards of quitting is almost endless, including improving immediate and long-term health, saving money, and feeling better about yourself. You can also stop worrying about quitting and set a good example for others.

Roadblocks: What are the potential obstacles to quitting? Are you worried about withdrawal symptoms, weight gain, or lack of support? How can these barriers be overcome?

Repetition: Revisit your reasons for quitting and strengthen your resolve until you are ready to prepare a plan. Most people make several attempts to quit before they succeed. Relapsing once does not mean that you will never succeed.

Sources: Rigotti, N. A., J. E. Lee, and H. Wechsler. 2000. U.S. college students' use of tobacco products. *Journal of the American Medical Association* 284(6): 699–705; Fiore, M. C., et al. 2000. *Treating Tobacco Use and Dependence.* Clinical Practice Guidelines. Rockville, Md.: U.S. Department of Health and Human Services.

Free telephone quitlines are emerging as a popular strategy to help people stop smoking. Quitlines are staffed by trained counsellors who help each caller plan a personal quitting strategy, usually including a combination of nicotine replacement therapy, changes in daily habits, and emotional support. Counsellors provide printed materials that match the smoker's needs and schedule phone counselling sessions for key days after a smoker quits. Smokers can schedule sessions to fit their schedule, and some quitlines may provide stop-smoking medications at reduced prices. Almost all smokers make more than one attempt to stop before they succeed in quitting for good; and quitline counsellors can help smokers understand what leads to relapse, review their reasons for wanting to quit, and make a better plan for the next attempt. The goal is for smokers to find a support system and techniques that work for them. Visit Health Canada's Web site for toll-free quitlines in most provinces and territories.

Most smokers in the process of quitting experience both physical and psychological effects of nicotine withdrawal, and exercise can help with both. For many smokers, their tobacco use is associated with certain times and places—following a meal, for example. Resolving to walk after dinner instead of lighting up provides a distraction from cravings and eliminates the cues that trigger a desire to smoke. In addition, many people worry about weight gain associated with quitting. Although most ex-smokers do gain a kilogram or so, at least temporarily, incorporating exercise into a new tobacco-free routine lays the foundation for healthy weight management. The health risks of adding a kilogram are far outweighed by the risks of continued smoking; it's estimated that a smoker would have to gain 35–45 kilograms to equal the health risks of smoking a pack a day.

As with any significant change in health-related behaviour, giving up tobacco requires planning, sustained effort, and support. It is an ongoing process, not a one-time event. The Behaviour Change Strategy describes one set of steps that some successful quitters follow.

Smoking Cessation Products

Each year, tens of thousands of Canadians visit their doctors in the hope of finding a drug that can help them stop smoking. Although pharmacological options are limited, the few available drugs have proved successful.

Champix (Varenicline)

The newest smoking cessation drug, marketed under the name Champix, works in two ways: It reduces nicotine cravings, easing the withdrawal process, and it blocks the pleasant effects of nicotine. The drug acts on neurotransmitter receptors in the brain.

Six clinical trials, which included more than 3600 long-term, chronic smokers, demonstrated that Champix is an effective smoking cessation aid. In one of the studies, nearly 25% of Champix users stopped smoking for a full year. Results varied with the dosage and duration of treatment.

Unlike most smoking cessation products currently on the market, Champix is not a nicotine replacement. For this reason, smokers may be advised to continue smoking for the first few days of treatment, to avoid withdrawal and to allow the drug to build up in their system. The approved course of treatment is 12 weeks, but the duration and recommended dosage depend on several factors, including the smoker's general health and the length and severity of his or her nicotine addiction.

Side effects reported with Champix include nausea, headache, vomiting, sleep disruptions, and change in taste perception. People with kidney problems or who take certain medications should not take Champix, and it is not recommended for women who are pregnant or nursing. In early 2008, Health Canada issued a public health advisory warning that some Champix users had experienced adverse reactions, such as behavioural changes, agitation, depression, suicidal thoughts, and attempted suicide. Anyone taking Champix should immediately notify his or her doctor of any sudden change in mood or behaviour.

Zyban (Bupropion)

Bupropion is an antidepressant (prescribed under the name Wellbutrin) as well as a smoking cessation aid (prescribed under the name Zyban). As a smoking cessation aid, bupropion eases the symptoms of nicotine withdrawal and reduces the urge to smoke. Like Champix, it acts on neurotransmitter receptors in the brain.

Bupropion is not a nicotine replacement, so the user may need to continue smoking for the first few days of treatment. A nicotine replacement product, such as a patch or gum, may be recommended to further ease withdrawal symptoms after the user stops smoking.

Bupropion users have reported an array of side effects, but they are rare. Side effects may be reduced by changing the dosage, taking the medicine at a different time of day, or taking it with or without food. Bupropion is not recommended for people with specific physical conditions or who take certain drugs. Zyban and Wellbutrin should not be taken together.

Nicotine Replacement Products

The most widely used smoking cessation products replace the nicotine that the user would normally get from tobacco. The user continues to get nicotine, so withdrawal symptoms and cravings are reduced. Although still harmful, nicotine replacement products provide a cleaner form of nicotine, without the thousands of poisons and tars produced by burning tobacco. Less of the product is used over time, as the need for nicotine decreases.

Nicotine replacement products come in several forms, including patches, gum, lozenges, nasal sprays, and inhalers. They are available in a variety of strengths and can be worked into many different smoking cessation strategies. Most are available without a prescription.

The nicotine patch is popular because it can be applied and forgotten until it needs to be removed or changed, usually every 16 or 24 hours. Placed on the upper arm or torso, it releases a steady stream of nicotine, which is absorbed through the skin. The main side effects are skin irritation and redness. Nicotine gum and nicotine lozenges have the advantage of allowing the smoker to use them whenever he or she craves nicotine. Side effects of nicotine gum include mouth sores and headaches; nicotine lozenges can cause nausea and heartburn. Nicotine nasal sprays and inhalers are available only by prescription.

Although all these products have proven to be effective in helping users stop smoking, experts recommend them only as one part of a complete smoking cessation program. Such a program should include regular professional counselling and physician monitoring.

Kicking the Tobacco Habit

You can look forward to a longer and healthier life if you join the millions of Canadians who have quit using tobacco. The steps for quitting described below are discussed in terms of the most popular tobacco product in Canada—cigarettes—but they can be adapted for all forms of tobacco.

Gather Information

Collect personal smoking information in a detailed journal about your smoking behaviour. Write down the time you smoke each cigarette of the day, the situation you are in, how you feel, where you smoke, and how strong your craving for the cigarette is, plus any other information that seems relevant. Part of the job is to identify patterns of smoking that are connected with routine situations (for example, the coffee break smoke, the after-dinner cigarette, the tension-reduction cigarette). Use this information to discover the behaviour patterns involved in your smoking habit.

Make the Decision to Quit

Choose a date in the near future when you expect to be relatively stress free and can give quitting the energy and attention it will require. Don't choose a date right before or during finals week, for instance. Consider making quitting a gift: Choose your birthday as your quit date, for example, or make quitting a Father's Day or Mother's Day present. You might also want to coordinate your quit date with a friend—a fellow tobacco user who wants to quit or a nonsmoker who wants to give up another bad habit or begin an exercise program. Tell your friends and family when you plan to quit. Ask them to offer encouragement and help hold you to your goal.

Decide which approach to quitting will work best for you. Will you go cold turkey, or will you taper off? Will you use nicotine patches or gum? Will you join a support group or enlist the help of a friend? Prepare a contract for quitting, as discussed in Chapter 1. Set firm dates and rewards, and sign the contract. Post it in a prominent place.

Prepare to Quit

One of the most important things you can do to prepare to quit is to develop and practice nonsmoking relaxation techniques. Many smokers find that they use cigarettes to help them unwind in tense situations or to relax at other times. If this is true for you, you'll need to find and develop effective substitutes. It takes time to become proficient at relaxation techniques, so begin practicing before your quit date. Refer to the detailed discussion of relaxation techniques in Chapter 3.

Other things you can do to help prepare for quitting include the following:

- Make an appointment to see your physician.

- Ask about OTC and prescription aids for tobacco cessation and whether one or more might be appropriate for you.

- Make a dentist's appointment to have your teeth cleaned the day after your target quit date.

- Start an easy exercise program, if you're not exercising regularly already.

- Buy some sugarless gum. Stock your kitchen with low-calorie snacks.

- Clean out your car, and air out your house. Send your clothes out for dry cleaning.

- Throw away all your cigarette-related paraphernalia (ashtrays, lighters, etc.).

- The night before your quit day, get rid of all your cigarettes. Have fun with this—get your friends or family to help you tear them up.

- Make your last few days of smoking inconvenient: Smoke only outdoors and when alone. Don't do anything else while you smoke.

Quitting

Your first few days without cigarettes will probably be the most difficult. It's hard to give up such a strongly ingrained habit, but remember that many other Canadians have done it—and you can, too. Plan and rehearse the steps you will take when you experience a powerful craving. Avoid or control situations that you know from your journal are powerfully associated with your smoking (see the table). If your hands feel empty without a cigarette, try holding or fiddling with a small object, such as a paper clip or pencil.

Social support can also be a big help. Arrange with a friend to help you with your weak moments, and call him or her whenever you feel overwhelmed by an urge to smoke. Tell people you've just quit. You may discover many inspiring former smokers who can encourage you and reassure you that it's possible to quit and lead a happier, healthier life. Find a formal support group to join if you think it will help.

Maintaining Nonsmoking

The lingering smoking urges that remain once you've quit should be carefully tracked and controlled because they can cause relapses if left unattended. Keep track of these urges in your journal to help you deal with them. If certain situations still trigger the urge for a cigarette, change something about the situation to break past associations. If stress or boredom causes strong smoking urges, use a relaxation technique, take a brisk walk, have a stick of gum, or substitute some other activity for smoking.

Don't set yourself up for a relapse. If you allow yourself to get overwhelmed at school or work or to gain weight, it will be easier to convince yourself that now isn't the right time to quit. This is the right time. Continue to practise time-management and relaxation techniques. Exercise regularly, eat sensibly, and get enough sleep. These habits will not only ensure your success at remaining tobacco-free but also serve you well in stressful times throughout your life. In fact, former smokers who have quit for at least three months report reduced stress levels, probably because quitting smoking lowers overall arousal.

Watch out for patterns of thinking that can make nonsmoking more difficult. Focus on the positive aspects of not smoking, and give yourself lots of praise—you deserve it. Stick with the schedule of rewards you developed for your contract.

Keep track of the emerging benefits that come from having quit. Items that might appear on your list include improved stamina, an increased sense of pride at having kicked a strong addiction, a sharper sense of taste and smell, no more smoker's cough, and so on. Keep track of the money you're saving by not smoking, and spend it on things you really enjoy. And if you do lapse, be gentle with yourself. Lapses are a normal part of quitting. Forgive yourself, and pick up where you left off.

Strategies for Dealing with High-Risk Smoking Situations

Cues and High-Risk Situations	Suggested Strategies
Awakening in morning	Brush your teeth as soon as you wake up. Take a shower or bath.
Drinking coffee or tea	Do something else with your hands. Drink another beverage instead.
Eating meals	Sit in nonsmoking sections of restaurants. Get up from the table right after eating, and start another activity. Brush your teeth right after eating.
Driving a car	Have the car cleaned when you quit smoking. Chew sugarless gum or eat a low-calorie snack. Take public transportation or ride your bike. Turn on the radio and sing along.
Socializing with friends who smoke	Suggest nonsmoking events (movies, theatre, shopping). Tell friends you've quit and ask them not to smoke around you, offer you cigarettes, or give you cigarettes if you ask for them.
Drinking alcohol	Try to take a nonsmoker with you, or associate with nonsmokers. Let friends know you've just quit. Moderate your intake of alcohol (it can weaken your resolve).
Encountering stressful situations	Practise relaxation techniques. Take some deep breaths. Get out of your room or house. Go somewhere that doesn't allow smoking. Take a shower, chew gum, call a friend, or exercise.

Source: Strategies adapted with permission from *Postgraduate Medicine* 90(1), July 1991.

McGraw Hill connect™

Practise and learn online with Connect. Connect allows you to practise important skills at your own pace and on your own schedule, with 24/7 online access to an eBook, practice quizzes, interactivities, videos, study tools, additional resources, and more.

SUMMARY

• Smoking is the largest preventable cause of ill health and death in the Canada. Nevertheless, millions of Canadians continue to use tobacco.

• Regular tobacco use causes physical dependence on nicotine, characterized by loss of control, tolerance, and withdrawal. Habits can become associated with tobacco use and trigger the urge for a cigarette.

• People who begin smoking are usually imitating others or responding to seductive advertising. Smoking is associated with low education level and the use of other drugs.

• Tobacco smoke is made up of hundreds of different chemicals, including some that are carcinogenic or poisonous or that damage the respiratory system.

• Nicotine acts on the nervous system as a stimulant or a depressant. It can cause blood pressure and heart rate to increase, straining the heart.

• Cardiovascular disease is the most widespread cause of death for cigarette smokers. Cigarette smoking is the primary cause of lung cancer and is linked to many other cancers and respiratory diseases.

• Cigarette smoking is linked to ulcers, impotence, reproductive health problems, dental diseases, and other conditions. Tobacco use leads to shorter life expectancy and to a diminished quality of life.

• The use of spit tobacco leads to nicotine addiction and is linked to oral cancers.

• Cigars, pipes, clove cigarettes, and bidis are not safe alternatives to cigarettes.

• Environmental tobacco smoke (ETS) contains high concentrations of toxic chemicals and can cause headaches, eye and nasal irritation, and sinus problems. Long-term exposure to ETS can cause lung cancer and heart disease.

• Infants and young children take in more pollutants than adults do; children whose parents smoke are especially susceptible to respiratory diseases.

• Smoking during pregnancy increases the risk of miscarriage, stillbirth, congenital abnormalities, premature birth, and low birth weight. SIDS, behaviour problems, and long-term impairments in development are also risks.

• The overall cost of tobacco use to society includes the cost of both medical care and lost worker productivity.

• Individuals and groups can use many avenues to act against tobacco use. Nonsmokers can use social pressure and legislative channels to assert their rights to breathe clean air.

• Giving up smoking is a difficult and long-term process. Although most ex-smokers quit on their own, some smokers benefit from stop-smoking programs, OTC and prescription medications, and support groups.

FOR MORE INFORMATION

BOOKS

Canadian Cancer Society. 2007. *One Step at a Time: For Smokers Who Want to Quit.* Toronto: Canadian Cancer Society. Provides information on how to quit smoking, what not to do, and how to help a smoker quit.

Heart and Stroke Foundation. 2005. *Just Breathe: Becoming and Remaining Smoke Free.* Ottawa: Heart and Stroke Foundation. Provides information on heart disease associated with smoking as well as the benefits of becoming smoke free.

Government of Ontario. 2008. *Quit: You Have It in You.* Ottawa: Queen's Printer for Ontario. Provides information for quitters on how to quit smoking, the benefits of cessation, and links to other resources.

Program Training and Consultation Centre. 2003. *Smoke-Free Homes.* Toronto: Government of Ontario. Provides information on how to make your home smoke free.

ORGANIZATIONS, HOTLINES, AND WEB SITES

The Internet addresses listed here were accurate at the time of publication.

Alberta Health Services: Beyond the ABCs of Tobacco. Provides information and links on smokeless tobacco products and the amount of money tobacco companies spend advertising their products.
http://www.albertahealthservices.ca/AddictionsSubstanceAbuse/hi-asa-beyond-abcs-tobacco.pdf

Canadian Cancer Society: The Tobacco Act: An Overview. Provides information on current tobacco legislation, youth and tobacco, and national partnerships in tobacco control.

http://www.cancer.ca

Health Canada: Canadian Tobacco Use Monitoring Survey. Provides information and statistics on current and past tobacco use in Canada.

http://www.hc-sc.gc.ca/hc-ps/tobac-tabac/research-recherche/stat/index-eng.php

Health Canada: Second-Hand Smoke. Provides information on the impact of second-hand smoke on Canadians.

http://www.hc-sc.gc.ca/hc-ps/tobac-tabac/second/index-eng.php

Non-Smokers' Rights Association. Provides a wide variety of information on the control of tobacco products.

http://www.nsra-adnf.ca/cms/index.cfm

Physicians for a Smoke-Free Canada. Provides information and links for tobacco facts, research papers, second-hand smoke, policies, and the legislation of tobacco products.

http://www.smoke-free.ca

Public Health Agency of Canada: Chronic Obstructive Pulmonary Disease. Provides information and links on COPD and smoking.

http://www.phac-aspc.gc.ca/cd-mc/crd-mrc/copd-mpoc-eng.php

Smoke-Free Living: Resources for Teachers. Provides information on youth smoking habits and smoking in grade schools and ways for teachers to include this information in their curriculum.

http://www.toronto.ca/health/smokefree/prevention/youth_teachers.htm

World Health Organization: Tobacco-Free Initiative. Promotes the goal of a tobacco-free world.

http://www.who.int/tobacco/en

World No Tobacco Day. Provides information on the annual worldwide event to encourage people to quit smoking, and general information about tobacco use and testimonials of ex-smokers.

http://www.who.int/tobacco/communications/events/wntd/en/

Youth Smoking Survey. Provides information and statistics on current and past youth tobacco use in Canada.

http://www.yss.uwaterloo.ca

See also the listings for Chapters 7, 8, and 14.

SELECTED BIBLIOGRAPHY

Canadian Lung Association. 2010. *Smoking and Tobacco* (http://www.lung.ca/protect-protegez/tobacco-tabagisme_e.php; retrieved May 3, 2011).

Collot, N. (writer/dir.). 2009. *The Tobacco Conspiracy*. Montreal: National Film Board of Canada [documentary].

Crow, M. E. 2005. The human rights responsibilities of multinational tobacco companies. *Tobacco Control* 14(2): 14–18.

D'Avernas, J. R., et al. 1997. *Cigarette Packaging and Event Marketing Increases the Attractiveness of Smoking: A Study of Youth*. Toronto: Ontario Tobacco Research Unit.

Daynard R. 2003. Why tobacco litigation? *Tobacco Control* 12: 1–2.

Edwards, R. 2004. ABCs of smoking cessation: The problem of tobacco smoking. *British Medical Journal* 328(7433): 217–219.

Fagerstrom, K. 2002. The epidemiology of smoking: Health consequences and benefits of cessation. *Drugs* 62 (2): 1–9.

Fair Air Association of Canada. 2006. *McGuinty Government's Addiction to Anti-Smoking Lobby Will Result in Smuggling, Job and Business Losses, Tax Hikes and Drastic Revenue Shortfalls* [press release] (http://www.smokersclubinc.com/modules.php?name=News&file=article&sid=2440; retrieved May 3, 2011).

Health Canada. 2006. *Tobacco Control Program, Supplementary Tables, CTUMS Annual 2006 (February–December 2006)* (http://www.hc-sc.gc.ca/hc-ps/tobac-tabac/research-recherche/stat/_ctums-esutc_2006/ann-table5-eng.php; retrieved May 3, 2011).

Health Canada. 2007. *Federal Tobacco Control Strategy* (http://www.hc-sc.gc.ca/hl-vs/tobac-tabac/res/news-nouvelles/ftcs-sflt_e.html; retrieved January 26, 2008).

Health Canada. 2007. *Youth Smoking Survey 2006–2007* (http://www.hc-sc.gc.ca/hl-vs/tobac-tabac/research-recherche/stat/_survey-sondage_2006–2007/result-eng.php; retrieved December 12, 2009).

Makomaski Illing, E. M., and M. J. Kaiserman. 2004. Mortality attributable to tobacco use in Canada and its regions. *Canadian Journal of Public Health* 95(1): 38–44.

Johnson, E. O., and S. P. Novak. 2009. Onset and persistence of daily smoking: The interplay of socioeconomic status, gender, and psychiatric disorders. *Drug and Alcohol Dependence* 104: S50–S57.

Kelton, M. H., and M. S. Givel. 2008. Public policy implications of tobacco industry smuggling through Native American reservations into Canada. *International Journal of Health Services* 38(3): 471–487.

Leatherdale, S. T. 2005. Predictors of different cigarette access behaviours among occasional and regular smoking youth. *Canadian Journal of Public Health* 96(5): 348–352.

McKennitt, D. 2007. A smoking prevention program for Aboriginal youth. *First Peoples Child and Family Review* 3(2): 52–55.

Ontario Tobacco Research Unit. 2006. Toward smoke-free Ontario strategy objectives, 2005–2006. *Special Reports: Monitoring and Evaluation Series, 2005–2006* 12(1). Toronto: Ontario Tobacco Research Unit.

Olser, M., et al. 1999. Gender and determinants of smoking cessation: A longitudinal study. *Preventive Medicine* 29(1): 57–62.

Perez, C. E. 2004. Second-hand smoke exposure: Who's at risk? *Health Reports* 16(3): 19–36.

Physicians for a Smoke-Free Canada. 2003. *Tobacco in Canada* (http://www.smoke-free.ca/pdf_1/TOBACCOINCANADA2003.pdf; retrieved May 3, 2011).

Reading, J., and Y. Allard. 1999. *The Tobacco Report: Report of the FNIRHS*. Ottawa: First Nations and Inuit Health Survey National Steering Committee.

Science Daily. 2009. *Smoking Gun: Just One Cigarette Has Harmful Effects on the Arteries of the Young and Healthy* (http://www.sciencedaily.com/releases/2009/10/091027085300.htm; retrieved May 3, 2011).

Shields, M. 2005. The journey to quitting smoking. *Health Reports* 16(3): 19–36.

Shields, M. 2007. Smoking-prevalence, bans and exposure to second hand smoke. *Health Reports* 18(3): 67–85.

Statistics Canada. 2010. *Canadian Tobacco Use Monitoring Survey, 2008* (http://www.hc-sc.gc.ca/hl-vs/tobac-tabac/research-recherche/stat/_ctums-esutc_2008/wave-phase-1_summary-sommaire-eng.php; retrieved January 6, 2010).

Wardman, D., and Khan, N. 2004. Smoking-attributable mortality among British Columbia's First Nations populations. *International Journal of Circumpolar Health* 63: 81–92.

Wardman, D., and Khan, N. 2005. Registered Indians and tobacco taxation: A culturally appropriate strategy? *Canadian Journal of Public Health* 96: 451–453.

World Health Organization. 2008. *The Global Tobacco Crisis* (http://www.who.int/tobacco/mpower/mpower_report_tobacco_crisis_2008.pdf; retrieved September 27, 2008).

Practise and learn online with Connect.

AGING: A VITAL PROCESS

17

LOOKING AHEAD>>>>>

AFTER READING THIS CHAPTER, YOU SHOULD BE ABLE TO

- Describe practical considerations of older adults and caregivers, including housing, finances, health care, communication, and transportation

- List strategies for healthful aging

- Explain the physical, social, and mental changes that may accompany aging and discuss how people can best confront these changes

TEST YOUR KNOWLEDGE

1. **Women do not need to take preventive measures against osteoporosis until after menopause.**
   True or false?

2. **What is the leading cause of vision loss in Canada?**
   a. glaucoma
   b. cataracts
   c. age-related macular degeneration (AMD)

3. **On average, a woman will spend more time caring for an aging relative than raising children.**
   True or false?

4. **For which of the following reasons is exercise beneficial for older people?**
   a. protects against osteoporosis
   b. maintains alertness and intelligence
   c. prevents falls

5. **Alcohol abuse is rare among older adults.**
   True or false?

ANSWERS

1. **FALSE.** Everyone—but especially women—needs to pay attention to diet and exercise in younger years to build bone mass.

2. **C.** According to the Canadian National Institute for the Blind, age-related macular degeneration affects approximately 1 million Canadians and is the leading cause of vision loss in Canada.

3. **TRUE.** The average woman will spend 17 years raising children and 18 years caring for an aging relative.

4. **ALL THREE.** Even for people over 80, exercise can improve physical functioning and balance and reduce falls and injuries.

5. **FALSE.** Alcohol abuse affects about 10% of older adults. It often goes undetected because its symptoms may mimic those of other conditions, such as Alzheimer's disease.

ging is the process of becoming older, a process that is genetically determined but profoundly affected by a person's environment. Your grandparents or great-grandparents may be examples of how these two determinants play a role in the aging process.

Aging does not begin at some specific point in life, and there is no precise age at which a person becomes "old." Rather, aging is a normal process of development that occurs throughout life. It happens to everyone, but at different rates for different people. Some people are old at 25, and others are still young at 75.

Although youth is not entirely a state of mind, your attitude toward life and your attention to your health significantly influence the satisfaction you will get from life. This is especially true when new physical, mental, and social challenges occur in later years. If you optimize wellness during young adulthood, you can exert great control over the physical and mental aspects of aging, and you can better handle your response to events that might be out of your control.

This chapter discusses the aging process and describes some of the major effects increasing age can have on your life.

AGING AND LIFE EXPECTANCY

Life expectancy is the average length of time we can expect to live. It is calculated by averaging mortality statistics, the ages at death of a group of people over a certain period. Between 2005 and 2007, life expectancy for the total Canadian population was 80.7 years. Women have a longer life expectancy than men (see the box "Why Do Women Live Longer?"). Life expectancy also varies among ethnic groups; reasons for these differences include socioeconomic, genetic, and lifestyle factors.

Life expectancy in Canada increased dramatically in the twentieth century, as described in Chapter 1. This does not mean that every Canadian lives longer now than in 1900; rather, far fewer people die young now, because childhood and infectious diseases are better controlled and diet and sanitation are much improved.

How long can humans expect to live in the best of circumstances? It now seems possible that our maximum potential **lifespan** is 100–120 years. Our **health span**, by contrast, is the period of life when we are generally healthy and free from chronic or serious disease. The major difference between lifespan (how long you live) and health span (how long you stay healthy) is freedom from chronic or disabling disease. As we've seen throughout this text, failure to achieve a positive health span results to some degree from destructive environmental and behavioural factors—factors over which we can exert considerable control. Longevity appears to be influenced very little by genetics. Studies of identical twins and other research suggest that lifespan is only about 3% heritable, meaning that the age at which a person's parents die has only a 3% effect on that person's age at death.

Long life does not necessarily mean a longer period of disability, either. People often live longer because they have been well longer. A healthy old age is very often an extension of a healthy middle age. However, behaviour changes cannot extend the maximum human lifespan, which seems to be built into our genes.

Aging is associated with several changes, both physical and psychological (many of these changes are discussed later in the chapter). No one really knows how and why people change as they get older. Different theories claim that aging is caused by accumulated injuries from ultraviolet light, wear and tear on the body, by-products of metabolism, and so on. Other theories view aging as a predetermined, genetically programmed process. No theory, however, sufficiently explains all the changes of the aging process. Aging is complex and varies in how it affects different people and even different organs. Most gerontologists (scientists who study aging and its effects) feel that aging is the cumulative result of the interaction of many lifelong influences, including heredity, environment, culture, diet, exercise and leisure, past illnesses, and many other factors.

Life in an Aging Canada

As life expectancy increases, a larger proportion of the population will be in their later years. This change will necessitate new government policies and changes in our general attitudes toward older adults.

Canada's Aging Population

People over 65 were a minority in the Canadian population at almost 14% of the total population in 2006. As the baby boomers age, the older adult population is expected to

QUESTIONS FOR CRITICAL THINKING AND REFLECTION

Have you ever thought about growing old? Is it a topic that you have discussed with others, or is it one that you avoid? What do you think are the most important dimensions of wellness for older adults? What health behaviours will you focus on as you move from youth to middle age to old age? What behaviour change strategies might be helpful?

Why Do Women Live Longer?

Women live longer than men in most countries around the world, even in places where maternal mortality rates are high. In Canada, women on average can expect to live about five years longer than men (see table at right). Worldwide, among people over age 100, women outnumber men about nine to one.

The reason for the gender gap in life expectancy is not entirely understood but may be influenced by biological, social, and lifestyle factors. Estrogen production and other factors during a woman's younger years may protect her from early heart disease and from age-related declines in the pumping power of the heart. Women may have lower rates of stress-related illnesses because they cope more positively with stress by seeking social support.

The news for women is not all good, however, because not all their extra years are likely to be healthy years. They are more likely than men to suffer from chronic conditions, such as arthritis and osteoporosis. Women's longer lifespan, combined with the facts that men tend to marry younger women and that widowed men remarry more often than

widowed women, means there are many more single older women than men. Older men are more likely to live in family settings, whereas older women are more likely to live alone. Older women are also less likely to be covered by a pension or to have retirement savings, so they are more likely to be poor.

Increased male mortality can be traced in part to higher rates of unhealthful behaviours, such as smoking and alcohol and drug abuse. Testosterone production may be partly responsible in that it is linked to aggressive and risky behaviour and to unhealthy cholesterol levels. Men have much higher rates of death than women from car crashes and other unintentional injuries, firearm-related deaths, homicide, suicide, AIDS, and early heart attack. Gender roles that promote risky behaviour among young men are a factor in many of these causes of death. Indeed, among people who have made it to age 65, the gender longevity gap is smaller.

Social and behavioural factors may be more important than physiological causes in explaining the gender gap; for example, among the Amish, a religious sect that has strict rules against smoking and drinking,

men usually live as long as women. This suggests that the longevity gap could be substantially narrowed through lifestyle changes.

Life Expectancy in Canada

Year	Men	Women
At birth		
1971	69.6	76.6
1991	74.6	81.0
2000–2002	77.0	82.0
2005–2007	78.3	83.0
At age 65		
1971	13.9	17.7
1991	15.8	20.0
2000–2002	17.0	20.5
2005–2007	18.1	21.3

Sources: Statistics Canada. 2000. *Report on the Demographic Situation in Canada* (http://www.statcan.gc.ca/pub/91-209-x/91-209-x2000000-eng.pdf; retrieved May 19, 2010); Statistics Canada. 2010. *Table 1: Life Expectancy at Birth and at Age 65 by Sex, Canada* (http://www.statcan.gc.ca/daily-quotidien/100223/t100223a1-eng.htm; retrieved May 19, 2010).

---

reach 6.7 million in 2021 and 9.2 million (nearly one in four Canadians) in 2041. The fastest growth is occurring among the oldest Canadians. In 2001, more than 430,000 Canadians were 85 years of age or older—more than twice as many as in 1981, and more than twenty times as many as in 1921. The proportion of Canadians ages 85 or older is expected to grow to 1.6 million in 2041, representing 4% of the overall population (Figure 17.1 on p. 530). According to Statistics Canada projections, an unprecedented event will take place in or around the year 2015: Older adults will outnumber children in Canada.

Today, low fertility rates (1.5 children per woman currently versus 3 or more children per woman in the mid-1940s to the 1960s), longer life expectancy, and the effects of the baby boom generation are some of the factors contributing to Canada's aging population (see the box "Baby Boomers: Redefining Age and Retirement" on p. 531).

The enormous increase in the aging population is markedly affecting our stereotypes of what it means to grow old. The misfortunes associated with aging—frailty, forgetfulness, poor health, isolation—occur in fewer people in their sixties and seventies and are shifting instead to burden the very old, those over 85.

According to Statistics Canada, the financial situation of older adults in Canada has improved over the past quarter century. In many cases, the living expenses of older adults are lower after retirement because they no longer support children and have fewer work-related expenses; they also consume and buy less food. They are more likely to

life expectancy The average length of time a person is expected to live.

lifespan A theoretically projected length of life based on the maximum potential of the human body in the best environment.

health span The period of life when a person is generally healthy and free from chronic or serious disease.

TERMS

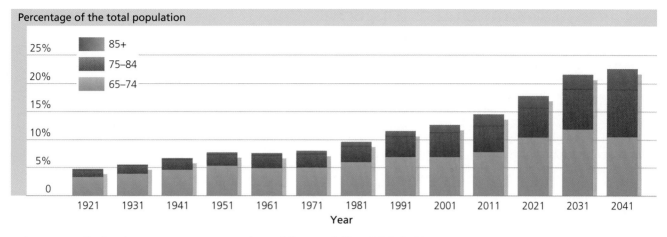

Percentage of the total population

FIGURE 17.1   Seniors by age group as a percentage of the population, 1921–2041.

Source: Canada's Aging Population. Public Health Agency of Canada, 2002. Reproduced with the permission of the Minister of Health, 2011.

continue practising their expertise for years after retirement: Thousands of retired consultants, teachers, technicians, and craftspeople work until their middle and late seventies. They also receive government assistance, including the **Old Age Security (OAS) pension**, and often have greater net worth from lifetime savings. Unfortunately, the highest incidence of low-income among older adults in Canada occurs among women who live alone.

As the aging population increases proportionately, however, the number of older people who are ill and dependent rises. Additionally, the need for medications, medical equipment, and health services—and the costs associated with them—are often substantial. On average, older Canadians visit physicians much more frequently than younger Canadians. In 2003, 67% of older men and 68% of older women visited a medical doctor three times or more. Older adults are also hospitalized more frequently and require at least twice as many prescription drugs as the general population. In Canada, insurance coverage often makes the difference in terms of disease prevention or access to health services. In 2003, about 80% of older Canadians indicated that they were insured for prescription medications. However, there were significant differences in insurance coverage for medications by provinces. For example, only about half of older adults living in Saskatchewan and 60% of those in Manitoba reported that they had their medications covered by insurance, compared with 86% in Nova Scotia and 90% in Alberta.

Health care policy planners hope that rising medical costs for older adults will shrink dramatically through education and prevention. Health care professionals, including **gerontologists** and **geriatricians**, are beginning to practise preventive medicine, just as pediatricians do. They advise older people about how to avoid and, if necessary, how to manage diseases and disabilities. In Canada, most older people have at least one chronic condition; many have more than one. Table 17.1 lists some of the most commonly reported conditions among older adults in Canada.

Table 17.1	Percentage of Older Canadians with Chronic Conditions, 2003	
Condition		**Percentage**
Arthritis/rheumatism		47.3%
Cataracts/glaucoma		24.7%
Back problems		24.1%
Heart disease		19.8%
Diabetes		13.5%
Thyroid condition		12.9%

Source: Gilmour, H., and J. Park. 2005. Dependency, chronic conditions and pain in seniors. *Health Reports* (16 Suppl.): 21–31 (http://www.statcan.gc.ca/pub/82-003-s/2005000/pdf/9087-eng.pdf; retrieved May 22, 2010).

Family and Community Resources for Older Adults

With help from friends, family members, and community services, people in their later years can remain active and independent. According to the 2001 census, 93% of Canadians over the age of 65 live in private households, either alone or with others. Only 7% live in institutional settings, such as hospitals or nursing homes, but among those over age 85, 32% live in institutional residencies (Figure 17.2 on p. 532 shows the breakdown by sex).

The living arrangements of older Canadians appear to be related to the overall well-being of these individuals. Although many factors influence a person's level of happiness, compared with older adults who live with a spouse or other family members, those living alone are less likely to describe themselves as very happy. In 2003, more than half (53%) of older Canadians between the ages of 65 and 74 who were living with their spouse described themselves as very happy, compared with 39% of those living alone and 37% of those in other types of living arrangements.

Baby Boomers: Redefining Age and Retirement

If you are a postsecondary student age 18–24, chances are good that one or both of your parents are members of the *baby boom* generation—people born between 1947 and 1966. Chances are also good that the boomers in your life will reach retirement age in the next decade or two. That doesn't mean, however, that they'll actually retire.

Living Longer, Living Younger

In general, baby boomers are living longer than their parents did. As a result, the average boomer's retirement period is longer. Near the beginning of the twentieth century, the average 65-year-old Canadian could expect to live another 13 years; today, that number has been extended to about 20 years. And it's

becoming increasingly common for people to live into their eighties and nineties. Boomers "live younger" than their parents, too, meaning they tend to be healthier than their parents and enjoy better long-term prospects for good health.

Redefining Notions of Age

What are baby boomers doing with all that extra time and health? As it turns out, they have big plans for retirement, including retiring early and continuing an active lifestyle. Baby boomers don't necessarily consider age 60 or 65 to be the start of their "golden years." As they reach age 60 and beyond, boomers are reinventing themselves and their lives, leaving long-held notions of aging in the dust.

A Shift in Thinking

Traditional views of retirement are starting to change, primarily because of the cost of retiring. Most Canadians do not save enough money to fund 20 or more years of leisure time. A 2010 Royal Bank of Canada (RBC) survey revealed that almost 40% of Canadians over the age of 50 retired with some form of debt, and one-quarter entered retirement with a mortgage.

Younger workers, especially baby boomers, don't necessarily see retirement as being very attractive. In fact, according to an RBC Poll conducted in 2009, 31% of Canadians who were still working said that they would never retire. Some older adults prefer to continue working, and many volunteer their time to good causes, further their education, or even start a new career.

A 2007–2008 Fidelity Canadian Retirement Survey showed that more than two-thirds of working baby boomers have no plans to downsize their lifestyles in retirement. In fact, the majority of these individuals plan to maintain or even increase their standard of living in retirement. This plan has led many older Canadians to practise what experts call *revolving or cycling retirement*: periods of work interspersed with extended periods of leisure. Following this strategy, older people can work only as required to support their lifestyle. When not working, they can pursue other interests.

Of course, this scenario can play out only if people stay relatively healthy. Although older Canadians are fitter than ever, continued good health is not a given. If current positive trends continue, however, baby boomers may be just the first of many generations not only to live longer but to put off retirement altogether.

THINKING ABOUT THE ENVIRONMENT

Both the natural and human-made environments pose many threats to the well-being of older adults.

Particulate air pollution and ozone, for example, aggravate breathing-related conditions, such as asthma and chronic obstructive pulmonary disease (COPD). In older people with such disorders, even brief exposure to dirty air can result in hospitalization. Indoor air can be just as hazardous, especially if it contains lingering mould or dust particles.

Environmental factors can be a special concern for older adults with diabetes. When a person with diabetes is exposed to hot weather, for example, the body can lose its ability to regulate its temperature—a condition that can be fatal. Air pollution can affect the ability of the blood vessels of a person with diabetes to control blood flow. Several types of air pollution have been associated with an increased risk of cardiovascular problems in people with diabetes.

For more information on the environment and environmental health, see Chapter 21.

Family Involvement in Caregiving Studies show that in about three out of four cases, a spouse, a grown daughter, or a daughter-in-law assumes a caregiving role for older relatives. With more parents living into their eighties and with fewer children per family, many people, especially women, will face the dilemma of how best to care for an aging relative. Recent surveys indicate that the average woman will spend about 17 years raising children and 18 years caring for an aging relative.

Old Age Security (OAS) pension   A monthly benefit available to Canadians 65 years of age and older who have lived in Canada for at least 10 years; financed through taxes paid by Canadians.

gerontologist   A person who studies the biological, psychological, and social phenomena associated with aging and old age.

geriatrician   A physician specializing in the diseases, disabilities, and care of older adults.

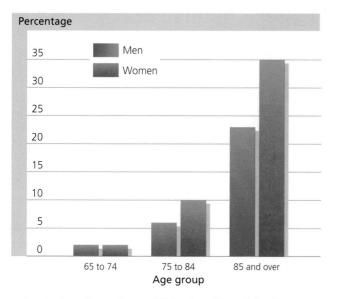

Percentage

<table>
<tr><td></td><td>Men</td><td>Women</td></tr>
</table>

FIGURE 17.2   **Percentage of older Canadians living in institutions, by age group and sex, 2001.**

Source: Turcotte, M., and G. Schellenberg. 2007. *A Portrait of Seniors in Canada, 2006,* p. 139 (http://www.statcan.gc.ca/pub/89-519-x/89-519-x2006001-eng.pdf; retrieved May 26, 2010).

Caregiving can be rewarding, but it is also hard work. If the experience is stressful and long-term, family members may become emotionally exhausted. Corporations are increasingly responsive to the needs of their employees who are family caregivers by providing helpful services, such as referrals, flexible schedules, and leaves. Professional health care advice is another critical part of successful home care. Caregivers need to give special consideration to such issues as hearing and vision loss, which can make an older adult feel disconnected or isolated, and dementia, which can make caregiving an extremely challenging prospect.

The caregiver must work with the older person's doctors and pharmacists to ensure that medication is available and taken as prescribed. (Studies show that older adults commonly skip their cholesterol and blood pressure medications, for example.) The caregiver may need to acquire a legal status called *power of attorney*, which enables him or her to make decisions about the patient's medical and personal care, as well as financial matters.

The best thing a family can do is talk honestly about the obligations, time, and commitment required by caregiving. Families should also explore the community resources and professional assistance that may be available to reduce the stress in this difficult job.

Other Living and Care Options   If living together is not possible for aging parents and adult children, other living and care options are available. Retirement communities are an option for individuals in good health and with a good income who want to maintain home ownership. Other types of facilities are available for people who need more assistance with daily living.

Community Resources   Community resources are available to help older adults remain active and in their own homes. Typical services include the following:

- *Senior centres or adult day care centres* provide meals, social activities, and health care services for those unable to be alone during the day.
- *Homemaker services* offer housekeeping, cooking, errand running, and escorting to appointments.
- *Visiting nurses* provide basic health care.
- *Household services* perform household repairs.
- *Friendly visitor or daily telephone reassurance services* provide contacts, medication and other reminders, and friendly conversation for older people who live alone.
- *Home food delivery services* provide meals to home-bound people.
- *Adult day hospital care* provides day care plus physical therapy and treatment for chronic illnesses.
- *Low-cost legal aid* helps manage finances and health care.
- *Transportation services* offer rides at low rates.
- *Case management* helps seniors navigate confusing health care services.

Additional information about services for older adults can be found in the phone book or on government Web sites, including Service Canada (http://www.servicecanada.gc.ca) and Seniors Canada (http://www.seniors.gc.ca).

Transportation   Older drivers usually have safe driving records compared with young adults because they tend to be more cautious; however, the number of crashes in the older age group is increasing and those crashes are more likely to be fatal. This trend is often explained by higher rates of illness, medication use, and related impairments. The decision to stop driving is an extremely difficult one for older adults, their family members, and their physicians. In Canada, most provinces and territories require physicians to report patients who are medically unfit to drive. Other regulations relating to driver's licences held by older adults vary across jurisdictions. In Ontario, for example, the Senior Driver Renewal Program requires that adult drivers ages 80 years and over complete a vision test and a knowledge test, and take part in a group education session every two years. Because of changes in vision or other health problems, some older drivers may be required to give up their licence before they feel ready. Many older adults report that the loss of a driver's licence, and the loss of independence it brings, is one of the most severe hardships they face.

Government Aid

Financial well-being is an essential component of health, wellness, and security for all individuals, including older adults. As stated in the 2005 document *Planning for Canada's Aging Population,* "income is one of the most important health determinants and the basis of an individual's ability to access appropriate housing and transportation required

to maintain independence; nutritious and sufficient food to maintain health; and non-insured medical services and supports such as medication and home support."

The federal government helps older Canadians through several programs, including the OAS program and the Canada Pension Plan (CPP) or Quebec Pension Plan (QPP).

The OAS pension is governed by Canada's Old Age Security Act, which came into effect in 1952. This program is Canada's largest public pension program and is financed solely from tax revenues collected by the government. Benefits paid under this act fall into several categories, including the basic OAS pension, the Guaranteed Income Supplement (GIS), the Allowance, and the Allowance for the Survivor. The OAS pension is a monthly benefit available to most Canadians ages 65 and over, regardless of employment history or retirement status. In 2010, the maximum amount was $516.96 per month. The GIS is an additional benefit for Canadians with little or no income other than the OAS. The Allowance and Allowance for the Survivor were established in response to the difficulties experienced by widows and by couples living on one pension. The Allowance provides a monthly benefit to low-income Canadians ages 60–64 whose spouse or common-law partner receives an OAS pension. The Allowance for the Survivor provides money to low-income Canadians ages 60–64 whose spouse or common-law partner has died.

The CPP and QPP are an earnings-related social insurance system that provides a retirement pension to Canadians as early as 60 years of age. This program provides benefits to Canadians who have contributed to the plan and who have retired or developed a disability. According to the Government of Canada, the CPP/QPP is designed to replace about 25% of an individual's earnings from employment, up to a maximum amount. For example, in 2010, the maximum CPP amount that a Canadian could receive was $934.17 per month.

Many older Canadians may also have contributed to private pensions and savings, such as Registered Pension Plans (RPPs) and Registered Retirement Savings Plans (RRSPs). In most cases, people have determined how much money they will need in retirement and contributed accordingly. Tax deductions on RPPs and RRSPs are the primary ways that the Canadian government assists individuals in saving for retirement. In Canada, the vast majority of retirement income is received from private pensions, while the remainder is typically composed of income from RRSPs.

Additional government programs for older Canadians who may be eligible include International Pension Benefits (for older adults who have lived or worked in another country), the Assisted Living Program (for First Nations members living on-reserve who have functional limitations because of age, disability, or health problems), and the Home Adaptations for Seniors Independence program (for older adults who are homeowners or landlords and who want to make specific home adaptations).

Between 1980 and 2006, the proportion of older Canadians living with a low income decreased from about

QUESTIONS FOR CRITICAL THINKING AND REFLECTION
What do you want your life to be like when you are old? Do you hope to retire or keep working indefinitely? Where would you like to live? How much time do you spend thinking about these questions? Have you done any planning yet for older age?

21% to 5%—a rate lower than most other industrialized countries. This decline has been attributed—in part—to the effectiveness of Canada's retirement income system. For example, one of the many factors that has contributed to the rising incomes of older Canadians has been the growing number of Canadians collecting CPP/QPP. CPP/QPP were established in 1966 and the first cohort of Canadians to receive full benefits turned 65 in 1976. With the aging of the Canadian population, the proportion of older adults eligible for full CPP/QPP benefits has increased. Between 1980 and 2003, the percentage of Canadian men over age 65 receiving CPP/QPP increased from 68.6% to 95.8%.

An even greater increase occurred among Canadian women as a result of their growing participation in the labour force; between 1980 and 2003, the share of Canadian women over age 65 receiving income from CPP/QPP increased from 34.8% to 85.8%. Despite this increase, financial planning for retirement is especially critical for women. Canadian women are still at a greater risk of having a low income in old age, reflecting the fact that many women have lower-paying jobs, work part-time, or work primarily in the home during their childbearing years. Women should investigate their retirement plans and take charge of their finances to be sure they will be provided for as they get older.

QUICK STATS

39% of Canadians over the age of 50 retire with some form of debt.

—RBC Retirement Myths and Realities Poll, 2010

GENERATING VITALITY AS YOU AGE

As we age, physical and mental changes occur gradually, over a lifetime. Biological aging includes all the normal, progressive, irreversible changes to the body that begin at birth and continue until death. Psychological aging and social aging usually involve more abrupt changes in circumstance and emotion: relocating, changing homes, losing a spouse and friends, retiring, having a lower income, and changing roles and social status. These changes represent opportunities for growth throughout life.

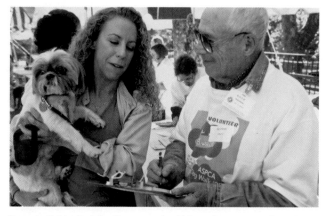

Some individuals defy all preconceived ideas about age and continue to live vigorous and productive lives into their seventies, eighties, and beyond.

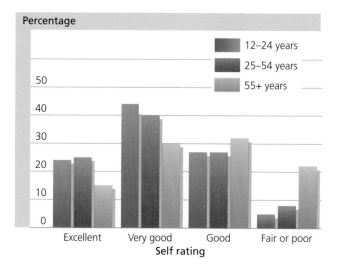

FIGURE 17.3 **Self-rated health of Canadians, 2005.**

Source: Statistics Canada. 2006. *CANSIM Table 105-0422: Self-Rated Health, by Age Group and Sex, Household Population Aged 12 and Over, Canada, Provinces, Territories, Health Regions (June 2005 Boundaries) and Peer Groups, Every 2 Years* (http://www4.hrsdc.gc.ca/.3ndic.1t. 4r@-eng.jsp?iid=10#M_3; retrieved May 19, 2010).

Not all of them happen to everybody, and their timing varies, partly depending on how we have prepared for our later days. Some people never have to leave their homes and appear to be in good health until the day they die. Others have tremendous adjustments to make—to entirely new surroundings with fewer financial resources, to new acquaintances, to the changing physical condition of their bodies and new health problems, and possibly to loneliness and loss of self-esteem.

Successful aging requires preparation. People need to establish good health habits in their teens and twenties. During their twenties and thirties, they usually develop important relationships and settle into a particular lifestyle. By their mid-forties, they generally know how much money they need to support the lifestyle they've chosen. At this point, and perhaps even earlier, they must assess their financial status and perhaps adjust their savings to continue enjoying that lifestyle after retirement. In their mid-fifties, they need to reevaluate their financial and retirement plans and may want to think about retirement housing. In their seventies and beyond, they need to consider ways of sharing their legacy with the next generation. Throughout life, people should cultivate interests and hobbies they enjoy, both alone and with others.

What Happens as We Age?

In comparison to younger age groups, a large number of older Canadians describe themselves as being in fair or poor health (Figure 17.3). Many of the characteristics associated with aging are not due to aging at all. Rather, they are the result of the neglect and abuse of our bodies and minds. These assaults lay the foundation for later psychological problems and chronic conditions, such as arthritis, heart disease, diabetes, hearing loss, and hypertension. We sacrifice our health by smoking, having poor nutrition, overeating, abusing alcohol and drugs, bombarding our ears with excessive noise, and exposing our bodies to too much ultraviolet radiation from the sun. We also jeopardize our bodies through inactivity, encouraging our muscles

and even our bones to wither and deteriorate. And we endure abuse from the toxic chemicals in our environment.

But even with the healthiest behaviour and environment, aging inevitably occurs. It results from biochemical processes we don't yet fully understand. The physiological changes in organ systems are caused by a combination of gradual aging and impairment from disease. Because of redundancy in most organ systems, the body's ability to function is not affected until damage is fairly extensive. Studies of healthy people indicate that functioning remains essentially constant until after age 70. Further research may help pinpoint the causes of aging and aid in the development of therapies to repair damage to aging organs.

Life-Enhancing Measures: Age-Proofing

You can prevent, delay, lessen, or even reverse some of the changes associated with aging through good habits. Simple things you can do daily will make a vast difference to your level of energy and vitality—your overall wellness. The following suggestions have been mentioned throughout this text. But because they are profoundly related to health in later life, we highlight them here.

Challenge Your Mind Numerous studies show that older adults who stay mentally active have a lower risk of developing dementia. Reading, doing puzzles, learning language, and studying music are good ways to stimulate the brain. The more complex the activity, the more protective it may be.

Develop Physical Fitness Exercise significantly enhances both psychological and physical health. A 2006 study showed that older adults who burned extra calories

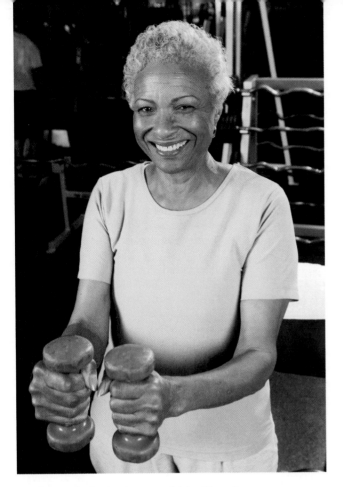
Regular exercise is a key to successful, healthy aging.

through daily activity had a much lower mortality rate than their peers who did not exercise. The positive effects of exercise include the following:

- Lower blood pressure and healthier cholesterol levels
- Better protection against heart attacks and an increased chance of survival should one occur
- Sustained or increased lung capacity
- Maintenance of strength, flexibility, and balance
- Protection against osteoporosis and type 2 diabetes
- Increased effectiveness of the immune system
- Maintenance of mental agility and flexibility, response time, memory, and hand-eye coordination

The stimulus that exercise provides also seems to protect against the loss of **fluid intelligence**, the ability to find solutions to new problems. Fluid intelligence depends on rapidity of responsiveness, memory, and alertness. Individuals who exercise regularly are also less susceptible to depression and dementia.

Regular physical activity also fends off *sarcopenia*, which is age-related loss of muscle mass, strength, and function (see Chapter 6). The weaker a person becomes, the less he or she can do; this condition can rob someone of self-sufficiency and lead to greater dependence on others. The muscle wasting that occurs in sarcopenia also leads to

weight gain because muscle burns more calories than fat, even at rest.

Regular physical activity is essential for healthy aging. The Canadian Physical Activity Guidelines for Older Adults—65 Years & Older recommend that people over the age of 65 should accumulate at least 150 minutes of moderate- to vigorous-intensity aerobic physical activity each week, in increments of at least 10 minutes each. These guidelines also suggest that older adults should engage in strength training activities that use major muscle groups at least twice per week. It is also recommended that people with poor mobility should perform physical activities that focus on balance and preventing falls. Older individuals who have been sedentary should be encouraged to become more active. It's never too late to start exercising. Even in people over 80, endurance and strength training can improve balance, flexibility, and physical functioning and reduce the potential for dangerous falls (see the box "Falls Among Older Adults" on p. 536 for more about falls).

Eat Wisely Good health at any age is enhanced by eating a varied diet full of nutrient-rich foods. Follow the recommendations in *Eating Well with Canada's Food Guide* to get enough essential nutrients while maintaining a healthy weight (Chapter 5). For many adults, that means eating more fruits, vegetables, and whole grains while eating fewer foods high in saturated and trans fats and added sugars. Additional recommendations for older adults include the following:

- Take a vitamin D supplement. Health Canada recommends that in addition to following *Eating Well with Canada's Food Guide*, adults over the age of 50 should take a daily vitamin D supplement of 400 IU.
- Make sure that you are getting an adequate amount of calcium from foods and supplements. According to Osteoporosis Canada, the daily calcium requirement for Canadians over the age of 50 is 1500 milligrams.
- Consume foods rich in dietary fibre and drink plenty of water to help prevent constipation, which may occur in up to 20% of older adults. A diet rich in whole grains, vegetables, and fruits can meet the recommended goals for fibre.
- Pay special attention to food safety; older adults tend to be more susceptible to food-borne illness (see Chapter 5).

Maintain a Healthy Weight Weight management is especially difficult if you have been overweight most of your life. A sensible program of expending more calories

fluid intelligence The ability to develop a solution when confronted with a new problem.

TERMS

Falls Among Older Adults

According to Health Canada, the primary cause of injury among older Canadians is falls. The 2005 *Report on Seniors' Falls in Canada* provides a wealth of information related to injuries and falls among older Canadians, including the following statistics:

• Close to 62% of injury-related hospitalizations for older adults are the result of falls.

• The rate of fall-related injuries among Canadians older than 65 years of age is nine times as great as among those younger than 65 years of age.

• Some 40% of admissions to nursing homes occur as a result of falls by older adults.

• Falls cause more than 90% of hip fractures in older adults; 20% of these older adults die within a year of the fracture.

In Canada, women typically sustain more injuries from falls and have higher rates of fall-related hospitalizations. Older women are also at greater risk than older men for breaking a bone as a result

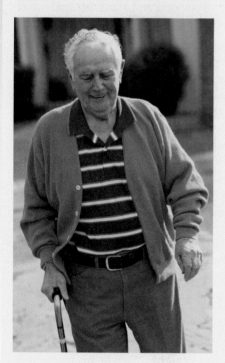

of a fall, in part because of lower bone density after menopause and higher rates of osteoporosis.

Among older Canadians, fall-related injuries not only threaten health, independence, and quality of life but can also lead to institutionalization and even death. Even if a fall does not result in an injury, it can result in fear, as well as a reduction in daily activities (such as regular exercise), both of which can negatively affect health and function and increase the risk for future falls.

Preventing Fall-Related Injuries

Although it is obvious that preventing falls and fall-related injuries is essential for older adults to remain active, healthy, and independent, it is not as easy as telling people to be careful. Fall-related risk factors are numerous and complex, and they typically interact on a number of levels, including biological and medical, behavioural, environmental, and socioeconomic:

• *Biological and medical risk factors* include age, physical disability, muscle weakness, poor fitness levels, and the presence of diseases, such as heart disease, osteoporosis, diabetes, and arthritis.

• *Behavioural risk factors* include risky behaviours (such as climbing up an insecure ladder), the use of multiple medications, and inadequate diet and exercise.

• *Environmental risk factors* include home hazards, such as poorly placed furniture. Almost half of all falls among older adults occur at home in the bathroom and on the stairs. Outside the home, environmental risk factors can include potholes in sidewalks and roads and poor lighting. Institutional hazards can include poorly designed buildings and noncompliance with safety and building standards, codes, or regulations.

• *Socioeconomic risk factors* include low income levels, which may affect an older adult's access to safe housing and appro-

priate health and social services. Additionally, food security issues can affect nutritional status and increase the susceptibility to falls and fall-related injuries.

Costs and Savings Associated with Falls

Fall-related injuries among older Canadians have been estimated to cost $2.8 billion a year for expenses related to hospitalization, medication, and treatment and rehabilitation. The Public Health Agency of Canada has estimated that a 20% reduction in falls could result in 7500 fewer hospitalizations and 1800 fewer older Canadians with permanent disabilities. These decreases would result in a savings of approximately $138 million annually.

Promising Practices

A number of prevention strategies have been shown to be effective in reducing falls and fall-related injuries among older adults in home, community, and institutional settings. These include regular physical activity, routine medical assessments and physician visits, healthy eating, appropriate home and environment modifications, proper footwear, and information about falls prevention being given to older adults. To reduce or eliminate the burden of fall-related injuries among older Canadians, additional research is needed to identify the effectiveness (including the cost effectiveness) of specific falls-prevention interventions alone and in combination.

Sources: Public Health Agency of Canada. 2006. *Healthy Aging in Canada: A New Vision, A Vital Investment, from Evidence to Action* (http://www.phac-aspc.gc.ca/seniors-aines/alt-formats/pdf/publications/pro/healthy-sante/haging_newvision/vision-rpt_e.pdf; retrieved February 18, 2011); Public Health Agency of Canada. 2005. *Report on Seniors' Falls in Canada* (http://www.phac-aspc.gc.ca/seniors-aines/alt-formats/pdf/publications/pro/injury-blessure/seniors_falls/seniors-falls_e.pdf; retrieved February 18, 2011).

through exercise, cutting calorie intake, or a combination of both will work for most people who want to lose weight, but there is no magic formula. Obesity is not physically healthy, and it leads to premature aging (see Chapter 4). Rising rates of obesity can be seen among Canadians of all ages, including older adults. According to Statistics Canada, the incidence of obesity among Canadians ages 75 or older increased from 11% in the late 1970s to 24% in 2004; among those ages 65–74, it increased from 20% to 25%.

Control Drinking and Overdependence on Medications
Alcohol abuse ranks with depression as a commonly hidden health problem, affecting 6%–10% of older adults. (The ability to metabolize alcohol decreases with age.) The problem is often not identified because the effects of alcohol or drug dependence can mimic disease, such as Alzheimer's disease. Signs of potential alcohol or drug dependence include unexplained falls or frequent injuries, forgetfulness, depression, and malnutrition. Older people who retire or lose a spouse are especially at risk. Problems can be avoided by not using alcohol to relieve anxiety or emotional pain and not taking medication when safer forms of treatment are available.

Don't Smoke The average pack-a-day smoker can expect to live about 13–14 years less than a nonsmoker. Furthermore, smokers suffer more illnesses that last longer, and they are subject to respiratory disabilities that limit their total vigour for many years before their death. Premature balding, skin wrinkling, and osteoporosis have been linked to cigarette smoking. Smokers at age 50 often look 10 years older.

Schedule Physical Examinations to Detect Treatable Diseases
When detected early, many diseases, including hypertension, diabetes, and many types of cancer, can be successfully controlled by medication and lifestyle changes. Regular testing for **glaucoma** after age 40 can prevent blindness from this eye disease. Recommended immunizations, including those for influenza, can protect you from preventable infectious diseases. (See Chapters 4 and 7–9 for screening and immunization guidelines.)

Recognize and Reduce Stress Stress-induced physiological changes increase wear and tear on your body. Cut down on the stresses in your life. Don't wear yourself out through lack of sleep, substance abuse or misuse, or overwork. Practise relaxation, using the techniques described in Chapter 3. If you contract a disease, consider it your body's attempt to interrupt your life pattern; reevaluate your lifestyle, and perhaps slow down.

The health behaviours you practise *now* are more influential in determining how long and how well you will live than your behaviours at a later age. Retiring from your life's occupation with a physically healthy body will allow far more options for enjoying yourself than will retiring with frail health or disabilities. Preventable poor health drains finances, emotions, and energy and contributes to poor psychological health. By enhancing your wellness today, you're ensuring some wellness for the future.

DEALING WITH THE CHANGES OF AGING

The changes that occur with aging have repercussions that must be grappled with and resolved. Just as you can act now to prevent or limit the physical changes of aging, you can also begin preparing yourself psychologically, socially, and financially for changes that may occur later in life. If you have aging parents, grandparents, and friends, the following information may give you insight into their lives and encourage you to begin cultivating appropriate and useful behaviours now.

Planning for Social Changes

Retirement marks a major change in the second half of life. As Canadians' longevity has increased, people have begun spending a larger proportion of their lives—an average of 20 years or more if they retire at age 65—in retirement. This has implications for reestablishing important relationships, developing satisfying interests outside work, and saving for an adequate retirement income. People who have well-developed leisure pursuits adjust better to retirement than those with few interests outside work.

Changing Roles and Relationships   Changes in social roles are a major feature of middle age. Children become young adults and leave home, putting an end to daily parenting. Parents experiencing this empty-nest syndrome must adapt to changes in their customary responsibilities and personal identities. And although retirement may be a desirable milestone for most people, it may also be viewed as a threat to prestige, purpose, and self-respect—the loss of a valued or customary role—and will probably require some adjustment.

Retirement and the end of child rearing also bring about changes in the relationship between marriage partners. The amount of time a couple spends together will increase and activities will change. Couples may need a period of adjustment, in which they get to know each other as individuals again. Discussing what types of activities each partner enjoys can help couples set up a mutually satisfying routine of shared and independent activities.

Increased Leisure Time   Although retirement confers the advantages of leisure time and freedom from deadlines, competition, and stress, many people do not know how to enjoy their free time. If you have developed diverse interests, retirement can be a joyful and fulfilling period of your life. It can provide opportunities for expanding your horizons by giving you the chance to try new activities, take classes, and meet new people. Volunteering in your community can enhance self-esteem and allow you to be a contributing member of society (see the box "Help Yourself by Helping Others").

The Economics of Retirement   Retirement is usually accompanied by a new economic situation. It may mean a severely restricted budget or possibly even financial disaster if you don't take stock of your finances and plan ahead. The majority of older Canadians live with fixed sources of income, such as pensions. In fact, in 2005, the OAS program and CPP made up roughly 44% of older adults' total incomes. It is vital to plan for an adequate retirement income, and this financial planning should begin early in life. People in their twenties and thirties should estimate how much money they need to support their standard of living, calculate their projected income, and begin a savings program. The earlier people begin such a program, the more money they will have at retirement.

> QUICK STATS
>
> In 2006, the median income for Canadians ages 65 and older was **$20,800**.
>
> —National Seniors Council, 2009

Adapting to Physical Changes

As described earlier in the chapter, people can do many things to avoid or minimize the effects of the physical

The retirement years can be the best part of life, socially, with increased opportunities to meet and interact with new and different people.

changes associated with aging. But although some age-related changes in physical functioning are preventable, others are inevitable, and successful aging involves anticipating and accommodating all of these changes.

Menopause   The natural—and inevitable—process of menopause usually occurs during a woman's forties or fifties. The ovaries gradually stop functioning, estrogen levels drop, and eventually menstruation ceases. Several years before a woman stops menstruating, her periods usually become irregular, and she may experience hot flashes, vaginal dryness, sleep disturbances, and mood swings. This time, called *perimenopause*, can be troublesome for many women.

During the 1990s, about one-third of menopausal women used hormone therapy (HT) to alleviate the symptoms of menopause and possibly prevent chronic diseases, such as cardiovascular disease (CVD) and osteoporosis. Many experts believed that HT would substantially reduce a woman's risk for CVD because estrogen has a favourable influence on blood lipids and overall cardiovascular health. The benefits of HT came into serious question, however, when a large-scale HT study (part of the Women's

Help Yourself by Helping Others

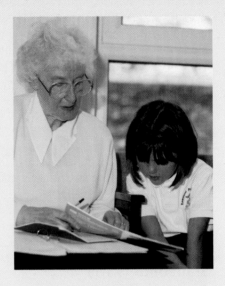

Choosing to help others—whether as a volunteer for a community organization or through spontaneous acts of kindness— can enhance emotional, social, spiritual, and physical wellness. Surveys and studies indicate that the sense of purpose and service and the feelings of generosity and kindness that go with helping others may be as important a consideration for wellness as good nutrition and regular exercise. Volunteer activities result in many of the same benefits as regular exercise, such as increased energy and vitality. Older adults who volunteer have higher levels of emotional and social wellness and lower rates of death.

In a survey of volunteers from all fields, helpers reported the following benefits:

• Helper's high—physical and emotional sensations, such as sudden warmth, a surge of energy, and a feeling of euphoria that occur immediately after helping

• Feelings of increased self-worth, calm, and relaxation

• A perception of greater physical health

• Fewer colds and headaches, improved eating and sleeping habits, and some relief from the pain of chronic diseases, such as asthma and arthritis

Just how might helping benefit the health of the helper? By helping others, we focus on things other than our own problems, and we get a special kind of attention from the people we help. Helping others can be effective at banishing a bad mood or a case of the blues. Helping others can also expand our perspective and enhance our appreciation for our own lives. Helping may benefit physical health by providing a temporary boost to the immune system and by combating stress and hostile feelings linked to the development of chronic diseases.

Helping others doesn't require a huge time commitment or a change of career. To get the most out of helping, keep the following guidelines in mind:

• *Make contact.* Choose an activity that involves personal contact.

• *Help as often as possible.* If your schedule allows, volunteer at least once a week. Any amount of time helping is better than none.

• *Make helping voluntary.* Voluntary helping has positive results, whereas obligatory helping situations can actually increase stress.

• *Volunteer with others.* Working with a group enables you to form bonds with other helpers who can support your interests and efforts. The health benefits of volunteering are strongest for people who otherwise have low levels of social interaction.

• *Focus on the process, not the outcome.* We can't always measure or know the results of our actions.

• *Practise random acts of kindness.* Smile, let people go ahead of you in line, pick up litter, and so on.

• *Adopt a pet.* Several studies suggest that pet owners enjoy better health, perhaps by feeling needed or by having a source of unconditional love and affection.

• *Avoid burnout.* Recognize your own limits, pace yourself, and try not to feel guilty or discouraged. Take pride in being a volunteer or caregiver.

Health Initiative) was halted in 2002, after a significant number of participants developed cardiovascular problems. This decision led many physicians to stop recommending HT for menopausal women. Newer data, however, are reopening the debate about HT. For example, a 2006 study published in the *Journal of Women's Health* reported that women who started HT near the beginning of menopause had a significantly lower risk of heart disease than women who did not take hormones. No benefit was found for women who started HT at older ages. Thus, age and the number of years a woman has been in menopause before starting therapy may be key considerations. A 2009 report released by the Society of Obstetricians and Gynaecologists of Canada (SOGC) reiterated that because of an increased risk of cardiac problems, health professionals should exercise caution when starting HT for women who have existing risk factors for CVD and who are more than a decade after menopause. Currently, the Heart and Stroke Foundation of Canada recommends that women do not use HT for the sole purpose of preventing heart disease or stroke.

Perhaps one of the greatest concerns related to the use of HT is the association between duration of use and breast cancer risk. Research has shown that women who have used HT for more than five years face an increased risk of breast cancer. According to the SOGC, this increased risk is similar to (or less than) that associated with other risk factors for breast cancer, including early puberty, late menopause, being older than 30 at the time of first pregnancy, not breastfeeding, being overweight, failing to exercise regularly, and consuming excessive amounts of alcohol. Research has also shown that the risk of breast cancer returns to normal levels after a woman stops using HT.

Researchers are studying variations in the timing, duration, and composition of HT to see if these changes will improve its effects on health. HT is effective for controlling severe menopausal symptoms, and it has been shown to reduce the risk of bone fractures and colon cancer. It may also be associated with a small increase in the risk of ovarian cancer. Decisions about HT should be made by individual women in consultation with their physicians, taking into account their overall health. The SOGC recommends that physicians prescribe HT at the lowest dose and for the shortest duration necessary to treat moderate to severe menopause symptoms.

Drugs called selective estrogen-receptor modulators (SERMs) mimic estrogen's effects on some body tissues while blocking its effects on others. Researchers hope to develop SERMs that provide estrogen's beneficial effects without the risks associated with HT. Phytoestrogens, plant-based substances similar to estrogen, may provide the protective effects of estrogen without its drawbacks. Black cohosh and vitamin E are also being studied.

Lifestyle strategies to reduce or manage menopause-related problems include many of the healthy habits discussed throughout the text: stop smoking, exercise, eat a healthy diet, lose excess weight, and perform relaxation techniques regularly.

Hearing Loss   Although not inevitable, the loss of hearing is a common physical change that can have a particularly strong effect on the lives of older adults. Some people lose their hearing slowly as they age—a condition known as *presbycusis*. Hearing loss affects a person's ability to interact with others and can lead to depression and a sense of isolation. Hearing loss should be assessed and treated by a health care professional; in some cases, hearing can be completely restored by dealing with the underlying cause of hearing loss. In other cases, hearing aids may be prescribed.

Protect your hearing by avoiding exposure to noises above 90 decibels, such as lawn mowers, motorcycles, gun shots, and loud music (Chapter 21). Wear ear plugs when you must be around loud noises, limit your time of exposure, and stay as far as possible from the sound's source.

Vision Changes   Vision usually declines with age. For some individuals this can be traced to physical conditions, such as glaucoma or **age-related macular degeneration (AMD)**, that can be treated medically. For others, the effects of a decline in vision can be managed by using strategies to make the most of remaining vision.

Glaucoma is caused by increased pressure within the eye cause by a buildup of fluid. The optic nerve can be damaged by this increased pressure, resulting in a loss of side vision and, if untreated, blindness. Medication can relieve the pressure by decreasing the amount of fluid produced or by helping it drain more efficiently. Laser and conventional surgery are other options. Glaucoma affects approximately 1 in 100 Canadians over the age of 40; because it often has no symptoms, however, it is estimated that only half of all individuals with glaucoma know that they have it. Old age, nearsightedness, being of African or Hispanic descent, and having a family history of glaucoma are some of the known risk factors for this disease.

AMD is a slow disintegration of the *macula*, the tissue at the centre of the retina where fine, straight-ahead detail is distinguished. AMD affects approximately 1 million Canadians—more than breast cancer, prostate cancer, Parkinson's disease, or Alzheimer's disease combined—and is the leading cause of vision loss in Canada. Losing this vision makes it difficult to read, drive, or perform other close-up activities. Risk factors for AMD are age, gender (women may be at higher risk than men), smoking, elevated cholesterol levels, and family history. Some cases of AMD can be treated with laser surgery. Both glaucoma and AMD can be detected with regular screening.

Vision can also be affected by conditions that are products of aging. By the time they reach their forties, many people have developed **presbyopia**, a gradual decline in the ability to focus on objects close to them. This occurs because the lens of the eye no longer expands and contracts as readily. **Cataracts**, a clouding of the lens caused by lifelong oxidation damage (a by-product of normal body chemistry), may dim vision by the sixties.

Arthritis   Approximately 4 million Canadian adults are estimated to have some form of **arthritis**. This degenerative disease causes joint inflammation leading to chronic pain, swelling, and loss of mobility. Its warning signs include swelling, pain, redness, warmth, tenderness, changes in joint mobility, early-morning stiffness, and unexplained weight loss, fever, or weakness in combination with joint pain.

There are more than 100 different types of arthritis; osteoarthritis (OA) is by far the most common. (Rheumatoid arthritis, an autoimmune disorder, is described in

Age-related macular degeneration (AMD) makes many daily tasks difficult or impossible. This photo shows how things look to someone with AMD.

Chapter 9.) In a person with OA, the cartilage that caps the bones in joints wears away, forming sharp spurs (Figure 17.4). It most often affects the hands and weight-bearing joints of the body—knees, ankles, and hips.

Strategies for reducing the risk of arthritis and, for those who already have OA, for managing it, include exercise, weight management, and avoidance of heavy or repetitive muscle use. Exercise lubricates joints and strengthens the muscles around them, protecting them from further damage. Swimming, walking, and tai chi are good low-impact exercises; knitting and crocheting are excellent for the hands. Maintaining an appropriate weight is important to avoid placing stress on the hips, knees, and ankles. Assistive devices, such as kitchen utensils and repair tools with large handles, can also help.

It is also important to visit a physician as soon as arthritis symptoms occur so appropriate treatment can be started to reduce pain and swelling, keep joints moving safely, and prevent further joint damage. If joints are severely damaged and activity is limited, surgery to repair or replace joints may be considered, but medication is usually the first treatment. Many people with OA take medication to relieve inflammation and reduce pain. A number of medications are used to treat arthritis in Canada. These include pain medications, such as acetaminophen, nonsteroidal anti-inflammatory drugs (NSAIDs), corticosteroids, and disease-modifying anti-rheumatic drugs (DMARDs). The newest class of medications used to treat arthritis are biologic response modifiers ("biologics"), which help to reduce inflammation and joint damage. Additionally, new and innovative medications for individuals with OA are being developed and will be offered in the future.

Osteoporosis   As described in Chapter 5, osteoporosis is a condition in which bones become dangerously thin and fragile over time. Fractures are the most serious consequence of osteoporosis; up to 20% of all people who suffer a hip fracture die within a year. Other problems associated with osteoporosis are loss of height and a stooped posture caused by vertebral fractures, severe back and hip pain, and breathing problems caused by changes in the shape of the skeleton.

Osteoporosis affects about 2 million Canadians; one in four women and at least one in eight men over the age of 50 are living with osteoporosis. Women are at greater risk than men for osteoporosis because they have 10%–25% less bone in their skeleton. As they lose bone mass with age, women's bones become dangerously thin sooner than men's bones (although more men will probably develop osteoporosis in the future as they live into their eighties and nineties). Bone loss accelerates in women during the first 5–10 years after the onset of menopause because of the drop in estrogen production. (Estrogen improves calcium absorption and reduces the amount of calcium the body excretes.) Although black women have higher bone density and fewer fractures than white or Asian women, they are still at significant risk of developing osteoporosis; this may be due, in part, to a vitamin D deficiency (caused by high levels of melatonin). Other risk factors include a family history of osteoporosis, early menopause (before age 45), abnormal or irregular menstruation, a history of anorexia, and a thin, small

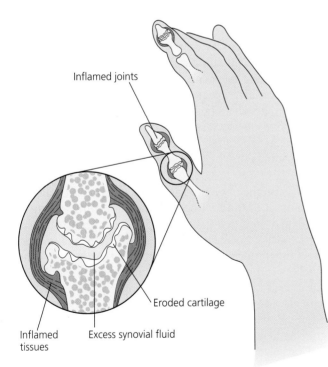

Inflamed joints

Eroded cartilage

Inflamed tissues

Excess synovial fluid

FIGURE 17.4   Osteoarthritis. When cartilage wears away within a joint, sharp spurs form and the amount of fluid increases, causing pain and swelling.

Source: Clayman, C. (ed.). 1995. *The Human Body: An Illustrated Guide to Its Structure, Function, and Disorders.* New York: DK.

TERMS

age-related macular degeneration (AMD)   A deterioration of the macula (the central areas of the retina) that leads to blurred vision and sensitivity to glare; some cases can lead to blindness.

presbyopia   The inability of the eyes to focus sharply on nearby objects, caused by the loss of elasticity of the lens that occurs with advancing age.

cataracts   Opacity of the lens of the eye that impairs vision and can cause blindness.

arthritis   Inflammation of a joint or joints, causing pain and swelling.

frame. Thyroid medication, corticosteroid drugs for arthritis or asthma, and long-term use of certain contraceptives can also have a negative effect on bone mass.

Preventing osteoporosis requires building as much bone as possible when you are young and then maintaining it as you age. Diet and exercise play key roles. Weight-bearing aerobic activities must be performed regularly throughout life to have lasting effects. Strength training improves bone density, muscle mass, strength, and balance, protecting against both bone loss and falls, a major cause of fractures. Even for people in their seventies, low-intensity strength training has been shown to improve bone density.

Two other lifelong strategies for reducing the effects of osteoporosis are avoiding tobacco use and managing depression and stress. Smoking reduces the body's estrogen levels and is linked to earlier menopause and more rapid postmenopausal bone loss. Some women with depression experience significant bone loss. Researchers have not identified the reason, but it may be linked to increases in the stress hormone cortisol.

Bone mineral density testing is the most accurate diagnostic test for osteoporosis and can be used to gauge an individual's risk of fracture and help determine if treatment is needed. Below-normal bone density may be classified as *osteopenia*, which is usually treated with exercise and nutrition. A greater loss of bone mass is classified as full-blown osteoporosis and is often treated with medications.

Handling Psychological and Mental Changes

Many people associate old age with forgetfulness, and slowly losing your memory was once considered an inevitable part of growing old. However, we now know that most older adults in good health remain mentally alert and retain their full capacity to learn and remember new information. Occasional confusion or forgetfulness may indicate only a temporary information overload, fatigue, or response to medications. Many people become more intelligent as they become older and more experienced.

Dementia A syndrome consisting of a wide range of symptoms, including loss of memory, judgment and reasoning, and changes in mood and behaviour, **dementia** affects about 1.5% of Canadians. In fact, it has been estimated that 1 in 11 Canadians over the age of 65 has some form of dementia. Early symptoms include slight disturbances in a person's ability to grasp the situation he or she is in. As dementia progresses, memory failure becomes apparent, and the person may forget conversations, the events of the day, or how to perform simple tasks. It is important to have any symptoms evaluated by a health care professional because some of the more than 50 known causes of dementia are treatable (for example, depression, dehydration, malnutrition, vitamin B12 deficiency, alcoholism, and misuse of medications).

The two most common forms of dementia among older people—**Alzheimer's disease** and multi-infarct dementia—are irreversible. Alzheimer's disease is characterized by changes in brain nerve cells. Multi-infarct dementia results from a series of small strokes or changes in the brain's blood supply that destroy brain tissue. Even for the incurable forms of dementia, however, treatment can improve an affected person's quality of life (see the box "Alzheimer's Disease").

Evidence suggests that some cases of dementia are hereditary, but experts say genetics are not always a sure sign that a person will develop the disease. You can also take lifestyle steps to help ward off dementia, such as controlling weight and blood pressure, eating a balanced diet (including adequate B vitamins and omega-3 fatty acids), exercising, practising stress reduction techniques, maintaining social contacts, and cultivating a variety of mental pursuits, such as doing crossword puzzles. Strong evidence links the Mediterranean diet with reduced risk of Alzheimer's disease.

Grief Another psychological and emotional challenge of aging is dealing with grief and mourning. Aging is associated with loss—the loss of friends, peers, physical appearance, possessions, and health. Grief is the process of getting through the pain of loss, and it can be one of the loneliest and most intense times in a person's life. It can take a year or two or more to completely come to terms with the loss of a loved one. (See Chapter 18 for more information about responses to loss and how to support a grieving person.)

Unresolved grief can have serious physical and psychological or emotional health consequences and may require professional help. Signs of unresolved grief include hostility toward people connected with the death (physicians or nurses, for example), talking about the death as if it

Alzheimer's Disease

IN FOCUS

Alzheimer's disease (AD) is a fatal brain disorder that causes physical and chemical changes in the brain. As the brain's nerve cells are destroyed, the system that produces the neurotransmitter acetylcholine breaks down, and communication among parts of the brain deteriorates. Autopsies reveal that the interiors of the affected neurons are filled with clusters of proteins known as *tangles*: the spaces between the neurons are filled with protein deposits called *amyloid plaques*.

Approximately half a million Canadians have Alzheimer's disease or a related dementia, and that number is expected to more than double in the next 25 years, as more people live into their eighties and nineties. AD usually occurs in people over 60 but can occur in people as young as 40.

Symptoms

The first symptoms of AD are forgetfulness and inability to concentrate. A person may have difficulty performing familiar tasks at home and work and have problems with abstract thinking. As the disease progresses, people experience severe memory loss, especially for

recent events. They may vividly remember events from their childhood but be unable to remember the time of day or their location. Depression and anxiety are also common.

In the later stages, people with AD are disoriented and may even hallucinate; some experience personality changes—becoming very aggressive or very docile. Eventually, they lose control of physical functioning and are completely dependent on caregivers. On average, a person will survive eight years after the development of the first symptoms.

Causes

Scientists do not yet know what causes Alzheimer's disease. Age is the main risk factor, although about 10% of cases seem tied to inherited gene mutations. Inherited familial AD generally strikes people before age 65, while the more common late-onset AD occurs in people 65 and older. Some evidence suggests that many of the same factors that affect heart disease risk also apply to AD. In women, low levels of estrogen in the brain may contribute to AD. A mutation of the protein apolipoprotein E, which can destroy neural cells, may be a cause of the disease in some people.

A great deal of research is focusing on the role of a peptide molecule known as amyloid-beta, which may play a role in the development of plaques in the brain. Scientists are looking for genetic factors that cause certain people to develop high levels of amyloid-beta. Some evidence links excess amyloid-beta production to obesity.

People who regularly take nonsteroidal anti-inflammatory drugs (NSAIDs) like ibuprofen (often to control arthritis) and people who regularly consume fish rich in omega-3 fatty acids appear to have lower rates of AD, indicating a possible protective effect of substances that reduce inflammation. Some studies indicate that vitamin E and other antioxidants may reduce risk for AD or slow

the progress of the disease, suggesting that oxidative stress caused by free radicals may also play a role.

Diagnosis and Treatment

Currently, the only certain way to diagnose AD is to examine brain tissue during an autopsy. In most cases, physicians use a combination of medical history, neurological and psychological tests, physical exams, blood and urine tests, and a brain-imaging scan. Good early results have also been seen by using a test that measures levels of a specific protein in spinal fluid; less invasive blood tests to measure the same proteins are under development.

For people with mild to moderate AD, several drugs can provide modest improvements in memory. Some medications help maintain cognitive function by inhibiting the breakdown of the neurotransmitter acetylcholine but do not alter the course of the disease. Thecholinesterase inhibitors include Aricept (donepezil), Exelon (rivastigmine), and Reminyl (galantamine). Another medication called Ebixa (memantine hydrochloride) has been conditionally approved by Health Canada for people with moderate to advanced AD, pending the results of more studies to verify its effectiveness.

Scientists are also developing new treatments to slow the production of amyloid-beta or to block its effects on brain cells. Other medicines now under investigation may stop Alzheimer's progress before it can cause too much damage. People with AD may also be prescribed antidepressant or antianxiety medications.

Sources: Alzheimer Society of Canada. 2009. *Ebixa (Also Known as Memantine Hydrochloride)* (http://www.alzheimer.ca/english/treatment/treatments-ebixa.htm#drugapproval; April 30, 2011); Alzheimer Society of Canada. 2010. *Key Facts About Alzheimer's Disease and Related Dementia* (http://www.alzheimer.ca/english/disease/stats-intro.htm; April 30, 2011).

Suicide Among Older Canadians

One group of Canadians is more likely to commit suicide than any other. From mass media accounts, you might imagine this group to be adolescents; according to Health Canada, however, men over the age of 80 have the highest suicide rate among Canadians.

Why is this so? One possible explanation is that because men generally have greater power and status in our society, aging and retirement represent a relatively greater loss for them. Older women, perhaps more accustomed to lesser status, may not be as threatened by the loss of economic and social power. Another theory is that men tend to have weaker social ties than women, and as they retire their increasing social isolation leads to depression and suicide. Indeed, depression is probably the single most significant factor associated with suicidal behaviour in older adults. Men who commit suicide are more likely to have a physical illness and be widowed or divorced.

Although Canadian women are more likely than men to attempt suicide, the rates are equal at 70 years of age and beyond, at which point more men than women are hospitalized for suicide attempts.

In contrast to younger Canadians, suicidal attempts among older adults—both male and female—are more likely to result in completed suicides. This may be because older adults choose more lethal methods to end their lives, and they are also more likely to be physically frail and thus not able to recover from self-inflicted injury. Social isolation also contributes to the increased likelihood of death among older adults by reducing the chance that they will be found by others in the time needed to receive medical attention.

See Chapter 2 for more on risk and protective factors for suicide.

Source: Canadian Mental Health Association, Ontario. n.d. *Seniors and Suicide* (http://www.ontario.cmha.ca/seniors.asp?cID=6336; retrieved April 30, 2011).

occurred yesterday, and unrealistic or harmful behaviour (such as giving away all of one's own belongings). Many people become depressed after the loss of a loved one or when confronted with retirement or a chronic illness. But after a period of grieving, people are generally able to resume their lives.

Depression   Unresolved grief can lead to depression, a common problem in older adults (see Chapter 2). If you notice the signs of depression in yourself or someone you know, consult a mental health professional. A marked loss of interest in usually pleasurable activities, decreased appetite, insomnia, fatigue, and feelings of worthlessness are signs of depression. Listen carefully when an older friend or relative complains about being depressed; it may be a request for help. Suicide rates are relatively high among older adults, and depression should be taken seriously (see the box "Suicide Among Older Canadians," above).

Changes in the Public's View of Aging

Aging people may be one of our least used and least appreciated resources. (For another view, see the box "Aboriginal Seniors in Canada: The Role of the Elder.") How can we use the knowledge and productivity of our growing numbers of older citizens, particularly those who are retiring early?

To start, we must change our thinking about what aging means. We must learn to judge productivity rather than age. Capacity to function should replace age as a criterion for usefulness. An example of this is the recent abolishment of mandatory retirement in many jobs across most of Canada, allowing Canadians to work beyond the age of 65. Instead of singling out 65 as a magic number, we are now starting to consider ages 50–75 as the third quarter of life. Changes occur around 50 that signal a new era: Children are usually grown and gone, and a person has often achieved a level in career, earnings, and accomplishments that meets his or her ambitions. The upper end of the quarter is determined by the fact that most people today are vigorous, in good health, mentally alert, and capable of making a productive contribution until they are at least in their seventies.

Aging can have benefits, but they don't come automatically. They require planning and wise choices earlier in life. One octogenarian, Russell Lee, founder of a medical clinic in California, perceived the advantages of aging as growth: "The limitations imposed by time are compensated by the improved taste, sharper discretion, sounder mental and aesthetic judgment, increased sensitivity and compassion, clearer focus—which all contribute to a more certain direction in living…. The later years can be the best of life for which the earlier ones were preparation."

Aboriginal Seniors in Canada: The Role of the Elder

The ancient wisdom, the traditions, rituals, languages and cultural values were passed on and carried forward. In this process, a primary role was played by the Elders, the Old Ones, the Grandmothers and Grandfathers. As individuals especially knowledgeable and experienced in the culture, they were seen as those most closely in touch with the philosophical teachings of life lived in harmony with the Creator and creation.

—Royal Commission on Aboriginal Peoples, 1996

Older adults are revered in many Aboriginal cultures for their knowledge and experiences, and the integral role that they play in the vitality and well-being of their families, communities, and nations. Aboriginal people view Elders as key sources of traditional knowledge, wisdom, and cultural continuity. In a sense, Elders are experts on life. Their expertise may depend on the nature of their experience, but in one way or another it involves some aspect of traditional knowledge and culture or an interpretation of their experience in traditional terms. They must also be able to communicate that learning to others. Although age is part of being an Elder, it is not the only part. As one Ojibway traditional teacher described it, "Some people say that it isn't a matter of age, but to a certain extent it is when you have experienced enough of the stages

of life that you can look back and reflect on them.... Some people have been able to do it more completely than others. When you're 35, you're only about halfway, so you can't talk about all of life, not from experience."

Aboriginal seniors have lived through many changes in their communities, and they are often considered an important link to the teachings of the past. It is not surprising that many people recognized as Elders have lived through difficult times, both personally and politically. Some have had problems with the law, with alcohol, with family separation; some have seen such things happen to others. What they have in common is the fact that they learned something from those experiences, that they turned to the traditional culture for understanding, support and healing, and that they are committed to helping others, especially those of similar background.

It is clear that Aboriginal seniors play an important role in passing Aboriginal culture and languages on to the next generation. The 2001 *Aboriginal Peoples Survey* (APS) conducted by Statistics Canada revealed that about 1 in 10 Aboriginal children received help learning an Aboriginal language from community Elders. For many Aboriginal children, spending time with Elders on a regular basis has a beneficial outcome. An analysis of participation in extracurricular activities of Aboriginal children living

off-reserve revealed that although sports are the most popular extracurricular activities, time spent with Elders ranked second. The 2001 APS also found that about half (47%) of the Aboriginal children who spent time with Elders four times or more a week were reported to be doing very well in school. Among those who rarely or never spent time with Elders, 38% did very well.

In the Aboriginal community, an Elder is not a figurehead or a symbol but someone who is actively involved in the community. A primary role of the Elder is to express the best of tradition and to bring that tradition forward into current times. Although many definitions of an Elder exist, perhaps the most appropriate description is one that has been advanced by the Elders themselves: "We are helpers, that is the highest level we can be. We are part of the family."

Sources: Stiegelbauer, S. M. 1996. What is an Elder? What do Elders do? First Nations Elders as teachers in culture-based urban organizations. *Canadian Journal of Native Studies* 16(1): 37–66 (http://www2.brandonu.ca/library//CJNS/16.1/Stiegelbauer.pdf; retrieved May 26, 2010); Turcotte, M., and G. Schellenberg. 2007. *A Portrait of Seniors in Canada, 2006* (http://www.statcan.gc.ca/pub/89-519-x/89-519-x2006001-eng.pdf; retrieved May 26, 2010); Royal Commission on Aboriginal Peoples. 1996. *The Report of the Royal Commission on Aboriginal Peoples.* Ottawa: Minister of Supply and Services Canada.

QUESTIONS FOR CRITICAL THINKING AND REFLECTION

Have you watched someone you know grow old? How did the aging process affect that person? In what ways did the person's physical and mental health change? In what ways were you affected, as you watched him or her age?

McGraw Hill connect™

Practise and learn online with Connect. Connect allows you to practise important skills at your own pace and on your own schedule, with 24/7 online access to an eBook, practice quizzes, interactivities, videos, study tools, additional resources, and more.

SUMMARY

• People over 65 form a minority in Canada, but their status is improving. The proportion of older adults in Canada is expected to grow substantially over the next few decades, reaching nearly one in four Canadians in 2041.

• Family and community resources can help older adults stay active and independent.

• Government aid to older Canadians includes the Old Age Security pension, the Guaranteed Income Supplement, the Allowance and Allowance for the Survivor, the Canadian Pension Plan/Quebec Pension Plan, and tax deductions on Registered Pension Plans and Registered Retirement Savings Plans.

• Retirement can be a fulfilling and enjoyable time of life for those who adjust to their new roles, enjoy participating in a variety of activities, and have planned ahead for financial stability.

• People who take charge of their health during their youth have greater control over the physical and mental aspects of aging.

• Biological aging takes place over a lifetime, but some of the other changes associated with aging are more abrupt.

• A lifetime of interests and hobbies helps maintain creativity and intelligence.

• Exercise and a healthy diet throughout life enhance physical and psychological health.

• Alcohol abuse is a common but often hidden problem, as is overdependence on medications. Tobacco use not only shortens life but also may cause severe health impairment for many years.

• Regular physical examinations help detect conditions that can shorten life and make old age less healthy.

• Stress increases wear and tear on the body; getting enough sleep, avoiding drugs, and practising relaxation help reduce stress.

• Successful aging involves anticipating and accommodating physical changes and limitations.

• Slight confusion and forgetfulness are not signs of a serious illness; however, severe symptoms may indicate Alzheimer's disease or another form of dementia.

• Resolving grief and mourning and dealing with depression are important tasks for older adults.

• Older adults can be role models for the successful integration of life's experiences and the ability to adapt to challenges.

FOR MORE INFORMATION

BOOKS

Beers, M. H. 2005. *Merck Manual of Health and Aging: The Complete Home Guide to Healthcare and Healthy Aging for Older People and Those Who Care About Them.* New York: Ballantine. Provides information on the fundamentals of aging and preventive care.

Johns Hopkins Medical Center. 2007. *The Johns Hopkins Medical Guide to Health After 50.* New York: Black Dog & Leventhal. A practical guide to healthy aging for all wellness dimensions.

Lazarus, R. S., and B. N. Lazarus. 2006. *Coping with Aging.* New York: Oxford. Explores the experience of aging from the standpoint of the individual.

National Institute on Aging. 2006. *Fitness Over Fifty: An Exercise Guide from the National Institute on Aging,* book and DVD ed. New York: Hatherleigh Press. A practical guide to physical activity and exercise, with specific guidelines for safe exercise for older adults.

Weil, A. 2007. *Healthy Aging: A Lifelong Guide to Your Physical and Spiritual Well-Being.* New York: Anchor. One of America's best-known complementary care physicians discusses the aging process and explains methods for maintaining health during the latter years of life.

ORGANIZATIONS AND WEB SITES

The Internet addresses listed here were accurate at the time of publication.

Alliance for Aging Research. A nonprofit organization supporting medical and psychological research on aging.
  http://www.agingresearch.org

Alzheimer Society of Canada. Provides research and news, and offers tips for caregivers and patients on the causes and treatment of Alzheimer's disease and related dementias.
  http://www.alzheimer.ca

The Arthritis Society. Provides information about arthritis, programs and services, and research updates.

http://www.arthritis.ca

Canadian National Institute for the Blind. Provides information, resources, and research about eye conditions, care, and safety. Also provides vision support services and works to protect and promote the vision health of all Canadians.

http://www.cnib.ca

CARP. Provides information on all aspects of aging, including health promotion, health care, and retirement planning.

http://www.carp.ca

Menopauseandu.ca. Provides information about menopause symptoms and treatments.

http://www.menopauseandu.ca

Osteoporosis Canada. Provides information on the causes, prevention, detection, and treatment of osteoporosis.

http://www.osteoporosis.ca

Public Health Agency of Canada, Division of Aging and Seniors. Provides information on matters related to healthy aging, including the prevention and control of disease and injury among older Canadians.

http://www.publichealth.gc.ca/seniors

Seniors Canada (Government of Canada). Provides a wide range of information about resources and services for older adults and caregivers in Canada, including financial matters and health and wellness.

http://www.seniors.gc.ca

Society of Obstetricians and Gynaecologists of Canada. Provides information, research, and resources related to women's health issues and clinical practice guidelines.

http://www.sogc.org

SELECTED BIBLIOGRAPHY

Alzheimer Society of Canada. 2005. *Alzheimer's Disease: Related Dementias* (http://www.alzheimer.ca/english/disease/dementias-intro.htm; retrieved May 20, 2010).

Alzheimer Society of Canada. 2009. *Alzheimer Treatment: Drug Treatments* (http://www.alzheimer.ca/english/treatment/treatments-ebixa.htm#drugapproval; retrieved May 20, 2010).

Alzheimer Society of Canada. 2009. *Rising Tide: the Impact of Dementia on Canadian Society* (http://www.alzheimer.ca/docs/RisingTide/Rising%20Tide_Full%20Report_Eng_FINAL_Secured%20version.pdf; retrieved May 20, 2010).

Alzheimer Society of Canada. 2010. *Alzheimer's Disease: Statistics* (http://www.alzheimer.ca/english/disease/stats-intro.htm; retrieved May 20, 2010).

Anderson, K., et al. 2005. Depression and the risk of Alzheimer's disease. *Epidemiology* 16(2): 233–238.

Arnold, W. 2006. Singapore acts as haven for stem cell research. *New York Times,* 17 August.

Arthritis Society. 2004. *ArthroScope: Revealing the Impact of Arthritis on the Lives of Canadians* (http://www.arthritis.ca/local/files/resources%20for%20advocates/arthroscope/ArthroScope_English.pdf; retrieved May 28, 2010).

Buys, Y. M. 2008. World Glaucoma Day, March 6, 2008—What can you do? *Canadian Journal of Ophthalmology* 43: 1–3 (http://www.jgh.ca/uploads/PatientVisitor/international_glaucoma_day.pdf; retrieved May 18, 2010).

Canadian Institute for Health Information. 2010. *Nearly Two-Thirds of Seniors Using Five or More Types of Prescription Drugs* (http://www.cihi.ca/CIHI-ext-portal/internet/en/document/types+of+care/pharmaceutical/release_18mar2010; retrieved May 29, 2010).

Canadian Institutes of Health Research. 2007. *Updated Guidelines for Human Pluripotent Stem Cell Research, June 29, 2007* (http://www.cihr-irsc.gc.ca/e/34460.html; retrieved May 18, 2010).

Canadian Mental Health Association. n.d. *Seniors and Suicide* (http://www.ontario.cmha.ca/seniors.asp?cID=6336; retrieved May 19, 2010).

Canadian National Institute for the Blind. 2009. *Age-Related Macular Degeneration (AMD)* (http://www.cnib.ca/en/your-eyes/eye-conditions/amd/Default.aspx; retrieved May 20, 2010).

Canadian Ophthalmological Society. 2008. *Glaucoma* (http://www.eyesite.ca/english/public-information/eye-conditions/pdfs/Glaucoma_e.pdf; retrieved May 29, 2010).

Canadian Society for Exercise Physiology. 2011. *Canadian Physical Activity Guidelines for Older Adults—65 Years & Older* (http://www.csep.ca/CMFiles/Guidelines/CSEP-InfoSheets-older%20adults-ENG.pdf; May 1, 2011).

CBC News Canada. 2009. *Mandatory Retirement Fades in Canada* (http://www.cbc.ca/canada/story/2009/08/20/mandatory-retirement-explainer523.html; retrieved May 30, 2010).

Centre for Addiction and Mental Health. 2009. *Responding to Older Adults with Substance Use, Mental Health and Gambling Challenges* (http://www.camh.net/Publications/Resources_for_Professionals/Older_Adults/rtoa_alcohol_problems.html; retrieved May 30, 2010).

Cirillo, D., et al. 2005. Effect of estrogen therapy on gallbladder disease. *Journal of the American Medical Association* 293(3): 330–339.

Cushman, M., et al. 2004. Estrogen plus progestin and risk of venous thrombosis. *Journal of the American Medical Association* 292: 1573–1580.

Ettinger, B., et al. 2004. Effects of ultra-low-dose transdermal estradiol on bone mineral density: A randomized clinical trial. *Obstetrics and Gynecology* 104(3): 443–451.

Evans, M. L., et al. 2004. Management of postmenopausal hot flushes with venlafaxine hydrochloride: A randomized, controlled trial. *Obstetrics and Gynecology* 105(1): 161–166.

Federal, Provincial, and Territorial Ministers Responsible for Seniors. 2005. *Planning for Canada's Aging Population.* Ottawa: Division of Aging and Seniors, Public Health Agency of Canada.

Gilmour, H., and Park, J. 2005. Dependency, chronic conditions and pain in seniors. *Health Reports* (16 Suppl.) (http://www.statcan.gc.ca/pub/82-003-s/2005000/pdf/9087-eng.pdf; retrieved May 22, 2010).

Government of Canada. 2009. *Canada's Aging Population: Seizing the Opportunity, Special Senate Committee on Aging Final Report* (http://www.parl.gc.ca/40/2/parlbus/commbus/senate/com-e/agei-e/rep-e/AgingFinalReport-e.pdf; retrieved May 26, 2010).

Government of Canada. 2009. *Report of the National Seniors Council on Low Income Among Seniors* (http://www.seniorscouncil.gc.ca/eng/research_publications/low_income/2009/hs1_9/page05.shtml#base_2; retrieved May 26, 2010).

Harvard Medical School. 2006. Minding your mind: 12 ways to keep your brain young with proper care and feeding. *Harvard Men's Health Watch* 10(10): 1–4.

Health Canada. 2002. *A Report on Mental Illness in Canada* (http://www.phac-aspc.gc.ca/publicat/miic-mmac/pdf/men_ill_e.pdf; retrieved May 1, 2011).

Health Canada. 2003. *Arthritis in Canada: An Ongoing Challenge* (http://www.phac-aspc.gc.ca/publicat/ac/pdf/ac_e.pdf; retrieved May 25, 2010).

Health Canada. 2004. *Aboriginal Health* (http://www.hc-sc.gc.ca/hcs-sss/delivery-prestation/fptcollab/2004-fmm-rpm/fs-if_02-eng.php; retrieved May 24, 2010).

Health Canada. 2009. *Vitamin D: Recommendations and Review Status* (http://www.hc-sc.gc.ca/fn-an/nutrition/vitamin/vita-d-eng.php; retrieved May 19, 2010).

Heyn, P. C., et al. 2008. Endurance and strength training outcomes on cognitively impaired and cognitively intact older adults: A meta-analysis. *Journal of Nutrition, Health and Aging* 12(6): 401–409.

Jager, R. D., et al. 2008. Age-related macular degeneration. *New England Journal of Medicine* 258(24): 2606–2617.

Kado, D. M., et al. 2005. Homocysteine versus the vitamins folate, B6, and B12 as predictors of cognitive function and decline in older high-functioning adults: MacArthur Studies of Successful Aging. *American Journal of Medicine* 118(2): 161–167.

Kolata, G. 2006. Live long? Die young? Answer isn't just in genes. *New York Times,* 31 August.

Lanza, R., and N. Rosenthal. 2004. The stem cell challenge. *Scientific American,* June.

Mayo Clinic. 2005. Beyond menopause: Life after estrogen. *Mayo Clinic Health Letter Supplement,* February.

Mayo Clinic. 2006. Osteoporosis: Treatments for men and women. *Mayo Clinic Health Letter* 24(6): 4–5.

National Seniors Council. 2009. *Report of the National Seniors Council on Low Income Among Seniors* (http://www.seniorscouncil.gc.ca/eng/research_publications/low_income/2009/hs1_9/page01.shtml; retrieved May 20, 2010).

Mudge, A. M., et al. 2008. Exercising body and mind: An integrated approach to functional independence in hospitalized older people. *Journal of the American Geriatrics Society* 56(4): 630–635.

Nelson, H. D., et al. 2006. Nonhormonal therapies for menopausal hot flashes: Systematic review and meta-analysis. *Journal of the American Medical Association* 295(17): 2057–2071.

Ontario Ministry of Health and Long-Term Care. 2009. *Seniors' Care: Overview of Care Options* (http://www.health.gov.on.ca/english/public/program/ltc/3_overview.html; retrieved May 24, 2010).

Ontario Ministry of Transportation. 2010. *Senior Drivers in Ontario* (http://www.mto.gov.on.ca/english/dandv/driver/senior/index.shtml; retrieved May 30, 2010).

Osteoporosis Canada. 2010. *Calcium Requirements: How Much Calcium Do We Need?* (http://www.osteoporosis.ca/index.php/ci_id/5535/la_id/1.htm; retrieved May 20, 2010).

Osteoporosis Canada. 2010. *Facts and Statistics* (http://www.osteoporosis.ca/index.php/ci_id/8867/la_id/1.htm; retrieved May 20, 2010).

Public Health Agency of Canada. 2002. *Canada's Aging Population* (http://www.phac-aspc.gc.ca/seniors-aines/alt-formats/pdf/publications/public/various-variee/papier-fed-paper/fedpager_e.pdf; retrieved May 25, 2010).

Public Health Agency of Canada. 2003. *Arthritis in Canada: An Ongoing Challenge* (http://www.phac-aspc.gc.ca/publicat/ac/ac_3e-eng.php#fig2_5; retrieved May 28, 2010).

Public Health Agency of Canada. 2005. *Report on Seniors' Falls in Canada* (http://www.phac-aspc.gc.ca/seniors-aines/alt-formats/pdf/publications/pro/injury-blessure/seniors_falls/seniors-falls_e.pdf; retrieved February 18, 2011);

Public Health Agency of Canada. 2006. *Healthy Aging in Canada: A New Vision, A Vital Investment, From Evidence to Action* (http://www.phac-aspc.gc.ca/seniors-aines/alt-formats/pdf/publications/pro/healthy-sante/haging_newvision/vision-rpt_e.pdf; retrieved February 18, 2011)

Public Health Agency of Canada. 2010. *Life with Arthritis in Canada: A Personal and Public Health Challenge* (http://www.phac-aspc.gc.ca/cd-mc/arthritis-arthrite/lwaic-vaaac-10/9-eng.php#Int6; retrieved February 18, 2011).

RBC Royal Bank. 2010. *RBC Retirement Myths and Realities Poll, April 2010* (http://www.rbcroyalbank.com/redefine/index.html; retrieved May 22, 2010).

Rosengren, A., et al. 2005. Body mass index, other cardiovascular risk factors, and hospitalization for dementia. *Archives of Internal Medicine* 165(3): 321–326.

Scarmeas, N., et al. 2006. Mediterranean diet, Alzheimer disease, and vascular mediation. *Archives of Neurology* 63: 1709–1717.

Service Canada. 2010. *Canada Pension Plan* (http://www.servicecanada.gc.ca/eng/isp/pub/factsheets/retire.shtml#a1; retrieved May 28, 2010).

Service Canada. 2010. *Old Age Security (OAS) Payment Rates* (http://www.servicecanada.gc.ca/eng/isp/oas/oasrates.shtml#note; retrieved May 29, 2010).

Service Canada. 2010. *Overview of the Old Age Security Program* (http://www.servicecanada.gc.ca/eng/isp/oas/oasoverview.shtml; retrieved May 28, 2010).

Society of Obstetricians and Gynaecologists of Canada. n.d. *Menopause-andu.ca: Hormone Therapies* (http://www.menopauseandu.ca/therapies/hormone-therapies_e.aspx; retrieved May 25, 2010).

Society of Obstetricians and Gynaecologists of Canada. 2008. *Menopause-andu.ca: Hormone Therapy Fact Sheet* (http://www.menopauseandu.ca/factsheets/HT08.pdf; retrieved May 25, 2010).

Society of Obstetricians and Gynaecologists of Canada. 2009. Menopause and osteoporosis update 2009. *Journal of Obstetrics and Gynaecology Canada* 31(1 Suppl.) (http://www.sogc.org/media/pdf/advisories/Meno-Osteo-Update_JOGC-Jan_09.pdf; retrieved May 25, 2010).

Sorrell, J. M. 2008. As good as it gets? Rethinking old age. *Journal of Psychosocial Nursing and Mental Health Services* 46(5): 21–24.

Stiegelbauer, S. M. 1996. What is an Elder? What do Elders do? First Nations Elders as teachers in culture-based urban organizations. *Canadian Journal of Native Studies* 16(1): 37–66 (http://www2.brandonu.ca/library//CJNS/16.1/Stiegelbauer.pdf; retrieved May 26, 2010).

Statistics Canada. 2000. *Report on the Demographic Situation in Canada* (http://www.statcan.gc.ca/pub/91-209-x/91-209-x2000000-eng.pdf; retrieved May 19, 2010).

Statistics Canada. 2001. *2001 Census of Canada* (http://www.statcan.gc.ca/pub/89-519-x/89-519-x2006001-eng.pdf; retrieved May 26, 2010).

Statistics Canada. 2005. *Population Projections for Canada, Provinces and Territories: Highlights* (http://www.statcan.gc.ca/pub/91-520-x/00105/4095095-eng.htm; retrieved May 26, 2010).

Statistics Canada. 2006. *CANSIM Table 105-0422: Self-Rated Health, by Age Group and Sex, Household Population Aged 12 and Over, Canada, Provinces, Territories, Health Regions (June 2005 Boundaries) and Peer Groups, Every 2 Years* (http://www4.hrsdc.gc.ca/.3ndic.1t.4r@-eng.jsp?iid=10#M_3; retrieved May 19, 2010).

Statistics Canada. 2007. 2006 Census: Age and sex. *The Daily,* July 17 (http://www.statcan.gc.ca/daily-quotidien/070717/dq070717a-eng.htm; retrieved May 26, 2010).

Statistics Canada. 2007. A portrait of seniors. *The Daily,* February 27 (http://www.statcan.gc.ca/daily-quotidien/070227/dq070227b-eng.htm; retrieved May 25, 2010).

Statistics Canada. 2009. *Widowhood: Consequences on Income for Senior Women* (http://www.statcan.gc.ca/pub/11-621-m/11-621-m2004015-eng.htm; retrieved May 26, 2010).

Statistics Canada. 2010. Deaths, 2007. *The Daily,* February 23 (http://www.statcan.gc.ca/daily-quotidien/100223/dq100223a-eng.htm; retrieved May 19, 2010).

Statistics Canada. 2010. *Table 1: Life Expectancy at Birth and at Age 65 by Sex, Canada* (http://www.statcan.gc.ca/daily-quotidien/100223/t100223a1-eng.htm; retrieved May 19, 2010).

Suicide Information and Education Centre. 1998. *Suicide Among the Aged* (http://www.suicideinfo.ca/csp/assets/alert28.pdf; retrieved May 1, 2011).

Turcotte, M., and G. Schellenberg. 2007. *A Portrait of Seniors in Canada, 2006* (http://www.statcan.gc.ca/pub/89-519-x/89-519-x2006001-eng.pdf; retrieved May 26, 2010).

Tufts University. 2006. Pendulum swings on estrogen and women's heart health risk. *Tufts University Health & Nutrition Letter* 24(3): 1–2.

U.S. Department of Health and Human Services. 2004. *Bone Health and Osteoporosis: A Report of the Surgeon General.* Washington, D.C.: U.S. Department of Health and Human Services.

Ward, E. M. 2006. A weekly to-do list to help delay or prevent dementia. *Environmental Nutrition* 29(5): 2.

Welland, D. 2006. Keeping an eye on your diet may help save your sight. *Environmental Nutrition* 29(5): 1, 6.

Whitmer, R. A., et al. 2005. Midlife cardiovascular risk factors and risk of dementia in late life. *Neurology* 64(2): 277–281.

Wilson, R. S., et al. 2005. Proneness to psychological distress and risk of Alzheimer disease in a biracial community. *Neurology* 64(2): 380–382.

Wolfe, M. S. 2006. Shutting down Alzheimer's. *Scientific American* 294(5): 72–79.

World Health Organization. 2004. Glaucoma is second leading cause of blindness globally. *Bulletin of the World Health Organization* 82(11): 811–890 (http://www.who.int/bulletin/volumes/82/11/feature1104/en/; retrieved May 22, 2010).

Yaffe, K., et al. 2004. The metabolic syndrome, inflammation, and risk of cognitive decline. *Journal of the American Medical Association* 292(18): 2237–2242.

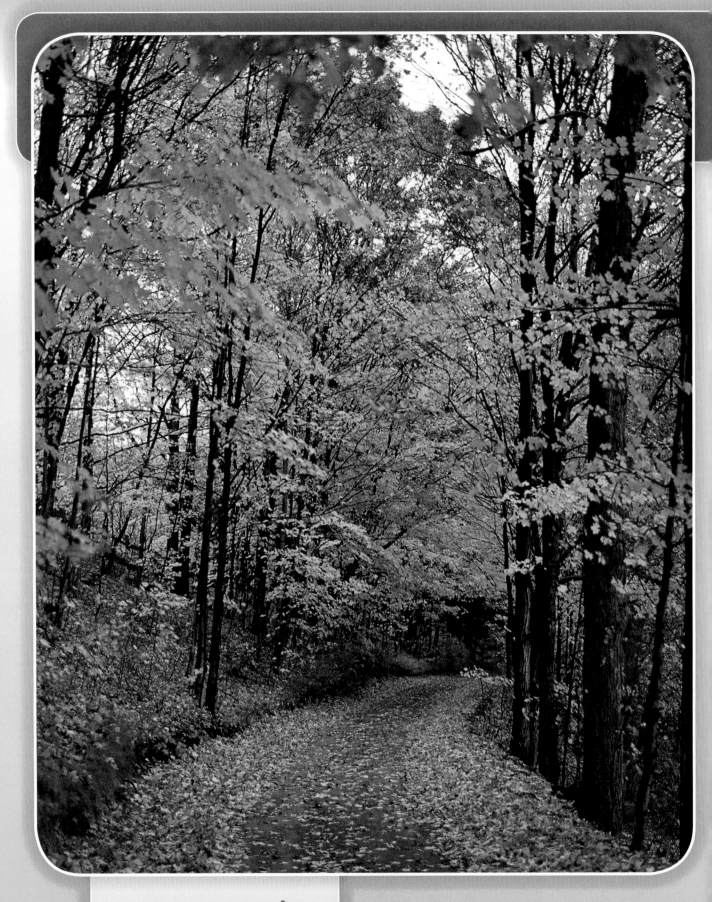

DYING AND DEATH

LOOKING AHEAD>>>>>

AFTER READING THIS CHAPTER, YOU SHOULD BE ABLE TO

- Identify the physical, mental, social, behavioural, and spiritual dimensions of dying and death

- Describe various ways of defining death and the components of a mature concept of death

- Understand personal considerations in preparing for death, including making a will, assessing choices for end-of-life care, and making arrangements for a funeral or memorial service

- Describe the experience of living with a life-threatening illness and list ways to support a person who is dying

- Explain the grieving process and how support can be offered to adults and children who have experienced a loss

TEST YOUR KNOWLEDGE

1. **More than half of Canadians die without leaving a will.**
   True or false?

2. **If you die in a car crash, your organs will automatically be donated to people waiting for transplants.**
   True or false?

3. **Approximately how many people are on the waiting list for an organ transplant in Canada?**
   a. 1000
   b. 4000
   c. 11,000

4. **Physician-assisted suicide is illegal in all provinces and territories in Canada.**
   True or false?

5. **The best way to help a friend who is grieving is to distract her or him from the loss by talking about sports, gossip, or other light topics.**
   True or false?

ANSWERS

1. **TRUE.** In such cases, the deceased person's estate is distributed according to provincial or territorial law, which may not reflect what the person would have wanted.

2. **FALSE.** For your organs to be donated, you must have authorized it before your death (for example, by completing an organ donor card), *and* the donation must be authorized by relatives at the time of your death.

3. **B.** In 2008, 4330 Canadians were on the waiting list for an organ transplant, and 215 people died while waiting for a needed organ. The number of patients waiting for organs is several times greater than the number of organs donated each year.

4. **TRUE.** The Criminal Code of Canada states that physician-assisted suicide (PAS) is illegal in all parts of Canada, with penalties of up to 14 years in prison.

5. **FALSE.** Most people who are grieving need to talk about their loss, and a friend who will let them talk freely is very valuable. The best strategy is simply to be a good listener.

Whether it is a powerful earthquake devastating Haiti, a man in a crowded restaurant having a heart attack, or an old woman dying peacefully with her family close by, images of death are easy to envision. Nevertheless, very rarely do we think about the inevitability of death in our own lives. Accepting and dealing with death are important tasks that present unique challenges to our sense of self, our relationships with others, and our understanding of the meaning of life itself.

Although times of pain and distress may accompany the dying process, facing death also presents an opportunity for growth and affirmation of the preciousness of simple aspects of our daily lives. The way we choose to confront death can greatly influence how we live our lives.

This chapter discusses some of the many questions surrounding the end of life. The following sections explain steps everyone can take to make their own death a bit easier for their loved ones and describes tasks you may need to consider in preparing for your own passing. This chapter also examines the process of grieving and provides advice that can help in dealing with the death of a loved one.

UNDERSTANDING DEATH AND DYING

Ultimately, there is no completely satisfying answer to the question of why death exists. When we look at the big picture, we see that death promotes variety through the evolution of species. The average human life is long enough to allow us to reproduce and ensure that our species continues. Yet it is brief enough to allow for new genetic combinations, thereby providing a means of adaptation to changing conditions in the environment. From the perspective of species survival, the cycle of life and death makes sense.

From a personal point of view, however, death challenges our emotional and intellectual security. We may acknowledge the fact that all living things eventually die and that this is nature's way of renewal, but this recognition offers little comfort when death touches our own lives. Questions about the meaning of death and what happens when we die are central concerns of the great religions and philosophies. Some promise a better life after death. Others teach that everyone is evolving toward perfection or divinity, a goal reached after successive rounds of death and rebirth. Some suggest that it is not possible to know what happens—if anything—after death and that any judgment about life's worth must be made on the basis of satisfactions or rewards that we create for ourselves in our lifetime.

It is worth noting that, even in modern secular societies, religion plays a major role in shaping our attitudes and behaviours toward death. Religion offers solace to the extent that it suggests some meaning in dying. The mourning ceremonies associated with various religious practices ease the pangs of grief for many people. Dying and death are more than biological events; they have social and spiritual dimensions. Our beliefs—religious or philosophical—

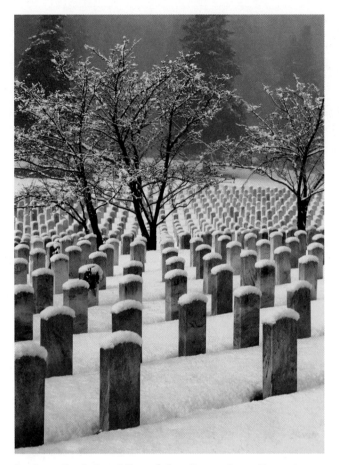

Death awaits all of us at the end of our lives, and accepting and dealing with death are difficult but important tasks.

can be a key to how we relate to the prospect of our own death as well as the deaths of others.

Death forces us to puzzle out an understanding of its meaning in our lives. We may choose not to think about some issues, such as the possibility of an afterlife, but we cannot keep from facing the reality of dying and death. Regardless of our explanations or efforts to minimize its effects, death can be challenging and painful—both to the person who is dying and to those left behind. However, it also offers an opportunity for remarkable growth and a deepening appreciation of relationships and the myriad aspects of life itself.

Defining Death

Traditionally, death has been defined as cessation of the flow of vital body fluids. This occurs when the heart stops beating and breathing ceases. These traditional signs are adequate for determining death in most cases. However, the use of respirators and other **life-support systems** in modern medicine allows some body functions to be artificially sustained. In such cases, making a determination of death requires the presence or absence of a physical response other than heartbeat or breathing. The concept of **brain death** was developed to determine whether a person is alive or dead when the traditional signs are inadequate because of supportive medical technology.

Brain death is assessed in clinical settings and has been defined as the complete and irreversible cessation of all neurological activity. According to standards published by a Harvard Medical School committee, brain death involves four characteristics: (1) lack of receptivity and response to external stimuli, (2) absence of spontaneous muscular movement and spontaneous breathing, (3) absence of observable reflexes, and (4) absence of brain activity, as signified by a flat **electroencephalogram (EEG)**. The Harvard criteria require a second set of tests to be performed after 24 hours have elapsed, and they exclude cases of hypothermia (body temperature below 32°C) and situations involving central nervous system depressants, such as barbiturates. In Canada, the legal definition of brain death includes the standard of "according to accepted medical practice," a potentially problematic scenario given that practices and policies often differ from hospital to hospital.

In contrast to **clinical death**, which is determined by either the cessation of heartbeat and breathing or the criteria for establishing brain death, **cellular death** refers to a gradual process that occurs when heartbeat, respiration, and brain activity have stopped. It encompasses the breakdown of metabolic processes and results in complete nonfunctionality at the cellular level. In a biological sense, therefore, death can be defined as the cessation of life because of irreversible changes in cell metabolism.

The way in which death is defined has potential legal and social consequences in a variety of areas, including criminal prosecution, inheritance, taxation, treatment of the corpse, and even mourning. It also affects the practice of organ transplantation, because some organs—hearts, most obviously—must be harvested from a human being who is legally determined to be dead. Timing is critical in removing a heart from someone who has been declared dead and transplanting it into a person whose life can thereby be saved. Safeguards are necessary to ensure that the determination of death occurs without regard to any plans for subsequent transplantation of the deceased's organs.

Learning About Death

Our understanding of death changes as we grow and mature, as do our attitudes toward it. Very young children view death as an interruption and an absence, but their lack of a mature time perspective means that they do not understand death as final and irreversible. A child's understanding of death evolves greatly from about age five to age nine. During this period, most children come to understand that death is final, universal, and inevitable. A child who consciously recognizes these facts is said to possess a **mature understanding of death**. This understanding of death is further refined during the years of adolescence and young adulthood by considering the impact of death on close relationships and contemplating the value of religious or philosophical answers to the enigma of death.

Based on work done by Mark Speece and Sandor Brent, a formal statement of the empirical, or observable, facts about death includes four components:

1. *Universality.* All living things eventually die. Death is all inclusive, inevitable, and unavoidable (although unpredictable with respect to its exact timing).

2. *Irreversibility.* Organisms that die cannot be made alive again.

3. *Nonfunctionality.* Death involves the cessation of all physiological functioning or signs of life.

4. *Causality.* The occurrence of death has biological reasons.

It is important to add, however, that individuals who possess a mature understanding of death commonly hold nonempirical ideas about it as well. Such nonempirical ideas—that is, ideas not subject to scientific proof—deal mainly with the notion that human beings survive in some form beyond the death of the physical body. What happens to an individual's personality after he or she dies? Does the self or soul continue to exist after the death of the physical body? If so, what is the nature of this afterlife? Developing personally satisfying answers to such questions, which involve what Speece and Brent term **noncorporeal continuity**, is also part of the process of acquiring a mature understanding of death.

TERMS

life-support systems   Medical technologies, such as the respirator, that allow vital body functions to be artificially sustained.

brain death   A medical determination of death as the cessation of brain activity indicated by various diagnostic criteria, including a flat EEG reading.

electroencephalogram (EEG)   A record of the electrical activity of the brain (brain waves).

clinical death   A determination of death made according to accepted medical criteria.

cellular death   The breakdown of metabolic processes at the level of the cell.

mature understanding of death   The recognition that death is universal and irreversible, that it involves the cessation of all physiological functioning, and that there are biological reasons for its occurrence.

noncorporeal continuity   The notion that human beings survive in some form after the death of the physical body.

Denying Versus Accepting Death

Understanding death in a mature fashion does not imply that we never experience anxiety about the deaths of those we love or about the prospect of our own death. The news of a friend's or loved one's serious illness can shock us into an encounter with mortality that creates a need to cope not only with the painful reality of our friend's or loved one's illness but also with our own eventual death. Our ability to find meaning and comfort in the face of mortality depends not only on our having an understanding of the facts of death but also on our attitudes toward it.

Many people seek to avoid any thought or mention of death. The sick and old are often isolated in hospitals and nursing homes. Relatively few Canadians have been present at the death of a loved one. Where the reality of death is concerned, "out of sight, out of mind" often appears to be the rule of the day. Instead of facing death directly, we tend to amuse ourselves with unrealistic portrayals on television and movie screens.

The fictitious deaths of characters we barely know do not cause us to confront the reality of death as it is experienced in real life. Moreover, such faked death is often presented as reversible. Children watch a daily fare of superhuman heroes, invincible to bullets and other weapons. In their games, they reenact these false ideas about death—falling down dead and jumping up again unharmed. Cartoons and video games present death in a two-dimensional world where one can die and then be reborn to play another day.

Although some commentators characterize the predominant attitude toward death in North America as "death denying," others are reluctant to generalize so broadly. People often maintain conflicting or ambivalent attitudes toward death. Those who come to view death as a relief or release from insufferable pain may have at least a partial sense of welcoming death. Few people wholly avoid or wholly welcome death. Problems can arise, however, when avoidance or denial fosters the notion that death happens to others, but not to you or me. (For another perspective, see the box "*El Día de los Muertos*: The Day of the Dead.")

PLANNING FOR DEATH

Acknowledging the inevitability of death allows us to plan for it. Adequate planning can help ensure that a sudden, unexpected death is not made even more difficult for survivors. Even when death is not sudden, individuals with a debilitating illness may become unable to make decisions. Many decisions can be anticipated, considered, and discussed with close relatives and friends.

Basic tasks in planning for death include making a will, anticipating medical care needs and expressing preferences for end-of-life care, considering whether to become an organ donor, and helping survivors plan tasks that will be carried out after we die. It is reasonable to begin such planning during the university years and to periodically review and revise your decisions throughout life.

Making a Will

Surveys indicate that about half of adult Canadians have made a will. Whatever the reason, dying without a will can lead to unnecessary hardships for survivors, even when an estate is modest in size.

A **will** is a legal instrument expressing a person's intentions and choices for the disposition of his or her property after death. It is a declaration of how the **estate**—that is, money, property, and other possessions—will be distributed after death. During the life of the **testator** (the person making the will), a will can be changed, replaced, or revoked. On the testator's death, it becomes a legal instrument governing the distribution of the testator's estate.

When a person dies **intestate**—that is, without having left a valid will—property is distributed according to rules set up by the province or territory. The failure to execute a will may result in a distribution of property that is not compatible with a person's wishes or best suited to the interests and needs of heirs. In making a will, it is generally advisable to involve close family members to prevent problems that can arise when actions are taken without the knowledge of those who will be affected.

Individuals can also help family members by completing a *testamentary letter*; this document includes information about an individual's personal affairs, such as bank accounts, credit cards, the location of documents and keys, the names of professional advisers, the names of people who should be notified of the death, and so on.

Considering Options for End-of-Life Care

An appropriate balance in end-of-life care may involve a combination of home care, hospital stays, and hospice or palliative care. By becoming aware of our options, we and our families are empowered to make informed, meaningful choices.

Home Care Many people express a preference to be cared for at home during the end stage of a terminal illness. An obvious advantage of home care is the fact that the dying person is in a familiar setting, ideally in the company of family and friends. For home care to be an option, however, support generally must be provided not only by family and friends, but also by skilled, professional caregivers.

QUESTIONS FOR CRITICAL THINKING AND REFLECTION

What situations or events make you think seriously about your own mortality? Is this something you consider often, or do you avoid thinking about death? What has influenced your willingness or reluctance to think about death?

El Día de los Muertos: The Day of the Dead

In contrast to the solemn attitude toward death so prevalent in North America, an entirely different and even ironic attitude is more common among Mexicans. In the Mexican worldview, death is another phase of life, and those who have passed into it remain accessible. Ancestors are not forever lost, nor is the past dead. This sense of continuity has its roots in the culture of the Aztecs, for whom regeneration was a central theme. When the Spanish came to Mexico in the sixteenth century, their beliefs about death, along with symbols, such as skulls and skeletons, were absorbed into the native culture.

Mexican artists and writers confront death with humour and even sarcasm, depicting it as the inevitable fate that all—even the wealthiest—must face. At no time is this attitude toward death livelier than at the beginning of each November on the holiday known as *Día de los Muertos*, "the Day of the Dead." This holiday coincides with All Souls' Day, the Catholic commemoration of the dead, and represents a unique blending of indigenous ritual and religious dogma.

The celebration in honour of the dead typically spans two days—one day devoted to dead children, one to adults. It reflects the belief that the dead return to Earth in spirit once a year to rejoin their families and partake of holiday foods prepared especially for them. The fiesta usually begins at midday on October 31, with flowers and food—candies, cookies, honey, milk—set out on altars in each house for the family's dead. The next day, family groups stream to the graveyards, where they have cleaned and decorated the graves of their loved ones, to celebrate and commune with the dead. They bring games, music, and special food. People sit on the graves, eat, sing, and talk with the departed ones. Tears may be shed as the dead are remembered, but mourning is tempered by the festive mood of the occasion.

During the season of the dead, graveyards and family altars are decorated with yellow candles and yellow marigolds—the "flower of death." In some Mexican villages, yellow flower petals are strewn along the ground, connecting the graveyard with all the houses visited by death during the year.

Keeping death in the forefront of consciousness may provide solace to the living, reminding them of their loved ones and assuring them that they themselves will not be forgotten when they die. Yearly celebrations and remembrances may help people keep in touch with their past, their ancestry, and their roots. The festive atmosphere may help dispel the fear of

death, allowing people to look at it more directly. Although it is possible to deny the reality of death even when surrounded by images of it, such practices as *Día de los Muertos* may help people face death with more equanimity.

Sources: Adapted from DeSpelder, L., and A. Strickland. 2007. *The Last Dance*, 8th ed. New York: McGraw-Hill; Azcentral. 2000. *Día de los Muertos* (http://www.azcentral.com/rep/dead; retrieved September 14, 2006); Puente, T. 1991. Día de los Muertos. *Hispanic*, October; Milne, J. 1965. *Fiesta Time in Latin America*. Los Angeles: Ward Ritchie Press.

Home care is a full-time job, and it is not always possible to provide a sufficient level of care in the home. Success depends on adequate preparation and commitment. When a patient requires sophisticated medical procedures, does not have access to qualified caregivers, or intends to be an organ donor, institutional care may be more appropriate. When suitable, however, home care is arguably the most satisfying option for care as a person's life comes to a close. In 2004, approximately 30% of Canadians died at home (about 10% died in nursing homes, and about 60% died in hospitals).

will   A legal instrument expressing a person's intentions and wishes for the disposition of his or her property after death.

estate   The money, property, and other possessions belonging to a person.

testator   The person who makes a will.

intestate   Referring to the situation in which a person dies without having made a legal will.

Hospital-Based Palliative Care Although hospitals are primarily organized to provide short-term intensive treatment for acute injury and illness, they are also adopting the principles of **palliative care** for patients who require comprehensive care at the end of life. Unlike acute care, which involves taking active measures to sustain life, palliative care focuses on controlling pain and relieving suffering by caring for the physical, psychological, spiritual, and existential needs of the patient. Although the emphasis is generally placed on comfort care, palliative therapies can be combined with cure-oriented treatment approaches in some cases. In all cases, the goal of palliative care is to achieve the best possible quality of life for patients and their families.

Hospice Palliative Care As a comprehensive program of care offering a set of services designed to support terminally ill patients and their families, **hospice** is a well-known form of palliative care. Although the term *hospice* sometimes refers to a freestanding medical facility to which terminally ill patients are admitted, Canada has few of these facilities, and consequently, most hospice care takes place in patients' homes with family members as primary caregivers. Entering hospice care usually means affiliating with a hospice program—that is, arranging to receive the services of a local hospice. Such hospices are generally community-based organizations that coordinate a range of palliative care services that may be provided in nursing homes and hospitals, as well as in patients' homes.

Hospice (and palliative care generally) involves a team-oriented approach to care that typically includes physicians, nurses, social workers, home health aides, pharmacists, chaplains, physical and occupational therapists, and trained volunteers. This team-oriented approach seeks to provide state-of-the-art care to prevent or relieve pain and other distressing symptoms, as well as to offer emotional and spiritual support to both patient and family.

Hospice care allows many people to choose where they die, a comforting fact for patients and families. In addition to helping patients achieve a peaceful death, an important gift of hospice care is the potential to help patients and families discover how much can be shared at the end of life through personal and spiritual connections.

Deciding to Prolong Life or Hasten Death

The decision to limit treatment, to stop doing everything that can be done, is often a difficult one for patients and their families. Many people owe their lives to the advanced

medical technologies now available. Yet a medical stance that strives to keep people alive by all means and at any cost is increasingly being questioned.

Modern medicine can keep the human organism alive despite the cessation of normal heart, brain, respiratory, or kidney function. But should a patient without any hope of recovery be kept alive by means of artificial life support? At what point does such treatment become futile? What if a patient has fallen into a **persistent vegetative state**, a state of profound unconsciousness, lacking any sign of normal reflexes and unresponsive to external stimuli, with no reasonable hope of improvement?

Ethical questions about a person's right to die became prominent in Canada in the early 1990s, with the landmark case of Sue Rodriguez. Rodriguez, a 42-year-old woman from British Columbia, suffered from amyotrophic lateral sclerosis (ALS), or Lou Gehrig's disease. She fought for the right to die with the assistance of a physician, taking her case through the British Columbia court system and eventually to the Supreme Court of Canada. She argued that the Canadian ban on physician-assisted suicide (PAS) violated the Constitution by dismissing her rights of personal autonomy as outlined in the Charter of Rights and Freedoms. In 2003, the Supreme Court of Canada denied her request, ruling in a five-to-four decision that society's obligation to respect human life outweighed her rights to exercise control over her own death.

Withholding or Withdrawing Treatment The right of a competent patient to refuse unwanted treatment is now generally established in both law and medical practice. The consensus is that no medical or ethical distinction exists between withholding (not starting) a treatment and withdrawing (stopping) a treatment once it has been started. The choice to forgo life-sustaining treatment involves refusing treatments that would be expected to extend life. The right to refuse treatment remains constitutionally protected even when a patient is unable to communicate. Although specific requirements may vary, all provinces authorize some type of written advance directive to honour the decisions of individuals unable to speak for themselves but who have previously recorded their wishes in an appropriate legal document. (Advance directives are discussed later in this chapter.)

The practice of withholding or withdrawing a treatment that could potentially sustain life is sometimes termed **passive euthanasia**, although many people consider this term a misnomer because it tends to confuse the widely accepted practice of withholding or withdrawing treatment with the generally unacceptable and unlawful practice of taking active steps to cause death. It can be argued that passive euthanasia is not euthanasia at all, but rather letting nature take its course. This distinction is sometimes phrased as the difference between "killing" and "allowing to die."

Assisted Suicide and Active Euthanasia In contrast to withdrawing or withholding treatment, assisted suicide

> ## QUICK STATS
>
> Only **16%–30%** of Canadians who die have access to or receive hospice palliative care services.
>
> —Canadian Institute for Health Information, 2007

and active euthanasia refer to practices that intentionally hasten the death of a person. Although some ethicists argue that the constitutional basis for the right to refuse treatment provides the same basis for a right to active euthanasia, this argument has not been accepted by the Supreme Court of Canada or by health care practitioners.

In **physician-assisted suicide (PAS)**, a physician provides lethal drugs or other interventions—at the patient's request—with the understanding that the patient plans to use them to end his or her life. The patient administers the fatal dose.

In Canada, PAS is illegal in all provinces and territories. In the United States, Oregon was the first state to legalize PAS. The Death with Dignity Act was passed by Oregon voters in 1994 and, after surviving judicial challenges, was reaffirmed in 1997. During its first nine years of implementation, 292 people were reported to have legally committed suicide with the assistance of their physicians. Specific quality-of-life concerns among these individuals included decreasing ability to participate in activities that make life enjoyable, losing control of bodily functions, and physical suffering. In March 2009, Washington became the second U.S. state to legalize PAS. Less than one year later (as of February 2010), at least 36 individuals had died after ingesting the lethal medication prescribed by a physician.

In the Netherlands, PAS has been legal since 1993. It is also legal in Switzerland, where more than 100 British people have travelled to end their lives. One such man was British conductor Sir Edward Downes. In 2009, Downes, though not dying of a disease, chose to die with his terminally ill wife in a double assisted suicide that took place in a Swiss clinic.

An issue of importance related to PAS is the concept of **double effect** in the medical management of pain. The doctrine of double effect states that a harmful effect of treatment, even if it results in death, is permissible if the harm is not intended and occurs as a side effect of a beneficial action. Sometimes the dosages of medication needed to relieve a patient's pain (especially those in the end stage of some diseases) must be increased to levels that can cause respiratory depression, resulting in the patient's death. Thus, the relief of suffering, the intended good effect, may have a potential bad effect, which is foreseen but is not the primary intention. It is generally accepted that such medication for pain, even if it hastens death, is not physician-assisted suicide if the intent is to relieve suffering.

Unlike physician-assisted suicide, **active euthanasia** is the intentional act of killing someone who would otherwise suffer from an incurable and painful disease. Active euthanasia can be involuntary, nonvoluntary, or voluntary. *Involuntary euthanasia* (or involuntary active euthanasia) refers to the ending of a patient's life by a medical practitioner without the patient's consent. The most notorious example of this is the medical killing programs of the Nazi regime. *Nonvoluntary euthanasia* occurs when a surrogate decision maker (not the patient) asks a physician for

assistance to end another person's life. *Voluntary euthanasia* (also known as voluntary active euthanasia) is the intentional termination of life at the patient's request by someone other than the patient. In practice, this generally means that a competent patient requests direct assistance to die, and he or she receives assistance from a qualified medical practitioner. Voluntary active euthanasia is legal in Belgium and the Netherlands but is unlawful in North America. Taking active steps to end someone's life is a crime—even if the motive is mercy.

Many people believe that the emphasis on a right to die results from inattention to the needs of the dying by the health care system. The advocates of hospice and palliative care have highlighted the need for adequate pain management, not only for patients with terminal illness but also for all patients with untreated or undertreated pain and suffering. Increasingly, pain is being viewed as a "fifth vital sign," one that should be added to the four vital signs—temperature, pulse, respiration, and blood pressure—now recorded and assessed as a standard part of patient care.

Unfortunately, tremendous variation exists among health care providers with respect to assessing and managing pain adequately. In 2002, the World Health Organization (WHO) published a number of recommendations for palliative care programs. In general, it is recommended that all countries develop and implement palliative care programs aimed at improving the quality of life of terminally ill patients and their families. In addition to psychosocial and spiritual support, the WHO emphasizes the need for palliative care programs that provide adequate pain relief.

palliative care   A form of medical care aimed at reducing the intensity or severity of a disease by controlling pain and other discomforting symptoms.

hospice   A program of care for dying patients and their families.

persistent vegetative state   A condition of profound unconsciousness in which a person lacks normal reflexes and is unresponsive to external stimuli, lasting for an extended period with no reasonable hope of improvement.

passive euthanasia   The practice of withholding (not starting) or withdrawing (stopping) treatment that could potentially sustain a person's life, with the recognition that, without such treatment, death is likely to occur.

physician-assisted suicide (PAS)   The practice of a physician intentionally providing, at the patient's request, lethal drugs or other means for a patient to hasten death with the understanding that the patient plans to use them to end his or her life.

double effect   A situation in which a harmful effect occurs as an unintended side effect of a beneficial action, such as when medication intended to control a patient's pain has the unintended result of causing the patient's death.

active euthanasia   A deliberate act intended to end another person's life; voluntary active euthanasia involves the practice of a physician administering—at the request of a patient—medication or some other intervention that causes death.

TERMS

It is suggested that all countries with available resources should ensure that national pain relief and palliative care guidelines are adopted by health care professionals at all levels of care.

Completing an Advance Directive

To make your preferences known about medical treatment, you need to document them through a written **advance directive**. In a general sense, an advance directive is any statement made by a competent person about choices for medical treatment should he or she become unable to make such decisions or communicate them at some time in the future.

Two forms of advance directives are legally important. First is the **instructional directive**, or living will, which enables individuals to provide instructions about the kind of medical care they want to receive if they become incapacitated or otherwise unable to participate in treatment decisions. Many people believe that living wills are appropriate only for stating a desire to forgo life-sustaining procedures or to avoid medical heroics when death is imminent; indeed, most standard forms for completing a living will reflect this purpose. In fact, however, a living will can be drafted to express very different ideas about the kinds of treatment a person would or would not want, and they can be written to cover various contingencies.

The second important form of advance directive is the **proxy directive**, which is also known as a *durable power of attorney for health care*. This document makes it possible to appoint another person to make decisions about medical treatment if you become unable to do so. This person, also known as a **substitute decision maker**, may be a family member, close friend, or attorney with whom you have discussed your treatment preferences. The proxy is expected to act in accordance with your wishes as stated in an advance directive or as otherwise made known. Some provinces allow individuals to appoint more than one proxy, so it is important to look into the details in your provincial or territorial legislation. A proxy should be asked in advance whether he or she is willing to take on the responsibility of making potentially difficult decisions for you, and he or she must also be capable of making these decisions.

For advance directives to be of value, you must do more than complete the paperwork. Discuss your wishes ahead of time with caregivers and family members as well as with your proxy and physician.

Becoming an Organ Donor

A human body is a valuable resource. Of all the advances in medical techniques for helping patients who were formerly beyond recovery, perhaps the best known is the transplantation of human organs. Yet the demand for organs continues to drastically outpace the number of organ donations. Each week about five Canadians die because not enough organs are available. In 2008, more than 4000 Canadians were on the waiting list for organ transplants, and 215 people died before receiving a transplant. In the coming decades, the need for transplants in Canada is expected to increase by 150%, whereas the number of available organs is expected to increase by only 12%. For a visual display of the projected need, supply, and shortage of organs for transplantation in Canada, see Figure 18.1.

The number of organ donors in Canada remains fairly consistent each year (about 14 organ donors per million population); however, this rate is low in comparison to many other countries. A report by Urban Futures entitled *Donation Matters: Demographics and Organ Transplants in Canada, 2000–2040* has outlined some interesting statistics that help to explain this trend. For example, it is suggested that Canada's low rate of organ donation is not from a lack of generosity but, rather, because of better health practices. According to this report, Canadians live healthier lifestyles and receive better health care than individuals in many other nations. Further, the report documents that Canada's death rate from automobile accidents is 50% of what it is in Spain and the United States, and deaths from

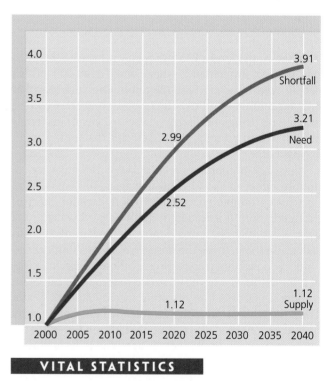

VITAL STATISTICS

FIGURE 18.1   The projected need, supply, and shortfall of organs for transplantation in Canada. The continuation of current demographic trends (declining birth and death rates and an aging population), combined with the rapidly growing need for transplants and projected organ donation rates, will lead to an ever-widening shortfall between the need for, and supply of, organs for transplantation.

Source: Baxter, D., and J. Smerdon. 2000. *Donation Matters: Demographics and Organ Transplants in Canada, 2000–2040.* The Urban Futures Institute. Vancouver: Canada (http://www.lhsc.on.ca/Patients_Families_Visitors/MOTP/Organ_and_Tissue_Donation/Report46.pdf; retrieved June 10, 2010).

gunshot wounds in Canada are three times lower than in the United States. These authors also point out that Canadians are more likely to receive timely and effective treatment for strokes and aneurysms than people in many other countries. In combination, it is suggested that these health practices and trends limit the number of potential organ donors in Canada.

If you decide to become a donor, the first step is to complete an **organ donor ID card**; alternatively, you can indicate your decision on your driver's licence or health card (depending on your province or territory), or simply write out your instructions on a piece of paper and sign it. Some provinces and territories, including British Columbia and Yukon, have an organ donor registry that residents can join. Because relatives are called on to make decisions about organ and tissue donation at the time of a loved one's death, your second step is to discuss your decision with your family and to complete an **organ donor notification card**. If your family does not know your wishes, they are likely to refuse organ donation. In a 2005 survey, 92% of respondents said they would donate a family member's organs if they knew that was what their loved one wanted. For more information about organ donation, see the box "What Can Be Done About the Shortage of Organ Donors?" on p. 560.

Planning a Funeral or Memorial Service

Funerals and memorial services are rites of passage that commemorate a person's life and acknowledge his or her passing from the community. Funerals and memorials allow survivors to support one another as they cope with their loss and express their grief. The presence of death rites in every human culture suggests that they serve innate human needs.

Disposition of the Body   When a death occurs, one of the immediate concerns of survivors is the disposition of the corpse. Although corpses must be disposed of for sanitary reasons, the disposition of a body is surrounded by a web of social, cultural, religious, psychological, and interpersonal considerations.

People generally have a preference about the final disposition of their body. For most Canadians, the choice is either burial or cremation. *Burial* usually involves a grave dug into the soil or entombment in a mausoleum. *Cremation* involves subjecting a body to intense heat, thereby reducing its organic components to a mineralized skeleton. The remaining bone fragments are then usually put through a cremulator, which reduces them to a granular state, often referred to as ashes (which actually resemble coarse coral sand). Cremated remains can be buried, placed in a columbarium niche, put into an urn kept by the family or interred in an urn garden, or scattered at sea or on land. If the body is to be viewed during a wake or will be present at the funeral, **embalming** is generally done.

Arranging a Service   In commemorating a person's life and death, the choice of last rites may involve a traditional funeral ceremony or a simple memorial service. Whereas the casketed body is typically present at a funeral, it is not at a memorial service. In some cases, both a funeral and a memorial service are held, the former occurring within a few days after death and the latter being held sometime later (perhaps in a different town where the deceased had a large social network). Although it is becoming more common for individuals and families to express a preference for no services, bereaved relatives and friends can derive important benefits from having an opportunity to honour the deceased and express their grief through ceremony.

Decisions about your last rites are ideally made with a view to the needs and wishes of your survivors. It can be worthwhile to consider such decisions early in life, so you can gather information about options and discuss plans with family members (see the box "A Consumer Guide to Funerals" on p. 562). Religious and cultural or ethnic traditions play a major role in shaping the way people honour their dead. The diversity of life and death in Canada calls

TERMS

advance directive   Any statement made by a competent person about his or her choices for medical treatment should he or she become unable to make such decisions or communicate them in the future.

instructional directive   A type of advance directive that allows individuals to provide instructions about the kind of medical care they want to receive if they become unable to participate in treatment decisions.

proxy directive   A type of advance directive that allows an individual to appoint another person as an agent in making health care decisions in the event he or she becomes unable to participate in treatment decisions; also known as a *durable power of attorney for health care*.

substitute decision maker   The agent appointed by a person to act on his or her behalf by means of a proxy directive.

organ donor ID card   A consent form authorizing the use of the signer's body parts for transplantation or medical research on his or her death.

organ donor notification card   A signed card indicating an individual's wishes for organ donation in the event of his or her death; to be given to the signer's loved ones so that they know of (and can honour) his or her decision.

embalming   The process of removing blood and other fluids and replacing them with chemicals to disinfect and temporarily slow deterioration of a corpse.

What Can Be Done About the Shortage of Organ Donors?

Since the first organ, a kidney, was successfully transplanted in 1954, the transplanting of organs into people whose organs have failed has become almost commonplace. As transplant techniques and other medical care have improved, however, an acute shortage of available organs has developed.

Sources of Organs and Tissues

Organs and tissues for transplant have several sources.

• *Self-donation* (*autograft*). This type of transplant involves taking part of the patient's own tissue and using it to replace damaged tissue in another area. An example is moving skin from the thigh to replace skin elsewhere that has been burned. Autografts are free from rejection problems (described below) but are not a source of replacement organs.

• *Deceased donor* (*cadaveric transplant*). A typical scenario for cadaveric transplant involves a young person who is injured and brain dead but whose other organs are still functioning. Rejection is a serious problem, and attempts are made to match donors and recipients in terms of blood and immune factors.

• *Living donor*. Organs from siblings, parents, and other close relatives are less likely than cadaveric transplants to be

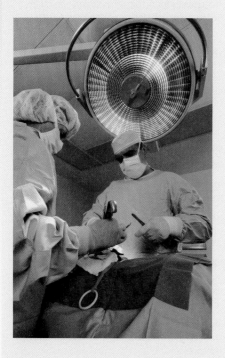

rejected by the body of the recipient. Because of their own need, living donors can donate only bone marrow, liver lobes, lung lobes, and kidneys.

• *Animal donor* (*xenotransplantation*). The supply of animal organs is potentially much greater than the supply of human organs, but xenotransplantation has both ethical and scientific problems. Organ rejection is very likely, and scientists fear the introduction of animal viruses into humans.

Rejection occurs when a patient's body recognizes a transplanted organ as foreign and the immune system attacks and destroys it. Autografts are almost always successful, and tissues or organs transplanted from close relatives are the next best alternative. To help prevent rejection, transplant recipients often must take powerful drugs to suppress their immune systems.

Causes of the Organ Shortage

Many reasons exist for the current shortage of donor organs. First, more people are now waiting for transplants because new technologies and drugs are keeping people with serious health problems alive longer. Another reason is that fewer brain-dead donors are available because seat belts and motorcycle helmets have reduced injury deaths.

The current consent system may contribute to shortages. Families of recently deceased patients must give their consent for the patient's organs to be donated. According to a 2006 Ipsos Reid survey, only 54% of Canadians carry documentation that indicates they want to donate their organs in the event of their death, and close to four in ten Canadians have not talked to their family members about organ donation. Families are more likely to refuse donation if they don't know the deceased's wishes or if they don't understand or trust the organ transplantation system.

Possible Solutions to the Organ Shortage

All Canadian provinces and territories have their own organ donation legislation. However, several possible solutions to the donor organ shortage have been

adopted or are being considered across Canada and worldwide:

• Use of unsuitable hearts, which would not typically be used for transplant, to serve as a temporary "bridge" in emergency situations until another heart becomes available

• Splitting of one liver into two pieces for transplant into two patients

• Education initiatives to encourage people to talk with their families and complete organ donor cards; in Ontario, for example, some high school students take part in an education program called One Life...Many Gifts, which teaches young people about the need for donation and the success of transplantation

• Financial or other incentives for families of donors

• Adoption of a system of presumed consent, in which organs are donated unless the family denies permission

• Xenotransplantation, with pigs as a possible source for transplant organs

• Greater use of devices, such as heart pacemakers and insulin pumps, that replace organ functions

• Development of bioartifical organs, which are made up of both genetically engineered living cells and mechanical components

• Use of stem cells, which could eventually be used to replace cells in damaged or diseased organs

Other strategies have focused on hospital policy, legislation, and recognition for the donor's family. In 1997, Bill C202 was approved, which designates the last week of April as National Organ and Tissue Donor Awareness Week across Canada.

Source: Some information is based on London Health Sciences Centre. 2007. Organ and Tissue Donation (http://www.lhsc.on.ca/ Patients_Families_Visitors/MOTP/Organ_ and_Tissue_Donation/index.htm).

for a diversity of rites. A meaningful funeral or memorial service can be designed in many ways.

Making at least some plans ahead of time and discussing the options with family members can help reduce the burden on survivors who find themselves facing a number of tasks and decisions once death occurs (see the box "Tasks for Survivors" on p. 563).

COPING WITH DYING

There is no one right way to live with or die of a life-threatening illness. Every disease has its own set of problems and challenges, and each person copes with these problems and challenges in his or her own way. Much of the suffering experienced by people with a life-threatening illness comes from overwhelming feelings

of loss on all levels. Besides the emotional havoc, they usually have concerns about medical care, loss of income, hospitalization, and physical pain. How a person copes with such an experience is likely to reflect his or her personality and life history, as well as the nature of family relationships and patterns of interaction in the person's wider social environment.

Awareness of Dying

Living with an illness that is life threatening and incurable can be described as a living-dying experience. From the time discomforting symptoms are first noticed and a person's worst fears confirmed by a diagnosis, through the ups and downs of treatment, and on to the final days or hours of life, hope and honesty are often delicately balanced—honesty to face reality as it is, hope for a positive outcome. The object of hope changes. The early hope that the symptoms are not really serious gives way to hope that a cure is possible. When the illness is deemed incurable, hope for more time arises. As time begins to run out, the hope changes to a pain-free death, a "good death" (see the box "In Search of a Good Death" on p. 564).

Psychiatrist Avery Weisman described this process of coping as involving **middle knowledge**, with patients and their families seeking a balance between sustaining hope and acknowledging the reality. Maintaining a sense of self-worth, setting goals and striving to reach them, engaging in fruitful interactions with the environment— all these reflect a coping strength that sustains the will to live fully despite a bleak prognosis.

The Tasks of Coping

In her 1969 book *On Death and Dying*, Elisabeth Kübler-Ross suggested that the response to an awareness of imminent death involves five psychological stages: denial, anger, bargaining, depression, and acceptance. The notion that these five stages occur in a linear progression has since become a kind of modern myth of how people *ought* to cope with dying. Unfortunately, this can lead to the idea that it is a person's task to move sequentially through these stages, one after another, and that if this is not accomplished, the person has somehow failed. In fact, however, Kübler-Ross said that individuals go back and forth among the stages during an illness, and different stages can occur simultaneously.

The stage-based model devised by Kübler-Ross more than four decades ago has been a stimulus toward a better understanding of how people cope with dying. The notion of stages, however, has been deemphasized in favour of

middle knowledge   A state of knowing when a person both acknowledges the reality of a threatening situation and maintains hope for a positive outcome.

TERMS

A Consumer Guide to Funerals

Funerals are a consumer product. They are also among the most expensive purchases consumers will ever make. A traditional funeral with a casket costs about $6000, and many funerals cost $10,000 or more. When no preplanning has been done, as often occurs, family members have to make decisions under time pressure and in the grip of strong feelings. As a result, they may make poor decisions and spend more than they need to.

To avoid these problems, many Canadian consumers are now making funeral arrangements in advance, comparing prices and services so they can make well-informed purchasing decisions. Many people see funeral planning as an extension of will and estate planning. It is also possible to prepay some or all of the expenses involved.

To ensure that you make the best possible decisions, follow these guidelines:

• *Plan ahead.* Think about what type of funeral you want— simple or elaborate, public or private, religious or secular. Do you want your funeral to be held in a house of worship, a funeral home, or a private setting? Also think about the disposition of the body—do you want your remains to be buried or cremated?

• *Shop around.* Look for a funeral home that has a good reputation, and compare prices from at least two funeral homes. Ask friends for recommendations, and consider whether the funeral home is likely to be in business for many more years.

• *Ask for a price list.* In most provinces and territories, funeral homes and cemeteries are required to provide families with a detailed cost breakdown of all the products and services they provide. This will enable you to select only those services you require and can afford.

• *Decide on the goods and services you want.* Basic services include planning the funeral and coordinating arrangements with the cemetery or crematory. The price of a casket can easily account for half the total cost of an average funeral service.

Prices range from a few hundred dollars for a cloth-covered casket to thousands of dollars for a metal or hardwood casket. You may have to ask to see less expensive caskets, since these are often not on display at funeral homes. Discount casket stores have also opened in some Canadian cities.

• *Consider your options.* In Canada, funeral and burial regulations vary depending on the province or territory. Generally, embalming is not legally required; however, it may be required when transferring remains to another province or territory, or out of the country (unless it is contrary to religious beliefs). In many cases, except in Alberta and Ontario, unless you give instructions to the contrary, funeral homes will automatically go ahead with embalming and charge you for it.

• *Resist pressure to buy goods and services you don't really want or need.* Funeral directors are required to inform you that you need buy only those goods and services you want.

• *Choose a cemetery carefully.* In choosing a cemetery, consider its location; its religious affiliation, if any; the types of monuments allowed; and cost. Visit the cemetery to make sure it's suitable, and ask for a copy of the cemetery's rules and regulations.

• *Commit it to paper.* Once you have made decisions, put them in writing, give copies to family members, and keep a copy accessible. It's a good idea to review your decisions every few years and revise them if necessary.

• *Ask for help.* If you need help dealing with a funeral home, contact your provincial or territorial consumer affairs office or funeral service regulator.

Source: Canada's Office of Consumer Affairs. 2009. *Canadian Consumer Handbook 2008–2009.* Ottawa: Industry Canada (http://consumer. ic.gc.ca/eic/site/oca-bc.nsf/vwapj/cchandbook2008_eng.pdf/$FILE/ cchandbook2008_eng.pdf; retrieved June 11, 2010). Reproduced with the permission of the Minister of Public Works and Government Services, 2011.

highlighting the tasks that deserve attention in coping with a life-threatening illness. Charles Corr, for example, distinguishes four primary dimensions in coping with dying:

1. *Physical:* Satisfying bodily needs and minimizing physical distress
2. *Psychological:* Maximizing a sense of security, self-worth, autonomy, and richness in living
3. *Social:* Sustaining significant relationships and addressing the social implications of dying
4. *Spiritual:* Identifying, developing, or reaffirming sources of meaning and fostering hope

Contemplating these dimensions gives us a framework for considering the specific tasks that need to be addressed in coping with dying. In addition to an *acute* phase initiated by the diagnosis, a *chronic* phase of living with the disease, and a *terminal* phase that involves coping with impending death, two other phases are sometimes reached: First, a *prediagnostic* phase, during which a person suspects the illness and may seek medical attention; and, second, a *recovery* phase following a cure or remission of a previously life-threatening disease. Even as the threat of dying recedes into the background, however, some people need to cope with the fact that they have had a potentially terminal illness.

In addition, though, we must remember that a person's death is as unique as his or her life. Thus, although models can help us gain understanding, they need to be balanced by paying attention to the dying person's own unfolding *life* story. Each person's pathway through life-threatening illness is determined by many factors, such as the specific disease and its course, his or her personality, and the available supportive resources.

People who apparently cope best with life-threatening illness often exhibit a fighting spirit that views the illness not only as a threat but also as a challenge. These people

Tasks for Survivors

Some of the following tasks must be attended to soon after a death occurs, whereas others take weeks or months to complete. Many of these tasks, especially those that need to be dealt with in the first hours and days following the death, can be taken care of by friends and relatives of the immediate survivors.

• Prepare a list of relatives, friends, and colleagues, and telephone them about the death as soon as possible. Friends can help with notifications.

• Find out if the deceased left instructions for disposition of the body or for a funeral or memorial service.

• If no prior plan exists, contact a mortuary or memorial society for help in making arrangements. Clergy, friends, and other family members can be asked to help decide what is most appropriate.

• If flowers are to be omitted from the funeral or memorial service, choose an appropriate charity or other memorial to which gifts can be made.

• Write the obituary. Include the deceased's age, birth-place, cause of death, occupation, academic degrees, memberships, military service, accomplishments, names and relationships of nearest survivors, and the time and place of the funeral or memorial service.

• Arrange for family members or close friends to take turns welcoming mourners who come in person and responding to those who send or telephone their condolences.

• Ask friends to help coordinate the supplying of meals for the first few days following the death, as well as the management of other household tasks and child care, if necessary.

• Arrange hospitality for relatives and friends who are visiting from out of town.

• If a funeral ceremony is planned, choose the individuals who are to be pallbearers, and notify them that you would like their participation.

• Send handwritten or printed notes of acknowledgment to the people who have provided assistance or who have sent flowers, contributions, or their condolences.

• Notify the lawyer, accountant, and other personal representatives who will be helping to settle the deceased's estate.

• With the help of a lawyer or an accountant, review all insurance policies as well as other sources of potential death benefits, such as the Canada Pension Plan Death Benefit, military service, fraternal organizations, and unions.

• Review all debts, mortgages, and instalment payments. Some may carry clauses that cancel debt in the event of death. If payments must be delayed, contact creditors to arrange for a grace period.

---

strive to inform themselves about their illness and take an active part in treatment decisions. They are optimistic and have a capacity to discover positive meaning in ordinary events. Holding to a positive outlook despite distressing circumstances involves creating a sense of meaning that is bigger than the threat. In the context of life-threatening illness, this encompasses a person's ability to comprehend the implications an illness has for the future, as well as for his or her ability to accomplish goals, maintain relationships, and sustain a sense of personal vitality, competence, and power. Although life-threatening illness disrupts virtually all aspects of a person's life, there is a vital link between finding meaning and achieving a sense of mastery.

The Trajectory of Dying

Our expectations about dying may be quite different from what most people actually experience. The concept of a **trajectory of dying** is useful for understanding patients' experiences as they near death. Although sudden death from an unexpected cause—a massive heart attack or an accident, for example—is one type of dying trajectory, our focus here is on deaths that occur when there is fore-warning. Among these, some trajectories involve a steady and fairly predictable decline. This is the case with many cancers, which tend to follow the course of a progressive disease with a terminal phase. Other kinds of advanced, chronic illness involve a long period of slow decline marked by episodes of crisis, the last of which proves to be "suddenly" fatal.

We can also distinguish between different stages in a dying trajectory, namely, a period when a person is known to be terminally ill but is living with a life expectancy of perhaps weeks or months, possibly years, and a later period when dying is imminent and the person is described as actively dying. The way in which such trajectories are estimated—their duration and expected course—can affect both patients and caregivers and influence their actions. Deaths that occur out of time (too quickly or too slowly) may pose special difficulties.

When a person is actively dying, his or her death is expected to occur within hours or, at most, a few days. During the last phase of a fatal illness, a dying person may exhibit irregular breathing or shortness of breath, decreased

trajectory of dying   The duration and nature of a person's experience in approaching death as influenced by the underlying cause of dying.

TERMS

In Search of a Good Death

Participants in a recent study were asked to discuss the deaths of family members, friends, or patients and reflect on what made their deaths good or bad. From these discussions, six major themes emerged as components of a good death.

The first component was pain and symptom management. Many people fear dying in pain, and portrayals of bad deaths usually included inadequate pain management. Every health care provider in the study told regret-filled stories of patients who died in pain. Patients were concerned with pain control; when reassured that pain could be managed, they were less anxious.

The second component of a good death was clear decision making. Both providers and families feared entering a medical crisis without knowing the patient's preferences. Patients and families who had good communication with health care providers and had discussed treatment decisions ahead of time felt empowered, and providers felt they were giving good care. Although all uncertainty about end-of-life decisions cannot be eliminated, tolerance for uncertainty may increase if values and preferences are clarified.

The third component was preparation for death. Patients expressed satisfaction when they had time to prepare their wills and help plan their funeral arrangements. Many times, providers avoided end-of-life discussions to prevent their patients from losing hope, thus depriving them of

the opportunity to plan ahead. Patients and families also wanted to know what to expect during the illness and what physical and psychosocial changes would take place as death approached. It was important for providers and families to have reached some personal comfort with death so they felt prepared when death occurred.

The fourth component was completion, the opportunity to review life, to resolve conflicts, to spend time with loved ones, and to say goodbye. Participants confirmed the deep importance of spirituality or meaningfulness at the end of life. Many times, patients were able to view their experience of dying as part of a broader life trajectory and thus continue to grow emotionally and spiritually in their last days. The fifth component was contributing to others. Patients wanted to know that they still had something to offer to others, whether it was making someone laugh or lightening the load of someone closer to death. Many patients found that as they reflected on their lives, what they valued most was their personal relationships with family and friends, and they were anxious to impart this wisdom to others.

The sixth component of a good death was affirmation of the whole person. Patients appreciated empathic health care providers, and family members were comforted by those who treated their loved ones as unique and whole people, rather than as a disease. The quality of

dying is related to the acknowledgment that people die in character; that is, as an extension of who they have been in their lives. Health care providers also focused on their personal relationships with patients and family members as important to a satisfying death.

The study affirmed that most people think of death as a natural part of life, not as a failure of technology. Although the biomedical aspects of end-of-life care are crucial, they merely provide a point of departure toward a good death. When pain is properly managed and the practical aspects of dying are taken care of, patients and their families have the opportunity to address the important emotional, psychological, and spiritual issues that all human beings face at the end of life.

---

appetite and thirst, nausea and vomiting, incontinence, restlessness and agitation, disorientation and confusion, and diminished consciousness. These symptoms usually can be managed by skilled palliative care. Pain, if it is present, should be treated aggressively as part of a comprehensive approach to comfort care. Since most patients are more comfortable without eating or drinking at the end of life, forcing food or liquids is usually not beneficial. The stopping of eating and drinking has always been part of the last phase of a terminal condition. Near the time of death, relaxation of the throat muscles or secretions in the throat may cause the person's breathing to become noisy, resulting in a sound called the death rattle. Other signals may be noticeable as death draws closer. For example, the patient's extremities may feel cold to the touch; lips, fingers, and ears may appear bluish; urination becomes less frequent; or the ability to communicate may be lost. In the

final hours, purple blotches (mottling) may appear on the legs or arms. Simple steps—such as repositioning the patient, covering him or her with blankets, dimming the room's lighting, or just holding hands—can provide great relief and reassurance in the last moments. Just before death, the person may take a breath and sigh or shudder.

Supporting a Dying Person

People often feel uncomfortable in the presence of a person who is close to dying. What can we say? How should we act? It may seem that any attempt to be comforting could result only in words that are little more than stale platitudes. Yet we want to express concern and establish meaningful contact with the person who is facing death. In such circumstances, the most important gift we can bring is that of listening. Offering the dying person opportunities to speak

The simple act of listening can be extremely supportive to someone who is facing death.

openly and honestly about his or her experience can be crucial, even when such conversation is initially painful.

We tend to place dying people in a special category, but the reality is that their needs are not fundamentally different from anyone else's, although their situation is perhaps more urgent. Dying people need to know that they are valued, that they are not alone, that they are not being unfairly judged, and that those closest to them are also striving to come to terms with a difficult situation. As with any relationship, opportunities for growth exist on both sides.

Besides friends and family, the dying person may need other supportive resources. These may include counsellors and clergy. Many hospitals, hospices, and other health care providers sponsor programs for dying patients and their families, offering opportunities for them to share their concerns in a supportive and validating atmosphere. Programs of this kind can be located by asking hospital staff or other medical personnel. Local support groups can also be found in many cities.

COPING WITH LOSS

Even if we have not experienced the death of someone close, we are all survivors of losses that occur in our lives because of changes and endings. The loss of a job, the ending of a relationship, transitions from one school or neighbourhood to another—these are examples of the kinds of losses that occur in all our lives. Such losses are sometimes called little deaths and, in varying degrees, they all involve grief.

Experiencing Grief

Grief is the reaction to loss. It encompasses thoughts and feelings, as well as physical and behavioural responses. Mental distress may involve disbelief, confusion, anxiety, disorganization, and depression. The emotions that can be present in normal grief include not only sorrow and sadness, but also relief, anger, and self-pity, among others. Bereaved people experience a range of feelings, even conflicting ones. Recognizing that grief can involve many different feelings—not just sadness—makes us more able to cope with it. Common behaviours associated with grief include crying, searching for the deceased, and talking incessantly about the deceased and the circumstances of the death. Bereaved people may be restless, as if not knowing what to do with themselves. Physically, grief may involve frequent sighing, insomnia, and loss of appetite. Grief may also evoke a reexamination of religious or spiritual beliefs as a person struggles to make meaning of the loss. All such manifestations of grief can be present as part of one's total response to **bereavement**—that is, the event of loss.

Mourning is closely related to grief and is often used as a synonym for it. However, mourning refers not so much to the *reaction* to loss but to the *process* by which a bereaved person adjusts to loss and incorporates it into his or her life. How this process is managed is determined, at least partly, by cultural and gender norms for the expression of grief (see the box "Grief and Gender" on p. 566). Considered jointly, grief and mourning are the means to healing the pain of loss.

Tasks of Mourning   Experiencing grief is part of the process by which a bereaved person integrates a significant loss into his or her life. Psychologist William Worden has identified four tasks that must be attended to:

1. *Accepting the reality* of the loss

2. *Working through the pain* of grief

Grief and Gender

The loss of a loved one generates a broad range of reactions—physical, emotional, and behavioural. But do women and men react differently to the loss of someone close to them? Some clinicians say yes, and studies now support the idea that grief has different gender patterns.

Data suggest that a greater proportion of women may be vulnerable to the more distressing and disruptive symptoms characteristic of severe grief reactions. In general, women have a higher lifetime incidence and prevalence of depressive and anxiety disorders, so it is not surprising that at times of great stress, such as the loss of a loved one, these gender differences would be present.

In a study of gender differences in grief among parents who have lost a child, researchers found that compared with fathers, mothers showed greater feelings of being hurt, cheated, and depressed, while also revealing greater irritability and anger. The women also cried more,

experienced greater numbness and confusion, were more preoccupied with thoughts of the deceased, and felt more guilt both for having failed to prevent the death and for having survived. They also experienced more physical symptoms, such as insomnia and loss of appetite.

In a study of people who had lost a spouse, researchers similarly found that women had a higher level of emotional distress in reaction to loss. Women who lost a husband had higher levels of traumatic grief, depression, and anxiety than men who had lost a wife. These findings persisted at least two years following the death of the spouse.

Physiological factors contributing to these gender differences might include hormonal differences, subtle differences in brain chemistry or function, or genetic influences. Gender roles and cultural expectations also likely play a role. Women are often readier to express emotion and seek out social support and opportunities

to talk about loss, whereas men may be more reticent to admit to any psychological distress or allow the appearance of excessive emotionality.

3. *Adjusting to a changed environment* in which the deceased is absent

4. *Emotionally relocating the deceased* and moving on with life

Accomplishing the fourth task does not mean dishonouring the deceased's memory or denying normal feelings of connection that persist beyond death. Finding healthy ways to maintain bonds with the deceased is a testimony to the enduring strength of love. When this task is managed successfully, however, the bereaved is not stuck in the past. Making the journey of grief and attending to the various tasks along the way, we come to a place where we learn how to keep a special place for the deceased in our hearts and memories while moving forward with our lives.

The Course of Grief   Grieving, like dying, is highly individual. In the first hours or days following a death, a bereaved person is likely to experience overwhelming shock and numbness, as well as a sense of disbelief. There is often a period of denial—"No! This can't be true!"—especially if the death was unexpected. Consider the ways in which people die: the aged grandmother, dying quietly in her sleep; the young child pronounced "dead on arrival" after a bicycle crash; the despondent executive who commits suicide; a young soldier killed in battle; the chronically ill person who dies a lingering death. The cause or mode

of death—natural, accidental, homicide, or suicide—has an influence on how grief is experienced (see the box "Profound Trauma and Loss"). Even when a death is anticipated, grief is not necessarily diminished when the loss becomes real.

The sense of disorganization experienced by survivors during the early period of grief is set against the need to attend to decisions and actions surrounding the disposition of the deceased's body. As family and friends gather to offer mutual support, funeral ceremonies are held. Engaging in such activities promotes accepting the reality of the death and moving beyond the initial shock and numbness.

In its middle phase, the course of grief is characterized by anxiety, apathy, and pining for the deceased. The pangs of grief are felt as the bereaved person deeply experiences the pain of separation. There is often a sense of despair as a person repeatedly goes over the events surrounding the loss, perhaps fantasizing that somehow everything could be undone and be as it was before. During this period, the bereaved also begins looking toward the future and taking the first steps toward building a life without the deceased.

This can be a difficult time in grieving. Yet the bereaved often find themselves without the social support of the relatives and friends who were present during the initial period. Grief occurs within a particular social or cultural context, and individual grievers differ in their particular

Profound Trauma and Loss

Profoundly traumatic events—the earthquakes in Japan and Haiti, Hurricane Katrina, the 2004 tsunami in Southeast Asia, the terrorist attacks of September 11, 2001, the deaths and destruction resulting from the wars in Iraq and Afghanistan—all represent a category of loss far beyond normal comprehension. Experiencing traumatic loss in such extraordinary circumstances can cause severe and disruptive reactions in emotion and behaviour.

World War I veterans often developed psychological symptoms that collectively were described as shell shock. However, it was not until after the Vietnam War that the medical community became fully aware of how disruptive and enduring the psychological effects could be for those experiencing profound traumatic loss.

It is now widely recognized that significant psychological symptoms can follow when people experience loss in traumatic circumstances. Elements commonly seen in a customary reaction to grief, such as sadness, disbelief, crying, insomnia, and loss of appetite, are frequently exaggerated in the aftermath of profoundly traumatic events and will often include more pronounced symptoms, such as overwhelming distress, numbness, doubt, despair, guilt, and disabling depression and anxiety.

Depending on the severity of exposure and a person's underlying vulnerability, the symptoms can persist long after the original trauma. Memories and images of the event may suddenly pop into the victim's mind, causing anxiety, depression, and anger. Insomnia and nightmares can disrupt the sleep-wake cycle. The person may start avoiding everything that serves as a reminder of the event and, as a kind of self-protection, may begin to become numb, to lose all feelings. Such people may startle easily and have difficulty concentrating. Their work life, social life, and intimate relationships may become markedly impaired. People experiencing these severe symptoms are said to have posttraumatic stress disorder (PTSD), which can persist for months or years.

The events of September 11, 2001, are an example of a profound trauma that caused PTSD in affected people. As described in Chapter 2, PTSD symptoms

occurred among survivors, rescue workers, passersby, residents of Manhattan, and some people exposed to the events through repeated television images. Researchers who interviewed residents of Manhattan found that about 7.5% reported symptoms consistent with a diagnosis of PTSD and 9.7% reported symptoms consistent with new onset of depression; these numbers are about twice as high as the expected rates in surveys of this type. Among people who lived closest to the World Trade Center, the prevalence of PTSD was as high as 20%.

Many people experience disabling depression or anxiety but do not meet the full criteria for PTSD. More persistent and severe grief reactions, unexplained physical symptoms, and the increased use of alcohol and drugs are frequent occurrences for people who have undergone such trauma. In addition, family and interpersonal conflict and financial strain are commonly seen. All too frequently, in war or natural disasters, the primary wage earner of the family dies or the family's house and belongings are destroyed.

How long will an individual's symptoms last after experiencing an event like September 11 or witnessing a friend killed by a roadside bomb in Iraq? Many factors, such as the severity of the trauma, the individual's proximity to the event, and his or her emotional closeness to those who have died, can all play important roles in the magnitude and duration of the reaction to traumatic loss. In general, though, symptoms will

diminish with time, especially in the absence of new threats and traumatic losses. Studies of those who have developed full-blown PTSD suggest that approximately half of the cases resolve within two years but that nearly a third never fully recover.

Psychological support and treatment can greatly help many of those who suffer from disabling emotional symptoms in reaction to traumatic loss. Building on research and work done with Vietnam veterans in the 1970s and 1980s, clinicians have developed multiple therapeutic strategies involving group therapy, individual psychological support, and pharmacologic intervention to treat persistent symptoms.

Sources: Coker, A. L., et al. 2006. Social and mental health needs assessment of Katrina evacuees. *Disaster Management and Response* 4(3): 88–94; Watanabe, T., et al. 2006. Acute stress syndrome in a victim of the Indian Ocean Tsunami. *Psychiatry and Clinical Neurosciences* 60(5): 644; Galea, S., and H. Resnick. 2005. Posttraumatic stress disorder in the general population after mass terrorist incidents: Considerations about the nature of exposure. *CNS Spectrums* 10(2): 107–115; Galea, S., et al. 2002. Psychological sequelae of the September 11 terrorist attacks in New York City. *New England Journal of Medicine* 346(13): 982–987; Shuster, M., et al. 2001. A national survey of stress reactions after the September 11, 2001, terrorist attacks. *New England Journal of Medicine* 345(20): 1507–1512; Ornstein, R. D., and R. K. Pitman (section eds.). 2000. Trauma and post-traumatic stress disorder. In *Massachusetts General Hospital Psychiatry Update and Board Preparation*, 2nd ed., T. A. Stern and J. B. Herman (eds.). New York: McGraw-Hill.

styles of grieving. This leads to the recognition that there is no standard way of coping with loss. Colin Murray Parkes points to three main influences on a person's course of grieving:

1. The urge to look back, cry, and search for what is lost

2. The urge to look forward, explore the world that emerges out of the loss, and discover what can be carried forward from the past into the future

3. The social and cultural pressures that influence how the first two urges are inhibited or expressed

As these influences interact in various ways, at times the bereaved tries to avoid the pain of grief and at other times confronts it. The goal is to achieve a balance between avoidance and confrontation that facilitates coming to terms with the loss. Attaining this goal can be seen as an oscillation between what Margaret Stroebe and Henk Schut call loss-oriented and restoration-oriented mourning. From this perspective, looking at old photographs and yearning for the deceased are examples of loss-oriented coping, whereas doing what is needed to reorganize life in the wake of the loss—for example, learning to do tasks that the deceased had always managed, such as finances—is part of restoration-oriented coping.

In moving toward the restoration of a sense of well-being, the last phase of active grief involves resolution. The acute pain and emotional turmoil of grief subside. Physical and mental balance is reestablished. The bereaved becomes increasingly reintegrated into his or her social world. Sadness doesn't go away completely, but it recedes into the background. Although reminders of the loss stimulate active grieving from time to time, the main focus is the present, not the past. Adjusting to loss may sometimes feel like a betrayal of the deceased loved one, but it is healthy to engage again in ongoing life and the future (see the box "Coping with Grief").

Some people, however, have more trouble resolving their grief than others. Such people may get stuck in the grieving process for months or even years, sometimes becoming so burdened with loss that they lose the ability to cope with daily living. Experts call this long-term, unresolved grief *complicated grief* and describe it as truly debilitating. Complicated grief is most likely to occur when a person has lost a loved one in a sudden, violent manner (such as homicide) or experienced an untimely death (such as the loss of a child). Grief counselling or therapy can help people work through complicated grief.

Supporting a Grieving Person

In experiencing a significant loss, a person initially may feel and behave much like a frightened, helpless child. He or she may respond best to the kind of loving support that is given by a parent. A hug may be more comforting than any words. Also, because talking about a loss is an important way that survivors cope with the changed reality, simply listening can be very helpful. The key to being a good listener is to refrain from making judgments about whether the feelings expressed by a survivor are right or wrong, good or bad. The emotions, thoughts, and behaviours evoked by loss may not be the ones we expect, but they can nonetheless be valid and appropriate within a survivor's experience of loss.

Talking and crying, even yelling in rage, are among the ways of coping with intense feelings of grief. Bereaved persons should not be urged to hold back their feelings or to be strong and brave. Expressions of grief are healing. On the other hand, the bereaved need not pretend to grieve or exaggerate his or her feelings to satisfy others' expectations. Funerals and other ceremonies generally help survivors gain a sense of closure and begin to integrate a loss into their lives. For some, funerals are occasions of weeping and wailing; for others, stoic and subdued emotions are the rule. Different styles of mourning can be equally valid and appropriate.

Social support for the bereaved is as critical during the later course of grief as it is during the first days after a loss. In offering support, we can reassure them that grief is normal, permissible, and appropriate. They may also need permission to occasionally give themselves a break from grieving. As they move forward in life, the bereaved may need encouragement from others to face the world confidently. An extended need for support often continues through the first year or two of mourning. The first anniversary following a significant loss can be a time of renewed grieving when the support of others is important and appreciated. Knowing that others remember the loss and that they take time to touch base is usually perceived as very helpful.

Bereaved people also may want to share their stories and concerns through organized support groups, such as those for widows and widowers. Many support groups are organized around some specific type of bereavement. Others offer support to anyone who has suffered a loss. GriefShare, for example, is an international organization that offers support to individuals who are grieving the death of a loved one.

Helping Children Cope with Loss

Children tend to cope with loss in a healthier fashion when they are included as part of their family's experience of grief and mourning. Although adults may be uncomfortable about sharing potentially disturbing or painful news with children, a child's natural curiosity usually negates the option of withholding information. Sudden changes in family communication patterns without any explanation can alarm a child and create anxiety. When children are asked about their experiences of family crises involving death, many say that the most difficult times occurred when they did not know what was happening. Mounting

Coping with Grief

- Recognize and acknowledge the loss.
- React to grief by accepting and expressing it.
- Take time for nature's process of healing.
- Know that powerful, overwhelming feelings will change with time.
- Review and remember the relationship with the deceased.
- Share your pain by accepting support from others.
- Surround yourself with life: plants, animals, friends.

- Make use of mementos to promote your mourning, not to live in the past.
- Avoid major decisions, if possible, and give yourself time to readjust.
- Adapt to a new world without forgetting the old.
- Prepare for change, new interests, new friends, creativity, and growth.
- Reinvest in life.

Sources: The Centre for Living with Dying (554 Mansion Park Dr., Santa, Clara, CA 95054; 408-980-9801); Rando, T. A. 1993. *The Treatment of Complicated Mourning.* Champaign, Ill.: Research Press.

evidence shows that it is best to include children from the beginning—as soon as a terminal prognosis is made, for example—to help them understand what is happening. Children should spend time with the dying person, if possible, to learn, share, and offer and receive comfort. Such visits can be made under the guidance of a mental health professional, working with the child's best interests in mind, if deemed appropriate.

In talking about death with children, the most important guideline is to be honest. Set the explanation you are offering at the child's level of understanding. In general, it's advisable to keep the explanation simple, stick to basics, and verify what the child has understood from your explanation. A child's readiness for more details can usually be assessed by paying attention to his or her questions.

QUESTIONS FOR CRITICAL THINKING AND REFLECTION

Have you ever been in the position of being supportive to a bereaved person? What kind of support did he or she seem to appreciate most? Why do you think that was the case? How did the experience affect you?

COMING TO TERMS WITH DEATH

We may wish we could keep death out of view and not make a place for it in our lives. But this wish cannot be fulfilled. With the death of a beloved friend or relative, we are confronted with emotions and thoughts that relate not only to the immediate loss but also to our own mortality.

Our encounters with dying and death teach us that relationships are more important than things and that life offers no guarantees. In discovering the meaning of death in our own lives, we find that life is both precious and precarious.

Allowing ourselves to make room for death, we discover that it touches not only the dying or bereaved person and his or her family and friends but also the wider community of which we are all part. We recognize that dying and death offer opportunities for extraordinary growth in the midst of loss. Denying death, it turns out, results in denying life.

McGraw Hill connect™

Practise and learn online with Connect. Connect allows you to practise important skills at your own pace and on your own schedule, with 24/7 online access to an eBook, practice quizzes, interactivities, videos, study tools, additional resources, and more.

SUMMARY

- Although death makes rational sense in terms of species survival and evolution, there may be no completely satisfying answer to the question of why death exists from a personal point of view.

- Dying and death are more than biological events; they have social and spiritual dimensions.

- The traditional criteria for determining death focus on vital signs such as breathing and heartbeat. Brain death is characterized by a lack of physical responses other than breathing and heartbeat.

- Between ages five and nine, most children develop a mature understanding of death; that is, they come to understand death as final, universal, and inevitable.

- A mature understanding of death can include ideas about the survival of the human personality after death.

- Problems arise when avoidance or denial of death fosters the notion that it happens only to others.

- Many basic tasks in preparing for death can and should be accomplished while one is young.

- A will is a legal instrument that governs the distribution of a person's estate after death.

- End-of-life care may involve a combination of home care, hospital stays, and hospice or palliative care.

- Palliative care is devoted to making dying patients comfortable by controlling pain and relieving suffering.

- Hospice programs apply a team-oriented approach to caring for dying patients and their families with the goal of helping people live as fully as possible until the end of their lives.

- Exercising choices about end-of-life care can involve making decisions about prolonging life or hastening death.

- The practice of withholding or withdrawing potentially life-sustaining treatment is sometimes termed passive euthanasia.

- Physician-assisted suicide occurs when a physician provides lethal drugs or other interventions, at a patient's request, with the understanding that the patient plans to use them to end his or her life. Voluntary active euthanasia refers to the intentional ending of a patient's life, at his or her request, by someone other than the patient.

- Advance directives, such as living wills and health care proxies, are used to express one's wishes about the use of life-sustaining treatment.

- People can donate their bodies or specific organs for transplantation and other medical uses after death.

- For Canadians, the decision about what to do with the body after death usually involves either burial or cremation.

- Bereaved people usually benefit from participating in a funeral or memorial service to commemorate a loved one's death.

- Coping with dying involves physical, psychological, social, and spiritual dimensions.

- It is useful for patients and caregivers to understand the trajectory, or course, of dying.

- In offering support to a dying person, the gift of listening can be especially important.

- Grief encompasses thoughts and feelings, as well as physical and behavioural responses.

- Mourning, the process by which a person integrates a loss into his or her life, is determined partly by social and cultural norms for expressing grief.

- Children tend to cope with death in a healthier fashion when they are included in their family's experience of grief and mourning.

- Dying and death offer opportunities for growth in the midst of loss.

Today, Canadians as a whole are becoming more empowered and confident in their ability to solve personal health problems on their own. People who manage their own health care gather information and learn skills from a variety of resources; they solicit opinions and advice, make decisions, and take action. They know how to practise safe, effective self-care, and they know how to make decisions about professional medical care, whether conventional Western medicine or complementary and alternative medicine or both. The key to good decision making is using the best evidence to help you choose which actions to take regarding your health care. As the terms *complementary* and *alternative* imply, these forms of medicine can be used as complements or alternatives to conventional medicine.

This chapter will help you develop the skills both to identify and manage health issues and to make the conventional health care system combined with complementary and alternative options work effectively for you.

SELF-CARE

Effectively managing health and medical problems involves developing several skills. First, you need to learn to be a good observer of your own body and assess your symptoms. You also must be able to decide when to seek professional advice and when you can safely deal with the problem on your own. You need to know how to self-treat common medical problems safely and effectively. Finally, you need to know how to develop a partnership with physicians and other health care providers and how to carry out treatment plans.

Self-Assessment

Symptoms are often an expression of the body's attempt to heal itself. For example, the pain and swelling that occur after an ankle injury immobilize the injured joint to allow healing to take place. A fever may be an attempt to make the body less hospitable to infectious agents. A cough can help clear the airways and protect the lungs. Understanding what a symptom means and what is going on in your body helps reduce anxiety about symptoms and enables you to practise safe self-care that supports your body's own healing mechanisms.

Carefully observing symptoms also lets you identify those signals that suggest you need professional assistance. You should begin by noting when the symptom began, how often and when it occurs, what makes it worse, what makes it better, and whether you have any associated symptoms. You can also monitor your body's vital signs, such as temperature and heart rate. Medical self-tests for blood pressure, blood sugar, pregnancy detection, and urinary tract infections can also help you make a more informed decision about when to seek medical help and when to self-treat.

Knowing When to See a Physician

In general, you should see a physician for symptoms that you would describe as follows:

1. *Severe.* If the symptom is very severe or intense, medical assistance is advised. Examples include severe pains, major injuries, and other emergencies.
2. *Unusual.* If the symptom is peculiar and unfamiliar, it is wise to check it out with your physician. Examples include unexplained lumps, changes in a mole, problems with vision, difficulty swallowing, numbness, weakness, unexplained weight loss, and blood in sputum, urine, or stool.
3. *Persistent.* If the symptom lasts longer than expected, seek medical advice. Examples in adults include fever for more than five days, a cough lasting longer than two weeks, hoarseness lasting longer than three weeks, and a sore that doesn't heal within a month.
4. *Recurrent.* If a symptom tends to return repeatedly, medical evaluation is advised. Examples include recurrent headaches, stomach pains, and backache.

Sometimes a single symptom is not a cause for concern, but when the symptom is accompanied by other symptoms, the combination suggests a more serious problem. For example, a fever with a stiff neck might suggest something more serious, such as meningitis.

If you evaluate your symptoms and think that you need professional help, you must decide how urgent the problem is. If it is a true emergency, you should go (or call someone to take you) to the nearest emergency room (ER). Emergencies include the following:

- Major trauma or injury, such as head injury, suspected broken bone, deep wound, severe burn, eye injury, or animal bite
- Uncontrollable bleeding or internal bleeding, as indicated by blood in the sputum, vomit, or stool
- Intolerable and uncontrollable pain or severe chest pain
- Severe shortness of breath
- Persistent abdominal pain, especially if associated with nausea and vomiting
- Poisoning or drug overdose

CONVENTIONAL AND COMPLEMENTARY MEDICINE

LOOKING AHEAD>>>>>

AFTER READING THIS CHAPTER, YOU SHOULD BE ABLE TO

■ Explain the self-care decision-making process and discuss options for self-treatment

■ Describe the basic premises, practices, and providers of conventional medicine

■ Describe the basic premises, practices, and providers of complementary and alternative medicine

■ Explain how to communicate effectively with health care providers and to use their input when evaluating different types of treatment

■ Discuss how health care is paid for in Canada

TEST YOUR KNOWLEDGE

1. **The people most likely to use complementary and alternative medicine are those without a conventional primary care physician.**
   True or false?

2. **Which practice or interest is shared by both conventional Western medicine and complementary and alternative medicine?**
   a. careful observation of symptoms
   b. treatment with remedies derived from plants
   c. concern with the patient-physician relationship

3. **The sale and use of herbal remedies and dietary supplements, such as ginkgo biloba and St. John's wort, are not well regulated in Canada.**
   True or false?

4. **Generic drugs are generally less effective than brand-name drugs.**
   True or false?

ANSWERS

1. **FALSE.** The more often a person visits a conventional primary care physician, the more likely he or she is to use complementary and alternative medicine.

2. **ALL THREE.** Although profound philosophical differences exist between the approaches, they share many characteristics.

3. **FALSE.** Under Health Canada's Natural Health Products Regulations, all natural health products require a product licence before they can be sold. Once a product has been assessed and granted market authorization by Health Canada, the product label must have an eight-digit product licence number preceded by the letters NPN (Natural Product Number) or, in the case of a homeopathic medicine, by the letters DIN-HM (Drug Identification Number-Homeopathic Medicine).

4. **FALSE.** Price is often the only difference. The generic version of a drug has the same active ingredient as the brand-name drug, but it may have different inactive ingredients.

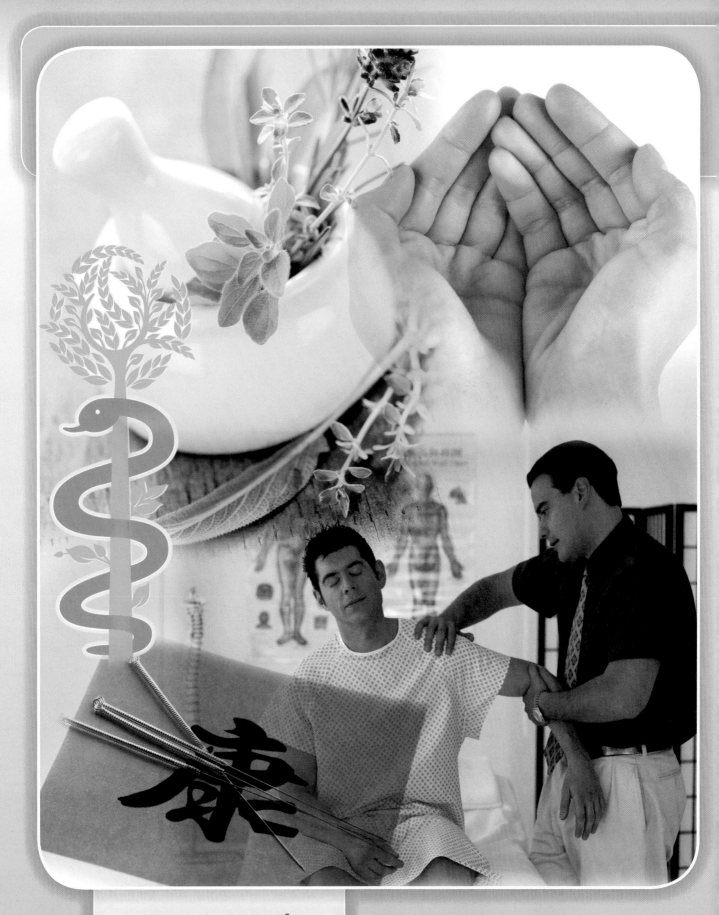

Jansen-van der Weide, M. C., et al. 2005. Granted, undecided, withdrawn, and refused requests for euthanasia and physician-assisted suicide. *Archives of Internal Medicine* 165(15): 1698–1704.

Kohara, H., et al. 2005. Sedation for terminally ill patients with cancer with uncontrollable physical distress. *Journal of Palliative Medicine* 8(1): 20–25.

Lipkin, K. M. 2006. Identifying a proxy for health care as part of routine medical inquiry. *Journal of General Internal Medicine,* 17 July [online early ed.].

London Health Sciences Centre. 2008. *Multi-Organ Transplant Program: Organ and Tissue Donation* (http://www.lhsc.on.ca/Patients_Families_Visitors/ MOTP/Organ_and_Tissue_Donation/index.htm; retrieved June 15, 2010).

Mayo Clinic. 2005. Advance directives: A plan for end of life. *Mayo Clinic Health Letter* 23(2): 6.

Melhem, N. M., et al. 2004. Traumatic grief among adolescents exposed to a peer's suicide. *American Journal of Psychiatry* 161(8): 1411–1416.

Natural Burial Co-operative. n.d. *Natural Burial in Canada* (http://natural-burial.coop/canada/; retrieved June 12, 2010).

Natural Burial Co-operative. n.d. *The Centre for Natural Burial* (http:// natural burial.coop/about-natural-burial/; retrieved June 10, 2010).

Onrust, S., et al. 2006. Predictors of psychological adjustment after bereavement. *International Psychogeriatrics,* 14 September, 1–15.

Oregon Department of Health and Human Services, Public Health Division. 2008. *"Death With Dignity Act" Annual Report: Year 9—2006 Summary* (http://www.oregon.gov/dhs/ph/pas/index.shtml; retrieved June 16, 2008).

Organ transplants. 2004. *Mayo Clinic Health Letter Supplement,* October.

Owen, A. M., et al. 2006. Detecting awareness in the vegetative state. *Science* 313(5792): 1402.

Patel, K. 2004. Euthanasia and physician-assisted suicide policy in the Netherlands and Oregon: A comparative analysis. *Journal of Health and Social Policy* 19(1): 37–55.

Pivar, I. L., and N. P. Field. 2004. Unresolved grief in combat veterans with PTSD. *Journal of Anxiety Disorders* 18(6): 745–755.

Rabow, M. W., J. M. Hauser, and J. Adams. 2004. Supporting family caregivers at the end of life. *Journal of the American Medical Association* 291(4): 483–491.

Rietjens, J. A., et al. 2004. Physician reports of terminal sedation without hydration or nutrition for patients nearing death in the Netherlands. *Annals of Internal Medicine* 141(3): 178–185.

Rietjens, J. A., et al. 2006. Terminal sedation and euthanasia: A comparison of clinical practices. *Archives of Internal Medicine* 166(7): 749–753.

Satel, S. 2006. Death's waiting list. *New York Times,* 15 May.

Schulz, R., et al. 2006. Predictors of complicated grief among dementia caregivers: A prospective study of bereavement. *American Journal of Geriatric Psychiatry* 14(8): 650–658.

Searight, H. R., and J. Gafford. 2005. Cultural diversity at the end of life: Issues and guidelines for family physicians. *American Family Physician* 71(3): 515–522.

Searle, J. 2010. Where there's a will (and maybe two), there's a way. *Canadian Business Journal* (http://www.canadianbusinessjournal.ca/legal/ march10_ legal/index.1.html; retrieved June 14, 2010).

Sepúlveda, C. et al. 2002. Palliative care: The World Health Organization's global perspective. *Journal of Pain and Symptom Management* 24(2): 91–96 (http://journals1.scholarsportal.info.proxy1.lib.uwo.ca:2048/tmp/ 6841733040255946677.pdf; retrieved June 14, 2010).

Shemie, S. D., et al. 2006. Brain arrest: The neurological determination of death and organ donor management in Canada. *Canadian Medical Association Journal* 174(6): S1–S12 (http://www.cmaj.ca/cgi/reprint/174/6/S1.pdf; retrieved June 14, 2010).

Siminoff, L. A., et al. 2006. Racial disparities in preferences and perceptions regarding organ donation. *Journal of General Internal Medicine* 21(9): 995–1000.

Organ Donation and Transplant Association of Canada. n.d. *The Organ Donation and Transplant Association of Canada* (http://www.organ donations.ca/ 62989%20Organ%20DTAC%20Bro_R3.pdf; retrieved June 14, 2010).

Organ Donation and Transplant Association of Canada. 2009. *Facts* (http:// organdonations.ca/facts; retrieved June 14, 2010).

Organ Donation and Transplant Association of Canada. 2009. *Become an Organ Donor!* (http://organdonations.ca/help/organdonor/; retrieved June 10, 2014).

Salvation Army. 2008. *Environmentally Friendly Burials* (http://www.salvation army.ca/2008/04/30/environmentally-friendly-burials/; retrieved June 11, 2010).

University of Toronto Joint Centre for Bioethics. *Living Will* (http://www. jointcentreforbioethics.ca/tools/documents/jcb_livingwill.pdf; retrieved June 15, 2010).

Washington State Department of Health. 2010. *Washington State Department of Health 2009 Death with Dignity Act Report* (http://www.doh.wa.gov/ dwda/forms/DWDA_2009.pdf; retrieved June 14, 2010).

Wijdicks, E. F., et al. 2006. Practice parameter: Prediction of outcome in comatose survivors after cardiopulmonary resuscitation (an evidence-based review): Report of the Quality Standards Subcommittee of the American Academy of Neurology. *Neurology* 67(2): 203–210.

Wilson, D. M., et al. 2009. The rapidly changing location of death in Canada, 1994–2004. *Social Science and Medicine* 68: 1752–1758.

BOOKS

Albom, M. 2005. *Tuesdays with Morrie: An Old Man, A Young Man, and Life's Greatest Lesson.* New York: Anchor. A young man reconnects with an old professor in his last months of life and learns some of the greatest lessons that life has to offer.

DeSpelder, L. A., and A. L. Strickland. 2009. *The Last Dance: Encountering Death and Dying,* 8th ed. New York: McGraw-Hill. A comprehensive and readable text highlighting a broad range of topics related to dying and death.

Shannon, J. B. 2006. *Death and Dying Sourcebook,* 2nd ed. Detroit: Omnigraphics. A wide-ranging discussion of topics relating to terminal illness, care for the dying, and the practical realities of death.

Turner, M. 2006. *Talking with Children and Young People about Death and Dying,* 2nd ed. London: Jessica Kingsley Publishers. A workbook designed to help parents explain death, loss, and grief to their children.

ORGANIZATIONS, HOTLINES, AND WEB SITES

The Internet addresses listed here were accurate at the time of publication.

The Dougy Center. Offers education about childhood bereavement and support groups for bereaved children.
http://www.dougy.org

Dying Well. A Web site focused on wellness through the end of life.
http://www.dyingwell.org

GriefNet. A site where you can communicate with others via email support groups in the areas of death, grief, and major loss.
http://www.griefnet.org

Grief Share. Offers group-based support to individuals who are grieving the death of a loved one.
http://www.griefshare.org

Growth House. Offers an extensive directory of Internet resources relating to life-threatening illness and end-of-life care.
http://www.growthhouse.org

Longwood College Library: Doctor Assisted Suicide—A Guide to Web Sites and the Literature. Information on physician-assisted suicide and links to related sites.
http://www.longwood.edu/library/suic.htm

Nolo Press: Wills and Estate Planning. Provides answers to questions about planning for death, from writing a basic will to organ donation.
http://www.nolo.com

On Our Own Terms: Public Broadcasting System. A companion Web site to the Bill Moyers PBS series on improving end-of-life care.
http://www.pbs.org/wnet/onourownterms

The following organizations provide information about organ donation and donor cards in Canada, as well as provincial or territorial information pertaining to organ donor requirements and registries.

Canadian Council for Donation and Transplantation
http://www.ccdt.ca
Canadian Association of Transplantation
http://www.transplant.ca
Canadian Society of Transplantation
http://www.cst-transplant.ca
The Organ Donation and Transplant Association of Canada
http://organdonations.ca
The Kidney Foundation of Canada
http://www.kidney.ca

Baxter, D., and J. Smerdon. 2000. *Donation Matters: Demographics and Organ Transplants in Canada, 2000–2040.* Vancouver: The Urban Futures Institute (http://www.lhsc.on.ca/Patients_Families_Visitors/MOTP/Organ_and_Tissue_Donation/Report46.pdf; retrieved June 10, 2010).

Bender, E. 2005. Palliative care. *Journal of the American Medical Association* 294(14): 1850.

Canadian Institute for Health Information. 2007. *Health Care Use at the End of Life in Western Canada.* Ottawa: CIHI.

Canada's Office of Consumer Affairs. 2009. *Canadian Consumer Handbook 2008–2009.* Ottawa: Industry Canada (http://consumer.ic.gc.ca/eic/site/oca-bc.nsf/vwapj/cchandbook2008_eng.pdf/$FILE/cchandbook2008_eng.pdf; retrieved June 11, 2010).

Canadian Press/Leger Marketing. 2001. *How Canadians View Paranormal Phenomena in This Halloween Season: Report* (http://www.legermarketing.com/documents/SPCLM/011022ENG.pdf; retrieved June 14, 2010).

Canadian Press/Leger Marketing. 2002. *Canadians and Death: Report* (http://www.legermarketing.com/documents/spclm/030113eng.pdf; retrieved June 14, 2010).

Canadian Red Cross. 2007. *Planning Your Legacy* (http://www.redcross.ca/article.asp?id=9043&tid=001; retrieved June 14, 2010).

Casarett, D., et al. 2005. Making difficult decisions about hospice enrollment: What do patients and families want to know? *Journal of the American Geriatrics Society* 53(2): 249–254.

CBC Digital Archives. 1993. *Sue Rodriguez and the Right-to-Die Debate* (http://archives.cbc.ca/politics/rights_freedoms/topics/1135/; retrieved June 15, 2010).

CBC News. 2008. *Green to the End: Environmentally Friendly Burials* (http://www.cbc.ca/news/goinggreen/green-burials.html; retrieved June 15, 2010).

CBC News. 2009. *Assisted Suicide: The Fight for the Right to Die* (http://www.cbc.ca/canada/story/2009/02/09/f-assisted-suicide.html; retrieved June 14, 2010).

Chochinov, H. M. 2006. Dying, dignity, and new horizons in palliative end-of-life care. *CA: A Cancer Journal for Clinicians* 56(2): 84–103.

Christ, G. H., and A. E. Christ. 2006. Current approaches to helping children cope with a parent's terminal illness. *CA: A Cancer Journal for Clinicians* 56(4): 197–212.

Collier, R. 2009. Euthanasia debate reignited. *Canadian Medical Association Journal* 181(8): 463–464 (http://canadianmedicaljournal.ca/cgi/reprint/181/8/463; retrieved June 14, 2010).

Smith Bucklin Corp. 2009. *Final 2007 Statistics and Projections to the Year 2025: 2008 Preliminary Data.* The Cremationist of North America 45(4): 6–15.

Donatelli, L. A., et al. 2006. Ethical issues in critical care and cardiac arrest: Clinical research, brain death, and organ donation. *Seminars in Neurology* 26(4): 452–459.

DuBois, J. M., and E. E. Anderson. 2006. Attitudes toward death criteria and organ donation among healthcare personnel and the general public. *Progress in Transplantation* 16(1): 65–73.

Field, N. P. 2006. Unresolved grief and continuing bonds: An attachment perspective. *Death Studies* 30(8): 739–756.

Gozalo, P. L., and S. C. Miller. 2006. Hospice enrollment and evaluation of its causal effect on hospitalization of dying nursing home patients. *Health Services Research,* 17 August [online early ed.].

GriefShare. n.d. *What Is GriefShare?* (http://www.griefshare.org/; retrieved June 10, 2010).

Harvard Medical School. 2005. Living wills and health care proxies. *Harvard Health Letter* 30(8): 1–3.

Health Law Institute, Dalhousie University. 2009. *Advance Directives* (http://as01.ucis.dal.ca/dhli/cmp_advdirectives/default.cfm?; retrieved June 15, 2010).

Health Law Institute, Dalhousie University. 2009. *Withholding and Withdrawal of Potentially Life-Sustaining Treatment* (http://as01.ucis.dal.ca/dhli/cmp_ww/default.cfm; retrieved June 15, 2010).

Ipsos Reid. 2006. *Canadians Willing to Donate Their Organs in the Case of Their Death* (http://www.marketwire.com/press-release/Canadians-Willing-to-Donate-their-Organs-in-the-Case-of-Their-Death-603162.htm; retrieved June 15, 2010).

- Loss of consciousness or seizure
- Stupor, drowsiness, or disorientation that cannot be explained
- Severe or worsening reaction to an insect bite or sting or to a medication, especially if breathing is difficult

If your problem is not an emergency but still requires medical attention, call your physician's office. Often you can be given medical advice over the phone without the inconvenience of a visit.

Self-Treatment

When confronted with a new symptom, many people try to find some pill or potion that will relieve or cure it. However, other self-treatment options are available.

Watchful Waiting   In most cases, your body itself can relieve your symptoms and heal the disorder. The prescriptions filled by your body's internal pharmacy are frequently the safest and most effective treatment, so patience and careful self-observation are often the best choices in self-treatment.

Nondrug Options   Nondrug options are often easy, inexpensive, safe, and highly effective. For example, massage, ice packs, and neck exercises may at times be more helpful than drugs in relieving headaches and other pains. Getting adequate rest, increasing exercise, drinking more water, eating more or less of certain foods, using humidifiers, and making changes in ergonomics when working at a desk are just some of the hundreds of nondrug options for preventing or relieving many common health problems. For a variety of disorders caused or aggravated by stress, the treatment of choice may be relaxation or other stress-management strategies (see Chapter 3 and the box "Expressive Writing and Chronic Conditions" on p. 578).

Self-Medication   Self-treatment with nonprescription medications is an important part of health care. Nonprescription or **over-the-counter (OTC) medications** are medicines that Health Canada, through the Food and Drug Act and the Therapeutic Products Programme, has determined are safe for use without a physician's prescription. More than 100,000 OTC drugs are on the market; about 60% of all medications are sold over the counter. During any six-month period, about two-thirds of Canadians use one or more OTC drugs.

Many OTC drugs are highly effective in relieving symptoms and sometimes in curing illnesses. In fact, many OTC drugs were formerly prescription drugs. More than 600 products sold over the counter today use ingredients or dosage strengths available only by prescription 20 years ago. However, with this increased consumer choice comes increased consumer responsibility for using OTC drugs safely. OTC drugs can be sold under a brand name, such as Tylenol, or in a generic form; generic drugs are the same as brand-name drugs in terms of quality, purity, effectiveness, and safety. Generic drugs have to meet the same Health Canada standards as their brand-name counterparts.

Consumers also need to be aware of the barrage of OTC drug advertising aimed at them. The implication of such advertising is that every symptom can and should be relieved by a drug. Although many OTC products are effective, others are unnecessary or divert attention from better ways of coping. Many ingredients in OTC drugs— perhaps 70%—have not been proven to be effective. And any drug has risks and side effects. The Drug Information and Research Centre is the leading Canadian provider of evidence-based drug information and the place to turn when you need information. See For More Information at the end of the chapter.

Follow these simple guidelines to self-medicate safely:

1. Always read labels and follow directions carefully. The information on most OTC and prescription drug labels appears in a standard format developed by Health Canada. Ingredients, directions for safe use, and warnings are clearly indicated, but if you have any questions, ask a pharmacist or another qualified health care provider before using a product. Your pharmacist and all health care providers should also know about all the OTC, prescriptions drugs, and natural health products you are taking. Use a chart, such as the one from Health Canada shown in Figure 19.1 on p. 579, to keep track of your medicines.

   The key to understanding and reading drug labels in Canada is learning about the Drug Identification Number (DIN). A DIN is a computer-generated eight-digit number assigned by Health Canada to a drug product before the drug is marketed. It uniquely identifies all authorized drug products sold in dosage form and is printed on the label of prescription and OTC drug products that are authorized for sale in Canada. The DIN identifies the manufacturer, product name, active ingredient(s), strength(s) of active ingredient(s), pharmaceutical form, and route of administration. Often, nonprescription and prescription drugs are packaged with what is called a monograph, a page containing detailed information for consumers.

2. Do not exceed the recommended dosage or length of treatment unless you discuss this change with your physician.

over-the-counter (OTC) medication   A medication or product that can be purchased by the consumer without a prescription.

Expressive Writing and Chronic Conditions

MIND/BODY/SPIRIT

The act of writing down feelings and thoughts about stressful life events has been shown to help people improve their health. In one recent study, people with asthma or rheumatoid arthritis were asked to write down their feelings about the most stressful event in their lives; they wrote for 20 minutes a day for three days. In follow-up exams four months later, nearly half of those who engaged in expressive writing experienced positive changes in their condition, such as improved lung function or reduced joint pain.

Investigators remain unsure why writing about our feelings has beneficial effects. It is possible that expressing feelings about a traumatic event helps people work through the event and put it behind them. The resulting sense of release and control may reduce stress levels and have positive physical effects, such as reduced heart rate and blood pressure and improved immune function. Alternatively, expressive writing may change the way people think about previous stressful events in their lives and help them cope with new stressors. What-

ever the cause, it's clear that expressive writing can be a safe, inexpensive, and effective supplement to the standard treatment of certain chronic illnesses.

What about the effects of expressive writing on otherwise healthy individuals?

Other studies have, in fact, found a similar benefit: People who wrote about traumatic experiences reported fewer symptoms, fewer days off work, fewer visits to the doctor, improved mood, and a more positive outlook.

If you'd like to try expressive writing to help you deal with a traumatic event, set aside a special time—15 minutes a day for four consecutive days, for example, or one day a week for four weeks. Write in a place where you won't be interrupted or distracted. Explore your very deepest thoughts and feelings and why you feel the way you do. Don't worry about grammar or coherence or about what someone else might think about what you're writing; you are writing just for yourself. You may find the writing exercise to be distressing in the short term—sadness and depression are common when dealing with feelings about a stressful event—but most people report relief and contentment soon after writing for several days. If you need help or guidance with expressive or journal writing, see For More Information at the end of the chapter.

---

3. Use caution if you are taking other medications or supplements, because OTC drugs and natural health products can interact with some prescription drugs. If you have questions about drug interactions, ask your pharmacist or another qualified health care provider *before* you mix medicines.

4. Try to select medications with one active ingredient rather than combination products. A product with multiple ingredients is likely to include drugs for symptoms you don't even have. Using single-ingredient products also allows you to adjust the dosage of each medication separately for optimal symptom relief with minimal side effects.

5. When choosing medications, try to buy **generic drugs**, which contain the same active ingredient as the brand-name product but generally at a much lower cost. (Brand-name and generic drugs are discussed in more detail later in the chapter.)

6. Never take or give a drug from an unlabelled container or in the dark when you can't read what the label says.

7. If you are pregnant or nursing or have a chronic condition, such as kidney or liver disease, consult your health care provider before self-medicating.

8. The expiration date marked on many medications is an estimate of how long the medication is likely to be safe and effective. If a medicine is more than a few years past its expiry date and you need to be certain that the medication is completely effective, buy new medication. You can dispose of old medicine by placing it in a sealed container with coffee grounds or cat litter, but the safest way to get rid of outdated medicines is to take them to a pharmacy or hospital. If you have any question about a medicine's expiration date, ask a pharmacist.

9. Store your medications and home medical care kit in a cool, dry place that is out of the reach of children (Figure 19.2).

10. Use special caution with Aspirin. Because of an association with a rare but serious problem known as Reye's syndrome, Aspirin or its generic counterpart, acetyl-salicylic acid (ASA), should not be used by children

TERMS

generic drug A drug that is not registered or protected by a trademark; a drug that does not have a brand name.

Use Medicines Safely

Use this chart to keep track of the medicines you are taking, including over-the-counter, natural health products and prescription drugs.

Name of Medicine	Dosage	Time when taken	Reason for taking

Family doctor's name: _____

Telephone number: _____

Name of pharmacy: _____

Telephone number: _____

Keep this chart up to date and share it with your doctor and pharmacist. Always use medicine as directed by your doctor or pharmacist. Know when to take it, how often, and for how long. Know when and under what conditions you should stop using a medicine, and what to do if you miss a dose.

Canada

FIGURE 19.1   Health Canada's medicine chart.   You can use this chart to keep track of the all the medicines you take. Make sure your pharmacist and all health care providers have a copy.

Source: Health Canada, 2005. Reproduced with the permission of the Minister of Health, 2011.

Closet
- Analgesic (relieves pain)
- Antacid (relieves upset stomach)
- Antibiotic ointment (reduces risk of infection)
- Antihistamine (relieves allergy symptoms)
- Antiseptic (helps stop infection)
- Fever reducer (adult and child)
- Hydrocortisone (relieves itching and inflammation)
- Decongestant (relieves stuffy nose and other cold symptoms)

Medicine Cabinet
- Adhesive bandages
- Adhesive tape
- Alcohol wipes
- Calibrated measuring spoon
- Disinfectant
- Gauze pads
- Thermometer
- Tweezers

FIGURE 19.2   Your home medical care kit.   A cool, dark, and dry place, such as the top of a linen closet, preferably in a locked container and out of a child's reach, is best for storing medicines. Showers and baths create heat and humidity that can cause some drugs to deteriorate rapidly. Use your bathroom medicine cabinet for supplies that aren't affected by heat and humidity.

Source: Lewis, C. 2000. Your medicine cabinet needs an annual checkup, too. *FDA Consumer*, March/April.

or adolescents who may have the flu, chicken pox, or
any other viral illness. Outdated Aspirin that has an
acidic odour should be discarded. Some people are
sensitive to the acidity of Aspirin; thus, some manufacturers coat Aspirin with an acid-resistant coating.
This means that the Aspirin is absorbed in the colon
rather than in the stomach. Enteric-coated Aspirin is
less potent than plain Aspirin and therefore perhaps
less effective among moderate- and high-risk patients
taking Aspirin daily to prevent heart attacks.

PROFESSIONAL CARE

When self-treatment is not appropriate or sufficient, you
need to seek professional medical care, whether by going
to a hospital emergency room, by scheduling an appointment with your physician, or by accessing some other
conventional health care. This system is a broad network
of professionals and organizations, including independent practitioners, health care providers, hospitals, clinics,
and public and private insurance programs.

In recent years, many Canadians have also sought health
care from practitioners of **complementary and alternative
medicine (CAM)**, defined as those therapies and practices

that do not form part of conventional, or mainstream,
health care and medical practices as taught in most Canadian medical schools and offered in most Canadian
hospitals. The most commonly used CAM therapies are
relaxation techniques, herbal medicine, massage, and
chiropractic (Table 19.1). People often use CAM therapies
in addition to their conventional medical treatments, but
many do not tell their physicians about it.

Consumers turn to CAM for a large variety of purposes
related to health and well-being, such as boosting their
immune system, lowering their cholesterol levels, losing
weight, quitting smoking, or enhancing their memory.
Studies suggest that people with chronic conditions,
including cancer, asthma, autoimmune diseases, and HIV
infection, are particularly likely to try CAM therapies. Despite their growing popularity, many CAM practices remain
controversial, and individuals need to be especially aware
of safety issues. In Canada, CAM products are regulated
by Health Canada's Natural Health Products division; in
2005, a nationwide survey administered by this division
determined that 71% of Canadians regularly take what
have become known as natural health products (NHPs):

- Vitamins and minerals
- Herbal remedies
- Homeopathic medicines
- Traditional medicines, such as traditional Chinese
  medicines (TCM)
- Probiotics
- Other products, such as amino acids and essential
  fatty acids

Through the Natural Health Products Directorate,
Health Canada ensures that all Canadians have ready access
to natural health products that are safe, effective, and of
high quality, while respecting freedom of choice and philosophical and cultural diversity. NHPs must be safe for
use as OTC products and not require a prescription to be
sold. Products requiring a prescription continue to be regulated under the Canadian Food and Drug Regulations. As
for specific CAM therapies, although some CAM practitioners are either regulated (e.g., chiropractors) or not
regulated (e.g., herbalists, homeopaths) in all provinces
and territories, others (e.g., naturopathic practitioners,
acupuncture/TCM practitioners) are regulated in some

Table 19.1 Demographics of Users of Complementary and Alternative Medicine in Canada and the United States

	Canada No. (%)	United States No. (%)
	70,884 (100)	16,400 (100)
Age, y		
15–19	4,449 (6)	1,590 (10)
20–44	34,053 (48)	8,026 (49)
45–64	19,019 (27)	4,339 (27)
≥65	13,363 (19)	2,445 (15)
Male	32,981 (47)	7,709 (47)
White	65,642 (93)	13,486 (82)
High school or higher	50,520 (72)	12,010 (74)
Residence[a]		
East	3,389 (5)	8,903 (54)
Central	40,128 (57)	3,569 (22)
West	27,367 (39)	3,687 (23)
Health status		
Excellent	16,437 (23)	4,951 (30)
Very good	26,988 (38)	4,872 (30)
Good	19,152 (27)	4,117 (25)
Fair	6,237 (9)	1,742 (11)
Poor	2,070 (3)	658 (4)
Problem with instrumental ADLs	8,282 (12)	632 (4)
Problem with ADLs	1,682 (2)	316 (2)
Service use in past 12 months		
MD/DO	56,035 (79)	10,894 (66)
Acupuncturist	800 (1)	101 (1)
Chiropractor	9,074 (13)	573 (4)
Homeopath/naturopath	906 (1)	73 (0.4)
Massage therapist	2,290 (3)	318 (2)
Any CAM provider	11,400 (16)	862 (5)
Only physician (MD or DO)	48,168 (68)	10,316 (63)
Only CAM provider	1,412 (2)	133 (1)
Both CAM and physician	9,979 (14)	729 (4)

Source: McFarland, B., et. al. 2002. Complementary and alternative medicine use in Canada and the United States. *American Journal of Public Health* 92(10): 1616–1618, Table 1, p. 1617 (retrieved from http://ajph.aphapublications.org/cgi/content/full/92/10/1616, May 31, 2011).

Note: ADLs = activities of daily living; CAM = complementary and alternative medicine (acupuncture, chiropractic, homeopathy/naturopathy, massage therapy); MD = doctor of medicine; DO = doctor of osteopathy.

[a] East = Atlantic Canada (including Nunavut) and Northeast and South U.S. census divisions; Central = Quebec and Ontario and Midwest U.S. census division; West = remaining Canadian provinces and territories and Western U.S. census division.

jurisdictions but not others. For Canadians seeking such therapies, this means that **evidence-based practice,** decision making, and decision analysis are very important (see the box "Evaluating Health News" on p. 584).

In the next sections of this chapter, we examine the principles and providers of both **conventional medicine**—the dominant medical system in North America and Europe, also referred to as standard Western medicine or biomedicine—and complementary and alternative medicine (also referred to as integrative medicine), paying particular attention to consumer issues.

CONVENTIONAL MEDICINE

Referring to conventional medicine as *standard Western medicine* draws attention to the fact that it differs from the various medical systems that have developed in China, Japan, India, and other parts of the world. Calling it *biomedicine* reflects conventional medicine's foundation in the biological and physical sciences.

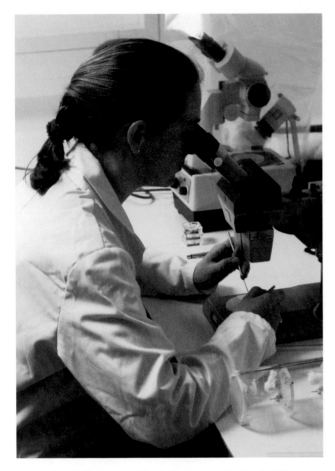

Conventional Western medicine is firmly grounded in scientific explanations resulting from the application of the scientific method to a question or problem.

Premises and Assumptions of Conventional Medicine

One of the important characteristics of Western medicine is the belief that disease is caused by identifiable physical factors. Western medicine identifies the causes of disease as pathogens (such as bacteria and viruses), genetic factors, and unhealthy lifestyles that result in changes at the molecular and cellular levels. In most cases, the focus is primarily on the physical causes of illness rather than on mental or spiritual imbalance.

Another feature that distinguishes Western biomedicine from other medical systems is the concept that every disease is defined by a certain set of symptoms and that these symptoms are similar in most patients suffering from this disease. Western medicine tends to treat illnesses as isolated biological disturbances that can occur in human beings, rather than as integral in some way to the individual with the illness.

Related to the idea of illness as the result of invasion by outside factors is the strong orientation toward methods of destroying pathogens or preventing them from causing serious infection. The public health measures of the nineteenth, twentieth, and twenty-first centuries—chlorination of drinking water, sewage disposal, food safety regulations, vaccination programs, education about hygiene, and so on—are an outgrowth of this orientation.

The implementation of public health measures is one way to control pathogens; another is the use of drugs and surgery. The discovery and development of sulpha drugs, antibiotics, and steroids in the twentieth century, along with advances in chemistry that made it possible to identify the active ingredients in common plant-derived remedies, paved the way for the current close identification of Western medicine with **pharmaceuticals** (medical drugs, both prescription and OTC). Western medicine also relies heavily on surgery and on advanced medical technology to discover the physical causes of disease and to correct, remove, or destroy them.

One technological innovation Canada will soon be implementing is the use of a health information highway. Infoway is a nonprofit organization that will collaborate with the provincial and territorial ministries of health, health care providers, and technology solution providers to accelerate the use of electronic health records (EHRs) in Canada. EHRs are secure electronic records of people's health history that can be accessed and shared through a network of client information management systems. With authorization from a patient, EHRs will enable health care professionals to view and update essential patient data, such as medications and X-rays and lab results. Some are skeptical about the use of this system, citing very real concerns about privacy issues for sensitive medical information.

Western medicine is based on the scientific method of obtaining knowledge and explaining health-related phenomena. Scientific explanations have these characteristics:

- *Empirical:* They are based on the evidence of the senses and on objective and systematic observation, often carried out under carefully controlled conditions; they must be capable of verification by others.
- *Rational:* They follow the rules of logic and are consistent with known facts.
- *Testable:* Either they are verifiable through direct observation or they lead to predictions about what should occur under conditions not yet observed.
- *Parsimonious:* They explain phenomena by using the fewest number of causes.
- *General:* They have broad explanatory power.
- *Rigorously evaluated:* They are constantly evaluated for consistency with the evidence and known principles, for parsimony, and for generality.
- *Tentative:* Scientists are willing to entertain the possibility that their explanations are faulty, based on new, better, or connected evidence.

The scientific method is both a way of acquiring knowledge and a way of thinking that involves approaching a problem by carefully defining its parameters, seeking out relevant evidence, and subjecting proposed solutions to rigorous testing.

Western medicine translates the scientific method into practice through the research process, a highly refined and well-established approach to exploring the causes of disease and ensuring the safety and efficacy of treatments. Research ranges from case studies—descriptions of a single patient's illness and treatment—to randomized controlled trials conducted on large populations.

The process of drug development is equally rigorous. Drugs are developed and tested through an elaborate course that begins with preliminary research in the lab and continues through trials with human participants, review and approval by Health Canada, and monitoring of the drugs' effects even after they are on the market.

When results of research studies are published in medical journals, a community of scientists, physicians, researchers, and scholars has the opportunity to read the findings and enter into a dialogue about the subject. Publication of research often prompts further research designed to replicate and confirm the findings, challenge the conclusions, or pursue a related line of thought or experiment. (For guidelines on how to interpret research when it is reported in the popular press, see the box "Evaluating Health News" on p. 584)

The Providers of Conventional Medicine

Since 1962, Canada has had a government-funded national health care system founded on the five basic principles of the Canada Health Act, namely, to provide a health care system that is (1) universally available to permanent residents, (2) comprehensive in the services it covers, (3) accessible without income barriers, (4) portable within and outside the country, and (5) publicly administered. Under this system, Canada's provinces and territories are responsible for administering their own health care plans and must provide residents with prepaid coverage for all medically necessary hospital and physician services. Coverage for other services, such as dental care, prescription drugs, optometric services, hearing aids, and home care, varies by province or territory. For example, Ontario has its own prescription drug plans, the Ontario Drug Benefit Program and the Trillium Drug Program, which help seniors and others in need with the high costs of prescription drugs. These differ from British Columbia's Fair Pharmacare Program and from Alberta's prescription drug plans, which are offered in conjunction with Blue Cross, a private insurer.

Conventional medicine is practised by a wide range of health care professionals in Canada. Several kinds of professionals are permitted to practise specific fields of medicine independently, including medical doctors, osteopath practitioners, podiatrists, optometrists, and dentists. Although every province and territory governs the qualifications and expectations of health care professionals, in general, health care professionals include the following:

- Registered nurses and registered psychiatric nurses
- Licensed practical nurses
- Medical laboratory technologists
- Medical laboratory technicians
- Respiratory therapists
- Medical radiation technologists
- Medical sonographers
- Audiologists/speech-language pathologists
- Physiotherapists
- Occupational therapists
- Dentists
- Dental hygienists and therapists
- Dental assistants
- Ergonomists
- Pharmacists
- Physicians

Medical doctors are practitioners who hold a doctor of medicine (MD) degree from one of 17 accredited Canadian medical schools. Their education in medicine has several stages: three to four years of premedical education in university, with an emphasis on the sciences; three to four years of medical school, which teaches basic medical skills and awards the MD degree; graduate medical study, called an internship, and residency and lasting from two to five years, during which a specialty (such as obstetrics) is chosen and studied and a medical licence is obtained. Medical certification and practice is regulated by each province and territory. MDs must pursue continuing medical education to keep abreast of advances in medical science.

Doctors of osteopathic medicine (DO) have received an undergraduate medical degree but their postgraduate training places special emphasis on musculoskeletal problems and manipulative therapy. MDs and DOs are the two types of "complete" physicians in the North America, meaning they are trained and licensed to perform surgery and prescribe medication. DOs are osteopathic graduates of medical schools, which emphasize training students to be primary care physicians and to practise a whole-person approach to medicine. According to the Canadian Osteopathic Association, despite a variety of business Web sites promoting training and certification in osteopathy within Canada, no government-recognized or accredited colleges of osteopathy exist in Canada. Only

pharmaceuticals Medical drugs, both prescription and over-the-counter.

medical doctor An independent practitioner who holds a doctor of medicine degree from an accredited medical school.

doctor of osteopathic medicine A medical practitioner who has graduated from a medical school in Canada or an osteopathic medical school in the United States; osteopathy incorporates the theories and practices of scientific medicine but focuses on musculoskeletal problems and manipulative therapy.

TERMS

Evaluating Health News

Health-related research is now described in popular newspapers and magazines rather than just in medical journals, meaning that more and more people have access to the information. Greater access is certainly a plus, but news reports of research studies may oversimplify or exaggerate both the results and what those results mean to the average person. Researchers do not set out to mislead people, but they must often strike a balance between reporting promising preliminary findings to the public, thereby allowing people to act on them, and waiting 10–20 years until long-term studies confirm (or disprove) a particular finding.

All this can leave you in a difficult position. You cannot become an expert on all subjects, capable of effectively evaluating all the available health news. However, the following questions can help you better assess the health advice that appears in the popular media:

1. *Is the report based on research or on an anecdote?* Information or advice based on one or more carefully designed research studies has more validity than one person's experiences.

2. *What is the source of the information?* A study published in a respected peer-reviewed journal has been examined by editors and other researchers in the field, people who are in a position to evaluate the merits of a study and its results. Many journal articles also include information on the authors and funders of research, alerting readers to any possible conflicts of interest. Research presented at medical meetings should be considered very preliminary because the results have not yet undergone a thorough prepublication review; many such studies are never published. It is also wise to ask who funded a study to determine whether any potential for bias exists. Information from government agencies (Health Canada and provincial or territorial government agencies) and national research organizations (such as Ipsos-Reid) are usually considered fairly reliable.

3. *How big was the study?* A study involving many subjects is more likely to yield reliable results than a study involving only a few subjects. Another important indication that a finding is meaningful is having several other studies yield the same results.

4. *Who were the participants involved in the study?* Research findings are more likely to apply to you if you share important characteristics with the participants in the study. For example, the results of a study on men over age 50 who smoke may not be particularly meaningful for a 30-year-old nonsmoking woman. Even less applicable are studies done in test tubes or on animals. Such research should be considered very preliminary in terms of its applicability to humans. Promising results from laboratory or animal research frequently cannot be replicated in human study subjects.

5. *What kind of study was it?* Epidemiological studies (which deal with the study of the causes, distribution, and control of disease in populations) use observation or interviews to trace the relationships among lifestyle, physical characteristics, and diseases. Although epidemiological studies can suggest links, they cannot establish cause-and-effect relationships. Clinical or interventional studies or trials involve testing the effects of different treatments on groups of people who have similar lifestyles and characteristics. They are more likely to provide conclusive evidence of a cause-and-effect relationship. The best interventional studies share the following characteristics:

   - *Controlled.* A group of people who receive the treatment is compared with a matched group of people (called a *control group*) who do not receive the treatment. The matched control group may receive an inert placebo or an established active treatment.

   - *Randomized.* The treatment and control groups are selected randomly.

   - *Double-blind.* Researchers and participants are unaware of who is receiving the treatment.

   - *Multicentre.* The experiment is performed at more than one institution.

   A third type of study, meta-analysis, involves combining the results of individual studies to get an overall view of the effectiveness of a treatment.

6. *What do the statistics really say?* First, are the results described as statistically significant? If a study is large and well designed, its results can be deemed statistically significant, meaning there is less than a 5% chance that the findings resulted from chance. Second, are the results stated in terms of relative or absolute risk? Many findings are reported in terms of relative risk—how a particular treatment or condition affects a person's disease risk. Consider the following examples of relative risk:

   - According to some estimates, taking estrogen without progesterone can increase a postmenopausal woman's risk of dying from endometrial cancer by 233%.

   - Giving AZT to HIV-infected pregnant women reduces prenatal transmission of HIV by about 90%.

   The first of these findings seems far more dramatic than the second—until you also consider absolute risk, the actual risk of the illness in the population being considered. The absolute risk of endometrial cancer is 0.3%; a 233% increase based on the effects of estrogen raises it to 1%, a change of 0.7%. Without treatment, about 25% of infants born to HIV-infected women will be infected with HIV; with treatment, the absolute risk drops to about 2%, a change of 23%. Because the absolute risk of an HIV-infected mother passing the virus to her infant (25%) is so much greater than a woman's risk of developing endometrial cancer (0.3%), a smaller change in relative risk translates into a much greater change in absolute risk.

7. *Is new health advice being offered?* If the media report new guidelines for health behaviour or medical treatment, examine the source. Government agencies and national research foundations usually consider a great deal of evidence before offering health advice. Above all, use common sense, and check with your physician before making a major change in your health habits based on news reports.

graduates of American colleges of osteopathic medicine accredited by the Canadian and American Osteopathic Associations are eligible for licensure in Canada. Some Canadian osteopaths are nonphysicians who practise osteopathic manual manipulation after graduation, with a diploma in osteopathic manual practice or DO(MP), from the Canadian College of Osteopathy, which has campuses in Toronto, Vancouver, and Halifax.

Podiatrists are practitioners who specialize in the medical and surgical care of the feet. In Canada, the only podiatric medical training is via the Michener Institute for Applied Health Sciences in Toronto. Graduates are called podiatrists or chiropodists (a primary care professional practising podiatric medicine who specializes in the assessment, management, and prevention of diseases and disorders of the foot), and they hold an advanced diploma of health sciences (podiatric medicine). In the United States, eight colleges and universities grant a doctor of podiatric medicine (DPM) degree; the length of training is similar to that of MDs. DPMs can prescribe drugs, perform surgery on the feet, and be licensed to practise in any province and territory in Canada.

Optometrists are primary health care providers trained to examine the eyes, detect eye diseases, and treat vision problems. Prospective optometrists must complete at least three years of prerequisite college or university courses, including those in mathematics and the physical and biological sciences, as well as a four- or five-year university doctor of optometry (OD) degree. To practise, graduates of the OD program must then satisfy the licensing requirements of a provincial or territorial college of optometry. Included in these requirements are the successful completion of a national examination (except in Quebec) and, typically, a province- or territory-specific jurisprudence examination. Canada has only two schools of optometry: one in Waterloo, Ontario, and one in Montreal, Quebec. Canadian optometrists are permitted to prescribe therapeutic pharmaceutical agents (drugs) in only seven jurisdictions nationally. Note that ophthalmologists have an MD followed by a specialization in ophthalmology; in essence, they are eye specialists who care for all types of eye problems and can perform eye surgery. An optician is a specialist in fitting eyeglasses and making lenses to correct vision problems. An optometrist performs eye examinations and writes prescriptions for corrective lenses; an optician fills that prescription.

Dentists specialize in oral hygiene, typically the care of the teeth and mouth. They are graduates of four-year dental schools in seven Canadian provinces and hold a doctor of dental surgery (DDS) degree; specialists (such as endodontists) receive additional education. Dentists can perform surgery and prescribe drugs within the scope of their training. Dental hygienists and dental assistants are trained dental professionals who are granted diplomas from a variety of community colleges and programs across the country.

In addition to these practitioners, millions of other trained health care professionals, known as **allied health care providers**, work in Canada. Some of them are licensed to work independently; others are permitted to work under medical supervision or medical referral. They include registered nurses (RNs), licensed vocational nurses (LVNs), physical therapists, social workers, registered dietitians (RDs), nurse practitioners, and certified nurse midwives.

Choosing a Primary Care Physician

Most experts believe it is best to have a primary care physician, someone who gets to know you, who coordinates your medical care, and who refers you to specialists when you need them. Primary care physicians include those certified in family practice, internal medicine, pediatrics, and gynecology. These physicians are able to diagnose and treat the vast majority of common health problems; they also provide many preventive health services. The best time to look for a physician is before you are sick.

At all ages, it is important for both men and women to obtain recommended health care screenings and immunizations. Preventive care throughout life is important to maximize wellness.

To select a physician, begin by making a list of possible choices. If your insurance, beyond Canada's national health care system, limits the type of health care providers you can see, check the plan's list first. Ask for recommendations from family, friends, co-workers, local medical societies, and the physician referral service at a local clinic or hospital. Some clinics provide brief biographies of physicians on staff who are taking new patients. If you have a particular health problem, you may want to identify physicians who are board-certified in appropriate specialties. In Canada, only the Royal College of Physicians and Surgeons can certify physicians and surgeons in medical specialties. When you have a list of possible physicians, find out if a consumer or other independent group has rated doctors in your area; this will help you check on the quality of care they provide.

Once you have the names of a few physicians you might want to try, call their offices to find out more information, such as the following:

- Is the physician accepting new patients?

podiatrist A practitioner who holds a doctor of podiatric medicine degree and specializes in the medical and surgical care of the feet.

optometrist A practitioner who holds a doctor of optometry degree and is trained to examine the eyes, detect eye diseases, and prescribe corrective lenses.

dentist A practitioner who holds a doctor of medical dentistry degree and who specializes in the prevention and treatment of diseases and injuries of the teeth, mouth, and jaws.

allied health care providers Health care professionals who typically provide services under the supervision or control of independent practitioners.

TERMS

- What are the office hours, and when is the physician or office staff available? What do patients do if they need urgent care or have an emergency?
- Which hospitals does the physician use?
- How many other physicians are available to cover when he or she isn't available, and who are they?
- How long does it usually take to get a routine appointment?
- Does the office send reminders about preventive tests, such as Pap tests?
- Does the physician (or a nurse or physician assistant) give advice over the phone for common problems?

Schedule a visit with the physician you think you would most like to use. During that first visit, you'll get a sense of how well matched you are and how well he or she might meet your medical needs. In 2002, Canadians made about 309 million visits to office-based physicians. Typically, females are viewed as more likely than males to visit a health care provider. Reproductive health care needs may be one reason for the difference, with women making doctor visits related to prenatal care and childbirth. Women of reproductive age may also need to make health care visits to obtain prescription contraceptives and have the necessary pelvic exam and Pap test. However, recent evidence in Canada suggests that physician visits and hospitalizations are comparable for both sexes when rates are adjusted to exclude reproductive issues.

Getting the Most Out of Your Medical Care

The key to making the health care system work for you lies in good communication with your physician and other members of the health care team. Studies show that patients who interact more with physicians and ask more questions enjoy better health outcomes. Canada's EHR system should help with cross-practitioner sharing of health information.

The Physician-Patient Partnership The physician-patient relationship is undergoing an important transformation. The image of the all-knowing physician and the passive patient is fading. What is emerging is a physician-patient *partnership*, in which the physician acts more like a consultant and the patient participates more actively. You should expect your physician to be attentive, caring, and able to listen and clearly explain things to you. You also must do your part. You need to be assertive in a firm but nonaggressive manner. You need to express your feelings and concerns, ask questions and, if necessary, be persistent. If your physician is unable to communicate clearly with you despite your best efforts, you probably need to change physicians.

Your Appointment with Your Physician Physicians are often pressed for time, so prepare for your visit ahead of time. Make a written list of your key concerns and questions, along with notes about your symptoms (when

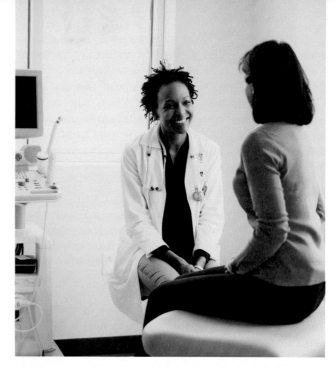

Good communication is a crucial factor in an effective physician-patient partnership.

they started, how long they last, what makes them better or worse, what treatments you have already tried, and so on). If you have questions you're uncomfortable about asking, practise discussing them ahead of time. Bring a list of all the medications you're taking—prescription, nonprescription, and herbal. Also bring any medical records or test results your physician may not already have.

Present your concerns at the beginning of the visit, to set the agenda. Be specific and concise about your symptoms, and be open and honest about your concerns. Share your hunches with your physician—your guesses can provide vital clues. Ask questions if you don't understand something. Let your physician know if you are taking any drugs, are allergic to any medications, are breastfeeding, or may be pregnant.

At the end of the visit, briefly repeat the physician's diagnosis, prognosis, and instructions. Make sure you understand your next steps, such as making another appointment, phoning for test results, watching for new symptoms, and so on. You may also want to ask about the possibility of using email for follow-up.

The Diagnostic Process The first step in the diagnostic process is the medical history, which includes your primary reason for the visit, your current symptoms, your past medical history, and your social history (job, family life, major stressors, living conditions, and health habits). Keeping up-to-date records of your medical history can help you provide your physician with key facts about your health (see the box "Personal Health Profile").

The next step is the physical exam, which usually begins with a review of vital signs: blood pressure, heart rate (pulse), breathing rate, and temperature. Depending

Personal Health Profile

General Information

Age: _____   Total cholesterol: _____   Blood pressure: _____/_____   Other: _____

Height: _____   HDL: _____   Triglycerides: _____   _____

Weight: _____   LDL: _____   Glucose: _____   _____

Blood type: _____

Medical Conditions

Check any of the following that apply to you and add other conditions that might affect your health and well-being.

_____ heart disease   _____ back pain   _____ depression, anxiety, or another psychological disorder

_____ lung disease   _____ arthritis   _____ major stressors

_____ diabetes   _____ allergies   _____ other injury or joint problem

_____ eating disorder   _____ asthma   _____ substance abuse problem

_____ other: _____   _____ other: _____

Medications/Treatments

List any drugs you are taking or any medical treatments you are undergoing. Include the name of the substance or treatment and its purpose. Include both prescription and OTC drugs and any vitamin, mineral, herb, or other dietary supplement you are taking.

_____   _____   _____

_____   _____   _____

Health Care Providers

Primary care physician: name _____   phone _____

Specialist physician: name _____   phone _____

   Condition treated: _____

Other health care provider: name _____   phone _____

   Condition treated: _____

To ensure that you get the most out of your medical care, you should also keep a record of your vaccinations and medical screening tests. Chapters 7–9 and 13 describe recommended vaccinations and screening tests for CVD, cancer, and STIs.

---

on your primary concern, your physician may give you a complete physical, or the exam may be directed to specific areas, such as your ears, nose, and throat.

Additionally, your physician may order medical tests to complete the diagnosis. Diagnostic testing provides a wealth of information to help solve medical problems. Physicians can order X-rays, biopsies, blood and urine tests, scans, and **endoscopies** to view, probe, or analyze almost any part of the body.

If your physician orders a test for you, be sure you know why you need it, what the risks and benefits of the test are for you, how you should prepare for it (for example, by fasting or discontinuing medications or herbal remedies), and what the test will involve. Also ask what the test results

mean, because no test is 100% accurate—**false positives** and **false negatives** do occur—and interpretation of some tests is subjective. Sometimes it is important to get a second opinion on a diagnosis.

TERMS

endoscopy   A medical procedure in which a viewing instrument is inserted into a body cavity or opening.

false positive   A test result that incorrectly detects a disease or condition in a healthy person.

false negative   A test result that fails to correctly detect a disease or condition.

Medical and Surgical Treatments Many conditions can be treated in a variety of ways; in some cases, lifestyle changes are enough. Make sure you know the possible risks and side effects of each treatment option, as well as the likelihood that it will improve your condition.

PRESCRIPTION MEDICATIONS In 2008, 453 million prescriptions were filled in the 10 Canadian provinces, up 7.1% over the previous year. That's about 14 prescriptions for each man, woman, and child in the country. Health Canada noted in 2002 that drug use among seniors was notably higher compared with the rest of the population; people over 65 take 40% of all medications dispensed. Thousands of lives are saved each year by antibiotics, insulin, and other drugs, but we pay a price for having such powerful tools. No specifically Canadian data are available regarding drug-related errors, also called *adverse drug events* or ADEs, but they do occur. ADEs happen for several reasons:

> QUICK STATS
>
> **Medications are given or prescribed in about 80% of physician office visits.**
>
> —Health Canada, 2003

• *Medication errors:* Physicians may overprescribe drugs, sometimes in response to pressure by patients (see the box "Medical Errors, Adverse Events, and Their Prevention"). Adverse effects can occur if a physician prescribes the wrong drug or a dangerous combination of drugs; such problems are especially prevalent for older adults, who typically take multiple medications. The risk of ADEs increases greatly with the number of medicines you take. At the pharmacy, patients may receive the wrong drug or may not be given complete information about drug risks, side effects, and interactions. Problems can occur because of a physician's poor handwriting, misinterpretation of an abbreviated drug name, or similarities between the names and packaging of different drugs.

> QUICK STATS
>
> **Prescription drug spending in Canada grew from 6% of total health care costs in 1977 to 14% in 2007.**
>
> —*Canadian Rx Atlas*, 2008

• *Off-label drug use:* Another potential problem is off-label use of drugs. Once a drug is approved by Health Canada for one purpose, it can legally be prescribed (although not marketed) for purposes not listed on the label. A recent study revealed that about 20% of medications are prescribed for off-label use; three-quarters of those prescriptions are made with little or no evidence supporting such use. Many off-label uses are safe and supported by some research, but both consumers and health care providers need to take special care with off-label use of medications.

• *Online pharmacies:* Although convenient, some online pharmacies may sell products or engage in practices that are illegal in the offline world, putting consumers at risk for receiving adulterated, expired, ineffective, or counterfeit drugs. Consumers should avoid sites that prescribe drugs for the first time without a physical exam, sell prescription drugs without a prescription, or sell medications not approved by Health Canada. You should also avoid sites that do not provide access to a registered pharmacist to answer questions or that do not provide a Canadian address and phone number to contact if there's a problem. Some online services, such as Canadian Pharmacy Online and Online Canada Rx, not pharmacies themselves but provide access to pharmacy services from licensed pharmacies. Many experts recommend that consumers use online pharmacies only to obtain medicines prescribed by their usual health care provider.

• *Costs:* International Marketing Services Health estimates that Canadians spent $21.4 billion on prescription medications in 2008, up from $20.2 billion in 2007. Consumers may be able to lower their drug costs by using generic versions of medications (the dispensed volume for generic drugs grew by 15% in 2008); by joining a drug discount program sponsored by a company, an organization, or a local pharmacy; or by investigating reputable mail-order or Internet pharmacies.

Patients also share some responsibility for problems with prescription drugs. Many people don't take their medications properly, skipping doses, taking incorrect doses, stopping too soon, or not taking the medication at all. Consumers can increase the safety and effectiveness of their treatment by reading carefully all prescription labels (Figure 19.3 on p. 590) and all fact sheets, brochures, or monographs that come with the medication. Whenever a health care provider gives you a prescription, ask the following questions:

• Are there nondrug alternatives?

• What is the name of the medication, and what is it supposed to do, within what period of time?

• How and when do I take the medication, how much do I take, and for how long? What should I do if I miss a dose?

• What other medications, foods, drinks, or activities should I avoid?

• What are the side effects, and what do I do if they occur?

• Can I take a generic drug rather than a brand-name one?

• Is there written information about the medication?

The Canadian Institute for Health Information estimates that $750 million in extra health care spending is attributable to medical errors, as are 23,750 deaths per year and 1.1 million days in hospital. The Institute of Medicine (IOM) defines a *medical error* as "the failure to complete a planned action as intended or the use of a wrong plan to achieve an aim," and an *adverse event* as "an injury caused by medical management rather than by the underlying disease or condition of the patient."

Medical errors take many forms, including surgical mismanagement, such as removal of the wrong breast in a mastectomy operation; misdiagnosis leading to incorrect therapy; misinterpretation of or failure to order diagnostic tests; failure to act on abnormal test results; equipment failure; blood transfusion injuries; misinterpretation of physician orders leading to use of the wrong drug or an incorrect dosage; and hospital-acquired infections.

Medication Errors

The U.S. Food and Drug Administration defines a *medication error* as "any preventable event that may cause or lead to inappropriate medication use or patient harm while the medication is in the control of the health care professional, patient, or consumer." Such events may be related to practice, including prescribing and order communication, or to product labelling, packaging, dispensing, administration, and use. In the absence of Canadian studies, extrapolation from U.S. data suggests that approximately 700 Canadians die each year as a result of medication errors.

Hospital Errors

Hospital-acquired infections are the fourth-leading cause of death in Canada. Each year 220,000–250,000 hospital-acquired infections result in 8000–12,000 deaths. Between 35% and 50% of these hospital-acquired infections are preventable. Most infections are caused by bacteria that normally inhabit the skin and mucous membranes. The most common infections involve the urinary tract, surgical wounds, the respiratory tract, and skin. Proper handling of equipment and frequent handwashing by providers are the major ways to avoid such infections.

Prevention within the System

Fortunately, most errors are preventable. Major system improvements proposed in recent report include the following:

- *The application of standardized procedure and equipment guidelines.* For example, the error rate in anaesthesia was cut by a factor of seven when standardized protocols and equipment were used.

- *Medical rounds that include a pharmacist.* Adding a pharmacist to the team, reduces medication error rates by 66%.

- *The use of computer technology and barcodes.* In one hospital, wireless computer technology and barcoding reduced medication errors by 70%.

In 2001, the National Steering Committee on Patient Safety was created in Canada. One of the recommendations of this committee was the establishment of the Canadian Patient Safety Institute (CPSI). In 2003, the federal government announced the provision of $10 million annually to support patient safety initiatives, including the formation of the CPSI. The mandate of the CPSI is to provide "national leadership in building and advancing a safer Canadian health system." The CPSI's flagship program, Safer Healthcare Now, endorses and promotes six interventions whose implementation has the potential to reduce mortality and morbidity:

- *Rapid response teams:* To prevent deaths in patients who are progressively failing outside the intensive care unit

- *Improved care for acute myocardial infarction:* To prevent deaths among patients hospitalized for acute myocardial infarction by ensuring the reliable delivery of evidence-based care

- *Prevention of ADEs:* To reduce ADEs by using a medication reconciliation process

- *Prevention of central line–associated bloodstream infection:* To reduce central venous catheter-related bloodstream infection and deaths from that infection by using two sets of interventions called the *central line insertion bundle* and the *central line maintenance bundle*

- *Prevention of surgical site infection (SSI):* To prevent SSI and deaths from SSI by using four interventions known as the *SSI bundle* in all surgical patients

- *Prevention of ventilator-associated pneumonia (VAP):* To prevent VAP and deaths from VAP and other complications in patients on ventilators by using a set of interventions known as the *ventilator bundle*

Studies show that most medical errors are system related and not attributable to negligence or misconduct by individual providers. Patient participation and empowerment may be the best defences against medical errors.

As a patient, you can take the following steps to prevent medical errors:

- *Take all medications exactly as prescribed, for as long as prescribed.* If you don't understand why you are being given a medication, ask your physician or pharmacist to explain.

- *If you require hospitalization, select your hospital carefully.* Research has shown that patients who choose a hospital with extensive experience treating patients with their condition can expect better results and fewer complications.

- *When being discharged from a hospital, ask about any special care, precautions, medications, and other procedures that will be required on returning home.* Studies show that physicians assume patients understand more about their discharge instructions than they actually do.

- *If you have doubts about the care you're getting, recruit a patient advocate.* Choose someone who can give support and speak on your behalf to protect your rights, promote your interests, and assist you in making decisions. An advocate can be a close friend or family member who is tactful and able to take accurate notes.

- *If you require hospitalization, rely on a hospitalist.* A *hospitalist* is a physician who specializes in the care of hospitalized patients. Hospitalists focus on advocacy and safety, and help remedy the lack of continuity that occurs among hospital providers. Hospitalists manage a patient's course through the hospital, coordinate the providers and consultants, and stay in touch with the patient's family and primary care physician. Hospitalists help remedy many of the problems that lead to medical errors.

Question		Answer
1.	What is the name of the pharmacy?	Manitoba Pharmacy
2.	What is the address of the pharmacy?	204 Manitoba Street, Winnipeg, MB, M2B 2Y2
3.	What is the store number of the pharmacy?	Store: #0001
4.	What is the phone number of the pharmacy?	Phone: 204-204-2004
5.	What is the prescription number?	Rx: #2042042
6.	What is the physician's name?	Dr. Manitoba

MANITOBA Pharmacy
204 Manitoba Street
Winnipeg MB M2B 2Y2 Canada
Store # 0001   Phone: 204-204-2004

R# 2042042   Ref:0   Dr. Manitoba
Toba Man
TAKE 1 CAPSULE THREE TIMES DAILY UNTIL FINISHED (ANTIBIOTIC)

APO-AMOXI 500MG
AMOXICILLIN 500MG
RED/YEL/ELLIP/APO{500}   **APX**
30 CAP   14 Oct 2012   Total: 21.43   00628123

EDS

KEEP OUT OF REACH OF CHILDREN

Tx #24242424

Important: Take this medication for the prescribed duration.

Question		Answer
7.	What is the date that the prescription was filled?	October 14, 2012
8.	What is the name of the person for whom the drug is prescribed? (Prescription drugs should be used only by the person for whom the drugs were prescribed.)	Toba Man
9.	What is the brand name of this drug? (Various manufacturers or companies may make the same generic drug but will call it by their own brand or trade name.)	APO-Amoxi
10.	What is the name of the medication or the main ingredient?	Amoxicillin is the generic name for the drug.
11.	What is the strength of the medication?	500 mg
12.	What do the letters APX mean?	The letters indicate the manufacturer's/company's code.
13.	What does the number listed below the company code represent?	This number indicates the Drug Identification Number (DIN).
14.	How much is in the package?	30 cap (capsules)
15.	What are the directions or instructions for taking the medication?	Take 1 capsule three times daily until finished (antibiotic).
16.	Are there any cautions or warnings on the label?	Important: Take this medication for the prescribed duration. Keep out of reach of children.
17.	Do prescription drug labels often include any additional information that is not on this one?	Expiry date, refill information, and additional information, on stickers, such as Take with food.

FIGURE 19.3   Reading and understanding prescription medication labels.

Source: Manitoba Education, Citizenship and Youth. *Grade 11 Active Healthy Lifestyles: Manitoba Physical Education Curriculum Framework of Outcomes and a Foundation for Implementation.* Winnipeg, MB: Manitoba Education, Citizenship and Youth, 2008. Reprinted with permission. All rights reserved.

Remember to store your medications in a cool, dry place, out of direct light. Never share your prescription medications with anyone else, and never use an old prescription for a new ailment.

WEB OR INTERNET HEALTH INFORMATION   It is important to approach Web-based health information with some skepticism. The information superhighway is a tremendous technological boon but information presented on the Internet may or may not be true. Here are important questions to consider before you accept any Web-based health information:

- Who runs this site?
- Who pays for this site?
- What is the purpose of this site?
- Where does the information come from?
- What is the basis of the information?
- How is the information selected?
- How current is the information?
- How does the site choose links to other sites?
- What information about you, if any, does this site collect and why?
- How does the site manage its interactions with visitors?

SURGERY   The number of surgeries performed in Canadian hospitals increased by 17% between 1995–1996 and 2005–2006, and by another 5% in 2007, according to the Canadian Institute for Health Information. In hospitals across the country, more surgeries are being performed in an **outpatient** day surgery setting (an increase of 31% over 10 years), while inpatient surgeries have decreased by 17% over the past decade.

If a health care provider suggests surgery for any reason, ask the following questions:

- Why do I need surgery at this time?
- Are any nonsurgical options available, such as medicine or physical therapy?
- What are the risks and complications of the surgery?
- Can the operation be performed on an outpatient basis?
- What can I expect before, during, and after surgery?

QUESTIONS FOR CRITICAL THINKING AND REFLECTION

What sort of relationship do you have with your primary physician? Do you think he or she really understands your needs and is familiar enough with your history? What could you do to improve this relationship? Does your primary physician support the integrated use of complementary and alternative forms of medicine?

COMPLEMENTARY AND ALTERNATIVE MEDICINE

Although *CAM* is the term commonly used in the Western world, some health practitioners instead use the term *integrative medicine* to capture the notion of conceptualizing medicine as allopathic *and* complementary or alternative. Compared with conventional or allopathic medicine, CAM implies the concept of *along with* rather than *instead of*. Some health care practitioners phrase the approach to medicine as a question: "Do we treat the disease or do we treat the patient?" But the difference is more subtle. While conventional Western medicine tends to focus on the body, on the physical causes of disease, and on ways to eradicate pathogens to restore health, CAM tends to focus on an integration of mind, body, and spirit in seeking ways to restore the whole person to harmony so that he or she can regain health. Conventional medicine is based primarily on science, and CAM tends to be based on healing traditions and accumulated experience.

Many alternative medical systems with long-standing traditions have concepts and theories of medicine that once were very different from those of conventional Western medical thought. Some people consider all of CAM quackery and tell you that you can recognize a quack by his or her use of pseudoscientific language. However, the use of some phrases, such as "bringing into harmony with nature" or "enhancing the flow of vital energy" does not necessarily mean that a practitioner is a quack; rather, it may reflect this practitioner's different concept of health and healing.

You might have heard that there are only anecdotal testimonials to support the value of many forms of CAM and that because such reports do not constitute scientific proof of effectiveness, they are meaningless. Although it is correct that anecdotes and testimonials are not, by the standards of clinical trials in the experimental method, scientifically reliable evidence, that does not mean that they are meaningless. What is called anecdotal evidence may actually be a form of case report, a valuable and standard form of study in which a researcher describes a single patient, his or her medical history, the treatments administered, and the outcome of the case. Still, case reports alone are not sufficient to prove scientifically the effectiveness of a medical treatment. Caution is in order when choosing any mode of treatment—conventional or unconventional—that has not been scientifically evaluated for safety and effectiveness (see the box "Avoiding Health Fraud and Quackery" on p. 593).

The National Center for Complementary and Alternative Medicine (NCCAM) in the United States conventionally groups CAM practices into five domains: alternative medical

outpatient   A person receiving medical attention without being admitted to the hospital.

TERMS

systems, mind-body interventions, biological-based therapies, manipulative and body-based methods, and energy therapies (Figure 19.4). It is impossible to discuss all of these forms fully in a single chapter. Instead, what follows is a general introduction to the types of CAM available and a brief description of some of the more widely used ones.

Alternative Medical Systems

Many cultures elaborated complete systems of medical philosophy, theory, and practice long before the current biomedical approach was developed. In fact, Western (or allopathic or conventional) medicine is only about 150 years old; some medical systems—the Indian Ayurvedic system, for example—have been practised for thousands of years and are the only systems available to a large proportion of the world's population. The complete systems that are best known in the North America are probably traditional Chinese medicine (TCM), chiropractic, naturopathy, and homeopathy. Traditional medical systems have also been developed in many other regions of the world, including North, Central, and South America; the Middle East; India; Tibet; and Australia. In many countries, these medical approaches continue to be used today—frequently alongside Western medicine and quite often by physicians trained in Western medicine. Today, about two-thirds of Canadians use some form of CAM each year.

Alternative medical systems tend to have concepts in common. For example, the concept of life force or energy exists in many cultures. In TCM, the life force contained in all living things is called *qi* (sometimes spelled chi). Qi resembles the *vis vitalis* (Latin for "life force") of Greek, Roman, and European medical systems, and *prana* of ayurveda, the traditional medical system of India. Most traditional medical systems think of disease as a disturbance or imbalance not just of physical processes but also of forces and energies within the body, the mind, the spirit, and even within the larger environment. In TCM, for example, the principle of balance is expressed as yin and yang, which are opposites yet complement each other; many apparent, natural dualities—dark and light, female and male, low and high, cold and hot—are viewed in Chinese culture as manifestations of yin and yang (respectively). Disease is seen a disturbance of qi reflecting an imbalance between yin and yang. Treatment aims at reestablishing equilibrium, balance, and harmony.

Because the whole patient, rather than an isolated set of symptoms, is treated in most comprehensive alternative medical systems, it is rare that only a single treatment approach is used. Most commonly, multiple techniques and methods are employed and are continually adjusted according to the changes in the patient's health status that occur naturally or are brought about by the treatment.

Domain	Characteristics	Examples
Alternative medical systems	Involve complete systems of theory and practice that have evolved independently of and often long before the conventional biomedical approach	Traditional Chinese medicine; Kampo; ayurveda (India); Native American, Aboriginal, African, Middle-Eastern, Tibetan, Central and South American medical systems; homeopathy; naturopathy
Mind-body interventions	Employ a variety of techniques designed to make it possible for the mind to affect bodily function and symptoms	Meditation, certain uses of hypnosis, prayer, mental healing
Biological-based therapies	Include natural and biologically based practices, interventions, and products, many of which overlap with conventional medicine's use of dietary supplements	Herbal, special dietary, orthomolecular,* and individual biological therapies
Manipulative and body-based methods	Include methods that are based on manipulation and movement of the body	Chiropractic, osteopathy, massage therapy
Energy therapies	Focus on energy fields within the body (biofields) or from other sources (electromagnetic fields)	Qi gong, Reiki, therapeutic touch, bioelectromagnetic-based therapies

Orthomolecular therapies are treatments of diseases with varying, but usually high, concentrations of chemicals, including minerals (e.g., magnesium), hormones (e.g., melatonin), or vitamins.

FIGURE 19.4   The five domains of CAM practices.

Avoiding Health Fraud and Quackery

According to the U.S. Federal Trade Commission, North American consumers waste billions of dollars on unproven, fraudulently marketed, and sometimes useless health care products and treatments. Various estimates indicate that 2%–10% of every health care dollar spent in North America is lost to fraud. In Canada, health care spending was $183 billion in 2009. That would mean that the real cost of health care fraud could be as much as $18 billion each year. These figures represent enough money to drastically revitalize Canadian medicare and purchase more than 3000 magnetic resonance imaging (MRI) machines. In addition, people with serious medical problems may waste valuable time before seeking proper treatment. Worse yet, some of the products they're buying may cause serious harm. Health fraud is a business that sells false hope. It preys on people with diseases that have no medical cure and on people who want shortcuts to weight loss or improvements to personal appearance.

To check out a particular product, talk to a physician or another health care professional and to family members and friends. Be wary of treatments offered by people who tell you to avoid talking to others. Check with the Better Business Bureau in Canada (http://www.bbb.org/canada/) or a local legal office to see whether other consumers have lodged complaints about the product or the product's marketer. You can also check with the appropriate health professional group. For example, check with the Canadian Diabetes Association or the Canadian Arthritis Network, if the products are promoted for diabetes or for arthritis. Take special care with products and devices sold online; the broad reach of the Internet, combined with the ease of setting up and removing Web sites, makes online sellers particularly difficult to regulate.

If you think you have been a victim of health fraud or if you have an adverse reaction that you think is related to a particular supplement, you can report it to the Canadian Health Care Anti-fraud Association. You can report suspected health or health care fraud anonymously. One self-appointed guardian against fraud and staunch advocate of conventional and allopathic medicine is physician Stephen Barrett; he monitors via his Web site, http://www.quackwatch.com, a wide variety of issues that he labels as quackery. Although his viewpoint is heavily based on the "truth" of the experimental method only, his evidence is worth considering in any health-related decision-making process.

Traditional Chinese Medicine Traditional Chinese medicine (TCM) is based on highly abstract concepts; a sophisticated set of techniques and methods; and individualized diagnosis, treatment, and prevention. No identical diseases exist in TCM. Two patients with the same diagnosis in Western medicine will get different diagnoses in TCM and will be given different treatments. In TCM, the free and harmonious flow of qi produces health—a positive feeling of well-being and vitality in body, mind, and spirit. Illness occurs when the flow of qi is blocked or disturbed. TCM works to restore and balance the flow of blocked qi; the goal is not only to treat illnesses but also to increase energy, prevent disease, and support the immune system. In TCM, diagnosis of each individual is a an extensive, fourfold process of inspection, listening and smelling, inquiry, and palpation; palpation is always the last part of the process.

Two of the primary treatment methods in TCM are herbal remedies and acupuncture. Chinese herbal remedies number about 5800 and include plant products, animal parts, and minerals. Herbal remedies, like everything else, have yin and yang properties. When a disease is perceived to be due to a yin deficiency, remedies with more yin characteristics might be used for treatment. The use of a single medicinal botanical is rare in Chinese herbal medicine; rather, several different plants are combined in very precise proportions, often to make a tea or soup. For example, a remedy might include a primary herb that targets the main symptom, a second herb that enhances the effects of the primary herb, a third that lessens side effects, and a fourth that helps deliver ingredients to a particular body site.

Acupuncture works to correct disturbances in the flow of qi through the insertion of thin needles at appropriate points in the skin. Acupuncture needles are blunted unlike hypodermic needles; that is, inserting an acupuncture needle is like inserting a knitting needle into a skein of wool; the knitting needle does not puncture the wool and so too the acupuncture needle rarely draws blood. Qi is believed to flow through the body along several *meridians*, or pathways, and people have 12–15 meridians and at least 2000 acupuncture points located along these meridians. The certified acupuncturist targets the acupuncture point, based on the diagnosis, and the needle actually moves through body tissue to the designated point. The traditional method consists of inserting the needle and leaving it in place for 20–40 minutes. Other means of stimulating acupuncture points include heat, pressure (called **acupressure**), friction, suction, laser, or

---

traditional Chinese medicine (TCM) The traditional medical system of China, which views illness as the result of a disturbance in the flow of qi, the life force; therapies include acupuncture, herbal medicine, and massage.

acupuncture Insertion of thin needles into the skin at points along meridians, pathways through which qi is believed to flow.

acupressure The art and science of applying physical pressure on certain acupuncture points.

TERMS

THINKING ABOUT THE ENVIRONMENT

Several forms of alternative medicine, such as traditional Chinese medicine, rely heavily on remedies made from plant and animal parts. Although millions of people claim that these remedies are beneficial, their production now threatens the very existence of several species. Here are some examples:

- Today fewer than 10,000 tigers live in the wild (and about 5000 are being raised on farms). Despite their dwindling numbers and status as an endangered species, hundreds of tigers are poached every year. The carcasses are sold to purveyors of traditional medicine, who use tiger body parts in some of their remedies.

- Only a few thousand rhinoceros live in the wild today, but they continue to be poached for their horns, which are prized by traditional healers. Rhinos are classified as "critically endangered" and will disappear within a few years unless they are protected.

- Other species, such as seahorses, musk deer, and bears, are being harvested at rates that may put them at risk of extinction soon.

For more than a decade, environmentalists and wildlife protection officials worldwide have been calling for practitioners of traditional medicine to either stop using endangered plants and animals in their remedies, or to support farming of these species as an alternative to harvesting them from the wild. Progress is slow, but according to many organizations, such as the International Fund for Animal Welfare, practitioners have started responding positively.

For more information on the environment and environmental health, see Chapter 21.

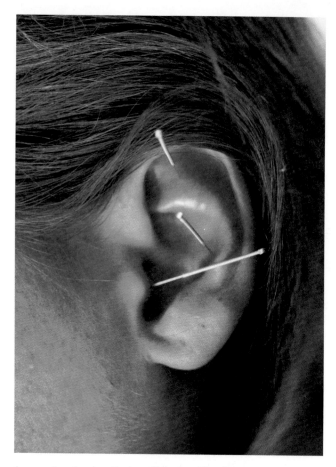

Acupuncture involves the insertion of needles at appropriate points in the skin to restore balance to the flow of qi.

QUICK STATS

About **54%** of Canadians have tried some form of CAM. Women are more likely than men to consult alternative practitioners.

—*National Population Health Survey,* **2001**

electric stimulation. The points chosen for acupuncture are highly individualized for each patient, and they change over the course of treatment as the patient's health status changes. In addition, acupuncture points are named, such as liver 12 or lung 7, but the names are not consistent with the anatomical location on the body. Lung 7, for example, is a site at the wrist.

The World Health Organization has identified more than 40 conditions for which acupuncture may be beneficial. At a recent conference called by the National Institutes of Health, a panel of experts analyzed the available infor-

mation on the scientific evidence for the efficacy of acupuncture in many of these conditions. These experts found evidence that acupuncture was effective in relieving nausea and vomiting after chemotherapy and pain after surgery, including dental surgery. Newer studies show that acupuncture may help relieve the painful symptoms of fibromyalgia and reduce the joint pain and stiffness of osteoarthritis. There is not yet enough evidence to show conclusively that acupuncture is effective for menstrual cramps, tennis elbow, carpal tunnel syndrome, asthma, or certain other conditions. Western researchers typically use a different framework for understanding the effects of acupuncture. For example, they might explain pain relief not in terms of qi but in terms of altering nervous system pathways and the release of hormones and neurotransmitters. Often, such explanations are framed in the context of anatomical acupuncture in efforts to add perceived Western precision to determining acupuncture's efficacy.

Very few negative side effects have been reported in conjunction with acupuncture. Nonetheless, problems can occur from the improper insertion and manipulation of needles and from the use of unsterile needles. If you consider acupuncture, you should ask your practitioner about the relative risks of the procedure and the safety practices he or she observes. Most provinces and territories regulate licensing for acupuncture practitioners, but requirements vary widely. Other regulated health care professionals, such as naturopaths, physicians, physiotherapists, chiropractors, dentists, and massage therapists, can perform acupuncture treatments when they fulfil educational requirements set up by their regulatory colleges. It is noteworthy that the school (philosophy and approach) and style of acupuncture differs depending on the training of the practitioner. TCM practitioners are trained at specific TCM-training colleges, such as the Academy of Clinical Chinese Medicine of Toronto, or at broad-based community colleges, such as the Grant MacEwan College in Edmonton.

Homeopathy   An alternative medical system of Western origin, **homeopathy** is based on two main principles: "Like cures like," and remedies become more effective with greater dilution. "Like cures like" summarizes the concept that a substance that produces the symptoms of an illness in a healthy person can cure the illness when given in very minute quantities. Modern vaccination is based on this same principle, although vaccinations are much more potent dosages than homeopathic remedies. Remedies containing very small quantities of a particular substance are obtained by repeatedly diluting the original solution. The extent of dilution varies, but the final extract is often so dilute that few, if any, of the original molecules are left in it. According to homeopathic thinking, such highly diluted extracts not only retain some form of biological activity but actually become more potent. As with all forms of CAM, the final dilution of remedy is based on the individual; therefore, it is very difficult to conduct scientific studies on one remedy when there is so much variation in dosage.

More than 1000 different substances (plant and animal parts, minerals, and chemicals) are used to prepare homeopathic remedies, and each of these substances is thought to have different effects at different dilutions. That means a homeopath must not only choose the correct remedy for a particular patient but also decide on the specific dilution of that remedy to achieve the desired effect.

As noted, and like other traditional systems of medicine, homeopathy constitutes a highly individualized form of therapy; that is, the treatment of each patient is determined by the overall condition of the patient rather than by specific signs and symptoms. To assess a patient's condition, homeopaths generally spend quite a bit of time talking with a patient and assessing his or her physical, psychological, and emotional health before deciding on the correct remedy at the proper dilution. This intensive interaction between the practitioner and the patient might play an important role in the success of the therapy. Indeed, critics of homeopathy often attribute its reported effectiveness to this nonspecific placebo effect (see the box "The Power of Belief: The Placebo Effect" on p. 596). However, when the results of 185 homeopathic trials were analyzed recently, it was concluded that the clinical effects of homeopathy could not be completely explained by the placebo effect. Homeopathy remains one of the most controversial forms of CAM.

Because of the extremely dilute nature of homeopathic remedies, it is generally assumed that they are safe. In Canada, the practice of homeopathic medicine is within provincial and territorial jurisdiction while the regulation of homeopathic medicines is federal. For example, in June 2007, Ontario passed the Homeopathy Act to regulate the practice of homeopathy. Homeopathic medicines, however, are regulated under the Natural Health Products Regulations, which came into force on January 1, 2004. These regulations are administered by the Natural Health Products Directorate branch of Health Canada. Remedies designed to treat many conditions, such as colds and headaches, can be sold over the counter; products that claim to treat serious conditions, such as heart disease, can be sold only by prescription.

Mind-Body Interventions

Mind-body interventions make use of the integral connection between mind and body and the effect each can have on the other. They include many of the stress-management techniques discussed in Chapter 3, including meditation, yoga, visualization, taijiquan, and biofeedback. Psychotherapy, support groups, prayer, and music, art, and dance therapy can also be thought of as mind-body interventions. In addition, the placebo effect is one of the most widely known examples of mind-body interdependence.

Some forms of **hypnosis** are considered to be CAM therapies. Hypnosis involves the induction of a state of deep relaxation during which the person is more suggestible (more easily influenced). While the individual is in such a hypnotic trance, the practitioner tries to help him or her change unwanted behaviour or deal with pain and other symptoms. Good evidence supports the effectiveness of relaxation techniques and hypnosis in reducing chronic pain stemming from a variety of medical conditions, although subsequent studies have cast some doubt on this conclusion. Hypnosis is sometimes used in smoking cessation programs and as a nondrug approach to anxiety disorders, such as phobias, and chronic conditions, such as irritable bowel syndrome. It has been shown to help some women deal with the pain of childbirth with less medication.

homeopathy   An alternative medical system that treats illnesses by giving very small doses of drugs that in larger doses would produce symptoms like those of the illness.

hypnosis   The process by which a practitioner induces a state of deep relaxation in which an individual is more suggestible; commonly used in cases of pain, phobia, and addiction.

TERMS

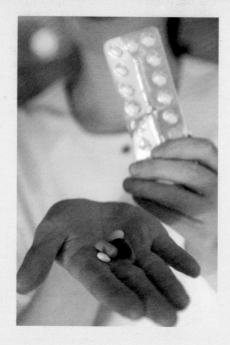

The Power of Belief: The Placebo Effect

A placebo is a chemically inactive substance or ineffective procedure that a patient believes is an effective therapy for his or her condition. Researchers frequently give placebos to the control group in an experiment testing the efficacy of a particular drug or other treatment. By comparing the effects of the actual treatment with the effects of the placebo, researchers can judge whether the treatment is effective.

The *placebo effect* occurs when a patient improves after receiving a placebo. In such cases, the effect of the placebo on the patient cannot be attributed to the specific actions or properties of the drug or procedure.

Researchers have consistently found that 30%–40% of all patients given a placebo show improvement. This result has been observed for a wide variety of conditions or symptoms, including coughing, seasickness, depression, migraines, and angina. For some conditions, placebos have been effective in up to 70% of patients. In some cases, people given a placebo even report having the side effects associated with an actual drug. Placebos are particularly effective when they are administered by a practitioner whom the patient trusts.

A clear demonstration of the placebo effect occurred in a recent study that examined the effectiveness of a drug used to treat benign enlargement of the prostate. The men who participated in the study were randomly assigned to one of two groups: One group received the medication; the other received a placebo, a look-alike dummy pill. More than half the men who got the placebo pills reported significant relief from their symptoms, including faster urine flow—despite the fact that men on the placebo actually experienced an *increase* in the size of their prostates.

How did the men in the study experience fewer symptoms despite no actual improvement in their condition? Researchers hypothesize that the patients' positive expectations of the medication's effects may have resulted in changes in nerve activity and muscle relaxation affecting the bladder, prostate, and urethra.

Studies on patients with depression and people with Parkinson's disease have found that treatment with an inactive placebo results in changes in brain function. Such changes in the electrical or chemical activity of the brain may help explain the placebo effect. Different forms of CAM are often criticized as being placebo-like in effect simply because the forms cannot be explained by the conventional scientific method. In efforts to counter this claim, studies have been done by using "sham" acupuncture; that is, a trained acupuncturist inserts needles in neutral points instead of normal treatment points; still, these studies are inconclusive at best.

The placebo effect can be exploited by unscrupulous people who sell worthless medical treatments to the scientifically unsophisticated public. But placebo power can also be harnessed for its beneficial effects. When a skilled and compassionate medical practitioner provides a patient with a sense of confidence and hope, the positive aspects of placebo power can boost the benefits of standard medical treatment. Whenever you swallow a pill, you swallow your expectations right along with the medication or herb; imagining how the pill is helping you can stimulate a positive placebo effect. Getting well, like getting sick, is a complex process. Anatomy, physiology, mind, emotions, and the environment are all inextricably intertwined. But the placebo effect does show that belief can have both psychological and physical effects.

Hypnosis can be used by medical professionals (MDs, DOs, DDSs) but is also offered by hypnotherapists. Physicians are certified by their own associations; however, hypnotherapy is not an insured physician service in Canada under the terms of the Medical Care Insurance Act of 1999. A certified clinical hypnotherapist must have a degree or advanced degree from an accredited university, be registered with a professional association approved by the province or territory where the hypnotherapist lives, and have a minimum of 50 class hours of training in hypnosis. There is little regulation of practitioners of other relaxation techniques, but it is very rare that adverse events result from such techniques. Many studies have shown that support groups, friendships, strong family relationships, and prayer can all have a positive impact on health.

Biological-Based Therapies

Biological-based therapies include substances derived from plant or animal origin. They consist primarily of herbal therapies or remedies, botanicals, extracts from animal tissues (such as shark cartilage), and dietary supplements. Herbal therapies are sometimes referred to as *materia medica*, Latin for "medical matter," a term that can include a much larger variety of compounds than just herbs (which are plants that die down at the end of a growing season and do not produce woody tissue). Some herbal remedies are not technically herbs; the leaves of the *Ginkgo biloba* tree are an example of a remedy commonly termed *herbal*. Other substances that constitute *materia medica* are algae, bacteria, fungi, and minerals. For traditional remedies that are of plant origin, many scientists prefer to use the term *botanicals*.

Herbal remedies are a major component of all indigenous forms of medicine; before the development of pharmaceuticals at the end of the nineteenth century, people everywhere in the world relied on materials from nature for pain relief, wound healing, and treatment of a variety of ailments. Herbal remedies are also a common element in most systems of traditional medicine. Much of the **pharmacopoeia** of modern scientific medicine originated in the folk medicine of native peoples, and many drugs used today are derived from plants.

A majority of botanical products are sold as natural health products, that is, in the form of tablets, pills, capsules, liquid extracts, or teas. Like foods, natural health products must carry ingredient labels (see Chapter 5). As with food products, it is the responsibility of the manufacturers to ensure that their natural health products are safe and properly labelled before marketing them. In Canada, the regulation of natural health products is governed and regulated by the Natural Health Products Directorate branch of Health Canada, and food regulations are regulated through the Canadian Food Inspection Agency.

Well-designed clinical studies have been conducted on only a small number of biologically based therapies. A few commonly used botanicals, their uses, and the evidence supporting their efficacy are presented in Table 19.2 on p. 598. Participants in clinical trials with St. John's wort, ginkgo, and echinacea experienced only minor adverse events. However, most clinical trials of this type last for only a few weeks, so the tests did not indicate whether it is safe to take these botanicals for longer times. They also didn't examine the effects of different dosages or how these therapies interact with conventional drugs.

Although most drug-herb interactions are relatively minor compared with conventional drug-drug interactions, some can be potentially serious. An example is the use of herbs that have anticoagulant (anticlotting) properties, such as ginkgo biloba, when used concurrently with the commonly prescribed anticoagulant Coumadin.

Studies have shown that most people do not reveal their use of CAM therapies to their conventional health care providers, an oversight that can have severe health consequences. Any herbs or drugs used in combination should be evaluated for safety by a knowledgeable health care provider, such as a pharmacist. See the box "Herbal Remedies: Are They Safe?" on p. 599.

Manipulative and Body-Based Methods

Touch and body manipulation are long-standing forms of health care. Manual healing techniques are based on the idea that misalignment or dysfunction in one part of the body can cause pain or dysfunction in that or another part; correcting these misalignments can bring the body back to optimal health.

Manual healing methods are an integral part of physical therapy and osteopathic medicine, now considered a form of conventional medicine. Other physical healing methods include massage, acupressure, Feldenkrais, Rolfing, and numerous other techniques. The most commonly used CAM manual healing method is **chiropractic**, a method that focuses on the relationship between structure, primarily of joints and muscles, and function, primarily of the nervous system, to maintain or restore health. An important therapeutic procedure is the manipulation of joints, particularly those of the spinal column. However, chiropractors also use a variety of other techniques, including exercise, patient education and lifestyle modification, nutritional supplements, and orthotics (mechanical supports and braces) to treat patients. They do not use conventional drugs or surgery.

Some **15%** or 4 million Canadians received chiropractic care in 2009.

—Chiropractic Canada, 2009

QUICK STATS

Chiropractors, or doctors of chiropractic, train for a minimum of four full-time academic years at accredited chiropractic colleges and can go on to postgraduate training in many countries. Although specifically listed by NCCAM as one of the manipulative and body-based methods of CAM, chiropractic is accepted by many health care and health insurance providers to a far greater extent than the other types of CAM therapies. Based on research showing the efficacy of chiropractic management in acute low-back pain, spinal manipulation has been included in most provincial and territorial guidelines for the treatment of this condition. In fact, electro-diagnostic tests show that chiropractic is effective in controlling back pain. Promising results have also been reported with the use of chiropractic techniques in treating neck pain and headaches.

A caution is in order regarding chiropractic: Spinal manipulation performed by a person without proper chiropractic training can be extremely dangerous. The

biological-based therapies CAM therapies that include biologically based interventions and products; examples include herbal remedies, extracts from animal tissues, and dietary supplements.

pharmacopoeia A collection of descriptions and formulas for drugs and medicinal preparations.

chiropractic A system of manual healing most frequently used to treat musculoskeletal problems; the primary treatment is manipulation of the spine and other joints.

TERMS

Botanical	Use	Evidence	Examples of Adverse Effects and Interactions
Cranberry (*Vaccinium macrocarpon*)	Prevention or treatment of urinary tract disorders	May eliminate and prevent bacteria from infecting the urinary tract	None known
Dandelion (*Taraxacum officinale*)	As a "tonic" against liver or kidney ailments	None yet	May cause diarrhea in some users; people with gallbladder or bile duct problems should not take dandelion
Echinacea (*Echinacea purpurea, E. angustifolia, E. pallida*)	Stimulation of immune functions; to prevent colds and flulike diseases; to lessen symptoms of colds and the flu	Some trials showed that it prevents colds and the flu and helps patients recover from colds faster	Might cause liver damage if taken over long periods of time (more than eight weeks); since it is an immune stimulant, it is not advisable to take it with immune suppressants (e.g., corticosteroids) or during chemotherapy
Evening primrose oil (*Oenothera biennis L.*)	Reduction of inflammation	Long-term supplementation effective in reducing symptoms of rheumatoid arthritis	None known
Feverfew (*Tanacetum parthenium*)	Prevention of headaches and migraines	The majority of trials indicate that it is more effective than placebo	Should not be used by people allergic to other members of the aster family; has the potential to increase the effects of warfarin and other anticoagulants
Garlic (*Allium sativum*)	Reduction of cholesterol	Short-term studies have found a modest effect	May interact with some medications, including anticoagulants, cyclosporine, and oral contraceptives
Ginkgo (*Ginkgo biloba*)	Improvement of circulation and memory	Improves cerebral insufficiency and slows progression of Alzheimer's disease and other types of senile dementia in some patients; improves blood flow in legs	Could increase bleeding time; should not be taken with nonsteroidal anti-inflammatory drugs or anticoagulants; gastrointestinal disturbance
Ginseng (*Panax ginseng*)	Improvement of physical performance, memory, immune function, and glycemic control in diabetes; treatment of herpes simplex 2	No conclusive evidence exists for any of these uses	Interacts with warfarin and alcohol in mice and rats, hence should probably not be used with these drugs; may cause liver damage
St. John's wort (*Hypericum perforatum*)	Treatment of depression	There is strong evidence that it is wort significantly more effective than placebo, is as effective as some standard antidepressants for mild to moderate depression, and causes fewer adverse effects	Known to interact with a variety of pharmaceuticals and should not be taken together with digoxin, theophylline, cyclosporine, indinavir, and serotonin-reuptake inhibitors
Saw palmetto (*Serenoa repens*)	Improvement of prostate health	Early studies showed that it may reduce mild prostate enlargement	Has no known interactions with drugs but should probably not be taken with hormonal therapies
Valerian (*Valeriana officinalis*)	Treatment of insomnia	Appears to help with sleep disorders	Interacts with thiopental and pentobarbital and should not be used with these drugs

Herbal Remedies: Are They Safe?

Consider the following research findings and advisories:

• St. John's wort interacts with drugs used to treat HIV infection and heart disease; the herb may also reduce the effectiveness of oral contraceptives, antirejection drugs used with organ transplants, and some medications used to treat infections, depression, asthma, and seizure disorders.

• Supplements containing kava kava have been linked to severe liver damage, and anyone who has liver problems or takes medications that can affect the liver are advised to consult a physician before using supplements that contain kava kava.

• In a sample of Ayurvedic herbal medicine products, 20% were found to contain potentially harmful levels of lead, mercury, or arsenic.

These findings highlight growing safety concerns about natural health products, which in 2010 had estimated sales of $ 1.4 billion in Canada.

Drug Interactions

Botanicals may decrease the effects of drugs, making them ineffective, or increase their effects, in some cases making them toxic. Most patients fail to tell their physicians about their use of herbal substances. Botanicals can also interact with alcohol, usually heightening alcohol's effects. Many manufacturers are offering new combinations of botanical preparations without empirical or scientific information about the interactions of the individual products.

Lack of Standardization

Natural health products must have labels that list the name and quantity of each ingredient. However, confusion can result because different plant species—with distinct chemical compositions and effects—may have the same common name. The content of herbal preparations is also variable. Botanicals are naturally grown products. Herb producers do not have complete control over natural processes any more than farmers have control over the vitamin content of fruit.

As an attempt toward standardization, herb producers have identified one or two substances that indicate quality; these substances should be listed on a product's label with their corresponding concentrations, lot numbers, and purity analysis data. Avoid any herbal product whose label is missing this information. Reputable retailers sell only products with this identifying information, and some send qualified inspectors to the site of production to verify the label information.

These self-imposed quality control measures have been adopted by reputable producers and retailers to increase consumer confidence and to help divert additional government-imposed regulation. Today, this level of disclosure and standardization is rarely seen in the production of healthy foods by the agricultural industry.

Canadian Chiropractic Association, listed in For More Information at the end of the chapter, can help you find a licensed chiropractor near you.

Energy Therapies

Energy therapies are forms of treatment that use energy originating either within the body (biofields) or from other sources (electromagnetic fields). Biofield therapies are based on the idea that energy fields surround and penetrate the body and can be influenced by movement, touch, pressure, or the placement of hands in or through the fields. **Qigong**, a component of TCM, combines movement, meditation, and regulation of breathing to enhance the flow of qi, improve blood circulation, and enhance immune function. **Therapeutic touch** is derived from the ancient technique of laying-on of hands; it is based on the premise that healers can identify and correct energy imbalances by passing their hands over the patient's body. **Reiki** is one form of therapeutic touch; it is intended to correct disturbances in the flow of life energy (ki is the Japanese form of the Chinese qi) and enhance the body's

healing powers through the use of 13 specific hand positions on the patient.

Bioelectromagnetics is the study of the interaction between living organisms and electromagnetic fields, both those produced by the organism itself and those produced by outside sources. The recognition that the body

energy therapies Forms of CAM treatment that use energy fields originating either within the body or from outside sources to promote health and healing.

qigong A component of traditional Chinese medicine that combines movement, meditation, and regulation of breathing to enhance the flow of qi, improve blood circulation, and enhance immune function.

therapeutic touch A CAM practice based on the premise that healers can identify and correct energy imbalances by passing their hands over the patient's body.

Reiki A CAM practice intended to correct disturbances in the flow of life energy and enhance the body's healing powers through the use of 13 hand positions on the patient.

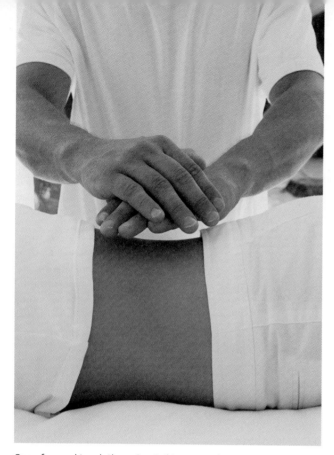

One of several touch therapies, Reiki massage has a spiritual, as well as physical, component.

produces electromagnetic fields has led to the development of many diagnostic procedures in Western medicine, including electroencephalography (EEG), electrocardiography (ECG), and nuclear magnetic resonance (NMR) scans.

Bioelectromagnetic-based therapies involve the use of electromagnetic fields to manage pain and to treat many conditions, such as asthma. Some indications suggest that the use of electromagnetic fields might be useful in the areas of bone repair, wound healing, nerve stimulation, immune system stimulation, and modulation of the neuroendocrine (nerve and hormonal) system. Although promising, the available research is still very limited and does not allow firm conclusions about the efficacy of these therapies.

Evaluating Complementary and Alternative Therapies

Because less information is available about complementary and alternative therapies, as well as less regulation of associated products and providers, it is important for consumers to take an active role when they are thinking about using them. It is difficult to appraise CAM methods by using research methods and standards that rely exclusively on traditional scientific, allopathic standards. Instead, decision analysis may provide a more practical framework for evaluating CAM. Decision analysis allows for an explicit estimate of how much evidence is enough evidence for decision making. To recommend a CAM therapy or treatment, the harmfulness of treatment must be lower than the harmfulness of the illness, multiplied by the probability that treatment will be successful. Thus, using decision analysis, we consider the effectiveness, potential harm, unintended side effects, and utility of any one therapy versus any other under consideration.

Working with Your Physician   If you are considering a CAM therapy, your first source of information should be your primary health care provider. Often, consumers are advised not to seek complementary therapies without first visiting a conventional health care provider for an evaluation and diagnosis of their symptoms. It's usually best to discuss and try conventional treatments that have been shown to be beneficial for your condition. If you are thinking of trying any alternative therapies, it is critically important to tell your physician to avoid any dangerous interactions with conventional treatments you are receiving. Areas to discuss with your physician or pharmacist include the following:

- *Safety:* Is there something unsafe about the treatment in general or for you specifically? Are there safety issues you should be aware of, such as drug-herb interactions?
- *Effectiveness:* Is there evidence-based research about the use of the therapy for your condition?
- *Timing:* Is the immediate use of a conventional treatment indicated?
- *Cost:* Is the therapy likely to be very expensive, especially in light of the potential benefit?

If appropriate, schedule a follow-up visit with your physician to assess your condition and your progress after a certain amount of time using a complementary therapy. Keep a symptom diary to more accurately track your symptoms and gauge your progress. (Some symptoms, such as pain and fatigue, are very difficult to recall with accuracy, so an ongoing symptom diary is an important tool.) If you plan to pursue a therapy against your physician's advice, you need to tell him or her.

For natural health products, particularly botanicals, pharmacists can also be an excellent source of information, if they are familiar with other medications you are taking.

Questioning the CAM Practitioner   You can also get information from individual practitioners and from schools, professional organizations, and licensing boards. Ask about education, training, licensing, and certification. If appropriate, check with provincial or territorial regulatory agencies to determine if any complaints have

TERMS

bioelectromagnetic-based therapies   CAM therapies based on the notion that electromagnetic fields can be used to promote healing and manage pain.

been lodged against the practitioner. Some guidelines for talking with a CAM practitioner include the following:

- Ask the practitioner why he or she thinks the therapy will be beneficial for your condition. Ask for a full description of the therapy and any potential side effects.

- Describe in detail any conventional treatments you are receiving or plan to receive.

- Ask how long the therapy should continue before it can be determined if it is beneficial.

- Ask about the expected cost of the treatment. Does it seem reasonable? Will your health insurance pay some or all of the costs?

If anything an alternative practitioner says or recommends directly conflicts with advice from your physician, discuss it with your physician before making any major changes in any current treatment regimen or in your lifestyle.

Doing Your Own Research You can investigate CAM therapies on your own by going to the library or doing research online, although caution is in order when using Web sites for the various forms of CAM. Erroneous information about CAM is rampant among unscientific and "pop" resources. A good place to start is the Cochrane Library, a research database for independent, high-quality evidence for health care decision making. Other excellent resources are Health Canada's Web site and the Natural Health Products Web site.

If possible, also talk to people with the same condition you have who have received the same treatment. Remember, though, that patient testimonials shouldn't be used as the sole criterion for choosing a therapy or assessing its safety and efficacy. Controlled scientific trials usually provide the best information and should be consulted whenever possible. The absence of documented danger is not the same thing as proof of safety. Quite often, people working in health food stores are only too willing to give advice and make recommendations, particularly about botanical products. Many of these people are not qualified to give this kind of advice. Ask about qualifications (training or education) before accepting recommendations from anyone. Perhaps more so than for any other consumer products and services, the use of CAM calls for consumer decision-making skills, critical thinking, and caution.

? QUESTIONS FOR CRITICAL THINKING AND REFLECTION
Have you ever considered using a complementary or alternative treatment? If so, was it in addition to conventional treatment, or instead of it? What kind of research did you do before having the treatment? What advice did your primary health care provider give you about it?

PAYING FOR HEALTH CARE

Health care spending in Canada reached $183 billion in 2009. Many factors contribute to the high cost of health care in our country, including the cost of advanced equipment and new technology, the expensive treatments for some illnesses, the aging of the population, the high earnings by some people in the health care industry, and the demand for profits by investors.

The Current System

Canada's national health insurance program, often referred to as medicare, is designed to ensure that all residents have reasonable access to medically necessary hospital and physician services, on a prepaid basis. Instead of having a single national plan, we have a national program that is composed of 13 interlocking provincial and territorial health insurance plans, all of which share certain common features and basic standards of coverage. Framed by the Canada Health Act, the principles governing our health care system are symbols of the underlying Canadian values of equity and solidarity.

The roles and responsibilities for Canada's health care system are shared between the federal and provincial or territorial governments. Under the Canada Health Act, our federal health insurance legislation, criteria and conditions are specified that must be met by the provincial and territorial health care insurance plans for them to qualify for their full share of the federal cash contribution, available under the Canada Health Transfer. Provincial and territorial governments are responsible for the management, organization, and delivery of health services for their residents.

Health Insurance

In 2007, out-of-pocket expenses by Canadians represented 15% of total health expenditure, or $23.4 billion. Private insurance accounted for 12%, or $19.5 billion. Thus, about 73% of total health care costs were paid by the provincial, territorial, and federal governments. Health insurance enables people to receive health care they might not otherwise be able to afford. Hospital care costs hundreds of dollars a day, and surgical fees can cost thousands. Health insurance is important for everyone, especially as health care costs continue to rise.

BEHAVIOUR CHANGE STRATEGY

Complying with Physicians' Instructions

Even though we sometimes have to entrust ourselves to the care of medical professionals, that doesn't mean we give up responsibility for our own behaviour. Following medical instructions and advice often requires the same kind of behavioural self-management that's involved in quitting smoking, losing weight, or changing eating patterns. For example, if you have an illness or injury, you may be told to take medication at certain times of the day, do special exercises or movements, or change your diet.

The medical profession recognizes the importance of patient adherence, or compliance, and encourages different strategies to support it, such as the following:

1. Use reminders placed at home, in the car, at work, on your computer screensaver, or elsewhere that improve follow-through in taking medication and keeping scheduled appointments. To help you remember to take medications:

   - Link taking the medication with some well-established routine, like brushing your teeth or eating breakfast.
   - Use a medication calendar, and check off each pill.
   - Use a medication organizer or pill dispenser.
   - Plan ahead; don't wait until the last pill to get a prescription refilled.

2. Use a journal and other forms of self-monitoring to keep a detailed account of health-related behaviours, such as pill taking, diet, exercise, and so on.

3. Use self-reward systems so that desired behaviour changes are encouraged, with a focus on short-term rewards.

4. Develop a clear image or explanation of how the medication or behaviour change will improve your health and well-being.

If these strategies don't help you stick with your treatment plan, you may need to consider other possible explanations for your lack of adherence. For example, are you confused about some aspect of the treatment?

Do you find the schedule for taking your medications too complicated, or do the drugs have bothersome side effects that you'd rather avoid? Do you feel that the recommended treatment is unnecessary or unlikely to help? Are you afraid of becoming dependent on a medication or that you'll be judged negatively if people know about your condition and treatment? An examination of your attitudes and beliefs about your condition and treatment plan can also help improve your compliance.

Practise and learn online with Connect. Connect allows you to practise important skills at your own pace and on your own schedule, with 24/7 online access to an eBook, practice quizzes, interactivities, videos, study tools, additional resources, and more.

SUMMARY

- Informed self-care requires knowing how to evaluate symptoms. It's necessary to see a physician if symptoms are severe, unusual, persistent, or recurrent.

- Self-treatment doesn't necessarily require medication, but OTC drugs can be a helpful part of self-care.

- Conventional medicine is characterized by a focus on the external, physical causes of disease; the identification of a set of symptoms for different diseases; the development of public health measures to prevent disease and of drugs and surgery to treat them; the use of rational, scientific thinking to understand phenomena; and a well-established research methodology.

- Conventional practitioners include medical doctors, doctors of osteopathic medicine, podiatrists, optometrists, and dentists, as well as allied health care providers.

- The diagnostic process involves a medical history, a physical exam, and medical tests. Patients should ask questions about medical tests and treatments recommended by their physicians.

- Safe use of prescription drugs requires knowledge of what the medication is supposed to do, how and when to take it, and what the side effects are.

- All surgical procedures carry risk; patients should ask about alternatives and get a second opinion from another physician.

- Complementary and alternative medicine (CAM) is defined as those therapies and practices that do not form part of conventional health care and medical practice as taught in most Canadian medical schools and offered in most Canadian hospitals.

- CAM is characterized by a view of health as a balance and integration of body, mind, and spirit; a focus on ways to restore the individual to harmony so that he or she can fight disease and regain health; and a body of knowledge based on accumulated experience and observations of patient reactions.

- Alternative medical systems, such as traditional Chinese medicine and homeopathy, are complete systems of medical philosophy, theory, and practice.

- Mind-body interventions include meditation, biofeedback, group support, hypnosis, and prayer.

- Biological-based therapies consist of herbal remedies, botanicals, animal-tissue products, and dietary supplements.

- Manipulative and body-based methods include massage and other physical healing techniques; the most frequently used is chiropractic.

- Energy therapies are designed to influence the flow of energy in and around the body; they include qigong, therapeutic touch therapies, and Reiki.

- Because less information available is about CAM and less regulation of its practices and providers, occurs, consumers must be proactive in researching and choosing treatments, using critical thinking and decision-analysis skills while exercising caution.

FOR MORE INFORMATION

BOOKS AND REPORTS

Chappell, N. L., and M. J. Penning. 2009. *Understanding Health, Health Care, and Health Policy in Canada: Sociological Perspectives.* Toronto: Oxford University Press. Examines topical issues, such as obesity, smoking, homelessness, AIDS, stress, and mental illness, from a sociological debate perspective and in the context of Canadian health policy.

Kliger, B., and R. Lee. 2004. *Integrative Medicine: Principles for Practice.* New York: McGraw-Hill. Integrates CAM with conventional medicine and is written primarily by physicians. This evidence-based and clinically authoritative guide often is used by family medicine and primary care providers.

Morgan, S., et al. 2008. *Canadian Rx Atlas,* 2nd ed. Vancouver: UBC Centre for Health Services and Policy Research. Provides the first-ever portrait of age-specific patterns of prescription drug use and costs across provinces. It breaks down nearly $20 billion in prescription drug spending by Canadians.

Romanow, R. (Commission on the Future of Health Care in Canada). 2002. *Building on Values: The Future of Health Care in Canada* (http://dsp-psd.pwgsc.gc.ca/Collection/CP32-85-2002E. pdf; retrieved June 1, 2011). Provides an important report of a comprehensive examination of health care in Canada. Its recommendations and findings reflect current thinking and initiatives about the future of health care in Canada.

Thompson, W. G. 2005. *The Placebo Effect and Health: Combining Science and Compassionate Care.* New York: Prometheus Books. Describes the placebo effect and how it may be used to benefit health.

Whorton, J. C. 2004. Nature *Cures: The History of Alternative Medicine in America.* New York: Oxford University Press. Provides a history of alternative medicine in the United States, including background information on many CAM therapies.

ORGANIZATIONS, HOTLINES, AND WEB SITES

The Internet addresses listed here were accurate at the time of publication.

CAMline. An evidence-based Web site on complementary and alternative medicine (CAM) for health care professionals and the public.
http://www.camline.ca

Canada Health Infoway. Information about electronic health records in Canada.
http://www.infoway-inforoute.ca/lang-en/about-ehr/what-is-ehr

Canada's Food and Drug Act. The statute about food, drugs, cosmetics, and therapeutic devices.
http://laws.justice.gc.ca/en/F-27/

Canadian Health Care Anti-fraud Association. Gives a voice to the public and private sector health care organizations interested in preventing fraud in the Canadian health care environment.
http://www.chcaa.org/report/

Canadian Chiropractic Association. Represents the chiropractic profession in Canada in collaboration with its provincial members.
http://www.ccachiro.org

Canadian Arthritis Network. The gateway to arthritis research and development in Canada.
http://www.arthritisnetwork.ca

Canadian Diabetes Association. Provides health care professionals and people with diabetes with education and services.
http://www.diabetes.ca

Canadian Institute for Health Information. A comprehensive site, in English and French, that provides information and resources for a wide variety of health issues.
http://www.cihi.ca

Canadian Patient Safety Institute. Performs a coordinating and leadership role across health sectors and systems, promotes leading practices and raises awareness with stakeholders, patients, and the general public about patient safety.
http://www.patientsafetyinstitute.ca

The Cochrane Library. A collaboration database for health care decision making.
http://www.thecochranelibrary.com

Drug Information and Research Centre. This site, owned by Ontario pharmacists, provides comprehensive information on evidence-based drug information for all of Canada.
http://www.dirc.ca

First Nations and Inuit Health Branch of Health Canada. A resource devoted to health issues and resources for Canada's indigenous populations.
http://www.hc-sc.gc.ca/ahc-asc/branch-dirgen/fnihb-dgspni/index-eng.php

Federal Publications Inc. A comprehensive listing of books, pamphlets, reports, and studies on health in Canada; covers the health care system, personal health, mental health, pregnancy and children, general issues, and statistical reports.
http://www.fedpubs.com/subject/health.htm

Health Canada Drug Product Database. Contains product specific information on drugs approved for use in Canada. The database is managed by Health Canada and includes human pharmaceutical and biological drugs, veterinary drugs, and disinfectant products. It contains approximately 18,000 products.
http://www.hc-sc.gc.ca/dhp-mps/prodpharma/databasdon/index-eng.php

Health Canada Compendium of Monographs. Helps speed the evaluation of the safety and efficacy of medicinal ingredients commonly used in natural health products. A monograph is a written description of particular elements on an identified topic.
http://www.hc-sc.gc.ca/dhp-mps/prodnatur/applications/licenprod/monograph/index-eng.php

Health Canada. The federal department responsible for helping Canadians maintain and improve their health, while respecting individual choices and circumstances.
http://www.hc-sc.gc.ca

International Association of Journal Writing. Promotes journal writing through expert advice, programs, and support.
http://www.iajw.org

Medwise Online. Advice on how to read Canadian OTC drug labels.
http://www.bemedwise.ca

Natural Health Products Directorate of Health Canada. Explains Canada's regulatory processes regarding vitamins and minerals, herbal products, homeopathic medicines and the like—products that have come to be known as natural health products.
http://www.hc-sc.gc.ca/dhp-mps/prodnatur/index-eng.php

Statistics Canada Health Data Tables and Maps. Database for almost all Canadian health indicators and measures.
http://www.statcan.gc.ca/pub/82-221-x/2008001/tbl-eng.htm

Quackwatch. Provides information on health fraud, quackery, and health decision making.
http://www.quackwatch.org

U.S. National Center for Complementary and Alternative Medicine. Provides general information packets, answers to frequently asked questions about CAM, consumer advice for safer use of CAM, research abstracts, and bibliographies.
http://nccam.nih.gov

SELECTED BIBLIOGRAPHY

Ernst, E. 2004. Prescribing herbal medications appropriately. *Journal of Family Practice* 53(12): 985–988.

Frazier, S. C. 2005. Health outcomes and polypharmacy in elderly individuals: An integrated literature review. *Journal of Gerontological Nursing* 31(9): 4–11.

Gan, T. J., et al. 2004. A randomized controlled comparison of electro-acupoint stimulation or ondansetron versus placebo for the prevention of postoperative nausea and vomiting. *Anesthesia and Analgesia* 99(4): 1070–1075.

Grzywaca, J. G., et al. 2008. Age-related differences in the conventional health care–complementary and alternative medicine link. *American Journal of Health Behavior* 32(6): 650–663.

Harden, B. L., and C. R. Harden. 1997. *Alternative Health Care: The Canadian Directory.* Toronto: Noble Ages Publishing.

Kaiser Family Foundation. 2005. *Trends and Indicators in the Changing Health Care Marketplace.* Menlo Park, Calif.: Kaiser Family Foundation.

Kondro, W. 2004. Canadian report quantifies the cost of medical errors. *The Lancet* 363(9426): 2059–2065.

Miller, F. G., et al. 2004. Ethical issues concerning research in complementary and alternative medicine. *Journal of the American Medical Association* 291(5): 599–604.

Progoff, I. 1992. *At a Journal Workshop: Writing to Access the Power of the Unconscious and Evoke Creative Ability.* New York: Tarcher.

Rappaport, K. (ed.). 1999. *Directory of Schools for Alternative and Complementary Health Care*, 2nd ed. Phoenix: Oryx Press.

Saper, R. B., et al. 2004. Heavy metal content of Ayurvedic herbal medicine products. *Journal of the American Medical Association* 292(23): 2868–2873.

Wahbeh, H., S. M. Elsas, and B. S. Oken. 2008. Mind-body interventions: Applications in neurology. *Neurology* 70(24): 2321–2328.

Practise and learn online with Connect.

PERSONAL SAFETY

LOOKING AHEAD >>>>>

AFTER READING THIS CHAPTER, YOU SHOULD BE ABLE TO

- Identify factors that contribute to unintentional injuries
- List the most common types of unintentional injuries and strategies for preventing them
- Describe factors that contribute to violence and intentional injuries
- Discuss different forms of violence and how to protect yourself from intentional injuries
- List strategies for helping others in an emergency situation

TEST YOUR KNOWLEDGE

1. **More Canadians are hospitalized each year through intentional acts of violence than through unintentional injuries (accidents).**
   True or false?

2. **You should not wear a seat belt because in a collision, your car might catch on fire or become submerged in water.**
   True or false?

3. **Your odds are greatest for being killed in which of the following?**
   a. a fire
   b. a fall
   c. a plane crash

4. **Talking on a cellphone while driving increases the risk of motor vehicle crashes.**
   True or false?

5. **About what percentage of sexual assaults against women are committed by strangers?**
   a. 15%
   b. 35%
   c. 65%

ANSWERS

1. **FALSE.** Far more people are injured each year through unintentional injuries than through intentional injuries. In 2004, 181,968 Canadians were hospitalized because of unintentional injuries, whereas 26,260 Canadians were hospitalized because of intentional injuries (suicide/self-harm or acts of violence).

2. **FALSE.** These kinds of crashes are rare, and the greatest danger is the impact that precedes them.

3. **B.** The odds of being fatally injured in a fall are estimated at about 1 in 200. The odds of being killed by fire are approximately 1 in 1167, and the odds of dying in a plane crash are 1 in 5552.

4. **TRUE.** Using a handheld or hands-free cellphone while driving decreases attentiveness and reaction time. A 20-year-old using a phone has the reaction time of a 70-year-old not using a phone.

5. **B.** In 2004, more than half of sexual assaults against women in Canada were committed by friends or acquaintances; 35% were committed by strangers.

Each year, thousands of Canadians die from injuries, and many more are temporarily or permanently disabled. In 2009, approximately one in seven (more than 4.1 million) Canadians ages 12 and older suffered an injury severe enough to limit their daily activities. The cost of injuries in Canada is high; in 2004, injuries resulted in 13,677 lives lost, more than 211,000 hospitalizations, more than 3 million emergency room visits, $10.7 billion in health care costs, and $19.8 billion in total economic costs. Injuries also cause emotional suffering for injured people and their families, friends, and colleagues.

Luckily, we can take many steps to reduce the risk of injuries. Engineering strategies, such as seat belts, can help lower injury rates, as can the passage and enforcement of safety-related laws, such as those requiring tamper-proof containers for over-the-counter (OTC) medications. Public education campaigns about risky behaviours, such as driving under the influence of alcohol or smoking in bed, can also help prevent injuries.

Ultimately, though, it is up to each person to take responsibility for his or her actions and make wise choices about safety behaviours. Many of the same sensible attitudes, responsible behaviours, and informed decisions that optimize your wellness can improve your chances of avoiding injuries. This chapter explains how you can protect yourself and those around you from becoming the victims of unintentional and intentional injuries.

DIFFERENTIATING INJURIES

Injuries can be intentional or unintentional. An **intentional injury** is one that is purposely inflicted, by ourselves or by another person. If an injury occurs when no harm is intended, it is considered an **unintentional injury**.

UNINTENTIONAL INJURIES

Unintentional injuries are the leading cause of death in Canada for people ages 1 to 44. Unintentional injuries include those related to motor vehicle crashes, falls,

drowning, fires, unintentional poisoning, sport, and other unintentional causes. (Note that public health officials prefer not to use the word *accidents* to describe unintentional injuries because it suggests events beyond human control. *Injuries* are predictable outcomes of factors that can be controlled or prevented.) Because unintentional injuries are so common, they account for more **years of potential life lost** than any other cause of death. In Canada, the greatest number of deaths occur in motor vehicle crashes, but the greatest number of hospitalizations occur because of falls (Table 20.1). In all these situations, the action you take can mean the difference between injury or death and no injury at all.

What Causes an Injury?

Most injuries are caused by a combination of human and environmental factors. Human factors are inner conditions or attitudes that lead to an unsafe state, whether physical, emotional, or psychological. Environmental factors are external conditions and circumstances, such as poor road conditions, a slippery surface, or the undertow of the ocean at the beach.

A common factor that leads to injuries is risk-taking behaviour. People vary in the amount of risk they tend to take in life; young men are especially prone to taking risks (see the box "Injuries Among Young Men"). Some people take risks to win the admiration of their peers; other people simply overestimate their physical abilities. Alcohol and drug use is another common risk factor that leads to many injuries and deaths.

Psychological and emotional factors can also play a part in injuries. People sometimes act on the basis of inadequate or inaccurate beliefs about what is safe or unsafe. For example, a person who believes that seat belts trap people in cars when a crash occurs and who therefore decides not to wear a seat belt is acting on an inaccurate belief. However, many people who have accurate infor-

---

TERMS

intentional injury An injury that is purposely inflicted, by either ourselves or another person.

unintentional injury An injury that occurs without harm being intended.

years of potential life lost The difference between an individual's life expectancy and his or her age at death.

motor vehicle injuries Unintentional injuries and deaths involving motor vehicles in motion, both on and off the highway or street; incidents causing motor vehicle injuries include collisions between vehicles and collisions with objects or pedestrians.

Table 20.1	Unintentional Injuries in Canada, 2004	
	Deaths	**Hospitalizations**
Motor vehicle incidents	3,067	30,932
Falls	2,225	105,565
Unintentional poisoning	944	7,060
Drowning	245	238
Fire/burns	233	2,002
Sport	<5	1,223
Other unintentional injuries	2,220	34,948

Source: SMARTRISK. 2009. *The Economic Burden of Injury in Canada.* Toronto: SMARTRISK, p. 2. Copyright 2009. ISBN 1-894828-50-X.

Injuries Among Young Men

Overall, rates of injury are highest among young adults and adults over age 65. Typically, injury rates are higher in males than in females—and the rate peaks among young adult males. In 2004, young men in Canada were particularly at risk of injury resulting from motor vehicle crashes, with those ages 20–24 experiencing the highest death rate, and those ages 15–19 experiencing the highest rates of hospitalization and permanent disability. Canadian men ages 25–64 were four times as likely as females in the same age range to die from a fall. With regard to intentional injuries, in 2004 Canadian males were almost three times as likely to die from suicide or self-harm as females, and males were also twice as likely as females to be killed as a result of violence.

Why do men, especially young men, have such high rates of injury? Gender roles may play a key part: Traditional gender roles for males may associate masculinity with risk-taking behaviour and a disregard for pain and injury, and risk-taking behaviour may be particularly common among young men. Men are more likely to drive dangerously, drink and drive, binge-drink, and use aggressive behaviour to control situations—all of which can lead to higher rates of fatal and nonfatal injury. Men may also have a lower perception of the risk of dangerous behaviours compared with women.

Traditional gender roles may also make it more difficult for men to admit to injury or emotional vulnerability. Physical injuries may worsen or become chronic if care is not sought promptly. Untreated depression can lead to suicide.

In addition, men may have greater exposure to some injury situations. Compared with women, men may drive more kilometres and be more likely to ride motorcycles, operate machinery, and have jobs associated with high rates of workplace injuries. They may be more likely to engage in sports and other recreational activities associated with high rates of injuries. Some researchers suggest that the male hormone testosterone may play a role in risky and aggressive behaviour. Differences in brain structure and activity may also influence how men and women respond to stressors and how quickly and to what degree they become verbally or physically aggressive in response to anger.

Further studies are needed to identify all the factors underlying excessive risk-taking among men and how these risk behaviours can be changed to lower the rates of fatal and nonfatal injury among men.

Sources: Centers for Disease Control and Prevention. 2004. Surveillance for fatal and nonfatal injuries—United States, 2001. *MMWR Surveillance Summaries* 53(SS7): 1–57; Courtenay, W. 1998. College men's health: An overview and a call to action. *Journal of American College Health* 46(6): 279–290; SMARTRISK. 2009. *The Economic Burden of Injury in Canada.* Toronto: SMARTRISK; World Health Organization. 2002. *Gender and Road Traffic Injuries.* Geneva: World Health Organization.

mation still decide to engage in risky behaviour. Young people often have unsafe attitudes, such as "I won't get hurt" or "It won't happen to me." Attitudes like those can lead to risk taking and ultimately to injuries.

Environmental factors leading to injury may be natural (weather conditions), social (a drunk driver), work related (defective equipment), or home related (faulty wiring). Making the environment safer is an important aspect of safety. Laws are often passed to try to make our environment safer; examples include speed limits on highways and workplace safety requirements.

Motor Vehicle Injuries

According to Transport Canada, an average of eight Canadians die in motor vehicle collisions every day, and many more are seriously injured. Worldwide, motor vehicle crashes kill 1.2 million and injure up to 50 million people each year, making motor vehicle injuries the 11th leading cause of death. Those most affected by motor vehicle crashes are people ages 15–24. It is more likely that your death will be caused by a motor vehicle crash than by any other type of unintentional or intentional injury. **Motor vehicle injuries** also result in the majority of cases of paralysis from spinal injuries, and they are a leading cause of severe brain injury in Canada.

Factors Contributing to Motor Vehicle Injuries

Common causes of motor vehicle injuries are speeding, aggressive driving, fatigue, inexperience, use of cellphones and other distractions, the use of alcohol and other drugs, and the incorrect use of seat belts and other safety devices.

SPEEDING According to Transport Canada, approximately 25% of all fatal motor vehicle crashes in Canada are caused by speeding. Eighty percent of speeding drivers in these fatal collisions are under the age of 45. As speed increases, momentum and the force of impact increase, and the time allowed for the driver to react (reaction time) decreases. Unless otherwise posted, the maximum speed limit

> **QUICK STATS**
>
> In 2004, unintentional injuries accounted for **88%** of the direct costs and **72%** of the indirect costs resulting from injury in Canada.
>
> —SMARTRISK, 2009

in Canada is typically 50 kilometres per hour in most cities and 80 kilometres per hour on most highways. Speed limits are posted to establish the safest maximum speed limit for a given area under ideal conditions; if visibility is limited or the road is wet, the safe maximum speed may be considerably lower.

AGGRESSIVE DRIVING Speeding is also a hallmark of aggressive drivers—those who operate a motor vehicle in an unsafe and hostile manner. Although it is difficult to define or measure, aggressive driving, also known as *road rage*, appears to be a growing problem for Canadians. In fact, some researchers have suggested that aggression is more common on the roads than in any other setting, for a number of reasons, including frustration, congestion, and anonymity. Canadian data from 2006 show that approximately 12% of Canadian drivers admitted to driving well over the speed limit, 9% admitted to regularly speeding up to get through a light, and 3% admitted to taking risks while driving. Other characteristics of aggressive driving include frequent, erratic, and abrupt lane changes; tailgating; running red lights or stop signs; passing on the shoulder; and blocking other cars trying to change lanes or pass. Aggressive drivers increase the risk of crashes for themselves and others. Injuries may also occur if aggressive drivers stop their vehicles and confront each other following an incident. For more on aggressive driving, take the quiz and review the strategies in the box "Are You an Aggressive Driver?"

FATIGUE AND SLEEPINESS Driving requires mental alertness and attentiveness. Studies have shown that sleepiness causes slower reaction time, reduced coordination and vigilance, and delayed information processing. Drowsiness can be caused by not getting enough hours of sleep, by sleep disorders that prevent sleep from being refreshing, or by disruptions caused by shift work that force people to sleep at odd hours. Research shows that even mild sleep deprivation causes a deterioration in driving ability comparable to that caused by a 0.05% blood alcohol concentration—a level considered hazardous when driving. Being awake for 18 hours can impair driving ability as much as drinking two alcoholic beverages.

CELLPHONES AND OTHER DISTRACTIONS Anything that distracts a driver can increase the risk of a motor vehicle injury. Several common causes of crashes, such as disregarding stop signs, have been linked to driver distraction. Distraction is a contributing factor in 25%–50% of all crashes. Cellphones are a widely documented source of distraction for drivers. A 2006 study showed that drivers who use

cellphones are nearly six times as likely to be involved in a crash as drivers who don't. The same study showed that sober drivers using cellphones can perform worse than drivers who are inebriated. Recently, Transport Canada conducted a one-week observational study in which it found that approximately 5.5% of Canadians were using a handheld cellphone while driving; in some urban areas, more than one in ten Canadians were observed using a cellphone while driving. Seven Canadian provinces (British Columbia, Saskatchewan, Ontario, Quebec, Prince Edward Island, Nova Scotia, and Newfoundland and Labrador) have banned handheld cellphone use while driving. Other provinces and territories are considering similar legislation (see the box "Cellphones and Distracted Driving" on p. 612).

ALCOHOL AND OTHER DRUGS Approximately one-third of Canadian drivers killed in car crashes have been drinking alcohol. More than 1000 Canadians die each year in alcohol-related crashes, some of whom have not been drinking themselves. Impaired driving is illegal in all provinces and territories; the legal limit for blood alcohol concentration (BAC) is 0.08%, but people can be impaired at much lower BACs. A driver with a BAC between 0.05% and 0.09% is nine times as likely to have a crash as a person who has not been drinking. The combination of fatigue and alcohol use increases the risk even further. Because alcohol affects reason and judgment as well as the ability to make fast, accurate, and coordinated movements, a person who has been drinking will be less likely to recognize that he or she is impaired.

Other substances also affect judgment and driving ability. A recent study found that hay fever sufferers who had taken diphenhydramine (an antihistamine found in OTC allergy medications, such as Benadryl) were as impaired as if they were legally drunk. Use of many OTC and all psychoactive drugs is potentially dangerous if you plan to drive (Chapters 14 and 15).

SEAT BELTS, AIR BAGS, AND CHILD SAFETY SEATS The improper use of seat belts, air bags, and child safety seats contributes to injuries and deaths in motor vehicle crashes. In Canada, the law requires that all drivers and passengers must wear seat belts at all times. About 93% of Canadians use seat belts; the 7% who choose not to wear them account for close to 40% of fatalities in car crashes. Of drivers not wearing a seat belt who have been killed in automobile crashes, an estimated 60%–70% would have survived if they had been wearing one. If you wear a combination lap and shoulder belt, your chance of surviving a crash is three to four times as likely as that of a person who doesn't wear one.

Some people think that if they are involved in a crash they are better off being thrown free of their vehicle. In fact, the chances of being killed are 25 times as great if you are thrown from a vehicle, whether it is due to injuries caused by hitting a tree or the pavement or by being hit by another vehicle. Seat belts not only prevent you

Are You an Aggressive Driver?

To find out if you are an aggressive driver, check any of the following statements that are true for you:

_____ I consistently exceed the speed limit; I'm often unaware of both my speed and the speed limit.

_____ I frequently follow closely behind the car in front of me.

_____ If I feel the car in front of me is going too slowly, I tailgate.

_____ I change lanes frequently to pass people.

_____ I seldom use my turn signal when changing lanes or turning.

_____ I often run red lights or roll through stop signs.

_____ I react to what I feel is another driver's mistake by cursing, shouting, or making rude gestures; by blocking a car from passing or changing lanes; by using high beams; or by braking suddenly in front of a tailgater.

_____ My personality changes and I become more competitive when I get behind the wheel.

_____ I often get angry or impatient with other drivers and with pedestrians.

_____ I would consider pulling over for a personal encounter with a bad driver.

Each of these statements is characteristic of aggressive drivers; the more items you checked, the greater your road rage. If you checked even one statement, consider taking some of the following steps to reduce your hostility behind the wheel:

• Allow enough time in your trip to reach your destination without speeding.

• Avoid driving during periods of heavy traffic.

• Don't drive when you are angry, tired, or intoxicated.

• Imagine that the other drivers are all people that you know and like. Be courteous and forgiving.

• Listen to soothing music or a book on tape, or practise a relaxation technique, such as deep breathing (see Chapter 3).

• Take a course in anger management.

Even if you control your own aggressive impulses, you may still encounter an aggressive driver on the road. The AAA Foundation for Traffic Safety recommends the following strategies:

• Avoid behaviours that may enrage an aggressive driver; these include cutting off cars when merging, driving slowly in the left lane, tailgating, and making rude gestures.

• If you make a mistake while driving, apologize. In surveys, the most popular and widely understood gestures for apologies include raising or waving a hand and touching or knocking the head with the palm of your hand (to indicate "What was I thinking?").

• Refuse to join in a fight. Avoid eye contact with an angry driver, and put distance between your car and his or her vehicle.

• If you think another driver is following you, call the police on a cellphone or drive to a public place.

Sources: New York State Department of Motor Vehicles. 2008. *Aggressive Driving* (http://www.nysgtsc.state.ny.us/aggr-ndx.htm; retrieved February 21, 2009); AAA Foundation for Traffic Safety. 1997. *Road Rage: How to Avoid Aggressive Driving.* Washington, D.C.: AAA Foundation for Traffic Safety.

---

from being thrown from the car at the time of the crash but also provide protection from the second collision: If a car is travelling at 100 kilometres per hour and hits another vehicle, the car stops first; then the occupants stop because they, too, are travelling at 100 kilometres per hour. The second collision occurs when occupants hit something inside the car, such as the dashboard or windshield. The seat belt stops the second collision from occurring and spreads the collision's force over the body.

In Canada, it is not mandatory for air bags to be installed in vehicles; however, when they are, they must meet specific safety requirements. Most new cars and light trucks have been equipped with dual air bags—one for the driver and one for the front passenger. Many vehicles also offer optional side air bags, which further reduce the risk of injury. Advanced air bag systems include risk-reduction technologies, such as sensors to detect crash severity, seat position, passenger size, and whether a passenger is wearing a seat belt. Although air bags provide supplementary protection in the event of a collision, most are useful only in head-on collisions. They also deflate immediately after inflating and therefore do not provide protection in collisions involving multiple impacts. Air bags are not a replacement for seat belts; everyone in a vehicle should buckle up.

Air bags deploy forcefully and can injure a child or short adult who is improperly restrained or sitting too close to the dashboard, although second-generation air bags are somewhat safer for children than the older devices. To ensure that air bags work safely, always follow these basic guidelines: Place infants in rear-facing infant seats in the back seat, transport children age 12 and under in the back

> **Seat belts save about 1000 lives each year in Canada.**
> —Transport Canada, 2010

> QUICK STATS

Cellphones and Distracted Driving

At any given moment, more than 5% of Canadian drivers are talking on their cellphones. As of February 2010, it was illegal to use handheld (not hands-free) cellphones while driving in British Columbia, Saskatchewan, Ontario, Quebec, Prince Edward Island, Nova Scotia, and Newfoundland and Labrador. According to the Canadian Automobile Association, drivers who cause a collision or who are observed driving unsafely while using a cellphone can be charged under a number of provincial, territorial, or federal laws, including dangerous driving, careless driving, and criminal negligence causing death or injury. Around the world, many countries have similar laws against the use of handheld cellphones while driving.

Available evidence indicates that use of a cellphone while driving can increase the risk of motor vehicle crashes. In a study using a driver-training simulator, cellphone users were about 20% slower to respond to sudden hazards than were other drivers, and they were about twice as likely to rear-end a braking car in front of them. Among young adult drivers who used a cellphone, reaction time was reduced to the level of a 70-year-old driver who was not using a phone. It is unclear, however, if bans, such as those in Canada and around the world, will help reduce the risk: Studies have not found much, if any, benefit in the use of headsets. It appears that the mental distraction of talking is a factor in crashes rather than holding the phone.

The safest strategy is not to use your phone while driving, even if you use a headset. For people who live in areas where cellphone use is legal while driving and who choose to use a phone, the following strategies may help increase safety:

• Be familiar with your phone and its functions, especially speed dial and redial.

• Store frequently called numbers on speed dial so you can place calls without looking at the phone.

• If your phone has voice-activated dialling, use it.

• Use a hands-free device so you can keep both hands on the steering wheel.

• Let the person you are speaking to know you are driving and be prepared to end the call at any time.

• Don't place or answer calls in heavy traffic or hazardous weather conditions.

• Don't take notes or look up phone numbers while driving.

• Time calls so that you can place them when you are at a stop.

• Never engage in stressful or emotional conversations while on the road. If you are discussing a complicated or emotional matter, pull off the road to complete your conversation.

Using text messaging and email is potentially even more distracting than talking on a cellphone. Currently, British Columbia, Saskatchewan, Ontario, Quebec, Nova Scotia, Prince Edward Island, and Newfoundland and Labrador prohibit text messaging while driving.

seat, always use seat belts or appropriate safety seats, and keep 25 centimetres between the air bag cover and the breastbone of the driver or passenger. If necessary, adjust the steering wheel or use seat cushions to ensure that an inflating air bag will hit a person in the chest and not in the face.

Another adjustment should be made for children who have outgrown child safety seats but are still too small for adult seat belts alone (usually ages four to eight). These children should be secured by using booster seats that ensure that the seat belt is positioned low across the waist. Transport Canada reports that 99 children ages 14 and under were killed in car crashes in 2007; another 11,737 were injured. According to Canadian car seat data, an estimated four out of five children are not properly restrained in their vehicles. A properly used child restraint will reduce the likelihood of a child being killed or injured in a collision by up to 75%. Canada's child restraint laws fall under the Motor Vehicle Safety Act, which includes regulations that apply to child and infant car seats and booster cushions.

The provincial and territorial governments also regulate child seat use, and individual municipalities enforce child seat laws through their local police services. Before driving with a child, make sure that you know the laws and regulations pertaining to child seat use; that you have an appropriate safety seat for the child's age, height, and weight; that the seat meets Canadian Motor Vehicle Safety Standards; that the seat is installed correctly; and that the child is properly secured in the seat.

In the rare event that individuals feel that air bags pose particular risks for them or their family members (for medical or other specific reasons), permission to install an on-off switch that temporarily disables the air bag can be applied for from Transport Canada. Air bags currently prevent far more injuries than they cause. A Transport Canada study of the years 1990–2000 revealed that 313 Canadian lives were saved by air bags during that period and that the economic benefits that can be attributed to the installation of air bags were $465.5 million.

Preventing Motor Vehicle Injuries Strategies for preventing motor vehicle injuries include the following:

- Obey the speed limit. If you have to speed to get somewhere on time, you're not allowing enough time.

- Always wear a seat belt. Fasten the lap belt, even if the vehicle has automatic shoulder belts. The shoulder strap should cross the collarbone, and the lap belt should fit low and snug across the hips and pelvic area. The shoulder strap should never be slipped under the arm or behind the back. Pregnant women should position the lap belt as low as possible on the pelvic area.

- Never drive under the influence of alcohol or other drugs, or ride with a driver who is.

- Keep your car in good working order.

- Always allow enough following distance. Use the three-second rule: When the vehicle ahead passes a reference point, count out three seconds. If you pass the reference point before you finish counting, drop back and allow more following distance.

- Always increase your following distance and slow down if weather or road conditions are poor.

- Choose highways rather than rural roads. Highways are typically safer because of better visibility, wider lanes, fewer surprises, and other factors.

- Always signal when turning or changing lanes.

- Stop completely at stop signs. Follow all traffic laws.

- Take special care at intersections. Look left, right, and then left again. Make sure you have time to complete your manoeuvre in the intersection.

- Don't pass on two-lane roads unless you're in a designated passing area and have a clear view ahead.

Motorcycles and Mopeds About 7% of the traffic fatalities in Canada in 2004 involved someone riding a motorcycle or a moped. In more than two-thirds of crashes involving a car and a motorcycle, the driver of the car is at fault. Injuries from motorcycle collisions are generally more severe than those involving automobiles because motorcycles provide little, if any, protection. Because head injuries are the major cause of death, the use of a helmet is critical for rider safety. Riders also need to know how to operate a motorcycle safely; operator error is a factor in 75% of fatal motorcycle crashes.

Moped riders face additional challenges. Mopeds usually have a maximum speed of 50–70 kilometres per hour and have less power for manoeuvrability, especially in an emergency. Moped riders should use caution and learn how to handle the vehicle in traffic.

Additional strategies for preventing motorcycle and moped injuries include the following:

- Wear light-coloured clothing, drive with your headlights on, and correctly position yourself in traffic.

- Develop the necessary skills. Lack of skill is a major factor in motorcycle and moped injuries. Skidding from improper braking is the most common cause of loss of control.

- Wear a helmet. Helmet use is required in all Canadian provinces.

- Protect your eyes with goggles, a face shield, or a windshield.

- Drive defensively, particularly when changing lanes and at intersections, and never assume that other drivers can see you.

Bicycles It has been estimated that bicycle crashes result in about 7500 serious injuries and 40 to 70 fatalities each year in Canada. According to researchers at the University of British Columbia, North American cyclists are 7 to 70 times as likely to be injured as people travelling in cars. Bicycle injuries result primarily from riders not knowing or understanding the rules of the road, failing to follow traffic laws, not having sufficient skill or experience to handle traffic conditions, or being intoxicated. Bicycles are considered vehicles; bicyclists must obey all traffic laws that apply to automobile drivers, including stopping at traffic lights and stop signs.

Head injuries are involved in about two-thirds of all bicycle-related deaths. British Columbia, New Brunswick, Nova Scotia, and Prince Edward Island have laws requiring cyclists of all ages to wear helmets. In Ontario and Alberta, the legislation applies to Canadians under the age of 18. Wearing a helmet reduces the risk of head injury by 85%, but according to a 2009 Statistics Canada report, only 36.5% of Canadian bicyclists ages 12 and over reported wearing a helmet regularly (see the box "Choosing a Bicycle Helmet" on p. 614). Safe cycling strategies include the following:

- Wear safety equipment, including a helmet, eye protection, gloves, and proper footwear. Secure the bottom of your pant legs with clips, and secure your shoelaces so they don't get tangled in the chain.

- Wear light-coloured, reflective clothing. Equip your bike with reflectors, and use lights, especially at night or when riding in wooded or other dark areas.

- Ride with the flow of traffic, not against it, and follow all traffic laws. Use bike paths when they are available.

- Ride defensively; never assume that drivers can see you. Be especially careful when turning or crossing at corners and intersections. Watch for cars turning right.

- Stop at all traffic lights and stop signs. Know and use hand signals.

- Continue pedalling at all times when moving (no coasting) to help keep the bike stable and to maintain your balance.

Choosing a Bicycle Helmet

Wearing a bicycle helmet can help you avoid serious head injury, brain damage, or even death in the event of a collision or fall. Helmets have a layer of stiff foam, which absorbs shock and cushions a blow to your head, covered by a thin plastic shell that will skid along the ground. For maximum protection, it's important to select a correctly fitting helmet. When you go shopping, remember the four S's: size, strap, straight, and sticker.

• *Size:* Try on several different sizes before making your selection; it may take several tries before you find the most comfortable fit. The helmet should be very snug but not overly tight on your head. Pads are usually provided to help adjust the fit. A good salesperson can also help you get the right fit. When the helmet is strapped onto your head, it should not move more than 2.5 centimetres in any direction, and you should not be able to pull or twist it off no matter how hard you try.

• *Strap:* Be sure that the chinstrap fits snugly under your chin and that the V in the strap meets under your ear. Avoid thin straps, which can be uncomfortable. Check to be sure that the buckle is strong and won't pop open and that the straps are sturdy.

• *Straight:* The helmet should sit straight on your head, not tilted back or forward. A rule of thumb is that the rim should be about two finger widths above your eyebrows (depending on the height of your forehead).

• *Sticker:* Look for a sticker or label that says the helmet meets safety standards. The sticker(s) should be from one or more of the following organizations: Canadian Standard Association (CSA), U.S. Consumer Product Safety Commission (CPSC), Snell Memorial Foundation, American National Standard Institute, American Society for Testing and Materials, British Standards Institute, or the Standards Association of Australia. If a helmet does not have a sticker from one of these organizations, it may not meet safety standards and should not be used.

You are more likely to wear your helmet if it is comfortable, so be sure that vents on the helmet provide airflow to promote cooling and sweat control. You will be safer with a brightly coloured helmet that makes you more visible to drivers, especially in rainy, foggy, or dark conditions. Reflective tape will also increase your visibility. Finally, a helmet is a good place to put emergency information (your name, address, and phone number, plus any emergency medical conditions and an emergency contact).

If you are involved in a crash, replace your helmet. Even if the helmet doesn't have any visible signs of damage, its ability to protect your head may be compromised.

Sources: Bicycle Helmet Safety Institute. 2009. *A Consumer's Guide to Bicycle Helmets* (http://www.helmets.org/guide.htm; retrieved February 21, 2009); Bicycle Helmet Safety Institute. 2007. *How to Fit a Bicycle Helmet* (http://www.helmets.org/.t.htm; retrieved February 21, 2009); Ministry of Transportation Ontario. 2010. *Frequently Asked Questions: Safety* (http://www.mto.gov.on.ca/english/faq/safety-test.shtml#BicycleHelmets2; retrieved July 1, 2010).

Pedestrians Pedestrians are no match for motor vehicles: 423 pedestrians were killed in Canada in 2004 (more than one each day), and another 2904 were hospitalized. Typically, the highest rates of death and injury occur among the very young and older adults. The majority of pedestrian deaths occur when people cross or enter the roadway between intersections. Alcohol intoxication plays a role in up to half of all adult pedestrian fatalities.

The following strategies can help prevent injuries when you're walking or jogging:

• Walk or jog in daylight.

• Wear light-coloured, reflective clothing.

• Face traffic when walking or jogging along a road, and follow traffic laws.

• Avoid busy roads or roads with poor visibility.

• Cross only at marked crosswalks and intersections.

• Don't use headphones while walking.

• Don't hitchhike; it places you in a potentially dangerous situation.

Home Injuries

A person's place of residence, whether a house, an apartment, a trailer, or a dormitory, is considered home. People spend a great deal of time at home and should feel that they are safe and secure there. However, home can be a dangerous place. Fatal **home injuries** can occur as a result of falls, fires, poisoning, and suffocation.

Falls In 2009, nearly 1.7 million Canadians—more than 40% of those who reported an injury—reported being injured in a fall. Falls are more common among women than men. Most deaths occurring from falls involve falling on stairs or steps or from one level to another. Falls also occur on the same level, from tripping, slipping, or stumbling. Alcohol is a contributing factor in many falls. Strategies for preventing falls include the following:

- Install handrails and nonslip surfaces in the shower and bathtub.

- Keep floors, stairs, and outside areas clear of objects or conditions that could cause slipping or tripping, such as ice, snow, electrical cords, and toys.

- Put a light switch by the door of every room so no one has to walk across a room to turn on a light. Use night lights in bedrooms, halls, stairs, and bathrooms.

- When climbing a ladder, use both hands. Never stand higher than the third step from the top. When using a stepladder, make sure the spreader brace is in the locked position. With straight ladders, set the base out 30 centimetres for every 120 centimetres of height.

- Don't use chairs to reach things.

- If small children are in the home, place gates at the top and bottom of stairs. Never leave a baby unattended on a bed or table. Install window guards to prevent children from falling out of windows.

Fires In Canada, 53,589 fires were reported in 2002, resulting in 304 deaths and 2547 injuries. Most of these fires occurred in the home; residential fires accounted for approximately 82% of Canada's fire-related fatalities. Most fires begin in the kitchen, living room, or bedroom. Careless smoking (and leaving an open flame unattended), cooking equipment, and heating equipment represent the three leading causes of home fires in Canada.

To prevent fires, it's important to dispose of all cigarettes in ashtrays and to never smoke in bed. Other strategies include proper maintenance of fireplaces, furnaces, heaters, chimneys, and electrical outlets, cords, and appliances. If you use a portable heater, keep it at least one metre away from curtains, bedding, or anything else that might catch fire. Never leave heaters on unattended.

It's important to be adequately prepared to handle fire-related situations. Plan at least two escape routes out of each room, and designate a location outside the home as a meeting place. For practice, stage a home fire drill; do it at night, as that's when most deadly fires occur.

Install smoke detectors on every level of your home. Your risk of dying in a fire is almost twice as high if you do not use them. Clean the detectors and check the batteries once a month, and replace the batteries at least once a year. Be sure that all residents are familiar with the sound of the smoke detector's alarm; when it goes off, take it seriously.

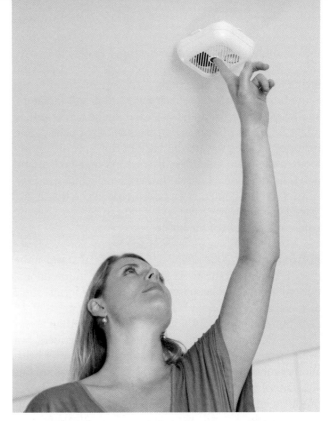

Install smoke detectors on every floor of your home, check them monthly, and replace the batteries at least once a year.

These strategies can help prevent injuries in a fire:

- Get out as quickly as possible, and go to the designated meeting place. Don't stop for a keepsake or a pet. Never hide in a closet or under a bed. Once outside, count heads to see if everyone is out. If you think someone is still inside the burning building, tell the firefighters. Never go back inside a burning building.

- If you're trapped in a room, feel the door. If it is hot or if smoke is coming in through the cracks, don't open it; use the alternative escape route. If you can't get out, go to the window and shout for help.

- Smoke inhalation is the main cause of death and injury in fires. To avoid inhaling smoke, crawl along the floor away from the heat and smoke. Cover your mouth and nose, ideally with a wet cloth, and take short, shallow breaths.

- If your clothes catch fire, don't run. Drop to the ground, cover your face, and roll back and forth to smother the flames. Remember: stop-drop-roll.

home injuries Unintentional injuries and deaths that occur in the home and on home premises to occupants, guests, domestic workers, and trespassers; falls, burns, poisonings, suffocations, drownings, and electrical shocks are examples.

TERMS

Although house fires cause the most deaths, hot water causes the most nonfatal burns. Set your water heater no higher than 49°C. Young children are particularly at risk of being burned. Place barriers around stoves and radiators, and keep young children out of the kitchen, where they might be burned by spills. Put pans on rear burners, and turn pot handles toward the back of the stove. Keep hot foods away from the edge of counters and tables, and don't put them on a tablecloth that a small child can pull. Always test the contents of a baby bottle; when bottles are heated in microwave ovens, the liquid can become scalding before the outside of the bottle gets very hot.

Poisoning   In 2004, there were 944 deaths and more than 7000 hospitalizations attributable to unintentional poisonings in Canada. Poisons come in many forms, some of which are not typically considered poisons. For example, even honey can be poisonous to children less than a year old. Medications are safe when used as prescribed, but overdosing or incorrectly combining medications with another substance may result in poisoning. Other poisonous substances include cleaning agents, petroleum-based products, insecticides and herbicides, cosmetics, nail polish and remover, and many houseplants. All potentially poisonous substances should be used only as directed and stored out of the reach of children.

The most common type of poisoning by gases is carbon monoxide poisoning. Carbon monoxide gas is emitted by motor vehicle exhaust and some types of heating equipment. The effects of exposure to this colourless, odourless gas include headache, blurred vision, and shortness of breath, followed by dizziness, vomiting, and unconsciousness. Carbon monoxide detectors (similar to smoke detectors) are available for home use; they should be used according to the manufacturer's instructions. To prevent poisoning by gases, have your furnace inspected yearly, use caution with any substance or device that produces potentially toxic fumes, and never operate a vehicle in an enclosed space.

Keep your local poison control hotline number near the phone or in another convenient location. A call to your regional poison information centre will allow you to speak with professionals who provide expert emergency advice 24 hours a day. If a poisoning does occur, it's important that you act quickly. Remove the poison from contact with the victim's eyes, skin, or mouth, or move the victim away from contact with poisonous gases. Call the poison control centre immediately for instructions; do not follow the emergency instructions on product labels because they may be incorrect. If you are unable to find the contact information for your local poison control centre, dial 911. Depending on the situation, you may be instructed to give the victim water to drink or to flush affected parts of the skin or eyes with water. Do not induce vomiting. If you are advised to go to an emergency room, take the poisonous substance or container with you.

Suffocation and Choking   Suffocation was the leading cause of death for Canadian infants less than one year of age in 2005. Children can suffocate if they put small items in their mouth, get tangled in their crib bedding, or get trapped in airtight appliances like old refrigerators. Keep small objects out of reach of children under age three, and don't give them hot dogs, popcorn, gum, hard candy, or raw carrots. Examine toys carefully for small parts that could come loose; don't give plastic bags or balloons to small children.

Adults can also become choking victims, especially if they fail to chew food properly, eat hurriedly, or try to talk and eat at the same time. Many choking victims can be saved with the **Heimlich manoeuvre**. The Canadian Red Cross recommends abdominal thrusts as the easiest and safest thing to do when an adult is choking. Individuals should never hit an adult on the back or give them a drink when they are choking; it could make the object more difficult to remove. According to St. John Ambulance, back blows in conjunction with chest thrusts are an acceptable procedure for dislodging an object from the throat of an infant.

Injuries Sustained During Leisure and Recreation Pursuits

Leisure activities encompass a large part of our free time, so it is not surprising that **leisure injuries** are a significant health-related problem in Canada. According to 2009 data from the *Canadian Community Health Survey*, taking part in sports or physical activity was the most frequent type of activity at the time of injury for Canadians over the age of 12. Key factors in leisure injuries include misuse of equipment, lack of experience and skill, use of alcohol or other drugs, and failure to use appropriate safety equipment. Specific safety strategies for activities associated with leisure injuries include the following:

- Don't swim alone, in unsupervised places, under the influence of alcohol, or for an unusually long time. Use caution when swimming in unfamiliar surroundings or in water colder than 21°C. Check the depth of water before diving. Make sure that residential pools are fenced and that children are never allowed to swim unsupervised.
- Always use a **personal flotation device** (also known as a life jacket) when on a boat.
- For all sports and recreational activities, make sure facilities are safe, follow the rules, and practise good

Safe in-line skating requires several pieces of gear, including a helmet and pads for the wrists, knees, and elbows.

sportsmanship. Develop adequate skill in the activity, and use proper safety equipment, including, where appropriate, a helmet, eye protection, correct footwear, and knee, elbow, and wrist pads.

- If using wheeled equipment, such as skateboards, snowboards, mountain bikes, or all-terrain vehicles, wear a helmet and other safety equipment, and avoid excessive speeds and unsafe stunts. Playground equipment should be used only for those activities for which it is designed.

- If you are active in excessively hot and humid weather, drink plenty of fluids, rest frequently in the shade, and slow down or stop if you feel uncomfortable. Danger signals of heat stress include excessive perspiration, dizziness, headache, muscle cramps, nausea, weakness, rapid pulse, and disorientation.

- Do not use alcohol or other drugs during recreational activities—such activities require coordination and sound judgment.

For more on exercise safety, see Chapter 6.

In-Line Skating Injuries   Millions of Canadians, young and old, enjoy in-line skating. Along with the increase in popularity of in-line skating has come a corresponding increase in the number of injuries that have resulted from this activity. Injuries to the wrist and head are most common; many occur because users do not wear appropriate

safety gear. Researchers estimate that more than one-third of all serious injuries could be prevented if all in-line skaters wore helmets and wrist and elbow protection.

To reduce your risk of being injured while in-line skating, wear a helmet, elbow and knee pads, wrist guards, a long-sleeved shirt, and long pants. Alcohol use appears to be a significant factor in in-line skating injuries that occur on university and college campuses. Because in-line skating involves skill, judgment, and coordination, it makes sense not to mix skating and drinking.

Scooter Injuries   Scooters are lightweight and have low-friction wheels for quickness and portability. Along with their skyrocketing popularity have come scooter-related injuries. The most common injuries are arm or hand fractures and dislocations, cuts and bruises, and sprains; most of these injuries involve children. Approximately 35% of the scooter-related injuries seen in Canadian children are fractures; 6% of all scooter-related injuries to children result in brain injury. Viewing scooters as toys more than as transportation may lead riders to ignore important safety precautions:

- Wear a helmet that meets bicycle helmet standards, along with knee and elbow pads.
- Be sure that handlebars, the steering column, and all nuts and bolts are securely fastened.
- Ride on smooth, paved surfaces away from motor vehicle traffic. Avoid streets and surfaces with water, sand, gravel, or dirt.
- Don't ride after dark.
- Closely supervise young children.

Work Injuries

The number of **work injuries** increased in Canada throughout the 1980s but has been declining since 1988. Despite these reduced rates, large numbers of Canadian workers are still being injured; in 2008 alone, 307,802 Canadians suffered work injuries, 1035 of which were fatal.

Heimlich manoeuvre   A manoeuvre developed by Henry J. Heimlich, MD, to help force an obstruction from the airway.

leisure injuries   Unintentional injuries and deaths that occur in public places or places used in a public way, not involving motor vehicles; includes most sports and recreation deaths and injuries; falls, drownings, burns, and heat and cold stress are examples.

personal flotation device   A device designed to save a person from drowning by buoying up the body while in the water.

work injuries   Unintentional injuries and deaths that arise out of and in the course of gainful work, such as falls, electrical shocks, exposure to radiation and toxic chemicals, burns, cuts, back sprains, and loss of fingers or other body parts in machines.

TERMS

Certain types of injuries, including injuries to muscles, tendons, ligaments, and joints, and musculoskeletal system and connective tissue diseases topped the list of injuries to Canadian workers in 2008. Not surprisingly, blue-collar workers tend to account for the majority of work-related injuries and illnesses, as their jobs usually involve long hours, shift work, and extensive manual labour and lifting. In 2007, Canadian workers in manufacturing, construction, and transport had the highest rates of work-related injuries; in contrast, workers in the financial sector held the lowest rate, with less than one injury per 1000 employees.

According to the *Canadian Community Health Survey*, health-related risk factors that have been linked to a higher risk of work-related injuries include having at least three chronic conditions, smoking daily, consuming large amounts of alcohol (at least five drinks per occasion, at least once a week), being obese (for women), and reporting high levels of personal life stress.

A large number of workplace injuries can be prevented. An improved understanding of the individual risk factors and work conditions that are linked to an increased risk of work injuries should aid in the development of effective prevention strategies. In addition to programs targeting smoking cessation, weight management, and stress reduction, it is also important that workplace safety programs be put in place for workers in high-risk occupations. Additionally, other risk factors, such as workplace hazards (also called **ergonomic hazards**), equipment design, and work schedules, should be routinely addressed (and modified, if necessary) by employers.

Back Injuries Back problems accounted for about 16% of all work injuries in 2003. Because many back injuries are the result of improper lifting technique, educating workers on the correct way to lift things is an important part of any comprehensive back injury prevention program (Figure 20.1).

- Avoid bending at the waist. Remain in an upright position and crouch down if you need to lower yourself to grasp the object. Bend at the knees and hips.

- Place feet securely about shoulder-width apart; grip the object firmly.

- Lift gradually, with straight arms. Avoid quick, jerky motions. Lift by standing up or pushing with your leg muscles. Keep the object close to your body.

- If you have to turn, change the position of your feet. Twisting is a common and dangerous cause of injury. Plan ahead so that your pathway is clear and turning can be minimized.

- Put the object down gently, reversing the steps for lifting.

QUICK STATS

4 out of 5 adults will experience at least one episode of back pain at some point in their lives.

—Statistics Canada, 2006

THINKING ABOUT THE ENVIRONMENT
Every year, thousands of people are killed and injured by weather-related events, such as floods and hurricanes. Earthquakes and tsunamis can cause massive destruction and loss of life while leaving thousands or even millions of people homeless and injured.

In January 2010, an earthquake measuring 7.0 on the Richter scale struck the Caribbean island of Haiti, killing more than 222,000 people and injuring countless others. Two years before, in May 2008, a cyclone struck Myanmar (formerly Burma), leaving nearly 135,000 people dead or missing. But weather emergencies usually are not on such a vast scale. For example, nine to ten Canadians die each year after being struck by lightning, almost always in isolated incidents. According to Environment Canada, about 80 tornadoes strike in Canada each year (mostly between May and September), causing an average of two deaths and 20 injuries annually.

For more information on the environment and environmental health, see Chapter 21.

FIGURE 20.1 Correct lifting technique. Stay upright, bending at the knees and hips.

Carpal Tunnel Syndrome

Carpal tunnel syndrome (CTS) is a repetitive strain injury characterized by pressure on the median nerve in the wrist. It is the most commonly reported work-related medical problem, accounting for about half of all upper limb work-related injuries. Women are about twice as likely as men to be affected by CTS.

The median nerve travels through the forearm to the hand through a tunnel in the wrist formed by the carpal (wrist) bones and associated tendons and covered by a ligament (see the figure). The median nerve can become compressed for a variety of reasons, including swelling of the surrounding tendons caused by pregnancy, diabetes, arthritis, or repetitive wrist motions during many activities, such as typing, cutting, or carpentry work. Symptoms of CTS include numbness, tingling, burning, or aching in the hand, particularly in the thumb and the first three fingers. The pain may worsen at night and may shoot up from the hand as far as the shoulder.

Many cases of carpal tunnel syndrome clear up on their own or with minimal treatment. Modification of the movement that is causing the problem

Carpal tunnel

Ligament

Tendon sheath

Tendons

Median nerve

Carpals

is critically important. For example, adjusting the height of a computer keyboard so that the wrists can be held straight during typing can help relieve

pressure on the wrists. CTS is often first treated by immobilizing the wrist with a splint during the night. People may also be given anti-inflammatory drugs or injections of cortisone in the wrist to reduce swelling. In a small percentage of severe cases, surgery to cut the ligament and reduce the pressure on the nerve may be recommended.

If you engage in activities that involve repetitive motions, such as typing or cutting, you can try some strategies to reduce your risk of developing CTS. Begin by modifying your work environment to reduce the stress on your wrists. Alternate activities and take frequent breaks to avoid spending long stretches of time engaged in the same motion.

Sources: Ly-Pen, D., et al. 2005. Surgical decompression versus local steroid injection in carpal tunnel syndrome: A one-year, prospective, randomized, open, controlled clinical trial. *Arthritis and Rheumatism* 52(2): 612–619; Carpal tunnel syndrome. 2002. *Journal of the American Medical Association* 288(10): 1310; American Academy of Orthopaedic Surgeons. 2007. *Ask an Orthopaedic Surgeon about Carpal Tunnel Syndrome* (http://orthoinfo.aaos.org/topic.cfm? topic=A00009; retrieved February 21, 2009).

QUESTIONS FOR CRITICAL THINKING AND REFLECTION

Think of one injury you have suffered. What were you doing when you were injured? Thinking back on the injury, was there anything you could have done to avoid or minimize it? How did the experience change your attitudes or behaviours?

Repetitive Strain Injuries Musculoskeletal injuries and disorders in the workplace include **repetitive strain injuries (RSIs)**. RSIs are caused by repeated strain on a particular part of the body. Repetition, force, awkward postures, and other stressors may contribute to RSIs. **Carpal tunnel syndrome** is one type of RSI that has increased in recent years because of increased use of computers, both at work and in the home (see the box "Carpal Tunnel Syndrome," above, for more information).

VIOLENCE AND INTENTIONAL INJURIES

Violence—the use of physical force with the intent to inflict harm, injury, or death on yourself or another—is a major public health concern in Canada. According to Statistics Canada, approximately one in five crimes reported to police in 2008 was violent. Worldwide, interpersonal

ergonomic hazards Workplace conditions that pose the risk of injury to the musculoskeletal system of the worker.

repetitive strain injury (RSI) A musculoskeletal injury or disorder caused by repeated strain on the hand, arm, wrist, or other part of the body; also called *cumulative trauma disorder (CTD)*.

carpal tunnel syndrome Compression of the median nerve in the wrist, often caused by repetitive use of the hands, such as in computer use; characterized by numbness, tingling, and pain in the hands and fingers; can cause nerve damage.

TERMS

violence is the third leading cause of death among people ages 15–44. Examples of types of violence are assault, homicide, sexual assault, domestic violence, suicide, and child abuse.

Factors Contributing to Violence

Most intentional injuries and deaths are associated with an argument or the committing of another crime. However, a great many forms of violence exist, and no single factor can explain all of them.

Social Factors   Rates of violence are not the same throughout society; they vary by geographic region, neighbourhood, socioeconomic level, and many other factors. According to 2008 police statistics, crime severity was highest in the Northern and Western regions of Canada. Neighbourhoods that are disadvantaged in status, power, and economic resources are typically the ones with the most violence. Rates of violence are also highest among young people and minority groups, people who have relatively little power.

People who feel they are a part of society (have strong family and social ties), who are economically integrated (have a reasonable chance at getting a decent job), and who grow up in areas with a feeling of community (good schools, parks, and neighbourhoods) are significantly less likely to engage in violence. Studies have shown that the environment on university and college campuses can contribute to violence. The nature of these campuses—transitory communities rather than permanent places where people work and live together over the long term—means that people have less incentive to cooperate and coexist amicably. Some campus groups even promote the ideas of bigotry and bias toward others, particularly toward individuals about whom they know little or with whom they have had little contact. Ignorance and insensitivity to differences can be precursors to acts of violence.

Violence in the Media   The mass media play a major role in exposing audiences of all ages to violence as an acceptable and effective means of solving problems. Children may view as many as 10,000 violent acts on television and in movies each year. Computer and video games also include many violent acts, leading to concern that children's exposure to violence will make them more accepting or tolerant of it. The consequences of violence are depicted much less frequently.

A 2005 study linked TV viewing to bullying among children. Researchers found that the more hours per day that a four-year-old spent watching TV, the more likely the child was to engage in bullying behaviour in later years. Factors that reduced the rate of bullying included cognitive stimulation, such as parents reading to a child, and emotional support and attention. It is thought that emotional support from parents helps children develop empathy, social competence, and self-regulation—skills

The victims of most types of violence are statistically likely to be young, poor, in a minority group, urban, and—except for sexual assault and domestic violence—male.

that enable them to deal with peers without resorting to aggressive or bullying behaviour.

Researchers have found that exposure to media violence at least temporarily increases aggressive feelings in children, making them more likely to engage in violent or fearful behaviour; the direct, short-term effects on teens and adults are less clear. It makes sense for parents to be aware of the potential influence of the media on their children. A child may not clearly understand the distinctions between the fantasy world portrayed in the media and the complexities of the real world. Parents should monitor the TV shows, movies, video games, music, and other forms of media to which children are exposed. Watching programs with children gives parents the opportunity to talk to children about violence and its consequences, to explain that violence is not the best way to resolve conflicts or solve problems, and to point out examples of positive behaviours, such as kindness and cooperation.

Gender   In most cases, violence is committed by men. Some researchers have suggested that the male hormone testosterone is in some way linked to aggressive behaviour. Others point to prevailing cultural attitudes about male roles (men as dominant and controlling) as an explanation for the high rate of violence among men. However, these theories do not explain why it is that violent men are more likely to live in Northern and Western Canada, belong to minority groups, be poor, and be young.

Women do commit acts of violence, including a relatively small but substantial number of spousal abuse and homicide cases. This fact has been used to argue that women have the same capacity to commit violence as men, but most researchers note substantial differences. Men often kill their wives as the culmination of years of violence or after stalking them; they may kill their entire family and themselves at the same time. Women virtually never kill in such circumstances; rather, they kill their husbands after repeated victimization or while being beaten.

Interpersonal Factors Although most people fear attack from strangers, the majority of sexual assault and murder victims are acquainted with their attacker. In many cases, crime victims and violent criminals tend to share certain characteristics—that is, they are likely to be young, male, in a minority group, and poor.

Alcohol and Other Drugs Substance abuse and dependence are consistently associated with interpersonal violence and suicide. Intoxication affects judgment and may increase aggression in some people, causing a small argument to escalate into a serious physical confrontation. On college and university campuses, alcohol is involved in about 95% of all violent crimes.

Assault

Assault is the use of physical force by a person or persons to inflict injury or death on another; homicide, aggravated assault, and robbery are examples of assault. Research indicates that the victims of assaultive injuries and their perpetrators tend to resemble one another in terms of ethnicity, educational background, psychological profile, and reliance on weapons.

Homicide

According to police statistics, 611 people were murdered in Canada in 2008, representing a 2% increase in the national homicide rate over the previous year. This rise was attributed to increases in homicide rates in Alberta and British Columbia, a large proportion of which was gang related. According to Canadian crime statistics, gang-related homicides have been on the rise since the early 1990s and in 2008 accounted for nearly one in four homicides. Many homicides are committed with a firearm, occur during an argument, and occur among people who know one another. Of all solved homicides in Canada in 2008, 41% were committed by an acquaintance, 19% were committed by a family member other than a spouse, 15% were committed by a spouse, and 9% were committed by someone known to the victim through a criminal relationship. The remaining 17% of victims were killed by a stranger. Wives are about three times as likely to be murdered as husbands, and when a wife kills her husband, it is usually in self-defence. In 2007, spousal homicide rates were highest for Canadians between the ages of 15 and 24 years.

Gang-Related Violence

Violence results from more than just the acts of individuals, as evidenced by the number of injuries and deaths resulting from gang activities. Gangs are most frequently associated with large cities, but gang activity also extends to the suburbs and even to rural areas. A 2008 article in the Royal Canadian Mounted Police magazine, *The Gazette*, suggests that gang members in Canada are increasingly "suburbanizing"; they are moving from large cities to outlying areas and neighbourhoods, and they are also moving from province to province.

According to a 2006 Criminal Intelligence Service Canada report, at least 11,000 Canadians under the age of 30 belong to street gangs. Many gangs control a particular territory and will oppose other gangs, as well as police and community efforts to eliminate them. Evidence also suggests that a growing number of gangs in Canada focus more on protecting economic markets than on protecting their turf. Additionally, a trend of "fluid gang affiliations" has become apparent, in which gangs or gang members join forces for a brief time to commit crimes, after which they disband. Gangs may be involved in illegal drug trade, extortion, and protection schemes. Gang members are more likely than those who are not gang members to possess weapons, and violence may result from conflicts over money, territory, or illegal activities.

Gangs are more common in areas that are poor and suffer from high unemployment, population density, and crime. Young gang members (and those who are at risk of joining gangs) tend to be from groups that endure the greatest levels of inequality and social disadvantage, and they are often drug users who are already involved in serious and violent crime. In Canada, Aboriginal youth are more vulnerable to gang recruitment and organized crime than non-Aboriginal youth. Often, gangs serve as a mechanism for companionship, self-esteem, support, and security; indeed, in some areas gang membership may be viewed as the only possible means of survival.

Hate Crimes

When bias against another person's race or ethnicity, national origin, religion, sexual orientation, age, profession, political beliefs, or disability motivates a criminal act, the offence is classified as a hate crime. Hate crimes may be committed against people or property. Those against people may include intimidation, assault, and even rape or murder. Crimes against property most frequently involve graffiti, the desecration of churches or synagogues, cross burnings, and other acts of vandalism or property damage.

About 890 hate-motivated crimes were reported in Canada in 2006; many more go unreported. Property-related crimes made up 52% of all incidents. Close to 40% of incidents were violent offences committed against a person; assault was the most common offence. One homicide and two attempted murders were also motivated by hatred in 2006. In total, race or ethnicity was cited as the main motivation in 61% of cases, religion in 27%, and sexual orientation in 10%.

Hate crimes may be extremely brutal acts perpetrated at random on total strangers by multiple offenders. In fact, the majority of violent hate crimes are committed by strangers. Suspects frequently are not identified, but police reports indicate that a substantial number of hate crimes in Canada are committed by youth ages 12–17 years. In 2006, victims of violent hate crimes were highest among Canadians ages 12–17 and 18–24. Hate crimes are sometimes, but not always, associated with fringe groups that have extremist ideologies, such as the Ku Klux Klan and neo-Nazi groups. The rapid growth of hate sites on the Internet is another area of concern.

Bullying

According to Public Safety Canada,* "Bullying is characterized by acts of intentional harm, repeated over time, in a relationship where an imbalance of power exists. It includes physical actions (punching, kicking, biting), verbal actions (threats, name calling, insults, racial or sexual comments), and social exclusion (spreading rumours, ignoring, gossiping, excluding)." In Canada, evidence suggests that on a weekly basis, 6% of students between the ages of 12 and 19 report bullying others, 8% report that they are victims of bullying, and 1% report that they bully others and are bullied. Although boys are more likely to bully and be bullied (usually in the form of a physical attack or aggressive behaviour), girls are more prone to indirect bullying in the form of social isolation and the spreading of rumours.

The consequences of bullying can be very serious. For example, research has shown that male victims are five times as likely to be depressed as their classmates, and female victims are three times as likely to be depressed. Victims of bullying are also more likely to display suicidal behaviours. Bullying behaviour during childhood is associated with later problematic behaviours. Evidence suggests that children who bully may become adolescents who sexually harass, become involved in delinquent or gang-related behaviours, or engage in dating violence. As adults, these individuals may also commit abuse or display harassment in the

workplace. The prevention of bullying among children and youth is an important factor for reducing the likelihood of future criminal activity among those who bully and in the development of confidence, self-esteem, and positive relationships among those who are bullied.

Workplace Violence

Close to 20% of the violent incidents (including sexual assault, robbery, and physical assault) reported by Canadians in 2004 occurred in the workplace. In more than 50% of these cases, workplace violence was committed against males (compared with 20% of cases involving female victims). About one-third of the incidents of workplace violence involved a victim who worked in social assistance or health care services. Another 14% involved individuals working in hotel or food services, and 11% involved victims working in educational services.

General crime-prevention strategies, including using surveillance cameras and silent alarms and limiting the amount of cash on hand, can help reduce workplace violence related to robberies. A highly stressed workplace is a risk factor in cases of violence between acquaintances or co-workers; clear guidelines about acceptable behaviour and prompt action after any threats or incidents of violence can help control this type of workplace violence.

Terrorism

Terrorism represents the most significant threat to Canada's national security. As Canada continues to play an active role in the worldwide fight against terror, it will undoubtedly face threats from terrorist organizations. Terrorism has been defined as the unlawful use of force or violence against people or property to intimidate or coerce a government, the civilian population, or any segment of it to further political or social objectives (see the box "Violence and Health: A Global View"). Terrorism can be either domestic, carried out by groups based in Canada, or international. It comes in many forms, including biological (see Chapter 9), chemical, nuclear, and cyber. Its intent is to promote helplessness by instilling fear of harm or destruction.

In response to the terrorist attacks in the United States on September 11, 2001, the Government of Canada enacted the Anti-terrorism Act. This act aims to combat terrorism at home and abroad through five main objectives: (1) preventing terrorists from getting into Canada; (2) protecting Canadians from terrorist acts; (3) using tools to identify, prosecute, convict, and punish terrorists; (4) keeping the Canada–U.S. border secure and open to trade; and (5) working with the international community to bring terrorists to justice and address the root causes of terrorism. Government efforts to prevent acts of terrorism include close work with law enforcement, intelligence,

---

* This section is based on *Bullying Prevention: Nature and Extent of Bullying in Canada* (http://www.publicsafety.gc.ca/res/cp/res/2008-bp-01-eng.aspx). Reproduced with the permission of the Government of Canada.

Violence and Health: A Global View

In 2002, the World Health Organization (WHO) issued its *World Report on Violence and Health*, which examines the magnitude and impact of violence throughout the world. Each year, more than 1.6 million people die from violent acts: Suicide claims a life every 40 seconds; homicide, every minute; and armed conflict, every two minutes. Violence is among the leading causes of death for people ages 15–44, accounting for 14% of deaths among males and 7% of deaths among females. Millions more victims of violence survive but are left with physical, psychological, and reproductive problems, including lost limbs, paralysis, depression, alcohol and drug abuse, sexual dysfunction, and sexually transmitted infections and other reproductive health problems. Beyond individual misery, violence has devastating social and economic consequences.

Interpersonal Violence

The WHO defines *interpersonal violence* as the intentional use of physical force or power, threatened or actual, against another person that is likely to result in injury, death, psychological harm, or deprivation. Each year, more than 500,000 people die from interpersonal violence, and more than 60 million children and older adults are maltreated. It's estimated that 10%–70% of women experience physical violence at the hands of an intimate partner during their lifetime; in addition, forced prostitution, child marriage, sexual trafficking, and female genital mutilation are prevalent in some areas of the world.

Worldwide, adolescents and young adults are the primary victims and perpetrators of interpersonal violence. Individual risk factors for violence highlighted in the WHO report include being young, male, and poor; being intoxicated; and having easy access to firearms. At the community and social levels, risk factors include low social capital (norms and networks that promote coordination and cooperation), high crime rates, rapid

social change, poverty, poor rule of law and corruption, gender inequality, firearm availability, and armed conflict.

Collective Violence

The WHO applies the term *collective violence* to violence inflicted by one group against another group to achieve political, economic, or social objectives. Collective violence includes armed conflict within or between nations; genocide, repression, and other human rights abuses; terrorism; and organized violent crime. Characteristics of countries with increased risk of violent conflict include long-standing tensions between groups, a lack of democratic processes, unequal access to power, unequal distribution and control of resources, and rapid demographic changes.

In the twentieth century, an estimated 191 million people—more than half of them civilians—lost their lives directly or indirectly as a result of armed conflict, and many more were injured. In addition to directly causing deaths and injuries, collective violence destroys

infrastructure and disrupts trade, food production, and vital services, thus setting the stage for famine, increased rates of infectious diseases, and mass movements of refugees. The resulting social turmoil also increases rates of interpersonal violence.

What Can Be Done?

The WHO report emphasizes that violence is neither an inevitable part of the human condition nor an intractable social problem. Rather, the wide variation in violence within and among nations over time suggests that violence is the product of a complex but modifiable set of social and environmental factors. Potential strategies to reduce violence include the following:

• Individual and relationship approaches to encourage healthy attitudes and behaviours, such as training in social, parenting, and relationship skills and conflict resolution; mentoring programs; and treatment for people who suffer from depression or who have inflicted abuse on partners or children

• Community-based efforts to raise public awareness and address local social and material causes of violence, such as creating safe places for children to play and adopting community policing

• Societal approaches to change underlying cultural, social, and economic factors, such as new laws and international treaties, policy changes to reduce poverty and inequality, efforts to change harmful social and cultural norms (for example, ethnic discrimination or gender inequality), and disarmament and demobilization programs in countries emerging from conflict.

Sources: World Health Organization. 2002. *The World Health Report 2002: Reducing Risks, Promoting Healthy Life.* Geneva: World Health Organization; World Health Organization. 2002. *World Report on Violence and Health.* Geneva: World Health Organization.

economic, and military communities to protect electric and water supply systems, transportation, gas and oil, emergency services, the computer infrastructure, and other systems.

One step you can take is to put together an emergency plan and kit for your family or household that can serve for any type of emergency or disaster (see the box "Emergency Preparedness"). See Chapters 2, 3, and 18 for advice on coping with the stress of terrorism or violence on campus, and recognizing post-traumatic stress disorder.

Family and Intimate Violence

Violence in families challenges some of our most basic assumptions about the family. Family violence generally refers to any rough and illegitimate use of physical force, aggression, or verbal abuse by one family member toward another. Such abuse may be physical or psychological in nature. According to Statistics Canada, an estimated 40,200 incidents of spousal violence, 53,400 cases of family-related assault against children, and 1938 incidents of family violence against older adults were reported in 2007.

Spousal Violence Approximately 83% of domestic violence victims in Canada are women. A substantial number of women who visit medical emergency rooms are there for injuries related to ongoing abuse. Violence against wives or intimate partners occurs at every level of society but is more common at lower socioeconomic levels. It occurs more frequently in relationships with a high degree of conflict—an apparent inability to resolve arguments through negotiation and compromise. About one-quarter of women report having been physically or sexually assaulted by an intimate partner, and more than half report having experienced some type of abuse—physical or psychological—in a relationship. In many cases, domestic violence continues for months or years. The problem of intimate violence is even apparent among young people; in 2007, the rate of spousal violence for female victims was highest among Canadian women ages 25–34.

At the root of much of this abusive behaviour is the need to control another person. Abusive partners are controlling partners. They not only want to have power over another person but also believe they are entitled to it, no matter what the cost to the other person. Abuse includes behaviour that physically harms, arouses fear, prevents a person from doing what she wants, or compels her to behave in ways she does not freely choose. Controlling people use a variety of psychological, emotional, and physical tactics to keep their partners bound to them. Early in a relationship, a person's tendency to be controlling may not be obvious (see the box "Recognizing the Potential for Abusiveness in a Partner" on p. 626).

In abusive relationships, the abuser (in most cases a man) usually has a history of violent behaviour, traditional

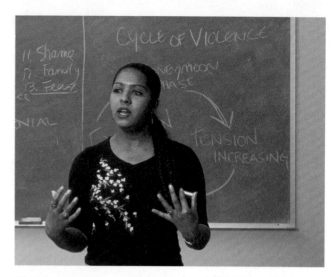

Education, counselling, and support can help the victims of family violence.

beliefs about gender roles, and problems with alcohol abuse. He has low self-esteem and seeks to raise it by dominating and imposing his will on another person. Research has revealed a three-phase cycle of battering, consisting of a period of increasing tension, a violent explosion, and a period of contriteness in which the man begs forgiveness and promises it will never happen again.

Abused women often stay in violent relationships for years. They may be economically dependent on their partners, feel trapped or fear retaliation if they leave, believe their children need a father, or have low self-esteem themselves. They may love or pity their husband, or they may believe they'll eventually be able to stop the violence. They usually leave the relationship only when they become determined that the violence must end. Shelters for abused women offer physical protection, counselling, support, and other assistance.

Many abusers are arrested, prosecuted, and imprisoned. Treatment programs are helpful in some cases but not all. Programs focus on stress management, communication and conflict-resolution skills, behaviour change, and individual or group therapy. A crucial factor in changing violent behaviour seems to be a partner's adamant insistence that the abuse must stop.

Stalking and Cyberstalking Spousal abuse is closely associated with **stalking**, also called **criminal harassment**, characterized by harassing behaviours, such as following or spying on a person and making verbal, written, or implied threats. In Canada, a total of 9080 criminal harassment incidents were reported to police in 2002; about 84% of stalkers were men. Approximately 31% of female victims were criminally harassed by current or former intimate partners, and 23% were stalked by a friend or an acquaintance. Research suggests that criminal harassment among

IN THE NEWS

Emergency Preparedness

In any given year, some part of Canada may be hit by an earthquake, flooding, tornadoes, or a mass power outage. These all-too-real situations—and the fear of potential threats, such as terrorist strikes or an outbreak of widespread violence—underscore the need for everyone to be prepared for an emergency. Two key elements of emergency preparedness are a well-stocked emergency supply kit and a well-reasoned emergency plan.

Emergency Supplies

An emergency supply kit should include everything you'll need to make it on your own for at least three days. You'll need nonperishable food, water, first aid supplies, essential medications, a battery-powered radio, toiletries, clothing, a flashlight or candles and matches, cash, keys, copies of important documents, and supplies for sleeping outdoors in any season or weather (blankets, sleeping bags, tent, and so on). Don't forget about special-needs items for infants, seniors, and pets.

In the case of certain types of terrorist attacks or industrial disasters, you may need supplies to "shelter in place"—to create a barrier between yourself and any dangerous airborne materials. These supplies might include filter masks or folded cotton towels that can be placed over the mouth and nose. Plastic sheeting and duct tape can be used to seal windows and doors.

You may want to create several kits of emergency supplies. The primary one would contain supplies for home use. Put together a smaller, lightweight version that you can take with you if you are forced to evacuate your residence and make kits for your car and office.

A Family or Household Plan

You and the members of your household may not be together when a disaster strikes. You should have a plan about where to meet and how to communicate. Choose at least two potential meeting places—one in your neighbourhood and one or more in other areas. Your community may also have set locations for community shelters.

Where you go may depend on the circumstances of the emergency situation. Use your common sense, and listen to the radio or television for instructions from emergency officials about whether to evacuate or stay in place. In addition, know all the transportation options in the vicinity of your home, school, and workplace; roadways and public transit may be affected, so keep walking shoes in your emergency kit.

Everyone in the household should also have the same emergency contact person to call, preferably someone who lives outside the immediate area. Local phone service may be significantly disrupted, so long-distance calls may be more likely to go through. Everyone should carry the relevant phone numbers and addresses at all times.

Check the emergency plans at any location where you or family members spend time, including schools and workplaces. For each location, know the safest place to be for different types of emergencies—for example, near load-bearing interior walls during an earthquake or in the basement during a tornado. Also know how to turn off water, gas, and electricity in case of damaged utility lines; keep the needed tools next to the shutoff valves.

Other steps you can take to help prepare for emergencies include taking a first aid class and setting up an emergency response group in your neighbourhood or building. More complete information about emergency preparedness is available from the following sources:

• Canadian Red Cross (http://www.red cross.ca)

• Government of Canada (http://www. GetPrepared.ca)

• Public Health Agency of Canada, Centre for Emergency Preparedness and Response (http://www.phac-aspc.gc.ca/ cepr-cmiu/index-eng.php)

---

female university or college students may be greater than that experienced by the general population. A stalker's goal may be to control or scare the victim or to keep her or him in a relationship. Most stalking episodes last a year or less.

The use of the Internet, email, chat rooms, and other electronic communications devices to stalk another person is known as **cyberstalking**. As with offline stalking, the majority of cyberstalkers are men, and the majority of targets are women, although there have been same-sex cyberstalking incidents. Online incidents of harassment

stalking (criminal harassment) Repeatedly harassing or threatening a person through such behaviours as following a person, appearing at a person's residence or workplace, leaving written messages or objects, making harassing phone calls, or vandalizing property; frequently directed at a former intimate partner.

cyberstalking The use of email, chat rooms, bulletin boards, or other electronic communications devices to stalk another person.

TERMS

Recognizing the Potential for Abusiveness in a Partner

You can't tell for sure whether someone will become abusive or violent toward an intimate partner, but there are warning signs that you can look for. (Remember that although most abusive relationships involve male violence directed at a woman, women can also be abusive, as can partners in a same-sex relationship. Because most abusers are male, the following material refers to the abuser as "he.") If you are concerned that a person you are involved with has the potential for violence, observe his behaviour, and ask yourself these questions:

• What is this person's attitude toward women? How does he treat his mother and his sister? How does he work with female students, female colleagues, or a female boss? How does he treat your female friends?

• What is his attitude toward your autonomy? Does he respect the work you do and the way you do it? Or does he put it down, tell you how to do it better, or encourage you to give it up? Does he tell you he'll take care of you?

• How self-centred is he? Does he want to spend leisure time on your interests or his? Does he listen to you? Does he remember what you say?

• Is he possessive or jealous? Does he want to spend every minute with you? Does he cross-examine you about things you do when you're not with him?

• What happens when things don't go the way he wants them to? Does he blow up? Does he always have to get his way?

• Is he moody, mocking, critical, or bossy? Do you feel as if you're walking on eggshells when you're with him?

• Do you feel you have to avoid arguing with him?

• Does he drink too much or use drugs?

• Does he refuse to use condoms or take other precautions for safer sex?

Listen to your own uneasiness, and stay away from any man who disrespects women, who wants or needs you intensely and exclusively, and who has a knack for getting his own way almost all the time.

If you are in a serious relationship with a controlling person, you may already have experienced abuse. Consider the following questions:

• Does your partner constantly criticize you, blame you for things that are not your fault, or verbally degrade you?

• Does he humiliate you in front of others?

• Is he suspicious or jealous? Does he accuse you of being unfaithful or monitor your email, mail, or phone calls?

• Does he track all your time? Does he discourage you from seeing friends and family?

• Does he prevent you from getting or keeping a job or attending school? Does he control your shared resources or restrict your access to money?

• Has he ever pushed, slapped, hit, kicked, bitten, or restrained you? Thrown an object at you? Used a weapon on you?

• Has he ever destroyed or damaged your personal property or sentimental items?

• Has he ever forced you to have sex or to do something sexually you didn't want to do?

• Does he anger easily when drinking or taking drugs?

• Has he ever threatened to harm you or your children, friends, pets, or property?

• Has he ever threatened to blackmail you if you leave?

If you answered yes to one or more of these questions, you may be experiencing domestic abuse. If you believe you or your children are in imminent danger, look in your local telephone directory for a women's shelter, or call 911. If you want information, referrals to a program in your area, or assistance, contact one of the organizations listed in For More Information at the end of the chapter.

Sources: Family Violence Prevention Fund. 2006. *It's Your Business.* San Francisco: Family Violence Prevention Fund; South Dakota Network Against Family Violence and Sexual Assault. 2005. *Are You in an Abusive Situation?* (http://www.sdnafvsa.com/abusive_relationship.php; retrieved June 16, 2008); National Coalition Against Domestic Violence. 2006. *2005 Domestic Violence Facts* (http://www.ncadv.org/files/DV_Facts.pdf; retrieved June 16, 2008).

or abuse are becoming more common and more serious, and in some cases, the perpetrator may be charged with criminal harassment. Depending on the activities involved, other charges (for example, unauthorized use of a computer) may also be appropriate. The impersonal nature of electronic communication may lower the barriers to harassment and threats, because a cyberstalker does not have to physically confront the victim, and this may make stalking more common. The popularity of online dating sites may also increase cyberstalking.

Cyberstalkers may send harassing or threatening emails or chat room messages to the target, or they may

encourage others to harass the person—for example, by impersonating the victim and posting inflammatory messages and personal information on bulletin boards or in chat rooms. Guidelines for staying safe online include the following:

• Never use your real name as an email username or chat room nickname. Select an age- and gender-neutral identity.

• Avoid filling out profiles for accounts related to email use or chat room activities with information that could be used to identify you.

- Do not share personal information in public spaces anywhere online or give it to strangers.
- Learn how to filter unwanted email messages.
- If you experience harassment online, do not respond to the harasser. Log off or surf elsewhere.

If you receive unwanted online contact, make it clear to that person that you want all contact to stop. If harassment continues, contact the harasser's Internet service provider (ISP) by identifying the domain of the stalker's account (after the "@" sign); most ISPs have an email address for complaints. Often, an ISP can try to stop the conduct by direct contact with the harasser or by closing his or her account. Save all communications for evidence, and contact your ISP and your local police department.

Violence Against Children Violence is also directed against children. In 2007, almost 53,400 Canadian children were the victims of assault, and about three in ten incidents were perpetrated by a family member. In approximately six out of ten cases of family violence directed toward children, a parent is identified as the abuser.

Parents who abuse children tend to have few social supports, to have mental health issues, to believe in physical punishment, to have a poor marital relationship, and to have been abused themselves (although many people who were abused as children do not grow up to abuse their own children). Poverty, unemployment, and social isolation are characteristics of families in which children are abused. External stressors related to socioeconomic and environmental factors are most closely associated with neglect, whereas stressors related to interpersonal issues are more closely associated with physical abuse. Single parents, particularly lone mothers, are at especially high risk for abusing their children. Very often one child, whom the parents consider different in some way, is singled out for violent treatment.

When child welfare services intervene in child-abuse situations, the goals are to protect the victims and to assist and strengthen the families. Successful programs emphasize education and early intervention, such as home visits to high-risk first-time mothers. Educational efforts focus on stress management, money management, job-finding skills, and information about child behaviour and development. Parents may receive counselling and be referred to substance-abuse treatment programs. Support groups are also effective for parents committed to changing their behaviour.

Elder Abuse It is estimated that 4%–10% of older adults in Canada are abused, exploited, or mistreated by someone who is supposed to be giving them care and protection. Most abusers are family members who are serving as caregivers.

Elder abuse can take many different forms: physical, sexual, or emotional abuse; financial exploitation; neglect; or abandonment. Elders who have lost some mental or physical functions and must rely on others for care are most at risk and may suffer malnutrition, dehydration, mismanaged medication, or infection from poor hygiene. Experts also cite a growing concern about self-neglect among older adults. This includes behaviour that threatens their own health or safety, and can include refusing to comply with doctors' orders or neglecting to eat a balanced diet.

Abuse often occurs when caring for a dependent adult becomes too stressful for the caregiver, especially if the elder is incontinent, has suffered mental deterioration, or is violent. Abuse may become an outlet for frustration. Many believe that the solution to elder abuse is support in the form of greater social and financial assistance, such as adult day care centres and education and public care programs.

Sexual Assault

Sexual coercion that relies on the threat and use of physical force or takes advantage of circumstances that render a person incapable of giving consent (such as when drunk) constitutes **sexual assault** or **rape**. In 1983, the Criminal Code of Canada was revised to replace the crimes labelled "rape" and "indecent assault" with three new sexual assault offences (levels 1, 2, and 3) which focus on the violent rather than sexual nature of the offence. However, the term *rape* is still commonly used throughout society. For example, coerced sexual activity in which the victim knows or is dating the rapist is often referred to as **date rape**, or *acquaintance rape*. Most sexual assault victims know their assailant, but less than one in ten sexual assault victims reports the crimes to police.

Any woman—or man—can be a victim of sexual assault, although females experience higher rates of sexual assault in Canada. According to the 2004 *General Social Survey (GSS)* on victimization, more than 512,000 Canadians ages 15 and older were the victims of sexual assault in the year before the survey. This survey also revealed that the rate of sexual assault for Canadians ages 15–24 was almost 18 times as great as the rate recorded for Canadians ages 55 years and older.

WHO COMMITS SEXUAL ASSAULT? Men who commit sexual assault may be any age and come from any socioeconomic group. Some offenders are exploiters in the sense that they

sexual assault (rape) The use of force to have sex with someone against that person's will.

date rape Sexual assault by someone the victim knows or is dating; also called *acquaintance rape*.

TERMS

assault on the spur of the moment and mainly want immediate gratification. Some attempt to compensate for feelings of sexual inadequacy and an inability to obtain satisfaction otherwise. Others are more hostile and sadistic and are primarily interested in hurting and humiliating a particular woman or women in general. Often, the offender is more interested in dominance, control, and power than in sexual satisfaction.

Most women are in much less danger of being sexually assaulted by a stranger than by a man they know or date. More than half of the sexual assaults reported in the 2004 GSS involved an offender who was a friend or an acquaintance; 35% of the reported sexual assaults involved a stranger.

Surveys suggest that as many as 25% of women have had experiences in which the men they were dating persisted in trying to force sex despite the women pleading, crying, screaming, or resisting. Most cases of date rape are never reported to the police, partly because of the subtlety of the crime. Usually no weapons are involved, and direct verbal threats may not have been made. Rather than being terrorized, the victim usually is attracted to the man at first. Victims of date rape tend to shoulder much of the responsibility for the incident, questioning their own judgment and behaviour rather than blaming the aggressor.

Sometimes husbands sexually assault their wives. According to Canadian police data, among the relatives accused in sexual assault cases in 2007, 4% were current or former spouses. A charge of sexual assault by a spouse can now be taken to court in Canada.

FACTORS CONTRIBUTING TO DATE RAPE Although the general status of women in society has improved, some people still hold the cultural belief that nice women don't say yes to sex (even when they want to) and that real men don't take no for an answer.

Men and women typically differ in their perception of romantic encounters and signals. In one study, researchers found that men interpreted women's actions on dates, such as smiling or talking in a low voice, as indicating an interest in having sex, whereas the women interpreted the same actions as just being friendly. Some men's thinking about forceful sex also tends to be unclear. One psychologist reports that men find "forcing a woman to have sex against her will" more acceptable than "raping a woman," even though the former description is the definition of rape.

Men who rape their dates tend to have certain attributes, including hostility toward women, a belief that dominance alone is a valid motive for sex, and an acceptance of sexual violence. They may feel that force is justified in certain circumstances, such as if they are sexually involved with a woman and she refuses to have sex, if the woman is known to have had sex with other men, or if the woman shows up at a party where people are drinking and taking drugs. The man often primes himself to force himself sexually on his date by drinking, which lowers his ordinary social inhibitions. Many university and college men who have committed date rape tried to seduce their dates by plying them with alcohol first.

DATE-RAPE DRUGS A 2006 study showed that drugs are a factor in more than 60% of sexual assaults and about 5% of victims are given date-rape drugs. Also called *predator drugs*, the drugs used in date rapes include flunitrazepam (Rohypnol), gamma hydroxybutyrate (GHB), and ketamine hydrochloride ("special K"). Rohypnol and GHB are not legally available in Canada, and ketamine is legally available only to veterinarians and physicians for medical use.

These drugs have a variety of effects, including sedation; if slipped surreptitiously into a drink, they can incapacitate a person within about 20 minutes and make her or him more vulnerable to assault. Rohypnol, GHB, and other drugs also often cause anterograde amnesia, meaning victims have little memory of what happened while they were under the influence of the drug. (See Chapter 14 for more on the effects of these and other psychoactive drugs.)

The makers of Rohypnol are modifying the pills so they will be a more noticeable colour and will dissolve more slowly, thereby reducing the likelihood that Rohypnol can be used as a date-rape drug; however, other drugs in powdered or liquid form can be slipped into drinks unnoticed. Some strategies, such as the following, can help ensure that your drink is not tampered with at a bar or party:

- Check with campus or local police to find out if drug-facilitated sexual assault has occurred in your area and, if so, where.

- Drink moderately and responsibly. Avoid group drinking and drinking games.

- Be wary of opened beverages—alcoholic or nonalcoholic—offered by strangers. When at an unfamiliar bar, watch the bartender pour your drink.

- Avoid drinking from punchbowls at bars, clubs, or raves.

- If an opened beverage tastes, looks, or smells strange, do not drink it. If you leave your drink unattended, such as when you dance or use the restroom, obtain a fresh drink when you return to your table.

- If you go to a party, club, or bar, go with friends. Have a prearranged plan for checking on each other visually and verbally. If you feel giddy or lightheaded, get assistance.

Both males and females can take actions that will reduce the incidence of acquaintance rape; see the box "Reducing Your Risk of Date Rape" for specific suggestions.

DEALING WITH A SEXUAL ASSAULT Experts disagree about whether a woman who is faced with a rapist should fight back or give in quietly to avoid being injured or to gain time in the hope of escaping. Some offenders say that if a woman had screamed or resisted loudly, they would have run; others report they would have injured or killed her. (If a rapist is carrying a weapon, most experts advise against fighting.) A woman who is sexually assaulted by a stranger is more likely to be physically injured than a woman assaulted by someone she knows. Each situation

Reducing Your Risk of Date Rape

Some experts have suggested that providing women with lists of do's and don'ts reinforces the belief that if a woman alters her behaviour, she will avoid being sexually assaulted. Although sexual assault is never the result of a woman's clothing or actions, it is important for men and women to consider some important safety information that could be useful in protecting themselves and others.

Guidelines for Women	Guidelines for Men
• Believe in your right to control what you do. Set limits, and communicate these limits clearly, firmly, and early. Say no when you mean no.	• Be aware of social pressure. It's OK to not score.
• Be assertive with someone who is sexually pressuring you. Men might interpret passivity as permission.	• Understand that no means no. Don't continue making advances when your date resists or tells you she wants to stop. Remember that she has the right to refuse sex.
• If you are unsure of a new acquaintance, go on a group date or double date. If possible, provide your own transportation.	• Don't assume sexy clothes and a flirtatious manner are invitations to sex, that previous permission for sex applies to the current situation, or that your date's relationships with other men constitute sexual permission for you.
• Remember that alcohol and drugs interfere with clear communication about sex.	• Remember that alcohol and drugs interfere with clear communication about sex.
• Use the statement that has proven most effective in stopping date rape: "This is rape, and I'm calling the police."	

is unique, and a woman should respond in whatever way she thinks best. If a woman chooses not to resist, it does not mean that she has not been sexually assaulted.

If you are threatened by a rapist and decide to fight back, here is what Women Organized Against Rape (WOAR) recommends:

- Trust your gut feeling. If you feel you are in danger, don't hesitate to run and scream. It is better to feel foolish than to be sexually assaulted.

- Yell—and keep yelling. It will clear your head and start your adrenaline going; it may scare your attacker and also bring help. Don't forget that an attacker is also afraid of pain and afraid of getting caught.

- If an attacker grabs you from behind, use your elbows to strike his neck, his sides, or his stomach.

- Try kicking. Your legs are the strongest part of your body, and your kick is longer than his reach. Kick with your rear foot and with the toe of your shoe. Aim low to avoid losing your balance.

- His most vulnerable spot is his knee; it's low, difficult to protect, and easily knocked out of place. Don't try to kick a rapist in the crotch; he has been protecting this area all his life and will have better protective reflexes there than at his knees.

- Once you start fighting, keep it up. Your objective is to get away as soon as you can.

- Remember that ordinary rules of behaviour don't apply. It's OK to vomit, act crazy, or claim to have a sexually transmitted infection (STI).

If you are sexually assaulted, tell what happened to the first friendly person you meet. Call the police, tell them you were sexually assaulted, and give your location. Try to remember as many facts as you can about your attacker; write down a description as soon as possible. Don't wash or change your clothes, or you may destroy important evidence. The police will take you to a hospital for a complete exam; show the physician any injuries. Tell the police simply, but exactly, what happened. Be honest, and stick to your story.

If you decide that you don't want to report the assault to the police, be sure to see a physician as soon as possible. You need to be checked for pregnancy and STIs.

THE EFFECTS OF SEXUAL ASSAULT Sexual assault victims suffer both physical and psychological injury. For most, physical wounds heal within a few weeks. Psychological pain may endure and be substantial. Even the most physically and mentally strong individuals are likely to experience shock, anxiety, depression, shame, and a host of psychosomatic symptoms after being victimized. These psychological reactions following sexual assault compose rape trauma syndrome, which is characterized by fear, nightmares, fatigue, crying spells, and digestive upset. (Rape trauma syndrome is a form of post-traumatic stress disorder; see Chapter 2.) Self-blame is very likely; society has contributed to this tendency by perpetuating the myths that women can actually defend themselves and that no one can be raped if she doesn't want to be. Fortunately, these false beliefs are dissolving in the face of evidence to the contrary.

Many organizations offer counselling and support to sexual assault victims. Look online or in the telephone directory under Sexual Assault or Rape Crisis Centre for a hotline number to call. Your campus may have counselling services or a support group.

Child Sexual Abuse   Child sexual abuse is any sexual contact between an adult and a child who is below the legal age of consent. Adults and older adolescents are able to coerce children into sexual activity because of their authority and power over them. Threats, force, or the promise of love, friendship, or material rewards may be used to manipulate a child. Sexual contacts are typically brief and usually consist of genital manipulation; genital intercourse is much less common.

Sexual abusers are usually male, heterosexual, and known to the victim. The abuser may be a relative, a friend, a neighbour, or another trusted adult acquaintance. Child abusers are often pedophiles, people who are sexually attracted to children. They may have poor interpersonal and sexual relationships with other adults and feel socially inadequate and inferior.

One highly traumatic form of sexual abuse is **incest**, sexual activity between people too closely related to legally marry. The most common forms of incest are father-daughter (which includes stepfather-stepdaughter) abuse, brother-sister abuse (usually an adolescent boy abusing a preadolescent girl), and uncle-niece abuse; mother-son sexual activity is rare. Adults who commit incest may be pedophiles, but they can also be sexual opportunists or people with poor impulse control and emotional problems.

Most sexually abused children are between ages 8 and 12 when the abuse first occurs. More girls are sexually abused than boys. The degree of trauma for the child can be very serious, but it varies with the type of encounters, their frequency, the child's age and relationship to the abuser, and the parents' response. Father-daughter abuse may be the most traumatic form, in part because it is a violation of the basic parent-child relationship and because the abuse tends to be more frequent.

Abused children may be depressed or moody, exhibit hyperactivity, play violently with others or with inanimate objects, talk nonsense, or unintentionally injure themselves.

Child sexual abuse is often unreported. Surveys suggest that as many as 27% of women and 16% of men were sexually abused as children. In Canada, more than 15,000 child maltreatment cases involved allegations of sexual abuse in 2003. It can leave lasting scars; victims are more likely to suffer as adults from low self-esteem, depression, anxiety, eating disorders, self-destructive tendencies, sexual problems, and difficulties in intimate relationships.

If you were a victim of sexual abuse as a child and feel it may be interfering with your functioning today, you may want to address the problem. A variety of approaches can help, such as joining a support group of people who have had similar experiences, confiding in a partner or friend, or seeking professional help.

Sexual Harassment   Unwelcome sexual advances, requests for sexual favours, and other verbal, visual, or physical conduct of a sexual nature constitute **sexual harassment** if such conduct explicitly or implicitly does any of the following:

- Affects academic or employment decisions or evaluations
- Interferes with an individual's academic or work performance
- Creates an intimidating, hostile, or offensive academic, work, or student living environment

Extreme cases of sexual harassment occur when a manager, professor, or other person in authority uses his or her ability to control or influence jobs or grades to coerce people into having sex or to punish them if they refuse. A hostile environment can be created by such conduct as making sexual gestures, displaying sexually suggestive objects or pictures, making derogatory comments and jokes, making sexual remarks about clothing or appearance, writing obscene letters, and touching or pinching. Sexual harassment can occur between people of the same or opposite sex.

Although sexual harassment is forbidden by law, many cases go unreported. If you have been the victim of sexual harassment, you may be able to take action to stop it. Be assertive with anyone who uses language or actions you find inappropriate. If possible, confront your harasser either in writing, over the telephone, or in person, informing him or her that the situation is unacceptable to you and you want the harassment to stop. Be clear. "Do not ever make sexual remarks to me" is an unequivocal statement. In addition to assertive communication, assemble a file or log documenting the harassment, noting the details of each incident and information about any witnesses who may be able to support your claims. You may discover others who have been harassed by the same person, which will strengthen your case. Then file a grievance

QUESTIONS FOR CRITICAL THINKING AND REFLECTION

Have you or anyone you know ever been the victim of a violent act? If so, what were the circumstances surrounding the event? What was the outcome? How did the event affect your life? In hindsight, what steps, if any, could have been taken to avoid or prevent the incident?

with the harasser's supervisor or employer, such as someone in the dean's office if you are a student or someone in the human resources office if you are an employee.

If your attempts to deal with the harassment internally are not successful, you can file an official complaint with your workplace human resources or equity office, or your provincial or territorial Human Rights Commission. You may also want to pursue legal action under local laws prohibiting employment discrimination. Very often, the threat of a lawsuit or other legal action is enough to stop the harasser.

What You Can Do About Violence

It is obvious that violence in our society is not disappearing and that it is a serious threat to our collective health and well-being. This is especially true on university and college campuses, which in a sense are communities in themselves but sometimes lack the authority or guidance to tackle the issue of violence directly (see the box "Staying Safe on Campus" on p. 632). Schools are now providing training for conflict resolution and are educating people about the diverse nature of our society, thereby encouraging tolerance and understanding. New programs are being developed at the grassroots level to deal with problems of violence directly.

As with any public health problem, one potential approach is to identify and target high-risk groups for intervention. Violence prevention programs currently focus on conflict-resolution training and the development of social skills. These measures have proven effective, but for behaviour change to be lasting, the focus of such programs must expand beyond individual intervention to include social and environmental factors.

PROVIDING EMERGENCY CARE

No matter how hard you try to avoid them, some injuries will inevitably occur. Therefore, it is important to prepare for situations in which you may need to provide emergency care for yourself or others. If you are prepared to help, you can improve someone else's chances of surviving or avoiding permanent disability.

A course in **first aid** can help you respond appropriately when someone is injured. One important benefit of first aid training is learning what *not* to do in certain situations. For example, a person with a suspected neck or back injury should not be moved unless other life-threatening conditions exist. A trained person can assess emergency situations accurately before acting.

Emergency rescue techniques can save the lives of people who are choking, who have stopped breathing, or whose hearts have stopped beating. As described earlier, the Heimlich manoeuvre is used when a victim is choking. Pulmonary resuscitation (also known as *rescue breathing, artificial respiration,* or *mouth-to-mouth resuscitation*) is used when a person is not breathing. Cardiopulmonary resuscitation (CPR) is used when a pulse cannot be found. Training is required before a person can perform CPR, and in 2005, significant changes were made to the guidelines for lay rescuer CPR. Courses are offered by the Canadian Red Cross, the Heart and Stroke Foundation of Canada, and St. John Ambulance Canada.

A new feature of some of these courses is training in the use of automatic external defibrillators (AEDs), which monitor the heart's rhythm and, if appropriate, deliver an electrical shock to restart the heart. Because of the importance of early use of defibrillators in saving heart attack victims, these devices are being installed in public places, including hockey arenas, airports, and many office buildings.

As a person providing assistance, you are the first link in the **emergency medical services (EMS) system**. Your responsibility may be to render first aid, provide emotional support for the victim, or just call for help. It is important to remain calm and act sensibly. The basic pattern for providing emergency care is check-call-care:

- *Check the situation:* Make sure the scene is safe for both you and the injured person. Don't put yourself in danger; if you get hurt too, you will be of little help to the injured person.

incest Sexual activity between close relatives, such as siblings or parents and their children.

sexual harassment Unwelcome sexual advances, requests for sexual favours, and other conduct of a sexual nature that affects academic or employment decisions or evaluations; interferes with an individual's academic or work performance; or creates an intimidating, hostile, or offensive academic, work, or student living environment.

first aid Emergency care given to an ill or injured person until medical care can be obtained.

emergency medical services (EMS) system A system designed to network community resources for providing emergency care.

TERMS

Staying Safe on Campus

University and college campuses can be the site of criminal activity and violence just as any other environment or living situation can be—and so they require the same level of caution and awareness that you would use in other situations. Two key points to remember: 80% of campus crimes are committed by a student against a fellow student, and alcohol or drug use is involved in 90% of campus felonies. Drinking or drug use can affect judgment and lower inhibitions, so be aware if you or another person is under the influence. Here are some suggestions for keeping yourself safe on campus:

• Don't travel alone after dark. Many campuses have shuttle buses that run from spots on campus, such as the library and recreation centre, to residence halls and other locations. Escorts are often available to walk with you at night.

• Be familiar with well-lit and frequently travelled routes around campus if you do need to walk alone.

• If you have a car, follow the usual precautions about parking in well-lit areas, keeping the doors locked while you are driving, and never picking up hitchhikers.

• Always have your keys ready as you approach your residence hall, room, and car. Don't lend your keys to others.

• Let friends and family members know your schedule of classes and activities so that you can create a buddy system.

• Be sure the doors and windows of your dorm room have sturdy locks, and use them.

• Don't prop open doors or hold doors open for nonstudents or nonresidents trying to enter your dorm. Be aware of nonresidents around your dorm. If someone says that he or she is meeting a friend inside, that person should be able to call the friend from outside the building.

• Keep valuables and anything containing personal information—credit cards, wallets, jewellery, and so on—hidden. Secure expensive computer and stereo equipment with cables so that it can't be easily stolen. Use a quality U-shaped lock whenever you leave a bicycle unattended.

• Be alert when using an ATM, and don't display large amounts of cash.

• Stay alert and trust your instincts. Don't hesitate to call the police or campus security if something doesn't seem or feel right.

• *Check the victim:* Conduct a quick head-to-toe examination. Assess the victim's signs and symptoms, such as level of responsiveness, pulse, and breathing rate. Look for bleeding and any indications of broken bones or paralysis.

• *Call for help:* Call 911 or a local emergency number.

• Identify yourself and give as much information as you can about the condition of the victim and what happened.

• *Care for the victim:* If the situation requires immediate action (no pulse, shock, etc.), provide first aid if you are trained to do so.

QUESTIONS FOR CRITICAL THINKING AND REFLECTION

What kinds of emergency training have you had? What kinds of skills do you have that would enable you to help someone who was hurt or trapped or needed some other kind of assistance?

Adopting Safer Habits

Why do you get injured? What human and environmental factors contribute to injuries? Identifying those factors is one step toward making your lifestyle safer. Changing unsafe behaviours before they lead to injuries is an even better way of improving your chances.

For the next 7–10 days, keep track of any mishaps you are involved in or injuries you receive, recording them on a daily behaviour record like the one shown in Chapter 1. Count each time you cut, burn, or injure yourself, fall down, run into someone, or have any other potentially injury-causing mishap, no matter how trivial. Also record any risk-taking behaviours, such as failing to wear your seat belt or bicycle helmet, drinking and driving, exceeding the speed limit, putting off home or bicycle repairs, and so on. For each entry (injury or incidence of unsafe behaviour), record the date, the time, what you were doing, who else was there and how you were influenced by him or her, what your motivations were, and what you were thinking and feeling at the time.

At the end of the monitoring period, examine your data. For each incident, determine both the human factors and the environmental factors that contributed to the injury or unsafe behaviour. Were you tired? Distracted? Did you not realize this situation was dangerous? Did you take a chance? Did you think this incident couldn't happen to you? Was visibility poor? Were you using defective equipment? Then consider each contributing factor carefully, determining why it existed and how it could have been avoided or changed. Finally, consider what preventive actions you could take to avoid such incidents or to change your behaviours in the future.

As an example, let's say that you usually don't wear a seat belt when you run local errands in your car and that several factors contribute to this behaviour: You don't really think you could be involved in a crash so close to home, you go only on short trips, you just never think to use it, and so on. One of the contributing factors to your unsafe behaviour is inadequate knowledge. You can change this factor by obtaining accurate information about auto crashes (and their usual proximity to a victim's home) from this chapter and from library or Internet research. Just acquiring information about motor vehicle crashes and seat belt use may lead you to examine your beliefs and attitudes about seat belts and motivate you to change your behaviour.

Once you're committed, you can use behaviour change techniques described in Chapter 1, such as completing a contract, asking family and friends for support, and so on, to build a new habit. Put a note or picture reminding you to buckle up in your car where you can see it clearly. Recruit a friend to run errands with you and to remind you about using your seat belt. Once your habit is established, you may influence other people—especially people who ride in your car—to use seat belts all the time. By changing this behaviour, you can reduce the chances that you or your passengers will suffer a serious injury or even die in a vehicle crash.

![Mc Graw Hill] connect™

Practise and learn online with Connect. Connect allows you to practise important skills at your own pace and on your own schedule, with 24/7 online access to an eBook, practice quizzes, interactivities, videos, study tools, additional resources, and more.

SUMMARY

- Injuries are caused by a dynamic interaction of human and environmental factors. Risk-taking behaviour is associated with a high rate of injury.

- Key factors in motor vehicle injuries include aggressive driving, speeding, a failure to wear seat belts, alcohol and drug intoxication, fatigue, and distraction.

- Motorcycle, moped, and bicycle injuries can be prevented by developing appropriate skills, driving or riding defensively, and wearing proper safety equipment, especially a helmet.

- Most fall-related injuries are a result of falls at floor level, but stairs, chairs, and ladders are also involved in a significant number of falls.

- Careless smoking and problems with cooking or heating equipment are common causes of home fires. Being prepared for fire emergencies means planning escape routes and installing smoke detectors.

- The home can contain many poisonous substances, including medications, cleaning agents, plants, and fumes from cars and appliances.

- Performing the Heimlich manoeuvre can prevent someone from dying by choking.

- Many injuries during leisure activities result from the misuse of equipment, lack of experience, use of alcohol, and a failure to wear proper safety equipment.

- Most work-related injuries involve extensive manual labour; back problems and repetitive strain injuries are common.

- Some of the factors contributing to violence in Canada include poverty, the absence of strong social ties, the influence of the mass media, cultural attitudes about gender roles, problems in interpersonal relationships, and alcohol and drug abuse.

- Types of violence include assault, homicide, gang-related violence, hate crimes, bullying, workplace violence, and terrorism.

- Assault and child abuse occur at every socioeconomic level. The core issue is the abuser's need to control other people.

- Most sexual assault victims are women, and most know their attackers.

- Child sexual abuse often results in serious trauma; usually the abuser is a trusted adult.

- Sexual harassment is unwelcome sexual advances or other conduct of a sexual nature that affects academic or employment performance or evaluations or that creates an intimidating, hostile, or offensive academic, work, or student living environment.

- Strategies for reducing violence include conflict-resolution training, social skills development, and education programs that foster tolerance and understanding among diverse groups.

- Steps in giving emergency care include making sure the scene is safe for you and the injured person, conducting a quick examination of the victim, calling for help, and providing emergency first aid.

FOR MORE INFORMATION

BOOKS

Becker, N. 2005. *Popular Mechanics Home Safety Handbook: Practical Tips for Safe Living*. Red Oak, Iowa: Popular Mechanics. Provides tips on living safely and how to prevent accidents and injuries in your home.

Dacey, J. S., and L. B. Fiore. 2006. *The Safe Child Handbook*. San Francisco: Jossey-Bass. A practical handbook for keeping your family safe and coping with the stress and fear associated with many real-world dangers.

Henry, J., H. Larson, and J. Rubin. 2007. *Home Emergency Pocket Guide*. Tigard, Ore.: Informed Publishing. A small, spiral-bound guide that provides critical information to help in dealing with a variety of emergencies.

MacPherson, J. 2003. *AAA Auto Guide: Driving Survival. How to Stay Safe on the Road*. Heathrow, Fl: AAA Publishing. Provides helpful strategies for choosing and maintaining a safe vehicle and for handling a variety of driving situations.

McGrew, J. 2005. *Think Safe: Practical Measures to Increase Security at Home, at Work, and Throughout Life.* Hilton Head Island, S.C.: Cameo Publications. A general guide to safety and crime and violence prevention.

National Safety Council. 2007. *Standard First Aid, CPR, and AED.* Itasca, Ill.: National Safety Council. An everyday guide to the most current first aid and emergency resuscitation techniques, with instructions for using automatic external defibrillators.

ORGANIZATIONS, HOTLINES, AND WEB SITES

The Internet addresses listed here were accurate at the time of publication.

Aboriginal Canada Portal. Provides resources, information (including health and social services information), and government programs in Canada for First Nations, Inuit, and Metis.

> http://www.aboriginalcanada.gc.ca

Canadian Automobile Association . Provides consumer information about all aspects of traffic safety.

> http://www.caa.ca

Canada Safety Council. Provides Canadians with safety training and resources, and delivers public awareness campaigns related to workplace safety, farm safety, summer safety, road safety, school safety, community safety and crime prevention, seniors' safety, and home fire safety.

> http://safety-council.org

Canadian Centre for Occupational Health and Safety. Provides information, tools, and resources related to workplace health and safety programs.

> http://www.ccohs.ca

Consumer Product Safety Commission. Provides information and advice about safety issues relating to consumer products.

> http://www.cpsc.gov

CyberAngels. Provides information on online safety and help and advice for victims of cyberstalking.

> http://www.cyberangels.org

Health Canada. Offers information on occupational health and safety and environmental and workplace health. Also provides links to resources statistics, educational materials, and support programs.

> http://www.hc-sc.gc.ca

Public Health Agency of Canada. Provides a wealth of credible and up-to-date information on a number of health-related topics in Canada, including infectious and chronic diseases.

> http://www.phac-aspc.gc.ca

Rape, Abuse, and Incest National Network. Provides guidelines for preventing and dealing with sexual assault and abuse.

> http://www.rainn.org

Safe Kids Canada. Provides information and resources for parents and professionals about reducing the risk of unintentional injuries among children and youth in Canada. Also offers a Safe Tip Line: 1-888-SAFE-TIP (723-3847).

> http://www.safekidscanada.ca

Shelternet.ca. An online resource for abused women and their children. Provides abused women with information and resources including a clickable map of shelters in Canada.

> http://www.shelternet.ca

Tolerance.Org: 10 Ways to Fight Hate on Campus. Offers suggestions for fighting hate and promoting tolerance; sponsored by the Southern Poverty Law Center.

> http://www.tolerance.org/campus/index.jsp

Transport Canada. Provides statistics and information about road and vehicle safety and regulations in Canada.

> http://www.tc.gc.ca

World Health Organization: Violence and Injury Prevention. Provides statistics and information about the consequences of intentional and unintentional injuries worldwide.

> http://www.who.int/violence_injury_prevention

The following sites provide statistics and background information on violence and crime in Canada:

> *Statistics Canada:* http://www.statcan.gc.ca/start-debut-eng.html
> *Royal Canadian Mounted Police:* http://www.rcmp-grc.gc.ca/index-eng.htm
> *Department of Justice Canada:* http://www.justice.gc.ca/eng/index.html

SELECTED BIBLIOGRAPHY

Association of Workers' Compensation Boards of Canada. 2010. *AWCBC-NWISP Statistical Summary Request Tables.* Sent via email to author on July 16, 2010.

Aultman-Hall, L., and M. G. Kaltenecker. 1999. Toronto bicycle commuter safety rates. *Accident Analysis and Prevention* 31(6): 675–686.

Brennan, S., and A. Taylor-Butts. 2008. Sexual assault in Canada: 2004 and 2007. *Canadian Centre for Justice Statistics Profile Series* 19 (http://www.statcan.gc.ca/pub/85f0033m/85f0033m2008019-eng.htm; retrieved July 3, 2010).

Browne, K. D., and C. Hamilton-Giachritsis. 2005. The influence of violent media on children and adolescents: A public-health approach. *Lancet* 365(9460): 702–710.

Canadian Automobile Association. n.d. *Driven to Distraction* (http://www.caa.ca/driventodistraction/home.html; retrieved June 26, 2010).

Carr, J. L. 2005. *American College Health Association Campus Violence White Paper.* Baltimore, Md.: American College Health Association.

CBC News. 2009. *Tornadoes* (http://www.cbc.ca/canada/story/2009/08/05/f-tornado.html; retrieved July 2, 2010).

CBC News Online. 2004. *In Depth: September 11. Canadian Casualties* (http://www.cbc.ca/news/background/sep11/cdncasualties.html; retrieved June 20, 2010).

Centers for Disease Control and Prevention. 2004. Impact of primary laws on adult use of safety belts—United States, 2002. *Morbidity and Mortality Weekly Report* 53(12): 257–260.

Centers for Disease Control and Prevention. 2005. Increase in poisoning deaths caused by nonillicit drugs. *Morbidity and Mortality Weekly Report* 54(2): 33–36.

Centers for Disease Control and Prevention. 2005. Unintentional non-fire-related carbon monoxide exposures—United States, 2001–2003. *Morbidity and Mortality Weekly Report* 54(2): 36–39.

Centre for Addiction and Mental Health. 2009. *Educating Students about Drug Use and Mental Health— Grade 9: Expectation 2* (http://www.camh.net/education/Resources_teachers_schools/Drug_Curriculum/Secondary/curriculum_gr9expect2.html; retrieved July 5, 2010).

Chettleburgh, M. C. 2008. Street gangs in Canada: The shape of things to come. *The Gazette* 70(2): 16–17 (http://www.rcmp-grc.gc.ca/gazette/vol70n2/gazette-vol70n2-eng.pdf; retrieved July 4, 2010).

College of Family Physicians of Canada. 2009. *Head Injuries: What to Watch for Afterward* (http://www.cfpc.ca/english/cfpc/programs/patient%20education/head%20injuries/default.asp?s=1; retrieved July 10, 2010).

Commission for Global Road Safety. 2008. *Global Road Safety Fact File* (http://www.fiafoundation.com/commissionforglobalroadsafety/fact.le/index.html; retrieved February 21, 2009).

Council of Canadian Fire Marshals and Fire Commissioners. 2007. *Annual Report 2002: Fire Losses in Canada* (http://www.ccfmfc.ca/stats/en/report_e_02.pdf; retrieved July 12, 2010).

Cummings, P., and F. P. Rivara. 2004. Car occupant death according to the restraint use of other occupants. *Journal of the American Medical Association* 291(3): 343–349.

Cummings, P., et al. 2006. Changes in traffic crash mortality rates attributed to use of alcohol, or lack of a seat belt, air bag, motorcycle helmet, or bicycle helmet, United States, 1982–2001. *Injury Prevention* 12(3): 148–154.

Dauvergne, M., K. Scrim, and S. Brennan. 2008. Hate crime in Canada. *Canadian Centre for Justice Statistics Profile Series* 17 (http://www.statcan.gc.ca/pub/85f0033m/85f0033m2008017-eng.pdf; retrieved July 4, 2010).

de Léséleuc, S. 2007. Criminal victimization in the workplace. *Canadian Centre for Justice Statistics* (http://www.statcan.gc.ca/pub/85f0033m/85f0033m2007013-eng.htm; retrieved July 14, 2010).

Department of Justice Canada. 2008. *The Anti-terrorism Act* (http://www.justice-canada.info/eng/antiter/press/info.html; retrieved July 5, 2010).

Department of Justice Canada. 2009. *Criminal Harassment: A Handbook for Police and Crown Prosecutors* (http://www.justice.gc.ca/eng/pi/fv-vf/pub/har/part1.html#cybstalk; retrieved July 14, 2010).

Environment Canada. 2010. *Lightning Detection* (http://www.weatheroffice.gc.ca/lightning/index_e.html; retrieved July 2, 2010).

Environment Canada. 2010. *Summer Hazards* (http://www.ec.gc.ca/meteo-weather/default.asp?lang=En&n=6C5D4990-1#Tornadoes; retrieved July 2, 2010).

Federal Bureau of Investigation. 2007. *Hate Crime Statistics, 2006.* Washington, D.C.: U.S. Department of Justice.

Foreign Affairs and International Trade Canada. 2003. *Backgrounder: Canada's Actions Against Terrorism Since September 11* (http://www.international.gc.ca/anti-terrorism/canadaactions-en.asp; retrieved July 5, 2010).

Foreign Affairs and International Trade Canada. 2010. *International Crime and Terrorism* (http://www.international.gc.ca/crime/terrorism-terrorisme.aspx?lang=engl; retrieved July 5, 2010).

Gorin, T. 2000. *A Rape Crisis Centre View of Rohypnol: How the Hype Tricks Raped Women.* Vancouver: Canadian Association of Sexual Assault Centres (http://www.casac.ca/content/rape-crisis-centre-view-rohypnol; retrieved July 5, 2010).

Government of Canada. 2008. *Canadian Laws and Safety* (http://www.goingtocanada.gc.ca/CIC/display-afficher.do?id=0000000000017&lang=eng; retrieved June 26, 2010).

Government of Canada. 2008. *Quick Facts on Elder Abuse in Canada. Elder Abuse: It's Time to Face the Reality* (http://www.seniors.gc.ca/c.4nt.2nt@.jsp?cid=145; retrieved June 26, 2010).

Graffunder, C. M., et al. 2004. Through a public health lens. Preventing violence against women: An update from the U.S. Centers for Disease Control and Prevention. *Journal of Women's Health* 13(1): 5–15.

Gray-Vickrey, P. 2004. Combating elder abuse. *Nursing* 34(10): 47–51.

Human Resources and Skills Development Canada. 2010. *Indicators of Well-Being in Canada: Work-Related Injuries* (http://www4.hrsdc.gc.ca/.3ndic.1t.4r@-eng.jsp?iid=20; retrieved July 13, 2010).

Infant and Toddler Safety Association (2009 Workshops). 2009. *Before You Turn the Key...Everything You Wanted to Know About Transporting Young Children, but Didn't Know You Needed to Ask.* Kitchener, ON.

Iudice, A., et al. 2005. Effects of prolonged wakefulness combined with alcohol and hands-free cellphone divided attention tasks on simulated driving. *Human Psychopharmacology* 20(2): 125–132.

Kilpatrick, D. 2004. Interpersonal violence and public policy: What about the victims? *Journal of Law, Medicine, and Ethics* 32(1): 73–81.

Krug, E. G. 2004. Injury surveillance is key to preventing injuries. *Lancet* 364(9445): 1563–1566.

Ministry of Transportation Ontario. 2010. *Frequently Asked Questions: Safety* (http://www.mto.gov.on.ca/english/faq/safety-test.shtml#BicycleHelmets2; retrieved July 1, 2010).

National Crime Prevention Centre, Public Safety Canada. 2007. *Youth Gangs in Canada: What Do We Know?* (http://www.publicsafety.gc.ca/prg/cp/bldngevd/_fl/2007-YG-1_e.pdf; retrieved July 4, 2010).

National Safety Council. 2008. *Injury Facts 2008.* Itasca, Ill.: National Safety Council.

National Traffic Safety Administration. 2007. *Traffic Safety Facts Research Note: Driver Cellphone Use in 2006—Overall Results.* Washington, D.C.: National Traffic Safety Administration.

Olson, C. M., et al. 2006. Association of first- and second-generation air bags with front occupant death in car crashes: A matched cohort study. *American Journal of Epidemiology* 164(2): 161–169.

Ontario Ministry of Transportation. 2010. *New and Alternative Vehicles* (http://www.mto.gov.on.ca/english/dandv/vehicle/emerging/; retrieved July 13, 2010).

Public Health Agency of Canada. 2008. *Leading Causes of Death and Hospitalization in Canada* (http://www.phac-aspc.gc.ca/publicat/lcd-pcd97/index-eng.php; retrieved July 1, 2010).

Public Health Agency of Canada. 2009. *Child and Youth Injury in Review, 2009 Edition: Spotlight on Consumer Product Safety* (http://www.phac-aspc.gc.ca/publicat/cyi-bej/2009/pdf/injrep-rapbles2009_eng.pdf; retrieved July 10, 2010).

Public Safety Canada, National Crime Prevention Centre. 2008. *Building the Evidence: Bullying Prevention* (http://www.publicsafety.gc.ca/res/cp/res/_fl/2008-BP-01-eng.pdf; retrieved February 19, 2011).

Ramage-Morin, P. L. 2008. Motor vehicle accident deaths, 1979 to 2004. *Health Reports* 19(3) (http://www.statcan.gc.ca/pub/82-003-x/2008003/article/10648-eng.pdf; retrieved July 13, 2010).

Reynolds, C. C. O., et al. 2009. The impact of transportation infrastructure on bicycling injuries and crashes: a review of the literature. *Environmental Health* 8: 47. doi:10.1186/1476-069X-8-47.

Silverman, J. G., A. Raj, and K. Clements. 2004. Dating violence and associated sexual risk and pregnancy among adolescent girls in the United States. *Pediatrics* 114(2): e220–225.

Safe Kids Canada. 2010. *Safe Scooter Riding* (http://www.safekidscanada.ca/Professionals/Safety-Information/Wheeled-Activities/Scooter-Riding/Safe-Scooter-Riding.aspx; retrieved July 2, 2010).

Safe Kids Canada. 2010. *Safety Information: Poison Prevention Tips* (http://www.safekidscanada.ca/parents/safety-information/poison-prevention/safety-tips/poison-prevention-tips.aspx; retrieved July 2, 2010).

Smart, R. G., and R. E. Mann. 2002. Deaths and injuries from road rage: Cases in Canadian newspapers. *Canadian Medical Association Journal* 167(7): 761–762 (http://www.cmaj.ca/cgi/reprint/167/7/761.pdf; retrieved July 10, 2010).

SMARTRISK. 2009. *The Economic Burden of Injury in Canada.* Toronto: SMARTRISK (http://www.smartrisk.ca/downloads/burden/Canada2009/EBI-Eng-Final.pdf; retrieved June 21, 2010).

Statistics Canada. 2006. *Musculoskeletal Diseases: Back Pain* (http://www.statcan.gc.ca/pub/82-619-m/2006003/4053542-eng.htm; retrieved July 2, 2010).

Statistics Canada. 2007. Study: Work injuries. *The Daily,* July 10 (http://www.statcan.gc.ca/daily-quotidien/070710/dq070710a-eng.htm; retrieved June 26, 2010).

Statistics Canada. 2009. *Family Violence in Canada: A Statistical Profile* (http://www.statcan.gc.ca/pub/85-224-x/85-224-x2009000-eng.htm; retrieved July 14, 2010).

Statistics Canada. 2009. Homicide in Canada: 2008. *The Daily,* October 28 (http://www.statcan.gc.ca/daily-quotidien/091028/dq091028a-eng.htm; retrieved July 13, 2010).

Statistics Canada. 2009. Police-reported crime statistics: 2008. *The Daily,* July 21 (http://www.statcan.gc.ca/daily-quotidien/090721/dq090721a-eng.htm; retrieved July 2, 2010).

Statistics Canada. 2010. *Bicycle Helmet Use, 2009* (http://www.statcan.gc.ca/pub/82-625-x/2010002/article/11274-eng.htm; retrieved July 13, 2010).

Statistics Canada. 2010. Canadian Community Health Survey: 2009. *The Daily,* June 15 (http://www.statcan.gc.ca/daily-quotidien/100615/dq100615b-eng.htm; retrieved July 4, 2010).

St. John Ambulance. 2010. *First aid for emergencies: Infants and children* (http://www.sja.ca/Canada/Documents/SJAPosteremergency(infant)v41English.pdf; retrieved June 23, 2010).

Strayer, D. L., et al. 2006. A comparison of the cellphone driver and the drunk driver. *Human Factors* 48(2): 381–391.

Thompson, R. S., et al. 2006. Intimate partner violence: Prevalence, types and chronicity in adult women. *American Journal of Preventive Medicine* 30(6): 447–457.

Although many environmental problems are complex and seem beyond the control of the individual, we have ways that we can make a difference to the future of the planet.

POPULATION GROWTH AND CONTROL

Throughout most of history, humans have been a minor pressure on the planet. About 300 million people were alive in the year AD 1; 1600 years later, the world population had increased gradually to a little more than 500 million. But then it began rising exponentially—zooming to 1 billion by about 1800, more than doubling by 1930, and then doubling again in just 40 years (Figure 21.1).

The world's population, currently about 6.6 billion, is increasing at a rate of about 76 million per year—150 people every minute. The United Nations projects that world population will reach 9.1 billion by 2050 and will continue to increase until it levels off above 10 billion in 2200. Virtually all of this increase is taking place in less-developed regions. In 1950, the more-developed regions accounted for 32% of the world's population; their share dropped to 20% in 2000 and is expected to further decline to 13% in 2050. Changes are also projected for the world's age distribution: The proportion of people age 60 and older will increase from 10% in 2000 to 22% in 2050, and by 2050 there will be more older persons than children.

This rapid expansion of population, particularly in the past 50 years, is generally believed to be responsible for most of the stress humans put on the environment. A large and rapidly growing population makes it more difficult to provide the basic components of environmental health discussed earlier, including clean and disease-free food and water. It is also a driving force behind many of the relatively more recent environmental health concerns, including chemical pollution, global warming, and the thinning of the atmosphere's ozone layer.

How Many People Can the World Hold?

No one knows how many people the world can support, but most scientists agree that a limit exists. A 2006 report from the United Nation's Convention on Biological Diversity states that the population's demand for resources already exceeds Earth's capacity by 20%. The primary factors that may eventually put a cap on human population are the following:

- *Food.* Enough food is currently produced to feed the world's entire population, but economic and sociopolitical factors have led to food shortages and famine. Food production can be expanded in the future, but better distribution of food will be needed to prevent even more widespread famine as the world's population continues to grow. For all people to receive adequate nutrition, the makeup of the world's diet may also need to change.

- *Available land and water.* Rural populations rely on trees, soil, and water for their direct sustenance, and a growing population puts a strain on these resources—forests are cut for wood, soil is depleted, and water is withdrawn at ever-rising rates. These trends contribute to local hardships and to many global environmental problems, including habitat destruction and species extinction (see the box "Natural Ecosystems and Biodiversity" on p. 642).

- *Energy.* Currently, most of the world's energy comes from nonrenewable sources: oil, coal, natural gas, and nuclear power. As nonrenewable sources are depleted, the world will have to shift to renewable energy sources, such as hydropower and solar, geothermal, wind, biomass, and ocean power. Supporting a growing population,

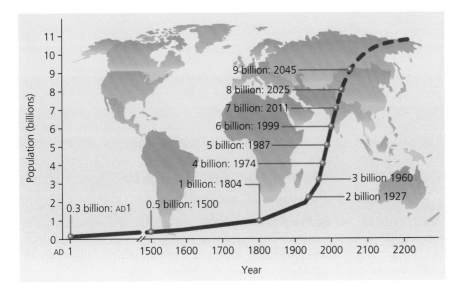

VITAL STATISTICS

FIGURE 21.1 World population growth.
The United Nations estimates that the world's population will continue to increase dramatically until it stabilizes above 10 billion people in 2200.

Source: United Nations Population Division. 2007. *World Population Prospects: The 2006 Revision.* New York: United Nations; U.S. Bureau of the Census.

Natural Ecosystems and Biodiversity

Our world supports an abundant variety of life. Scientists have identified some 1.75 million species, but they suspect that probably 10 million–80 million more exist.

Different environments generate diverse life strategies, so that each **ecosystem**—from desert to tropical rainforest—contains a unique, close-knit community of organisms, linked together in a **food chain** or web. Plants use sunlight and soil for their needs. In turn, they sustain herbivores (plant eaters), which may themselves succumb to predators. When predators and surviving herbivores die, they become food for scavengers, then insect larvae, and finally bacteria, which break them down into organic substances. These substances, drawn from the soil by plants, help maintain the cycle. A similar system, based on plankton, exists in the oceans. Disruption at any point in this intricate, balanced cycle can alter or destroy an entire ecosystem.

Natural ecosystems maintain the climate and the composition of the atmosphere, cycle water and nutrients, produce food, dispose of organic wastes, generate and maintain soils, control pests, and pollinate crops. Ecosystems also support biological diversity, or **biodiversity**, represented by both the millions of different species on Earth and the genetic diversity within these species.

Biodiversity is critical as the basis for the future evolution of new species and as a genetic bank from which humans can draw useful genetic material and compounds. Although thus far we have examined few of these resources, the ones

we have used provide many benefits, including medicines and pest and disease resistance for crops.

Human activity—driven by poverty and population growth in the developing world and excessive consumerism in the industrial nations—threatens biodiversity. In some cases, species and populations are being lost through direct action, such as the overharvesting of elephants, whales, and certain fish. In 2006, for example, an international team of researchers predicted the global collapse of seafood stocks in the world's oceans within 50 years if current fishing trends continue. In other cases, species and populations are lost indirectly, through habitat destruction.

The destruction of tropical rainforests, which are disappearing at the rate of almost half a hectare every second, is of particular concern. Rainforests cover only about 7% of the planet but are thought to harbour more than half the world's species. The World Conservation

Union's "red list" of animals in serious danger of extinction contains about 16,000 species, including the polar bear and hippopotamus. The red list now includes one in four mammals, one in eight birds, one-third of all amphibians, and 70% of the world's assessed plants.

Extinction is irreversible, and species are disappearing far faster (50–100 a day) than they can be identified and assessed for useful properties. The current extinction rate is up to 10,000 times as high as expected. Cutting down on greenhouse gasses and storing carbon dioxide could save many species from vanishing. Some scientists fear that humans are precipitating a wave of mass extinction so great that the diminished stock of species will not be an adequate base on which natural selection can work to rebuild biodiversity. Even if adequate, it could take more than 10 million years for biodiversity to be restored. And because of the many ties between organisms and the physical environment, mass extinction could also threaten the functioning of the entire biological world.

What can be done to maintain biodiversity? Canada has laws that protect specific endangered species, which by indirectly preserving natural communities help maintain biodiversity. International laws and conventions also protect certain rare species, although enforcement continues to be a problem. The Convention on Biological Diversity, for example, deals specifically with the issue of biodiversity. It commits countries to preserving and managing biological resources and to integrating plant and animal preservation into economic planning.

maintaining economic productivity, and preventing further environmental degradation will require both greater energy efficiency and an increased use of renewable energy sources.

• *Minimum acceptable standard of living.* The mass media have exposed the entire world to the North American lifestyle and raised people's expectations of living at a comparable level. But such a lifestyle is supported by levels of energy consumption that Earth cannot support worldwide. In 2002, Canada almost tied the United States for highest per capita energy consumption among the G8 nations (the eight most industrialized countries in the world). In contrast, Italy ranked last among the G8 countries;

Canadians consumed almost three times as much energy as Italians did. If all people are to enjoy a minimally acceptable standard of living, the population must be limited to a number that the available resources can support.

Factors That Contribute to Population Growth

Although it is apparent that population growth must be controlled, population trends are difficult to influence and manage. A variety of interconnecting factors fuel the current population explosion:

• *High fertility rates.* The combination of poverty, very high child mortality rates, and a lack of social provisions of every type is associated with high fertility rates in the developing world. Families may have to have more children to ensure that enough survive childhood to work for the household and to care for parents in old age. Most countries, both developed and developing, have experienced significant reductions in fertility as contraceptive use has increased. However, the majority of developing countries still have fertility levels that ensure substantial population growth. In a small number of countries, most of which are classified as least developed, fertility levels continue to be very high.

• *Lack of family planning resources.* Half the world's couples don't use any form of family planning.

• *Lower death rates.* Although death rates remain relatively high in the developing world, they have decreased in recent years because of public health measures and improved medical care.

Changes in any of these factors can affect population growth, but the issues are complex. Increasing death rates through disease, famine, or war might slow population growth, but few people would argue in favour of these as methods of population control. (The United Nations' population estimates project that there will be 344 million fewer people alive in 2050 than there would have been without deaths from HIV/AIDS.) Although the increased availability of family planning services is a crucial part of population management, cultural, political, and religious factors also need to be considered.

To be successful, population management must change the condition of people's lives, especially poverty, to remove the pressures for having large families. Research indicates that the combination of improved health, better education, and increased literacy and employment opportunities for women works together with family planning to decrease fertility rates. Unfortunately, in the fastest-growing countries, the needs of a rapidly increasing population use up financial resources that might otherwise be used to improve lives and ultimately slow population growth.

AIR QUALITY AND POLLUTION

Air pollution is not a human invention or even a new problem. The air is polluted naturally with every forest fire, pollen bloom, and dust storm, as well as with countless other natural pollutants. To these natural sources, humans have always contributed the by-products of their activities.

Air pollution is linked to a wide range of health problems; the very young and older adults are among those most susceptible to air pollution's effects. For people with chronic ailments, such as diabetes or heart failure, even relatively brief exposures to particulate air pollution increases the risk of death by nearly 40%. Recent studies have linked exposure to air pollution to reduced birth weight in infants, reduced lung capacity in teens, and atherosclerosis (thickening of the arteries) in adults.

Air Quality and Smog

Health Canada and Environment Canada have developed a new measure called the **Air Quality Health Index (AQHI)** to indicate whether air pollution levels pose a health concern for Canadians. The AQHI—not yet available in all regions across Canada—is calculated based on the relative risks of a mixture of air pollutants, including the following:

• *Nitrogen dioxide (NO_2).* NO_2 is a reddish-brown, highly reactive gas formed when nitric oxide combines with oxygen in the atmosphere; major sources include motor vehicles and power plants. In people with respiratory diseases, such as asthma, NO_2 affects lung function and causes symptoms, such as wheezing and shortness of breath. NO_2 exposure may also increase the risk of respiratory infections.

• *Particulate matter ($PM_{2.5}/PM_{10}$).* Particles of different sizes are released into the atmosphere from a variety of sources, including combustion of **fossil fuels**, crushing or grinding operations, industrial processes, and dust from roadways. PM can accumulate in the respiratory system, aggravate cardiovascular and lung diseases, and increase the risk of respiratory infections.

• *Ground-level ozone (O_3).* At ground level, ozone is a harmful pollutant; where it occurs naturally in the upper atmosphere, it shields Earth from the sun's harmful ultra-

QUESTIONS FOR CRITICAL THINKING AND REFLECTION

What is the population of your town or city? Does the number of people in your town make living there difficult or more enjoyable? In what ways? Do you believe your city or town has adequate infrastructure and resources to support its residents?

TERMS

ecosystem   The community of organisms (plants and animals) in an area and the nonliving physical factors with which they interact.

food chain   The transfers of food energy and other substances in which one type of organism consumes another.

biodiversity   The variety of living things on Earth, including all the different species of flora and fauna and the genetic diversity among individuals of the same species.

Air Quality Health Index (AQHI)   A Canadian measure of local air quality and what it means for health; uses a scale of 1–10+, as well as categories of low, moderate, high, or very high health risk.

fossil fuels   Buried deposits of decayed animals and plants that are converted into carbon-rich fuels by exposure to heat and pressure over millions of years; oil, coal, and natural gas are fossil fuels.

Smog tends to form over Toronto and other large cities for numerous reasons, including the tremendous amount of motor vehicle exhaust in the air.

violet rays. (The health hazards from the thinning of this protective ozone layer are discussed later in the chapter.) Ground-level ozone is formed when pollutants emitted by cars, power plants, industrial plants, and other sources react chemically in the presence of sunlight (photochemical reactions). Ozone can irritate the respiratory system, reduce lung function, aggravate asthma, increase susceptibility to respiratory infections, and damage the lining of the lungs. Short-term elevations of ozone levels have also been linked to increased death rates.

AQHI values range from 1 to 10+; the higher the AQHI, the greater the level of pollution and associated health danger. When the AQHI exceeds 7, the health risk is considered *high*, particularly for sensitive groups of people and then for everyone as AQHI values rise further. Depending on the AQHI value, precautionary health messages are provided. For example, when the AQHI is in the *very high* range (above 10), people with heart or breathing problems (as well as children and older adults) are encouraged to avoid strenuous activities outdoors, whereas the general population is encouraged to reduce or reschedule these activities.

The term **smog** was first used in the early 1900s in London, England, to describe the combination of smoke and fog. What we typically call smog today is a mixture of pollutants, with ground-level ozone being the key ingredient. Major smog occurrences are linked to the combination of several factors: heavy motor vehicle traffic, high temperatures, and sunny weather, which can increase the production of ozone. Pollutants are also more likely to build up in areas with little wind or where a topographic feature, such as a mountain range or valley, prevents the wind from pushing out stagnant air.

The Greenhouse Effect and Global Warming

The temperature of Earth's atmosphere depends on the balance between the amount of energy the planet absorbs from the sun (mainly as high-energy ultraviolet radiation) and the amount of energy radiated back into space as lower-energy infrared radiation. Key components of temperature regulation are carbon dioxide, water vapour, methane, and other **greenhouse gases**—so named because, like the glass panes in a greenhouse, they let through visible light from the sun but trap some of the resulting infrared radiation and reradiate it back to Earth's surface. This reradiation causes a buildup of heat that raises the temperature of the lower atmosphere, a natural process known as the **greenhouse effect** (Figure 21.2). Without it, the atmosphere would be far cooler and much more hostile to life.

There is growing consensus that human activity is causing **global warming**. The concentration of greenhouse gases is increasing because of human activity, especially the combustion of fossil fuels (Table 21.1). Carbon dioxide levels in the atmosphere have increased rapidly in recent decades. The use of fossil fuels pumps more than 20 billion metric tons of carbon dioxide into the atmosphere every year. Experts believe carbon dioxide may account for about 60% of the greenhouse effect. Analysis of ice core samples shows that carbon dioxide levels are now about 25% higher than at any other time in the last 650,000 years. In 2007, Canada was among the top 10 carbon-dioxide-emitting countries in the world; these 10 countries are responsible for about two-thirds of the world's total emissions of carbon dioxide. Deforestation, often by burning, also sends carbon dioxide into the atmosphere and reduces the number of trees available to convert carbon dioxide into oxygen.

In 2006, the National Research Council reported that the overall global temperature had increased 0.6°C during the twentieth century (Figure 21.3 on p. 647). Agreement is growing among scientists that temperatures will continue

FIGURE 21.2 The greenhouse effect.

1. **Energy from the sun warms Earth.** Most incoming solar radiation is absorbed by the atmosphere and Earth's surface; the rest gets reflected back into space.

2. **Earth radiates heat away as infrared energy.** Some of this energy is radiated into space, some is absorbed by the atmosphere, and some is reradiated back to Earth's surface by greenhouse gases in the atmosphere. This reradiated energy also warms Earth.

3. **Human activity is increasing the concentration of greenhouse gases in the atmosphere.** The concentration of these gases helps determine how much infrared radiation gets reflected back to Earth, so an increase in these gases can cause Earth's temperature to rise.

Table 21.1	Sources of Greenhouse Gases
Greenhouse Gas	**Sources**
Carbon dioxide	Fossil fuel and wood burning, factory emissions, car exhaust, deforestation
Chlorofluorocarbons (CFCs)	Refrigeration and air conditioning, aerosols, foam products, solvents
Methane	Cattle, wetlands, rice paddies, landfills, gas leaks, coal and gas industries
Nitrous oxide	Fertilizers, soil cultivation, deforestation, animal feedlots and wastes
Ozone and other trace gases	Photochemical reactions, car exhaust, power plant emissions, solvents

to rise, although estimates vary as to how much they will change. If global warming persists, experts say the impact may be devastating (see the box "Global Warming, Local Action" on p. 646). Possible consequences include the following:

- Increased rainfall and flooding in some regions, increased drought in others. Coastal zones, where half the world's people live, would be severely affected.

- Increased mortality from heat stress, urban air pollution, and tropical diseases. Deaths from weather events, such as hurricanes, tornadoes, droughts, and floods, might also increase.

- A poleward shift of about 150–550 kilometres in the location of vegetation zones, affecting crop yields, irrigation demands, and forest productivity.

- Increasingly rapid and drastic melting of Earth's polar ice caps. Arctic ice melts to some extent during the summer each year, but during the 2007 melting season, Arctic ice formations melted faster and farther than any other time since observations began. Experts predicted that as soon as 2030, the Arctic sea ice could melt away completely during the summer but would return in the winter months. Such extensive melting could mean increased flooding in the northern hemisphere, further changes in weather patterns, and the elimination of habitat for species that live in the Arctic.

smog Hazy atmospheric conditions resulting from increased concentrations of ground-level ozone and other pollutants.

greenhouse gas A gas (such as carbon dioxide) or vapour that traps infrared radiation instead of allowing it to escape through the atmosphere, resulting in a warming of Earth (the greenhouse effect).

greenhouse effect A warming of Earth caused by a buildup of carbon dioxide and certain other gases.

global warming An increase in Earth's atmospheric temperature when averaged across seasons and geographical regions.

TERMS

Global Warming, Local Action

At current rates of consumption, we are using up Earth's resources so rapidly that they may run out sooner than anyone expects. Some experts say that humankind is already outstripping the planet's biological capacity by 20%. Indeed, a 2006 report from the Worldwatch Institute says that if fast-growing nations, such as China and India, start using Earth's stores at the same rate as North America does, we will need the resources of *a second Earth* to keep everyone satisfied.

But this problem has a second, more urgent part—that is, the way all those resources (especially minerals, such as coal and oil) are being used. We use millions of metric tons of fossil fuel each year to power homes, cars, and factories. However unintentionally, we are also using them to destroy our planet.

Evidence of Global Warming

Ample evidence shows that global warming is a reality. Here are just a few examples:

• Scientists have been measuring atmospheric carbon dioxide (CO_2) levels for years and say the amount of CO_2 is continually rising. In 2005, atmospheric CO_2 measured 380 parts per million (ppm), compared with about 290 ppm in 1850. At least one expert estimates that atmospheric CO_2 could reach 900 ppm by 2100, with a corresponding rise in global temperature of 5°C–10°C.

• Glaciers and other large ice formations are melting at a quickening pace and shrinking measurably. The Greenland Ice Sheet, for example, is now melting at a rate of about 225 cubic kilometres each year. Such melting threatens to raise ocean levels around the world—possibly as much as 1–1.5 metres in the coming decades. In scenarios now envisioned, large swaths of coastline will be swamped and some small islands may disappear entirely.

• The World Health Organization says that ecological damage caused by human activities (such as burning fossil fuels and destroying forests and wetlands) is threatening our health. The WHO also predicts dramatic increases in disease during the next 50 years and that climate change could have catastrophic results in poor nations that already are unable to grow enough food or provide enough clean water for their people.

Despite the evidence, skepticism persists. Respected government agencies, such as the National Oceanic and Atmospheric Administration, NASA, and others, have declared global warming to be a real phenomenon and a threat to humanity, yet many elected government officials dismiss such claims as faulty or incomplete science. In other countries, too, political and business leaders put climate change in second place after economic development. And one key component of Western-style economic development is the burning of fossil fuels to power industry and transportation.

Who Is Responsible?

To some degree, we are all responsible for climate change, just as we all stand to suffer because of it. Scientists can calculate just how much each person, house, car, appliance, and factory contributes to global warming; they call this measure an "environmental footprint." The footprint's size is determined by the amount of greenhouse gases the source generates, either directly (such as a car or factory) or indirectly (such as an electric appliance, which runs on electricity produced by a fossil-fuel-burning power plant). Here are some examples:

• For every litre of gas your car burns, it releases more than two kilograms of CO_2 into the atmosphere. A mid-size car puts out more than 1350 kilograms of CO_2 per year; most SUVs put out about 2500 kilograms.

• A typical refrigerator is responsible for more than 900 kilograms of CO_2 annually. (The gas is actually released by a power plant; the amount is based on how much electricity the refrigerator uses.)

• A typical Canadian household consisting of two adults and two children in a 2500-square-foot home with one car will generate more than 27,000 kilograms of CO_2 per year.

Even though it isn't weightless, CO_2 is a gas. If you try to imagine how many CO_2 molecules it would take to make up a single pound, you can easily see why atmospheric CO_2 levels are increasing so rapidly.

What Is Being Done?

The need to slow climate change is undeniable and urgent. At the global level,

many governments are taking initiatives to slow the release of greenhouse gases. One result of these efforts is the Kyoto Protocol to the United Nations Convention on Climate Change, which took effect in 2005. Under the terms of this agreement, participating countries—including Canada—had to reduce greenhouse gas emissions by 2012 to an average of 5% below 1990 levels. In early 2010, Canada announced that it has committed, under the Copenhagen Accord, to a 17% reduction in greenhouse gas emissions (from 2005 levels) by 2020. Canada has also committed to working closely with the United States on climate and energy policies. In 2008, Canada joined other G8 countries in adopting a long-term target of cutting greenhouse gas emissions in half by 2050. Industries are slowly adapting, too, although some must be forced to reduce their greenhouse emissions. Many companies are investing in cleaner fuel technology and scrubbing their emissions before they enter the environment. Automakers are rapidly improving existing hybrid automobiles and making more models available, while focusing on the development of all-electric cars and hydrogen fuel cell technologies that virtually eliminate automotive pollution.

Individuals are making a difference, too. You can learn more about climate change and what it means to our future by checking out the organizations and Web sites listed in For More Information at the end of the chapter.

Global Temperature Change (°C)

— Annual mean
— Five-year mean

FIGURE 21.3   Trend in annual mean temperature.
This graph traces the trend in the annual mean temperature relative to the 1951–1980 mean value. A strong warming trend has occurred over the past 30 years.

Source: Goddard Institute for Space Studies. 2009. *GISS Surface Temperature Analysis, Global Temperature Trends: 2009 Summation* (http://data.giss.nasa.gov/gistemp/2007; retrieved February 19, 2009).

According to estimates from the U.S. Environmental Protection Agency (EPA), Earth's average surface temperature is likely to increase 1.1°C –6.4°C by the end of the twenty-first century (Figure 21.4). Warming will not be evenly distributed around the globe. Land areas will warm more than oceans in part because of water's ability to store heat. High latitudes will warm more than low ones in part because of the effects of melting ice. Most of North America, all of Africa, Europe, Northern and Central Asia, and most of Central and South America are likely to warm more than the global average.

Thinning of the Ozone Layer

Another air pollution problem is the thinning of the **ozone layer** of the atmosphere, a fragile, invisible layer about 16–48 kilometres above Earth's surface that shields the planet from the sun's hazardous ultraviolet (UV) rays. Since the mid-1980s, scientists have observed the seasonal appearance and growth of a hole in the ozone layer over Antarctica. More recently, thinning over other areas—including Canada, Scandinavia, the northern United States, Russia, Australia, and New Zealand—has been noted.

ozone layer   A layer of ozone molecules (O_3) in the upper atmosphere that screens out UV rays from the sun.

TERMS

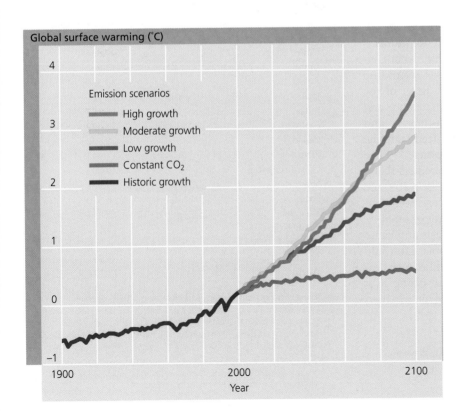

Global surface warming (°C)

Emission scenarios
— High growth
— Moderate growth
— Low growth
— Constant CO_2
— Historic growth

Year

FIGURE 21.4   Temperature projections to the year 2100 based on different greenhouse gas growth scenarios.
The orange line shows that temperatures would change only slightly if greenhouse gas emissions stopped rising.

Source: Environmental Protection Agency, 2007. *Future Temperature Changes* (http://www.epa.gov/climatechange/science/futuretc.html; retrieved February 19, 2009).

The ozone layer is being destroyed primarily by **chlorofluorocarbons (CFCs)**, industrial chemicals used as coolants in refrigerators and in home and automobile air conditioners; as foaming agents in some rigid foam products, including insulation; as propellants in some kinds of aerosol sprays (most such sprays were banned in Canada in the late 1970s); and as solvents. When CFCs rise into the atmosphere, winds carry them toward the polar regions. During winter, circular winds form a vortex that keeps the air over Antarctica from mixing with air from elsewhere. CFCs react with airborne ice crystals, releasing chlorine atoms, which destroy ozone. When the polar vortex weakens in the summer, winds richer in ozone from the north replenish the lost Antarctic ozone.

In the northern hemisphere, ozone levels have declined by about 10% since 1980, and certain areas may be temporarily depleted in late winter and early spring by as much as 40%. The largest and deepest ozone hole on record occurred in late September 2006, reaching 27.5 million square kilometres, considerably larger than the surface area of North America. The hole also had an unusual vertical extent, with nearly all the ozone between approximately 13 and 21 kilometres above Earth's surface destroyed.

Without the ozone layer to absorb the sun's UV radiation, life on Earth would be impossible. (UV radiation levels under the Antarctic hole were high enough to cause sunburn within seven minutes.) The potential effects of increased long-term exposure to UV light for humans include skin cancer, wrinkling and aging of the skin, cataracts and blindness, and reduced immune response. The United Nations Environment Programme predicts that a drop of 10% in overall ozone levels would cause a 26% rise in the incidence of nonmelanoma skin cancers. Some scientists blame ozone loss for many cases of melanoma.

UV light may interfere with photosynthesis and cause lower crop yields; it may also kill phytoplankton and krill, the basis of the ocean food chain. And because heat generated by the absorption of UV rays in the ozone layer helps create stratospheric winds, the driving force behind weather patterns, a drop in the concentration of ozone could potentially alter Earth's climate systems.

Worldwide production and use of CFCs have declined rapidly since the danger to the ozone layer was recognized. Industrialized nations agreed to eliminate CFC production and use by 2000, and limits have also been placed on other agents that destroy ozone. Metered-dose inhalers for several conditions, such as asthma, are the only significant commercial product to contain CFCs, and CFC-free inhalers are already available for some medications.

Ozone-depleting substances have very long lifetimes in the atmosphere, however, so despite these efforts, the ozone hole is not expected to recover until 2070. The gradual recovery is masked by annual variations caused by weather fluctuations over Antarctica.

Energy Use and Air Pollution

Canadians are large consumers of energy; however, Americans are the biggest energy consumers in the world (Table 21.2). North Americans use energy to create electricity, transport us, power our industries, and run our homes. About 32% of the energy we use in Canada comes from oil, followed by hydroelectricity (25%), natural gas (24%), and coal (10%). The remainder comes from nuclear power and renewable energy sources (such as wind and solar power).

Table 21.2	Primary Energy Consumption of Selected Countries, 2006
Country	**Total Consumption (quadrillion Btu*)**
United States	99.856
China	73.808
Russia	30.386
Japan	22.786
India	17.677
Germany	14.629
Canada	13.950
France	11.445
United Kingdom	9.802
South Korea	9.447
Spain	6.510
Australia	5.611
South Africa	5.177
Taiwan	4.569
Thailand	3.741
World Total	**472.274**

Source: Energy Information Administration. 2008. *International Total Primary Energy Consumption and Energy Intensity: Total Primary Energy Consumption (Quadrillion Btu): All Countries, 1980–2006* (http://www.eia.doe.gov/emeu/international/energyconsumption.html; retrieved August 10, 2010).

*Includes total consumption of petroleum, dry natural gas, and coal, and net hydroelectric, nuclear, geothermal, solar, wind, and wood and waste electricity; also includes net electricity imports.

TERMS

chlorofluorocarbons (CFCs) Chemicals used as spray-can propellants, refrigerants, and industrial solvents, implicated in the destruction of the ozone layer.

Energy consumption is at the root of many environmental problems, especially those relating to air pollution. Automobile exhaust and the burning of oil and coal by industry and by electric power plants are primary causes of smog, acid precipitation, and the greenhouse effect. The mining of coal and the extraction and transportation of oil cause pollution on land and in the water; coal miners often develop serious health problems related to their jobs. Nuclear power generation creates hazardous wastes and carries the risk of dangerous releases of radiation.

Two key strategies for controlling energy use are conservation and the development of nonpolluting, renewable sources of energy. Although the use of renewable energy sources has increased in recent years, renewables still supply only a small proportion of our energy, in part because of their cost. Some countries have chosen to promote energy efficiency by removing subsidies or adding taxes on the use of fossil fuels. This strategy is reflected in the varying prices drivers pay for gasoline. Despite recent increases in Canadian consumer gas prices, a growing number of Canadians are driving minivans and sport utility vehicles (SUVs). These vehicles tend to have low fuel economy; the largest SUVs increase greenhouse gas emissions by six or more metric tons per year in comparison with an average car.

Alternative Fuels   The Government of Canada and some provincial governments have encouraged researchers and automobile manufacturers to develop and use alternative fuels, such as ethanol. Ethanol, a form of alcohol, is a renewable transportation fuel produced from fermenting plant sugars, such as corn and wheat. Ethanol use reduces the amount of oil required to produce gasoline, reduces overall greenhouse gas emissions from automobiles, and supports the Canadian agricultural industry. In Canada, ethanol can be used in gasoline-powered automobiles made after the 1980s. Most of these vehicles can run on a mixture of 90% gasoline and 10% ethanol (known as E10), a fuel that is now available at many service stations across Canada. Another type of alternative fuel is E85, a mixture of 85% ethanol and 15% gasoline. E85 is currently used by some businesses with large vehicle fleets, but it is not yet commercially available in Canada. Ethanol has been mixed with gasoline for years in Canada, but several other countries (such as Brazil) use ethanol much more extensively.

Ethanol, however, has its critics, who say the alternative fuel may do more harm than good. For one thing, some reports show that corn-based ethanol requires more energy to produce than it yields when burned as fuel. Other reports dispute this point, and improvements in manufacturing processes may reduce the amount of energy required to make the fuel. Regardless, ethanol made from sugar cane and other plant matter may be far more energy-efficient, say some experts.

One huge potential drawback of ethanol is the diversion of corn crops from the food supply to produce the fuel. In 2007 and 2008, this practice was blamed for skyrocketing food prices and food shortages around the world, which led to food riots in several countries. The food-related concerns prompted the United Nations to call for a moratorium on food-based ethanol production until nonfood sources of alternative fuels could be developed.

Wind Power   Electricity from wind energy is one of the fastest-growing methods of electrical generation in the world. Kinetic energy from moving air is converted into electricity by wind turbines that are mounted in locations where there are favourable weather patterns. Wind turbines may be used individually but are often installed in groups to form wind farms or wind power plants. Electricity generated by wind farms may be used locally or placed on the electric grid to power homes and businesses farther away. Energy derived from wind can also be converted to hydrogen and used as a form of fuel for transportation or stored for subsequent power generation. Using wind energy reduces the environmental impact of generating electricity because it requires no fuel and does not produce pollution or greenhouse gases.

In response to emerging public health concerns about the potential health impact of noise generated by wind turbines, the chief medical officer of health in Ontario conducted a review of the scientific evidence on this topic. This 2010 report concluded that although some residents of homes located near wind turbines have reported various symptoms, such as dizziness, headaches, and sleep disturbance, research does not seem to support the existence of a direct link between wind turbine noise and negative health effects. More specifically, it was concluded that some people may find it bothersome, but the sound level from wind turbines is not sufficient to cause hearing impairment or other adverse health outcomes.

Hybrid and Electric Vehicles   A more positive trend has been the introduction of hybrid electric vehicles (HEVs). Hybrid vehicles use two or more distinct power sources to propel the vehicle, such as an on-board energy storage system (batteries, for example) and an internal combustion engine and electric motor. The hybrid vehicle typically realizes greater fuel economy than a conventional car does and produces fewer polluting emissions. Hybrids also tend to run with less noise than conventional vehicles. Several hybrid models are currently available in Canada but typically cost several thousand dollars more than their conventional gas-powered counterparts. Still, hybrids are gaining popularity with consumers and are being more commonly used in both corporate and government vehicle fleets.

Researchers hope that hybrid technology can be extended to all classes of vehicles and that North Americans can be convinced to use more fuel-efficient vehicles and to travel more frequently on public transportation, in carpools, or on foot.

Another type of alternative vehicle is all electric. In these vehicles, electricity is stored in battery packs and then converted into mechanical power that runs the vehicle.

After a given number of kilometres, the batteries must be recharged. These vehicles do not produce tailpipe emissions, but generators that produce the electricity for the batteries do emit pollutants.

Even when mass production begins, electric vehicles are expected to cost more than conventionally fuelled ones. Even with lower "fuel" and maintenance costs (electric vehicles have fewer moving parts than gas-powered cars), the lead-acid battery packs must be replaced every few years, adding to the overall cost of electric vehicles.

Indoor Air Pollution

Although most people associate air pollution with the outdoors, your home may also harbour potentially dangerous pollutants. Some of these compounds trigger allergic responses, and others have been linked to cancer. Common indoor pollutants include the following:

- *Environmental tobacco smoke (ETS)*, a human carcinogen that also increases the risk of asthma, bronchitis, and cardiovascular disease (see Chapter 16). In most Canadian provinces and territories, smoking is banned in almost all public places and workplaces. In others, indoor areas used by the public are smoke free except for certain enclosed and separately ventilated areas.
- *Carbon monoxide and other combustion by-products*, which can cause chronic bronchitis, headaches, dizziness, nausea, fatigue, and even death. Common sources in the home are woodstoves, fireplaces, kerosene heaters and lamps, and gas ranges. In poverty-stricken areas, especially in Asia and Africa, people commonly burn solid fuels, such as coal, for cooking and heating their homes. The WHO says the smoke and by-products from these indoor fires kill about 1.5 million people annually—mostly children.
- *Formaldehyde gas*, which can cause eye, nose, and throat irritation; shortness of breath; headaches; nausea; lethargy; and, over the long term, cancer. This gas can seep from certain construction materials, paints, floor finishes, permanent press clothing, and nail polish.
- *Biological pollutants*, including bacteria, dust mites, mould, and animal dander, which can cause allergic reactions and other health problems. These allergens are typically found in bathrooms, damp or flooded basements, humidifiers, air conditioners, and even some carpets and furniture.
- *Indoor mould*, the fuzzy black substance growing on shower tiles and damp basement walls, is an indoor pollutant not to be taken lightly. Even though more than 100 common indoor moulds have been classified as potentially hazardous to people, only a few are serious threats to human health. One of the most common of these is *Stachybotrys* mould, commonly known as toxic black mould. It is greenish black and appears slimy when wet. Toxic mould spores permeate the air and can cause health problems when inhaled, especially for people with asthma and other respiratory conditions.

Preventing Air Pollution

You can do a great deal to reduce air pollution. Here are a few ideas:

- Cut back on driving. Ride your bike, walk, use public transportation, or carpool in a fuel-efficient vehicle.
- Keep your car tuned up and well maintained. Use only unleaded gas, and keep your tires inflated at recommended pressures. To save energy when driving, avoid quick starts, stay within the speed limit, limit the use of air conditioning, and don't let your car idle unless absolutely necessary. Have your car's air conditioner checked and serviced by a station that uses environmentally friendly refrigerants.
- Buy energy-efficient appliances, and use them only when necessary. Run the washing machine, dryer, and dishwasher only when you have full loads, and do laundry in warm or cold water instead of hot; don't overdry your clothes. Clean refrigerator coils and clothes dryer lint screens frequently. Towel or air-dry your hair rather than using an electric dryer.
- Replace incandescent bulbs with compact fluorescent bulbs (not fluorescent tubes). For more information, see the box "Compact Fluorescent Light Bulbs."
- Make sure your home is well insulated with ozone-safe agents; use insulating shades and curtains to keep heat in during winter and out during summer. Seal any openings that produce drafts. In cold weather, put on a sweater and turn down the thermostat. In hot weather, wear lightweight clothing and, whenever possible, use a fan instead of an air conditioner to cool yourself.
- Plant and care for trees in your own yard and neighbourhood. Because they recycle carbon dioxide, trees work against global warming. They also provide shade and cool the air, so less air conditioning is needed.
- Before discarding a refrigerator, air conditioner, or humidifier, check with the waste hauler or your local government to ensure that ozone-depleting refrigerants will be removed before disposal. If you use a metered-dose inhaler, ask your physician if an ozone-safe inhaler is available for your medication.
- To prevent indoor air pollution, keep your house adequately ventilated, and buy some houseplants; they have a natural ability to rid the air of harmful pollutants.
- Keep paints, cleaning agents, and other chemical products tightly sealed in their original containers.
- Don't smoke, and don't allow others to smoke in your room, apartment, or home. If these rules are

Compact Fluorescent Light Bulbs

A good way to cut your home's energy use, lower your energy bills, and reduce your environmental footprint is by using energy-efficient light bulbs, commonly called *compact fluorescent light bulbs (CFLs)*.

According to Environment Canada, CFLs are cost efficient because they use 75% less energy than traditional incandescent light bulbs, and they last 10 times as long. Although CFLs initially cost more than regular light bulbs, over the long term they save you money. This is because they use less energy by requiring less electricity to produce light. For example, a 15-watt CFL is equivalent to a 60-watt incandescent light bulb.

Environment Canada says that if every Canadian home replaced one incandescent bulb with a CFL, the country would save more than $73 million in energy costs every year. It would also reduce greenhouse gas emissions by an amount equal to the output of 66,000 cars.

In spite of their positive attributes, compact fluorescent bulbs have a downside: They contain a gas that includes low-

pressure mercury and argon. If all the CFLs currently in use were disposed of in landfills, they could generate about almost 14,000 kilograms of mercury that could eventually leech into the groundwater system. For this reason, it is best to take your burned-out CFLs to a community recycling centre for proper disposal instead of tossing them in the trash.

Even though the amount of mercury in a single CFL is very small, you should take extra precautions when cleaning up a broken bulb. If a CFL breaks, shut off the central heating/air condition system, open a window, and clear all people and animals out of the room for at least 15 minutes. Put on rubber or latex gloves, and carefully pick up the large pieces of glass. Put the pieces in a glass jar that can be closed with a lid, or in a heavy-duty plastic bag that can be sealed. Gently sweep up the small pieces and dust by using a broom and dustpan.

You can use duct tape to pick up fine particles. Seal everything up (including your gloves) in the jar or bag, and take it to a recycling centre for disposal.

> ## QUESTIONS FOR CRITICAL THINKING AND REFLECTION
> What are your views on the issue of climate change? Do you believe it is a real problem or that it has been overly hyped by the media and some politicians? How do you support your views?

too strict for your situation, limit smoking to a single, well-ventilated room.

- Clean and inspect chimneys, furnaces, and other appliances regularly. Install carbon monoxide detectors.

WATER QUALITY AND POLLUTION

Few parts of the world have enough safe, clean drinking water, and yet few things are as important to human health.

Water Contamination and Treatment

In 2007, close to 90% of the water processed by Canada's drinking water plants came from surface water sources, such as lakes and rivers. In comparison with ground water, surface water is more likely to be contaminated with both organic matter and pathogenic microorganisms, so it is purified in water-treatment plants before being piped into the community. At treatment facilities, the water is

subjected to various physical and chemical processes, including screening, filtration, and disinfection (often with chlorine), before it is introduced into the water supply system. **Fluoridation**, a water-treatment process that reduces tooth decay by 15%–40%, was introduced into Canadian communities more than 60 years ago. However, as recently as 2007, less than half of the Canadian population had access to fluoridated water supplies.

In most areas of Canada, water systems have adequate, dependable supplies, are able to control waterborne disease, and provide water without unacceptable colour, odour, or taste. However, problems do occur. In 2000, approximately 2500 people became ill and seven died when drinking water in Walkerton, Ontario, was contaminated with *Escherichia coli* (*E. coli*) bacteria. Also, according to a report published in the *Canadian Medical Association Journal*, 1766 boil-water advisories were in effect across Canada in April 2008. Further, it was estimated that approximately 90 Canadians die each year from consuming contaminated water. Pollution by hazardous chemicals from manufacturing, agriculture, and household wastes is another concern. (Chemical pollution is discussed later in the chapter.) Worldwide, more than 2 million people, mostly children, die from water-related diseases each year.

---

fluoridation The addition of fluoride to the water supply to reduce tooth decay.

TERMS

Most communities in Canada draw on surface water for their drinking water supply. Unlike ground water, surface water is never free of contaminants and has to be treated before it is safe for people to drink.

Water Shortages

Water shortages are a growing concern in many regions of the world. Generally speaking, Canada is considered a *water-rich* country. Despite this abundance of water, shortages are a serious problem for regions of Canada where human demand outstrips the ability of natural water supplies to provide adequate water to all.

According to the WHO, 1 billion people do not have safe drinking water and 2.6 billion do not have access to basic sanitation. Less than 1% of the world's fresh water—about 0.007% of all the water on Earth—is readily accessible for direct human use.

Groundwater pumping and the diversion of water from lakes and rivers for irrigation are further reducing the amount of water available to local communities. In some areas, groundwater is being removed at twice the rate at which it is replaced. The Aral Sea, located in Kazakhstan and Uzbekistan, was once one of the world's largest inland seas. Since the 1960s, it has lost two-thirds of its volume to irrigation, and the exposed seabed is now as big as the Netherlands. People living in the area have experienced severe water and food shortages and increased rates of respiratory disease and throat cancer linked to dust storms

from the dry seabed. Because of agricultural diversions, the Yellow River ran dry in 1972 for the first time in China's 3000-year history, failing to reach the sea for 15 days that year; now, the dry period extends for more than half of each year. In Canada, more than half of the country's fresh water drains to the north, while 85% of the Canadian population lives within 300 kilometres of the Canada–U.S. border.

Sewage

Before the mid-nineteenth century, many people contracted serious diseases, such as typhoid, cholera, and hepatitis A, by direct contact with human feces, which were disposed of at random. Once the links between sewage and disease were discovered, practices began to change. People learned how to build sanitary outhouses and how to locate them so they would not contaminate water sources. As plumbing moved indoors, sewage disposal became more complicated. In rural areas, the **septic system**, a self-contained sewage disposal system, worked quite well. Today, many rural homes still rely on septic systems; however, many old tanks are leaking contaminants into the environment.

Different approaches became necessary as urban areas developed. Most cities have sewage-treatment systems that separate fecal matter from water in huge tanks and ponds and stabilize it so that it cannot transmit infectious diseases. Once treated and biologically safe, the water is released back into the environment. The sludge that remains behind is often contaminated with **heavy metals** and is handled as hazardous waste; if not contaminated, sludge may be used as fertilizer. If incorporated into the food chain, heavy metals, such as lead, cadmium, copper, and tin, can cause illness or death; therefore, these chemicals must be prevented from being released into the environment when sludge is burned or buried.

In addition to regulating industrial discharge, many cities have now begun expanded sewage-treatment measures to remove heavy metals and other hazardous chemicals. This action has resulted from many studies linking exposure to chemicals, such as mercury, lead, and *polychlorinated biphenyls* (PCBs), with long-term health consequences, including cancer and damage to the central nervous system. The technology to effectively remove heavy metals and chemicals from sewage is still developing, and the costs involved are immense.

Protecting the Water Supply

By reducing your own water use, you help preserve your community's valuable supply and lower your monthly water bill. By taking steps to keep the water supply clean, you reduce pollution overall and help protect the land, wildlife, and other people from illness. Here are some simple steps you can take to protect your water supply:

- Take showers, not baths, to minimize your water consumption. Don't let water run when you're not actively using it while brushing your teeth, shaving, or handwashing clothes. Don't run a dishwasher or washing machine until you have a full load.

- Install sink faucet aerators and water-efficient shower-heads, which use two to five times less water with no noticeable decrease in performance.

- Purchase a water-saver toilet, or put a displacement device in your toilet tank to reduce the amount of water used with each flush.

- Fix any leaky faucets in your home. Leaks can waste thousands of litres of water per year.

- Don't pour toxic materials, such as cleaning solvents, bleach, or motor oil down the drain. Store them until you can take them to a hazardous waste collection centre.

- Don't pour old medicines down the drain or flush them down the toilet. A 2007 report conducted on behalf of Environment Canada's National Water Research Institute revealed that samples of surface water used as a source of drinking water for Ontario residents were contaminated with detectable

QUESTIONS FOR CRITICAL THINKING AND REFLECTION
How would you describe the quality of the water where you live? Are there lakes or streams where you can safely swim or fish? What local information sources can you find about water quality in your area?

amounts of prescription and over-the-counter drugs, as well as triclosan (an antimicrobial agent found in many personal care products, such as soaps, toothpastes, and mouthwashes). Some medications enter the water system after human excretion into sewage systems, but many people flush old or unused medicines. Strategies are being developed to remove medicines from drinking water, but experts suggest that the drugs appear only in trace amounts and generally are not considered a health hazard. Still, it has been suggested that the best way to discard old medicines is to mix them with coffee grounds or cat litter, seal them in a container, and put them in the trash.

SOLID WASTE POLLUTION

Humans generate huge amounts of waste, which must be handled appropriately if the environment is to be kept safe.

Solid Waste

The bulk of the organic food garbage produced in Canadian kitchens is now dumped in the sewage system by way of the mechanical garbage disposal. The garbage that remains is not very hazardous from the standpoint of infectious disease because there is very little food waste in it, but it does represent an enormous disposal and contamination problem.

What's In Our Garbage? The average Canadian generates more than 380 kilograms of household waste every year. The biggest single component of household trash by weight is organic waste from kitchens and yards, followed by paper products, including newspapers, junk mail, and other paper fibres (Figure 21.5 on p. 654). Plastic, metals, and glass, as well as animal waste, textiles, tires, and wood, are other significant components. A relatively small percentage of the solid waste is toxic, although a new and growing

septic system A self-contained sewage disposal system, often used in rural areas, in which waste material is decomposed by bacteria.

heavy metal A metal with a high specific gravity, such as lead, copper, or tin.

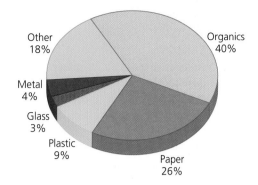

Other
18%

Organics
40%

Metal
4%

Glass
3%

Plastic
9%

Paper
26%

Note: The Other wastes category includes such materials as animal waste, textiles, tires, and wood.

FIGURE 21.5 Components of municipal solid waste, by weight, generated by Canadian households.

Source: Statistics Canada. 2005. *Human Activity and the Environment: Annual Statistics 2005* (http://www.statcan.gc.ca/pub/16-201-x/16-201-x2005000-eng.pdf; retrieved August 10, 2010).

source of toxic waste is the disposal of computer components in both household and commercial waste. Burning, as opposed to burial, reduces the bulk of solid waste, but it may release hazardous material into the air.

Solid waste is not limited to household products. Manufacturing, mining, and other industries all produce large amounts of potentially dangerous materials that cannot simply be dumped.

Disposing of Solid Waste The most common way to dispose of waste in Canada is to bury it in **sanitary landfill** disposal sites (Figure 21.6). Careful site selection and daily management are an essential part of this approach to disposal. The site is thoroughly studied to ensure that it is not near groundwater, streams, or any other source of water that could be contaminated by leakage from the landfill. In contrast to the garbage dumps used in previous generations, modern landfills are now designed with protective liners to control leachate (a toxic mixture of water and dissolved solids) and gas emissions. Layers of solid waste are regularly covered with thin layers of dirt until the site is filled. Some communities then plant grass and trees and convert the site into a park. Landfill is relatively stable; almost no decomposition occurs in the solidly packed waste.

Burying solid waste in landfills has several disadvantages. Much of this waste contains chemicals, ranging

95% of Canadian households had access to recycling in 2007; nearly all of those with access chose to recycle, but the extent of this recycling varied.

—Statistics Canada, 2007

from leftover pesticides to paints and oils, which should not be released indiscriminately into the environment. Despite precautions, buried contaminants sometimes leak into the surrounding soil and groundwater. Burial is also expensive and requires huge amounts of space.

Biodegradability *Biodegradation* is the process by which organic substances are broken down naturally by living organisms. Organic materials can be degraded either aerobically (with oxygen) or anaerobically (without oxygen). These organic materials—including plant and animal matter, substances originating from living organisms, or artificial materials similar in nature to plants and animals—are put to use by microorganisms. The term **biodegradable** means that certain products can break down naturally, safely, and quickly into the raw materials of nature, and then disappear back into the environment. Table 21.3 shows the amount of time required for different types of material to biodegrade.

Recycling Because of the expense and potential chemical hazards of any form of solid waste disposal, most communities in Canada encourage individuals and businesses to recycle their trash. In **recycling**, many kinds of waste materials are collected and used as raw materials in the production of new products. For example, waste paper can be recycled into new paper products, or an old bicycle frame can be melted down and used in the production of appliances. The number of recycling opportunities is almost limitless. These materials are not limited to paper, glass, and cans but also include other things, such as discarded tires and used oils. Recycling is a good idea for two reasons. First, it puts unwanted objects back to good use. Second, it reduces the amount of solid waste sitting in landfills, some of which takes decades to decay naturally. Even as recycling grows in popularity, however, the total amount of garbage Canadians generate will probably continue to rise as the population increases.

Discarded Technology A newer solid waste disposal problem involves the discarding of old computers, televisions, and other electronic devices. According to Environ-

Table 21.3	Biodegrading Times of Different Objects
Item	**Time Required to Biodegrade**
Banana peel	2–10 days
Paper	2–5 months
Rope	3–14 months
Orange peel	6 months
Wool sock	1–5 years
Cigarette butt	1–12 years
Plastic-coated milk carton	5 years
Aluminum can	80–100 years
Plastic six-pack holder ring	450 years
Glass bottle	1 million years
Plastic bottle	Forever

FIGURE 21.6   A sanitary landfill.

ment Canada, Canadians scrap about 140,000 metric tons of electronic waste each year. This "e-waste" is the fastest-growing portion of our waste stream. Junked electronic devices are toxic, hazardous waste because they contain varying amounts of lead, mercury, and other heavy metals.

The e-waste problem is expected to get worse because the Canadian Radio-television and Telecommunications Commission has mandated (in most areas of Canada) the transition to digital television broadcasting by 2011. Many consumers will throw out their old televisions to upgrade their sets for digital reception.

Reducing Solid Waste

By recycling more and throwing away less, you can conserve landfill space and put more reusable items back into service. Here are some ideas to help you reduce solid waste:

- Buy products with the least amount of packaging you can, or buy products in bulk (see the box "How to Be a Green Consumer" on p. 656). For example, buy large jars of juice, not individually packaged juice drinks. Buy products packaged in recyclable containers.

- Buy recycled or recyclable products. Avoid disposables; instead, use long-lasting or reusable products, such as refillable pens and rechargeable batteries.

- Avoid using foam or paper cups and plastic stirrers by bringing your own coffee mug and metal spoon to work or wherever you drink coffee or tea. Pack your lunch in reusable containers, and use a cloth or plastic lunch bag or a lunch box.

- To store food, use glass jars and reusable plastic containers rather than foil and plastic wrap.

- Recycle your newspapers, glass, cans, paper, and other recyclables. If you receive something packaged with foam pellets, take them to a commercial mailing centre that accepts them for recycling.

- Do not throw electronic items, batteries, or fluorescent lights into the trash. Check with your municipality for reuse, recycling, and disposal options, and donate old equipment to charitable organizations.

sanitary landfill   A disposal site where solid wastes are buried.

biodegradable   Refers to the ability of some materials to break down naturally and disappear back into the environment.

recycling   The use of waste materials as raw materials in the production of new products.

TERMS

How to Be a Green Consumer

It may seem like a hassle to consider the environmental impact of the things you buy, but a few simple choices can make a big difference without compromising your lifestyle. You can quickly and easily develop habits that direct your consumer dollar toward environmentally friendly products and companies.

• Remember the four Rs of green consumerism:

1. *Reduce* the amount of garbage and pollution you generate by consuming and throwing away less.

2. *Reuse* as many products as possible—either yourself or by selling them or donating them to charity.

3. *Recycle* all appropriate materials and buy recycled products whenever possible.

4. *Respond* by educating others about reducing waste and recycling, by finding creative ways to reduce waste and toxicity, and by making your preferences known.

• Choose products packaged in refillable, recycled, reusable containers or in readily recyclable materials, such as paper, cardboard, aluminum, or glass. Don't buy products that are excessively packaged or wrapped.

• Look for products made with the highest possible content of recycled paper, metal, glass, plastic, and other materials.

• Choose simple products containing the lowest amounts of bleaches, dyes, and fragrances. Look for organically grown foods and clothes made from organically grown cotton or another naturally coloured type of cotton.

• Buy high-quality appliances that have an Energy Star symbol from Natural Resources Canada's Office of Energy Efficiency, or some other type of certification indicating that they are energy- and water-efficient.

• Get a reusable cloth shopping bag. Don't bag items that don't need to be bagged. If you forget to bring your bag to the store, it doesn't matter much if you use a paper or plastic bag to carry your purchases home. What's important is that you reuse whatever bag you get.

• Don't buy what you don't need—borrow, rent, or share. Take good care of the things you own, repair items when they break, and replace them with used rather than new items whenever possible.

• Walk or bike when you can. If you must drive, do several errands at once to save energy and cut down on pollution.

• Look beyond the products to the companies that make them. Support those with good environmental records. If some of your favourite products are overpackaged or contain harmful ingredients, write to the manufacturer.

• Keep in mind that doing something is better than doing nothing. Even if you can't be a perfectly green consumer, doing your best on any purchase will make a difference.

Sources: Natural Resources Canada. 2010. *What Is Energy Star?* (http://oee.nrcan.gc.ca/residential/business/energystar/index.cfm?attr=4; retrieved August 10, 2010); U.S. Environmental Protection Agency. 2009. *Consumer Handbook for Reducing Solid Waste* (http://www.epa.gov/osw/wycd/catbook; retrieved February 19, 2009); Natural Resources Defense Council. 2009. *NRDC's Guide to Greener Living* (http:// www.nrdc.org/cities/living/gover.asp; retrieved February 19, 2009).

• Start a compost pile for your organic garbage (non-animal food and yard waste) if you have a yard. If you live in an apartment, you can create a small composting system by using earthworms, or take your organic wastes to a community composting centre.

• Stop junk mail. Canada Post suggests that if individuals would like to stop receiving unaddressed advertisements, such as coupons, flyers, catalogues, government mailings, and municipal notices, they can simply place a note in their mailbox stating that they do not want to receive this type of mail (http://www.canadapost.ca).

QUESTIONS FOR CRITICAL THINKING AND REFLECTION

What are your own waste-disposal habits like? Do you recycle everything you possibly can? Do you get rid of items that are still usable? Even if you are conscientious about the way you deal with waste, how could you improve your habits?

CHEMICAL POLLUTION AND HAZARDOUS WASTE

Chemical pollution is by no means a new problem. The ancient Romans were plagued by lead poisoning; industrial chemicals have claimed countless lives over the past few centuries.

Today, new chemical substances are constantly being introduced into the environment—as pesticides, herbicides, solvents, and hundreds of other products. More people and wildlife are exposed and potentially exposed to them than ever before. Many chemicals are harmless by themselves but become deadly in combination. Chemical pollutants have been responsible for several environmental disasters, including thousands of deaths and injuries among people in Bhopal, India, that occurred when a powerful chemical used in manufacturing the insecticide Sevin was released from a plant. Catastrophes illustrate the short-term potential for disaster, but the long-term health consequences may be just as deadly.

The problem of chemical pollution and hazardous waste was highlighted in Canada and the United States in the late 1980s when the International Joint Commission identified 43 areas of concern (AOCs) in the Great Lakes Basin area. Seventeen Canadian "pollution hot spots" were identified, two of which have since been fully restored. According to Environment Canada, clean up has been completed in an additional Canadian AOC, and it is now being monitored for recovery. In response to these environmental concerns, the Great Lakes Sustainability Fund was established in 2000 by Environment Canada and several other government departments to accelerate the work being carried out to restore the environmental quality of the remaining AOCs.

Asbestos

A mineral-based compound, asbestos was widely used for fire protection and insulation in buildings until the 1980s. Microscopic asbestos fibres can be released into the air when this material is applied or when it later deteriorates or is damaged. These fibres can lodge in the lungs, causing **asbestosis**, lung cancer, and other serious lung diseases. Similar conditions expose workers to risk in the coal mining industry, from coal and silica dust (black lung disease), and in the textile industry, from cotton fibres (brown lung disease). Working with asbestos is also the primary risk factor for **mesothelioma**.

Asbestos can pose a danger in homes and apartment buildings, about 25% of which are thought to contain some asbestos. Areas where it is most likely to be found are insulation around water and steam pipes, ducts, and furnaces; boiler wraps; vinyl flooring; floor, wall, and ceiling insulation; roofing and siding; and fireproof board.

Lead

Thanks to better preventive efforts, lead poisoning is not as serious a problem today as it was a few years ago. Researchers suggest that children under the age of three are most susceptible to the negative effects of lead. According to Health Canada, the blood levels of lead in Canadian children are generally low. Although no population-based studies have been conducted with Canadian children under the age of six, U.S. research shows that many children with unsafe lead levels in their blood live in poor, inner city areas (see the box "Poverty and Environmental Health" on p. 658). When lead is ingested or inhaled, it can damage the central nervous system, cause mental impairment, hinder oxygen transport in the blood, and create digestive problems. Severe lead poisoning may cause coma or even death. Neurological damage can be permanent.

Long-term exposure to low levels of lead may cause kidney disease; it can also cause build up in bones, where it may be released into the bloodstream during pregnancy or when bone mass is lost from osteoporosis.

Young children can easily ingest lead from their environment by picking up dust and dirt on their hands and then putting their fingers in their mouth. Lead-based paints are the chief culprit in lead poisoning of children. In Canada, lead was added to most household and industrial paints until the 1960s, and was eliminated from all paint in 1991 (although Canadian regulations have limited lead in most indoor paints since 1978). If your house or building was built before the 1970s, it is best to assume that it contains leaded paint. Although it is rare for houses built after this time to contain large quantities of leaded paint, some exceptions do exist. Some old pipes and faucets (typically in homes built before 1975) also contain lead, which can leach into water that has been sitting in pipes. For this reason, the Public Health Agency of Canada recommends letting tap water run until it is cold before using it for drinking, cooking, or preparing baby formula. Canadians are also advised not to use water from the hot water tap for drinking or cooking. Contact your local Public Health Department if you are concerned about lead levels in your home.

Pesticides

Pesticides are used primarily for two purposes: to prevent the spread of insect-borne diseases and to maximize food production by killing insects that eat crops. Both uses have risks as well as benefits. Take, for example, the pesticide DDT. Recognized as a powerful pesticide in 1939, DDT was extremely important in efforts to control widespread insect-borne diseases in tropical countries and increase crop yields throughout the world. In 1962, however, biologist Rachel Carson questioned the safety of DDT in her book *Silent Spring*, pointing out that the pesticide disrupts the life cycles of birds, fish, and reptiles. DDT also builds up in the food chain, increasing in concentration as larger animals eat smaller ones, a process known as **biomagnification**.

Poverty and Environmental Health

Residents of poor communities and those populated by minority group members are often exposed to more environmental toxins than residents of wealthier communities, and they are more likely to suffer from health problems caused or aggravated by pollutants.

Poor neighbourhoods are often located near highways and industrial areas that have high levels of air and noise pollution; they are also common sites for hazardous waste production and disposal. Residents of substandard housing are more likely to come into contact with lead, asbestos, carbon monoxide, pesticides, and other hazardous pollutants associated with peeling paint, old plumbing, poorly maintained insulation and heating equipment, and attempts to control high numbers of pests, such as cockroaches and rodents.

Poor people are more likely to have jobs that expose them to asbestos, silica dust,

and pesticides, and they are more likely to catch and consume fish contaminated with PCBs, mercury, and other toxins.

The most thoroughly researched and documented link among poverty, the environment, and health is lead poisoning in children. Many studies have shown that children of low-income black families are much more likely to have elevated levels of lead in their blood than are white children.

Asthma is another health threat that appears to be linked with both environmental and socioeconomic factors. Worldwide, the prevalence of asthma is growing by 50% every decade; it is the most common chronic disease among children, and most asthma-related deaths occur in lower income countries. Researchers are not sure what accounts for this increase but probable causes include household pollutants, pesticides, air pollution, cigarette smoke, and allergens, such as cockroaches. These risk factors are likely to cluster in poor areas where inadequate health care may worsen asthma's effects.

Despite its effectiveness as a pesticide, DDT was banned in Canada in 1985 because the costs associated with its use—to wildlife and potentially to humans—were too high. Most pesticide hazards to date have been a result of overuse, but concerns remain about the health effects of long-term exposure to small amounts of pesticide residues in foods, especially for children.

Mercury

A naturally occurring metal, mercury is a toxin that affects the nervous system and may damage the brain, kidneys, and gastrointestinal tract; increase blood pressure, heart rate, and heart attack risk; and cause cancer. Mercury slows fetal and child development and causes irreversible deficits in brain function. According to 2008 data from the Canadian Health Measures Survey, less than 1% of Canadian adults have blood mercury concentrations that exceed the maximum value set by Health Canada. Coal-fired power plants are the largest producers of mercury; other sources include mining and smelting operations and the disposal of consumer products containing mercury.

Mercury persists in the environment and, like pesticides, it is bioaccumulative. In particular, large, long-lived fish may carry high levels of mercury. Chapter 5 includes information on safe fish consumption; see the box "Gender and Environmental Health" for more on issues affecting pregnant women.

Hazardous chemicals accumulate in many homes, as well as in businesses and industrial sites.

Because of health concerns, many stores have replaced mercury thermometers with mercury-free alternatives. If a mercury thermometer breaks or is disposed of improperly, mercury can enter the environment; if it vaporizes into the atmosphere, it can be hazardous to health. To safely clean up mercury from a broken thermometer, increase ventilation in the room and pick up the mercury with an eyedropper or scoop up the beads with a piece of heavy paper. Dispose of it and any contaminated instruments by placing them in a plastic bag and taking them to an appropriate hazardous waste disposal site.

Gender and Environmental Health

Although many environmental health risks are shared by all, some risks disproportionately affect women or men. Women and men often have different roles and responsibilities with respect to family, community, and the workforce. These differences can determine the types of environmental hazards that individuals are exposed to and what the potential risks of those exposures are.

In many societies, women are more often involved in day-to-day activities associated with the environment, including food preparation, agricultural work, and tasks around the home. These activities can expose women to greater levels of indoor air pollution, water pollution, food-borne pathogens, agricultural chemicals, and waste contamination. Indoor pollutants, especially soot from burning wood, charcoal, and other solid fuels used for home heating and cooking, are a particular risk for women. Exposure to this particulate pollution increases the risk of respiratory diseases, lung cancer, and reproductive problems.

All humans are exposed to chemicals in air, food, and drinking water, and we all carry a body load of chemicals. Some of these chemicals bioaccumulate in our bones, blood, or fatty tissues. Women are smaller than men, on average, and have a higher percentage of body fat; so chemicals that accumulate in fatty tissue may pose a relatively greater risk for women. Conversely, men may be more likely to work in industries that involve significant occupational exposures to disease-related toxins; for example, coal miners have an increased risk of lung cancer (black lung disease).

Although any chemical exposure can be a concern for health, women face the added risk of passing pollutants to a developing fetus during pregnancy or to an infant through breastfeeding. Even relatively low exposure to pollutants can result in a significant chemical body load in an infant or young child because of their small body size. And because infants and children are still developing, the effects of chemical exposure can be significant and devastating. It is not unusual for dangerous environmental toxin exposures to be first recognized through noticeable effects on infants or children.

Reproductive risks are not limited to women and infants in developing parts of the world. Even in industrialized countries with strong environmental laws, infants and children are affected by such chemicals as lead and mercury. In 2005, American scientists announced that they had found elevated levels of the rocket fuel chemical perchlorate in human breast milk in amounts above the safe dose set by the National Academy of Sciences. Many other chemicals, including PCBs and pesticides, have already been found in breast milk.

Studies are ongoing to identify and reduce environmental hazards in Canada and throughout the world. However, many of the people most directly affected by environmental health problems—women, children, and people living in poor communities—have limited economic, social, and political power. It is important that everyone affected by environmental problems be given a voice in determining environmental policies.

Sources: Kirk, A. B., et al. 2005. Perchlorate and iodide in dairy and breast milk. *Environmental Science and Technology*, Web release, February 22; McCally, M., ed. 2002. *Life Support: The Environment and Human Health.* Cambridge, Mass.: MIT Press; Population Reference Bureau. 2002. *Women, Men, and Environmental Change: The Gender Dimensions of Environmental Policies and Programs.* Washington, D.C.: Population Reference Bureau.

Other Chemical Pollutants

The list of real and potential chemical pollution problems may well be as long as the list of known chemicals. To the preceding examples we can add recent concern about arsenic in drinking water, poisonous chemicals in plastic baby bottles, hormones in streams, and other by-products of our industrial age.

As mentioned earlier, hazardous wastes are also found in the home and should be handled and disposed of properly. They include automotive supplies (motor oil, antifreeze, transmission fluid), paint supplies (turpentine, paint thinner, mineral spirits), art and hobby supplies (oil-based paint, solvents, acids and alkalis, aerosol sprays), insecticides, batteries, computer and electronic components, and household cleaners containing sodium hydroxide (lye) or ammonia. These chemicals are dangerous when inhaled or ingested, when they contact the skin or the eyes, or when they are burned or dumped.

Many cities provide guidelines about approved disposal methods and have hazardous waste collection days. Look online or in the government pages of your phone book under Hazardous Waste or Waste Disposal.

Preventing Chemical Pollution

You can take steps to reduce the chemical pollution in your community. Just as important, by reducing and eliminating the number of chemicals in your home, you may save the life of a child or animal who might encounter one of those chemicals.

- When buying products, read the labels, and try to buy the least toxic ones available. Choose nontoxic nonpetrochemical cleansers, disinfectants, polishes, and other personal and household products.

- Dispose of your household hazardous wastes properly. If you are not sure whether something is hazardous or don't know how to dispose of it, contact your local environmental health office or health department. Don't burn garbage.

- Buy organic produce or produce that has been grown locally. Wash, scrub, and, if appropriate, peel fruits and vegetables. Consider eating less meat; animal products require more pesticides, fertilizer, water, and energy to produce.

QUESTIONS FOR CRITICAL THINKING AND REFLECTION

Are there any hazardous chemicals in your home, such as cleaning products, solvents, paint, or batteries? Would you know what to do if one of these chemicals spilled? How would you clean it up?

- If you must use pesticides or toxic household products, store them in a locked place where children and pets can't get to them. Don't measure chemicals with food-preparation utensils, and wear gloves whenever handling them.

- If you have your house fumigated for pest control, be sure to hire a licensed exterminator. Keep everyone, including pets, out of the house while the crew works and, if possible, for a few days after.

RADIATION POLLUTION

Many people are afraid of **radiation**, in part because they don't understand what it is. Basically, radiation is energy.

It can come in different forms, such as ultraviolet rays, microwaves, or X-rays, and from different sources, such as the sun, uranium, and nuclear weapons (Figure 21.7). These forms of electromagnetic radiation differ in wavelength and energy, with shorter waves having the highest energy levels.

Of most concern to health are gamma rays produced by radioactive sources. such as nuclear weapons, nuclear energy plants, and radon gas; these high-energy waves are powerful enough to penetrate objects and break molecular bonds. Although gamma radiation cannot be seen or felt, its effects at high doses can include **radiation sickness** and death; at lower doses, chromosome damage, sterility, tissue damage, cataracts, and cancer can occur. Other types of radiation can also affect health; for example, exposure to UV radiation from the sun or from tanning salons can increase the risk of skin cancer. The effects of some sources of radiation, such as cellphones, remain controversial.

Nuclear Weapons and Nuclear Energy

Nuclear weapons pose a health risk of the most serious kind to all species. Public health associations have stated that in the event of an intentional or unintentional discharge of these weapons, the casualties would run into the hundreds of thousands or millions. Reducing the stockpiles of nuclear weapons is a challenge and a goal for the twenty-first century.

Power-generating plants that use nuclear fuel also pose health problems. When **nuclear power** was first developed as an alternative to oil and coal, it was promoted as clean, efficient, inexpensive, and safe. In general, this has proven to be the case. Power systems in several parts of the world rely on nuclear power plants. However, despite all the built-in safeguards and regulating agencies, accidents in nuclear power plants do happen, many through human error (as at Chernobyl in Ukraine and Tokaimura in Japan), and the consequences of such accidents are far more serious than those of similar accidents in other types of power-generating plants. The 1986 fire and explosion at the Chernobyl nuclear power station in Ukraine caused hundreds of deaths and increased rates of genetic mutation and cancer; the long-term effects are not yet clear. The zone around Chernobyl has been sealed off to human habitation and could be unsafe for the next 24,000 years.

FIGURE 21.7 Electromagnetic radiation. Electromagnetic radiation takes the form of waves that travel through space. The length of the wave determines the type of radiation: The shortest waves are high-energy gamma rays; the longest are radio waves and extremely low frequency waves used for communication between aircraft, ships, and submarines. Different types of electromagnetic radiation have different effects on health.

An additional, enormous problem is disposing of the radioactive wastes these plants generate. They cannot be dumped in a sanitary landfill because the amount and type of soil used to cap a sanitary landfill are not sufficient to prevent radiation exposure. Deposit sites have to be developed that will be secure not just for a few years but for tens of thousands of years—longer than the total recorded history of human beings on this planet. To date, no storage method has been devised that can provide infallible, infinitely durable shielding for nuclear waste.

Medical Uses of Radiation

Another area of concern is the use of radiation in medicine, primarily the X-ray. The development of machines that could produce images of internal bone structures was a major advance in medicine, and applications abounded. Chest X-rays were routinely given to screen for tuberculosis, and children's feet were even X-rayed in shoe stores to make sure their new shoes fit properly. But, as is often the case, this new technology had disadvantages. As time passed, studies revealed that X-ray exposure is cumulative and that no exposure is absolutely safe.

Early X-ray machines are no longer used because of the high amounts of radiation they give off. Each new generation of X-ray machines has used less radiation more effectively. From a personal health point of view, no one should ever have a "routine" X-ray examination; each such exam should have a definite purpose, and its benefits and risks should be carefully weighed.

Radiation in the Home and Workplace

Recently, concern has grown about electromagnetic radiation associated with common modern devices, such as microwave ovens, computer monitors, cellphones, and even high-voltage power lines. These forms of radiation do have effects on health, but research results are inconclusive.

Another area of concern is **radon**, a naturally occurring radioactive gas found in certain soils, rocks, and building materials. When the breakdown products of radon are inhaled, they cling to lungs and bombard sensitive tissue with radioactivity. Among miners, exposure to high levels of radon has been shown to cause lung cancer; overall, it is the second-leading cause of lung cancer after smoking tobacco. Radon can enter a home by rising through the soil into the basement through dirt floors, cracks, and other openings.

In 2009, Health Canada, along with the Federal Provincial Territorial Radiation Protection Committee, recommended that Canadians take action if their homes contain an average annual radon concentration of more than 200 becquerels per cubic metre (Bq/m^3). If elevated levels of radon are found, the problem should be dealt with as soon as possible through such measures as sealing cracks or installing basement ventilation systems. More information is available at the Health Canada Web site or by emailing radon@hc-sc.gc.ca.

QUESTIONS FOR CRITICAL THINKING AND REFLECTION

Do you live in an area where radon is a problem? If so, has your home been checked for radon?

Avoiding Radiation

The following steps can help you avoid unneeded exposure to radiation:

- If your physician orders an X-ray, ask why it is necessary. Only get X-rays that you need, and keep a record of the date and location of every X-ray exam. Don't have a full-body CT scan for routine screening; the radiation dose of one full-body CT scan is nearly 100 times that of a typical mammogram.

- Follow Health Canada's recommendations for radon testing.

- Find out if there are radioactive sites in your area. If you live or work near such a site, form or join a community action group to get the site cleaned up.

NOISE POLLUTION

We are increasingly aware of the health effects of loud or persistent noise in the environment. Concerns focus on two areas: hearing loss and stress. Prolonged exposure to sounds above 80–85 **decibels** (a measure of the intensity of a sound wave) can cause permanent hearing loss (Figure 21.8 on p. 662). Hearing damage can occur after eight hours of exposure to sounds louder than 80 decibels. Regular exposure for longer than one minute to more than 100 decibels can cause permanent hearing loss. Children may suffer damage to their hearing at lower noise levels than adults.

radiation Energy transmitted in the form of rays, waves, or particles.

radiation sickness An illness caused by excess radiation exposure, marked by low white blood cell counts and nausea; possibly fatal.

nuclear power The use of controlled nuclear reactions to produce steam, which in turn drives turbines to produce electricity.

radon A naturally occurring radioactive gas emitted from rocks and natural building materials that can become concentrated in insulated homes, causing lung cancer.

decibel A unit for expressing the relative intensity of sounds on a scale from 0 for the average least perceptible sound to about 120 for the average pain threshold.

	180 — Rocket launch
Rifle shot	160 —
Jet engine	
	140 — Thunder overhead
Rock concert	
	120 — Pain threshold
Motorcycle	100 —
	Heavy traffic
	80 —
Vacuum cleaner	
	60 —
Birds singing	Normal conversation
	40 —
	Whispering
	20 —
Leaves rustling	
	0 — Faintest audible noise

Sound intensity or loudness
(decibels)

FIGURE 21.8 **The intensity of selected sounds.**

Two common sources of excessive noise are the workplace and large gatherings of people at sporting events and rock concerts. Federal and provincial or territorial governments set limits for noise in the workplace, but no common laws exist regulating noise levels at rock concerts, which can be much louder than most workplaces.

QUESTIONS FOR CRITICAL THINKING AND REFLECTION
How often do you listen to loud music? Do you ever use headphones? At what volume level do you like to listen? Do you think your listening habits pose a threat to your hearing? Would you let a child listen at the same volume level?

Here are some ways to avoid exposing yourself to excessive noise:

• Wear ear protectors when working around noisy machinery.

• When listening to music on a headset with a volume range of 1–10, keep the volume no louder than 6; your headset is too loud if you are unable to hear people around you speaking in a normal tone of voice. Earmuff-style headphones may be easier on the ears than earbuds, which are inserted into the ear canal. Experts warn that earbuds should not be used more than 30 minutes a day unless the volume is set below 60% of maximum; headphones can be used up to one hour.

• Avoid loud music. Don't sit or stand near speakers or amplifiers at a rock concert, and don't play a car radio or stereo so high that you can't hear the traffic.

• Avoid exposure to painfully loud sounds, and avoid repeated exposure to any sounds above 80 decibels.

YOU AND THE ENVIRONMENT

Faced with a vast array of confusing and complex environmental issues, you may feel overwhelmed and conclude that there isn't anything you can do about global problems. But this is not true. If everyone made individual changes in his or her life, the impact would be tremendous. (To assess your current lifestyle, refer to the box "Environmental Health Checklist.")

At the same time, it is important to recognize that large corporations and manufacturers are the ones primarily responsible for environmental degradation. Many of them have jumped on the environmental bandwagon with public relations and advertising campaigns designed to make them look good, but they haven't changed their practices nearly enough to make a difference. To influence them, people have to become educated, demand changes in production methods, and elect people to office who consider environmental concerns along with sound business practices.

Environmental Health Checklist

The following list of statements relates to your effect on the environment. Put a checkmark next to the statements that are true for you.

_____ I ride my bike, walk, carpool, or use public transportation whenever possible.

_____ I keep my car tuned up and well maintained.

_____ My residence is well insulated.

_____ Where possible, I use compact fluorescent bulbs instead of incandescent bulbs.

_____ I turn off lights and appliances when they are not in use.

_____ I avoid turning on heat or air conditioning whenever possible.

_____ I run the washing machine, dryer, and dishwasher only when they have full loads.

_____ I run the clothes dryer only as long as it takes my clothes to dry.

_____ I dry my hair with a towel rather than a hair dryer.

_____ I keep my car's air conditioner in good working order and have it serviced by a service station that recycles CFCs.

_____ When shopping, I choose products with the least amount of packaging.

_____ I choose recycled and recyclable products.

_____ I avoid products packaged in plastic and unrecycled aluminum.

_____ I store food in glass jars and waxed paper rather than plastic wrap.

_____ I take my own bag along when I go shopping.

_____ I recycle newspapers, glass, cans, and other recyclables.

_____ When shopping, I read labels and try to buy the least toxic products available.

_____ I dispose of household hazardous wastes properly.

_____ I take showers instead of baths.

_____ I take short showers and switch off the water when I'm not actively using it.

_____ I do not run the water while brushing my teeth, shaving, or handwashing clothes.

_____ My faucets have aerators installed in them.

_____ My shower has a low-flow showerhead.

_____ I have a water-saver toilet or a water displacement device in my toilet.

_____ I snip or rip plastic six-pack rings before I throw them out.

_____ When hiking or camping, I never leave anything behind.

Statements you have not checked can help you identify behaviours you can change to improve environmental health.

For an overall estimate of how much land and water your lifestyle requires, take the Ecological Footprint quiz at http://www.myfootprint.org.

Large-scale changes and individual actions complement each other. What you do every day does count. Following the suggestions throughout this chapter will help you make a difference in the environment. In addition, you can become a part of larger community actions to work for a healthier world:

• Share what you learn about environmental issues with your friends and family.

• Join, support, or volunteer your time to organizations working on environmental causes that are important to you.

• Contact your elected representatives and communicate your concerns. For guidelines on how to be heard, see the box "Making Your Letters Count" on p. 664.

TAKE CHARGE

Making Your Letters Count

It takes only a few minutes to write to an elected official, but it can make a difference on an environmental issue you care about. When elected officials receive enough letters or emails on an issue, it does influence their vote—they want to be re-elected, and your vote counts! To give your letter the greatest possible influence, use these guidelines:

• Use your own words and your own stationery.

• Be clear and concise. Keep your letter to one or two paragraphs, never more than one page.

• Focus on only one subject in each letter, and identify it clearly. Refer to legislation by its name or number.

• Request a specific action—vote a particular way on a piece of legislation, request hearings, support a bill—and state your reasons for your position.

• If you live or work in the official's district, say so.

• Courteous letters work best. Don't be insulting or unnecessarily critical.

You can send letters via regular mail; however, increased security screenings often delay delivery. You can email the minister of the environment at minister@ec.gc.ca. To locate the contact information for your local member of parliament, visit http://www.parl.gc.ca/Parlinfo/Compilations/HouseOf Commons/MemberByPostalCode.aspx.

SUMMARY

• Environmental health encompasses all the interactions of humans with their environment and the health consequences of those interactions.

• The world's population is increasing rapidly, especially in the developing world. Factors that may eventually limit human population are food, availability of land and water, energy, and minimum acceptable standard of living.

• Increased amounts of air pollutants are especially dangerous for children, older adults, and people with chronic health problems.

• Factors contributing to the development of smog include heavy motor vehicle traffic, hot weather, and stagnant air.

• Carbon dioxide and other natural gases act as a greenhouse around Earth, increasing the temperature of the atmosphere. Levels of these gases are rising through human activity; as a result, the world's climate could change.

• The ozone layer that shields Earth's surface from the sun's UV rays has thinned and developed holes in certain regions.

• Environmental damage from energy use can be limited through energy conservation and the development of non-polluting, renewable sources of energy.

• Indoor pollutants can trigger allergies and illness in the short term and cancer in the long term.

• Concerns with water quality focus on pathogenic organisms and hazardous chemicals from industry and households, as well as on water shortages.

• Sewage treatment prevents pathogens from contaminating drinking water; it often must also deal with heavy metals and hazardous chemicals.

• The amount of garbage is growing all the time; organic waste from kitchens and yards is the biggest component. Recycling can help reduce solid waste disposal problems.

• Potentially hazardous chemical pollutants include asbestos, lead, pesticides, mercury, and many household products. Proper handling and disposal are critical.

• Radiation can cause radiation sickness, chromosome damage, and cancer, among other health problems.

• Loud or persistent noise can lead to hearing loss and stress; two common sources of excessive noise are the workplace and rock concerts.

• Most health advances today must come from lifestyle changes and improvements in the global environment. The effects of personal changes made by every concerned individual could be tremendous.

FOR MORE INFORMATION

BOOKS

Ausenda, F. 2009. *Green Volunteers: The World Guide to Voluntary Work in Nature Conservation,* 7th ed. New York: Universe. Describes a variety of opportunities to volunteer for environmental causes in many different parts of the world.

Brown, M. J. 2007. *Building Powerful Community Organizations: A Personal Guide to Creating Groups That Can Solve Problems and Change the World.* Chicago: Long Haul Press. Provides advice for facing environmental (and other) challenges through local organizing and recruiting.

Cunningham, W. P., et al. 2007. *Environmental Science: A Global Concern,* 10th ed. New York: McGraw-Hill. A nontechnical survey of basic environmental science and key concerns.

Maslin, M., 2005. *Global Warming: A Very Short Introduction.* New York: Oxford University Press. A survey of the science and politics of global warming.

Nadakavukaren, A. 2005. *Our Global Environment: A Health Perspective,* 6th ed. Prospect Heights, Ill.: Waveland Press. A broad survey of major environmental issues and their effects on personal and community health.

ORGANIZATIONS, HOTLINES, AND WEB SITES

The Internet addresses listed here were accurate at the time of publication.

Canada's Action on Climate Change (Government of Canada). Provides information related to climate change and Canada's actions at home and abroad.
   http://www.climatechange.gc.ca

Earth Times. An international online newspaper devoted to global environmental issues.

http://www.earthtimes.org

Ecological Footprint. Calculates your personal ecological footprint based on your diet, transportation patterns, and living arrangements.

http://www.myfootprint.org

Student Environmental Action Coalition. A coalition of student and youth environmental groups.

http://www.seac.org

United Nations. Several U.N. programs are devoted to environmental problems on a global scale; the Web sites provide information on current and projected trends and on international treaties developed to deal with environmental issues.

http://www.un.org/popin (Population Division)

http://www.unep.org (Environment Programme)

Worldwatch Institute. A public policy research organization focusing on emerging global environmental problems and the links between the world economy and the environment.

http://www.worldwatch.org

Many national and international organizations are working on environmental health problems. A few of the largest and best known are listed below:

Greenpeace: 800-320-7183; http://www.greenpeace.org

Canadian Wildlife Federation: 800-563-9453; http://www.cwf-fcf.org

Nature Conservancy of Canada: 800-465-0029; http://www.nature conservancy.ca

Sierra Club of Canada: 888-810-4204; http://www.sierraclub.ca

World Wildlife Fund—Canada: 800-267-2632; http://www.wwf.ca

SELECTED BIBLIOGRAPHY

Abelsohn, A. R., and M. Sandborn. 2010. Lead and children: Clinical management for family physicians. *Canadian Family Physician* 56: 531–535.

Bell, M. L., et al. 2004. Ozone and short-term mortality in 95 U.S. urban communities, 1987–2000. *Journal of the American Medical Association* 292(19): 2372–2378.

Canadian Hearing Society. 2008. *The Canadian Hearing Society Position Paper on Noise Pollution* (http://www.chs.ca/en/items/chs-releases-position-paper-on-noise-pollution.html; retrieved August 10, 2010).

Canadian Lung Association. 2009. *Clean Air Must Be Top Priority Despite Tough Economy: Lung Association Survey* (http://www.lung.ca/media-medias/news-nouvelles_e.php?id=149; retrieved July 23, 2010).

Canada Mortgage and Housing Corporation. 2000. *Research Highlights: Ten Steps to a Cooler Planet. Technical Series 00-146* (http://www.cmhc-schl.gc.ca/publications/en/rh-pr/tech/00-146-E.htm; retrieved August 10, 2010).

Canada Mortgage and Housing Corporation. 2010. *Asbestos* (http://www.cmhc-schl.gc.ca/en/co/maho/yohoyohe/inaiqu/inaiqu_001.cfm; retrieved August 10, 2010).

Canadian Nuclear Safety Commission. 2009. *Nuclear Power Plants* (http://www.cnsc-ccsn.gc.ca/eng/about/regulated/powerplants/; retrieved August 10, 2010).

Canadian Radio-television and Telecommunications Commission. 2007. *Broadcasting Public Notice CRTC 2007-53: Determinations Regarding Certain Aspects of the Regulatory Framework for Over-the-Air Television* (http://www.crtc.gc.ca/Eng/archive/2007/pb2007-53.htm; retrieved August 10, 2010).

CDC National Center for Environmental Health. 2007. *Children's Blood Lead Levels in the United States* (http://www.cdc.gov/nceh/lead/research/kids-BLL.htm; retrieved February 19, 2009).

Centers for Disease Control and Prevention. 2006. Adult blood lead epidemiology and surveillance—United States, 2003–2004. *Morbidity and Mortality Weekly Report* 55(32): 876–879.

Centers for Disease Control and Prevention. 2006. Surveillance for waterborne disease and outbreaks associated with drinking water and water not intended for drinking—United States, 2003–2004. *Morbidity and Mortality Weekly Report* 55(SS12): 31–58.

Chief Medical Officer of Health Report. 2010. *The Potential Health Impact of Wind Turbines* (http://www.health.gov.on.ca/en/public/publications/ministry_reports/wind_turbine/wind_turbine.pdf; retrieved February 19, 2011).

Delworth-Bart, J. E., and C. F. Moore. 2006. Mercy mercy me: Social injustice and the prevention of environmental pollutant exposures among ethnic minority and poor children. *Child Development* 77(2): 247–265.

Dominici, F., et al. 2006. Fine particulate air pollution and hospital admission for cardiovascular and respiratory diseases. *Journal of the American Medical Association* 295(10): 1127–1134.

Eggertson, L. 2008. Investigative report: 1766 boil-water advisories now in place across Canada. *Canadian Medical Association Journal* 178(10): 1261–1263.

Energy Information Administration. 2005. *Impacts of Modeled Recommendations of the National Commission on Energy Policy.* Washington, D.C.: U.S. Department of Energy.

Energy Information Agency. 2009. *Gasoline and Diesel Fuel Update* (http://tonto.eia.doe.gov/oog/info/gdu/gasdiesel.asp; retrieved February 19, 2009).

Environment Canada. 2004. Any questions? *EnviroZone* 48 (http://www.ec.gc.ca/envirozine/english/issues/48/any_questions_e.cfm; retrieved July 22, 2010).

Environment Canada. 2009. *Backgrounder: Great Lakes Sustainability Fund* (http://www.ec.gc.ca/default.asp?lang=En&n=714D9AAE-1&news=57C0304D-4625-47F7-878C-0F73300E03C5; retrieved August 10, 2010).

Environment Canada. 2009. *Water—In Canada* (http://www.ec.gc.ca/eau-water/default.asp?lang=en&n=5EA1D86E-1; retrieved August 10, 2010).

Environment Canada. 2010. *Air Quality Health Index* (http://www.ec.gc.ca/cas-aqhi/default.asp?Lang=En; retrieved July 21, 2010).

Environment Canada. 2011. *Climate Change: Canada's Action on Climate Change* (http://www.climatechange.gc.ca/default.asp?lang=En&n=72F16A84-0; retrieved February 19, 2011).

Environment Canada. 2010. *Dichlorodiphenyltrichloroethane (DDT)* (http://www.ec.gc.ca/toxiques-toxics/Default.asp?lang=En&n=98E80CC6-1&xml=13272755-983C-4DF5-8EA2-E734EFC39869; retrieved August 10, 2010).

Environment Canada. 2010. *Great Lakes Sustainability Fund* (http://www.ec.gc.ca/raps-pas/default.asp?lang=En&n=F328E319-1; retrieved August 10, 2010).

Environment Canada. 2010. *Water Levels* (http://www.ec.gc.ca/indicateurs-indicators/default.asp?lang=en&n=7FAFC303-1; retrieved August 10, 2010).

Environmental Protection Agency. 2008. *Municipal Solid Waste: Basic Facts* (http://www.epa.gov.epaoswer/non-hw/muncpl/facts.htm; retrieved February 19, 2009).

Gauderman, W. J., et al. 2004. The effect of air pollution on lung development from 10 to 18 years of age. *New England Journal of Medicine* 351(11): 1057–1067.

Health Canada. 2009. *Environmental and Workplace Health: Government of Canada Radon Guideline* (http://www.hc-sc.gc.ca/ewh-semt/radiation/radon/guidelines_lignes_directrice-eng.php; retrieved August 10, 2010).

Health Canada. 2010. *Environmental and Workplace Health: Radon Frequently Asked Questions* (http://www.hc-sc.gc.ca/ewh-semt/radiation/radon/faq_fq-eng.php#health; retrieved August 10, 2010).

Health Canada. 2010. *Environmental and Workplace Health: Reducing Exposure to Lead* (http://www.hc-sc.gc.ca/ewh-semt/hazards-risques/lead-plomb/index-eng.php#plumbing; retrieved August 10, 2010).

International Energy Agency. 2009. *CO₂ Emissions from Fuel Combustion: Highlights, 2009 Edition* (http://www.iea.org/co2highlights/co2highlights.pdf; retrieved August 10, 2010).

International Joint Commission: Canada and United States. 2010. *Groundwater in the Great Lakes Basin: A Report to the International Joint Commission from the IJC Great Lakes Science Advisory Board* (http://www.ijc.org/php/publications/pdf/ID1637.pdf; retrieved August 10, 2010).

Kunzli, N., et al. 2005. Ambient air pollution and atherosclerosis in Los Angeles. *Environmental Health Perspectives* 113(2): 201–206.

Laden, F., et al. 2006. Reduction in fine particulate air pollution and mortality: Extended follow-up of the Harvard Six Cities study. *American Journal of Respiratory and Critical Care Medicine* 173(6): 667–672.

Ménard, M. 2009. *Canada, a Big Energy Consumer: A Regional Perspective.* Statistics Canada, Analysis in Brief: 11-621-M Number 23 (http://www.statcan.gc.ca/pub/11-621-m/11-621-m2005023-eng.htm; retrieved August 3, 2010).

NASA Goddard Institute for Space Studies. 2008. *Global Temperature Trends: 2007 Summation* (http://www.giss.nasa.gov/gistemp/2008; retrieved February 19, 2009).

National Academies. 2006. *Surface Temperature Reconstructions for the Last 2,000 Years.* Washington, D.C.: National Academies Press.

Natural Resources Canada. 2009. *Energy Efficiency Trends in Canada: 1990 to 2007* (http://oee.nrcan.gc.ca/publications/statistics/trends09/pdf/trends.pdf; retrieved August 10, 2010).

Natural Resources Canada. 2009. *Renewables: Wind Energy* (http://canmet-energy-canmetenergie.nrcan-rncan.gc.ca/eng/renewables/wind_energy.html; retrieved February 19, 2011).

Natural Resources Canada. 2010. *Freshwater: The Role and Contribution of Natural Resources Canada* (http://www.nrcan.gc.ca/sd-dd/pubs/h2o/int-eng.php; retrieved August 10, 2010).

Natural Resources Canada. 2010. *What Is Energy Star?* (http://oee.nrcan.gc.ca/residential/business/energystar/index.cfm?attr=4; retrieved August 10, 2010).

Natural Resources Canada, Office of Energy Efficiency. 2009. *Ethanol: What Is Ethanol?* (http://oee.nrcan.gc.ca/transportation/fuels/ethanol/ethanol.cfm; retrieved August 10, 2010).

Natural Resources Canada, Office of Energy Efficiency. 2009. *Research and Programs: Research* (http://oee.nrcan.gc.ca/transportation/fuels/ethanol/research.cfm?attr=16; retrieved August 10, 2010).

National Oceanic and Atmospheric Administration. 2008. *Billion Dollar U.S. Weather Disasters, 1980–2007* (http://www.ncdc.noaa.gov/oa/reports/billionz.html; retrieved February 19, 2009).

Ontario Ministry of the Environment. 2008. *My Environment: Household Waste* (http://www.ene.gov.on.ca/en/myenvironment/home/household-waste.php; retrieved August 10, 2010).

Parker, J. D., et al. 2005. Air pollution and birth weight among term infants in California. *Pediatrics* 115(1): 121–128.

Physicians for a Smoke-Free Canada. 2007. *Background on Protection from Second-Hand Smoke in Canada* (http://www.smoke-free.ca/pdf_1/ Q&A-smokefreecommunities1.pdf; retrieved August 10, 2010).

Public Health Agency of Canada. 2000. Waterborne outbreak of gastroenteritis associated with a contaminated municipal water supply, Walkerton, Ontario, May–June 2000. *Canada Communicable Disease Report* 26 (http://www.phac-aspc.gc.ca/publicat/ccdr-rmtc/00vol26/dr2620eb.html; retrieved July 22, 2010).

Rabb-Waytowich, D. 2009. Water fluoridation in Canada: Past and present. *Journal of the Canadian Dental Association* 75(6): 451–454 (http://www.cda-adc.ca/jcda/vol-75/issue-6/451.pdf; retrieved August 10, 2010).

Servos, M. R., et al. 2007. The presence of selected pharmaceuticals and the antimicrobial triclosan in drinking water in Ontario, Canada. *Water Quality Research Journal of Canada* 42(2): 130–137.

Statistics Canada. 2005. *Human Activity and the Environment: Annual Statistics 2005* (http://www.statcan.gc.ca/pub/16-201-x/16-201-x2005000-eng.pdf; retrieved August 10, 2010).

Statistics Canada. 2008. *Population Growth in Canada* (http://www.statcan.gc.ca/pub/91-003-x/2007001/4129907-eng.htm; retrieved July 21, 2010).

Statistics Canada. 2009. Survey of drinking water: 2005 to 2007. *The Daily,* December 9 (http://www.statcan.gc.ca/daily-quotidien/091209/dq091209a-eng.htm; retrieved August 10, 2010).

Trasande, L., P. J. Landrigan, and C. Schechter. 2005. Public health and economic consequences of methylmercury toxicity to the developing brain. *Environmental Health Perspectives* 28 (http://ehp03.niehs.nih.gov/article/fetchArticle.action?articleURI=info:doi/10.1289/ehp.7743; retrieved June 7, 2011).

United Nations Population Division. 2007. *World Population Prospects: The 2006 Revision.* New York: United Nations.

U.S. Department of Health and Human Services. 2005. *Surgeon General Releases National Health Advisory on Radon* (http://www.surgeongeneral gov/press releases/sg01132005.html; retrieved February 19, 2009).

U. S. Energy Information Administration. 2009. *Canada: Background* (http://www.eia.doe.gov/cabs/Canada/Background.html; retrieved August 10, 2010).

U.S. Environmental Protection Agency. 2007. *Superfund National Accomplishments Summary Fiscal Year 2007* (http://www.epa.gov/superfund/accomp/numbers07.htm; retrieved February 19, 2009).

Virtanen, J. K., et al. 2005. Mercury, fish oils, and risk of acute coronary events and cardiovascular disease, coronary heart disease, and all-cause mortality in men in eastern Finland. *Arteriosclerosis, Thrombosis, and Vascular Biology* 25(1): 228–233.

Wong, S. L., and E. J. D. Lye. 2008. Lead, mercury and cadmium levels in Canadians. *Health Reports* (http://www.statcan.gc.ca/pub/82-003-x/2008004/article/6500822-eng.pdf; retrieved August 10, 2010).

World Health Organization. 2005. *International Decade for Action: Water for Life 2005–2015* (http://www.who.int/water_sanitation_health/2005advocguide/en/index1.html; retrieved February 19, 2009).

World Health Organization. 2006. Cholera, 2005. *Weekly Epidemiological Record* 81(31): 297–308.

World Health Organization. 2006. *Fuel for Life: Household Energy and Health.* Geneva: WHO Press.

Worldwatch Institute. 2007. *Vital Signs 2007–2008.* New York: Norton.

World Health Organization. 2008. *Asthma. Fact Sheet No. 307* (http://www.who.int/mediacentre/factsheets/fs307/en/index.html; retrieved August 10, 2010).

NUTRITIONAL CONTENT OF POPULAR ITEMS FROM FAST-FOOD RESTAURANTS

Tim Hortons

	Serving size	Calories	Protein	Total fat	Saturated fat	Trans fat	Carbohydrate	Sugars	Fibre	Cholesterol	Sodium	Vitamin A	Vitamin C	Calcium	Iron
			g	g	g	g	g	g	g	mg	mg	% Daily Value			
Ham & Swiss Sandwich	262 g	390	23	12	5	0.2	49	4	3	45	1450	4	20	20	35
Turkey Bacon Club Sandwich	254 g	370	21	7	2	0	54	6	3	35	1410	0	20	2	30
BLT Sandwich	212 g	420	17	18	5	0	47	4	3	25	830	0	20	2	30
Chicken Caesar Sandwich	244 g	370	21	12	2	0.1	45	2	3	35	880	0	20	2	30
Chili	284 mL	300	26	19	7	1	17	4	4	90	1320	4	10	6	25
Coffee (1 cream, 1 sugar)	10 oz	75	1	3.5	2	0.1	9	9	0	15	15	2	0	2	0
Steeped Tea (1 milk, 1 sugar)	10 oz	50	1	1	0.5	0	10	0	0	5	20	2	0	4	0
Hot Chocolate	10 oz	240	2	6	5	0.2	45	38	2	0	360	0	0	2	15
French Vanilla Cappuccino	10 oz	250	4	8	7	0.1	41	31	1	5	240	0	0	10	2
Iced Cappuccino	10 oz	250	2	11	6	0.4	33	33	0	45	50	8	0	10	2
Apple Fritter Donut	95 g	300	4	11	5	0.1	49	16	2	0	350	0	4	4	20
Maple Dip Donut	62 g	210	4	8	3.5	0.1	32	9	1	0	190	0	0	2	10
Chocolate Glazed Donut	75 g	260	4	10	4.5	0.1	39	20	2	5	300	0	0	2	15
Boston Cream Donut	69 g	250	4	8	3.5	0.1	40	13	2	5	260	0	0	2	15
Sour Cream Glazed Timbit	19 g	90	1	4.5	2	0	12	7	0	5	65	0	0	0	2
Chocolate Glazed Timbit	19 g	70	1	2.5	1	0	10	5	0	0	75	0	0	0	4
Chocolate Chunk	52 g	230	2	9	6	0.1	35	19	1	20	260	8	0	2	10
Peanut Butter Cookie	52 g	280	6	16	7	0.1	27	16	2	20	260	8	0	2	8
Oatmeal Raisin Spice Cookie	52 g	220	3	8	5	0.1	35	21	1	25	200	8	0	2	8
Blueberry Muffin	115 g	340	5	11	2	0.2	53	25	2	40	570	0	0	4	10
Chocolate Chip Muffin	115 g	410	5	15	5	0.3	62	37	2	35	430	0	0	4	10
Fruit Explosion Muffin	122 g	360	5	11	2	0.2	56	27	2	40	580	0	4	4	10
Whole Grain Carrot Orange Muffin	115 g	370	5	13	2.5	0.2	59	30	4	25	470	50	4	4	15
Low Fat Double Berry Muffin	115 g	290	4	2.5	0.5	0.1	59	30	2	0	500	0	2	4	8
Plain Bagel	114 g	260	9	1.5	0.2	0	52	7	2	0	450	0	0	2	20
Sesame Seed Bagel	114 g	270	9	2.5	0.4	0	53	7	2	0	430	0	0	2	30
Everything Bagel	114 g	280	10	2	0.3	0	53	7	3	0	460	0	0	4	20
Cinnamon Raisin Bagel	114 g	270	10	1	0.2	0	55	12	3	0	350	0	0	4	20
Plain Cream Cheese	43 g	144	3	14	9	0.5	2	2	0	50	179	15	0	6	0
Cheese Croissant	75 g	320	10	20	10	0.4	25	3	2	25	440	4	0	15	0
Raisin Tea Biscuit	90 g	280	6	9	1.5	0.1	46	15	2	0	550	0	0	4	20
Cinnamon Roll–Frosted	119 g	470	4	25	12	0.2	59	22	2	0	380	2	0	4	20
Creamy Vanilla Yogurt with Berries	170 g	160	4	2.5	1.5	0	33	25	2	10	45	2	20	10	2

Source: http://www.timhortons.com/ca/pdf/nutrition-guide-can.pdf. Logos are registered trademarks of the TDL Marks Corporation and are used under licence to the TDL Group Corp. Used with permission.

KFC

	Serving size	Calories	Protein	Total fat	Saturated fat	Trans fat	Carbohydrate	Sugars	Fibre	Cholesterol	Sodium	Vitamin A	Vitamin C	Calcium	Iron
	g		g	g	g	g	g	g	g	mg	mg	% Daily Value			
Original Recipe Drumstick (Leg)	41	100	10	5	1	0	4	0	0	45	180	0	0	0	2
Original Recipe Thigh 1 piece	101	300	18	20	4	0.1	11	0	0	90	530	2	0	2	10
Classic Sandwich 1 sandwich	193	450	16	21	3.0	0.1	49	7	3	40	890	2	0	4	30
Toasted Wrap 1 sandwich	120	280	12	13	2.5	0	29	2	2	25	720	0	0	2	15
Big Crunch® 1 sandwich	256	590	28	27	3	0	58	7	4	60	1190	10	6	8	25
Spicy Big Crunch 1 sandwich	256	620	28	30	4	0	57	10	2	55	1310	10	6	8	25
Crispy Strips® 3 pieces	126	320	23	14	1	0.1	16	0	1	50	1120	0	2	2	10
Chicken Nuggets 4 nuggets	92	160	12	8	1.5	0	10	3	1	30	520	0	0	0	6
Popcorn Chicken® Small Size	142	525	21	34	3.0	0.2	24	0	1	75	1290	0	1	2	20
French Fries Individual size	113	340	3	17	1	0	44	0	4	0	770	0	2	2	6
Potato Salad Individual Size	125	200	2	9	1.5	0	25	6	2	15	460	8	10	2	4
Macaroni Salad Individual Size	125	190	3	9	1.5	0	23	4	1	20	650	8	2	0	6
Coleslaw Salad Individual Size	125	150	1.0	8	1.5	0	20	15	3	5	240	2	2	6	4

Source: http://www.kfc.ca/home/en/downloads/nutrition.pdf. ® Yum! Franchise I LP. Used under licence. © 2010 Yum! Restaurants International (Canada) Company. All rights reserved. The information contained in the table is for indicative purposes only and may not be a representation of current products and values.

Subway

	Serving size	Calories	Protein	Total fat	Saturated fat	Trans fat	Carbohydrate	Sugars	Fibre	Cholesterol	Sodium	Vitamin A	Vitamin C	Calcium	Iron	Calories from fat
	g		g	g	g	g	g	g	g	mg	mg	% Daily Value				
Ham Sandwich (6 inch)	219	280	15	4	1	0	47	6	3	15	730	8	20	6	15	35
Oven Roasted Chicken Sandwich (6 inch)	226	310	21	4.5	1.5	0	47	8	5	40	600	8	20	4	15	40
Subway Club® Sandwich (6 inch)	233	300	18	4	1	0	47	7	5	25	870	8	20	6	20	35
Turkey Breast Sandwich (6 inch)	219	280	16	3	1	0	46	7	5	20	790	8	20	6	15	25
Veggie Delite® Sandwich (6 inch)	162	230	8	2.5	0.5	0	44	6	5	0	310	8	20	4	15	20
Cold Cut Combo Sandwich (6 inch)	244	470	19	24	9	0.2	47	7	6	50	1120	8	20	15	20	230
Italian B.M.T.® Sandwich (6 inch)	237	450	21	19	8	0.5	47	7	5	50	1440	8	20	10	15	180
Meatball Marinara Sandwich (6 inch)	372	570	24	22	9	1	69	18	9	40	1420	40	45	15	25	200
Pizza Sub Sandwich (6 inch)	249	490	21	24	10	1	50	10	6	50	1640	15	25	20	20	210
Spicy Italian Sandwich (6 inch)	233	520	22	28	11	0.5	46	8	5	65	1720	10	20	35	20	250
Chocolate Chip Cookie	45	210	2	10	6	0.1	30	18	1	15	150	6	0	0	6	90
White Chip Macadamia Nut Cookie	45	220	2	11	5	0.1	29	18	1	15	160	6	0	2	4	100
Apple Pie	82	250	0	10	4	0.1	37	14	2	0	200	0	0	0	6	90
Bacon (2 strips)	9	40	3	3	1	0	0	0	0	10	150	0	0	0	0	25
Chipotle Southwest Sauce	21	90	0	9	1.5	0	2	1	0	10	220	0	0	0	0	80
Honey Mustard Sauce, Fat Free	21	30	0	0	0	0	7	5	0	0	140	0	0	0	0	2
House Sandwich Sauce	21	110	0	12	1.5	0	1	1	0	0	170	0	0	0	0	110
Mayonnaise (15 mL)	15	110	0	12	2	0.2	0	0	0	10	80	0	0	0	0	110
Ranch Dressing	21	110	0	11	2	0	1	1	0	5	200	0	0	0	0	100
Cheddar Cheese Product, Processed	11	40	2	3	2	0.2	0	0	0	10	200	0	0	6	0	30
Swiss Cheese	14	50	4	4	3	0.2	0	0	0	10	45	0	0	15	0	35

Source: http://world.subway.com/Countries/NutritionFiles/CanNutritionValues.pdf. The information contained in the table is for indicative purposes only and may not be a representation of current products and values. Used with permission.

McDonald's

	Serving size	Calories	Protein	Total fat	Saturated fat	Trans fat	Total carbohydrate	Sugars	Fibre	Cholesterol	Sodium	Vitamin A	Vitamin C	Calcium	Iron	% calories from fat
	g		g	g	g	g	g	g	g	mg	mg	% Daily Value				
Hamburger	100	250	12	9	3.5	0.5	31	6	2	25	528	0	2	10	15	40
Quarter Pounder®	169	410	24	19	7	1	37	8	3	65	730	2	4	15	20	41
Quarter Pounder® w/cheese	198	510	29	26	12	1.5	40	9	3	90	1190	10	4	30	25	45
Big Mac®	214	540	25	29	10	1.5	45	9	3	75	1040	6	2	25	25	48
Big N' Tasty®	206	460	24	24	8	1.5	37	8	3	70	720	6	8	15	25	47
Filet-O-Fish®	142	380	15	18	3.5	0	38	5	2	40	640	2	0	15	10	45
McChicken®	143	360	14	16	3	0	40	5	2	35	830	0	2	10	15	42
Medium French Fries	117	380	4	19	2.5	0	48	0	5	0	270	0	10	2	6	45
Chicken McNuggets® (6 pieces)	95	280	14	17	3	0	16	0	0	40	600	2	2	2	4	57
Chicken Select® Premium Breast Strips (5 pieces)	219	660	38	40	6	0	39	0	0	85	1680	0	6	4	8	55
Tangy Honey Mustard Sauce	43	70	1	2.5	0	0	13	9	0	5	170	0	0	0	1	29
Bacon Ranch Salad w/Grilled Chicken (w/o dressing)	321	260	33	9	4	12	5	5	3	1010	130	50	15	10	35	0
Caesar Salad w/Crispy Chicken (w/o dressing)	314	330	130	17	4.5	20	6	3	60	840	130	50	20	10	46	0
Newman's Own® Ranch Dressing (2 oz)	59	170	1	15	2.5	9	4	0	20	530	0	0	4	0	76	0
Egg McMuffin®	139	300	18	12	5	30	3	2	260	820	10	2	30	20	37	0
Sausage Biscuit w/ Egg	163	510	18	33	14	36	2	2	250	1170	6	0	8	20	57	0
Hotcakes (w/o syrup & margarine)	151	350	8	9	2	60	14	3	20	590	2	0	15	15	23	0
Fruit 'n Yogurt Parfait	149	160	4	2	1	31	21	1	5	85	0	15	15	4	13	0
Chocolate Triple Thick® Shake (475 mL)	444	580	13	14	8	102	84	1	50	250	20	0	45	10	21	1

Source: McDonald's Corporation, 2008. (http://www.mcdonalds.com). Used with permission from McDonald's Corporation. For the most current information, visit the McDonald's Web site (http://www.mcdonalds.ca/pdfs/NutritionFactsEN.pdf).

Wendy's

	Serving size	Calories	Protein	Total fat	Saturated fat	Trans fat	Total carbohydrate	Sugars	Fibre	Cholesterol	Sodium	Vitamin A	Vitamin C	Calcium	Iron	% calories from fat
	g		g	g	g	g	g	g	g	mg	mg	% Daily Value				
Classic Single® w/everything	226	430	25	20	7	1	39	9	2	75	870	8	8	4	25	42
Jr. Hamburger	98	230	13	8	3	0	27	5	1	30	490	0	0	2	20	30
Jr. Bacon Cheeseburger	136	320	17	16	6	0.5	26	5	1	50	670	10	6	10	20	44
Ultimate Chicken Grill Sandwich	211	320	28	7	1.5	0	36	8	2	70	950	6	10	4	20	19
Spicy Chicken Sandwich	223	440	28	16	2.5	0	46	6	3	60	1300	6	8	4	15	34
Homestyle Chicken Fillet Sandwich	226	430	25	16	2.5	0	48	6	2	45	1120	6	8	4	15	33
10 Piece Chicken Nuggets	150	460	24	30	6	0	24	0	0	70	1040	0	0	2	6	59
Caesar Side Salad (no toppings or dressing)	142	260	8	19	4	0	14	2	2	490	270	100	35	10	6	57
Mandarin Chicken® Salad w/grilled chicken fillet	402	540	31	25	3	0.5	50	31	5	65	1260	70	50	6	10	43
Southwest Taco Salad (no toppings or dressing)	520	640	30	39	16	1	44	12	9	110	1570	80	35	45	20	55
Creamy ranch dressing	64	200	1	20	3.5	0	4	2	0	15	400	0	0	4	2	87
Reduced fat creamy ranch dressing	64	90	1	7	1.5	0	6	3	1	10	400	0	0	6	2	70
Large French Fries	184	550	7	26	4	0	73	0	7	0	480	4	15	2	10	42
Sour Cream & Chive Baked Potato	308	320	8	4	2	0	63	4	7	10	50	4	60	8	15	11
Strawberry Frosty™ shake, small	325	390	7	11	7	0.5	67	58	0	35	170	2	2	22	6	26
Chili, small, plain	227	190	14	6	2.5	0	19	6	5	40	830	4	4	8	15	32
Crispy Chicken Nuggets™ (5)	75	230	12	15	3	0	12	0	0	35	520	0	0	0	2	59
Barbecue sauce (1 packet)	28	45	1	0	0	0	10	8	0	0	170	0	0	0	4	0
Vanilla Frosty™, medium	298	410	11	10	6	0.5	68	57	0	45	240	20	0	40	20	22

Source: Wendy's International, Inc., 2008. (http://www.wendys.com). Reproduced with permission from Wendy's International, Inc. The information contained in Wendy's International Information is effective as of July 30, 2008. Wendy's International, Inc., its subsidiaries, affiliates, franchises, and employees do not assume responsibility for a particular sensitivity or allergy (including peanuts, nuts or other allergies) to any food product provided in our restaurants. We encourage anyone with food sensitivities, allergies, or special dietary needs to check on a regular basis with Wendy's Consumer Relations Department to obtain the most up-to-date information.

Information on additional foods and restaurants is available online; see the Web sites listed in this appendix and the following additional sites: Starbucks: http://www.starbucks.com/menu/catalog/nutrition?drink=all#view_control=nutrition and http://www.starbucks.com/menu/catalog/nutrition?food=all#view_control=nutrition; Harvey's: http://harveys.ca/nutritionals/; Burger King: http://www.burgerking.ca/RTEContent/Document/nutritionalGuide_webFormat_Nov2009_2.pdf.

PHOTO CREDITS

Chapter One
p. 2, © Amana Productions/Getty Images; p. 6, dynamicgraphics/Jupiterimages; p. 11, Tony Anderson/Getty Images; p. 15, Jules Frazier/Getty Images; p. 17, © Brand X Pictures/PunchStock; p. 26, © Cindy Charles/PhotoEdit; p. 27, © Thomas Northcut/Digital Vision/Getty Images

Chapter Two
p. 32, LWA/Sharie Kennedy/Blend Images/Getty Images; p. 39, © Royalty-Free/Corbis; p. 40, © Purestock/PunchStock; p. 43, © PhotoAlto/Laurence Mouton/Getty Images; p. 45, © Monica Rodriguez/Riser/Getty Images; p. 46, © Ryan McVay/Photodisc/Getty Images; p. 49, © The McGraw-Hill Companies, Inc./Gary He, photographer; p. 50, © Ken Bank/Corbis; p. 53, © Paul Skelcher/Rainbow/Getty Images; p. 55, © Rob Melnychuk/JupterImages/Brand X/Alamy; p. 56, © SW Productions/PhotoDisc/Getty Images; p. 57, © David Harry Stewart/Stone/Getty Images

Chapter Three
p. 64, © The McGraw-Hill Companies, Inc./Gary He, photographer; p. 71, © The McGraw-Hill Companies, Inc./Gary He, photographer; p. 72, © Purestock/PunchStock; p. 74, Photodisc Collection/Getty Images; p. 75, © 3D4Medical.com/Getty Images; p. 76, © Tom Grill/Corbis; p. 78, © Tim Boyle/Getty Images; p. 79, © Scott Olson/Getty Images; p. 80, © PNC/PhotoDisc/Getty Images; p. 83, © The McGraw-Hill Companies, Inc./Lars Niki, photographer; p. 86, © ThinkStock/JupiterImages; p. 87, © Purestock/PunchStock

Chapter Four
p. 94, © Kelly Redinger/DesignPics; p. 99, © Julie Brown/Custom Medical Stock Photo; p. 103, TRBfoto/Getty Images; p. 106, © Serge Attal/Time Life Pictures/Getty Images; p. 107, © Royalty-Free/Corbis; p. 112, Jason Reed/Getty Images; p. 113, © Copyright 1997 IMS Communications Ltd/Capstone Design. All Rights Reserved; p. 114, Justin Sullivan/Staff/Getty Images; p. 115, Screenshot from The National Weight Control Association reprinted with permission; p. 120, © BananaStock/PunchStock

Chapter Five
p. 128, © Comstock/PunchStock; p. 132, © Onoky/Superstock; p. 137 (right), © Brand X Pictures/PunchStock; p. 145, © Royalty-Free/Corbis; p. 150, © BananaStock/PunchStock; p. 154, Eating Well With Canada's Food Guide, Health Canada. Reproduced with the permission of the Minister of Public Works and Government Services Canada, 2011; p. 157, © Royalty-Free/CORBIS; p. 160, © 2007 Canadian Diabetes Association and Dietitians of Canada; p. 162, © PhotoAlto/PunchStock; p. 164 (top), Twphoto/Corbis; p. 164 (middle), Used with permission of CFIA; p. 166, US FDA

Chapter Six
p. 176, Eyewire/Getty Images; p. 179, © Bob Daemmrich/PhotoEdit; p. 182, © Royalty-Free/Corbis; p. 189, Image Source/Getty Images; p. 194, Courtesy Robin Mouat; p. 195, © Tanya Constantine/Blend Images/Getty Images; p. 197, © Neil Tanner; p. 198, ©Hekimain Julien/Corbis Sygma

Chapter Seven
p. 208, CPimages.ca/Phototake; p. 214, © Barros & Barros/Photographer's Choice/Getty Images; p. 218, © Michael Krasowitz/Photographer's Choice/Getty Images; p. 219, © AP/Wide World Photos; p. 220, © Royalty-Free/Corbis; p. 222, © Jose Luiz Pelaez Inc./Blend Images/Getty Images; p. 227, © Paul Seheult/Eye Ubiquitous/Corbis

Chapter Eight
p. 242, CP PHOTO/Toronto Star - Bernard Weil); p. 248 (top), © Jose Luis Pelaez, Inc./Corbis; p. 248 (bottom), © The McGraw-Hill Companies, Inc./Christopher Kerrigan, photographer; p. 250, © Howard Sochurek/Corbis; p. 254, Karl Weatherly/Getty Images; p. 261, Chad Baker/Getty Images; p. 264, © James Leynse/Corbis; p. 270, Custom Medical Stock Photo

Chapter Nine
p. 276, © Stockdisc/PunchStock; p. 282, © Eye of Science/Photo Researchers, Inc.; p. 284, © Crack Palinggi/Reuters/Corbis; p. 287, © David Young-Wolff/PhotoEdit; p. 291, © Scott Camazine/Alamy; p. 293, © John Durham/Photo Researchers, Inc.; p. 298, © Michael Smith/Getty Images; p. 302, © Jack Fields/Corbis; p. 304, © SMC Images/The Image Bank/Getty Images; p. 305, Stop/Getty Images

Chapter Ten
p. 308, © Pinnacle Pictures/Photodisc/Getty Images; p. 312, © JLP/Jose L. Pelaez/Corbis; p. 314, © Blend Images/PunchStock; p. 315, © Mike Iannace/Corbis; p. 317, © Royalty Free/Corbis; p. 319, © Elie Bernager/ONOKY/Getty Images; p. 320, Steve Mason/Getty Images; p. 321, © Michael J. Doolittle/The Image Works; p. 324, © AP/Wide World Photos; p. 325, © Queerstock; p. 327, © Big Cheese Photo/PunchStock; p. 328, Photodisc Collection/Getty Images

Chapter Eleven
p. 334, © Stockbyte/Getty Images; p. 340, © Digital Vision/Getty Images; p. 341, © Thinkstock/JupiterImages; p. 344, © Veroniwue Krieger/DK Stock/Getty Images; p. 349, © Dex Image/PunchStock; p. 351, © Leigh Schindler/PhotoDisc/Getty Images; p. 352, ©Lee Schindler/Photo Disc/Getty Images; p. 354, Monica Lau/Getty Images; p. 355, © PhotoAlto/Sigrid Olsson/Getty Images; p. 359, © Joel Gordon; p. 360, © SIU Biomed Comm/Custom Medical Stock Photo

Chapter Twelve
p. 374, © Ariel Skelley/Blend Images/Getty Images; p. 380, © Comstock Images/PictureQuest; p. 383, Glowimages/Getty Images; p. 387, Sarah M. Golonka/Brand X Pictures/JupiterImages; p. 388, © Tissuepix/Photo Researchers Inc.; p. 390, © rubberball/Getty Images; p. 391, © Jose Luis Pelaez, Inc./Blend Images/Getty Images; p. 392, Blend Images/Getty Images; p. 403, © Bananastock/PictureQuest

Chapter Thirteen
p. 408, Win McNamee/Getty Images; p. 413, Ryan McVay/Getty Images; p. 416, Monkeybusinessimages/Dreamstime.com; p. 417, © Zoom (189) Friends-Campus Life/Imagemore/Getty Images; p. 429, Keith Brofsky/Getty Images; p. 431, © Joel Gordon; p. 435, William Nicklin/Getstock

Chapter Fourteen
p. 440, © travelib india/Alamy; p. 444, Egyuri/Dreamstime.com; p. 445, © AP/Wide World Photos; p. 448, Jose Azel/Aurora Photos; p. 449, © Brand X Pictures/PunchStock; p. 453, © The McGraw-Hill Companies, Inc./Gary He, photographer; p. 457, Rubberball/Getty Images; p. 461, Doug Menuez/Getty Images; p. 463, © BananaStock/JupiterImages/i2i/Alamy

Chapter Fifteen
p. 472, © Mitch Tobias/The Image Bank/Getty Images; p. 483, © Rachel Weill/UpperCut Images/Getty Images; p. 490, © Maren Caruso/Taxi/Getty Images; p. 491, © Purestock/Alamy

Chapter Sixteen
p. 498, © China Foto Press [2009] all rights reserved; p. 501, Kevin Palmer Photography; p. 504, © Chris Howes/Wild Places Photography/Alamy; p. 505, Credit Piksel/Dreamstime.com GetStock.com; p. 506, Steve Granitz/Contributor; p. 508, © Tim Wright/Corbis; p. 513, © Michael A. Keller/zefa/Corbis; p. 514, Goldminer/Dreamstime.com; p. 515, © Jeff Greenberg/The Image Works; p. 518, Stefanolunardi/Dreamstime.com

Chapter Seventeen
p. 526, BananaStock/Alamy; p. 531, © John Lund/Drew Kelly/Blend Images/Getty Images; p. 534, © Joel Gordon; p. 535, © Barry Austin/Digital Vision/Getty Images; p. 536, Steve Mason/Getty Images; p. 538, © Comstock/PunchStock; p. 539, © Photofusion Picture Library/Alamy; p. 540, © Joe McNally/Getty Images; p. 543, © Stockbyte/Getty Images; p. 544, © Peter Hince/Photographer's Choice/Getty Images

Chapter Eighteen
p. 550, Stockbyte/Getty Images; p. 552, © Tom Mareschal/Photographer's Choice/Getty Images; p. 555, © Macduff Everton/The Image Bank/Getty Images; p. 560, © Royalty-Free/Corbis; p. 564, © Royalty-Free/Corbis; p. 565, © Thinkstock/SuperStock; p. 566, © Johner Royalty Free/Getty Images; p. 567, THE CANADIAN PRESS/Paul Chiasson

Chapter Nineteen
p. 574 (hands), Givaga/Dreamstime.com; p. 574 (medicine symbol), Scusi/Dreamstime.com; p. 574 (acupuncture), Amaviael/Dreamstime.com; p. 574 (mortar and pestle), Elenathewise/Dreamstime.com; p. 574 (chiropractor), Creatas Images/PunchStock; p. 578, Meredith Heuer/Riser/Getty Images; p. 582, Andrew Wakeford/Getty Images; p. 586, © Thomas Barwick/Lifesize/Getty Images; p. 594, Jack Star/PhotoLink/Getty Images; p. 596, © P. Broze/ONOKY/Getty Images; p. 599, © Marc Schlossman/The Image Bank/Getty Images; p. 600, © Image Source/Getty Images

Chapter Twenty
p. 606, © Verity Smith/Brand X/Corbis; p. 612, © Ed Bock/UpperCut Images/Getty Images; p. 615, © Image Source Pink/Alamy; p. 617, Michej/Dreamstime.com; p. 618, Kenhurst/Dreamstime.com; p. 620, © Ruberball/SuperStock; p. 623, © Peter Turnley/Corbis; p. 624, © Marianne Todd/Getty Images; p. 625, © Rachel Epstein/PhotoEdit

Chapter Twenty-One
p. 638, Tobkatrina/Dreamstime.com; p. 640, U.S. Air Force photo by Tech. Sgt. James L. Harper Jr.; p. 642, © Digital Vision/Getty Images; p. 644, THE CANADIAN PRESS/Adrian Wyld; p. 646, Photodisc/Getty Images; p. 651, © Cameron Spencer/Getty Images; p. 652, © Brand X Pictures/PunchStock; p. 658 (top), © Mark Fiennes/Arcaid/Corbis; p. 658 (bottom), © Mira/Alamy

INDEX

A

ABCDE test, 256*f*
Aboriginal peoples
    AIDS, 425, 426
    alcohol consumption, 13*f*, 489
    Assisted Living Program, 533
    elders, 545
    health challenges faced by, 10–13
    HIV, 426
    nutritional guidelines, 157
    physical activity, 13*f*
    smoking, 501
    suicide and, 48
Aboriginal Peoples Survey (APS), 545
abortifacients, 361
abortion, 367–369
    defined, 367
    manual vacuum aspiration (MVA),
        368, 369
    medical abortion, 369
    methods of abortion, 368–369
    possible psychological effects, 369
    spontaneous abortion, 396
    suction curettage, 368, 368*f*, 369
    total induced abortions, by province and
        territory, 368*t*
absorption of alcohol, 475
academic stress, 75–76
Acamprosate, 488
Acceptable Macronutrient Distribution
    Ranges (AMDRs), 135, 136, 139
acceptance, 34–35, 311
access to health care
    disparities in, 11
    and wellness, 16
acetaldehyde, 476
acetylsalicylic acid (ASA), 578–580
    see also Aspirin
acne, 343
acquaintance rape, 627
    see also date rape
acquired immune deficiency syndrome
    (AIDS), 278, 411*t*, 413, 419–431
acquired immunity, 284, 285
acrylamide, 262
action stage, 22, 23
active euthanasia, 556–558
active immunity, 285
acupressure, 593–594, 595
acupuncture, 593–595
acute alcohol poisoning, 478
acute bacterial prostatitis, 346
added sugars, 153–154
addiction, 442–445
    see also addictive behaviour

addictive behaviour, 442–445
    addiction, 442–445
    characteristics of, 443
    compulsive buying or shopping, 445
    compulsive exercising, 444
    compulsive or pathological gambling, 444
    defined, 445
    development of addiction, 443
    examples, 444–445
    Internet addiction, 445
    people with addictions, characteristics of, 445
    sex and love addiction, 445
    work addiction, 444–445
additives
    in cigarettes, 507
    in food, 165
Adequate Intake (AI), 145
adipose tissue, 104–105
adolescents. *See* youth
adrenal androgens, 198
adrenal glands, 339
adult identity, 36–37
adults
    older adults. *See* older adults
    physical activity, 183*f*
    sexuality, 350
advance directive, 558, 559
adverse drug events (ADEs), 588, 589
adverse event, 589
advertising
    alcohol, 493
    tobacco, 506, 506*f*
African sleeping sickness, 301
age
    and fertility, 382
    and parenthood, 376
    and pregnancy, 377
    as risk factor, 4
age-proofing, 534–537
age-related macular degeneration (AMD),
    540, 541
aggression, and alcohol, 478–479
aggressive driving, 610, 611
agility, 180
aging
    see also older adults
    age-proofing, 534–537
    Alzheimer's disease, 542, 543
    arthritis, 540–541
    Canada's aging population, 528–530, 530*f*
    and cardiovascular disease (CVD), 220–221
    changes of aging, 537–544
    characteristics associated with, 534
    dementia, 542
    depression, 544
    and diet, 535

drinking and meditations, 537
early detection of diseases, 537
fluid intelligence, 535
and gender, 529
grief, 542–544
hearing loss, 540
helping others, 539
life-enhancing measures, 534–537
and life expectancy, 528–533
menopause, 538–540
mental changes, 542–544
osteoporosis, 541–542
perimenopause, 538
physical changes, 538–542
physical fitness, 534–535
preparation for, 534
psychological changes, 542–544
public's view of aging, 544
retirement, 538
and sexuality, 343–344
and smoking, 537
social changes, 537–538
stress, 537
vision changes, 540
and vitality, 533–537
weight management, 535–537
aging male syndrome, 344
agoraphobia, 45
air bags, 610–612
air pollution, 643–651
    energy use and, 648–650
    indoor air pollution, 650
    prevention, 650–651
air quality, 643–651
Air Quality Health Index (AQHI), 643–644
Al-Anon, 488
alarm stage, 72–73
Alateen, 488
alcohol
    Aboriginal peoples, 13*f*, 489
    absorption, 475
    actual servings, 474
    acute alcohol poisoning, 478
    advertising, 493
    and aggression, 478–479
    and aging, 537
    alcohol abuse, 485
    alcohol dependence, 485, 486
    alcohol-drug combinations, 478
    alcohol emergency, dealing with, 479
    alcohol-related injuries, 478
    alcoholic beverages, 474–475, 474*f*
    alcoholism, 485, 486–488
    binge drinking, 485–486, 485*t*
    blood alcohol concentration (BAC),
        475–477, 476*f*

essential hypertension, 214
essential nutrients, 130, 130t, 131
estate, 554, 555
Estimates Average Requirement (EAR), 145
estrogen, 222, 250, 339
estrogenic phase, 341
ethanol, 649
ethics
  and euthanasia, 557
  and right to die, 556
ethnic distribution of Canadian population, 9f
ethnic foods, 148
ethnicity
  see also diversity
  and body image, 120
  and cardiovascular disease (CVD), 221
  and genetic diseases, 380
  health disparities among ethnic minorities, 11
  overweight and obesity, 106
  and physical activity, 181
  and psychological disorders, 45
  and smoking, 501
  and wellness, 10–13
euphoria, 454
eustress, 72
euthanasia
  active euthanasia, 556–558
  involuntary euthanasia, 557
  nonvoluntary euthanasia, 557
  passive euthanasia, 556, 557
  voluntary euthanasia, 557
evaluation of health news, 584
evening primrose oil (Oenothera biennis L.),
    598t
evidence-based practice, 580, 581
excess body fat
  see also obesity; weight management
  factors contributing to, 103–108
  genetic factors, 103–104
  lifestyle factors, 105–107
  physiological factors, 104–105
  psychosocial factors, 107–108
  and wellness, 99–102
excessive noise, 661–662
excitement phase, 337
exercise
  Aboriginal peoples, 13f
  ACSM recommendations, 191t
  benefits of, 185–189
  and body composition, 186
  and body image, 112
  and cardiorespiratory functioning, 185
  and cardiovascular disease (CVD), 236
  common injuries and discomforts, 202t
  compulsive exercising, 444
  defined, 181
  disease prevention and management,
    187–188
  Guidelines for Healthy Eating, 147
  for health and fitness, 180–185
  health and fitness benefits, 191f
  health-related fitness, 178–180

immediate effects, 186f
isometric (static) exercises, 195
isotonic (dynamic) exercises, 195–196
long-term effects, 186f
and metabolism, 185
physical fitness, 178–180, 183–184
popularity of physical recreation activities,
    180t
during pregnancy, 395
program. See exercise program
resistance exercise, 195
as risk factor, 4
self-esteem, 112
skill-related fitness, 180, 181
special health concerns, 189
and stress management, 80–81
and total wellness, 182
and weight, 106–107
weight management, 111, 124
exercise machines, 196
exercise program, 190–199
  assessment of fitness, 202
  basic principles of physical training, 192
  cardiorespiratory endurance exercises,
    193–194
  consistency, 201
  cross-training, 203
  eating and drinking for exercise, 200–201
  first steps, 190–192
  flexibility exercises, 197–199
  getting started, 199–203
  individual differences, 192
  injury management, 202–203
  managing your fitness program, 201–203
  medical clearance, 190–192
  muscular strength and endurance, 195–197
  personal exercise program, 204
  phases, 201, 201f
  progressive overload, 192
  putting it all together, 199
  reversibility, 192
  selecting instructors, equipment, and
    facilities, 200
  selection of activities, 192
  specificity, 192
  staying on track, 199–203
  training in specific skills, 199
exhaustion stage, 73
expectations, 84, 313–314
exposure, 55
expressive writing, 578

F

fad diets, 112–114
fallopian tubes, 337
falls, 536, 615
false negatives, 587
false positives, 587
family disaster plan, 625
family health tree, 381
family history
  as risk factor, 4

and wellness, 15–16
family life
  caregiving, 531–532
  new parents, 328
  parenting, 328–330
  single parents, 330
  stepfamilies, 330
  successful families, 330–331
family life cycle, 329–330
family violence, 624–627
fat cells, 104–105
fat-free mass, 179
fat-soluble vitamins, 141t
fatigue, 295t
fats, 130, 130t, 133–136, 147, 153–154,
    233–234, 237, 262
fatty acids, 135f
feedback, 317
fellatio, 354, 355
female athlete triad, 102, 103
female condoms, 363–364, 364f
female infertility, 379–382
female reproductive tract cancers, 252–254
female sex organs, 336–337, 336f
female sexual maturation, 340–343
FemCap, 366, 367
fertility, 358, 359
  see also infertility
  and age, 382
  conception, 378–379
  and population growth, 643
  understanding fertility, 378–384
fertilization, 378, 379, 379f
fertilized egg, 378, 379
fetal alcohol spectrum disorder (FASD),
    394, 483
fetal alcohol syndrome (FAS), 483
fetal death, 396
fetal demise, 396
fetal development, 386–391
  see also pregnancy
  cross-sectional view of fetus, 389f
  diagnosis of abnormalities, 389–390
  fetal programming theory, 390–391
  first trimester, 387–389
  milestones, 388f
  second trimester, 389
  third trimester, 386f, 389
fetal programming theory, 390–391
fetus, 337, 377
fever, 295t
feverfew (Tanacetum parthenium), 598t
fibre, 114, 139–140, 235, 262
fight-or-flight reaction, 67, 68f, 72
financial concerns, 76
financial wellness, 6
finding help, 20–21
fires, 615–616
first aid, 631
First Nations people. See Aboriginal peoples
First Nations Regional Longitudinal Health
    Survey, 489

hangover, 478
hantavirus, 302
hardiness, 70
harm-reduction strategies, 466
hate crimes, 621–622
hatha yoga, 86
hazardous waste, 656–660
headache, 11, 76, 295t
health
    and alcohol, 477–484
    and body fat distribution, 102
    defined, 4
    determinants of health, 4, 4t
    and fats, 134
    and stress, 72–75
Health Canada, 53, 102, 114, 140, 145, 146,
    159, 161, 162, 165, 181, 214, 264, 342,
    390, 394, 403, 410, 416, 427, 461, 504,
    577, 588, 595, 597
Health Canada's medicine chart, 579f
health care costs, 601
health fraud, 593
health habits
    current health habits, 18–19
    motivation to change, 21–22
    readiness to change, 22–23
    and spiritual wellness, 38
    and wellness, 14–15
health information sources, 20
health insurance, 601
health journal, 25f
health promotion, 4
health-related fitness, 178–180
health-related research, 584
health span, 528, 529
healthy eating objective, 8
healthy for life, 28
healthy weights objective, 8
hearing loss, 540
heart, 210–211, 211f, 212f
Heart and Stroke Foundation of Canada, 226
heart attack, 11, 225–228, 226t
    see also myocardial infarction (MI)
heart attack warning signs, 228
heart disease
    see also cardiovascular disease (CVD)
    and exercise, 189
    and heart attack, 225–228
heart valve disorders, 233
heartbeat, 211
heavy metals, 653
Hegar's sign, 385
height, and gender, 11
height-weight charts, 97
Heimlich manoeuvre, 616, 617
Helicobacter pylori, 292
helper T cells, 281, 311
helping others, 539
hematologist, 247
hemochromatosis, 380
hemolytic uremic syndrome, 161
hemorrhagic stroke, 229, 231f

hepatitis, 298–299, 299
Hepatitis A, 285t
hepatitis A (HAV) virus, 162, 298
Hepatitis B, 285t
hepatitis B, 411t, 431–432
hepatitis B (HBV) virus, 298
hepatitis C virus (HCV), 298
herbal supplements, 114, 159–161
herbal therapies, 596–597, 598t, 599
heredity
    see also genetics
    and cancer, 259–261
    family health tree, 381
    and wellness, 15–16
heroin, 454
herpes simplex, 394
    see also genital herpes
herpes simplex virus (HSV) types 1 and 2,
    298, 418
herpesviruses, 296–298
heterosexual, 323, 351
hierarchy of needs, 34–35, 34f
high, 453
high blood pressure. See hypertension
high-density lipoproteins (HDL), 134, 187, 216
highly active antiretroviral therapy (HAART),
    428
hippocampus, 75
histamine, 281
HIV antibody tests, 425–426, 429
HIV infection, 421–423
    see also human immunodeficiency virus
        (HIV) infection
HIV positive, 426, 427
HIV transmission, 423–424, 424f
H1N1 flu pandemic, 297
Home Adaptations for Seniors Independence
    Program, 533
home care, 554–555
home injuries, 614–616
home medical care kit, 579f
homeopathy, 592, 595
Homeopathy Act, 595
homeostasis, 67
homeostatic resilience, 70
homicide, 621
homocysteine, 223
homophobia, 324
honest communication, 42
honesty, 313
hormonal methods, 357
hormone therapy (HT), 343, 538–539
hormones
    see also specific hormones
    defined, 66
    and excess body fat, 104
    and high birth weight, 391
    and reproductive life cycle, 339–344
    sex hormones, 339–344
    sexual differentiation, 340
    stress hormones, 82
hospice, 556, 557

hospital errors, 589
hostility, 218, 220
household disaster plan, 625
HPV vaccine, 285t
HSV 1 and 2. See herpes simplex virus (HSV)
    types 1 and 2
human behaviours, 303
human chorionic gonadotropin (HCG),
    384, 385
human immunodeficiency virus (HIV)
    infection, 419–431
    antivirals, 427–428, 428f
    around the world, 420, 420t
    asymptomatic stage, 423
    and casual contact, 424
    CD4 T cells, 422, 423
    chronic asymptomatic stage, 423
    chronic symptomatic stage, 423
    defined, 419
    diagnosis, 425–426
    direct contact with infected blood,
        423–424
    epidemiology of, 411t
    general pattern of untreated HIV infection,
        422f
    HIV antibody tests, 425–426, 429
    HIV education program, 431
    HIV positive, 426, 427
    and immune system, 278
    life cycle of HIV, 428f
    mother-to-child transmissions, 394–395,
        424
    opportunistic (secondary) infections, 422,
        423, 428
    people living with HIV, 2009, 421f
    populations of special concern, 424–425
    and pregnancy, 378
    primary/acute infection phase, 422
    protection from, 430–431
    reporting, 426–427
    sexual activity, 430, 430f
    sexual contact, 423
    symptoms, 425
    transmissions of virus, 423–424, 424f
    treatment, 427–428
    vaccine, 428–430
human papillomavirus (HPV), 300, 411t,
    415–418
human sexuality. See sexuality
humour, 41t, 84–85
"Hunger Winter," 391
hybrid electric vehicles (HEVs), 649
hydrocodone, 456
hydrogenation, 133–134
hydrostatic (underwater) weighing, 99
hymen, 336–337, 337
hyperactivity, 132
hypertension, 187, 189, 213–215
Hypertension Canada, 213
hypertrophic cardiomyopathy (HCM),
    232, 233
hypertrophy, 217

hypnosis, 595–596
hypnotherapy, 596
hypnotics, 54
hypothalamus, 339
hysterectomy, 357

I

identical twins, 379
identity
    adult identity, 36–37
    gender identity, 348–349
identity crisis, 37
immune function, 188
immune response, 11, 282–284, 283f
immune system, 280–288
    allergies, 167, 286–288
    and cancer, 303
    chemical barriers, 280
    contagion, 284
    defined, 281
    described, 280–284
    food allergies, 167
    immune response, 282–284, 283f
    immunity, 284
    immunization, 284–286, 285t
    immunological defenders, 281
    inflammatory response, 281–284
    physical barriers, 280
    and stress, 73, 74
    supporting your immune system, 304–305
    symptoms, 284
    vaccines, 284–286
immunity, 284, 285, 305
    see also immune system
immunization, 284–286, 285, 285t
immunoglobulin E (IgE), 286
immunological defenders, 281
impotence, 511
in-line skating injuries, 617
in vitro fertilization (IVF), 382, 383
incest, 630, 631
income, and health disparities, 11, 13
incomplete proteins, 131–132
incontinence, 252, 253
incubation, 284, 285
Indian Ayurvedic system, 592
Indian cuisine, 148
indirect transmission, 279
indoor air pollution, 650
indoor mould, 650
induction chemotherapy, 267
induction of labour, 397
indulgent parents, 329
infant mortality, 397–398, 398f
infants. See children
infatuation, 312
infections
    see also infectious disease; specific infections
    body piercing, 299
    breaking the chain, 280
    chain of infection, 278–280, 278f
    common types of infection, 288, 288t

defined, 279
emerging infectious diseases, 301–303
and immune system, 278
preconception care, 377
during pregnancy, 394–395
systemic infection, 280, 281
tattoos, 299
infectious agents, 223
infectious disease
    see also infections; specific infectious
        diseases
    contributing factors, 303
    cycle, 278
    defined, 7
    Ebola, 302
    emerging infectious diseases, 301–303
    environmental factors, 302
    Escherichia coli 0157:H7, 302
    hantavirus, 302
    history of, 6
    infections of concern, 301–302
    pathogens, and associated diseases, 289f
    rotavirus, 302
    severe acute respiratory syndrome (SARS),
        302
    West Nile virus, 302
infertility, 379–384
    emotional response to, 383–384
    environmental factors, 382
    female infertility, 379–382
    impotence, and smoking, 511
    male infertility, 382
    treatment, 382–384
    understanding infertility, 378–384
inflammation, 221
inflammatory response, 281–284
influenza, 285t, 295–296, 297
ingested chemicals, 263–264
inhalants, 455t, 462–463, 463f
injectable contraceptives, 361
injection drug use, 450–451
injection drug users (IDU), 426
injuries
    back injuries, 618
    causes, 608–609
    differentiating, 608
    emergency care, 631–632
    home injuries, 614–616
    intentional injury, 608, 619–631
    leisure injuries, 616–617
    management of, 202–203
    motor vehicle injuries, 608, 609–614
    prevention of, 188
    repetitive strain injuries (RSIs), 619
    safer habits, 633
    unintentional injury, 608–619, 608t
    work injuries, 617–619
    years of potential life lost, 608
injury management, 202–203
injury prevention, 188
inner-directed, 35
inorganic micronutrients, 142

insect stings, 286
Insite, 423–424
insoluble fibre, 139
insomnia, 82, 83
Institute of Medicine, 135, 139, 140, 146
instructional directive, 558, 559
insulin resistance, 222–223
intake goals, 136
Integrated Pan-Canadian Healthy Living
    Strategy, 7–8, 9t
integrated prenatal screening (IPS), 390, 391
integration, 38
integrative medicine, 591
    see also complementary and alternative
        medicine (CAM)
intellectual wellness, 5, 182
intentional injury, 608, 619–631
    see also injuries
interfaith and intrafaith partnerships, 321
interferons, 282
interleukins, 282
intermittent explosive disorder (IED), 43
internal stressors, 78–79
International Agency for Research on
    Cancer, 482
International Marketing Services Health, 588
International Pension Benefits, 533
Internet
    addiction, 445
    cyberstalking, 624–627
    health information, 591
    pharmacies, 588
    relationships, 322
    safety, 625–627
    weight-loss programs, 117
Internet addiction, 445
interpersonal stress, 76
interpersonal violence, 623
interpersonal wellness, 5, 182
intersexed individuals, 348
intestate, 554, 555
intimacy
    capacity for intimacy, 35
    development of intimacy, 37
    and relationships, 311–312
intimate relationships, 311, 320–326
    see also marriage
    co-habitating relationship, 321–323, 323f
    common law relationship, 321–323, 323f
    dating, 320–321
    and health, 327
    interfaith and intrafaith partnerships, 321
    living together, 321–323
    online relationships, 322
    partner selection, 320
    same-sex partnerships, 323–325
intimate violence, 624–627
intoxication, 442, 445, 449–450, 475
intracerebral hemorrhage, 229, 231f
intracytoplasmic sperm injection (ICSI), 383
intrauterine device (IUD), 361–362
intrauterine insemination, 382, 383

small-for-date, 397
small-for-gestational age, 397
SMART goals, 24–25
smog, 644, 645
smoking
    see also tobacco use
    additional concerns, 511–512
    advertising, 506, 506*f*
    and aging, 537
    among ethnic populations, 501
    bidis, 514
    and cancer, 248, 248*f*, 261–262, 510
    and cardiovascular disease (CVD),
        212–213, 236, 509–510
    chronic bronchitis, 511
    chronic obstructive pulmonary disease
        (COPD), 510–511
    cigarette tar, 507
    cigars, 513–514
    clove cigarettes, 514
    cosmetic concerns, 512
    counterproductive coping strategy, 87
    court cases, 517
    cumulative effects, 512
    deaths attributable to, 500*f*
    dental diseases, 512
    diminished physical senses, 512
    economic costs, 512
    effects of, 508–514, 509*f*
    emphysema, 511
    environmental factors, 517
    environmental tobacco smoke (ETS),
        515, 516
    gender differences, 11
    genetic factors, 503
    health hazards, 507–508
    impotence, 511
    inhalation, results of, 507–508
    injuries, 512
    levels, among Canadians, 10*t*
    "light" cigarettes, 508
    long-term effects, 509–512
    low-tar cigarettes, 508
    lung cancer, 510, 510*f*, 515
    mainstream smoke, 515
    in the media, 505–506
    menthol cigarettes, 508
    nicotine addiction, 502
    nonsmokers, effects on, 514–517
    "occasional smokers," 500
    and other drug use, 501–502
    pipes, 513–514
    preconception care, 377
    during pregnancy, 394, 515–516
    quitting, 519–523, 519*t*
    rates, 500
    reasons for smoking, 502–506
    and religion, 504
    reproductive health problems, 512
    respiratory damage, 511, 511*f*
    as risk factor, 4
    self-assessment, 503

short-term effects, 509*f*
sidestream smoke, 507
smokers, 500–502, 500*t*
smoking cessation products, 521
social and psychological factors, 502–503
starting to smoke, 504–506
taking action, 518
tobacco smoke, 507–508
ulcers, 511
and vitamin C, 146
and young people, 501
sneezing, 295*t*
sober sex, 356
social anxiety, 59
social factors
    and cardiovascular disease (CVD), 218–219
    psychoactive drugs, 454
    smoking, 502–503
    violence, 620
social influences, 27
social isolation, 219
social networks, 77–78
social phobia, 44
social stressors, 77–78
social support
    and spiritual wellness, 38
    and stress management, 79–80
    supportive individuals, 22
social wellness, 5
social withdrawal, 53
social workers, 58
Society of Obstetricians and Gynaecologists
    of Canada (SOGC), 377, 378, 390, 395,
    401, 402, 415, 539
socioeconomic status
    and cardiovascular disease (CVD), 219
    and health, 11
    and HIV infection, 427
    nutritional guidelines, 157
    and obesity, 107
sodium, 143*t*, 151, 235
soft drinks, 107
solid fats, 153–154
solid waste pollution, 653–656
soluble (viscous) fibre, 139
somatic nervous system, 69
sonogram, 389–390
sore throat, 295*t*
sources of health information, 20
soy protein, 235
soy sauce, 264
speaking, 318
special health concerns
    exercise, 189
    nutritional guidelines, 159
specific phobia, 44
specificity, 192
Speece, Mark, 553
speed, 180
speeding, 609–610
sperm, 336, 337, 378
spermicide, 364–365, 366–367

sphygmomanometer, 213
spinal manipulation, 597–599
spiritual wellness, 5–6, 38, 39
spirituality, and drug abuse, 450
spirochete, 289
spit (smokeless) tobacco, 512–513
sponge, 366, 367
spontaneous abortion, 396
spousal violence, 624, 626
squamous cell carcinomas, 255
St. John's wort (*Hypericum perforatum*),
    51, 598*t*
stability, 38
Stachybotrys mould, 650
stages of change model, 22, 24*f*
staging, 245
stalking, 624–627
standard drink, 474, 475*t*
standard of living, minimum acceptable, 642
standard Western medicine, 581
    see also conventional medicine
staphylococcus, 290–291, 291
Staphylococcus aureus (MRSA), 161–162,
    291
state dependence, 459
static exercises, 195
Statistics Canada, 214, 402, 451, 613
stealth diseases, 416
stem cell transplants, 267–268
stem cells, 268, 269
stepfamilies, 330
stereotyping, 9
sterilization, 357
steroids, 198
stillbirth, 396
stillborn, 396
stimulants, 54, 198, 455*t*, 457–460
stimulus, 55
STIs. *See* sexually transmitted infections
    (STIs)
stomach cancer, 258
stomach flu, 162
strength training exercises, 195
strep throat, 290
streptococcus, 290
Streptococcus pneumoniae, 290
stress
    see also stressor
    and aging, 537
    allostatic load, 73
    behavioural symptoms, 70*t*
    and the brain, 75
    burnout, 77
    and cardiovascular disease (CVD), 218
    and culture, 70
    daily hassles, 75
    defined, 66
    and discrimination, 78
    distress, 72
    emotional symptoms, 70*t*
    and the environment, 72
    eustress, 72

World No Tobacco Day, 518
world population growth, 641–643, 641*f*
World Report on Violence and Health, 623
writing, 578

X

X-rays, 661
xenotransplantation, 560

Y

Yasmin, 342
Yaz, 342
years of potential life lost, 608
yeast infection, 300, 346
Yerba mate, 116*t*
Yersinia enterocolitica, 162
yoga, 86
youth
   HIV, 427
   mature understanding of death, 553
   nutritional guidelines, 156
   physical activity, 181*f*, 183*f*
   sexuality, 350
   and smoking, 501, 504–505, 505*f*
Youth Smoking Survey, 504, 517

Z

zinc, 143*t*, 156
Zyban (bupropion), 521
zygote intrafallopian transfer (ZIFT),
   382, 383